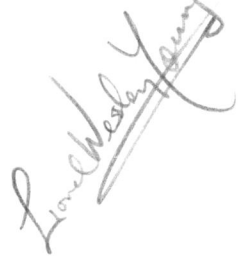

ULTRASONOGRAPHY OF INFANTS AND CHILDREN

ULTRASONOGRAPHY OF INFANTS AND CHILDREN

Rita Littlewood Teele, M.D.
Radiologist and Ultrasonologist
Department of Radiology
Children's Hospital

Associate Professor of Radiology
Harvard Medical School

Consultant in Neonatal Radiology
Brigham and Women's Hospital
Boston, Massachusetts

Jane Chrestman Share, M.D.
Radiologist and Ultrasonologist
Department of Radiology
Children's Hospital

Instructor in Radiology
Harvard Medical School

Consultant in Neonatal Radiology
Brigham and Women's Hospital
Boston, Massachusetts

W.B. SAUNDERS COMPANY
Harcourt Brace Jovanovich, Inc.
Philadelphia   London   Toronto   Montreal   Sydney   Tokyo

W. B. SAUNDERS COMPANY
Harcourt Brace Jovanovich, Inc.

The Curtis Center
Independence Square West
Philadelphia, PA 19106

Library of Congress Cataloging-in-Publication Data

Teele, Rita L. (Rita Littlewood)
Ultrasonography of infants and children / Rita Littlewood Teele, Jane Chrestman Share.

p. cm

ISBN 0–7216–8775–X

1. Children—Diseases—Diagnosis.   2. Diagnosis, Ultrasound.   I. Share, Jane Chrestman.   II. Title.

[DNLM: 1. Ultrasonic Diagnosis—in infancy & childhood. WS 141 T258u]

RJ51.U45T44 1991

618.92′007543—dc20

DNLM/DLC   90–9123

Editor: Lisette Bralow
Designer: Maureen Sweeney
Production Manager: Ken Neimeister
Manuscript Editor: Anne Ostroff
Illustration Coordinator: Peg Shaw
Page Layout Artist: Dorothy Chattin
Indexer: Helene Taylor

Ultrasonography of Infants and Children   ISBN 0–7216–8775–X

Copyright © 1991 by W. B. Saunders Company.

All rights reserved. No part of this publication may be reproduced or transmitted in any form or by any means, electronic or mechanical, including photocopy, recording, or any information storage and retrieval system, without permission in writing from the publisher.

Printed in the United States of America.

Last digit is the print number: 9   8   7   6   5   4   3   2   1

To the men in our lives:
David W. Teele, Donald S. Share, and John A. Kirkpatrick, Jr.

FOREWORD

We're not sure how many people read the foreword in a book. We hope you will read this one because it includes all the other "authors" who were involved in producing the volume you are holding. This book was an international affair. I, Rita L. Teele, was given the opportunity to spend 10 months in New Zealand between 1988 and 1989 while my husband was on sabbatical there. Writing a book seemed to be the answer to the problem of keeping me out of trouble, and it allowed me to have an excuse for enrolling our youngest child in the wonderful day care program at the University of Otago in Dunedin. Jane C. Share, in the meantime, took over the total responsibility for ultrasonography at Children's Hospital and collected the cases that were needed to illustrate the text. In New Zealand, I was helped by some very special people: Ruth Henderson, who expertly typed sheets of manuscript in record time and deserves credit for being able to read my handwriting with no experience in doing so; the ultrasonographers at Dunedin Public Hospital, who contributed their expertise: Leanne Bardwell, Sue Verwey, Averlea Duncan, and Cathy Sorensen; the radiologists, who became new colleagues and are now old friends: Drs. Sue Craw, Lewis Beale, D. Ross Smith, Neil Morrison, and Gillian Morris; and Professor Terence Doyle, who found an office for me and allowed me to work in his department. The registrars in the Department of Radiology at Dunedin Public Hospital, University of Otago, were willing readers of rather preliminary chapters: Drs. Tim Buckenham, Sally Chartres, Richard Farris, and Russell Taylor. There was help from Mr. Ian Stewart, Mr. Jeff Robinson, Dr. Phil Silva, and Professor Graham Mortimer, who kept my husband occupied so that I could work on the book! Alison Stewart and Clasina Robinson arranged housing and helped supply us with the necessities of life for our stay there.

After arriving back in Boston with pounds of paper and reference cards, it was time to put everything together. The two technologists with whom we work at Children's Hospital are responsible for most of the images in this book. They do beautiful studies every day on children who are sick, cranky, or just plain truculent; they are hard-working artists, and there is no way to thank them adequately—not only for helping with the book but, more important, for helping in the diagnostic evaluation of more than 7000 patients a year. We are almost afraid to divulge their names for fear of having them enticed away from us! Linda Masters and Donna Duncan, we hope we will be working with you for many years to come. Other contributors included Rosemary Frasso Jaramillo, our "apprentice technologist," and Drs. Kathleen Murray, James Meyer, Barbara Dangman, Kate Nimkin, April Preston, and Richard Braverman, who performed many of the portable studies. Jim Brewer made copies of selected films, in addition to his regular workload of running the darkroom. All of the photographic work was produced by Don Sucher, who, with the help of his son Aaron, had to deal with hundreds of postage stamp–sized images and print them the right way up—not an easy feat with ultrasonograms. We appreciate his tolerance of our prolonged project and thank him for his craftsmanship.

Miriam Geller, librarian in the Department of Radiology at Children's Hospital, was responsible for keeping us up to date with references and helping us to find the citations when we couldn't remember where we'd seen them. She was also in charge of the taxi service that brought Dr. Share to work for our early morning sessions during the winter months!

Secretaries are also unsung heroines and heroes. Susan McCarron Briggs never thought she would see so many references on ultrasonography. Judith Cohen helped us pull together the pieces by typing the tables and the legends for the figures—and then retyping them with our modifications.

A Department of Radiology is a reflection of the clinical services in a hospital; we are fortunate in working with some of the best pediatric surgeons and physicians in the world, and we benefit every day from their skill. Many have been instrumental in providing us with clinical information about their patients that we could include in the legends. Dr. Robert Shamberger should have his name in capital letters in this regard. Drs. Craig Lillehei, Joseph Vacanti, Jay Wilson, Jay Schnitzer, Dennis Lund, Judah Folkman, Angelo Eraklis, Neil Feins, and Samuel Schuster, and their chief, Dr. Hardy Hendren, are valued colleagues and have helped us immeasurably. The orthopedic surgeons, James Kasser, Michael Millis, Frank Rand, John Emans, Peter Waters, and their chief, John Hall, have worked with us in developing the orthopedic applications of ultrasonography, the most recent ultrasonic frontier. Much of the time, pediatric ultrasonography is renal ultrasonography. The Division of Urologic Surgery, headed by Dr. Alan Retik, includes Arnold Colodny, Stuart Bauer, James Mandell, Craig Peters, and their fellows. We value the working relationship with these surgeons that has been fostered by Dr. Robert Lebowitz, urologic radiologist extraordinaire and also a member of the division of urologic surgery. Our other radiologic colleagues have also had to bear with our project, and they have done so with great tolerance. Drs. Clif Harris, Bob Wilkinson, N. Thorne Griscom, Fredric Hoffer, Judy Estroff, Valerie Mandell, Diego Jaramillo, Roy Strand, Pat Barnes, Ted Treves, and Lorcan O'Tuama have been supportive and encouraging. Dr. Fred Hoffer is a master of many trades, including ultrasonography, and he performed many of the interventional procedures mentioned in the book. Dr. Judy Estroff works with us part time and also contributed illustrations. Our radiologist-in-chief is John A. Kirkpatrick, Jr. Without his support and encouragement, we would never have finished this project. For those of you who know him, we need not explain why he is included in the dedication of this book.

At W.B. Saunders Company, our editor was Lisette Bralow, who drew the line only when we asked for marbling on the end papers and who was the model of restraint as we passed several of our deadlines. Her assistant is Beth Bond. Ken Neimeister was the production manager; Anne Ostroff, a very patient copy editor; Peg Shaw, the coordinator of illustrations; Carolyn Naylor, the assistant general manager in the production department; Maureen Sweeney, the designer; Dorothy Chattin, the page layout artist; and Nancy Murphy, the marketing manager.

You, the reader, will appreciate that this book is different in format from the usual medical textbook. We have organized the chapters to reflect the clinical concerns that result in a child's being referred for ultrasonography. Included are not only the expected ultrasonographic findings for a specific disease or problem but also the pitfalls. Some of our opinions are undoubtedly biased, but they are tempered by over 15 years of experience in one of the busiest pediatric hospitals in the United States. The references that we have listed at the conclusion of each chapter are not all cited within the text, but they are included to allow the reader an easy foray into an area of interest.

Writing a book is much harder than having a baby. Gestational age seems to be dreadfully prolonged with books! We've saved our biggest thank you's for the last. We deeply appreciate the forbearance of our husbands throughout the past 2 years. Not only did they tolerate early mornings—5:50 A.M. on a digital clock is permanently imprinted on the retina of one David W. Teele—but they tolerated the late nights that we spent with computers and with photographic prints, which were used as carpeting for the Shares' apartment. The Teele children think that "book" is the forbidden four-letter word. Sarah, Elinor, Katharine, and Benjamin can now have back the use of the computer.

We hope that you, the reader, will learn as much from this book as we did from writing it and that children everywhere will benefit in some small way from our efforts.—Rita L. Teele

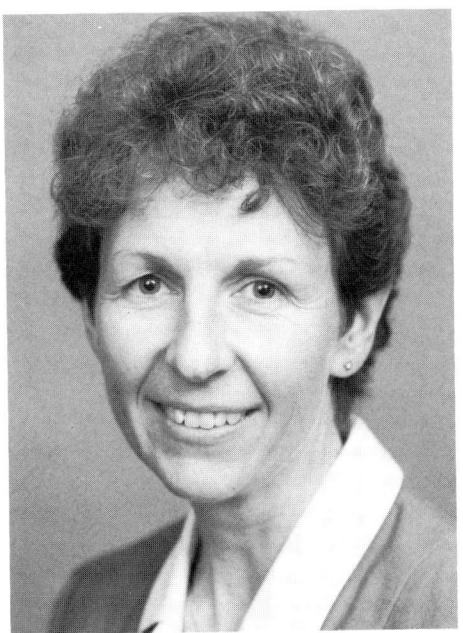

Rita Teele

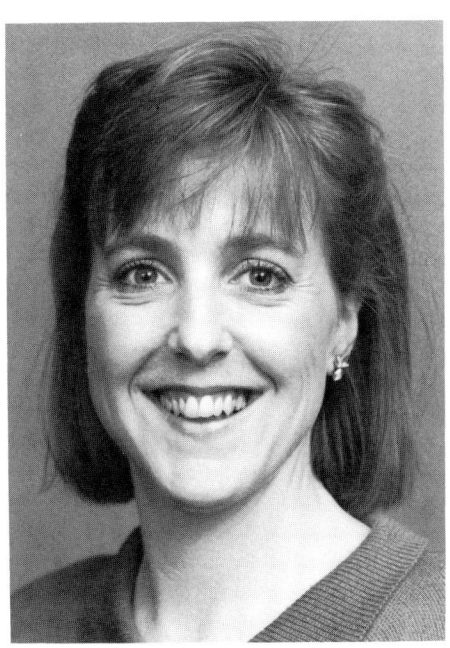

Jane Share

CONTENTS

CHAPTER 1
CRANIAL ULTRASONOGRAPHY 1

CHAPTER 2
SPINAL ULTRASONOGRAPHY AND INTRAOPERATIVE NEUROSONOGRAPHY 57

CHAPTER 3
THE FACE AND NECK 73

CHAPTER 4
THE CHEST 91

CHAPTER 5
THE EXTREMITIES 109

CHAPTER 6
RENAL SCREENING 137

CHAPTER 7
INFECTION OF THE URINARY TRACT 193

CHAPTER 8
ABDOMINAL MASSES 214

CHAPTER 9
ENDOCRINOLOGIC ULTRASONOGRAPHY 317

CHAPTER 10
RECURRENT ABDOMINAL PAIN 343

CHAPTER 11
INTRA-ABDOMINAL INFLAMMATION 346

CHAPTER 12
GASTRODUODENAL ULTRASONOGRAPHY 357

CHAPTER 13
BLUNT ABDOMINAL TRAUMA 364

CHAPTER 14
ASCITES AND OTHER ABDOMINAL PROBLEMS 372

CHAPTER 15
PANCREATITIS AND PANCREATIC MASSES 389

CHAPTER 16
THE SPLEEN 405

CHAPTER 17
THE LIVER 416

CHAPTER 18
HEPATIC TRANSPLANTATION 452

CHAPTER 19
PARENCHYMAL RENAL DISEASE 462

CHAPTER 20
RENAL TRANSPLANTATION 477

INDEX 491

ULTRASONOGRAPHY OF INFANTS AND CHILDREN

COLOR PLATE SECTION

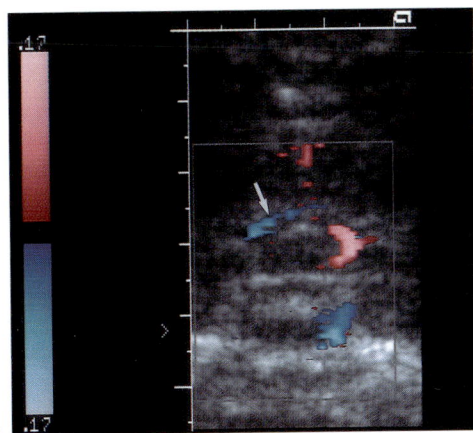 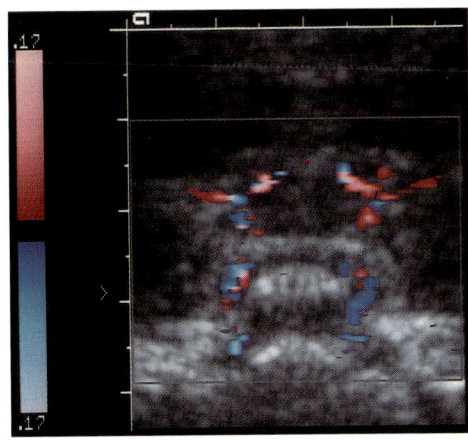

Plate I. These two views, of the anterior portion of the circle of Willis at the base of the brain, are of a baby who underwent extracorporeal membrane oxygenation (ECMO) for respiratory failure, which was precipitated by aspiration of meconium. Because the right carotid artery was used for cannulation during the procedure, flow to the right-sided anterior and middle cerebral arteries was via the left carotid and basilar arteries. Therefore, the flow in the right anterior communicating artery was *away* from the transducer (arrow, **A**). There was no detectable flow in the right carotid siphon. When the baby was taken off the ECMO circuit, the right carotid artery was reanastomosed, and the arterial circulation was restored to normal (**B**).

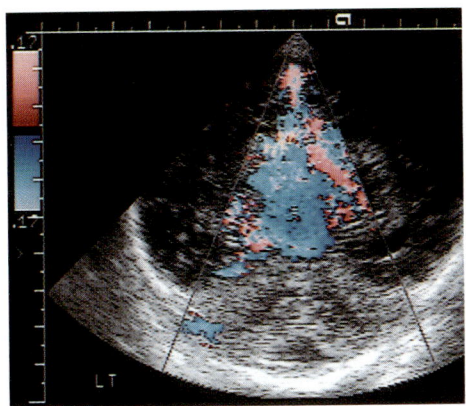 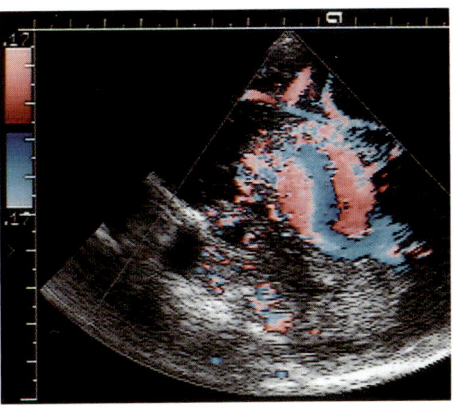

Plate II. Coronal (**A**) and midline sagittal (**B**) scans of the brain show swirling flow in a venous aneurysm, posterior to the third ventricle and part of a generalized malformation of cerebral vasculature. This baby had presented in congestive heart failure without underlying structural cardiac disease. He died after attempts at embolization.

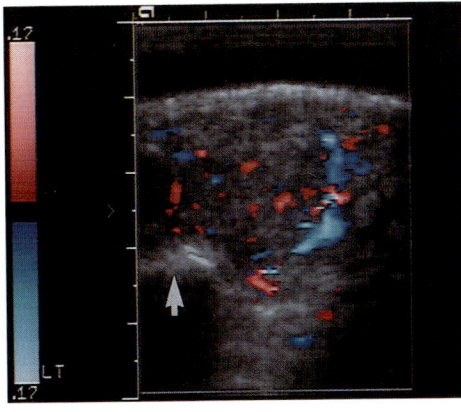

Plate III. The face is a common site for the development of vascular malformation and hemangioma. Often it is difficult, on clinical examination alone, to discriminate between them. This child has had a mass near the left parotid gland since birth. The mass has both arterial and venous flow within it and a moderate amount of stroma. It is regressing with age and therefore is likely to be a hemangioma rather than an arteriovenous malformation. A lymphatic malformation (cystic hygroma, lymphangioma) usually has large cystic spaces that are silent on Doppler ultrasonograms. A venous malformation is compressible and demonstrates only venous signal on Doppler ultrasonogram. Arrow = mandible.

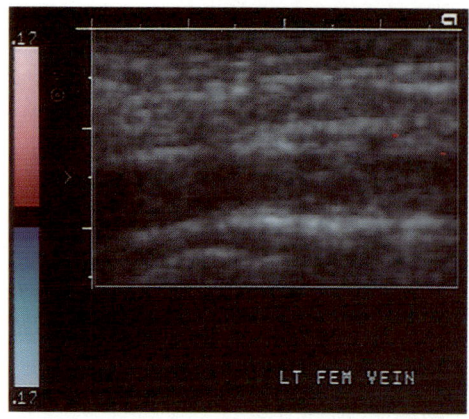 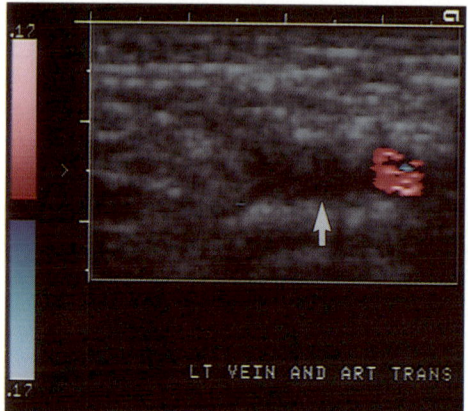

Plate IV. Color Doppler ultrasonography is not necessary for examination of patients suspected of having deep venous thrombosis, but it helps in quickly localizing the vessels. The femoral vein normally produces an obvious signal. The thrombosed vein is devoid of color **(A)**. When compressed, as on the transverse scan **(B)**, the vein does not flatten (arrow). The red signal is from the adjacent femoral artery.

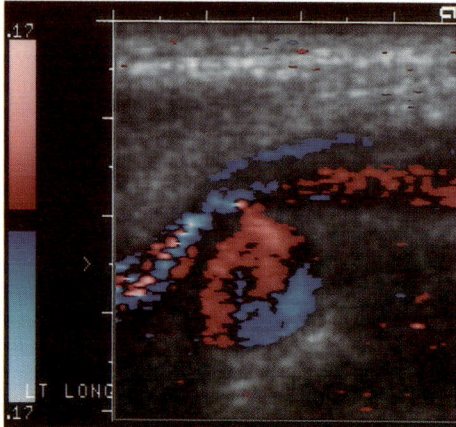 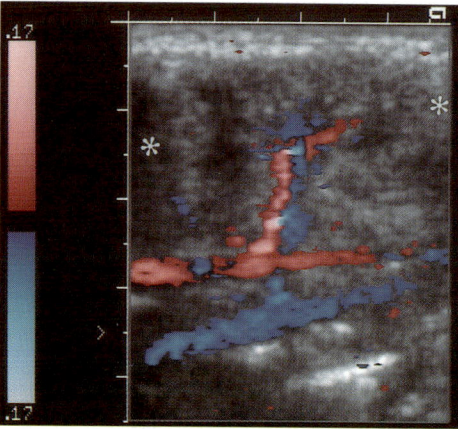

Plate V. This adolescent boy had suffered an accidental gunshot wound to the leg 1 year before this scan was performed. His shattered tibia was reconstructed with internal reduction and external fixation, and he regained his mobility. When he re-presented with a pulsatile mass in the popliteal fossa, the color Doppler examination demonstrated the presence of a pseudoaneurysm. This was removed, and the popliteal artery repaired. Note the yin/yang sign of circular flow in the pseudoaneurysm.

Plate VI. Coronal scan of the left kidney in a neonate born at 30 weeks' gestational age easily demonstrates the normal renal arterial (red) and venous (blue) flow with the corresponding great vessels. Asterisks mark upper and lower renal borders.

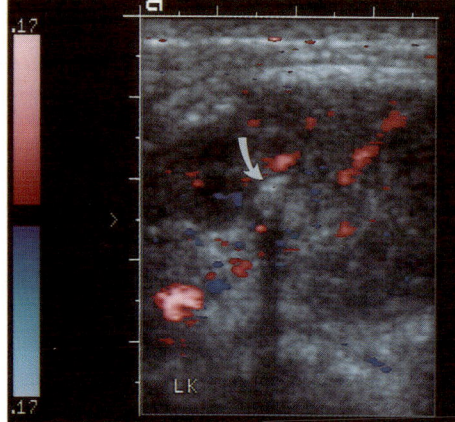

Plate VII. This baby, whose scans show renal venous thrombosis, presented with a left-sided flank mass and hematuria. Arterial flow (red) entering the kidney is apparent, but there is no flow exiting the kidney. A shadowing thrombus (arrow) is present in the renal vein.

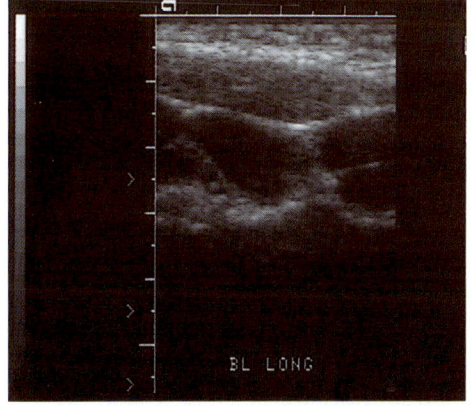
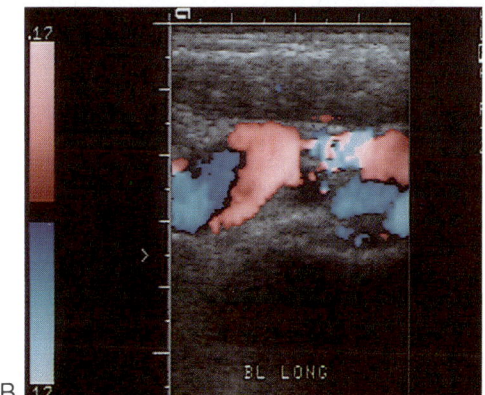
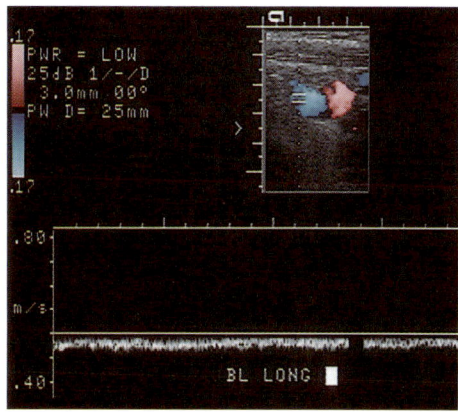

Plate VIII. These three scans are longitudinal midline views of the pelvis in a boy whose Ewing sarcoma of the ilium was treated with radiation and chemotherapy after surgery. The large lucent tubular structure is a collateral vessel (**A** and **B**). Pulsed Doppler ultrasonogram shows that it has a venous signal (**C**). Any unusual cystic mass in the abdomen or pelvis should be evaluated with color or pulsed Doppler ultrasonography, or both, in order to determine whether it is vascular in origin.

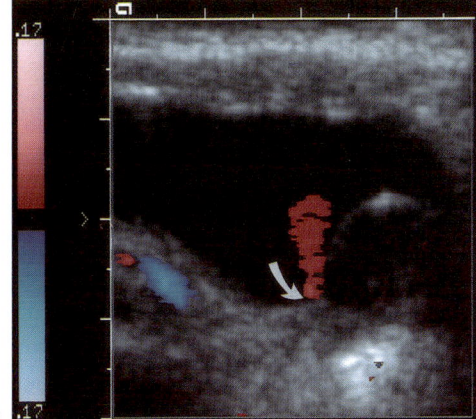
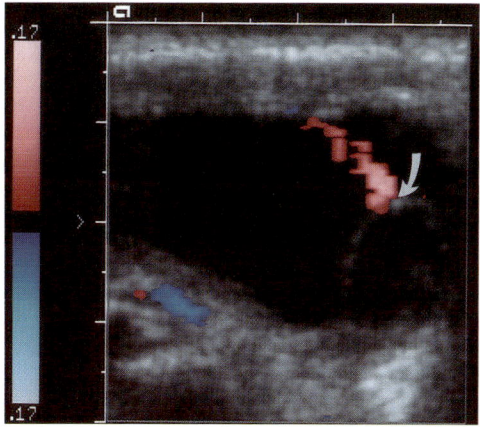

Plate IX. Color flow does not necessarily imply vascular flow. The ability of color Doppler ultrasonography to demonstrate ureteral jets is well known. In this child, the normal right-sided ureteral orifice (arrow, **A**) is unaffected by the adjacent left-sided ureterocele. The ureter from the lower pole of the duplex left kidney exits (arrow, **B**) on the mound of the ureterocele because its tunnel is distorted by the adjacent anomaly. The ureterocele is the distal termination of the obstructed ureter from the upper pole.

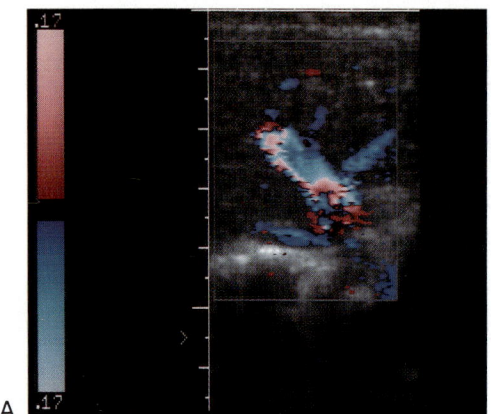 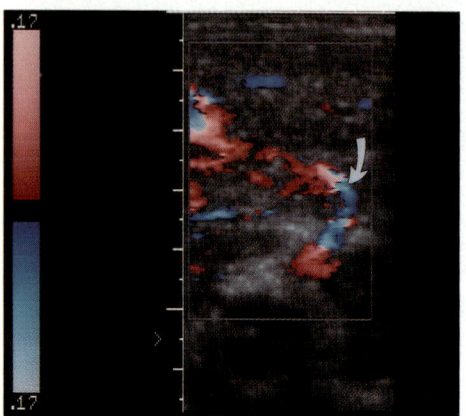

Plate X. Two scans show the vascular supply and drainage from an arteriovenous malformation (AVM) that effectively replaced the liver in this newborn girl. She presented in respiratory distress, and it was originally thought that congenital heart disease was a cause of her symptoms. The cardiologists diagnosed the hepatic anomaly when they saw turbulent flow entering the right atrium from a distended inferior vena cava. The transverse view just below the diaphragm **(A)** shows the large hepatic veins with the middle dilated out of proportion to the others. The other transverse scan **(B)** demonstrates the dilated hepatic artery (arrow), which carries the major arterial supply to the AVM in the liver. Two separate angiographic procedures allowed embolization of multiple vessels that supplied the liver, but baby died because similar malformations involved other abdominal viscera.

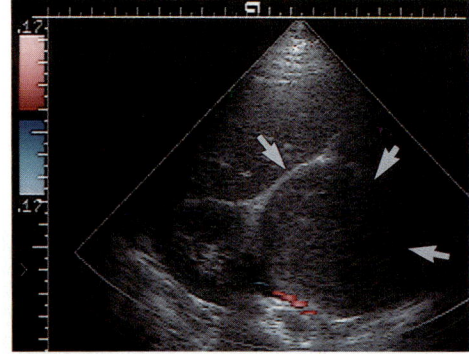 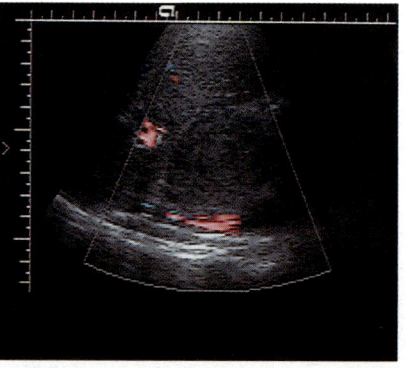

Plate XI. Transverse **(A)** and longitudinal **(B)** views of the upper abdomen show a large avascular mass sandwiched between the inferior vena cava and the portal vein. These scans localize the mass to the head of the pancreas. The patient was a 16-year-old girl who presented to the emergency room with symptoms of mild abdominal discomfort. She was quite obese; no mass was palpable. Ultrasonography was requested to rule out cholelithiasis. Computed tomography (CT) scans confirmed the presence and location of the mass as shown on ultrasonography and revealed no other abnormalities. A cystadenocarcinoma of the head of the pancreas was removed during Whipple procedure.

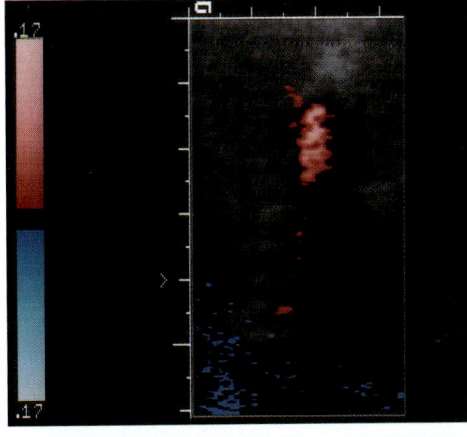

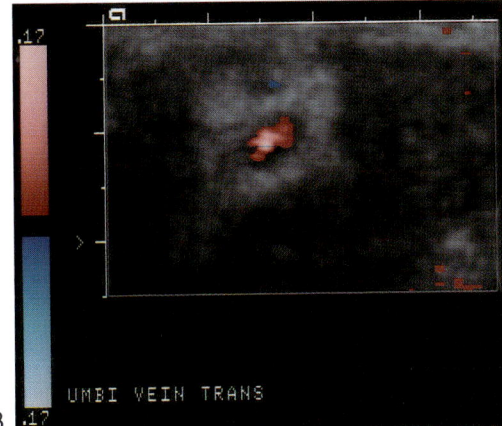
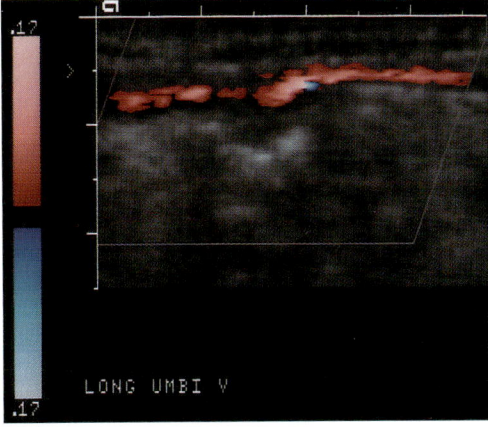

Plate XII. The umbilical vein was patent in this 3-year-old boy, who developed cirrhosis of the liver after prolonged therapy with intravenous hyperalimentation. Flow in the left portal vein **(A)** was hepatopetal, but it exited the liver via the ligamentum teres **(B)** to the umbilical vein **(C)**. Scans shown are transverse views of the left portal vein and the ligamentum teres; the patent umbilical vein is shown in a longitudinal view.

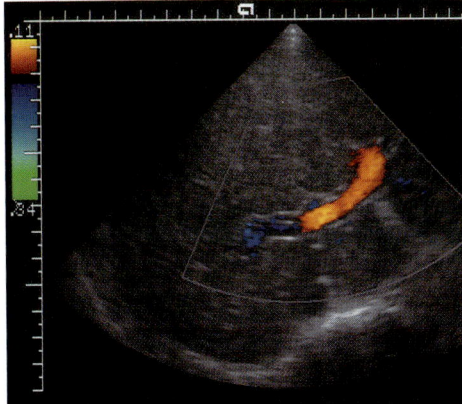
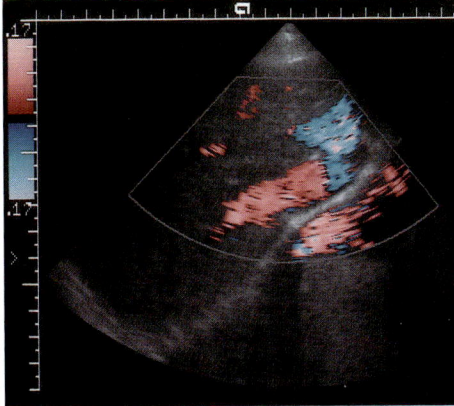

Plate XIII. The normal portal vein and hepatic artery are both hepatopetal in their course. In color Doppler imaging, both color signals may combine to produce one track of color entering the liver. Note that on this transverse scan, the left portal vein is orange because flow is moving toward the transducer. In the right portal vein, flow is moving away from the transducer and thus is coded as blue.

Plate XIV. The normal hepatic veins are shown in this upright view of the upper inferior vena cava. Because blood in the right hepatic vein is flowing toward the transducer, its color signal is red. The left and middle hepatic veins have combined and show a blue signal because their flow of blood is away from the transducer.

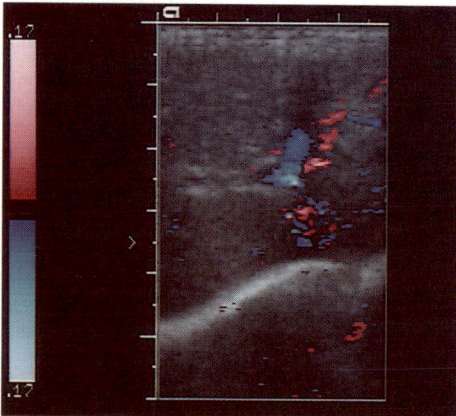

Plate XV. Severe portal hypertension has resulted in reversal of portal venous flow, demonstrated on this transverse scan. The blue signal is from blood in the left portal vein flowing away from the transducer in a hepatofugal course. The red signal is from blood in the left hepatic artery.

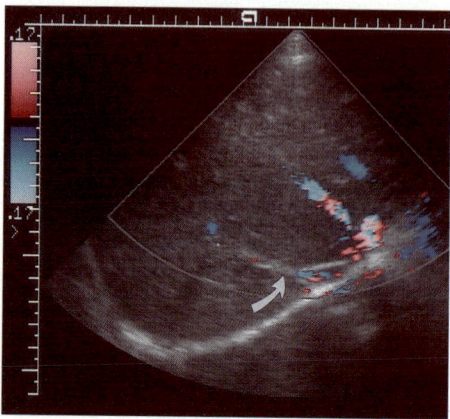

Plate XVI. Compare this scan of a boy who has Budd-Chiari syndrome with the normal scan shown in Plate XIV. The hepatic veins are small in caliber, and the flow is disordered in comparison with normal. Only the right hepatic vein connected to the inferior vena cava, and this connection was narrow (arrow). The left and middle hepatic veins joined the right via a circuitous collateral vein within the liver. We assume that the diagnosis is of a venous dysgenesis that prevented normal development of the draining hepatic veins. Tests of liver function had persisted in remaining mildly abnormal when he was taken off drugs that treated his hyperactivity. Ultrasonography revealed the venous abnormality, which was treated, unsuccessfully, with catheterization and balloon dilatation of the right hepatic vein.

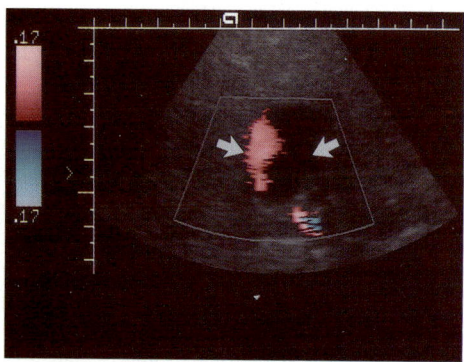

Plate XVII. Longitudinal scan of the portal vein shows a color signal from only half the vessel (arrows). This patient, who had undergone hepatic transplantation, was developing portal venous thrombosis in the graft. He died shortly after this study was done.

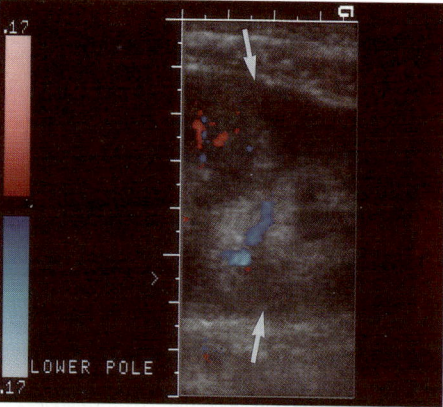

Plate XVIII. Longitudinal scan of a transplanted kidney, performed within 24 hours of surgery, shows no color signal from the lower pole. This portion of the kidney was supplied by a separate renal artery that thrombosed after surgery. Note also the relative lucency of the parenchyma of the lower pole from the acute ischemia. Arrows mark the boundary between vascular and avascular portions.

CHAPTER 1

CRANIAL ULTRASONOGRAPHY

TECHNIQUE

Most of our patients who require cranial ultrasonography are premature babies, and most neurosonography is therefore performed in the special care nursery. It is always easier to move an ultrasound unit to the bedside than to move a sick baby with the attendant equipment. This investment of time outside the department—both for equipment and for personnel—requires good planning. Nurses in the intensive care nursery appreciate being called in advance of the study. An intravenous line, which enters the scalp over the fontanelle, means that either the line is sacrificed or the examination is postponed. The sick neonate requires multiple interventive procedures, and stress to the infant should be kept to a minimum; for example, we try not to do scans directly after the baby has been fed because manipulation predisposes the baby to vomit, and nutrition is too crucial to lose. On entering the nursery, we check in with the nursing staff, pick up the requisition, and follow the routine gowning/washing procedure. Ideally, the requisition should list the baby's gestational age, age in days, and birth weight. In a teaching hospital, this allows collection of worthwhile demographic data. The reality is that true gestational age is difficult to ascertain unless the baby is the result of in vitro fertilization! Information regarding the mother's last menstrual period is notoriously unreliable when it is obtained second- or third-hand. Results of ultrasonography in the first trimester may or may not be available. The Dubowitz score, a clinical assessment of gestational age, is inaccurate for babies of very low birth weight. It is therefore important, if tabulating gestational age, that one notes the source of the information. As a corollary, when one is reading the medical literature, it is critical to know how gestational age was ascertained in studies of premature neonates.

There is often little room for a large ultrasound unit between monitors, ventilators, and incubators. The nurses need access to the baby at all times. The machine should be plugged in, warmed up, and set up with the identifying data before the baby is disturbed. Good cleansing of the transducer and of one's hands is the last step before one opens the incubator. Heat shields and oxygen hoods should be moved out of the way; oxygen by mask can be substituted. A cloth under the baby's head saves the bedding from being ruined by the coupling gel. If good access through a porthole in the incubator is available, the study can be done without heat lamps. If the door is completely open, blankets or heat lamps are needed to keep the baby warm. The added light from lamps reduces the examiner's visual acuity; they should be aimed at the baby and not at the viewing screen.

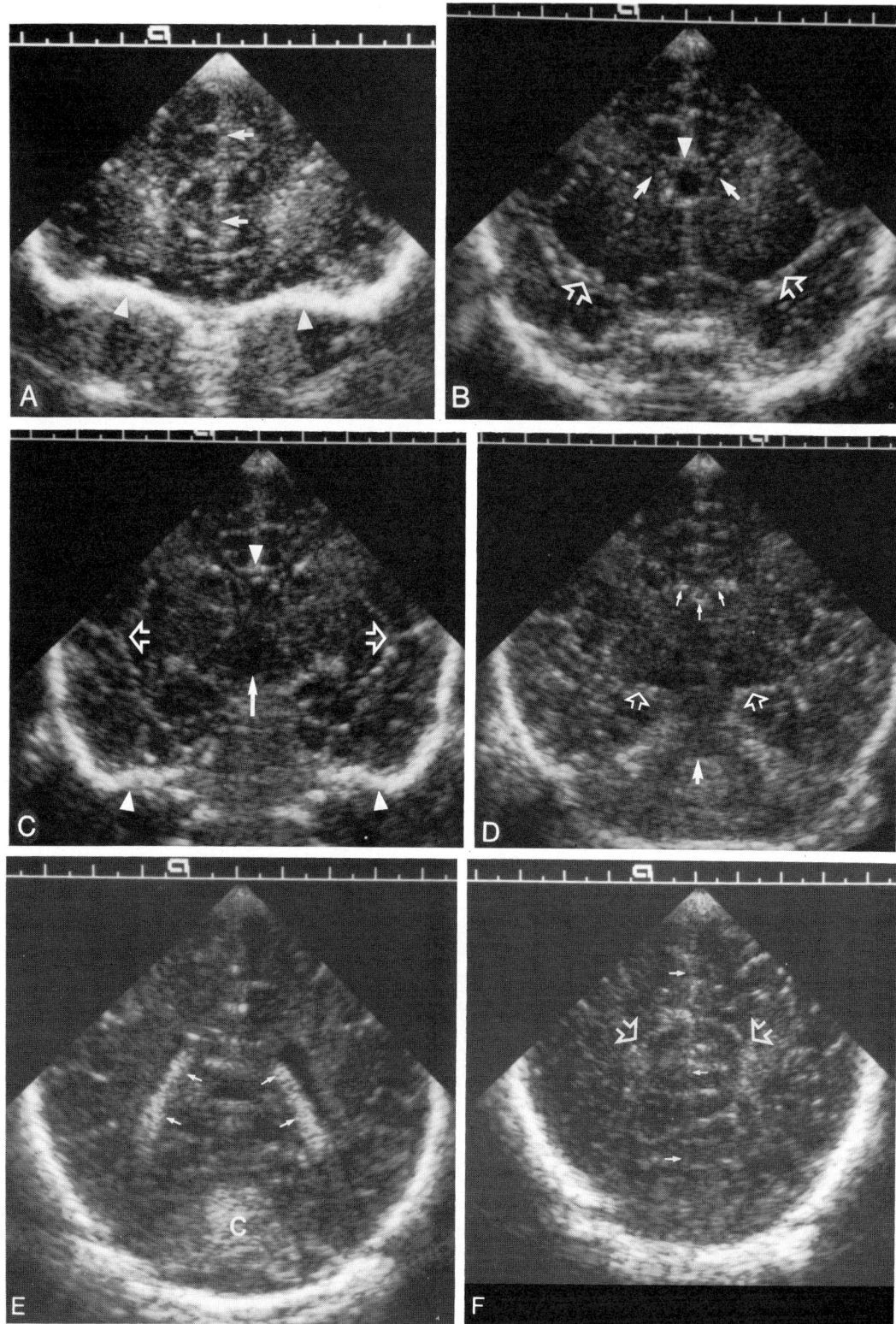

Figure 1–1 See legend on opposite page

To have comparable examinations, we follow a protocol that gives us a minimum of six coronal scans and six sagittal scans for each baby. Abnormalities are studied in detail with extra views. Using the anterior fontanelle as an acoustic window, and viewing the brain in the coronal plane, we sweep the transducer from anterior to posterior. By convention, the right side of the brain is displayed on the left side of the screen. Because the fontanelle is variable in size and covered with variable amounts of hair, the smaller the transducer, the easier the access. The coronal scans are not truly coronal but angled from the fulcrum of the anterior fontanelle. The most posterior section, therefore, is actually an axial view of the parietal and occipital cortex. The six standard views and the anatomic landmarks that define each section are

1. Orbital roofs (Fig. 1–1A): longitudinal, intracerebral fissure; frontal cortex; frontal gyri.
2. Pentagon view (Fig. 1–1B): five-sided star formed from internal carotid, middle cerebral, and anterior communicating arteries; anterior horns of lateral ventricles; genu of corpus callosum; basal ganglia; subependymal germinal matrix; tips of temporal lobes.
3. Third ventricle (Fig. 1–1C): foramen of Monro; choroid plexus of lateral and third ventricles; basal ganglia and thalami; bodies of lateral ventricles; temporal lobes.
4. Fourth ventricle (Fig. 1–1D): bodies of lateral ventricles; quadrigeminal plate and cistern; medulla; fourth ventricle; cerebellar hemispheres; cisterna magna.
5. Trigones (Fig. 1–1E): choroid plexus in lateral ventricles; periventricular white matter; parietal and occipital cortex.
6. Over the top (Fig. 1–1F): occipital horns of lateral ventricles; parietal and occipital cortex; centrum semiovale.

For the six sagittal sections, two views of midline are followed by a parasagittal scan of the right lateral ventricle; a steep parasagittal scan of right frontal, parietal and temporal cortex; a parasagittal scan of the left lateral ventricle; and a steep parasagittal scan of left frontal, parietal, and temporal cortex (Fig. 1–2). With this format, the films from sequential scans can be hung side by side on a viewbox and changes in ventricular size easily appreciated.

More points regarding technique are as follows. (1) Know your neuroanatomy. (2) The base of the skull must be perfectly symmetric on coronal scans. The transducers now allow such good resolution that on angled coronal scans, normal fiber tracts on one side appear different from those on the other and simulate pathology (Fig. 1–3). (3) Check pulsation of vessels; especially compare middle cerebral arteries. (4) On sagittal midline scans, establish a plane of section in line with the cavum septum pellucidum if it is present (or with the third ventricle if not) and with the fourth ventricle. If this seems difficult, look at the baby instead of the screen, and line up the transducer with the baby's nose. (5) To get views of an entire lateral ventricle, move the transducer to the side of the fontanelle *opposite* the ventricle of interest, and angle it back toward the ventricle. This allows access through the maximal diameter of the fontanelle. Because the lateral ventricle is not in a truly sagittal plane, the posterior edge of the transducer must be more lateral than the anterior edge. (6) If possible, consign to another person the tasks of changing films,

Figure 1–1. Normal coronal scans in a baby born at term. **A** shows the most anterior of the routine views. Arrows mark the longitudinal intracerebral fissure. Arrowheads mark orbital roofs. Note the symmetric blush from fibers that pass anterior to the anterior horns of the lateral ventricles in each cerebral hemisphere. **B** is the "pentagon view." Anterior horns of the lateral ventricles, when normal, are slitlike (arrows). Arrowhead marks the genu of the corpus callosum. The cavum septum pellucidum is the central lucency below the corpus callosum. Middle cerebral arteries in sylvian fissures are marked by open arrows. **C** is a coronal scan at the level of the foramen of Monro. The floor of the middle cranial fossa is marked by lower arrowheads. The third ventricle is a vertical lucent slit (arrow) inferior to the choroid plexus. Upper arrowhead marks the corpus callosum. Sylvian fissures are Y-shaped interfaces bilaterally (open arrows). In **D**, the normal fourth ventricle (large arrow) is an interface between the two cerebellar hemispheres. The choroid plexus in the roof of third and floor of the lateral ventricles is marked by small arrows. The posterior choroidal artery (open arrows) marks the superior margin of the temporal lobe. In **E**, this coronal view is the most valuable in the evaluation of periventricular white matter around the trigones of the lateral ventricles. The choroid plexus (arrows) is evident in each lateral ventricle. The cerebellum (C) is echogenic in the posterior fossa. **F** is the sixth view in the series and is close to an axial view. The centrum semiovale is a symmetric, echogenic blush in each cerebral hemisphere (open arrows), equidistant from the longitudinal fissure (small arrows).

4 / CRANIAL ULTRASONOGRAPHY

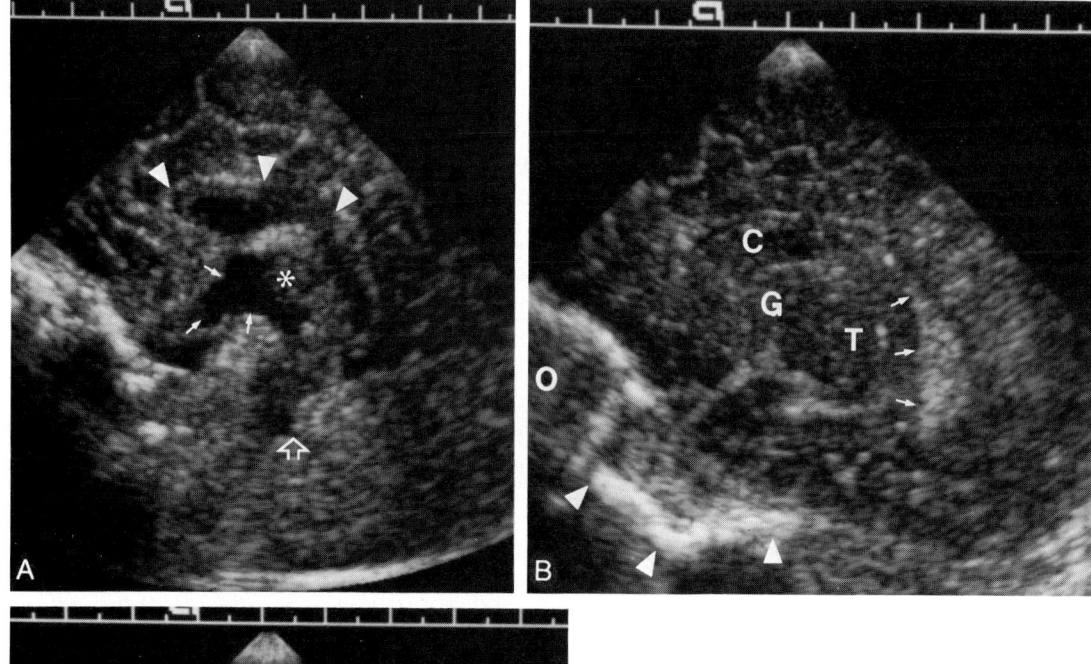

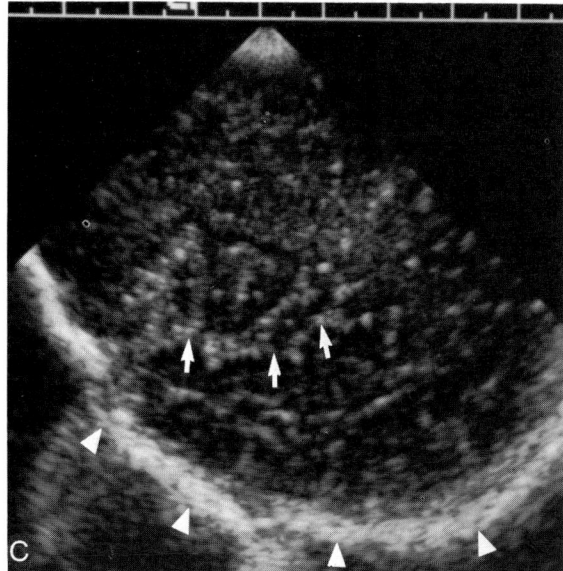

Figure 1–2. Normal sagittal scans. **A** shows the midline sagittal view. The third ventricle (small arrows) is outlined by cerebrospinal fluid tracking anteriorly around the massa intermedia of the thalamus (asterisk). Arrowheads mark the corpus callosum; the open arrow marks the fourth ventricle. **B** is a sagittal scan of the normal lateral ventricle. Note the head of the caudate (C), the basal ganglia (G), and the thalamus (T). The choroid plexus lies along the floor of the lateral ventricle (arrows). Arrowheads outline the base of the skull. O = orbit. **C** is a steep parasagittal scan of the frontal, parietal, and temporal cortex. The sylvian fissure is outlined with arrows. Arrowheads outline the base of the skull.

modifying gain and slope settings, and squirting gel. (7) When in doubt, use more gel!

Many radiologists videotape procedures performed outside the department. This is a perfectly reasonable approach; real-time scanning, vicarious or not, is preferable to reliance on static views alone. The staff in the neonatal care unit appreciate being notified of the results of a study as soon as possible. Changes in management of a baby may need to take place, and, equally important, parents like to be kept informed of the results of examinations. We feel that cranial scans of babies in the intensive care units should be done without their parents present. Scans that show a large intraparenchymal hemorrhage in a baby's brain are obviously abnormal to the layperson. Seeing the actual picture is extremely upsetting to the parents. Also, all information regarding a neonate's clinical condition should be given by just one or two caregivers. One can hardly feign ignorance regarding the scans if one is performing them. On the other hand, the nurses, house staff, and neonatologists ben-

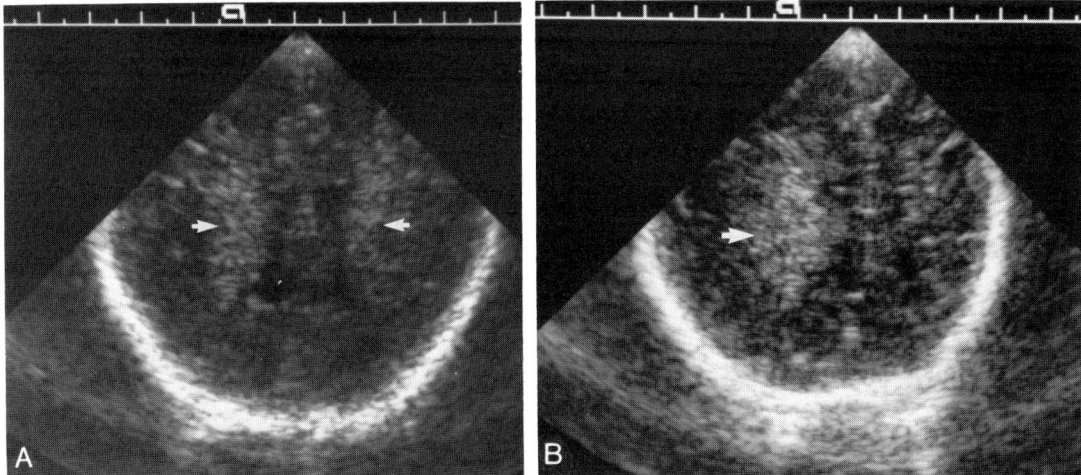

Figure 1–3. There is normally an echogenic blush (arrows) on both sides of the longitudinal cerebral fissure (**A**). This represents the centrum semiovale, which is the coronal view of the corona radiata. Note that if the transducer is angled in relation to the base of the skull, then normal fiber tracks on one side are more or less parallel to the beam, and the blush (arrow) is asymmetric (**B**).

efit from seeing the study as it is done, particularly when a subtle abnormality is present.

When babies come to the department for cranial ultrasonography, no preparation, such as sedation, is needed. Parents usually accompany their children, and we explain the study to them, emphasizing that we are looking at cranial anatomy and *not* potential intelligence. These are babies who generally are well and are referred because of craniomegaly or who are having follow-up scans after having graduated from the intensive care units. Their parents are better able to cope in this situation. If the baby is inconsolable, it may help to feed the child during the study or let a parent hold the child. The fontanelle generally stays palpably patent in the baby up to 6 months of age and longer in those born prematurely. Even in older infants, there remains enough of a window through which to measure the lateral ventricles, although views of parenchyma and the posterior fossa are limited. In early infancy the posterior fontanelle may be a site of access, but it is usually small, and the views obtained are not as easy to orient. However, abnormality of the posterior fossa can be amplified with such scans and matched more easily with computed tomography (CT) scans. Axial scans through the thin temporal bone add little to the study except in cases of extra-axial collections of fluid, which can often be visualized best in this plane, and in Doppler studies of the middle cerebral arteries.

THE PREMATURE INFANT
Clinical Background

Screening for intracranial hemorrhage (ICH), specifically germinal matrix hemorrhage and intraventricular hemorrhage, is the most common request that we receive from the neonatal nursery. Babies between 26 and 32 weeks of gestational age (weighing 880 to 1830 g) are at particular risk for ICH. Large studies of premature infants show the prevalence of ICH, as determined by ultrasonography or CT, to be 29 to 48 percent of the populations studied (van de Bor et al., 1987; Anderson et al., 1988). In a combined study from the nurseries of three Boston hospitals, 38 percent of 328 babies weighing less than 1751 g had ICH as determined by ultrasonography (Kuban et al., 1986).

Infants with ICH may have subtle or no neurologic signs. According to two prospective studies, the clinical diagnosis of hemorrhage was made in 50 percent (Lazzara et al., 1980) and 75 percent (Dubowitz et al., 1981) of babies subsequently shown to have ICH on imaging. Retrospective studies indicate that the clinical diagnosis is made less often, in about one third of cases (Szymonowicz et al., 1984). Apnea and bradycardia, hypotension, drop in hematocrit, and changes in findings of neurologic examination are clues to ICH but do not specify the intracranial events. The baby may exhibit signs and symptoms that appear with alarming speed after a large intracranial hemorrhage. In our experience, however, this result is much less common than gradual clinical deterioration. Longitudinal studies of premature infants have shown that approximately 50 percent of infants with ICH experience the onset of hemorrhage in the first 24 hours after birth. Onset of hemorrhage occurs in 90 percent of affected babies by 72 hours (Partridge et al., 1983). Of importance is that progression of the ultrasonographic abnormalities may occur in babies shown to have ICH early in their clinical course. Levene and de Vries (1984) reported that 17 of 126 infants with intracranial hemorrhage had extension of their abnormality, usually within 3 days of initial diagnosis. In another study, more than 40 percent of infants had worsening scans (Partridge et al., 1983).

Why should premature babies be at high risk for ICH? There are both anatomic and physiologic reasons. The germinal matrix, a highly vascular nest of neuroblasts, occupies the region adjacent to the developing caudate nucleus until the middle of the third trimester, at which time it involutes. The germinal matrix is a developmental watershed because its arterial supply is from both anterior and middle cerebral arteries. Its capillary bed is atypical in that the vessels are large, irregular, and loosely lined with endothelium. The region that it occupies is exquisitely sensitive to hypoxia, acidosis, changes in blood pressure, coagulative state, and possibly other variables. The extracranial physiologic problems of the premature neonate—respiratory distress and mechanical ventilation; cardiac dysfunction or patent ductus arteriosus; metabolic derangements and poor nutrition—contribute to disturb intracranial homeostasis.

The following hypothetical situation of a baby sustaining an acute pneumothorax provides a model with which to appreciate the chain of events that culminate in hemorrhage. A small premature baby who has hyaline membrane disease is being ventilated with positive pressure when pulmonary interstitial air acutely ruptures into the pleural space. The baby becomes acutely hypertensive, the ipsilateral lung cannot collapse because of interstitial air, and the mediastinum shifts into the opposite hemithorax, thereby compromising the other lung. The increased intrapleural pressure from the pneumothorax prevents normal venous return to the right side of the heart. The cardiac output drops, and the baby becomes hypotensive and acidotic. Because the vascular supply of the germinal matrix is pressure passive, it is subjected to a fluctuating cerebral blood flow from the initial hypertension and subsequent hypotension. The cells of the germinal matrix, which have a high requirement for oxygen, suffer both from low oxygen tension in the blood and from acidosis. Vascular flow is further slowed by the impedance to venous return in the chest, and at some critical point, blood bursts from the vascular network into the gelatinous matrix. Fibrinolytic activity in the region prevents some of the clotting mechanisms from functioning. Blood accumulates in a subependymal blister and then bursts through the ependymal lining of the adjacent ventricle.

In fact, acute pneumothorax is one of the known triggers of ICH in premature babies, and its occurrence is adequate reason to perform cranial ultrasonography even after the first 5 days of life, when most instances of ICH have occurred.

Because both germinal matrix and intraventricular hemorrhages can be recognized easily on ultrasonograms of good quality, we have tended in the past to focus on hemorrhage to the exclusion of the rest of the brain. It has become apparent that hemorrhage in the germinal matrix is the proverbial tip of the iceberg: such hemorrhage is a sign that the premature brain has suffered an insult. The neurologic prognosis of premature babies with hemorrhage is better correlated with the degree of injury to the brain, when it can be measured, than with the severity of intraventricular hemorrhage. The problem in imaging is in evaluating the degree of parenchymal injury. The same physiologic event or events that promote germinal matrix hemorrhage undoubtedly affect other areas of brain. In addition, expansion of the lateral ventricle with blood under pressure may change the ipsilateral circulation to periventricular tissue, specifically by affecting the venous drainage (Volpe, 1989b).

Hypoxic ischemic insults are, according to most neuropathologists and clinicians, responsible for periventricular damage to white matter in the premature brain. This damage is called periventricular leukomalacia (PVL). This descriptive term refers to the appearance of the involved brain on gross examination. PVL simply means areas of soft white spots that represent necrosis. They are usually distributed around ventricular trigones and near the foramen of Monro. These areas are border zones between posterior and middle circulations and between middle and anterior circulations, respectively. PVL particularly affects the premature infant; in contrast, the full-term infant exhibits different histopathologic responses to hypoxic-ischemic insult.

Hypoxic-ischemic injury resulting in PVL appears to follow a course of coagulation necrosis, astrocytic degeneration, microglial reaction, proliferation of astrocytes, and endothelial hyperplasia with or without superimposed hemorrhage (Banker and Larroche, 1962). A hemorrhage may be subtle and petechial in appearance or gross, extending outward to involve adjacent gray matter. If necrosis is severe and the ependymal lining of the adjacent ventricle ruptures, the hemorrhage evolves into a porencephalic cyst as it heals. Diffuse necrotic regions with adjacent intact ventricular ependyma result in cystic encephalomalacia: multiple small cysts replacing white matter in the periventricular regions. Over time, these cysts may shrink and disappear on ultrasonographs, but glial scarring and impaired myelination remain (de Vries, Wigglesworth, et al., 1988). The degree of ischemia required to produce PVL may vary, depending on the state of development of periventricular vessels. This variation is primarily a function of gestational age (de Reuck, 1971). Premature infants may be spared generalized cortical necrosis because of the presence of bridging leptomeningeal vessels (Brett, 1983). Mortality rates in those babies with extensive intraparenchymal hemorrhage is high, and of the survivors, almost 100 percent have neurologic, particularly motor, deficits (Monset-Couchard et al., 1988; Nwaesei et al., 1988; Zorzi et al., 1988).

Ultrasonography is insensitive to subtle ischemic damage in the brain, especially when involvement is symmetric. Studies of autopsies of premature infants suggest that ultrasonography misses at least 25 percent of those with PVL (de Vries, Wigglesworth, et al., 1988; Carson et al., 1990). Abnormal results of scans, at term or when a baby is discharged from an intensive care nursery, are strongly predictive of later neurodevelopmental abnormalities, but normal scan results are not predictive of a normal outcome (Nwaesei et al., 1988). Another study revealed a 62 percent rate of false-negative scans; only 11 of 39 abnormal hemispheres (hypoxic-ischemic injury but no hemorrhage) were identified on ultrasonography before the babies' deaths (Hope et al., 1988).

The ultrasonographic literature has been less than uniform in its definition of PVL, and many published reports have had little or no neuropathologic correlation to support the ultrasonographic findings. Unfortunately, there is also confusion with another term: "periventricular intraventricular hemorrhage." Most authors use this latter term to describe hemorrhage in the periventricular germinal matrix associated with intraventricular extension. In the literature on cranial ultrasonography, it is worth paying careful attention to the definitions used in a paper and to the correlative histopathology offered in proof of a particular observation. We support the use of the descriptive term "intraparenchymal echogenicity" (IPE), rather than assigning a pathologic diagnosis to an ultrasonographic finding. Research with magnetic resonance imaging (MRI) and positron-emission tomography (PET) is being directed toward evaluation of the early changes in hypoxic-ischemic encephalopathy of the premature baby. Clinical research is ongoing for groups of babies, identified as having IPE on ultrasonography, who survive into childhood.

Cranial Ultrasonography of Premature Infants

When doing an ultrasonographic study of a premature baby, one should follow the routine series of scans and obtain extra views if an abnormality is evident. Specific areas of interest in this population are (1) the region of the germinal matrix that corresponds to the region of the caudate nucleus but also extends back along the subependymal border of the lateral ventricle; (2) the size and contents of the lateral, third, and fourth ventricles; and (3) cerebral parenchyma, particularly in the peritrigonal area and near the foramen of Monro. The brain changes dra-

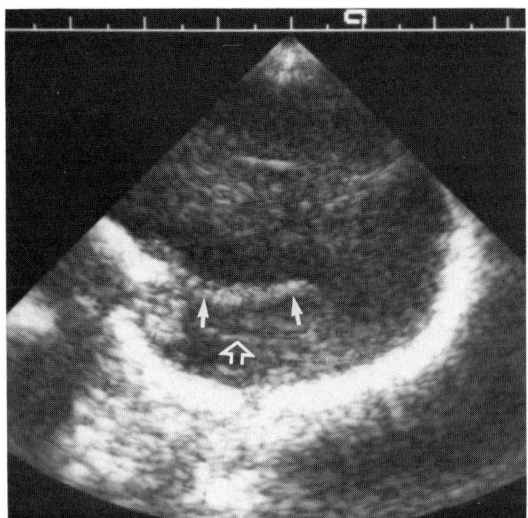

Figure 1–4. Steep parasagittal scan of the temporal lobe in a baby who is only 26 weeks of gestational age. Note the relatively smooth, featureless brain in comparison with Figure 1–2C. The sylvian fissure is present (arrows). There is early development of the superior temporal sulcus (open arrow).

matically in its appearance during the second and third trimesters with the development of sulci and gyri (Fig. 1–4).

Screening studies are done after the 3rd day of postnatal life, and we routinely study those babies who are born younger than 33 weeks of gestation. In a large study from The Netherlands, gestational age was better correlated with intraventricular hemorrhage than was birth weight (van de Bor et al., 1987). If a baby has had initial instability, unexplained drop in hematocrit, coagulopathy, change in neurologic status, or unexplained episodes of apnea and bradycardia, we do the study on demand. The neonate who has sustained tension pneumothorax at any age is also studied at the request of the clinicians because this insult predisposes even the older premature infant to hemorrhage.

The germinal matrix, being a very vascular network, may in normal, very premature babies (aged 25 to 28 weeks) be slightly more echogenic than adjacent brain tissue, which at this stage has the consistency of jelly. In older premature infants, the germinal matrix is inseparable in appearance from the caudate nucleus. It becomes quite echogenic when it contains a hemorrhage. We rely heavily on the "pentagon view," which presents the vasculature from the circle of Willis as a five-sided star. This coronal section cuts across the major portion of germinal matrix. Asymmetry in echogenicity just inferior to the lateral ventricles usually represents hemorrhage. This can be confirmed with sagittal views because any echogenicity anterior to the foramen of Monro is abnormal (Fig. 1–5). The choroid plexus, a thick echogenic band that hugs the floor of the lateral ventricles, passes through the foramen to cling to the roof of the third ventricle.

Small amounts of intraventricular blood can be identified if the choroid is asymmetrically very irregular or if there is echogenicity extending back into occipital horns (Fig. 1–6). Neuropathologic studies suggest that coincident hemorrhage in the choroid plexus is present in 25 percent of premature infants with other sources of intraventricular hemorrhage (Armstrong, unpublished data cited by Volpe, 1987). With ultrasonography we cannot differentiate an intrinsic hemorrhage of the choroid plexus from a clot that adheres to the choroid. There are three pitfalls to avoid: (1) children with meningomyelocele and Arnold-Chiari II malformation often have a lumpy, bumpy choroid plexus (Fig. 1–7); (2) in a very immature baby, 24–27 weeks old, lateral ventricles, including occipital horns, may normally be filled with choroid; and (3) in any baby, parasagittal scans may cut the calcar avis in such a way that it appears to be an intraventricular echogenic mass—that is, a clot (Fig. 1–8; DiPietro et al., 1985).

Grading intraventricular hemorrhage has been popular with many physicians, but there are drawbacks to its use. First, there are several grading systems, and one has to know the definitions of each and know which is being used in an institution or by a physician or a nurse. The original system of grading intraventricular hemorrhage was, in fact, based on CT scans and not on ultrasonograms. Grade IV hemorrhage was originally thought to represent an extension of the intraventricular hemorrhage into the brain, but now it is recognized as a sign of primary parenchymal involvement. Hemorrhage into the ventricles is part of a dynamic, not static, situation, and depending on the time of the scan, the grade may change. Babies, however, tend to get labeled as "a grade I" or "a grade IV," and the label sticks with no subtleties attached. Grading systems do not allow detailed description of the parenchymal abnormalities that, as discussed previously, are likely the most important findings on

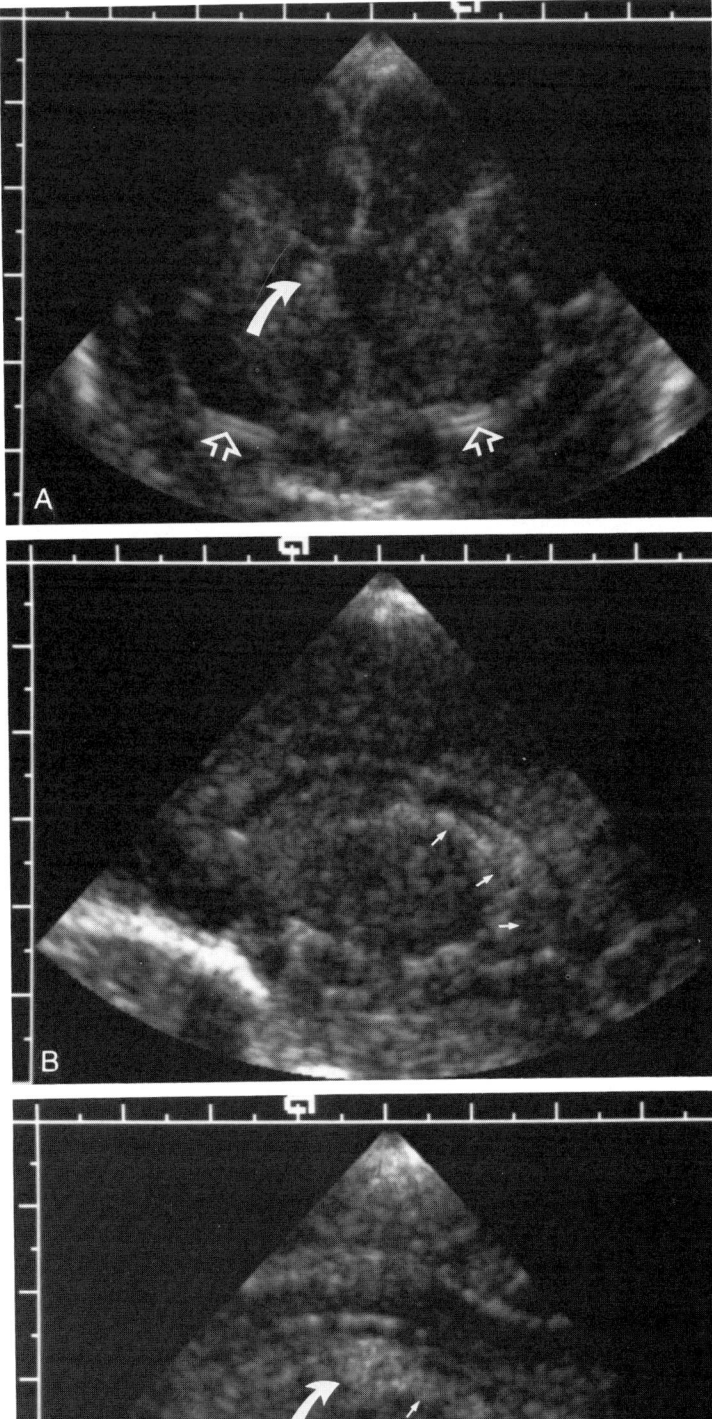

Figure 1–5. Coronal scan (**A**) of this 28-week-old baby who weighed 1550 g shows right-sided hemorrhage in the germinal matrix. There is asymmetry of parenchymal echogenicity (large arrow) just inferior to the anterior horns of the lateral ventricles. The central lucency is the normal cavum septum pellucidum. Open arrows mark the middle cerebral arteries. On the parasagittal scans of the lateral ventricles, note the asymmetry in echogenicity just anterior to the caudothalamic groove. The normal left side is shown in **B**. The small hemorrhage in the right germinal matrix (large arrow) is shown in **C**. Small arrows mark the choroid plexus in the body and the trigone in each lateral ventricle.

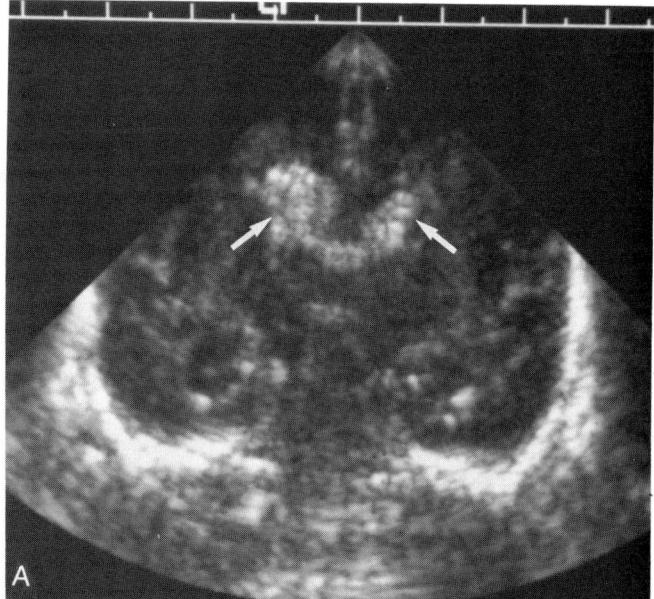

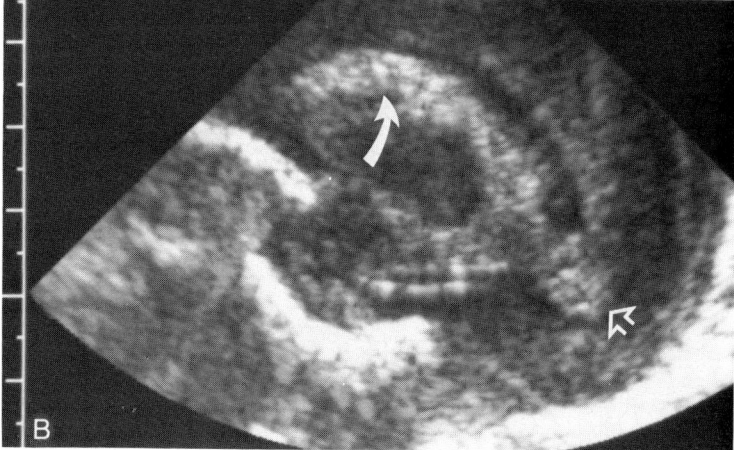

Figure 1-6. This baby, born at 26 weeks of gestation, has hemorrhage in both lateral ventricles (arrows, **A**). The sagittal view of the left lateral ventricle (**B**) shows echogenicity (large arrow) extending anterior to the caudothalamic notch. Often, it is difficult to discern which portion represents intraventricular blood and which represents hemorrhage in the germinal matrix. Note that the occipital horn is filled with blood (open arrow). The choroid plexus does not usually extend this far into the occipital horn.

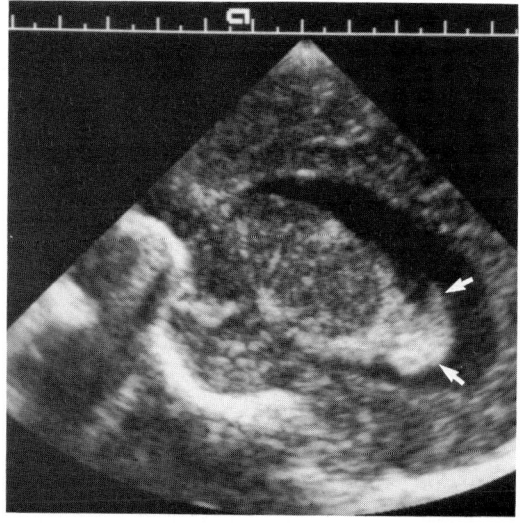

Figure 1-7. Arnold-Chiari II malformation associated with meningomyelocele is present in this baby. The lumpy choroid plexus (arrows) in the trigone on this parasagittal view is typical of such babies and does not represent bleeding associated with the choroid.

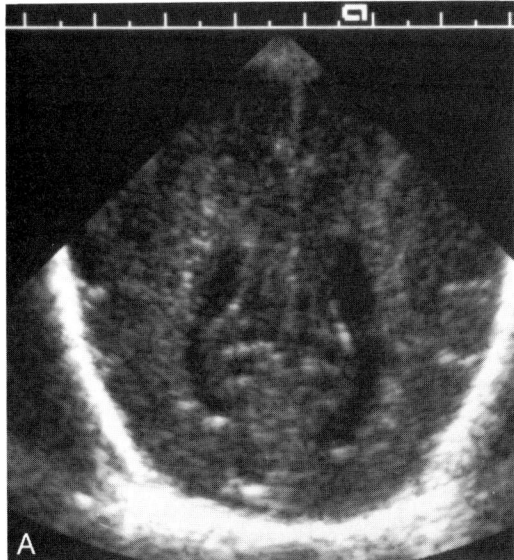

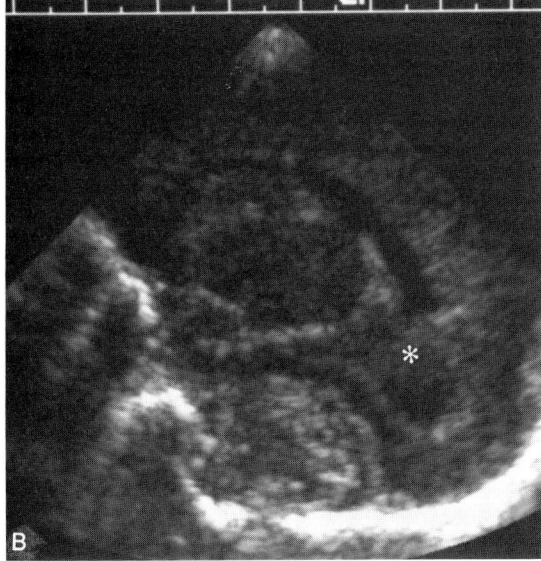

Figure 1–8. Occipital horns of the lateral ventricles are usually more prominent in premature babies than in babies born at term (A). If one obtains an angled sagittal section through the ventricle (B) the calcar avis (asterisk) may appear as a mass within the atrium of the lateral ventricle.

scans. Therefore, our approach has been to avoid grading and to use a worksheet for each baby each time a cranial scan is performed. Data are collected in a descriptive but quantitative manner, both for immediate clinical management and for follow-up. This type of worksheet is very useful in research protocols in which large groups of babies are being studied because the entries can be transferred to a computer (Fig. 1–9; Kuban and Teele, 1984).

When large amounts of blood distend the ventricular system, the plane between the hemorrhagic germinal matrix and the blood-filled ventricle becomes indistinguishable (Fig. 1–10). Blood in the third ventricle produces an echogenic line on coronal scans and an echogenic band anterior to the massa intermedia on sagittal scan (Fig. 1–11). Interestingly, it is unusual to detect blood in the fourth ventricle even in massive intraventricular hemorrhage. Blood exits the ventricular system through the foramina of Luschka and Magendie. On sagittal scans, blood in the adjacent cisterna magna softens the normally sharp cerebellar contour. Actually, on scans of a baby who has had a severe intraventricular hemorrhage, all of the interfaces throughout the brain appear less sharp; this is likely a reflection of the more global insult to the brain.

On sagittal scans of the normal premature

12 / CRANIAL ULTRASONOGRAPHY

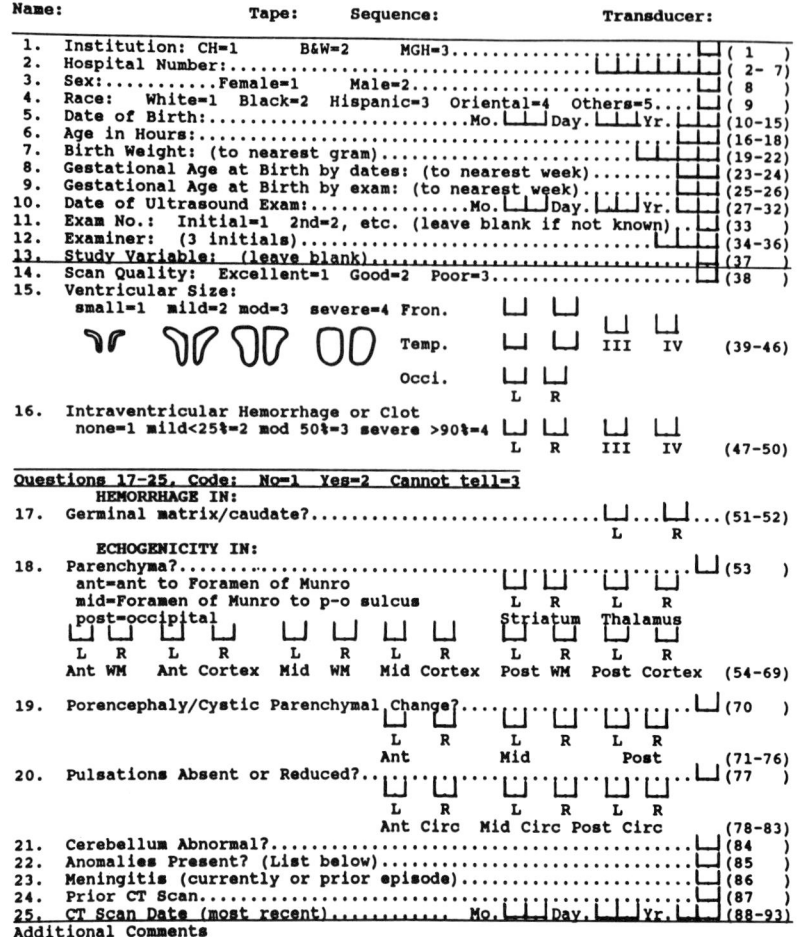

Figure 1-9. Worksheet used to collect data on babies undergoing cranial ultrasonography. (Adapted from Kuban K, Teele RL: Rationale for grading intracranial hemorrhage in premature babies. Pediatrics 1984; 74:358-363.)

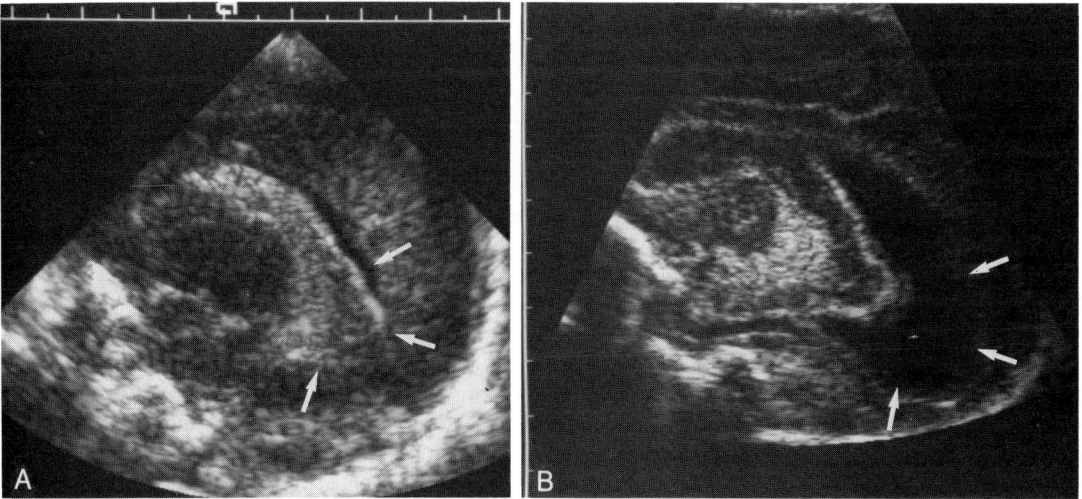

Figure 1-10. When blood fills the lateral ventricle, it forms a cast of the ventricle (**A**) that tends to persist as ventricular dilatation occurs (**B**). Arrows outline the occipital horn on these parasagittal scans, which were done 7 days apart.

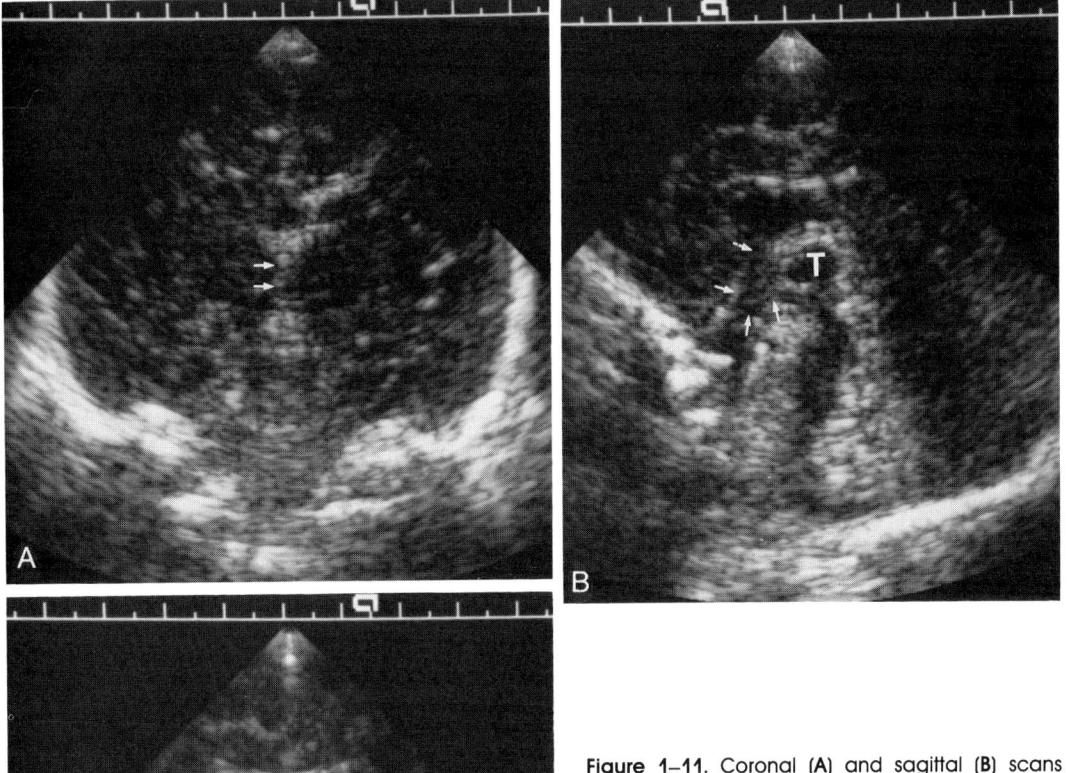

Figure 1-11. Coronal (A) and sagittal (B) scans show the typical appearance of blood in the third ventricle. Rather than a lucent slit extending in the midline inferior to the lateral ventricles, the blood-filled third ventricle is an echogenic line (arrows) on the coronal scan. On the sagittal scan the blood is an echogenic band (arrows) anterior to the massa intermedia (T). When the blood (probably from hemorrhage in the choroid plexus) resolves, the third ventricle again contains clear CSF (arrows) (C).

baby, a periventricular blush around the trigone of each lateral ventricle and also around the tip of the frontal horns is apparent. This blush represents normal interfaces produced by reflection of the ultrasonic beam from radiating neuronal fibers and accompanying blood vessels of the corona radiata (DiPietro et al., 1986). Scans through a patent posterior fontanelle show no peritrigonal blush because the ultrasonic beam is parallel, rather than perpendicular, to the fibers (Fig. 1–12). Steeply angled coronal scans show the maximal blush from the white matter of the corona radiata, which extends to the peripheral gray matter in parietal and occipital lobes. The last coronal scan in the routine series is almost an axial section of the brain. The corona radiata, when viewed in this steep coronal plane, is termed the "centrum semiovale."

How does one recognize a pathologic IPE? An asymmetric blush is abnormal; thus careful coronal scanning is essential. Sagittal scans are difficult to compare unless one can use a "split-screen" function to compare identical views. The beam of sound must

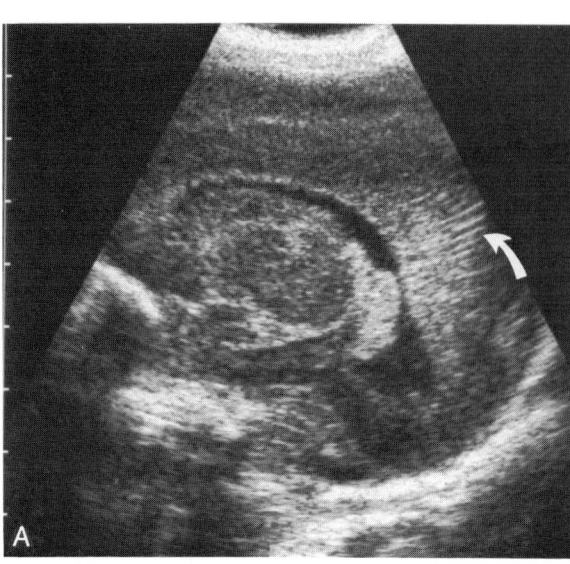 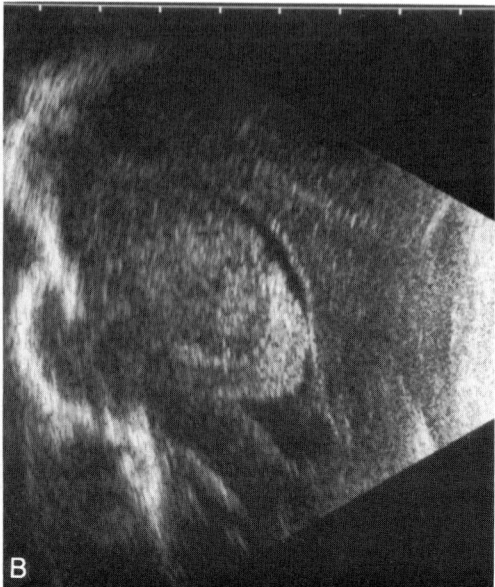

Figure 1-12. Scanning through the anterior fontanelle typically results in a peritrigonal blush (arrow) on the sonograms because the beam of sound is perpendicular to the radiating fibers (A). If one scans through the posterior fontanelle as B, the ultrasonic beam is parallel to the fibers, and there is no resultant interface and thus no periventricular blush.

intersect each hemisphere in the same plane. A pathologic IPE is coarse, is occasionally irregular in outline, and fails to conform to the fine paint-brush appearance of the normal blush. It can be identified both on coronal and sagittal views and through anterior and posterior fontanelle (Fig. 1-13). Usually, but not invariably, intraventricular hemorrhage accompanies the parenchymal insult. Over time, intraparenchymal echogenicities follow four separate evolutions: fading and disappearing altogether; association with generalized ventricular dilatation, which is likely ex vacuo; fading or cavitating with gradual development of a porencephalic cyst, which communicates with the lateral ventricle in the same area; or replacement with a matrix of cystic spaces, so-called cystic encephalomalacia (Fig. 1-14). These changes take weeks to evolve. If only a single set of scans, rather than a sequence of studies, is available, interpretation is quite difficult. Babies who have intraventricular hemorrhage that distends the ventricles generally have outcomes similar to those with documented IPE and therefore likely have parenchymal damage that is obscured or silhouetted by the adjacent ventricular blood (Garfinkel et al., 1988).

It is apparent that survivors of prematurity for whom IPE was noted on ultrasonograms form the major group at risk for cerebral palsy (used to describe any type of neuromotor disability) or impaired development quotient (a measure that includes intelligence), or both. Extensive periventricular cystic encephalomalacia is an extremely poor prognostic sign.

There is one area of injury that has escaped much notice, on both ultrasonographic and CT scans. Intracerebellar hemorrhage is probably more common than is realized. Perlman (1983) cited studies of premature infants, 15 to 25 percent of whom were, at autopsy, found to have cerebellar hemorrhage. Results from autopsy are, of course, skewed to the population with the most severe abnormalities, but it appears that these hemorrhages are being missed in surviving infants with great regularity. There is a germinal matrix in the subependymal area in the cerebellum that likely responds to similar insults and in similar fashion, as does the germinal matrix adjacent to the lateral ventricles. Blood may extrude into the cerebellum from a distended, obstructed fourth ventricle or, more likely, may be the result of venous infarction. Ultrasonography has been diagnostic in isolated cases of intracerebellar hemorrhage (Perlman, 1983; Reeder, 1982). Visualizing an echogenic hemorrhage in the normally echogenic cerebellum is difficult, but it is impor-

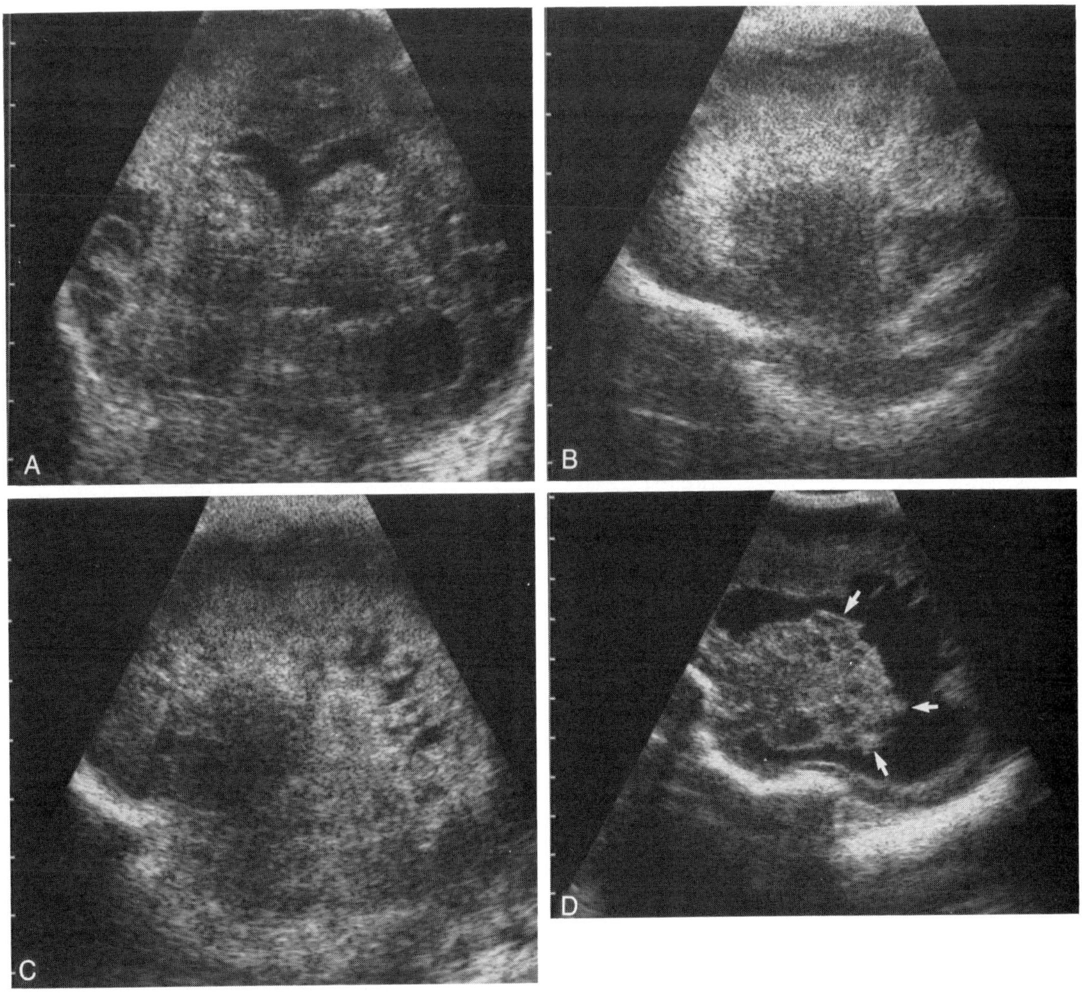

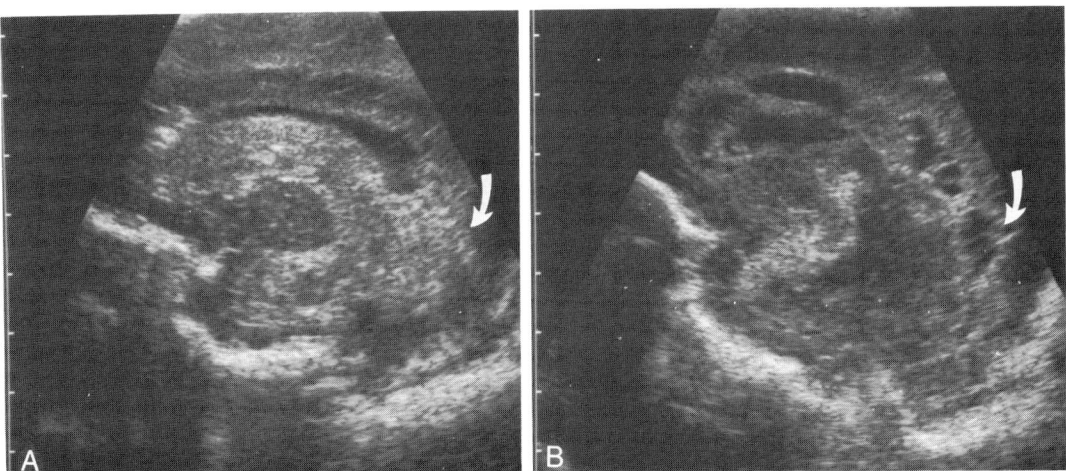

Figure 1-13. Coronal (**A**) and right parasagittal (**B**) views show extensive right-sided periventricular echogenicity and intraventricular hemorrhage in this baby, who was 32 weeks of gestational age and weighed 1600 g. Over the next week, cavitations appeared within the periventricular blush (**C**). Several weeks later, these cavitations coalesced, and because the ependymal lining was not intact, porencephaly resulted. Note on the last parasagittal scan (**D**) the irregular contour of the lateral ventricle. There is a residual clot (arrows) associated with the choroid plexus.

Figure 1-14. Parasagittal view of the left lateral ventricle (**A**) shows blood that forms a cast of the lateral ventricle and is indistinguishable from echogenicity involving the adjacent peritrigonal parenchyma (arrow). Nine days later (**B**), cavitations (arrow) were evident within the damaged brain.

16 / CRANIAL ULTRASONOGRAPHY

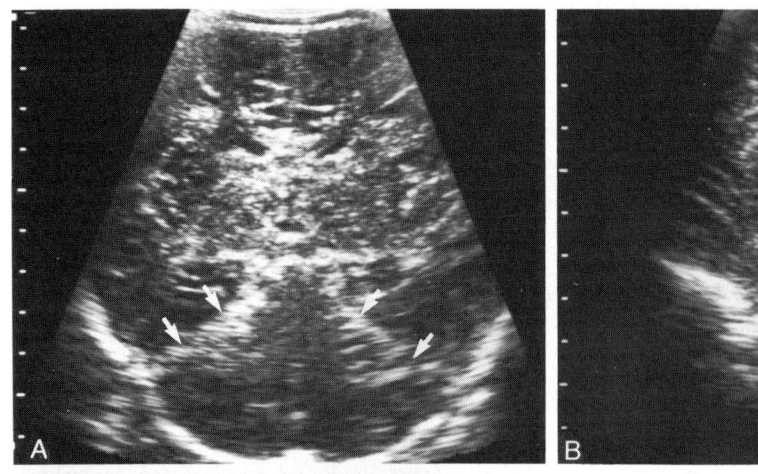

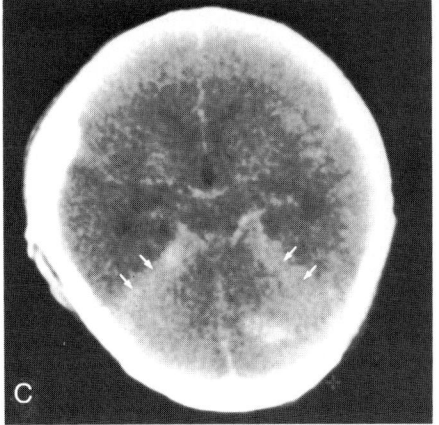

Figure 1–15. No normal cerebellar tissue could be identified on coronal (A) and midline sagittal (B) scans of the brain in this baby, who was comatose after cardiac arrest associated with congenital heart disease. CT scan (C) followed immediately and showed infarction of the cerebellum as well as profound bihemispheric edema. Arrows mark level of tentorium. Asterisk in (B) marks the third ventricle.

tant to think of the diagnosis and look for any asymmetry in the cerebellar contour and parenchymal pattern. Both the premature infant and the infant born at term after a difficult delivery are at risk for this complication. We scanned one baby who had infarction of the cerebellum secondary to low cardiac output resulting from congenital heart disease (Fig. 1–15).

Close follow-up of babies who have had ICH is essential. Clinical signs may be absent, and measurements of head circumference tend to lag at least 1 week behind the development of ventricular dilatation. Therefore, we schedule scans for 4 to 5 days after the initial diagnosis of ICH (1) to assess any progression of hemorrhage, (2) to document degree of ventricular dilatation, and (3) to search again for parenchymal abnormalities that may have become apparent or developed since prior scans. Scans are performed on request if there is acute deterioration in the baby's condition before the scheduled follow-up study. If the follow-up scan is unchanged or ICH is clearing, we wait 7 to 10 days before another study. By this point, our major interest is in the degree of intracranial ventricular dilatation. In a longitudinal study of babies who had intraventricular hemorrhage, 13 percent developed ventriculomegaly (Dykes et al., 1989). Of note is the fact that posthemorrhagic ventriculomegaly occurred almost exclusively (92 percent of instances) in those babies who had had distention of ventricles with hemorrhage or associated parenchymal damage (Fig. 1–16).

Babies with hemorrhage in the germinal matrix alone have a good prognosis: ventricular dilatation rarely follows, and neurologic outcome, at least for the short term, appears little affected. The glial precursors, destroyed in the hemorrhage, would have contributed to myelination of axons, and the effect of their absence may be delayed and difficult to measure without very detailed neurologic testing. The echogenicity from hemorrhage in the germinal matrix may fade with time or may leave behind a small subependymal

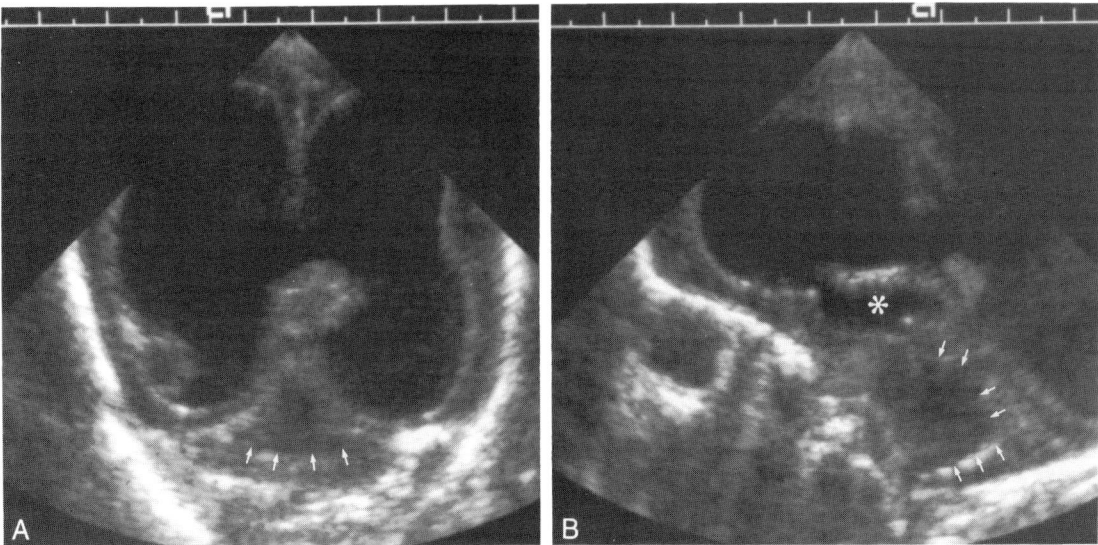

Figure 1–16. This baby was born prematurely with her twin at 26 weeks of gestational age after maternal cocaine abuse. She had severe intracranial hemorrhage associated with distention of the lateral ventricles at the outset of her course. The follow-up scans done 1 month later show hugely dilated lateral ventricles as well as dilated fourth ventricle (arrows) on the coronal scan **(A)**. The sagittal scan **(B)** shows dilated third ventricle (asterisk) and debris-filled massively enlarged fourth ventricle (arrows).

cyst (Fig. 1–17). The small periventricular, subependymal cysts that we occasionally find on scans of newborn infants may represent the sequelae of hemorrhage in utero or may be a normal phase or "variant" of the maturation of the germinal matrix, which early in intrauterine life surrounds the lateral ventricles (Keller et al., 1987).

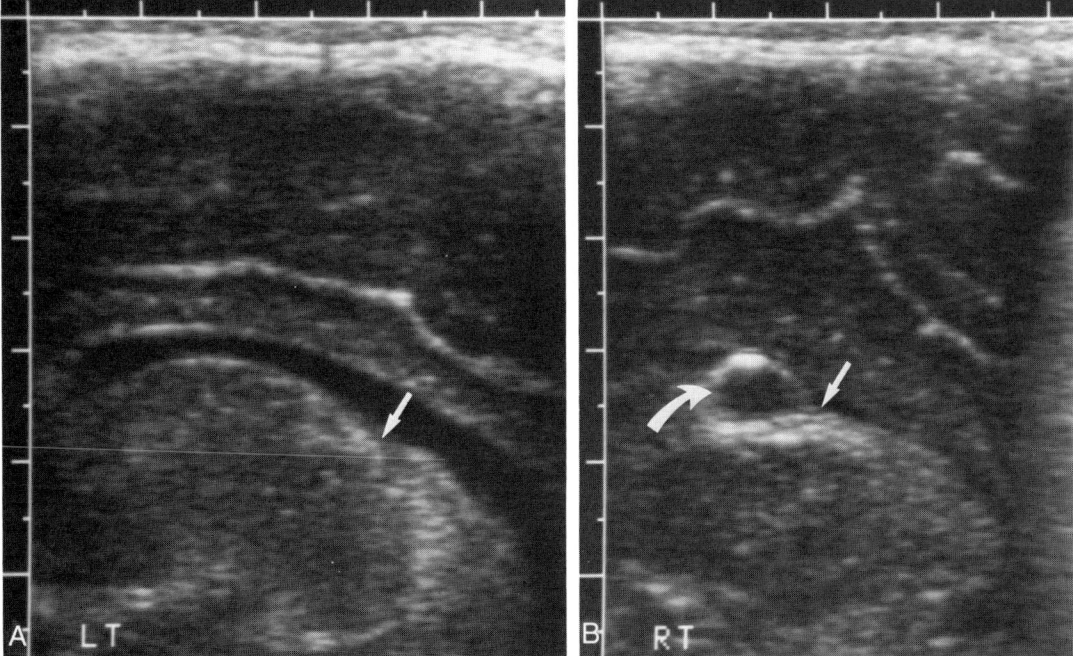

Figure 1–17. Parasagittal scan of the normal anterior horn, left lateral ventricle **(A)** is shown for comparison with the abnormal right side **(B)**. A small cyst (curved arrow) was present 3 weeks after documentation of hemorrhage in the right germinal matrix. The caudothalamic notch is marked on each side by the straight arrow.

The causes of ventricular dilatation are incompletely understood. Blood around the cisterns—having exited the foramina of Magendie and Luschka—may clot and plug cisterns and foramina. This is the "clogged plumbing" analogy: cerebrospinal fluid (CSF) manufactured by the choroid plexus cannot drain, and therefore the ventricular system dilates. Blood over the brain may contribute to the obstruction by interfering with resorption of CSF through the subarachnoid villi. It is also theoretically possible that there is increased production of CSF that cannot be handled adequately. Finally, there is the situation in which the ventricles fill in space left vacant by brain tissue destroyed by ischemia.

Of note is that intraventricular blood, for whatever reason, seems to be more harmful than blood that arises from the subarachnoid space. Babies with primary subarachnoid hemorrhage have only a small chance of developing ventriculomegaly (Leblanc and O'Gorman, 1980). We have been avoiding the term "hydrocephalus"; in most textbooks and medical parlance, hydrocephalus implies not only ventricular enlargement but also CSF under increased pressure. Ultrasonic scans can give reliable information only regarding the size of the ventricles; they cannot measure the pressure of CSF. Together with clinical evaluation (head circumference, appearance of fontanelle, neurologic status) and quantitative information (such as pressure sensors on anterior fontanelle), degree of obstruction, if present, can be inferred. In our practice, absolute measurements of ventricular size have been less useful than comparison of serial scans (for which landmarks are kept identical) and the presence or absence of fourth ventricular dilatation. Dilatation of the fourth ventricle occurs when there is obstruction to flow of CSF distal to it, either at the foramina or in the subarachnoid space (Fig. 1–16). There are cyclic spells of enthusiasm to use serial lumbar punctures and withdrawal of CSF to treat babies who have ventriculomegaly. Decompression of the ventricles with such a procedure can be documented with pre- and posttreatment ultrasonic scans. One can infer that there is communication between the ventricular system and the lumbar subarachnoid space if the ventricles shrink (Fig. 1–18). Failure of decompression indicates noncommunicating, obstructive ventriculomegaly and is a more pressing indication for neurosurgical evaluation and possibly shunting by intraventricular catheter. Intraventricular shunting in the small premature baby carries a high rate of morbidity; thus there is an increasing reliance on medical management for the rare baby who has progressive posthemorrhagic hydrocephalus (Dykes et al., 1989). As an example

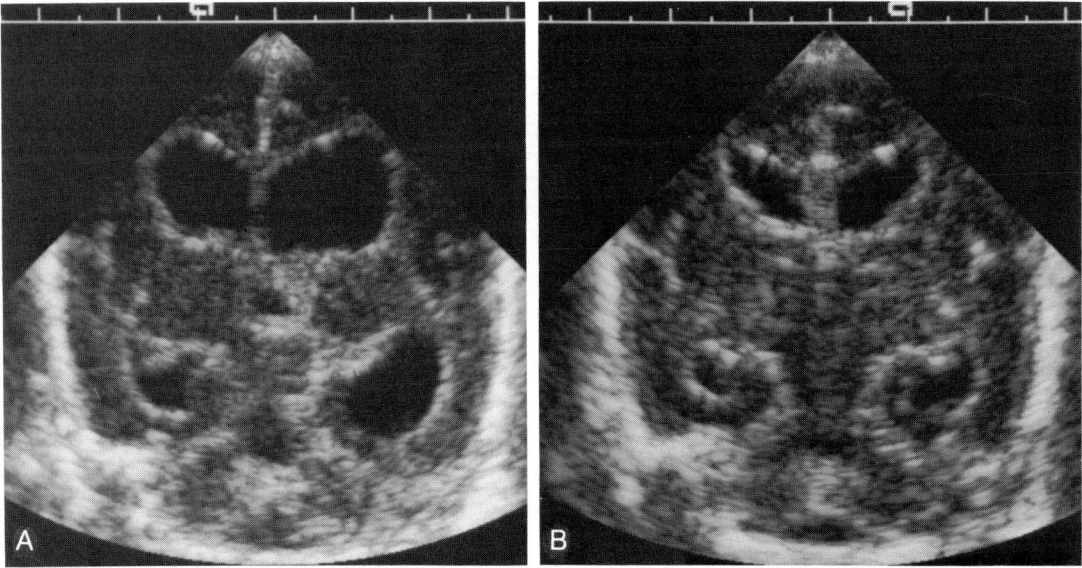

Figure 1–18. Three weeks after intraventricular hemorrhage **(A)**, the ventricular system was dilated in this baby, who was having episodes of apnea and bradycardia. Coronal scans **(B)** followed lumbar puncture and documented decompression of the ventricular system after the procedure.

of one complication, it appears that the combination of prior intraventricular hemorrhage and repeated revisions of a shunt increases the risk of the occluded or "trapped" fourth ventricle (Coker and Anderson, 1989).

Ultrasonograms are tailored to answer specific clinical questions after a prematurely born neonate reaches 2 weeks of age. We do not have a schedule of routine scans, partly because staff in our nursery transfer babies to their "home" hospitals when they have passed the stage of needing intensive care. Ideally, each premature baby for whom an intracranial abnormality is found on early scans has a study before discharge, and the results of this study travel with him or her. Longitudinal studies that have been reported indicate that careful neurologic examination coupled with ultrasonic studies at or near term can be used to predict neurologic outcome (Nwaesei, 1988). *Any* baby who has had moderate to severe intracranial hemorrhage must be watched carefully because there is a small group who, after a benign initial course, develop ventriculomegaly months after discharge from the intensive care nursery (Perlman et al., 1990).

THE BABY BORN AT TERM

Asphyxia Neonatorum

Perinatal asphyxia of the baby born at term is still a depressingly common event in spite of advances in obstetric care, perinatal monitoring, and neonatal care. Incidence of asphxia was 6 per 1000 live-born babies delivered over 4 years in a busy obstetric hospital (Levene et al., 1985). The authors commented that previous data from the same busy maternity service indicated that there had been no change in incidence over 10 years. Intrauterine growth retardation was present in 25 percent of asphyxiated infants, which suggests that the diagnosis is associated not only with difficult or breech delivery, maternal infection, and prolonged rupture of membranes, but with prenatal factors as well.

If one reviews the literature of asphyxia neonatorum, one realizes how imprecisely the definition of asphyxia has been applied. Avery (1989) defined asphyxia as the condition resulting from the baby's inability to exchange oxygen and carbon dioxide. The organ of gas exchange, before delivery, is the maternal placenta. The neonatal lungs replace placental function after the umbilical cord is ligated. Asphyxia results in hypercapnia and hypoxemia, which if prolonged result in metabolic acidosis. Since 1953, when the Apgar score* was introduced, heavy reliance has been placed on the score as a marker of perinatal asphyxia. The realization that the score, particularly 1 minute after birth, was poorly sensitive as a marker of asphyxia led to many articles advocating more accurate assessment of neonatal asphyxia. There is little question, specifically in the United States, that malpractice litigation focusing on childbirth has stimulated more precise definition of fetal asphyxia. A committee report from the American Academy of Pediatrics in 1986 defined perinatal asphyxia as an Apgar score of 0 to 3 at 10 minutes after birth, early neonatal seizures, and prolonged hypotonia. The report further stated that absence of metabolic acidemia in blood from the umbilical artery in the cord makes the diagnosis of asphyxia unlikely.

Hypoxia is not equivalent to ischemia. Ischemia is defined as impaired perfusion of tissue. Research with animal models has been directed toward separating the pathology and biochemistry of hypoxia and ischemia. In the asphyxiated neonate, both mechanisms probably contribute to damage the immature brain. The hyphenated term "hypoxic-ischemic encephalopathy," which lumps the two etiologic factors with the outcome, is used in most clinical references. If we refer to the pathologic descriptions of neonatal injury that result from cerebral hypoxia-ischemia, we find that we have rediscovered with imaging what the neuropathologists have known for some time. As cataloged by Brett (1983), hypoxic-ischemic injury results in four pathologic patterns. (1) Neuronal necrosis affects neurons of the cerebral and cerebellar cortex; extent of necrosis ranges from loss of hippocampal and Purkinje cells to gross shrinkage of gyri. (2) Status marmoratus is symmetric marbling of the basal ganglia that occurs, particularly in the caudate nucleus and putamen, secondary to neuronal loss and subsequent gliosis. (3) Watershed infarcts affect the brain in boundary zones between circulations. (4) Periven-

---

*Apgar = heart rate, respiratory effort, muscle tone, reflex irritability, and color, each scored 0, 1, or 2. Total possible score is 10.

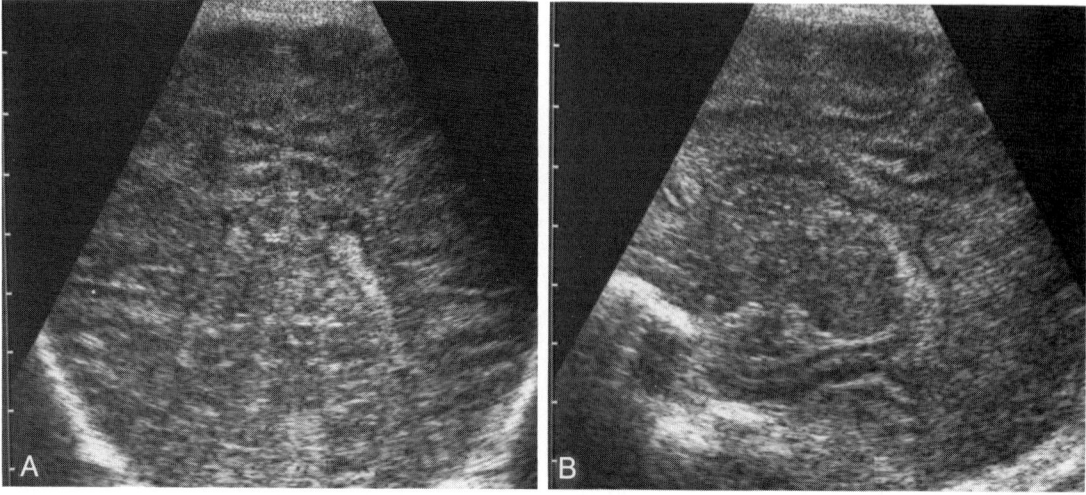

Figure 1–19. Diffuse edema is apparent on the coronal (A) and parasagittal (B) views of the left lateral ventricle. This baby, who was born at 40 weeks of gestational age, had Apgar scores of 1 and 3 five and ten minutes after birth. Edema of the brain was confirmed by computed tomography (CT) scans. At 6 months of age, the baby had developmental delay, microcephaly, and spastic quadriplegia. At 10 months of age, blindness was diagnosed.

tricular leukomalacia is infarcted white matter typically at the outer angles of lateral ventricles (see section on "The Premature Infant"). We now discuss the ultrasonographic correlates of these neuropathologic features.

Ultrasonic scans of recently asphyxiated infants often show increased parenchymal echogenicity associated with small ventricles (Fig. 1–19; Babcock, 1983). The pattern of echogenicity is coarser than that present in the much rarer situation of infiltrative disorders of brain. Cerebral edema is likely responsible for increased parenchymal echogenicity in asphyxiated infants and probably reflects shifts of water between intra- and extracellular spaces. It is not necessarily a sign of increased intracranial pressure. As in the premature infant, ultrasonography is not as sensitive a technique as we would like it to be, and a normal scan in no way rules out the presence of significant ischemic damage. If there is extensive neuronal necrosis, later scans show the prominent sulci and large ventricles of atrophy.

The ultrasonic findings of status marmoratus have been reported (Kreusser et al., 1984; Hertzberg et al., 1987; Voit et al., 1987).

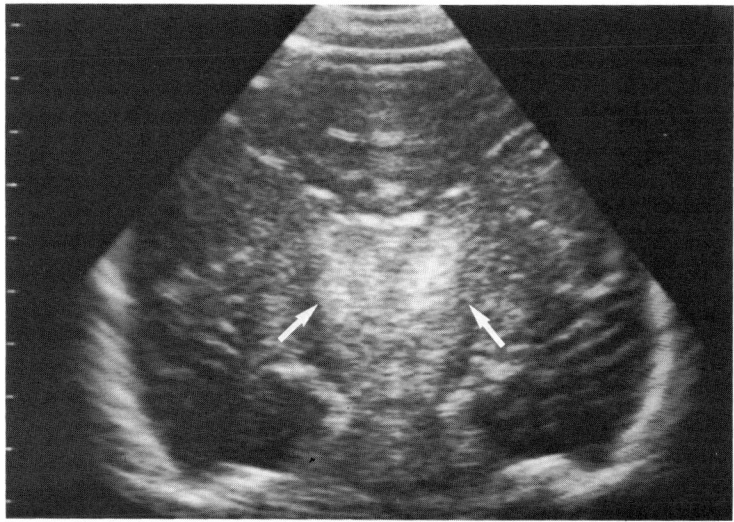

Figure 1–20. These echogenic areas (arrows) were identified when ultrasonograms followed accidental asphyxia in a previously healthy 4½-month-old whose head got caught between the railings of her crib. The baby was too unstable to transport to the CT scanner until 3 days after the accident. CT scans confirmed the abnormalities in basal ganglia as regions of necrosis. Tonsillar herniation ensued, and the baby died 11 days after the accident.

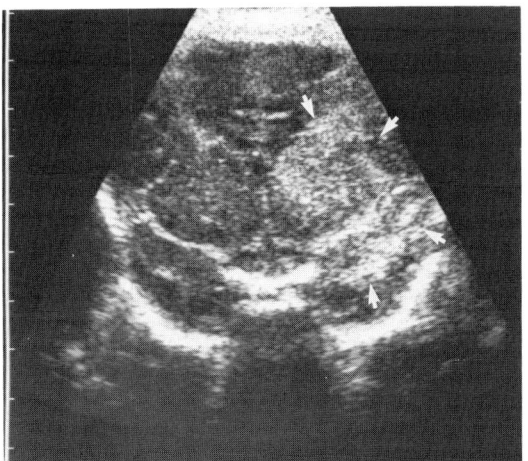

Figure 1–21. Coronal scan shows echogenicity (arrows) in the distribution of the left middle cerebral artery, probably from infarct secondary to embolus. The baby had transposition of the great arteries and had undergone multiple attempts at atrial balloon septostomy. She had a documented clot within the superior vena cava. We assume that some clot broke free to become an embolus, which traveled via the right ventricle to the aorta and then to the left carotid and middle cerebral artery.

Strikingly echogenic areas in thalami and basal ganglia are present in babies whose neurologic outcome includes dystonia, severe mental retardation, and microcephaly (Fig. 1–20).

With watershed and larger infarcts, ultrasonography may show localized areas of increased parenchymal echogenicity. These correlate with areas of low-density on CT (Figs. 1–21, 1–22; Martin et al., 1983). Decreased or absent flow in the region may be suggested on real-time examination. This is one situation in which Doppler ultrasonography is very helpful because it can establish the presence or absence of arterial flow. Bleeding into areas of infarct may occur. Hemorrhage into the brain results in more striking echogenicity on ultrasonography than does ischemia alone (Fig. 1–23).

Babies born at term and who have withstood difficult deliveries are also at risk for subdural hemorrhage. Tentorial laceration, falcial tears, and occipital osteodiastasis cause rupture of adjacent or bridging venous sinuses or veins. The diagnosis of subdural hemorrhage is supported when frankly bloody CSF is obtained from lumbar puncture. Of note is that in one busy neonatal unit, a study of routine lumbar punctures showed the "traumatic tap" to be rare. Of babies with blood in CSF specimens, 92 percent had intracranial blood shown on the CT scan that followed (Volpe, 1987). CT scanning is the modality of choice in this situation if at all possible. Ultrasonography is not reliable for identifying and quantifying blood

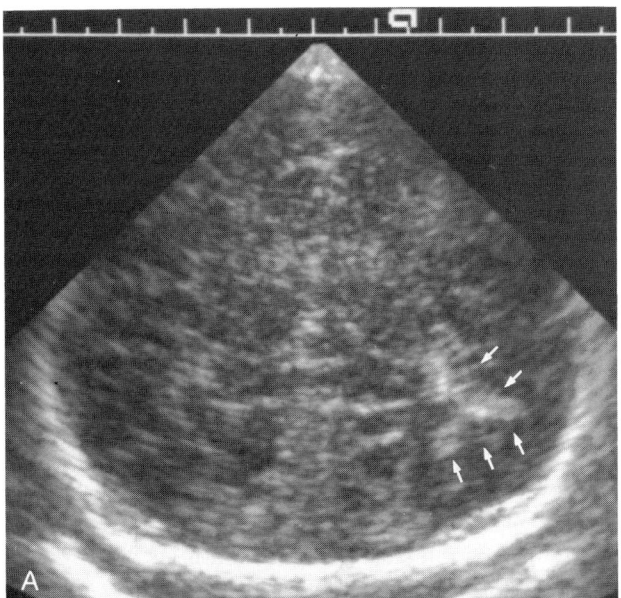
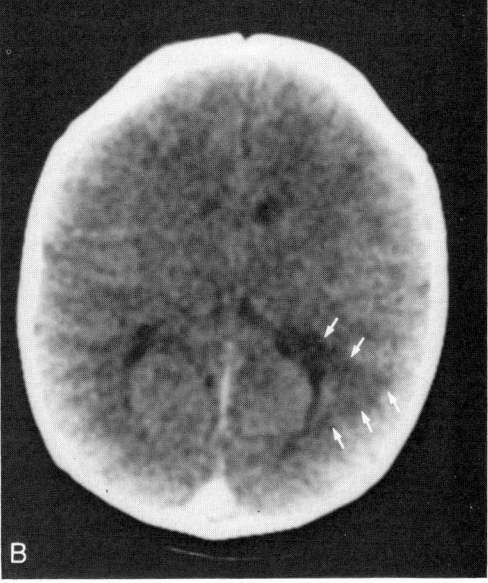

Figure 1–22. A 2-day-old baby who was born at term was transferred from another hospital when he had generalized seizures. The coronal scan (**A**) showed an unusual echogenicity on the left (arrows). CT scan (**B**) followed within hours and showed a similar area of abnormality, low in density (arrows). The etiology of this infarct is unknown.

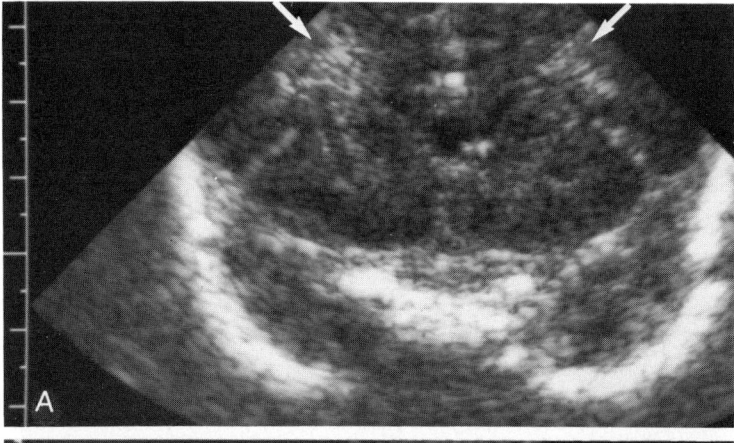
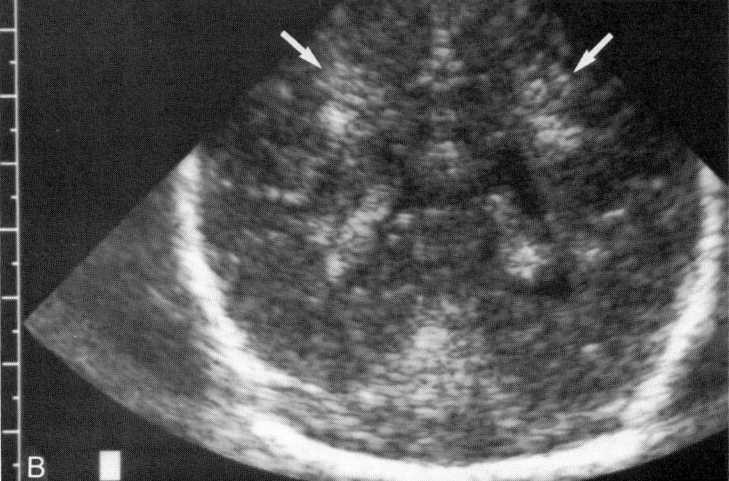

Figure 1-23. The periventricular echogenicity (arrows) shown on two coronal views (A and B) represents areas of bleeding secondary to severe hypertension caused by renal arterial thrombosis.

in the posterior fossa (von Gontard et al., 1988; de Campo, 1989). A large collection of blood in the posterior fossa has to be drained surgically, and this must be done expeditiously if the brain stem and the cerebellum are compromised (Tanaka et al., 1988). Subdural hematoma over the cerebral convexity may be associated with underlying parenchymal hematoma. Management is usually conservative; percutaneous drainage of the collection or craniotomy is reserved for babies who have signs of increased intracranial pressure.

Ultrasonography occasionally reveals the presence of subdural collection. Specific features include an echogenic extracerebral collection, shift of midline structures, and compression of the ipsilateral ventricle if the collection is large and supratentorial; poor definition of cerebellar hemispheres if the collection is infratentorial; and, on occasion, underlying parenchymal echogenicity, which represents cerebral contusion (Fig. 1–24).

Term babies who have had hypoxic-ischemic insult or trauma during birth are also at risk for intraventricular hemorrhage. Neuropathologic material indicates that these usually originate in the choroid plexus and then spread through the ventricular system. Remnants of the germinal matrix are present in the caudothalamic area, the hippocampus, and the ventricular trigones. Therefore, there is also the rare baby born at term who may have a hemorrhage in the germinal matrix (Hayden et al., 1985).

In summary, ultrasonography of the asphyxiated baby should include (1) an estimation of overall parenchymal echogenicity (normal or increased), (2) meticulous comparison of right and left hemispheres to enable identification of localized parenchymal abnormalities, (3) assessment of ventricular size and sulcal detail, (4) comparison of vascular pulsation between hemispheres, and (5) careful inspection of the posterior fossa.

Although we have listed the ultrasonic

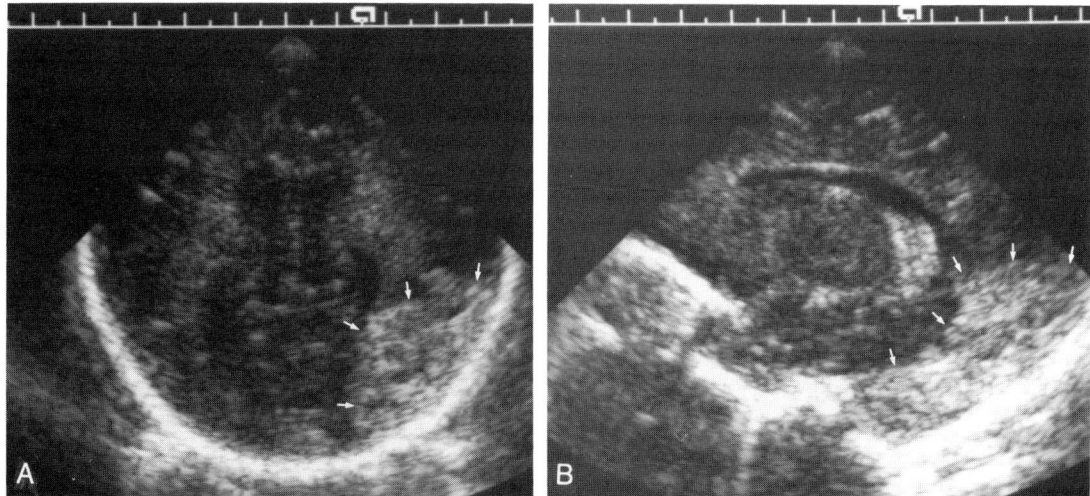

Figure 1-24. Thrombocytopenia was the only pre-existing problem in this baby who was born at 34 weeks of gestational age. The echogenicity (arrows) shown on the coronal (A) and sagittal (B) scans proved to be hemorrhage that was both intracerebral and subdural.

features of asphyxia neonatorum, the reality is that we currently rely on CT scanning to evaluate affected infants if they can be transported to the scanner. CT is better able to show blood in subarachnoid and subdural spaces, including the posterior fossa, where surgical intervention may be needed. CT can provide quantitative estimates of density of brain, and it is not limited by a small fontanelle. Follow-up studies can be compared easily because technical factors stay constant. MRI has the potential of providing even more elegant studies of cerebral insult; it can show the process of normal myelination and the abnormal progression that follows asphyxia. Phosphorus nuclear magnetic resonance spectroscopy has also been used as an investigative tool in evaluating asphyxiated babies (Hope et al., 1984). In spite of diagnostic advances in imaging and therapeutic maneuvers in neonatology, there has been little change in final outcome. We have refined the diagnosis and prognosis but have, as yet, been unable to reverse the devastating neurologic sequelae of perinatal hypoxic-ischemic encephalopathy.

The Baby Treated with ECMO

There is a special group of babies who should be discussed separately under the general heading of asphyxia neonatorum. These children are for multiple reasons—including meconium aspiration, severe hyaline membrane disease, diaphragmatic hernia, and persistent pulmonary hypertension of the neonate—candidates for extracorporeal membrane oxygenation (ECMO). This technique allows circulatory bypass of the lungs by means of two external cannulas. One is placed into the right atrium through the right internal jugular vein, and the other into the aortic arch through the right common carotid artery. The vessels cephalad from the insertion sites are ligated; therefore, venous flow exits the brain through the left jugular vein, and arterial flow is supplied by the left carotid artery and the two vertebral arteries (Plate I). The venous cannula draws returning systemic venous blood into the membrane oxygenator, which then returns oxygenated blood to the aortic arch through the arterial cannula. Because of the extracorporeal circuit, the blood must be heparinized. Thus three insults are presented to the baby's brain: a change in vascular supply and egress, heparinization of the perfusing blood, and the hypoxic situation that precipitated application of ECMO.

In our early experience with this technique, candidates for ECMO were those who had severe pulmonary hypoplasia secondary to diaphragmatic hernia. The babies were positioned supine with their heads turned to the left to allow good visualization of the cannulas. This group of babies had a high rate of intracranial hemorrhage in comparison

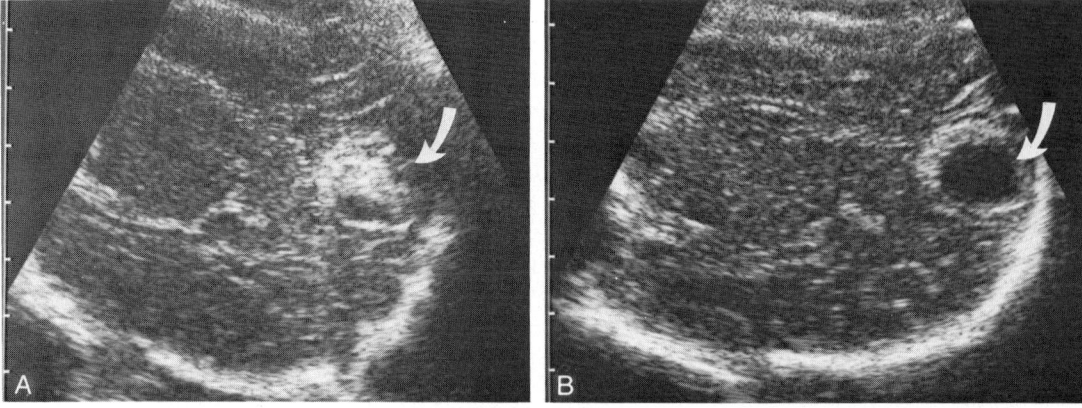

Figure 1–25. Sagittal scans (A and B) of the left hemisphere show evolution of hemorrhagic parieto-occipital infarct (arrow) that occurred the day after cannulas were removed. Scan B followed scan A by 10 days. The baby had been placed on extracorporeal membrane oxygenation (ECMO) because of congenital diaphragmatic hernia. We assume that a clot, which broke off the aortic cannula, was carried by left carotid flow to the brain.

with babies in our later experience. We believe that there were at least two reasons for this: the severity of the pulmonary hypoplasia was, in many cases, uncorrectable, and the twisted neck likely prevented adequate venous drainage through the remaining jugular vein. Many variables changed during the more widespread use of this technique in both our and other institutions. Currently most of the candidates for ECMO are babies who have normally developed lungs that have suffered an acquired insult. With maintenance of the face-upward position, refinements in cannulas and equipment, and considerable experience on the part of physicians, nurses, and respiratory therapists, an intracranial hemorrhage is now a rare occurrence. All candidates have a full ultrasonographic study before they are placed on ECMO; virtually all have normal scans. We may, however, be missing small collections of extra-axial blood and ischemia too subtle to recognize. After a baby has been started on ECMO, our current protocol calls for cranial ultrasonography every other day unless the clinical situation warrants more frequent studies. We routinely obtain scans after decannulation. One baby in our study group developed left-sided parenchymal hemorrhage after manipulation of the cannulas. We postulate that a clot from the arterial cannula, as the cannula was with-

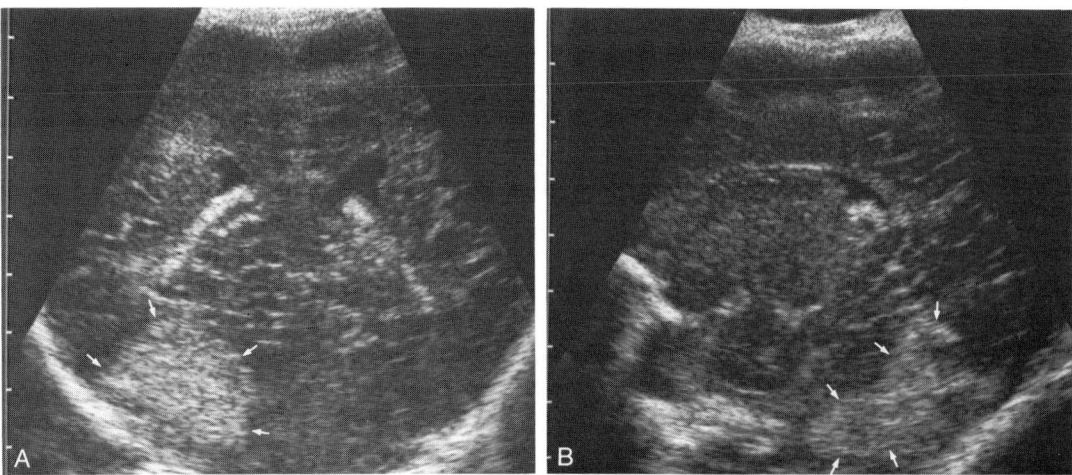

Figure 1–26. Coronal (A) and sagittal (B) scans show an echogenic region (arrows) that represents a hemorrhage in the right temporo-occipital area. This baby had been placed on ECMO because of diaphragmatic hernia. Despite heroic efforts by hospital staff, the baby died at the age of 9 days, 2 days after the scan was obtained.

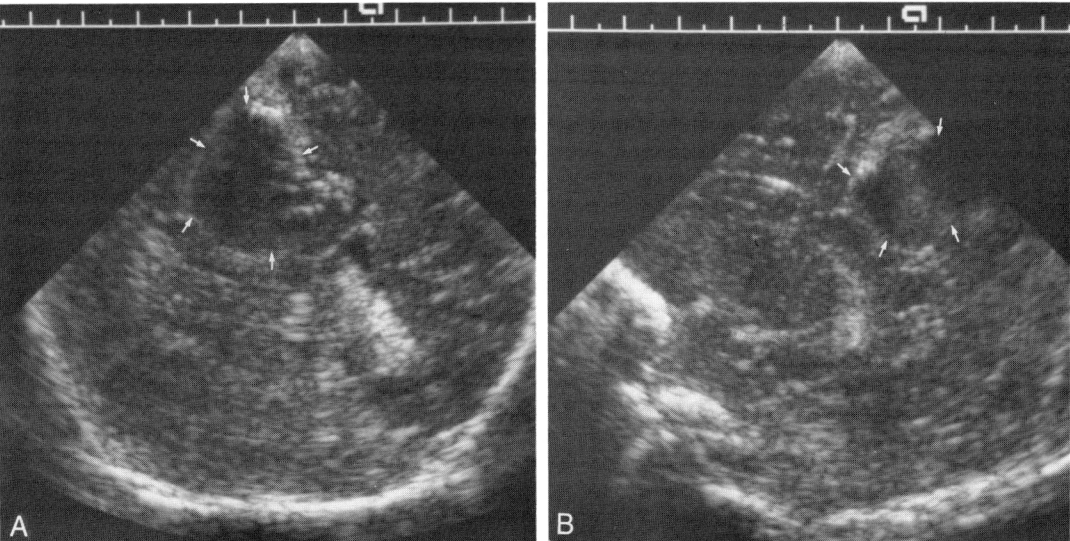

Figure 1–27. Coronal (A) and parasagittal (B) scans show an intracranial hemorrhage that evolved into this area of relative echolucency (arrows) 5 days after the baby was placed on ECMO for congenital diaphragmatic hernia. At the time of ultrasonographic study, this was interpreted as intraparenchymal hemorrhage. However, autopsy showed it to be subdural in location. This difficulty in differentiating between extracerebral and intracerebral hemorrhage should always be considered when lesions are peripheral in location.

drawn, reached the left hemisphere through the left carotid artery (Fig. 1–25).

Several series of ultrasonographic studies in babies receiving ECMO have been published (Babcock et al., 1989; Luisiri et al., 1988; Slovis et al., 1988; Taylor GA, et al., 1987a; Taylor GA, et al., 1987b; Taylor GA, et al., 1988; Taylor GA, et al., 1989a; Taylor GA, et al., 1989b). None are comparable because techniques differ among centers, because severity and type of initial illness vary among patients, and because experience of physicians differs. Slovis and colleagues (1988) reported that the frequency of ICH decreased from 72 to 13 percent as they gained experience. Luisiri and associates (1988) cited a 25 percent incidence of abnormal results of scans: PVL, bleeding from the choroid plexus, cerebral edema, and infarction were noted as complications (Figs. 1–26, 1–27).

Cranial Doppler Ultrasonography

The literature regarding cranial Doppler ultrasonography in premature and term babies is confusing, at times contradictory, and at best incomplete. In a comparison of studies, it is apparent that equipment, methodology, and selection of subjects varies widely. There is concern from some quarters that levels of power needed to perform intracranial duplex Doppler ultrasonography may be too high for its routine use (KJW Taylor, 1987). However, others have not obtained informed consent when using this method in a clinical setting (Seibert et al., 1989). It is safe to state only that cranial Doppler ultrasonography is still new, that it is usually a research tool in most centers, and that clinical decisions based solely on results of studies with the method are to be discouraged. In early studies, researchers used continuous-wave Doppler ultrasonography and those studies cannot be compared with current situations, in which color and duplex Doppler ultrasonography is used.

Prospective studies of normal asymptomatic neonates are scarce, and their sample sizes are small. It is, of course, especially difficult to find "normal" premature babies. Published results indicate that the velocity of blood in intracranial arteries increases progressively with age (Horgan et al., 1989; Deeg and Rupprecht, 1989). In two studies, resistive index [(peak systolic velocity − end-diastolic velocity)/peak systolic velocity] fell with increasing gestational age (Horgan et al., 1989; Seibert et al., 1989). Resistive index did not change with age in a third study (Deeg and Rupprecht, 1989). Mean resistive index in healthy infants is 75 percent, but the standard deviation is very large. Antegrade diastolic flow is present in all normal infants of all gestational ages. The presence of patent ductus arteriosus results in low velocity or reversed diastolic flow (Fig. 1–28; Lipman, 1982).

True velocity can be calculated only when the angle between the Doppler pulse and the axis of the insonated vessel is known. Color Doppler ultrasonography is very helpful in allowing visualization of the vessel's direction so that the angle of insonation (theta) can be measured accurately. The anterior cerebral artery is easily interrogated through the anterior fontanelle, as are the basilar artery and the internal carotid artery. The middle and posterior cerebral arteries have to be examined through a transcranial approach in order that the angle between ultrasonic beam and artery be as little as possible (Horgan et al., 1989).

Duplex scanning of the venous drainage of the neonatal brain has been reported. Winkler and Helmke (1989) used data from 49 healthy infants, 30 to 42 weeks of gestational age, to calculate velocities within individual veins and to characterize patterns of flow. These authors also reported changes in velocities of flow within arteries when transfontanellar scanning was performed with heavy pressure on the transducer—an important technical artifact.

Much of the early interest in intracranial Doppler ultrasonography was centered on premature babies who were at risk for intracranial hemorrhage. It does appear that there is variability in the velocity of cerebral arterial flow during the first 12 hours of life and that this variability decreases over the next 48 hours. Furthermore, intubated babies whose respiratory efforts are asynchronous with the ventilator have significantly greater variability of cerebral arterial velocities (Rennie et al., 1987). Interestingly, intermittent patterns of flow in venous drainage also have been associated with adverse outcome (Winkler and Helmke, 1989).

In general, the more severe an intracranial hemorrhage is, the more likely the mean resistive index is to be elevated in the affected premature baby. However, because of the large standard deviation, there is no statistical significance between babies who have intracranial hemorrhage and those who are normal (Seibert et al., 1989).

Studies of asphyxiated infants have yielded contradictory results, probably because of associated confounding variables such as patent ductus arteriosus, myocardial ischemia,

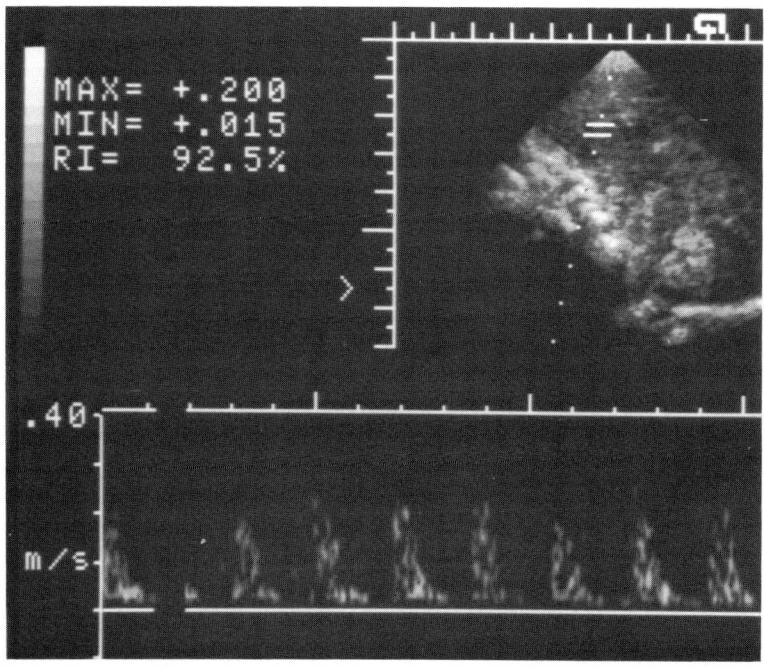

Figure 1–28. Virtually no antegrade diastolic flow is evident on these scans. The resistive index of anterior cerebral artery was calculated to be 92.5 percent. Patent ductus arteriosus was documented on cardiac echography.

and differences in degrees of cerebral edema between subjects. A markedly increased resistive index (>120 percent) on serial examinations is a poor prognostic sign considered indicative of sustained increased intracranial pressure (Glasier et al., 1989; Hassler et al., 1988; Couture et al., 1987). Increased intracranial pressure associated with subdural effusion or hydrocephalus, or both, appears to increase the resistive index by compression of the intracranial vessels, thus increasing impedance. Drainage of CSF by tapping or shunting resulted in a significant decrease in resistive index in one study of affected patients (Seibert et al., 1989).

Radiologists have learned—somewhat belatedly—that the physiologic images from duplex Doppler ultrasonography are not quite as easy to interpret as the anatomic images from the same cross-section. Research in the 1990s should yield more information and define the practical and safe applications for this most difficult of examinations.

The Baby Who Has Meningitis

Meningitis is a clinical diagnosis, and imaging is necessary only for babies who do not respond promptly to appropriate management and the correct antimicrobial therapy. Because the anterior fontanelle is gradually obliterated as a scanning window over the 1st year of life, we are limiting the discussion of meningitis to that which occurs before 1 year of age.

In most infants, infection of the CSF is preceded by, or coincident with, sepsis. Bacterial seeding of the choroid plexus, which has a substrate rich in glycogen and is therefore an ideal culture medium, occurs through the arteries. In neuropathologic studies of babies dying early in the course of their disease, exudate is most prominent in the stroma of the choroid plexus. Contamination of the ventricular system leads to ependymitis. Borne along by the flow of CSF, bacteria infect the subarachnoid spaces and stimulate an inflammatory response by the meninges. The inflammation affects bridging and cortical blood vessels, particularly the veins. Phlebitis occurs in arachnoidal, subependymal, and cortical veins. Venous occlusion results in areas of hemorrhagic infarction that may extend from the peripheral cerebral cortex to the underlying white matter. In summary, acute changes of bacterial meningitis include ventriculitis, arachnoiditis, vasculitis, infarction, cerebral edema, and encephalopathy. Parenchymal damage follows a pattern similar to that seen in hypoxic-ischemic injury.

Complications of meningitis include severe increase in intracranial pressure, ventriculitis with walled-off pockets of infection as the ependyma proliferates and glial bridges form, acute hydrocephalus from inflammatory obstruction at any level of the ventricular system or subarachnoid spaces, and a mass (abscess, infarct, and subdural effusion). These complications are clinically manifested by seizures, full fontanelle, increasing head circumference, change in mental status, and focal neurologic deficits. There are some clinical facts of which the ultrasonographer should be aware. Subdural effusions are much less common in the neonatal group than in older infants. This likely reflects different bacteriology between groups: group B streptococcus is responsible for approximately 35 percent of cases of meningitis in very young babies; *Haemophilus influenzae* is more common in the older group. Brain abscess, in the absence of meningitis, is often *unassociated* with fever. Severe cerebral necrosis, and resultant cystic encephalomalacia, is characteristic of infection with *Proteus, Pseudomonas, Paracolobactrum,* or *Citrobacter* species. *Serratia marcescens* causes fulminating hemorrhagic necrosis of brain (Volpe, 1987). Candidal infection typically affects babies of low birth weight who have a history of prolonged intravenous catheterization, poor nutrition, and prolonged therapy with broad-spectrum antibiotics. If *Candida* is cultured from the blood, there is a 60 percent or higher chance that the central nervous system is infected (Bozynski et al., 1986). A baby who has meningitis on the 1st day of life may have had transplacental infection with *Listeria monocytogenes*.

Because the clinical picture may not be as clear as the textbooks suggest, ultrasonographers may find themselves scanning a baby before the diagnosis of intracranial infection has been made on clinical grounds. As one performs the study, one should recall the pathophysiology as described earlier and search for the ultrasonographic correlates. (1) Is the ventricular fluid clear to the ultrasonic beam, or is it subtly or overtly echogenic? (2) Is the choroid plexus lumpy, hazy in outline,

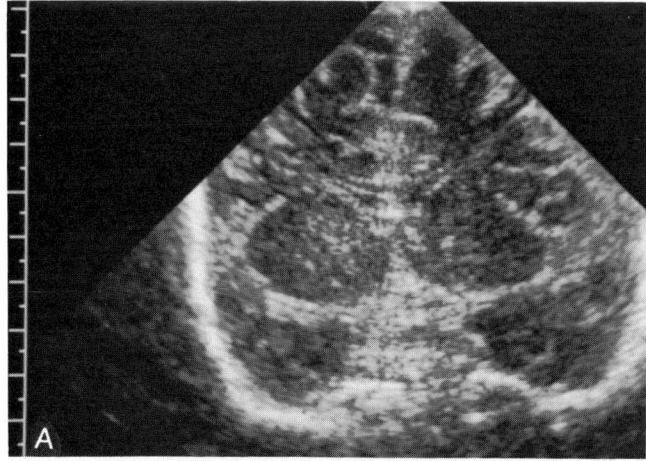
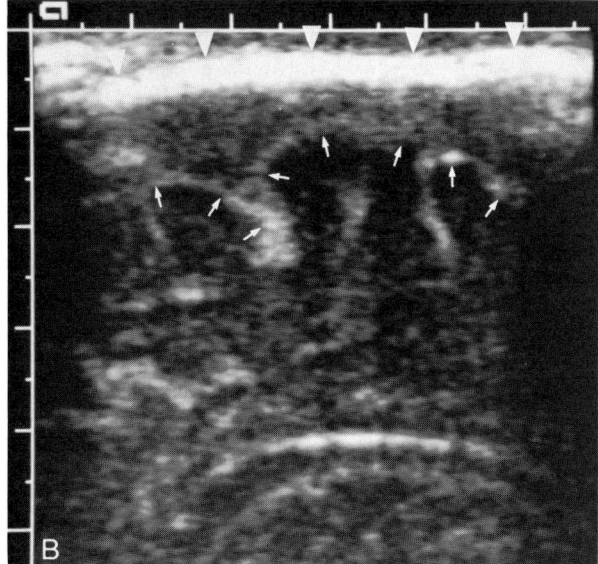

Figure 1-29. Extra-axial fluid in this 4-month-old baby is shown on a coronal sector scan (A) as thickened sulci. Sagittal scan with linear array transducer (B) shows echogenic fluid beneath the skull (arrowheads) surrounding the gyri, which are outlined by arrows. *Haemophilus influenzae* was cultured from CSF obtained by lumbar puncture.

or enlarged? (3) Are the ventricles of normal size? (4) Are the sulci thickened or prominent? (5) Is there extra-axial fluid? (6) Is the parenchyma normal throughout? (Figs. 1–29, 1–30, 1–31.) To find collections of extra-axial fluid (Cremin et al., 1984) and the increased echogenicity of gyral infarction (Babcock and Han, 1985), one must use high-frequency transducers that have good resolution in the near field. Axial scans through the temporal bone may be helpful to evaluate the subdural space if the fontanelle is too small to allow steeply angled coronal views of this area (Fig. 1–32).

Ultrasonographic scans are abnormal in only 62 percent of patients with acute symptoms of meningitis, and many abnormal results of scans are nonspecific (Han et al., 1985). Therapy should be based on clinical examination and on results from cultures of blood and CSF. For babies who have an established diagnosis of meningitis but are responding poorly to treatment, ultrasonography or CT can be used to evaluate complications (Fig. 1–33). The ability to show perfusion and enhancement of cerebral parenchyma from intravenous contrast material is, of course, available only with CT. Subdural effusions and their size and exact location are better demonstrated with CT but are usually not drained if there is neither midline shift nor clinical evidence of loculated infection. The ventricles or loculations within the ventricular system can be tapped under ultrasonic guidance when microbiologic examination of CSF or intrathecal administration of antibiotics is needed.

There is the special situation of congen-

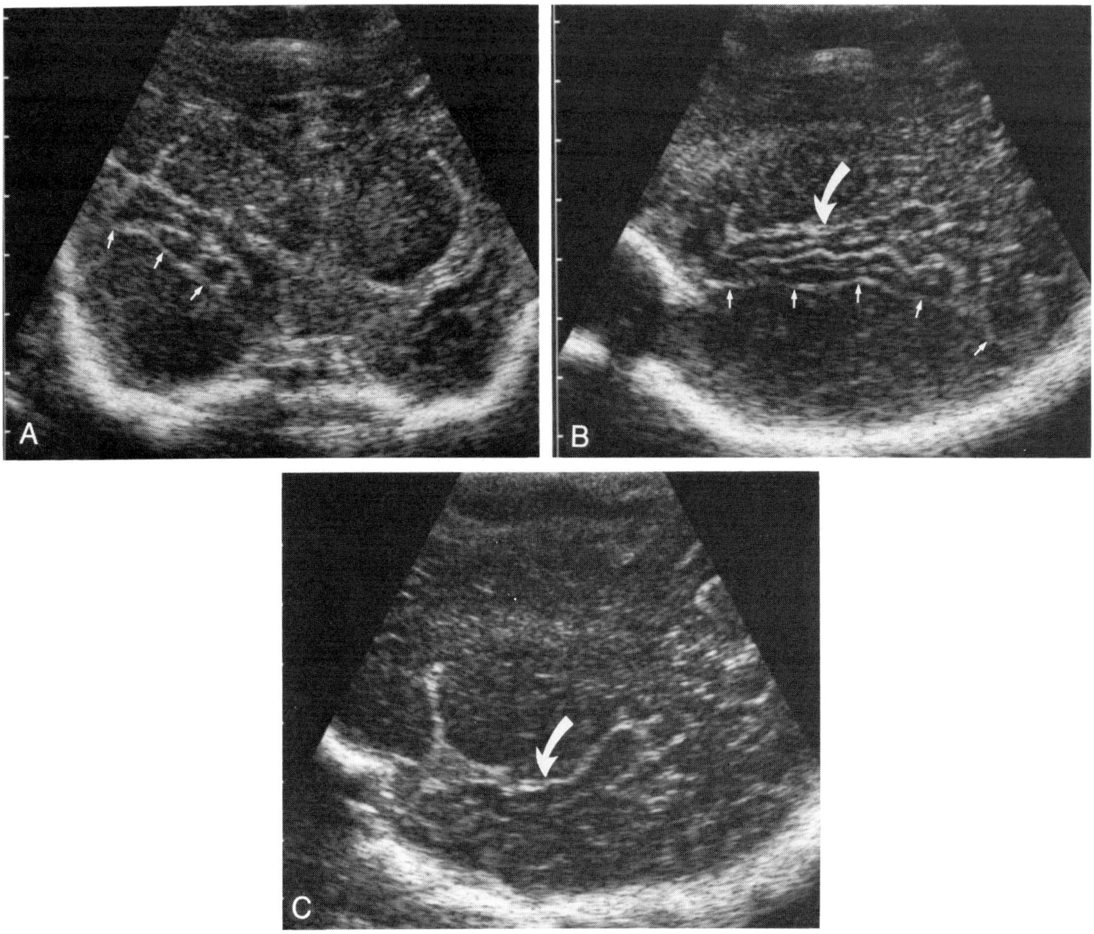

Figure 1-30. This 17-day-old boy had been diagnosed as having meningitis secondary to *Escherichia coli* shortly after birth when he was acutely febrile. He had been treated with appropriate antibiotics for 2 weeks. Because he was irritable, the house officers requested these ultrasonograms. The coronal view (A) shows distortion of the five-pointed star. The entire temporal lobe (arrows) is pushed superiorly by an echogenic subtemporal collection. This is easier to see on the parasagittal view of the temporal lobe (B). Small arrows mark the inferior extent of the temporal lobe, which has been elevated superiorly by a large subtemporal abscess. The normal left temporal lobe (C) is shown for comparison. Curved arrow in B and C marks the sylvian fissure.

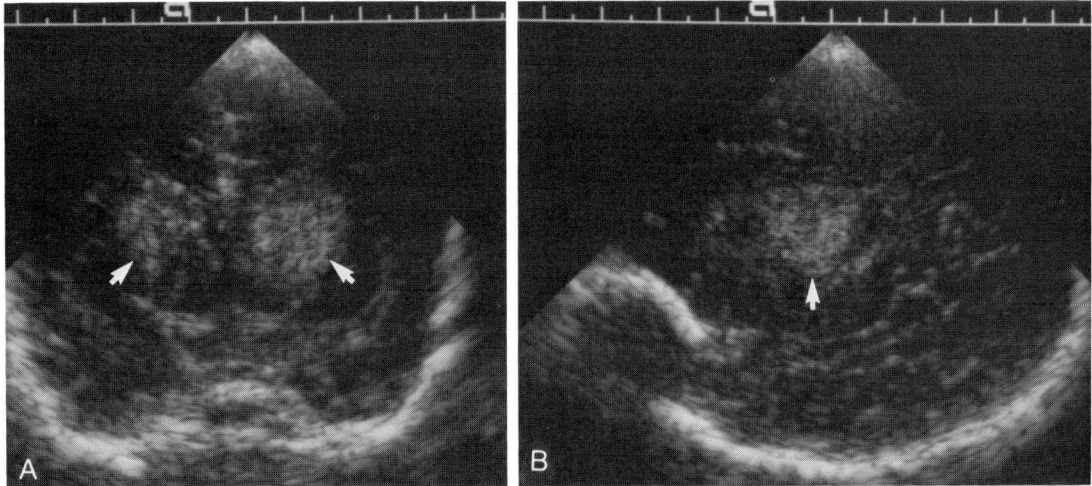

Figure 1-31. Echogenic areas in the basal ganglia (arrows on coronal scan [A] and left parasagittal scan [B]) were associated with Group B streptococcal meningitis in this 2-week-old baby. Parenchymal damage associated with meningitis follows a pattern similar to that seen in hypoxic-ischemic injury.

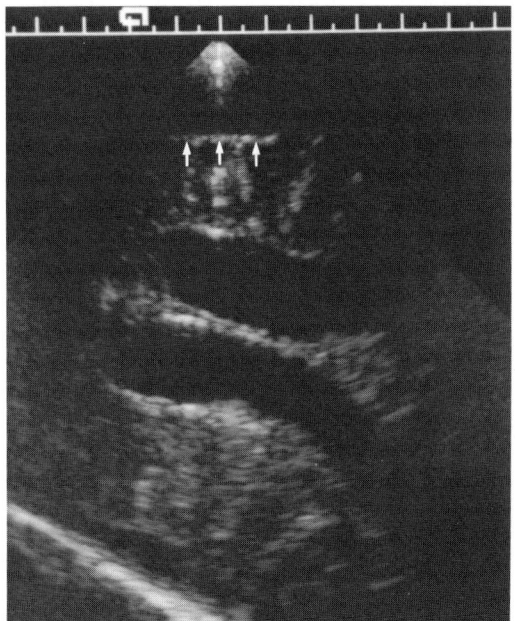

Figure 1–32. Axial scan with the transducer held against the coronal suture. It shows collection of fluid between the skull and the surface of the brain (arrows). This fluid was sterile. Note dilatation of lateral ventricles.

ital infection. The TORCH group of infectious agents (*t*oxoplasmosis; *o*ther, which includes syphilis; *r*ubella; *c*ytomegalovirus; and *h*erpes) is usually responsible for inflammatory intracranial events in utero. Mineralization and ultimately calcification result from inflammation and necrosis in both fetal and neonatal brains. The pattern of involvement is variable, depending on the severity of the infection and its timing in pregnancy. Periventricular cysts have been described in neonates who survived congenital rubella (Beltinger and Saule, 1988). Evidence of ventriculitis also has been shown on ultrasonography (Carey et al., 1987). Prominent linear densities in the basal ganglia have been demonstrated as correlating with mineralizing vasculopathy and to be associated with intrauterine infection, most notably cytomegalovirus (Fig. 1–34; Teele et al., 1988). Clumped, irregular periventricular calcification or dilatation of the ventricles, or both, in the absence of prior intracranial hemorrhage should raise the possibility of intrauterine infection (Grant et al., 1985; JL Frank, 1986). Many of the changes that we see pathologically, radiographically, and ultrasonographically are likely the result of ischemia and of subsequent attempts by the developing brain to repair the damage (Fig. 1–35). It is noteworthy that we have not as yet been able to document mineralizing vasculopathy or other distinct abnormalities in newborn babies who have been infected with the human immunodeficiency virus. Later in infancy, they may develop calcifications in basal ganglia, cerebral atrophy, and superimposed opportunistic infections or lymphoma (Epstein et al., 1988; Genieser et al., 1988).

The Dysmorphic Baby

Experienced pediatricians are quick to recognize a newborn dysmorphic baby. The ears may be a bit low set or rotated, the eyes may be positioned too closely or too far apart, and the shape and size of the head may be abnormal. In sum, the baby's appearance jars with the incredibly varied but normal faces of other babies in the nursery. There are often additional anomalies or findings present in the same child; for example, unusual cry, hypotonicity or hypertonicity, abnormal feet or hands, abnormal pattern of hair. The combination may be typical of a known syndrome or chromosomal abnormality, but most clinical impressions need confirmation from other studies. Radiologic and ultrasonographic evaluation is done as quickly as possible in such situations. The information gained is used immediately to plan further diagnostic evaluation and further care for the infant.

The ultrasonographer may encounter such bizarre anatomy when performing the cranial scans that it is imperative to obtain views in sequence and, wherever possible, establish the presence of normal landmarks. It is always most difficult to recognize what normal structure is missing. In the following outline, we therefore emphasize those features that may be absent on ultrasonography of the dysmorphic baby.

1. Judge the development of sulci and gyri for the baby's estimated gestational age.
2. Assess size and configuration of the ventricular system. The ventricular chambers are markers for anomalies affecting adjacent parenchyma.
3. Because midline structures are commonly abnormal in syndromic conditions, specifically identify longitudinal sulcus and falx, corpus callosum, septi pellucidi, vermis

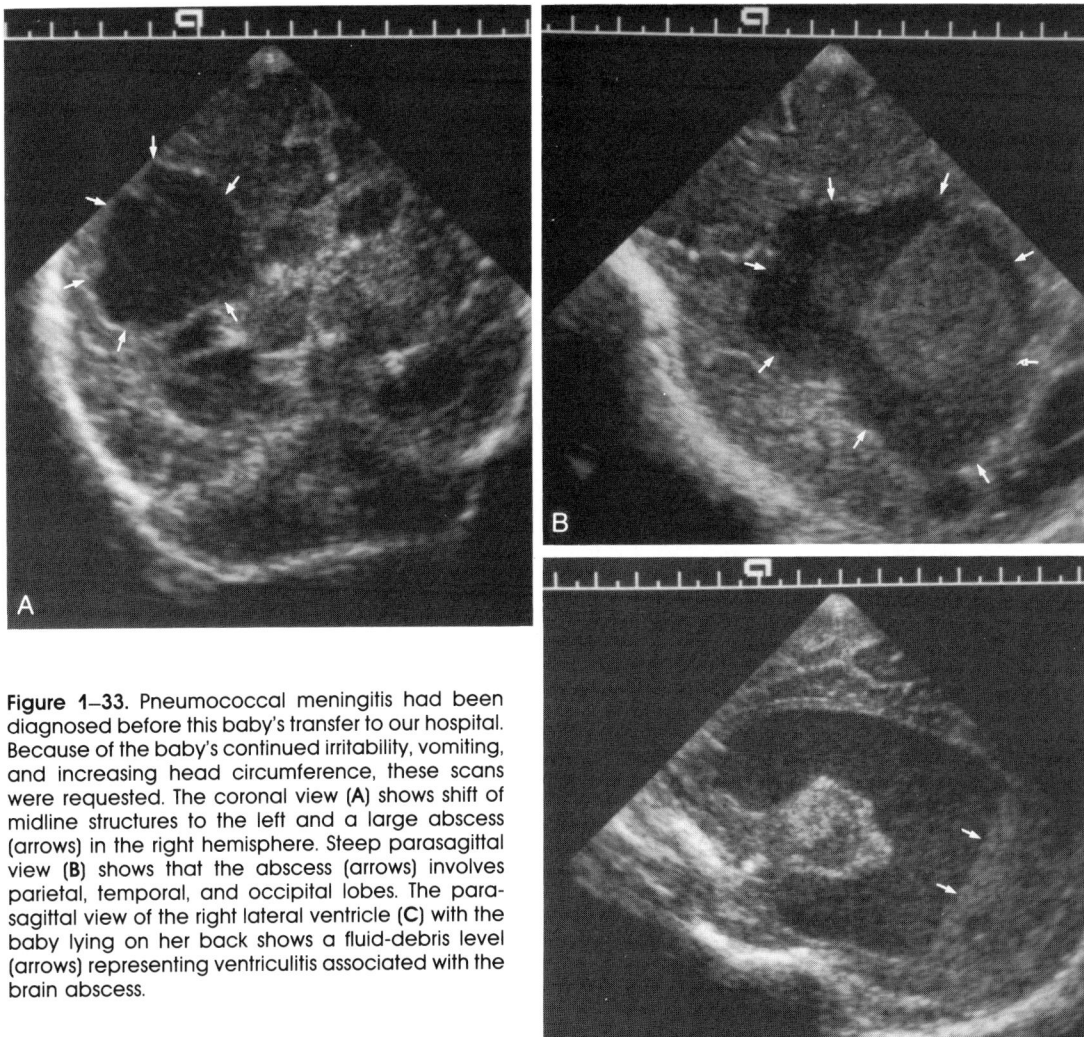

Figure 1-33. Pneumococcal meningitis had been diagnosed before this baby's transfer to our hospital. Because of the baby's continued irritability, vomiting, and increasing head circumference, these scans were requested. The coronal view (A) shows shift of midline structures to the left and a large abscess (arrows) in the right hemisphere. Steep parasagittal view (B) shows that the abscess (arrows) involves parietal, temporal, and occipital lobes. The parasagittal view of the right lateral ventricle (C) with the baby lying on her back shows a fluid-debris level (arrows) representing ventriculitis associated with the brain abscess.

of cerebellum, and total cerebellar volume and position. Midline facial anomalies—cleft lip and palate, hypotelorism, abnormal development of nose—are clues to the presence of midline cerebral defects.

4. Identify cystic or solid masses in relationship to ventricular system, parenchyma, and arachnoid space. Huge masses, cystic or solid, so distort the anatomy that their size is an impediment to diagnosis.

GYRAL ANOMALIES. Normal babies develop patterns of sulci and gyri along an established developmental pathway. In some pathologic studies, material from necropsies is used to mark the time of appearance of sulci according to gestational age (Worthen et al., 1986). Truly accurate gestational age of a subject may *not* have been acquired at the time of neuropathologic study. In addition, conceptual age is often interpreted as gestational (i.e., menstrual) age and vice versa. Thus there is overlap between babies established as "normal" in the literature that is not just biologic variability.

Micropolygyria is a reduction in size and increase in number of gyri. This may be difficult to appreciate with ultrasonography. Steep parasagittal scans, with the beam skimming the surface of the parietal and temporal lobes, may show this rare anomaly. Micro-

32 / CRANIAL ULTRASONOGRAPHY

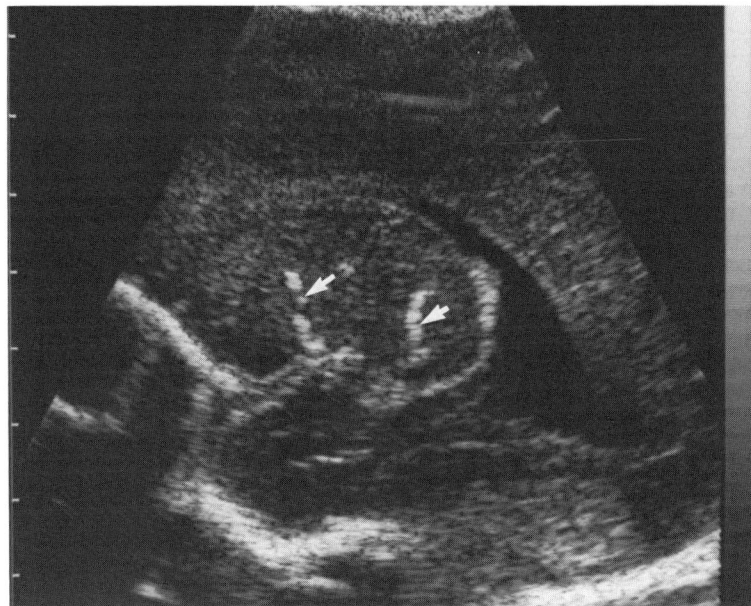

Figure 1–34. This baby died before an etiology was found to explain her echogenic, thalamic, and basal ganglia vasculature (arrows) shown on parasagittal scan of the lateral ventricle. Mineralizing vasculopathy was identified on neuropathologic examination.

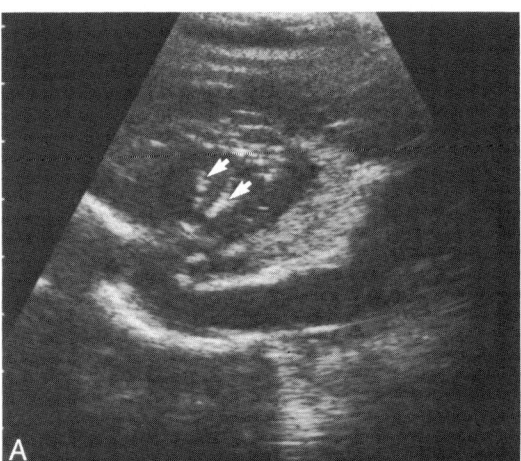

Figure 1–35. This baby died shortly after birth. Cytomegalovirus was cultured from the urine. The steep parasagittal view (**A**) through a very small anterior fontanelle showed echogenic vasculature (arrows) in the region of the basal ganglia and thalamus. There was irregular echogenicity around the ventricles, and on the sagittal scan (**B**), densely shadowing focus (arrow) was seen in the region of the cerebellum. The radiograph of the infant's skull and brain before necropsy (**C**) shows calcification within the brain. Calcification in the posterior fossa (arrow) was calcified cerebellum and corresponded to the abnormality seen in **B**.

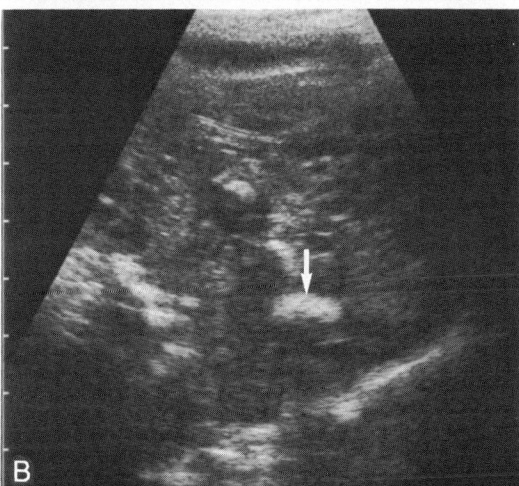
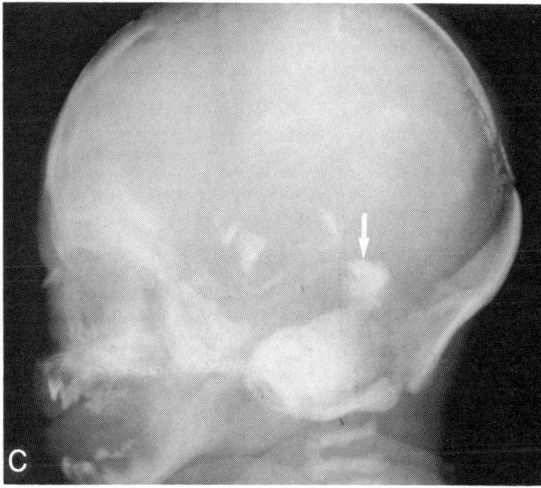

polygyria occurs at times with Arnold-Chiari II malformation.

Pachygyria (broad, sparse gyri) overlaps with agyria or lissencephaly (smooth brain), often in the same hemisphere. The brain is usually smaller than normal; the ratio of gray to white matter is increased because of an absolute decrease in the amount of white matter; ventricles may be enlarged; and corpus callosum may be absent. The baby typically has marked failure to thrive, and early death is common. On ultrasonography, the contour of the brain seems featureless; the sylvian, calcarine, and parieto-occipital fissures may be rudimentary; and the branching gyri are diminished in number or absent (Fig. 1–36; Motte et al., 1987).

Pathologic studies have shown abnormali-

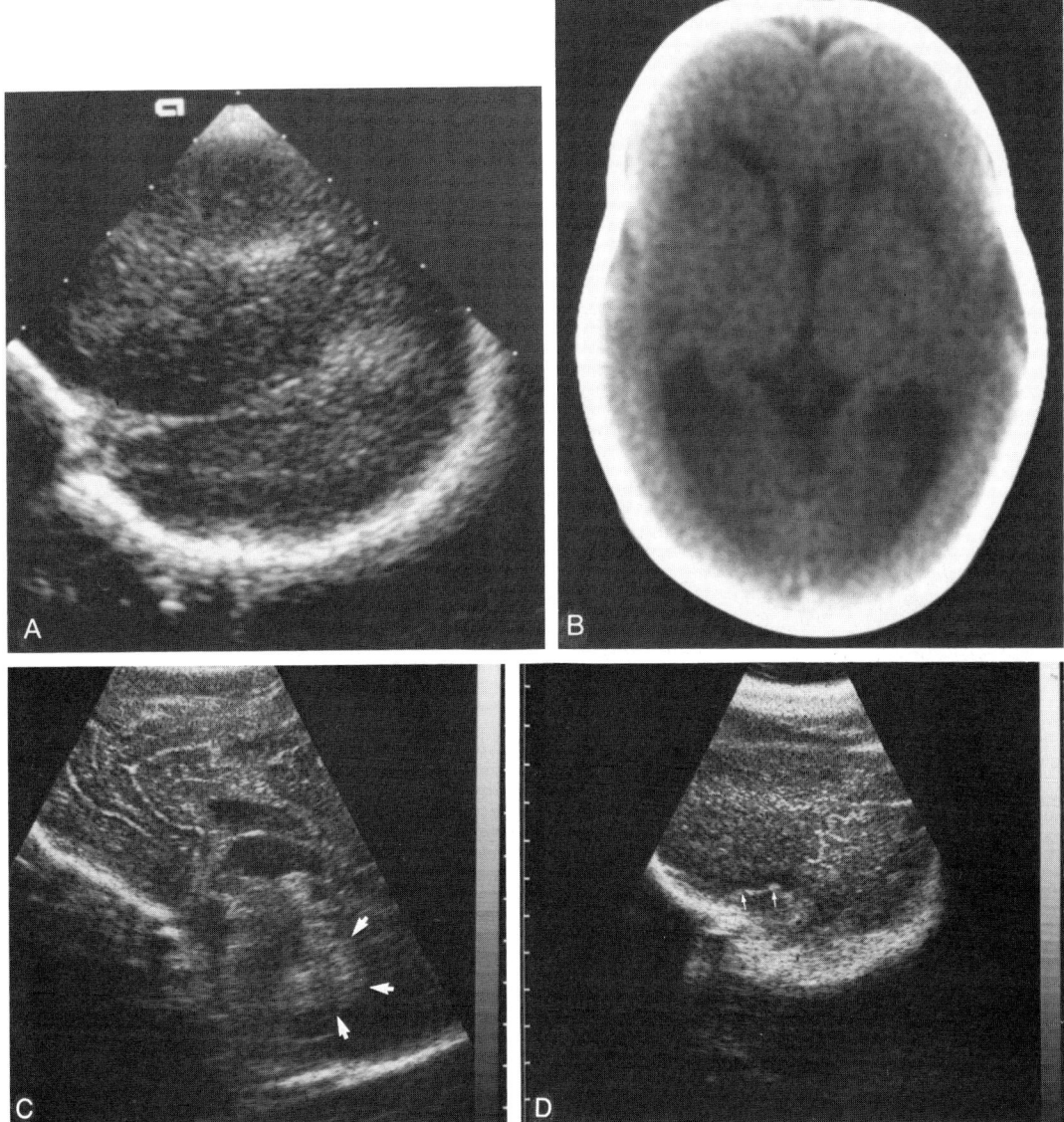

Figure 1–36. Sagittal ultrasonogram (A) of a baby who had severe failure to thrive shows diminished number of sulci and gyri. CT scan (B) confirms these findings. Final diagnosis was of lissencephaly associated with Miller-Dieker syndrome. C and D are midline and temporal sagittal scans from a baby who had Meckel-Gruber syndrome and who, at autopsy, had cerebellar hypoplasia (arrows, C) and lissencephaly. Cingulate and frontal sulci were present, but the sylvian fissure (arrows, D) was underdeveloped, and hemispheric surface was smooth (A and B courtesy of Diane Leighton and Vim Nayanar, Prince of Wales Hospital, Sydney, Australia.)

ties of folial patterns and nuclei in the cerebellum, but this may be inapparent on scans. Lissencephaly may occur as the primary feature of the Walker-Warburg and Miller-Dieker syndromes, or it may be present with other syndromes such as Meckel-Gruber and Zellweger.

One gyral anomaly occurs frequently in Down syndrome: superior position of the superior temporal sulcus. It is quite easy to identify this sulcus in the normal baby. In fact, in our experience, it is a good marker for gestational age of 26 weeks and is imaged by steep parasagittal scan of the temporal lobe.

The missing longitudinal sulcus is a feature of complex anomalies, specifically those classified under holoprosencephaly (see later section). The missing falx is typically a marker of holoprosencephaly in contradistinction to hydranencephaly.

ABSENCE OF CORPUS CALLOSUM. Absence may be partial or complete. The normal corpus callosum (genu, rostrum, splenium) is present on midline sagittal scans as a thin band of tissue looking rather like a Frisbee cut in cross-section. The superior edge is sharply demarcated by the pericallosal artery, in the pericallosal sulcus. The inferior edge is an interface with the fluid in the cavum septum pellucidum. On coronal scans, the corpus callosum is best demonstrated anterior to the foramen of Monro, where its superior and inferior borders are perpendicular to the beam of sound (Fig. 1–37). When it is absent, the anterior horns of the lateral ventricles are lateral to their normal position, and occipital horns are prominent. The remnants of callosal commissural fibers form the bundles of Probst, fiber tracts that run parallel and medial to lateral ventricles and may be seen as lobular masses on coronal scans. When no callosal bridge is present, sulci extend in a more vertical direction. They converge on the roof of the third ventricle, which may extend farther cephalad than normal (Fig. 1–38; Babcock, 1986; Hernanz-Schulman et al., 1985). Cortical heterotopia is frequently associated with agenesis of the corpus callosum, but we have not, to date, recognized this associated anomaly on ultrasonograms. Both lipoma of the corpus callosum and midline cyst can be identified when either is present (Fig. 1–39). Arachnoidal cysts are associated with agenesis of the corpus callosum, as is the Dandy-Walker malformation (Fig. 1–40). Callosal agenesis by itself is not a major clinical problem; it is

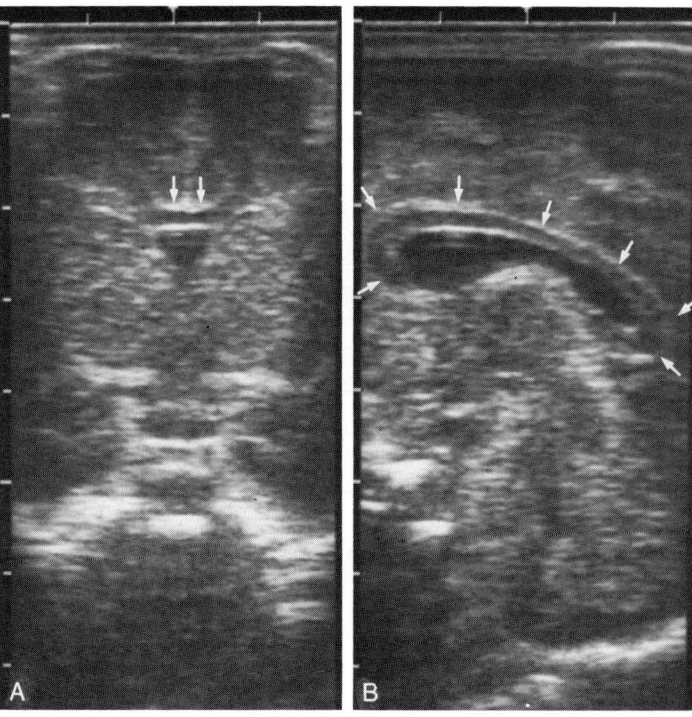

Figure 1–37. The corpus callosum is best viewed on coronal scans (**A**) anterior to the foramen of Monro. It is a thin band of tissue outlined superiorly by the sulcus of the pericallosal artery (arrows) and inferiorly by the cavum septum pellucidum. On the sagittal scan (**B**) the corpus callosum (arrows) is sharply outlined. This baby's sulci were undeveloped because he was 26 weeks of gestational age.

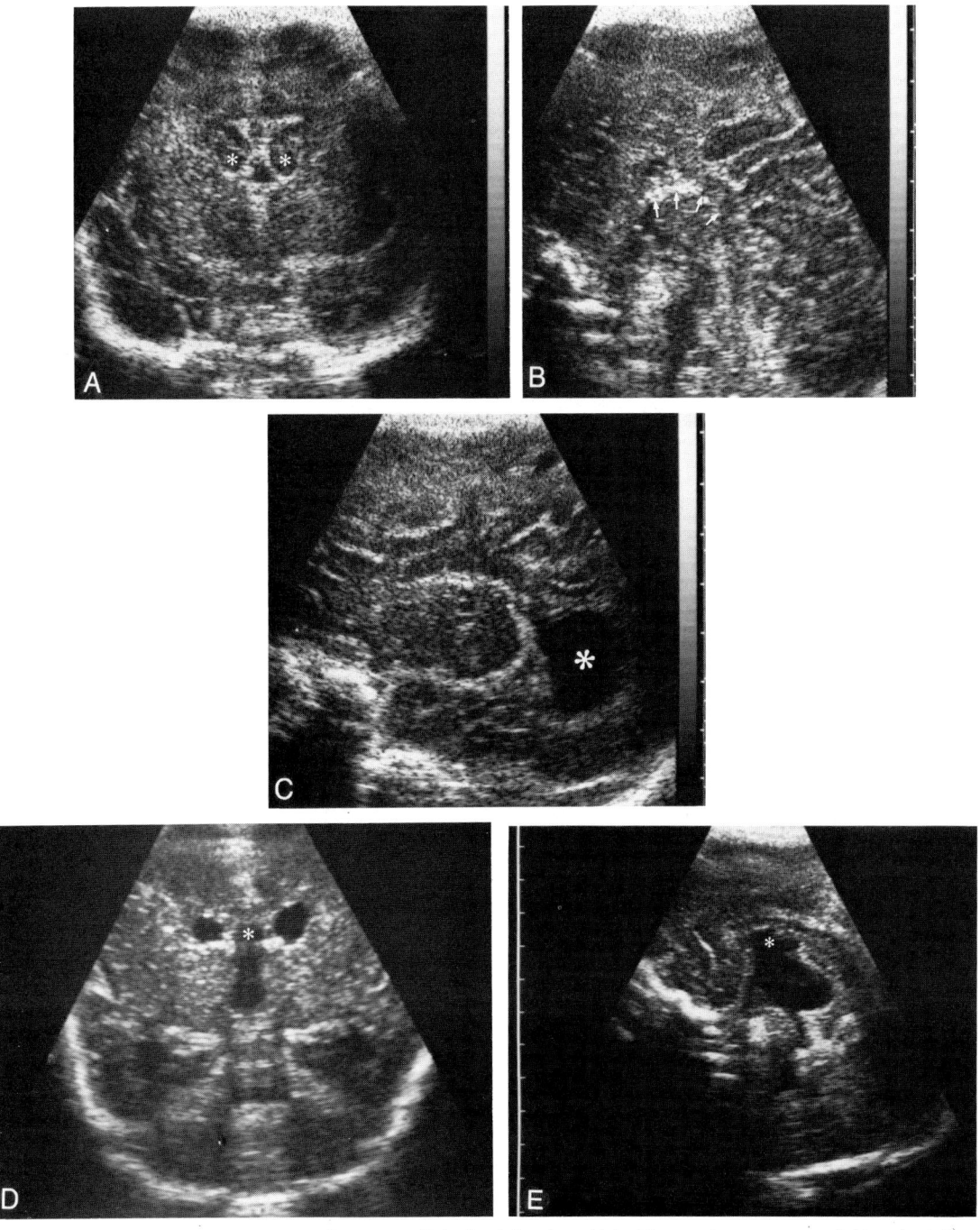

Figure 1–38. Agenesis of the corpus callosum results in the lateral ventricles' becoming more parallel in orientation. Bundles of Probst (asterisks) represent callosal tissue medial to the lateral ventricles (A). The sulci converge in a vertical direction on the roof of the third ventricle (arrows) on the sagittal scan (B). The occipital horn of lateral ventricle (asterisk) is usually prominent (C). In another baby, who presented at 2 months of age with failure to thrive, agenesis of corpus callosum shown on coronal (D) and midline sagittal (E) scans is accompanied by lissencephaly and dorsal extension of the third ventricle (asterisk). Agenesis may be part of a much more extensive cranial anomaly.

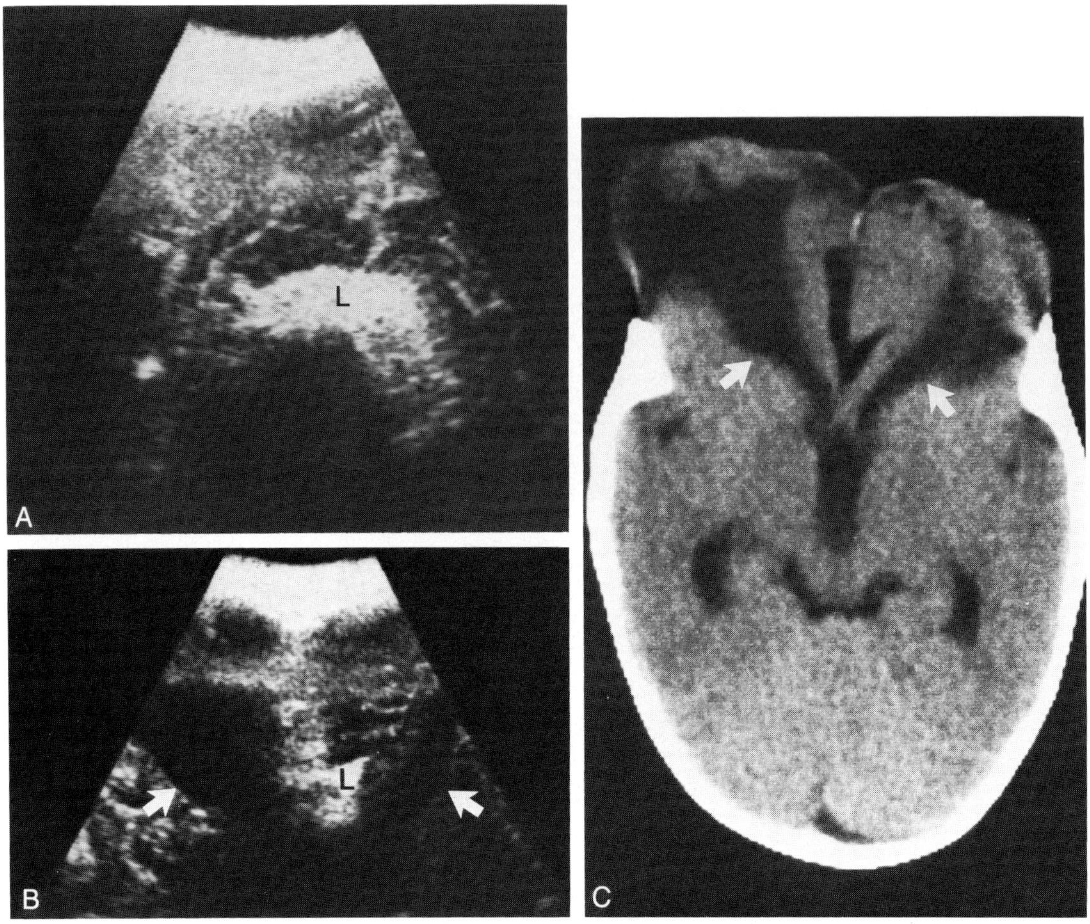

Figure 1–39. Sagittal midline scan (A) demonstrates lipoma of the corpus callosum (L), which casts such an acoustic shadow that definition of inferior structures is lost. The coronal scan (B) catches the anterior horns of the lateral ventricles (arrows). L = lipoma. The ultrasonogram corresponds in orientation to the CT scan (C) where anterior horns are also indicated by arrows. This patient had anterior encephalocele associated with agenesis of the corpus callosum and lipoma. (From Hernanz-Schulman M, Dohan FC Jr, Jones T, et al: Sonographic appearance of collosal agenesis: Correlation with radiologic and pathologic findings. AJNR 1985; 6:361–368.)

the associated anomalies that are the cause of mild to marked neurodevelopmental retardation.

ABSENCE OF SEPTI PELLUCIDI. This anomaly may be overlooked if attention to midline structures is cursory. One child, who had this anomaly with its associated mild lateral ventricular dilatation, was referred to us for "follow-up hydrocephalus" after an abnormal result on a prenatal scan. Part of the spectrum of septo-optic dysplasia (de Morsier syndrome), this malformation appears to include schizencephaly (clefting of the parietal lobe of the cerebrum; Kuban et al., 1989). The septi pellucidi are absent, optic nerves may be hypoplastic, and the hypothalamus is variably abnormal (Fig. 1–41). Babies may present with hypoglycemia, neonatal seizures, or other evidence of hypothalamic dysfunction. Schizencephaly has appeared in a number of these patients. If a large enough cleft is present, it should be recognizable on careful scanning of the lateral ventricular wall.

ABSENCE OF CEREBELLAR VERMIS (DANDY-WALKER MALFORMATION). Now commonly diagnosed by obstetric ultrasonography, this malformation appears to be the result of partial or complete agenesis of the cerebellar vermis and subsequent ballooning of the fourth ventricle, which then presents as a cystic mass in the posterior fossa. Cerebellar hemispheres are variably hypoplastic. Ultrasonography of this malformation is directed toward establishing that a cystic mass in the posterior fossa is an en-

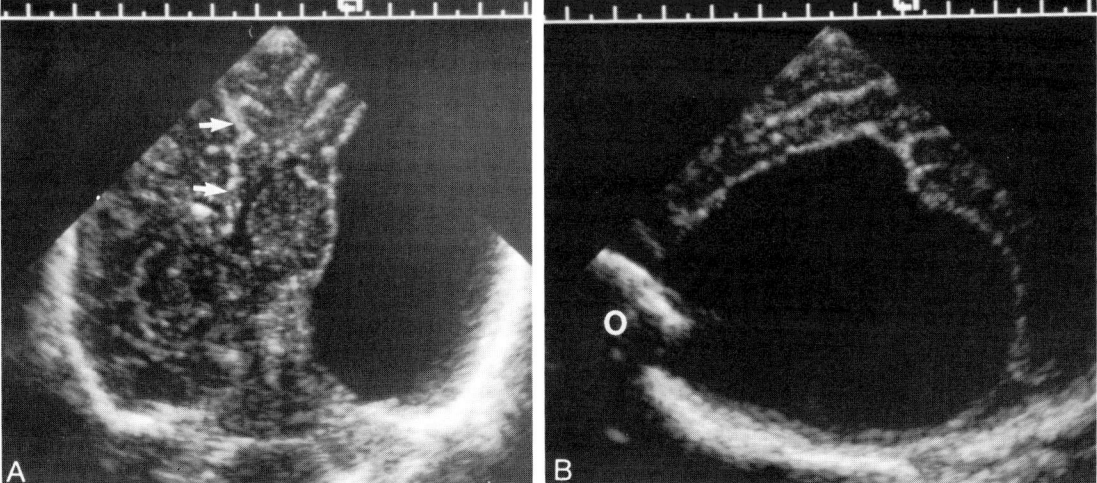

Figure 1–40. Partial agenesis of the corpus callosum was associated with a subtemporal arachnoid cyst in this baby who presented with increasing head circumference. The coronal scan (**A**) through the anterior fontanelle shows distortion of the brain from the large left-sided subtemporal arachnoid cyst. Longitudinal fissure is marked with arrowheads. Parasagittal scan (**B**) shows the anteroposterior extent of the subtemporal arachnoid cyst. O = orbit.

larged fourth ventricle, as opposed to a subarachnoid cyst, which displaces brain stem and cerebellum anteriorly. Coronal scans are best for showing the relationship of the ballooned fourth ventricle to the cerebellar hemispheres if they are present (Fig. 1–42).

Mass effect of the cyst results in expansion of the posterior fossa, and this can be appreciated on plain radiographs of the skull. Obstruction of normal flow of CSF results in dilatation of third and lateral ventricles in most cases. Other cranial anomalies, such as agenesis of corpus callosum, gyral abnormalities, and cortical heterotopia, may be present. Goldston syndrome is the association of Dandy-Walker malformation and cystic renal disease.

ABSENCE OF MIDLINE STRUCTURES (HOLOPROSENCEPHALY). Encompassing a spectrum of related anomalies, this term generally describes the failure of the embryonic forebrain to cleave in two. Absence of

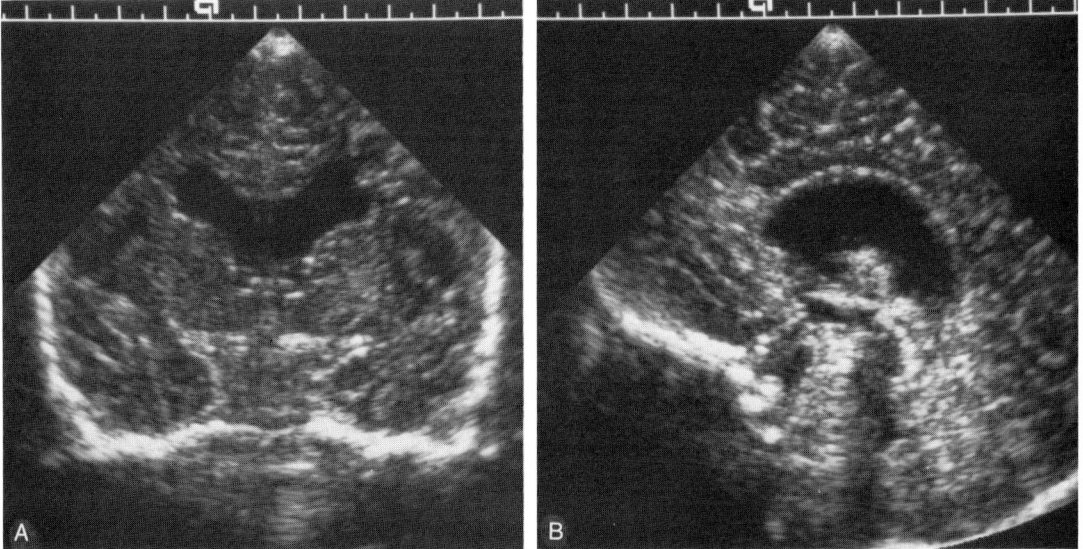

Figure 1–41. Absence of the septi pellucidi is obvious on anterior coronal (**A**) and midline sagittal (**B**) scans.

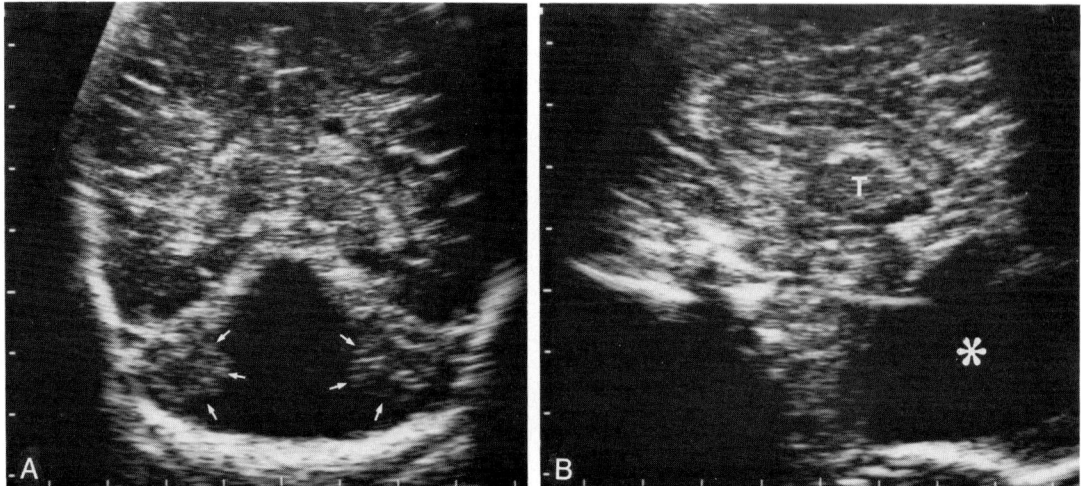

Figure 1–42. Dandy-Walker malformation is diagnosed by coronal (**A**) and sagittal (**B**) scans through the posterior fossa. The cerebellar vermis is absent. The fourth ventricle bulges posteriorly as a cystic mass that outlines each cerebellar hemisphere (arrows). On midline sagittal scan, the posterior fossa is filled by fluid (asterisk). T = massa intermedia of thalamus.

olfactory bulbs and tracts on neuropathologic examination is characteristic of even the mildest forms; hence the genesis of the older term "arrhinencephaly," which is still occasionally used in the literature. The most severe form of holoprosencephaly is termed "alobar." The brain is small and spherical in shape, gyri are underdeveloped, and on coronal scans the ventricular system is represented by a single, upside-down-U-shaped chamber that surrounds fused thalami. The falx is absent (Fig. 1–43). The association of facial malformations with holoprosencephaly has supported the theory that a faulty embryonic interaction among notochordal plate, neuroectoderm, oral plate, and olfactory placodes is responsible for the extensive anomalies. Cyclopia, ethmocephaly (single, double, or absent proboscis), premaxillary agenesis (ocular hypotelorism, flat nose, median cleft lip), and cebocephaly (ocular hypotelorism, nose with single nostril) are associated with alobar holoprosencephaly. Less severe or no facial dysmorphia is associated with lobar

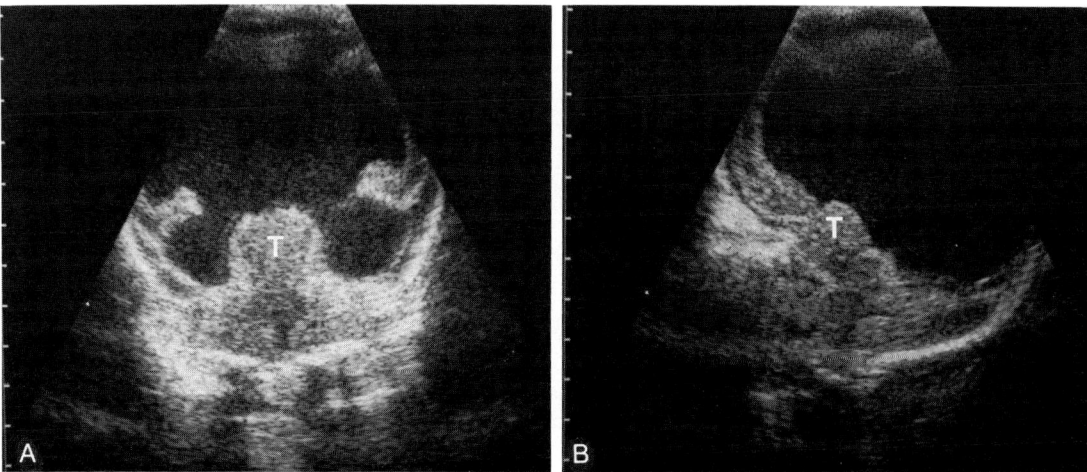

Figure 1–43. This baby was born at 37 weeks of gestation. She had fused eyelids, and a single midline proboscis. Coronal (**A**) and midline sagittal (**B**) scans of the brain showed a single ventricle surrounding fused thalami (T). Very little cerebral cortex was present. The baby died shortly thereafter of respiratory insufficiency. Pathologic examination confirmed alobar holoprosencephaly and trisomy 13.

(mild) or semilobar (moderate) forms (McGahan et al., 1990).

Lobar holoprosencephaly belongs to the spectrum of other midline anomalies (Fig. 1–44; Poe et al., 1989). Because the presence or absence of olfactory bulbs and tracts cannot be determined with ultrasonography, separation of mild lobar holoprosencephaly from absence of corpus callosum or septi pellucidi is difficult. The range of expression of the disorder between lobar and alobar forms demonstrates varying degrees of cerebral hypoplasia, ventriculomegaly, and variability in fusion of basal ganglia, thalami, or both and is termed "semilobar." The definitions of holoprosencephaly vary, depending on whether the reported series are from clinicians, pathologists, or radiologists. The ultrasonographer should show the anatomy in detail and characterize the scan as either demonstrating typical alobar holoprosencephaly or showing no, mild, or moderate anomalies in the midline. Implications of severe anomalies are significant: chromosomal deletions 18p− and 13q− and trisomies 13 and 18 are associated with holoprosencephaly.

ABSENT VASCULATURE (HYDRANENCEPHALY). Intrauterine insult to normal cerebral arterial flow with complete occlusion of internal carotid arteries is theorized to be the cause of hydranencephaly. The telencephalon fails to develop or is destroyed, and a bag of CSF is all that remains above the tentorium (Fig. 1–45). Coronal scans on such sad babies often fail to show the falx cerebri, which is usually present, because the scanning plane is parallel to the interface from the falx. Axial scanning, therefore, or "off-center" coronal or sagittal scans should be used to identify the falx. Ventricular dilatation in alobar holoprosencephaly, which has a different etiology and different genetic implications, also occasionally results in a hugely dilated sac, but the falx is absent. The differential diagnosis between severe obstructive hydrocephalus and hydranencephaly is less easy. In some babies who have had hydranencephaly, the fluid has been diffusely echogenic, which suggests that it is high in protein content. In those with severe obstructive hydrocephalus, CT scanning allows more accurate measurement of uniformity and thickness of cerebral mantle than does ultrasonography.

VENTRICULOMEGALY. In the absence of meningomyelocele, simple obstructive ventriculomegaly, diagnosed on postnatal scans, is usually secondary to intraventricular blockage of CSF at the aqueduct of Sylvius (Volpe, 1987). Aqueductal stenosis probably occurs later in gestation (15 to 17 weeks) than do other cranial malformations. It is less likely to be associated with other intra- or

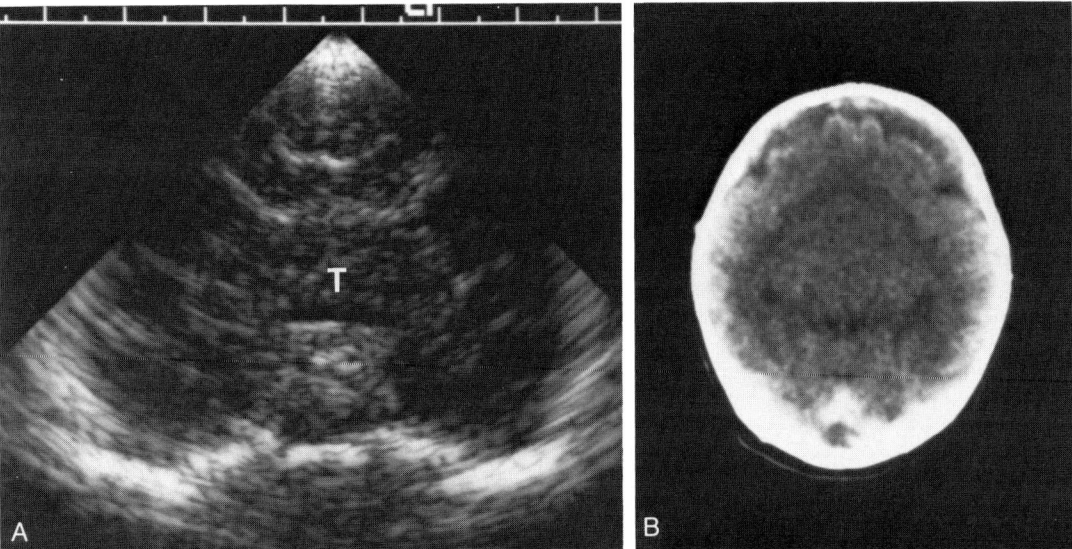

Figure 1–44. Chromosomal analysis showed this baby girl to have trisomy 13. Microcephaly and hypotelorism were obvious at birth. Lateral ventricles were present, but the basal ganglia and thalami (T) appear fused (A). The CT scan (B) showed the same findings. This is considered to be semilobar holoprosencephaly.

Figure 1–45. A shows the difficulty in differentiating hydranencephaly, severe hydrocephalus, and severe alobar holoprosencephaly. No identifiable cerebral tissue is evident above the midbrain. The CT scan that followed **(B)** confirmed absence of any cerebral mantle, and hydranencephaly was diagnosed.

extracranial anomalies. Babies with aqueductal stenosis survive to term more often than do babies with more complex anomalies. Occlusion or stenosis may occur in isolation, may be associated with X-linked inheritance, or may be secondary to intrauterine infection or hemorrhage. Scans reveal a normal fourth ventricle but dilatation of the lateral and third ventricles (Fig. 1–46). An enlarged fourth ventricle implies more distal obstruction at the outlet of the fourth ventricle, in the subarachnoid space, or at the arachnoid villi.

The Arnold-Chiari II malformation virtually always accompanies meningomyelocele; it is variable in its clinical presentation. Babies with thoracolumbar and lumbar lesions have a higher likelihood of significant ventriculomegaly than do babies with lesions at other sites (90 percent versus 60 percent; Charney et al., 1985).

Depending on the population and on the medical and surgical management, 80 to 90 percent of babies ultimately need ventricular shunting (McLone et al., 1982; Charney et al., 1985). In the Arnold-Chiari II malformation, the cerebellar vermis is elongated and the cerebellum is oval rather than spherical in shape. The medulla and upper spinal cord may be kinked, and intraventricular blockage to flow of CSF may be caused by obstruction at the level of the aqueduct. Sagittal midline scans, done with care to include the anterior edge of occipital bone, are most revealing. The cerebellar tissue extends down to, or through, the foramen magnum; the cisterna magna is obliterated. The third ventricle is more capacious than usual: it appears as though its posterior wall were being pulled back and down. The massa intermedia, outlined by fluid fore and aft, is prominent. The fourth ventricle is often difficult to outline

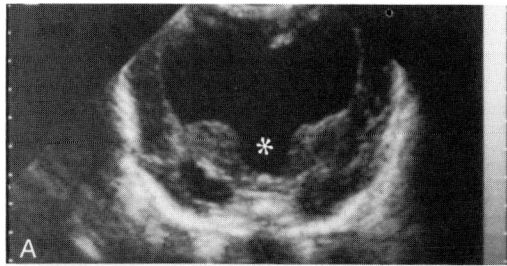

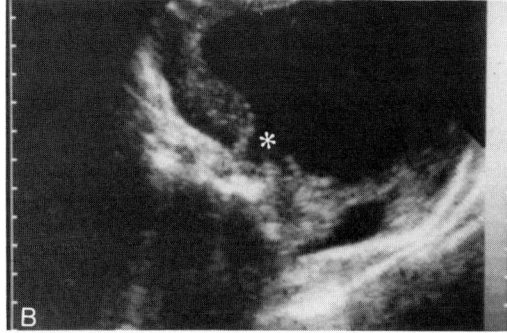

Figure 1–46. Aqueductal stenosis may be diagnosed on scans done in utero, as was the case for this baby. The lateral and third (asterisk) ventricles are dilated on coronal **(A)** and midline sagittal **(B)** scans. The fourth ventricle is normal in size.

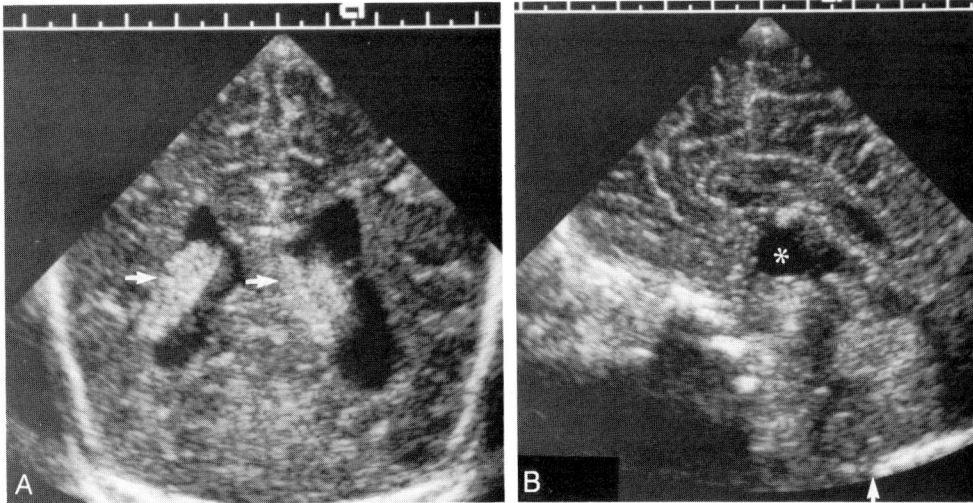

Figure 1–47. Coronal (A) and sagittal (B) scans of this baby were done shortly after his birth. He had been diagnosed at 25 weeks of gestational age as having a thoracolumbar meningomyelocele. The coronal scan shows very mild dilatation of the lateral ventricles. Note the choroid plexus (arrows), which flopped to the dependent side of the lateral ventricles as the infant lay on his right side. His third ventricle (asterisk, B) is mildly dilated. The cerebellum, which extends to the edge of the occipital bone (arrow), obliterates the cisterna magna. Ultrasonography was used in following this child over the next 4 months. His ventricular dilatation stayed mild, and therefore no shunting was performed.

because of the distortion of the brain stem (Figs. 1–47, 1–48).

Ultrasonography may not be able to discriminate level of obstruction—aqueduct versus posterior fossa—but therapy does not depend on this discrimination. Therapy (i.e., ventricular shunting) depends on the degree of lateral ventricular dilatation, its rate of change after birth, and associated neurologic abnormalities. Of infants who develop significant hydrocephalus in association with meningomyelocele, 80 percent exhibit clinical signs of increasing intracranial pressure within the first 6 weeks of life (Stein and Schut, 1979). After a shunt has been placed, ultrasonography is an easy method with which to document the location of the tip. If a child does poorly after surgery, common

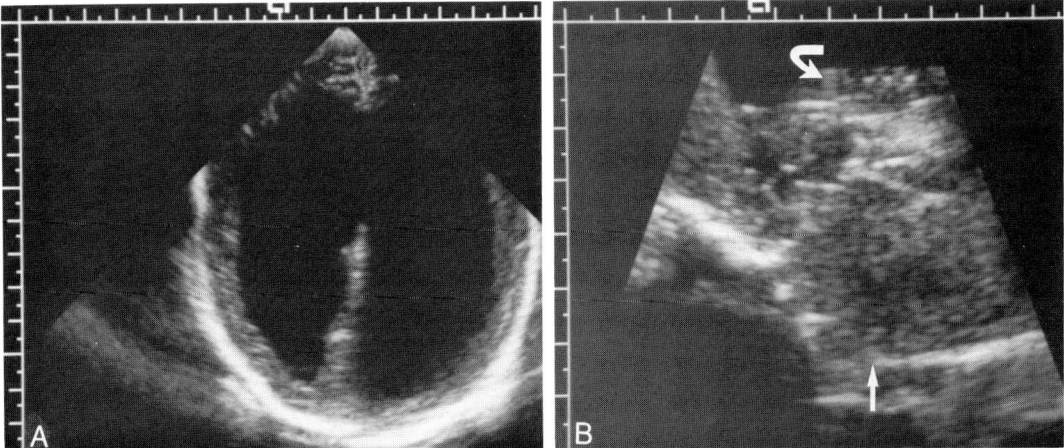

Figure 1–48. Severe hydrocephalus was associated with lumbar meningomyelocele in this baby. When the back was closed, a shunt was placed. The coronal scan (A) shows the severe dilatation of both lateral ventricles. The sagittal midline scan (B) shows the tip of the shunt (curved arrow). Note the poor delineation of structures in the midbrain and the posterior fossa. A normal fourth ventricle cannot be delineated. There is no cisterna magna. The edge of the occipital bone is marked by a straight arrow.

42 / CRANIAL ULTRASONOGRAPHY

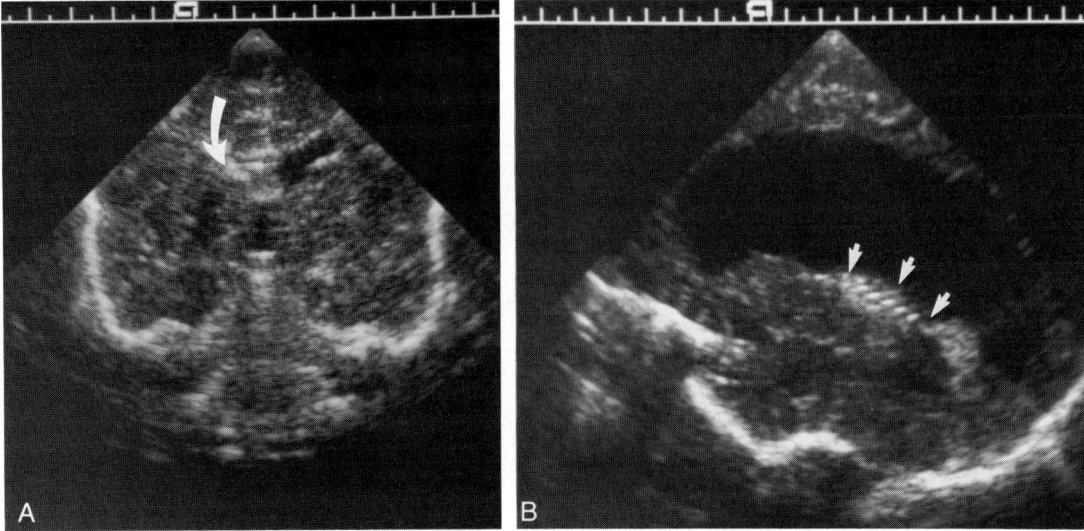

Figure 1–49. The original postoperative scans on this baby with meningomyelocele and Arnold-Chiari II malformation showed decompression of the ventricular system. The shunt, in the right lateral ventricle on this coronal scan (**A**), is a faintly shadowing focus (arrow). Eight months later, the baby was reevaluated when head circumference began crossing normal growth curves. The parasagittal scan of the right lateral ventricle at that time (**B**) shows the shunt tubing surrounded by the choroid plexus (arrows). The choroid plexus had blocked the side holes, preventing drainage of CSF.

complications attributable to the shunt include its obstruction by a clot or by the choroid plexus (Fig. 1–49). The tip should be in the anterior horn of the lateral ventricle but occasionally is found on ultrasonography to be within the parenchyma of the brain (Fig. 1–50).

One can achieve scans of the cervicomedullary junction by scanning over the posterior neck, above the arch of C-1. However, landmarks are difficult to recognize and inconstant, depending on the degree of flexion or extension of the neck (Fig. 1–51). Tissue-equivalent stand-off allows better resolution.

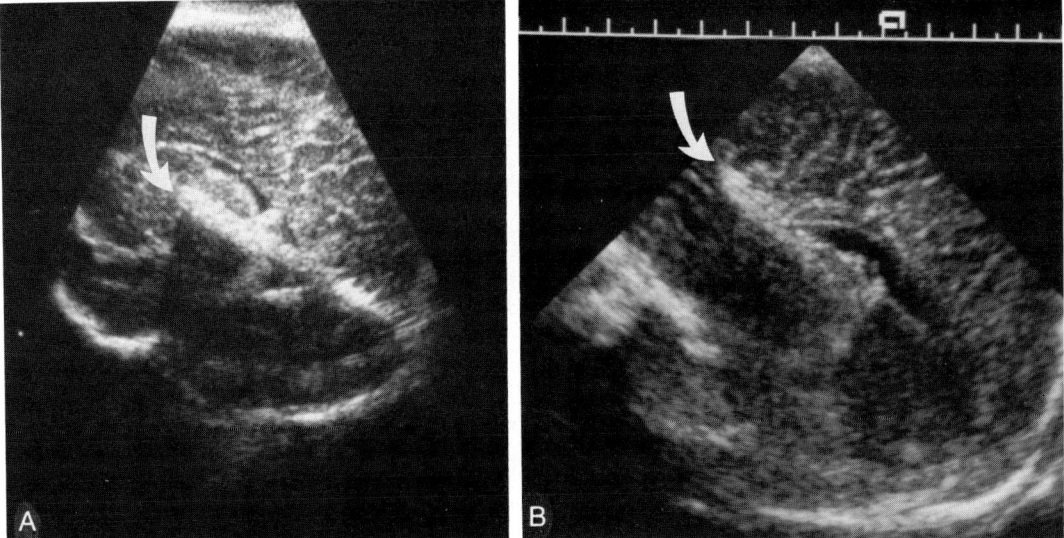

Figure 1–50. Parasagittal scan (**A**) shows the tip of a ventricular shunt (arrow) in the basal ganglia. In another baby (**B**) the ventricular shunt ends in the frontal cortex (arrow).

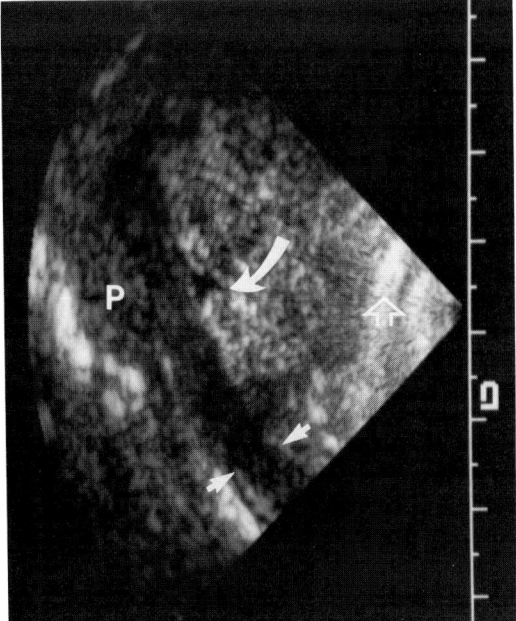

Figure 1–51. Sagittal scan of the upper neck demonstrates the Arnold-Chiari II malformation. It was performed while the baby was lying on her side with her neck flexed. Note the fourth ventricle (curved arrow), cerebellar tissue extending below the occipital bone (open arrow), and the relatively echolucent cervical cord (straight arrows). P = pons.

Table 1–1. CAUSES OF VENTRICULOMEGALY IN INFANTS AND CHILDREN

Location of Abnormality	Type of Abnormality
Arachnoid villi	failure to develop obstruction by hemorrhage or infection

Subarachnoid spaces	meningitis
	hemorrhage • previous IVH
	            • traumatic
	            • AVM

Fourth ventricular outlet and fourth ventricle	meningitis, including TB Arnold-Chiari II malformation Dandy-Walker malformation arachnoidal cyst in posterior fossa neoplasm previous IVH
Aqueduct	ependymitis • pyogenic • mumps genetic (X-linked obstruction) Arnold-Chiari II malformation aneurysm, vein of Galen mesencephalic tumor or AVM neuroectodermal tumor "disuse" atrophy after shunt arachnoidal cyst previous IVH
Third ventricle	pinealoma neoplasm arachnoidal cyst
Foramen of Monro	ventriculitis neoplasm, tuberous sclerosis cyst of choroid plexus
Lateral ventricles	papilloma of choroid plexus neoplasm

IVH = intraventricular hemorrhage. AVM = arteriovenous malformation. TB = tubercular.

Scans of the cervical cord may show central cavitation. Hydromyelia (dilatation of central canal) and syringomyelia (cavitation adjacent to, but often communicating with central canal) are associated with the Arnold-Chiari II malformation, as is cerebellar tonsillar herniation.

In any baby with ventriculomegaly, baseline scans should be performed with careful attention to landmarks because follow-up studies often are needed to assess change in ventricular size with time. If ventriculomegaly is identified at any time in the baby's development, scans are directed toward identifying which ventricles are dilated, quantifying degree of dilatation, evaluating extra-axial spaces to the limits of the technique, and identifying a cause for the dilatation. Causes of ventriculomegaly are listed in Table 1-1.

This section began with a discussion centered on the dysmorphic child. However, significant intracranial anomalies may occur in a child who otherwise looks and seems perfectly normal and who has apparently normal chromosomes. Children who are diagnosed on their mothers' obstetric scans as having an anomaly are becoming more frequent visitors to our department. Parents are justifiably upset when told of a possible intracranial abnormality in their baby, and if the baby survives, scanning is repeated as soon as possible after birth to allow confirmation of a diagnosis or to further define an anomaly.

There are two situations in which normal development or variants have been labeled anomalies: the fluid-filled cavum septum pellucidum has been mistaken as a cystic mass, as have cysts of the choroid plexus. The

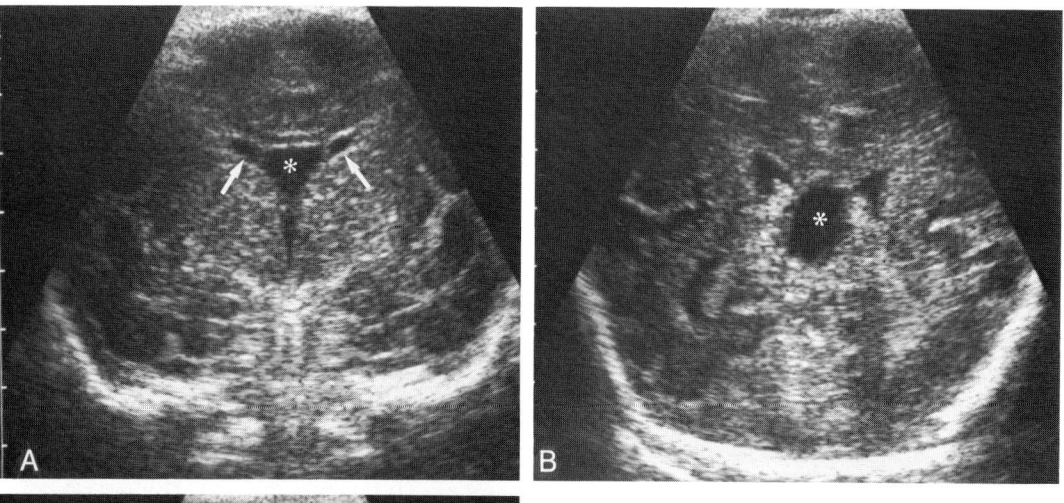

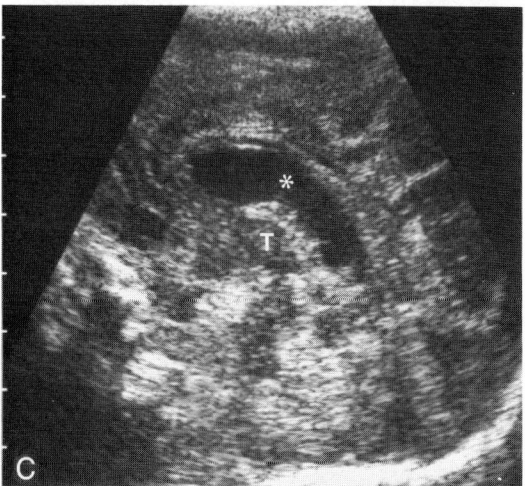

Figure 1-52. Anterior coronal scan (A) shows the cavum septum pellucidum (asterisk) between the two anterior horns of the lateral ventricles (arrows). The corpus collusum is the thin band of tissue immediately superior to the cavum. The normal third ventricle is a fine linear lucency immediately inferior to the cavum septum pellucidum. Angled coronal scan (B) at the level of the trigones of the lateral ventricles shows posterior extension of the cavum septum pellucidum (asterisk), which is termed "cavum vergae." The midline sagittal scan (C) shows the fluid-filled cavum (asterisk) extending posteriorly below the corpus callosum. The cavum should not be mistaken for enlargement of the third ventricle or a cystic mass. T = massa intermedia of thalamus.

cavum septum pellucidum is filled with fluid and present in virtually all babies at the beginning of the third trimester. It often extends far posteriorly, under the corpus callosum, earning the term "cavum vergae." By 3 months after birth, this potential space disappears in 50 percent of the population. It persists, but is variable in size, in 20 percent of children and adults, and it disappears sometime after age 3 months in 30 percent. On steep coronal scans, the cavum vergae may be mistaken for a dilated third ventricle, but the sagittal scan in midline shows its close relationship to the undersurface of the corpus callosum (Fig. 1–52). Differentiating the cavum velum interpositum (upward and forward extension of the cistern of the quadrigeminal plate) from the cavum vergae is an academic exercise and really proved only with axial sections on CT scanning.

Choroidal cysts are occasionally noted on prenatal studies. Most seem to involute and disappear. There are only two situations in which their identification is important. First is the rare complication of obstruction, by the cyst, of the foramen of Monro (Fig. 1–53). Second, multiple cysts have been associated with chromosomal abnormalities (Fakhry et al., 1985; Chitkara et al., 1988).

In summary, ultrasonography is extremely valuable in the assessment of the dysmorphic baby and in characterizing anomalies that are discovered incidentally on prenatal or postnatal scans. When should CT or MRI scan-

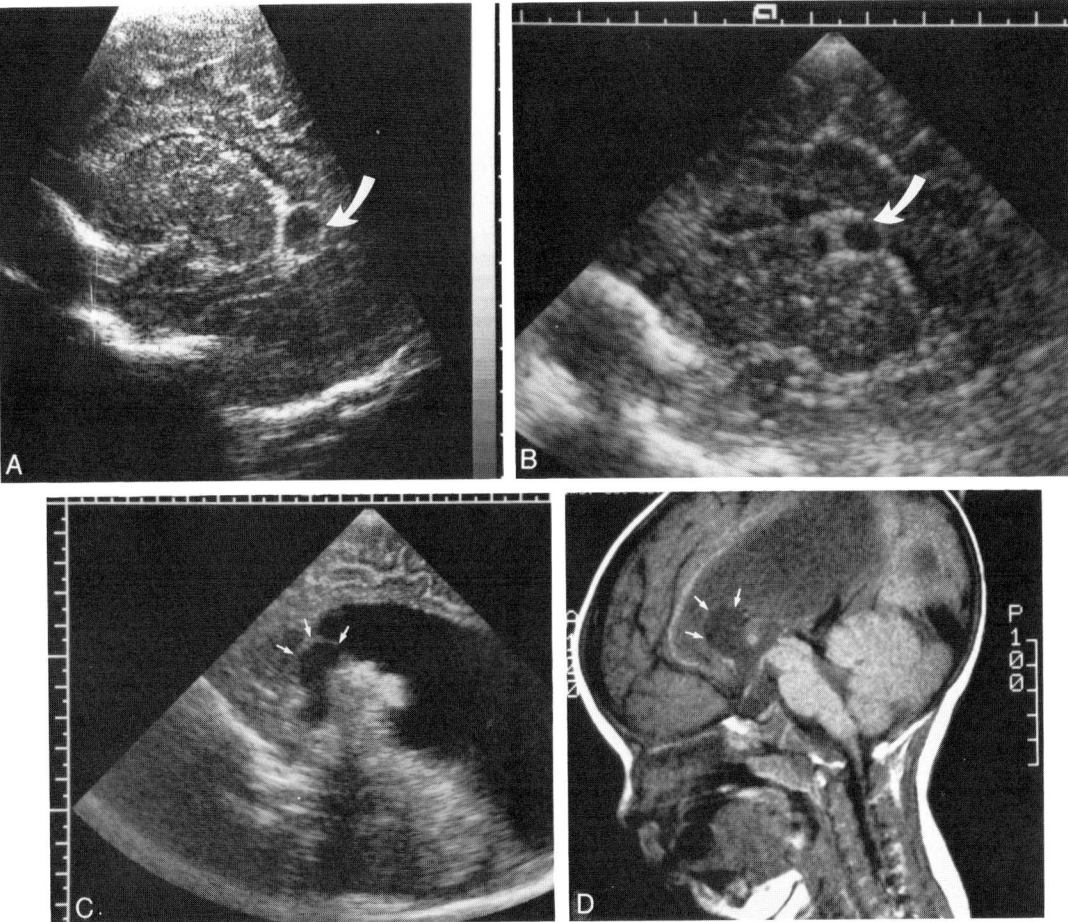

Figure 1–53. Sagittal scans in two different babies show choroidal cyst in the trigone (A) and choroidal cysts near the caudothalamic groove (B). These generally are of no clinical significance and disappear spontaneously. C is a scan of a 6-month-old baby girl who was examined after cranial circumference appeared to be increasing too rapidly for age. The midline sagittal sonogram demonstrated a cyst (arrows) that appeared to be obstructing the lateral ventricles, thereby causing hydrocephalus. The cyst was also evident on MRI scanning (arrows, D) that followed. We assume that it arose from the choroid plexus at the level of the foramen of Monro.

ning be added to the evaluation? (1) To differentiate between hydranencephaly and severe hydrocephalus; (2) to further investigate complex malformations (MRI, especially, can show abnormalities of gray and white matter that are beyond the capability of ultrasound); (3) when the fontanelle is too small for effective examination; and (4) when the referring physician or surgeon cannot feel comfortable with ultrasonography alone. With time and experience on the part of the clinicians, "confirmatory" studies will be needed in only the unusual cases.

Congenital Neoplasm

Congenital intracranial neoplasms, defined as tumors present at birth or discovered in the first 12 months of life, are extremely rare but may present as cranial enlargement in an otherwise normal baby. In one study of 35 children with such enlargement who were less than 1 year of age, 49 percent had astrocytoma. Neuroectodermal tumors, papillomas of choroid plexus, and miscellaneous other tumors and cysts each accounted for 17 percent of all masses (Chuang and Harwood-Nash, 1986). In general, however, neuroectodermal tumors may constitute 33 to 67 percent of the total number (Buetow et al., 1990; Takaku et al., 1978).

The gliomas may be supratentorial or infratentorial in location. Medulloblastoma has a particular affinity for cerebellar vermis and may obstruct aqueduct or fourth ventricle. Supratentorial astrocytomas have usually been echogenic, or of mixed cystic and solid pattern, when scanned (Han et al., 1984). Differentiation between types of tumors is best left to the pathologist. However, neuroectodermal tumors tend to be midline and large and contain cystic spaces and calcifications. Because the baby comes to medical attention by virtue of an increasing head size or symptoms of increased intracranial pressure, it is not surprising that obstructive ventriculomegaly is present in virtually all cases (Fig. 1–54).

The tubers of tuberous sclerosis may be microscopic, but they occasionally reveal themselves as irregularities of the lateral ventricular wall or shadowing foci if they are calcified. Tubers may undergo malignant change (usually later in childhood and adolescence) or may be large enough to obstruct the flow of CSF. Adenoma sebaceum usually

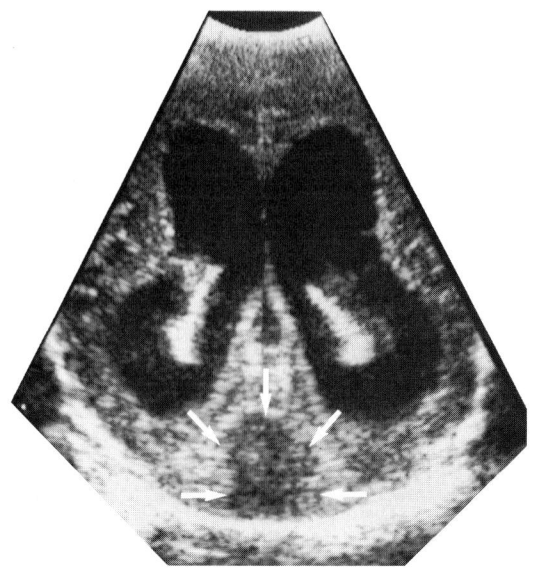

Figure 1–54. At 2 weeks of age, this full-term infant was noted to have increasing head circumference associated with full anterior fontanelle. Scans showed ventricular dilatation associated with a mass (arrows) in the posterior fossa. Of note was the simultaneous development of a left axillary mass. This was biopsied and proved to be neuroepithelioma of peripheral nerve. The tumor in the posterior fossa was treated with palliative therapy but did not respond; it actually increased in size over the next 3 to 4 weeks. The baby died at 7 weeks of age. The final diagnosis was of primitive neuroectodermal tumor.

develops after onset of seizures so that an affected baby may be seen in ultrasonography before the diagnosis is established (Fig. 1–55).

Lipoma of the corpus callosum is a very echogenic mass in the midline, often associated with callosal agenesis and other anomalies. Its appearance is characteristic, predominantly because of its location, but its lipomatous nature is easily confirmed by CT scanning (Fig. 1–39). Lipoma of the corpus callosum and intracranial dermoids are associated with the Goldenhar syndrome (oculoauriculovertebral dysplasia; Beltinger and Saule, 1988). The exact genesis of fatty tissue in the midline is a matter of speculation. Persistence of primitive meningeal tissue that matures into adipose tissue is cited as a possibility (Fisher and Cremin, 1988).

Other intracranial masses that present in infancy are usually cystic, and most are classified as arachnoidal cysts. Their etiology is poorly understood. A primary fault associated with the developing leptomeninges has been considered responsible for "congenital"

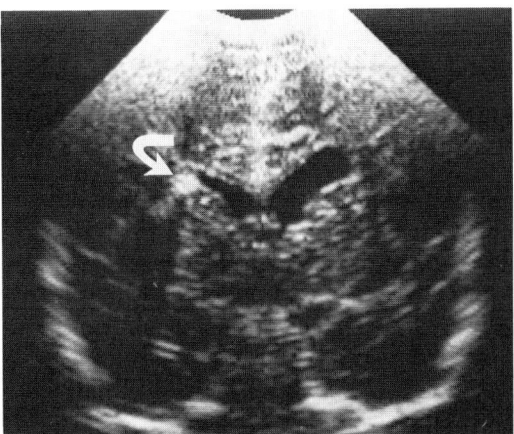

Figure 1–55. The original scans of this baby were renal ultrasonograms. He had presented with renomegaly. When macroscopic cysts were evident in both kidneys, scans of the brain through a still-patent fontanelle were performed. They showed small shadowing masses adjacent to the ventricles, typical of tuberous sclerosis. The coronal scan shows a single shadowing focus (arrow).

cysts. "Acquired" cysts have been blamed on previous hemorrhage, trauma, or infection. It is interesting that choroid-plexus–like material has been found in congenital arachnoidal cysts (Meizner et al., 1988). This would explain solid material, which might be seen along the wall of the cyst, as well as an increase in size of the cyst. In order of decreasing frequency, the temporal fossa, suprasellar region, posterior fossa, and quadrigeminal plate are the most common sites for arachnoidal cyst (Fig. 1–56; Armstrong et al., 1983). Those cysts that are centrally located may obstruct the adjacent ventricle or aqueduct (Fig. 1–57). Temporal cysts may be relatively silent; asymmetry of the middle fossa may be the only radiographic evidence of their existence. Differentiation of arachnoidal cysts in the posterior fossa from the Dandy-Walker malformation depends on identification of the cerebellar vermis, hemispheres, and fourth ventricle. Arachnoidal cysts do not communicate with the fourth ventricle (Fig. 1–58).

Arachnoidal cysts are a component of some of the malformation syndromes such as callosal agenesis and the Arnold-Chiari II malformation. Midline dorsal cysts associated with holoprosencephaly and callosal agenesis are likely different in etiology and are related to the dysgenetic ventricular system rather than to the leptomeninges (Fig. 1–59).

A colloid cyst of the third ventricle is attached to the choroid or the roof of the third ventricle. It is a condition found in adults, and to date we know of no babies with this lesion. The lining cells are ciliated, and the contents of the cyst are mucinous. The position of the cyst causes obstruction to CSF at the foramen of Monro. An ultrasonogram would be expected to show a spherical mass, which is mildly echogenic, because of the colloidal nature of its contents.

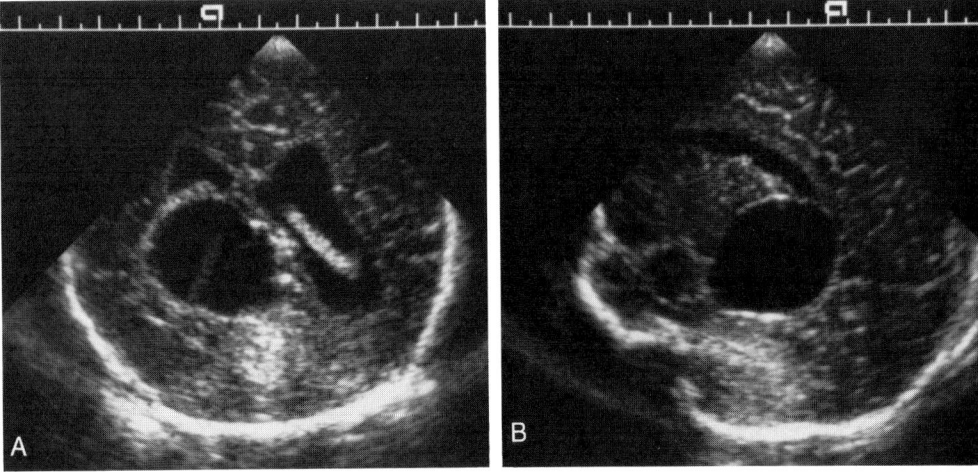

Figure 1–56. Prenatal diagnosis of an intracerebral cystic mass prompted this baby's referral to our hospital. A cystic mass to the right of the midline, possibly originating from the quadrigeminal plate cistern, is apparent on these coronal (A) and right parasagittal (B) scans. The mass, presumed to be an arachnoidal cyst, caused mild ventricular dilatation. However, because ventriculomegaly stayed stable over the next year, no shunting was performed and at 1½ years of age, the baby was developing normally.

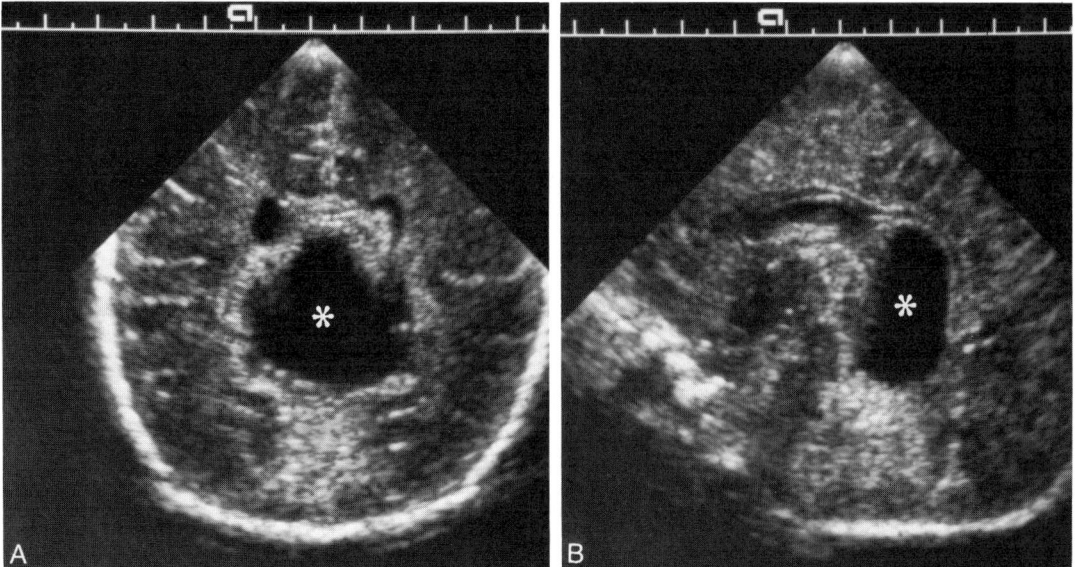

Figure 1–57. Prenatal ultrasonography had shown hydrocephalus in this baby. At birth, ventricular dilatation shown by CT scanning prompted ventriculoperitoneal shunting. Coronal (**A**) and sagittal (**B**) scans of the brain after shunting show decompression of the lateral ventricles. There is a midline arachnoid cyst (asterisk) whose separation from the cavum vergae is obvious because it deforms the splenium of the corpus callosum.

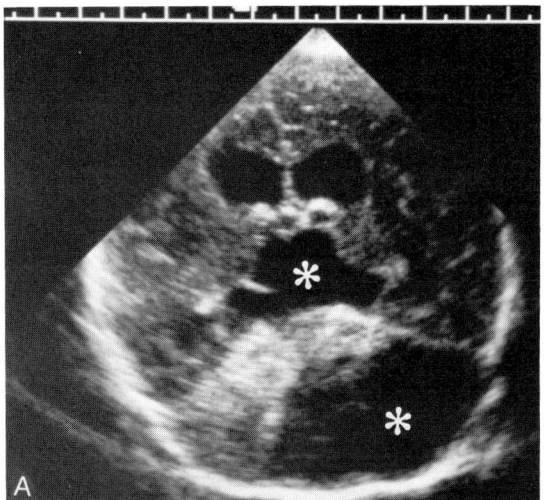

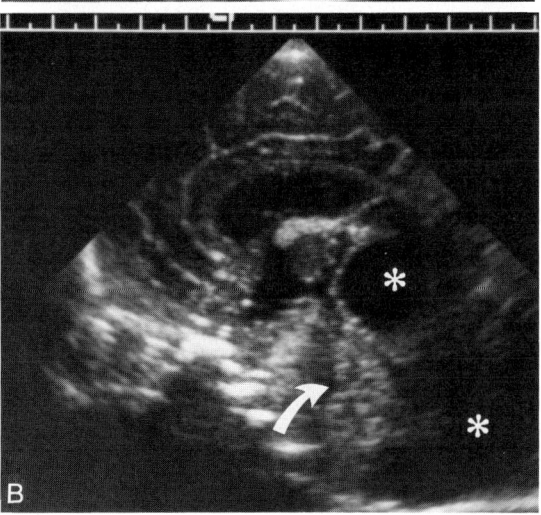

Figure 1–58. This baby had an extensive arachnoid cyst (asterisks) that involved the posterior fossa as well as extending above the tentorium. It is eccentric and associated with dilatation of the lateral ventricles and the third ventricle on coronal (**A**) and midline sagittal (**B**) scans. It deforms the cerebellum, but the vermis is intact. The fourth ventricle (arrow) is not communicating with the cyst. This is the differentiating feature between an arachnoidal cyst of the posterior fossa and Dandy-Walker malformation. Because of the ventriculomegaly that gradually increased, the baby had the cyst shunted to the peritoneal cavity.

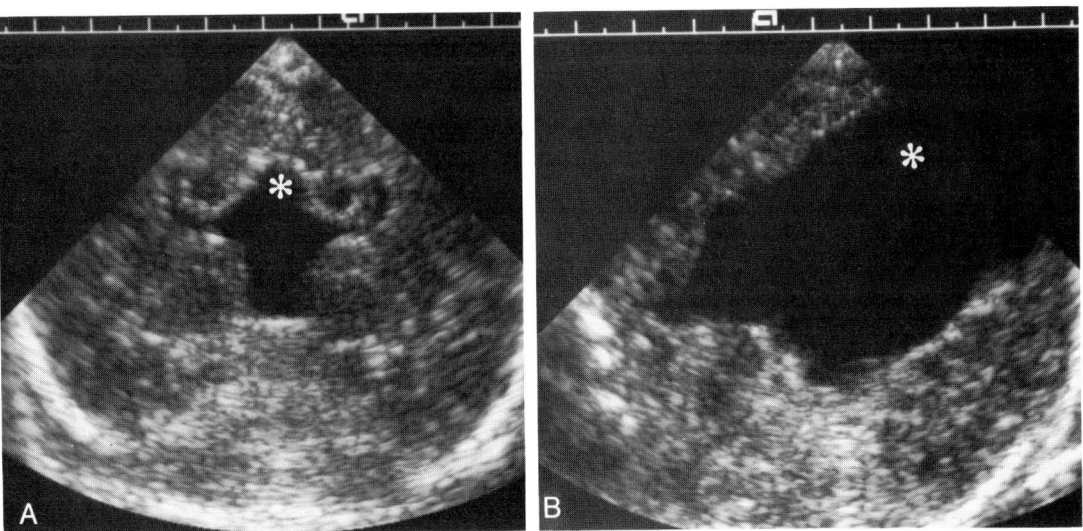

Figure 1–59. The midline dorsal cyst (asterisk) as shown on anterior coronal (A) and midline sagittal (B) scans is related to agenesis of the corpus callosum.

The Baby Who Has Craniomegaly

The pediatrician relies on signposts of normal development—feeding, smiling, rolling over, sitting, crawling, and so forth—along with measurements of head circumference to judge a baby's cerebral development. Because the neurologic examination of the young infant is only a gross measure of higher cortical function, clinical signs of insidious hydrocephalus are often subtle or absent. For the pediatrician who is faced with a baby whose measurements of head circumference are crossing growth curves on the standard charts, ultrasonography is an ideal method with which to evaluate intracranial anatomy. Most of the babies who have large heads are brought into the hospital by large-headed parents, and the macrocranium is genetically determined.

Most of the babies with macrocrania have a normally structured brain, mild ventricular prominence, and a capacious subarachnoid/subdural space (Fig. 1–60). This appearance has earned the unfortunate label "benign subdurals of infancy." The usual pediatric response to the word "subdural" is to consider it as secondary to infection or trauma. "Benign macrocrania" is a preferable term, as it avoids the connotation that these subdural collections are abnormal. No other imaging is needed for these babies unless they continue to cross growth curves on the charts of normal head circumference or have neurologic findings. Then, repeat ultrasonography should be performed, with CT or MRI to follow if ventricular size is increasing without obvious cause or if abnormalities of parenchyma are suspected. There are some babies whose subdural space continues to increase and who require shunting to decompress the ventricular system.

There are rare storage diseases of the brain that cause craniomegaly because of an increase in parenchymal volume. Obvious neurologic dysfunction commonly accompanies these conditions. The differential diagnosis of diffuse infiltrating process includes leukodystrophy, lipidosis, mucopolysaccharidosis, Canavan disease, and Alexander disease. For most infiltrative disorders, the biochemical assays of blood and clinical signs and symptoms are diagnostic. Biopsy of the brain is needed in some situations. Ultrasonic findings reported for Alexander disease have been mildly dilated lateral ventricles, diffusely echogenic brain, and poor delineation of sulci and anatomic detail (Harbord and LeQuesne, 1988).

In summary, any baby with macrocrania or evidence of increased intracranial pressure is scanned with the following checklist in mind. (1) Is the anatomy normal? (2) Is the parenchyma normal? (3) If ventriculomegaly is present, which ventricles are affected? (4) Is there a mass? (5) Is the subarachnoid space widened but clear, or is it abnormally echogenic, thereby suggesting hemorrhage or in-

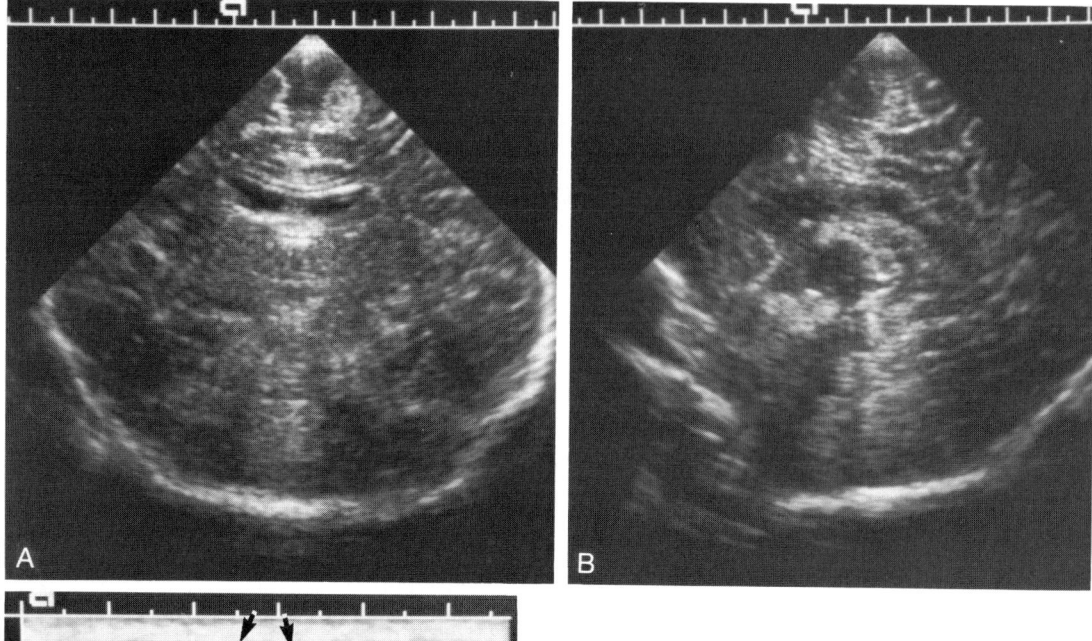
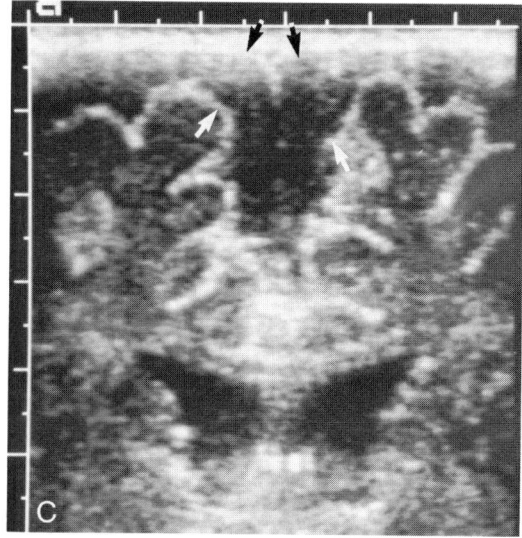

Figure 1–60. Ventriculomegaly as shown on the coronal scan (**A**) is mild. The midline sagittal scan (**B**) is normal with no evidence of mass. This baby presented at 4 months of age because his pediatrician was concerned that the baby's head was too large for his age. The coronal scan (**C**) performed with linear array transducer shows capacious subdural space. The average width (arrows) is approximately 8 mm. These scans are typical of benign macrocrania.

fection? (6) If the brain is dysgenetic, what other organs (e.g., kidneys) should be scanned?

The Baby Who Has Unexplained Cardiac Failure

In our nursery, the rare neonate who has had aneurysm of the vein of Galen, or a more global arteriovenous malformation, has presented with cardiac failure. It is usually after the echocardiogram is done and pronounced normal that attention (and the stethoscope) has shifted away from the chest to the liver and brain, the most common extracardiac sites of arteriovenous shunts. On the echocardiograms there has typically been a signpost to the brain in the form of a dilated superior vena cava. The affected babies whom we have examined have had large shunts, and their entire brains have been part of the arteriovenous malformation.

The texture of the brains in these babies has not been normal; they have had the diffuse increase in echogenicity and muddy appearance that are associated with diffuse ischemia. Undoubtedly, the vascular steal has rendered the cerebral hemispheres hypoxic (Fig. 1–61). With real-time or Doppler ultrasonography, swirling blood within the draining venous sinuses is obvious (Fig. 1–

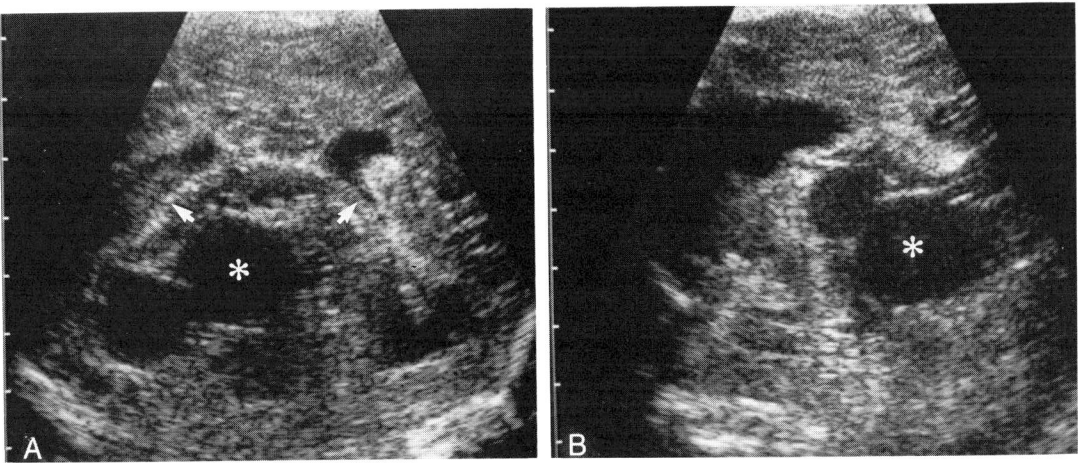

Figure 1-61. Coronal (A) and right parasagittal (B) scans show poor delineation of normal cerebral anatomy. The lateral ventricles (arrows) are splayed by a complex cystic mass (asterisk) that represents marked enlargement and tortuosity of the vein of Galen, which was being directly supplied by arterial branches.

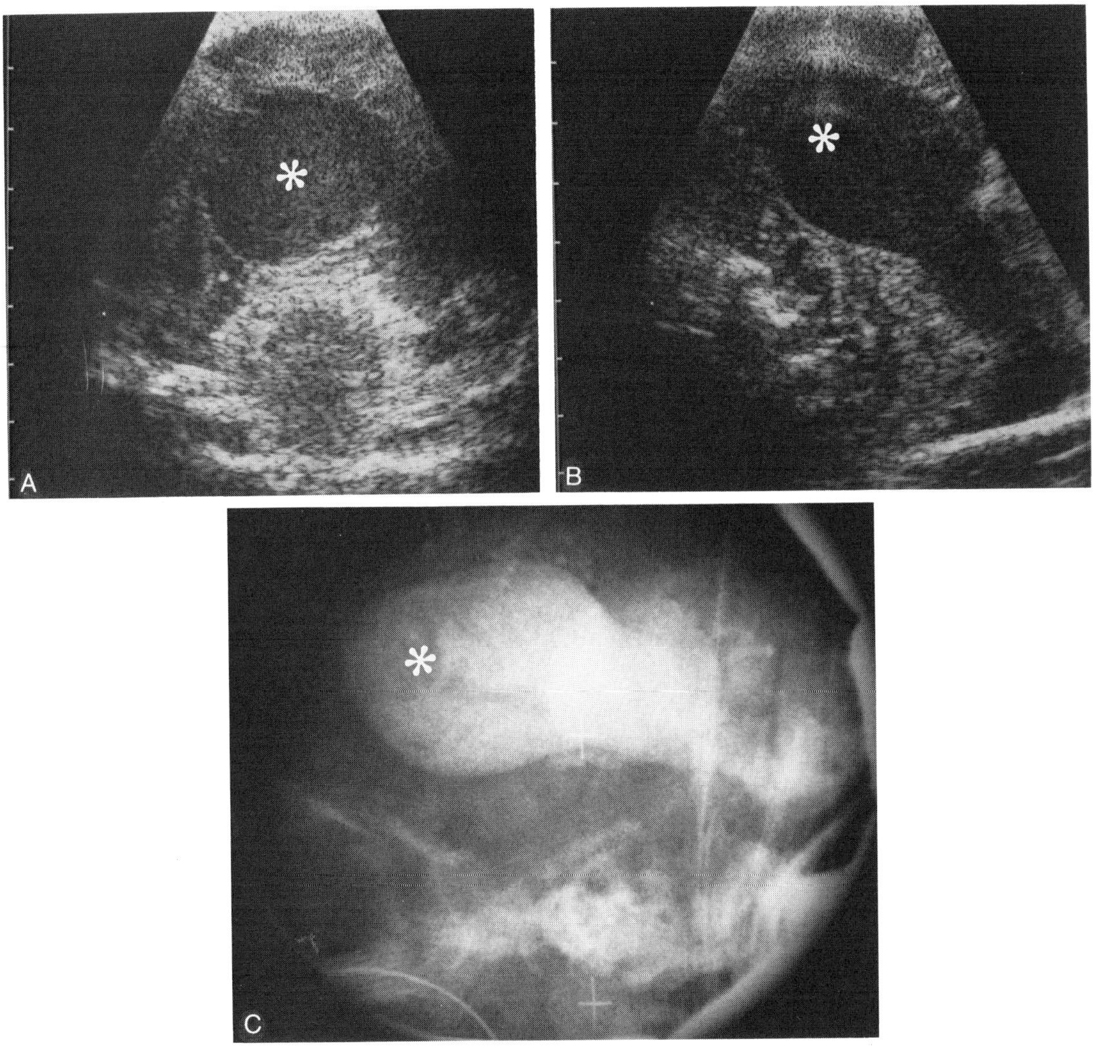

Figure 1-62. Swirling blood in an aneurysmal central draining vein was evident in real-time examination of this baby. The coronal scan (A) shows the central dilated vein (asterisk). The echogenicity resulted from the abnormal flow within it. The sagittal scan (B) was matched with the subsequent spot film obtained from cineangiographic study (C). This baby died of cardiac failure associated with the high output state.

62; Plate II). Variable degrees of ventricular dilatation occur when the aneurysmal veins compress the third ventricle or aqueduct. Treatment of huge shunts is palliative.

Any "cyst" in the locale of the vein of Galen, which is directly posterior to the third ventricle, should be scrutinized with Doppler ultrasonography, if available. CT with contrast can substitute for the Doppler method in making the diagnosis of vascular structure versus avascular cyst.

REFERENCES

General

Grant EG, Tessler F, Perrella R: Infant cranial sonography. Radiol Clin North Am 1988; 26:1089–1110.

Koeda T, Ando Y, Takashima S, et al: Changes in the lateral ventricle with the head position: Ultrasonographic observation. Neuroradiology 1988; 30:315–318.

Larroche JC: Development of the nervous system in early life. Part II. The development of the central nervous system during intrauterine life. In Falkner F (ed): Human Development. Philadelphia: WB Saunders, 1966; pp 257–276.

Levene MI: Cerebral ultrasound and neurological impairment: Telling the future. Arch Dis Child 1990; 65:469–471.

Murphy NP, Rennie J, Cooke RWI: Cranial ultrasound assessment of gestational age in low birthweight infants. Arch Dis Child 1989; 64:569–572.

The Premature Infant: Intraventricular Hemorrhage

Allan WC: Intraventricular hemorrhage. J Child Neurol 1989; 4:S12–S22.

Anderson GD, Bada HS, Sibai BM, et al: The relationship between labor and route of delivery in the preterm infant. Am J Obstet Gynecol 1988; 158:1382–1390.

Blumhagen JD, Mack LA: Abnormalities of the neonatal cerebral ventricles. Radiol Clin North Am 1985; 23:13–27.

Bozynski ME, Nelson MN, Genaze D, et al: Cranial ultrasonography and the prediction of cerebral palsy in infants weighing less than or equal to 1200 grams at birth. Dev Med Child Neurol 1988; 30:342–348.

Cohen HL, Haller JO, Pollack A: Ultrasound of the septum pellucidum. Recognition of evolving fenestrations in the hydrocephalic infant. J Ultrasound Med 1990; 9:377–383.

Coker, SB, Anderson CL: Occluded fourth ventricle after multiple shunt revisions for hydrocephalus. Pediatrics 1989; 83:981–985.

Darrow VC, Alvord EC Jr, Mack LA, et al: Histologic evolution of the reactions to hemorrhage in the premature human infant's brain. A combined ultrasound and autopsy study and a comparison with the reaction in adults. Am J Pathol 1988; 130:44–58.

Dincsoy MY, Kim YM, Siddiq F, et al: Intracranial hemorrhage in small-for-gestational-age neonates: Comparison with weight-matched appropriate-for-gestational-age infants. Clin Pediatr 1988; 27:21–26.

DiPietro MA, Brody BA, Teele RL: The calcar avis: Demonstration with cranial ultrasound. Radiology 1985; 156:363–364.

Dolfin T, Skidmore MB, Fong KW, et al: Incidence, severity and timing of subependymal and intraventricular hemorrhages in preterm infants born in a perinatal unit as detected by serial real-time ultrasound. Pediatrics 1983; 71:541–546.

Dubowitz LMS, Levene MI, Morante A, et al: Neurologic signs in neonatal intraventricular hemorrhage: A correlation with real-time ultrasound. J Pediatr 1981; 99:127–133.

Dykes FD, Dunbar B, Lazzara A, et al: Posthemorrhagic hydrocephalus in high-risk preterm infants: Natural history, management, and long-term outcome. J Pediatr 1989; 115:504–505.

Gaisie G, Roberts MS, Bouldin TW, et al: The echogenic ependymal wall in intraventricular hemorrhage: Sonographic-pathologic correlation. Pediatr Radiol 1990; 20:297–300.

Garfinkel E, Tejani N, Boxer HS, et al: Infancy and early childhood follow-up of neonates with periventricular or intraventricular hemorrhage or isolated ventricular dilation: A case controlled study. Am J Perinatol 1988; 5:214–219.

Hill A, Shackleford GD, Volpe JJ: A potential mechanism of pathogenesis for early post hemorrhage hydrocephalus in the premature newborn. Pediatrics 1984; 73:19–21.

Hokazono Y, Yokochi K, Ohtani Y, et al: A premature infant with a bilateral thalamostriatal hemorrhage: Brain imaging and pathology. Acta Paediatr Jpn Overseas Ed 1987; 29:867–871.

Kirks DR, Bowie JD: Cranial ultrasonography of neonatal periventricular/intraventricular hemorrhage: Who, how, why and when? Pediatr Radiol 1986; 16:114–119.

Kuban K, Teele RL: Rationale for grading intracranial hemorrhage in premature babies. Pediatrics 1984; 74:358–363.

Kuban KCK, Levinton A, Krishnamoorthy KS, et al: Neonatal intracranial hemorrhage and phenobarbital. Pediatrics 1986; 77:443–450.

Lazzara A, Ahmann P, Dykes F, et al: Clinical predictability of intraventricular hemorrhage in preterm infants. Pediatrics 1980; 65:30–34.

Leblanc R, O'Gorman AM: Neonatal intracranial hemorrhage: A clinical and serial computerized tomographic study. J Neurosurg 1980; 53:642–651.

Levene MI, de Vries L: Extension of neonatal intraventricular hemorrhage. Arch Dis Child 1984; 59:631–636.

Levene MI, Starte DR: A longitudinal study of post haemorrhagic ventricular dilatation in the newborn. Arch Dis Child 1981; 56:905–910.

Partridge JC, Babcock DS, Steichen JJ, et al: Optimal timing for diagnostic cranial ultrasound in low-birth-weight infants: Detection of intracranial hemorrhage and ventricular dilation. J Pediatr 1983; 102:281–287.

Pinto J, Paneth N, Kazam E, et al: Interobserver variability in neonatal cranial ultrasonography. Pediatr Perinat Epidemiol 1988; 2:43–58.

Rumack CM, Manco-Johnson ML, Manco-Johnson MJ, et al: Timing and course of neonatal intracranial hemorrhage using real-time ultrasound. Radiology 1985; 154:101–105.

Stewart A, Hope PL, Hamilton P, et al: Prediction in very preterm infants of satisfactory neurodevelopmental progress at 12 months. Dev Med Child Neurol 1988; 30:53–63.

Szymonowicz W, Schafler K, Cussen LJ, et al: Ultrasound and necropsy study of periventricular hemorrhage in preterm infants. Arch Dis Child 1984; 59:637–642.

Tzogalis D, Fawer CL, Wong Y, et al: Risk factors associated with the development of peri-intraventricular haemorrhage and periventricular leukomalacia. Helv Paediatr Acta 1989; 43:363–376.

van de Bor M, Verloove-Vanhorick SP, Brand R, et al: Incidence and prediction of periventricular-intraventricular hemorrhage in very preterm infants. J Perinat Med 1987; 15:333–339.

Volpe JJ: Neurology of the Newborn (2nd ed). Philadelphia: WB Saunders, 1987, pp. 311–361.

Volpe JJ: Intraventricular hemorrhage in the premature infant—Current concepts. Part II. Ann Neurol 1989a; 25:109–116.

Ischemic Parenchymal Injury in Premature Brain

Amato M, Gambon R, Von Muralt G, et al: Neurosonographic and biochemical correlates of periventricular leukomalacia in low-birth-weight infants. Pediatr Neurosci 1987; 13:84–89.

Banker BQ, Larroche JC: Periventricular leukomalacia of infancy. A form of neonatal anoxic encephalopathy. Arch Neurol 1962; 7:386–410.

Bernert G, Göttling A, Rosenkranz A, et al: Hemorrhagic and hypoxic-ischemic intracranial lesions in neonates diagnosed by realtime sonography: Incidence and short-term outcome. Padiatr Padol 1988; 23:25–37.

Brett EM: Paediatric Neurology. New York: Churchill Livingstone, 1983.

Carson SC, Hertzberg BS, Bowie JD, et al: Value of sonography in the diagnosis of intracranial hemorrhage and periventricular leukomalacia: A postmortem study of 35 cases. AJR 1990; 155:595–601.

de Reuck J: The human periventricular arterial blood supply and the anatomy of cerebral infarctions. Europ Neurol 1971; 5:321–334.

de Vries LS, Dubowitz LM, Pennock JM, et al: Extensive cystic leucomalacia: Correlation of cranial ultrasound magnetic resonance imaging and clinical findings in sequential studies. Clin Radiol 1989; 40:158–166.

de Vries LS, Regev R, Dubowitz LM, et al: Perinatal risk factors for the development of extensive cystic leukomalacia. Am J Dis Child 1988; 142:732–735.

de Vries LS, Regev R, Pennock JM, et al: Ultrasound evolution and later outcome of infants with periventricular densities. Early Hum Dev 1983; 16:225–233.

de Vries LS, Regev R, Connell JA, et al: Localized cerebral infarction in the premature infant: An ultrasound diagnosis correlated with computed tomography and magnetic resonance imaging. Pediatrics 1988; 81:36–40.

de Vries LS, Wigglesworth JS, Regev R, et al: Evolution of periventricular leukomalacia during the neonatal period and infancy: Correlation of imaging and postmortem findings. Early Hum Dev 1988; 17:205–219.

DiPietro MA, Brody BA, Teele RL: Peritrigonal echogenic "blush" on cranial sonography: Pathologic correlates. AJR 1986; 146:1067–1072.

Goldstein RB, Filly RA, Hecht S, et al: Noncystic "increased" periventricular echogenicity and other mild cranial sonographic abnormalities: Predictors of outcome in low birth weight infants. JCU 1989; 17:553–562.

Grant EG: Sonography of the premature brain: Intracranial hemorrhage and periventricular leukomalacia. Neuroradiology 1986; 28:476–490.

Hope PL, Gould SJ, Howard S, et al: Precision of ultrasound diagnosis of pathologically verified lesions in the brains of very preterm infants. Dev Med Child Neurol 1988; 30:457–471.

Keller MA, DiPietro MA, Teele RL, et al: Periventricular cavitations in the first week of life. AJNR 1987; 8:291–295.

Low JA, Froese AF, Galbraith RS, et al: The association of fetal and newborn metabolic acidosis with severe periventricular leukomalacia in the preterm newborn. Am J Obstet Gynecol 1990; 162:977–981.

Monset-Couchard M, de Bethmann O, Radvanyi-Bouvet MF, et al: Neurodevelopmental outcome in cystic periventricular leukomalacia (CPVL) (30 cases). Neuropediatrics 1988; 19:124–131.

Nwaesei CG, Allen AC, Vincer MJ, et al: Effect of timing of cerebral ultrasonography on the prediction of later neurodevelopmental outcome in high-risk preterm infants. J Pediatr 1988; 112:970–975.

Ogino T, Kanda Y, Kawakita A et al: Ultrasonographic findings in periventricular leukomalacia in the newborn: two cases associated with early onset group B Streptococcal sepsis. Acta Paediatr Jpn Overseas Ed 1988; 30:89–93.

Paneth N, Rudelli R, Monte W, et al: White matter necrosis in very low birth weight infants: Neuropathologic and ultrasonographic findings in infants surviving six days or longer. J Pediatr 1990; 116:975–984.

Perlman JM, Lynch B, Volpe JJ: Late hydrocephalus after arrest and resolution of neonatal post-hemorrhagic hydrocephalus. Dev Med Child Neurol 1990; 32:725–729.

Schellinger D, Grant EG, Manz HJ, et al: Intraparenchymal hemorrhage in preterm neonates: A broadening spectrum. AJR 1988; 150:1109–1115.

Szymonowicz W, Schafler K, Cussen LJ, et al: Ultrasound and necropsy study of periventricular haemorrhage in preterm infants. Arch Dis Child 1984; 59:637–642.

Tzogalis D, Fawer CL, Wong Y, et al: Risk factors associated with the development of peri-intraventricular haemorrhage and periventricular leukomalacia. Helv Paediatr Acta 1989; 43:363–376.

Volpe JJ: Edward B. Neuhauser lecture. Current concepts of brain injury in the premature infant. AJR 1989b; 153:243–251.

Zorzi C, Angonese I, Zaramella P, et al: Periventricular intraparenchymal cystic lesions: Critical determinant of neurodevelopmental outcome in preterm infants. Helv Paediatr Acta 1988; 43:195–202.

Asphyxia Neonatorum

Avery ME: Respiration around the time of birth. In Avery ME, First RL (eds): Pediatric Medicine. Baltimore: Williams and Wilkins, 1989, p. 154.

Babcock DS, Ball W Jr: Postasphyxial encephalopathy in full-term infants: Ultrasound diagnosis. Radiology 1983; 148:417–423.

Fischer AQ, Anderson JC, Shuman RM: The evolution of ischemic cerebral infarction in infancy: a sonographic evaluation. J Child Neurol 1988; 3:105–109.

Hayden CK Jr, Shattuck KE, Richardson CJ, et al: Subependymal germinal matrix hemorrhage in full-term neonates. Pediatrics 1985; 75:714–718.

Hernanz-Schulman H, Cohen W, Genieser NB: Sonography of cerebral infarction in infancy. AJR 1988; 150:897–902.

Hertzberg BS, Pasto ME, Needleman L, et al: Postasphyxial encephalopathy in term infants: Sonographic demonstration of increased echogenicity of the thalamus and basal ganglia. J Ultrasound Med 1987; 6:197–202.

Hope PL, Costello AM, Cady EB, et al: Cerebral energy metabolism studied with phosphorus NMR spectroscopy in normal and birth-asphyxiated infants. Lancet 1984; 2:366–370.

Kreusser KL, Schmidt RE, Shackelford GD, Volpe JJ:

Value of ultrasound for identification of acute hemorrhagic necrosis of thalamus and basal ganglia in an asphyxiated term infant. Ann Neurol 1984; 16:361–363.

Lacey DJ, Terplan K: Intraventricular hemorrhage in full-term neonates. Develop Med Child Neurol 1982; 24:332–337.

Levene MI, Kornberg J, Williams THC: The incidence and severity of post-asphyxial encephalopathy in full-term infants. Early Hum Dev 1985; 11:21–26.

Martin DJ, Hill A, Fitz CR, et al: Hypoxic/ischaemic cerebral injury in the neonatal brain. A report of sonographic features with computed tomographic correlation. Pediatr Radiol 1983; 13:307–312.

Voit T, Lemburg P, Neuen E, et al: Damage of thalamus and basal ganglia in asphyxiated full-term neonates. Neuropediatrics 1987; 18:176–181.

Posterior Fossa Hemorrhage

de Campo M: Neonatal posterior fossa haemorrhage: A difficult ultrasound diagnosis. Australas Radiol 1989; 33:150–153.

Grant EG, Schellinger D, Richardson JD: Real-time ultrasonography of the posterior fossa. J Ultrasound Med 1983; 2:73–87.

Perlman JM, Nelson JS, McAlister WH, Volpe JJ: Intracerebellar hemorrhage in a premature newborn: Diagnosis by real-time ultrasound and correlation with autopsy findings. Pediatrics 1983; 71:159–162.

Reeder JD, Setzer ES, Kaude JV: Ultrasonographic detection of perinatal intracerebellar hemorrhage. Pediatrics 1982; 70:385–386.

Tanaka Y, Sakamoto K, Kobayashi S, et al: Biphasic ventricular dilatation following posterior fossa hematoma in the full-term neonate. J Neurosurg 1988; 68:211–216.

von Gontard A, Arnold D, Adis B: Posterior fossa hemorrhage in the newborn—diagnosis and management. Pediatr Radiol 1988; 18:347–348.

Extracorporeal Membrane Oxygenation (ECMO)

Babcock DS, Han BK, Weiss RG, et al: Brain abnormalities in infants on extracorporeal membrane oxygenation: Sonographic and CT findings. AJR 1989; 153:571–576.

Crombleholme TM, Adzick NS, deLorimier AA, et al: Carotid artery reconstruction following extracorporeal membrane oxygenation. Am J Dis Child 1990; 144:872–874.

Luisiri A, Graviss ER, Weber T, et al: Neurosonographic changes in newborns treated with extracorporeal membrane oxygenation. J Ultrasound Med 1988; 7:429–438.

Mitchell DG, Merton DA, Graziani LF, Desai HJ, et al: Right carotid artery ligation in neonates: Classification of collateral flow with color Doppler imaging. Radiology 1990; 175:117–123.

Slovis TL, Sell LL, Bedard MP, et al: Ultrasonographic findings (CNS, thorax, abdomen) in infants undergoing extracorporeal oxygenation therapy. Pediatr Radiol 1988; 18:112–117.

Taylor GA, Fitz CR, Miller MK, et al: Intracranial abnormalities in infants treated with extracorporeal membrane oxygenation: Imaging with US and CT. Radiology 1987a; 165:675–678.

Taylor GA, Glass P, Fitz CR, et al: Neurologic status in infants treated with extracorporeal membrane oxygenation: Correlation of imaging findings with developmental outcome. Radiology 1987b; 165:679–682.

Taylor GA, Fitz CR, Glass P, et al: CT of cerebrovascular injury after neonatal extracorporeal membrane oxygenation: Implications for neurodevelopmental outcome. AJR 1989a; 153:121–126.

Taylor GA, Fitz CR, Kapur S, et al: Cerebrovascular accidents in neonates treated with extracorporeal membrane oxygenation: Sonographic-pathologic correlation. AJR 1989b; 153:355–361.

Taylor GA, Short BL, Glass P, et al: Cerebral hemodynamics in infants undergoing extracorporeal membrane oxygenation: Further observations. Radiology 1988; 168:163–167.

Doppler Ultrasonography

Anderson JC, Mark JR: Intracranial arterial duplex Doppler waveform analysis in infants. Childs Nerv Syst 1988; 4:144–148.

Bode H, Eden A: Transcranial Doppler sonography in children. J Child Neurol 1989; 4(Suppl):68–76.

Bode H, Sauer M, Pringsheim W: Diagnosis of brain death by transcranial Doppler sonography. Arch Dis Child 1988; 63:1474–1478.

Chadduck WM, Seibert JJ, Adametz J, et al: Cranial Doppler ultrasonography correlates with criteria for ventriculoperitoneal shunting. Surg Neurol 1989; 31:122–128.

Chadduck WM, Seibert JJ: Intracranial duplex Doppler: Practical uses in pediatric neurology and neurosurgery. J Child Neurol 1989; 4(Suppl):77–86.

Couture A, Veyrac C, Baud C, et al: New imaging of cerebral ischaemic lesions. High frequency probes and pulsed Doppler. Ann Radiol 1987; 30:452–461.

Deeg KH: Colour flow imaging of the great intracranial arteries in infants. Neuroradiology 1989; 31:40–43.

Deeg KH, Rupprecht T: Pulsed Doppler sonographic measurement of normal values for the flow velocities in the intracranial arteries of healthy newborns. Pediatr Radiol 1989; 19:71–78.

Deeg KH, Rupprecht T, Zeilinger G: Dopplersonographic classification of brain edema in infants. Pediatr Radiol 1990; 20:509–514.

Evans DH, Levene MI, Shortland DB, et al: Resistance index, blood flow velocity, and resistance-area product in the cerebral arteries of very low birth weight infants during the first week of life. Ultrasound Med Biol 1988; 14:103–110.

Fischer AQ, Livingstone JN 2d: Transcranial Doppler and real-time cranial sonography in neonatal hydrocephalus. J Child Neurol 1989; 4:64–69.

Glasier CM, Seibert JJ, Chadduck WM, et al: Brain death in infants: Evaluation with Doppler US. Radiology 1989; 172:377–380.

Grolimund P, Seiler RW: Age dependence of the flow velocity in the basal cerebral arteries—a transcranial Doppler ultrasound study. Ultrasound Med Biol, 1988; 14:191–198.

Hassler W, Steinmetz H, Gawlowski J: Transcranial Doppler ultrasonography in raised intracranial pressure and in intracranial circulatory arrest. J Neurosurg 1988; 68:745–751.

Horgan JG, Rumack CM, Hay T, et al: Absolute intracranial blood-flow velocities evaluated by duplex Doppler sonography in asymptomatic preterm and term neonates. AJR 1989; 152:1059–1064.

Lipman B, Serwer GH, Brazy JE: Abnormal cerebral

hemodynamics in preterm infants with patent ductus arteriosus. Pediatrics 1982; 69:778–781.
Mitchell DG, Merton D, Needleman L, et al: Neonatal brain: Color Doppler imaging. Part I. Technique and vascular anatomy. Radiology 1988; 167:303–306.
Mitchell DG, Merton D, Desai H, et al: Neonatal brain: Color Doppler imaging. Part II. Altered flow patterns from extracorporeal membrane oxygenation. Radiology 1988; 167:307–310.
Pfannschmidt J, Jorch G: Transfontanelle pulsed Doppler measurement of blood flow velocity in the internal jugular vein, straight sinus, and internal cerebral vein in preterm and term neonates. Ultrasound Med Biol 1989; 15:9–12.
Rennie JM, South M, Morley CJ: Cerebral blood flow velocity variability in infants receiving assisted ventilation. Arch Dis Child 1987; 62:1247–1251.
Seibert JJ, McCowan TC, Chadduck WM et al: Duplex pulsed Doppler US versus intracranial pressure in the neonate: Clinical and experimental studies. Radiology 1989; 171:155–159.
Taylor KJW: A prudent approach to Doppler US. Radiology 1987; 165:283–284.
van Bel F, den Ouden L, van de Bor M, et al: Cerebral blood-flow velocity during the first week of life of preterm infants and neurodevelopment at two years. Dev Med Child Neurol 1989; 31:320–328.
van Bel F, van de Bor M, Baan J, et al: Blood flow velocity pattern of the anterior cerebral arteries. Before and after drainage of posthemorrhagic hydrocephalus in the newborn. J Ultrasound Med 1988; 7:553–559.
van Bel F, van de Bor M, Stijnen T, et al: Cerebral blood flow velocity pattern in healthy and asphyxiated newborns: A controlled study. Eur J Pediatr 1987; 146:461–467.
Winkler P, Helmke K: Duplex-scanning of the deep venous drainage in the evaluation of blood flow velocity of the cerebral vascular system in infants. Pediatr Radiol 1989; 19:79–90.
Winkler P, Helmke K, Mahl M: Major pitfalls in Doppler investigations: Part II. Low flow velocities and colour Doppler applications. Pediatr Radiol 1990; 20:304–310.
Wong WS, Tsuruda JS, Liberman RL, et al: Color Doppler imaging of intracranial vessels in the neonate. AJR 1989; 152:1065–1070

Meningitis and Congenital Infection

Babcock DS, Han BK: Sonographic recognition of gyral infarction in meningitis. AJR 1985; 144:883–886.
Beltinger C, Saule H: Sonography of subependymal cysts in congenital rubella syndrome. Eur J Pediatr 1988; 148:206–207.
Bozynski ME, Naglie RA, Russell EJ: Real-time ultrasonographic surveillance in the detection of CNS involvement in systemic candida infection. Pediatr Radiol 1986; 16:235–237.
Butt W, Mackay RJ, de Crespigny LC, et al: Intracranial lesions of congenital cytomegalovirus infection detected by ultrasound scanning. Pediatrics 1985; 73:611–614.
Carey BM, Arthur RJ, Houlsby WT: Ventriculitis in congenital rubella: Ultrasound demonstration. Pediatr Radiol 1987; 17:415–416.
Cremin BJ, Lipinski KJ, Sharp JA, et al: Ultrasonic detection of subdural collections. Pediatr Radiol 1984; 14:191–194.

Epstein LG, Sharer LR, Goudsmit J: Neurological and neuropathological features of human immunodeficiency virus infection in children. Ann Neurol 1988; 23(Suppl):19–23.
Frank JL: Sonography of intracranial infection in infants and children. Neuroradiology 1986; 28:440–451.
Frank LM, White LE: Neurosonographic features of central nervous system infections in infancy and childhood. J Child Neurol 1989; 4(Suppl):41–51.
Genieser NB, Hernanz-Schulman M, Krasinski K, et al: Pediatric AIDS. In Federle MP, et al (eds): Radiology of AIDS. New York: Raven Press, 1988, 131–142.
Grant EG: Neurosonography of the Pre-Term Neonate. New York: Springer Verlag, 1986.
Grant EG, Williams AL, Schellinger D, Slovis TL: Intracranial calcification in the infant and neonate: evaluations by sonography and CT. Radiology 1985; 157:63–68.
Han BK, Babcock DS, McAdams L: Bacterial meningitis in infants: Sonographic findings. Radiology 1985; 154:645–650.
Hill A, Shackelford GD, Volpe JJ: Ventriculitis with neonatal bacterial meningitis: Identification by real-time ultrasound. J Pediatr 1981; 99:133–136.
Kirpekar M, Abriri MM, Hilfer C, et al: Ultrasound in the diagnosis of systemic candidiasis (renal and cranial) in very low birth weight premature infants. Pediatr Radiol 1986; 16:17–20.
Rosenberg HK, Levine RS, Stoltz K, et al: Bacterial meningitis in infants: Sonographic features. AJNR 1983; 4:822–825.
Stannard MW, Jimenez JF: Sonographic recognition of multiple cystic encephalomalacia. AJNR 1983; 4: 1111–1114; AJR 1983; 141:1321–1324.
Teele RL, Hernanz-Schulman M, Sotrel A: Echogenic vasculature in the basal ganglia of neonates: A sonographic sign of vasculopathy. Radiology 1988; 169:423–427.
Theophilo F, Burnett A, Jucá Filho G, et al: Ultrasound-guided brain abscess aspiration in neonates. Childs Nerv Syst 1987; 3:371–374.
Volpe JJ: Neurology of the Newborn (2nd Ed). Philadelphia: WB Saunders, 1987, 547–635.
Wilson DA, Nguyen DL, Marshall K: Sonography of brain abscesses complicating Citrobacter neonatal meningitis. Am J Perinatol 1988; 5:37–39.

Dysmorphic Brain

Babcock DS: Sonographic demonstration of lissencephaly (agyria). J Ultrasound Med 1983; 2:465–466.
Babcock DS: Sonography of congenital malformations of the brain. Neuroradiology 1986; 28:428–439.
Barkovich AJ, Norman D: MR imaging of schizencephaly. AJR 1988; 150:1391–1396.
Bell WO, Sumner TE, Volberg FM: The significance of ventriculomegaly in the newborn with myelodysplasia. Childs Nerv Syst 1987; 3:239–241.
Beltinger C, Saule H: Imaging of lipoma of the corpus callosum and intracranial dermoids in the Goldenhar syndrome. Pediatr Radiol 1988; 18:72–73.
Benacerraf BR: Fetal central nervous system anomalies. Ultrasound Quarterly 1990; 8:1–42.
Bosnjak V, Besenski N, Della-Marina BM, et al: Ultrasonography in hereditary degenerative diseases of the cerebral white matter in infancy. Neuropediatrics 1988; 19:208–211.
Charney EB, Weller SC, Sutton LN, et al: Management

of the newborn with myelomeningocele: Time for a decision-making process. Pediatrics 1985; 75:58–64.

Chitkara U, Cogswell C, Norton K, et al: Choroid plexus cysts in the fetus: A benign anatomic variant or pathologic entity? Report of 41 cases and review of the literature. Obstet Gynecol 1988; 72:185–189.

Edwards BO Jr, Fischer AQ, Flannery DB: Joubert syndrome: Early diagnosis by recognition of the behavioral phenotype and confirmation by cranial sonography. J Child Neurol 1988; 3:247–249.

Fakhry J, Schechter A, Tenner MS, et al: Cysts of the choroid plexus in neonates: Documentation and review of the literature. J Ultrasound Med 1985; 4:561–563.

Fisher RM, Cremin BJ: Lipoma of the corpus callosum: Diagnosis by ultrasound and magnetic resonance. Pediatr Radiol 1988; 18:409–410.

Harbord MG, LeQuesne GW: Alexander's disease: Cranial ultrasound findings. Pediatr Radiol 1988; 18:341–343.

Hernanz-Schulman M, Dohan FC Jr, Jones T et al: Sonographic appearance of callosal agenesis: Correlation with radiologic and pathologic findings. AJNR 1985; 6:361–368.

Inagaki M, Ando Y, Mito T, et al: Comparison of brain imaging and neuropathology in cases of trisomy 18 and 13. Neuroradiology 1987; 29:474–479.

Kuban KCK, Teele RL, Wallman J: Septo-optic-dysplasia-schizencephaly. Radiographic and clinical features. Pediatr Radiol 1989; 19:145–150.

McGahan JP, Ellis W, Lindfors KK, et al: Congenital cerebrospinal fluid-containing intracranial abnormalities: A sonographic classification. J Clin Ultrasound 1988; 16:531–544.

McGahan JP, Nyberg DA, Mack LA: Sonography of facial features of alobar and semilobar holoprosencephaly. AJR 1990; 154:143–148.

McLone DG, Czyzewski D, Raimondi AJ, et al: Central nervous system infections as a limiting factor in the intelligence of children with myelomeningocele. Pediatrics 1982; 70:338–342.

Motte J, Gomes H, Morville P, et al: Sonographic diagnosis of lissencephaly. Pediatr Radiol 1987; 17:362–364.

Noetzel MJ: Myelomeningocele: Current concepts of management. Semin Perinatol 1989; 16:311–329.

Poe LB, Coleman LL, Mahmud F: Congenital central nervous system anomalies. Radiographics 1989; 9:801–826.

Roland EH, Flodmark O, Hill A: Neurosonographic features of Aicardi's syndrome. J Child Neurol 1989; 4:307–310.

Shackelford GD: Neurosonography of hydrocephalus in infants. Neuroradiology 1986; 28:452–462.

Stein SC, Schut L: Hydrocephalus in myelomeningocele. Child's Brain 1979; 5:413–419.

Weese-Mayer DE, Smith KM, Reddy JK, et al: Computerized tomography and ultrasound in the diagnosis of cerebro-hepato-renal syndrome of Zellweger. Pediatr Radiol 1987; 17:170–172.

Worthen NJ, Gilbertson V, Lau C: Cortical sulcal development seen on sonography: Relationship to gestational parameters. J Ultrasound Med 1986; 5:153–156.

Craniomegaly, Intracranial Masses

Armstrong EA, Harwood-Nash DC, Hoffman H, et al: Benign suprasellar cysts: The CT approach. AJNR 1983; 4:163–166.

Babcock DS, Han BK, Dine MS: Sonographic findings in infants with macrocrania. AJR 1988; 150:1359–1365.

Buetow PC, Smirniotopoulos JG, Done S: Congenital brain tumors: A review of 45 cases. AJR 1990; 155:587–593.

Chitkara U, Cogswell C, Norton K, et al: Choroid plexus cysts in the fetus: A benign anatomic variant or pathologic entity? Report of 41 cases and review of the literature. Obstet Gynecol 1988; 72:185–189.

Chuang S, Harwood-Nash D: Tumors and cysts. Neuroradiology 1986; 28:463–475.

Fakhry J, Schechter A, Tenner MS, et al: Cysts of the choroid plexus in neonates: Documentation and review of the literature. J Ultrasound Med 1985; 4:561–563.

Han BK, Babcock DS, Oestreich AE: Sonography of brain tumors in infants. AJR 1984; 143:31–36.

Hurst RW, McIlhenny J, Park TS, et al: Neonatal craniopharyngioma: CT and ultrasonographic features. J Comput Assist Tomogr 1988; 12:858–861.

Krul JM, Gooskens RH, Ramos L, et al: Ultrasound detection of a choroid plexus papilloma of the third ventricle. J Neuroradiol 1987; 14:179–182.

Meizner I, Barki Y, Tadmor R, et al: In utero ultrasonic detection of fetal arachnoid cyst. J Clin Ultrasound 1988; 16:506–509.

Odell JM, Allen JK, Badura RJ, et al: Massive congenital intracranial teratoma: A report of two cases. Pediatr Pathol 1987; 7:333–340.

Schellhas KP, Siebert RC, Heithoff KB, et al: Congenital choroid plexus papilloma of the third ventricle: Diagnosis with real-time sonography and MR imaging. AJNR 1988; 9:797–798.

Strassburg HM, Sauer M, Weber S, et al: Ultrasonographic diagnosis of brain tumors in infancy. Pediatr Radiol 1984; 14:284–287.

Takaku A, Kodama N, Ohara N, et al: Brain tumour in newborn babies. Child's Brain 1978; 4:365–375.

Intracranial Vascular Malformation

Abbitt PL, Hurst RW, Ferguson RD, et al: The role of ultrasound in the management of vein of Galen aneurysms in infancy. Neuroradiology 1990; 32:86–89.

McCord FB, Shields MD, McNeil A, et al: Cerebral arteriovenous malformation in a neonate: Treatment by embolisation. Arch Dis Child 1987; 62:1273–1275.

O'Donnabhain D, Duff DF: Aneurysms of the vein of Galen. Arch Dis Child 1989; 64:1612–1617.

Miscellaneous

Jordan GD, Jarrett RV, Garcia J: Central nervous system air embolism in respiratory distress syndrome: Considerations for patient survival. Am J Perinatol 1989; 6:80–83.

Williams CE, Gordon A, Arthur RJ: "Pseudocatheter" due to inadvertent ventricular catheter placement. Pediatr Radiol 1988; 18:353–354.

CHAPTER 2

SPINAL ULTRASONOGRAPHY AND INTRAOPERATIVE NEUROSONOGRAPHY

The temptation, when one begins to perform spinal ultrasonography, is to look for the instantly recognizable conus medullaris. It is more useful to begin by evaluating the vertebral bodies, making sure that they are all present, that there is no segmental anomaly, and that L2 is located. Any previous radiographs should be reviewed; an anomaly of vertebral segmentation or sacral dysgenesis is occasionally found only in retrospect. Because anomalies, when present, may affect several levels, the ultrasonographic examination should include the entire spinal canal. The spinal cord is scanned in its entirety, its pulsation (or lack thereof) noted, and the location of the conus medullaris established. The thecal sac, epidermal soft tissues, and masses, if present, are then mapped out.

NORMAL SPINE AND CONTENTS

Sagittal scans of the upper spinal canal are improved by the use of standoff material between the flexed neck and the linear array transducer. The foramen magnum casts a shadow across the most superior portion of the spinal canal and cord, but just below the foramen magnum, one can identify the echogenic focus of the arch of C1 and the poorly echogenic peg of the odontoid as it sits on the C2 vertebral body (Fig. 2–1). The spinal cord is a hypoechoic band, thickest in the cervical region, thinnest in the thorax, and delineated by anterior and posterior hyperechoic borders. A variably intense echo, which is anterior in the upper region of the spinal cord and becomes more central in the lower cord, had been attributed to the central canal until Nelson and colleagues published their paper in 1989. They showed, quite convincingly, that the central echogenicity arises from the interface between the myelinated ventral white commissure and the central portion of the anterior median fissure. The central canal in normal babies is, in fact, overgrown with glial fibrils and is variably present at different levels.

The anterior and posterior borders of the cord are prominent because their interface is with subarachnoid fluid. The thecal sac is defined both anteriorly and posteriorly by another strikingly echogenic line, which probably represents the arachnoid-dural layer. As the spinal canal curves posteriorly

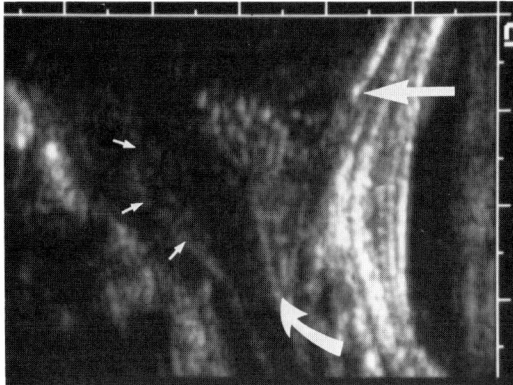

Figure 2–1. Sagittal views of the cervicomedullary junction are best achieved when the baby's neck is flexed and a tissue-equivalent standoff pad is used. This baby has Arnold-Chiari II malformation. The straight large arrow points to the edge of the occipital bone. The pons is outlined with small arrows. The curved large arrow marks the inferior extent of cerebellar tissue.

at the lumbosacral junction, this perpendicular interface is lost, and the termination of the thecal sac at S2 is often poorly defined (Fig. 2–2; Gusnard et al., 1986).

Because the level of termination of the conus medullaris is so crucial to the discussion of a tethered spinal cord, vertebral bodies must be counted. It is easiest to identify sacral vertebrae first and then to count from the bottom up. Additional help from other landmarks is available: the top of the iliac crests is usually at L4, and the tip of the last rib is normally at L2. The conus medullaris should not extend below the disc between L2 and L3 at any age (Wilson and Prince, 1988). The spinal cord should be in the center of the canal in the lumbar region; tethering tends to pull it dorsally. The roots of the cauda equina fill in the lower thecal sac with linear echoes and help define the tapered

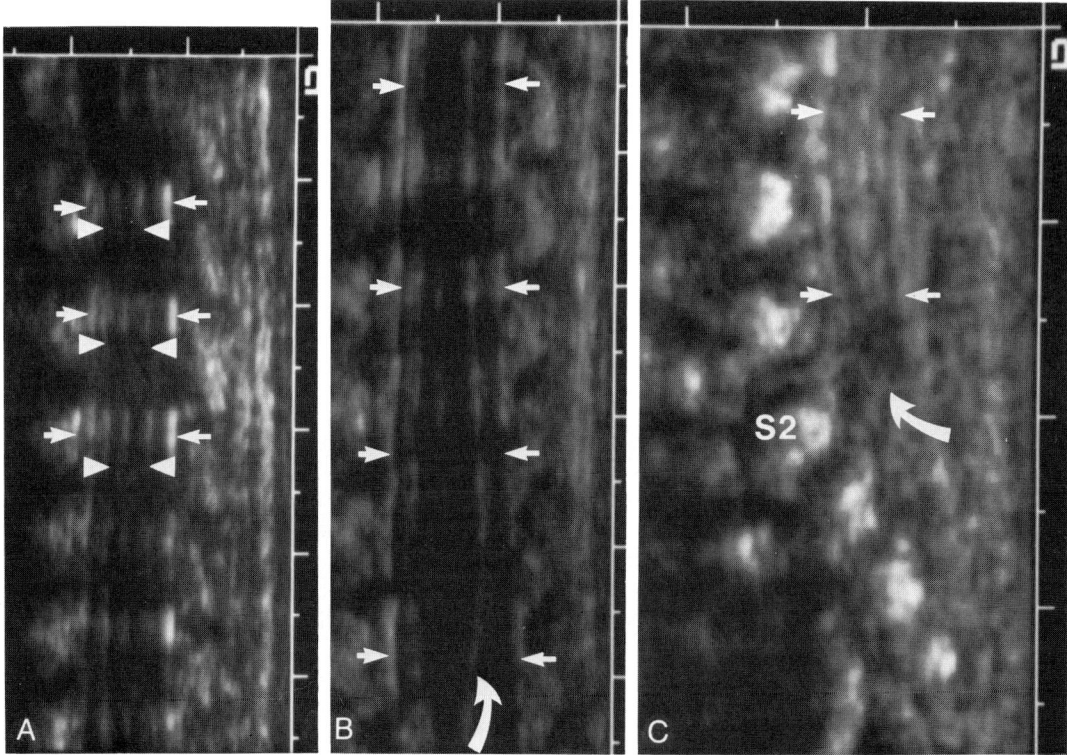

Figure 2–2. This longitudinal scan of the thoracic canal (A) shows the borders of the thecal sac (arrows) and the borders of the spinal cord (arrowheads). Note the central echogenicity from the interface between the myelinated ventral white commissure and the central anterior median fissure. The sagittal scan of the lumbar region (B) again shows the thecal sac (straight arrows) and the anterior and posterior borders of the relatively echolucent spinal cord. The central echogenicity is seen in part as a dotted line. The conus medullaris (curved arrow) is the bulbous swelling of the distal part of the spinal cord. Its termination should never extend below the disc between L2 and L3. The termination of the thecal sac (curved arrow) at the level of S2 is often difficult to delineate (C). The cauda equina fill the thecal sac in its sacral portion. S2 = second sacral vertebra. Straight arrows mark the lateral margin of the thecal sac.

conus medullaris (Fig. 2–3). The normal filum terminale is typically indistinguishable from the adjacent cauda equina. The anterior spinal artery is a single pulsatile focus in the anterior median fissure. Posterior spinal arteries are smaller dorsal reflectors on the posterolateral surface of the cord. The rhythmic pulsation of the cord can be captured with M-mode ultrasonography.

The best scans of the neural canal are achieved in the newborn. The age of the baby dictates what proportion of the vertebral skeleton is ossified (Gusnard et al., 1986). In general, we rarely obtain satisfactory scans after the baby reaches 12 weeks of age. Before that time, the posterior elements are predominantly cartilaginous, and one can position the transducer just off center of the posterior spinous processes to obtain excellent sagittal views of the spinal canal and its contents. In an award-winning paper on spinal sonography, Naidich and colleagues (1984) made the excellent suggestion that patients be examined with the upper body elevated in order that the normal subarachnoid sac, a hydromyelic cavity, or a meningocele be distended with cerebrospinal fluid (CSF). Flexion of the patient's lower body allows a wider acoustic window between posterior spinous processes.

Axial scans are used in a supporting role to normal or abnormal sagittal scans. Small degrees of angulation produce different views of a vertebral body with its own or adjacent lamina, transverse processes, and posterior spinal process. Transverse scans are useful for the comparison of muscles and other soft tissues and to show the central location of the cord within the spinal canal (Fig. 2–4).

Does ultrasonography preclude the need for other studies? A normal ultrasonographic examination of a newborn who has a deep sacral dimple is reassuring to clinicians. Magnetic resonance imaging (MRI) and computed tomography (CT) scanning are not universally available, and ultrasonography is a cheap and efficient method of screening. Identification of an anomaly expedites and guides further evaluation. Furthermore, ultrasonographic examination of the spine and paraspinal soft tissues can be extended to include the brain and kidneys. Arnold-Chiari malformation virtually always accompanies meningomyelocele. Neurologic control of the bladder is abnormal in many patients who have spinal dysraphism, and hydronephrosis

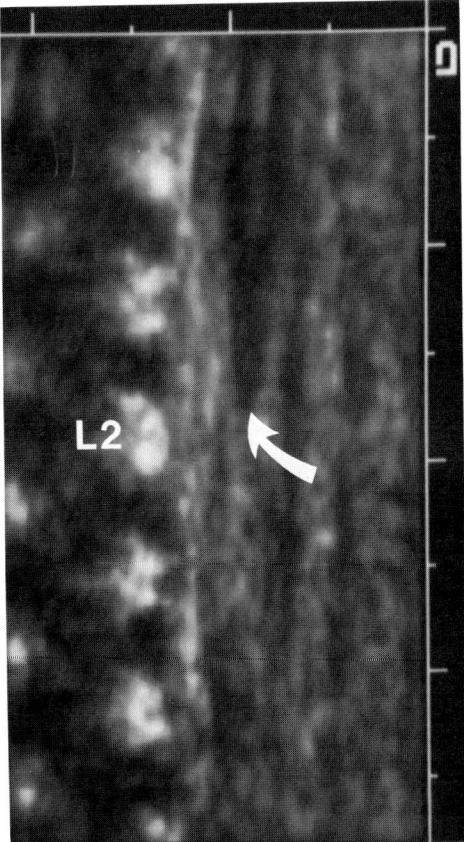

Figure 2–3. The tapered conus medullaris (curved arrow) is well defined by the echogenicity that represents the cauda equina within the thecal sac. L2 = second lumbar vertebra.

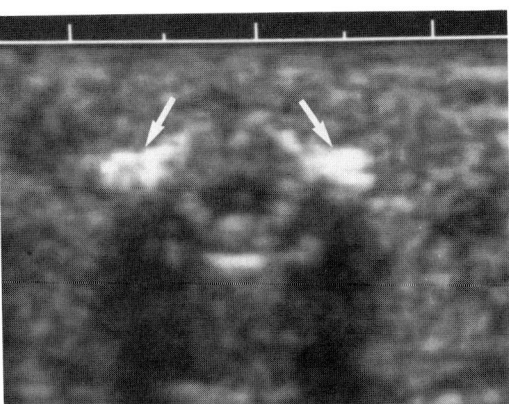

Figure 2–4. This transverse scan of the vertebral canal at the level of L1 shows the distal portion of the cord as a lucency within the thecal sac. The central echogenicity is the small dot. The transverse processes (arrows) extend laterally from the midline. Note that the cord is centrally positioned within the canal.

may result from retention of urine or vesicoureteral reflux, or both. For the older child, MRI or CT scanning of the spine is far superior to ultrasonography because the posterior elements are ossified. Some neural anomalies can be imaged in part when they are associated with failure of fusion of posterior vertebral elements. There are situations in which ultrasonography can provide information quickly—showing the cystic versus lipomatous nature of a subcutaneous mass, for instance—but for most patients older than 3 months, ultrasonography alone cannot provide enough diagnostic information.

MYELODYSPLASIA: EMBRYOLOGY AND CLASSIFICATION

Embryologists have generated theories to explain anomalies of the spinal cord and its enveloping membranes, malformations that are included in the general term "myelodysplasia."

Insults to the embryo as it grows from 2 to 9 mm in length affect neuralation, the process by which ridges from the neural plate fuse into a tube. At this stage, the neural tissue is in contact with amniotic fluid and is not yet covered by ectoderm. By the time the embryo is 22 mm long, ectoderm has covered the neural tube. Malformations that occur during this period, the time in which the neural tube undergoes elongation and canalization, are covered by intact skin. During the next stage, as the embryo grows to 200 mm from crown to rump, retrogressive differentiation of tissue results in the disappearance of the embryonic tail. There are simultaneous formations of the ventricular terminalis (the terminal extension of the central canal in the conus medullaris), the filum terminale, and the coccygeal medullary vestige (the small ependymal rest that anchors the filum terminale to the coccyx).

Simple meningomyelocele results from a failure of normal neuralation. It is an open defect of the back in which both neural and meningeal tissue are exposed. The neural plate, having failed to fuse into a tube, is a plaque of disorganized tissue. The subarachnoid space ventral to the cord is typically enlarged, and the dysplastic cord bulges above the plane of surrounding skin and leaks CSF. The clinical appearances of malformations that occur during the second and third phases of neural development often overlap. The term "myelocystocele" is used to define cystic dilatation of the central canal. The protuberant sac is usually covered by skin. This rare lesion frequently coexists with cloacal exstrophy and vertebral anomalies. "Lipomeningomyelocele" is a subcutaneous fatty mass that traverses the dura by fibrous connection and leads to an intradural lipomatous mass and meningomyelocele. The subcutaneous mass is occasionally marked by a hairy patch, abnormal pigmentation, a nevus or a sinus tract. A "meningocele" is a prolapse of arachnoid and dura mater: this occurs dorsally, through unfused spinal processes, or ventrally, through a sacral defect (anterior, sacral meningocele). A meningocele is not necessarily associated with other anomalies of the neural tube.

Although these definitions allow a tidy framework from which to start, each baby with myelodysplasia is unique. When examining a child with suspected anomaly of the neural tube and meninges, one should be on the lookout for multiple variations of the disorder. The indications for spinal ultrasonography of the neonate are as follows:

1. Sacral agenesis (shallow intergluteal cleft, flat glutei)
2. Vertebral anomalies of lumbosacral region of the spine
3. Sacrococcygeal cleft or deep dimple
4. Mass, hairy patch, or abnormal pigmentation over lumbrosacral region
5. Abnormal neurologic examination of lower extremities
6. Abnormal rectum
7. Sacrococcygeal teratoma

ULTRASONOGRAPHY OF THE ABNORMAL SPINE

Absent or Abnormal Vertebrae

Absence of sacral vertebrae may be partial or complete. Complete absence, which can occur in association with maternal diabetes, results in a narrow spinal canal in which the cauda equina are crowded together. Hydromyelia may be present, but the cord usually terminates in the normal position. Anomalies of sacral vertebrae commonly coexist with imperforate anus. In some patients, spinal dysraphism coexists with anorectal malformation, and complete evaluation of these babies (who are commonly referred to ultrasonography for suspected renal anomaly) should include examination of the spine (Karrer et al., 1988).

Diastematomyelia affects eight times as many girls as boys and almost always coexists with widening of interpediculate distance, anomalies of segmentation, and narrowing of disc space at the level of the double spinal cord. If each cord is invested in dura, a bony, cartilaginous, or fibrous septum is present in 40 to 50 percent of patients. Hydromyelia is present, usually above the clefting, in 50 percent of patients (Schlessinger et al., 1986). In most cases, the hemicords reunite into one cord below the level of the vertebral anomaly. This is one situation in which careful axial scanning may show the anomaly to better advantage than sagittal scans. Hydromyelia may be so gross that the thinned cord may be overlooked and the cystic space misinterpreted as subarachnoid fluid.

Sacral Dimple

Pilonidal sinuses are epithelium-lined dimples overlying sacrum and coccyx. When the skin near the opening is moved toward the baby's head, the dimple deepens because the tract is coursing inferiorly. A superiorly directed tract associated with dermal sinus would cause the dimple to become more shallow during this maneuver. The pilonidal sinus is hyperechoic on ultrasound, is associated with the dorsal surface of the coccyx, and is not related to the spinal canal, which terminates above the tract (Naidich et al., 1984). Dermal sinuses are persistent adhesions between cutaneous and neural ectoderm. The more atypical the dimple, the more likely there is to be an underlying associated anomaly (Fig. 2–5). Fifty to 67 percent of sinuses extend into the spinal canal, and 60 percent are associated with deep dermoid or epidermoid cyst. Dermal sinuses may act as a conduit for infection and be discovered only after meningitis has supervened. The sinus may be demonstrated on parasagittal scans as an echogenic band extending anteriorly, but it is difficult to prove whether the sinus communicates with the spinal canal (Fig. 2–6; Naidich 1984). Likewise, associated dermoid or epidermoid may be small and indistinguishable among cauda equina. Metrizamide CT myelography or MRI is needed for these patients because the failure to make a correct diagnosis may lead to catastrophic meningitis or subdural or epidural abscess.

Meningomyelocele

A baby with overt open meningomyelocele does not need ultrasonographic evaluation of the area for three reasons: the neuropathology is similar in all cases, surgery is not altered by diagnostic imaging, and, most important, contamination of the sac must be avoided because infection of the subarachnoid space worsens prognosis. Neurologic deterioration occurring some time after surgery can be investigated with ultrasonography. Normal postoperative appearance is of a pulsatile cord lying low, but centrally, in the spinal cord, of disorganized but freely moving nerve roots, and of no intracanalicular mass. Retethering of cord by adhesions to site of surgery, hydrosyringomyelia, and dermoid, epidermoid, or lipoma may be identified on postoperative scanning in a symptomatic patient (Naidich et al., 1984). Because surgical changes in overlying soft tissues prevent good acoustic access, we commonly rely on MRI for postoperative imaging in symptomatic patients (Balasubramaniam et al., 1990).

Epithelialization of the meningomyelocele occurs if surgery is not performed. The associated deficiency of posterior spinous elements provides an acoustic window for "delayed" ultrasonographic evaluation in this situation.

Hydrosyringomyelia, diastematomyelia, or lipomata, or a combination of these three, coexist with meningomyelocele in 25 to 30 percent of patients (Glasier et al., 1990). *Hydromyelia* refers to dilatation of the spinal canal. *Syringomyelia* refers to a cavity within the cord. One can rarely differentiate the two on ultrasonography. The diameters of the thoracic and lumbar regions of the spinal cord in babies with meningomyelocele are significantly less than those of the normal neonate born at term (Glasier et al., 1990).

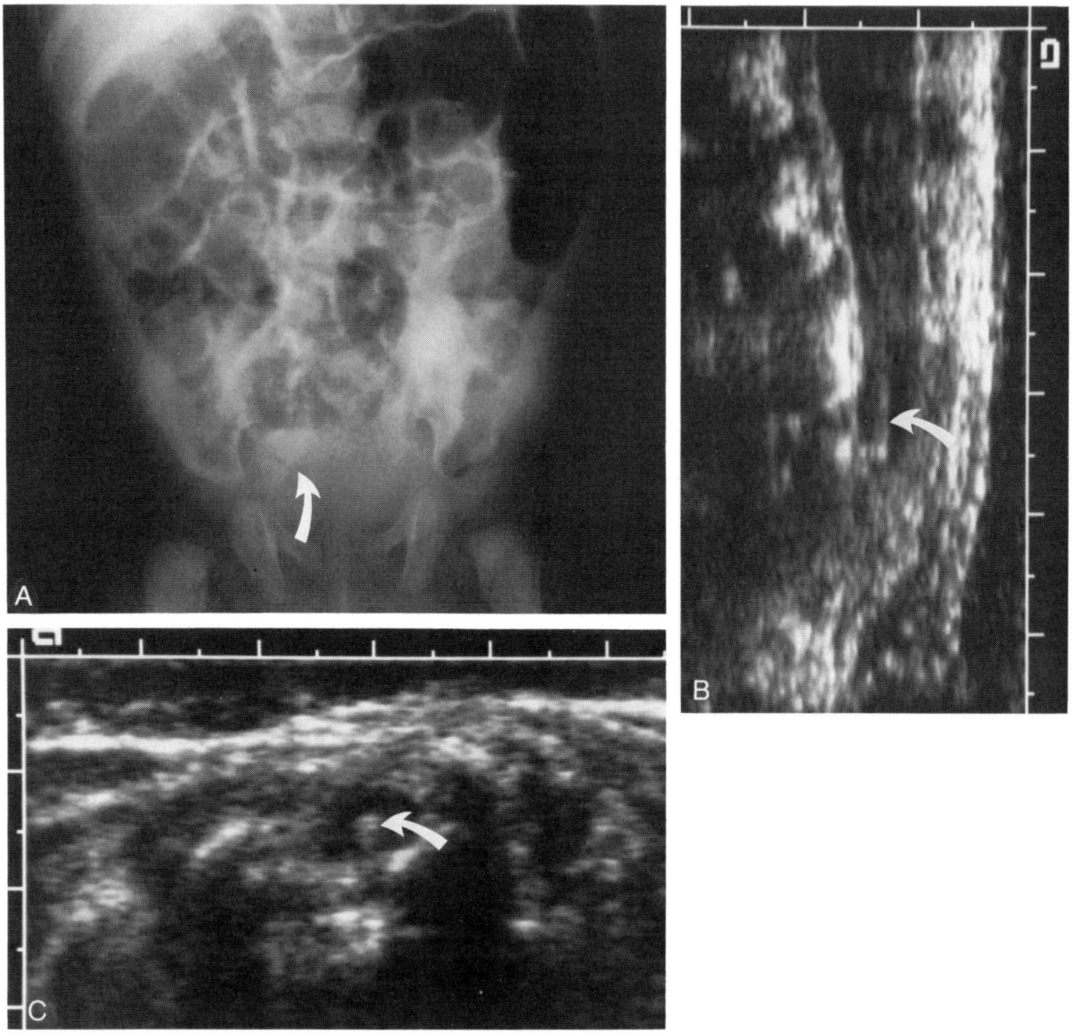

Figure 2-5. This baby was noted to have unusual prominence of the sacrum associated with deep dermal cleft. Plain film **(A)** shows the sacrum (arrow) deviating to the right. Longitudinal scans of the spinal canal showed the conus medullaris ending at L3. The distorted sacral thecal sac was filled with the cauda equina, and on both longitudinal **(B)** and axial **(C)** scans, an echogenic focus within the canal (arrow) was apparent. This fibrous stalk, a thickened filum associated with tethered cord, was confirmed by computed tomography (CT) scanning. Note how asymmetric the soft tissues appear on the axial scan because of the spinal anomaly.

The normal diameter of the cervical spinal cord is 5.0 ± 0.45 mm; that of the thoracic cord is 3.7 ± 0.44 mm; and that of the lumbar cord is 5.1 ± 0.44 mm (Kawahara et al., 1987).

Skin-Covered Soft Tissue Mass

Simple meningocele is an outpouching of the dural sac and is therefore a sonolucent mass, usually associated with local widening of the spinal canal (Fig. 2-7). Meningocele may be unassociated with other anomalies, but is usually one component of a more complex anomaly (Fig. 2-8). One case of anterior sacral meningocele coexisted with sacral intramedullary dermoid and tethered cord (Naidich et al., 1984). Lipomeningomyelocele is marked by dermal abnormality in many cases, but as a mass it is differentiated from teratoma by lying above, not below, the intergluteal crease (Fig. 2-9). Most lipomas are lumbosacral, quite echogenic, and poorly encapsulated (Fig. 2-10). They may reflect

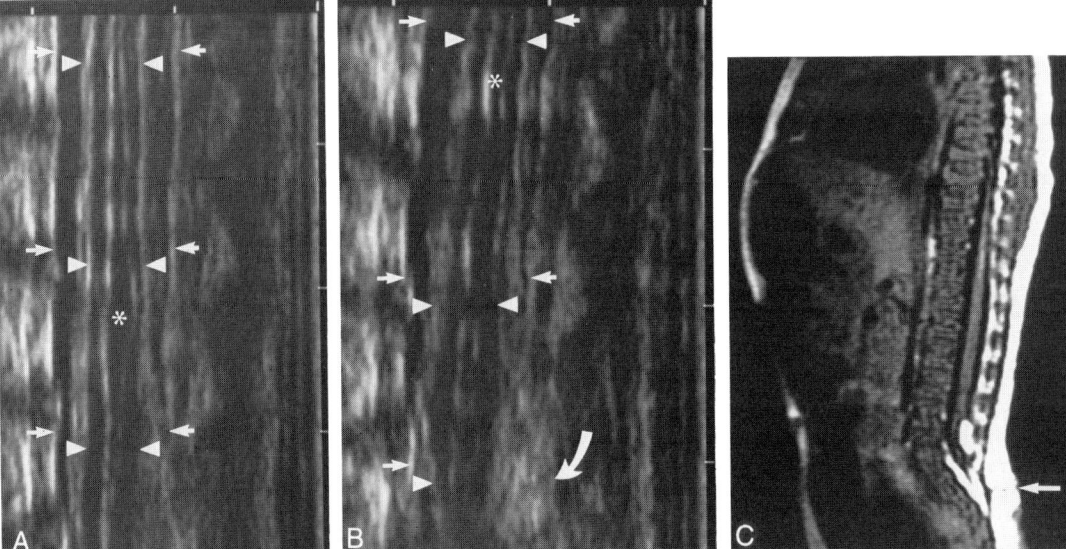

Figure 2–6. This child had a deep dimple over the lower spine, and the dimple appeared to course in a cephalad direction. Longitudinal scans of the lumbar spine (**A** and **B**) are oriented to match the subsequent magnetic resonance imaging (MRI) scan. (**C**). Note the presence of a syrinx (asterisk) within the cord. The thecal sac is outlined with arrows. Anterior and posterior borders of the cord are outlined with arrowheads. The cord extends well below the level of L2-L3 and is associated with a dorsal plaque of echogenicity (curved arrow, **B**) that represents fatty tissue. This is shown on the MRI scan as a high-signal (white) pad of abnormality dorsal to the spinal cord. The dermal sinus was not apparent on the sagittal ultrasonograms, but it can be traced on MRI scan (straight arrow, **C**).

sound so efficiently that identification of ventral structures is hindered. They extend into the spinal canal and onto the surface of the cord from the plane of subcutaneous fat. The cord may stay within the canal, tethered in a low position, or protrude through the posterior spinal defect with a meningocele to form part of the palpable mass (Fig. 2–11).

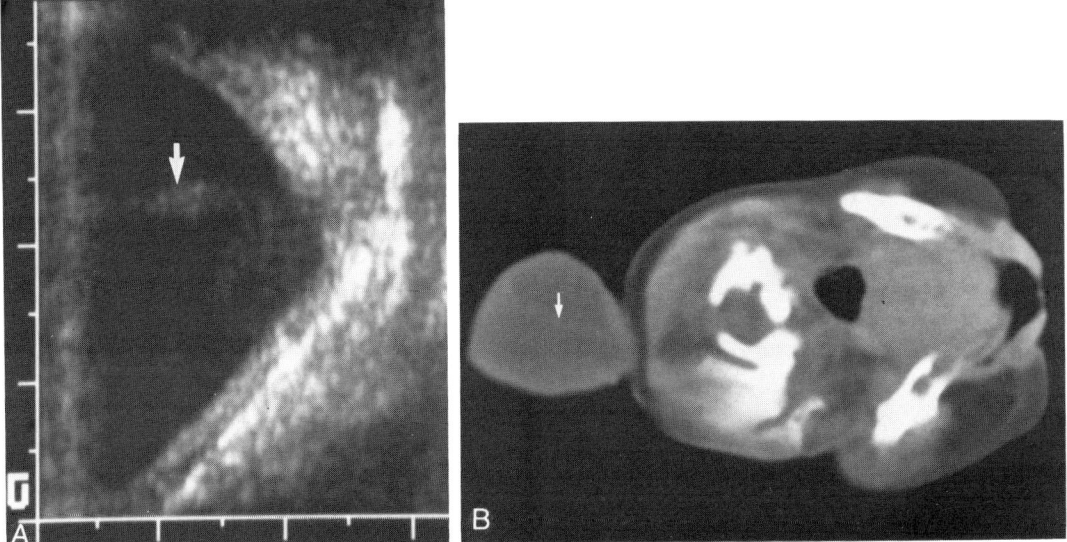

Figure 2–7. A pedunculated mass was evident over the neck of this newborn baby. The scan of this mass (**A**) showed it to be echo free with septation (arrow). (Other echogenicity shown on this scan is artifactual.) The scan is oriented to match the subsequent CT scan (**B**). The septation (arrow) is faintly apparent. The baby underwent resection of a meningocele. No neural tissue was present. The baby has since been asymptomatic.

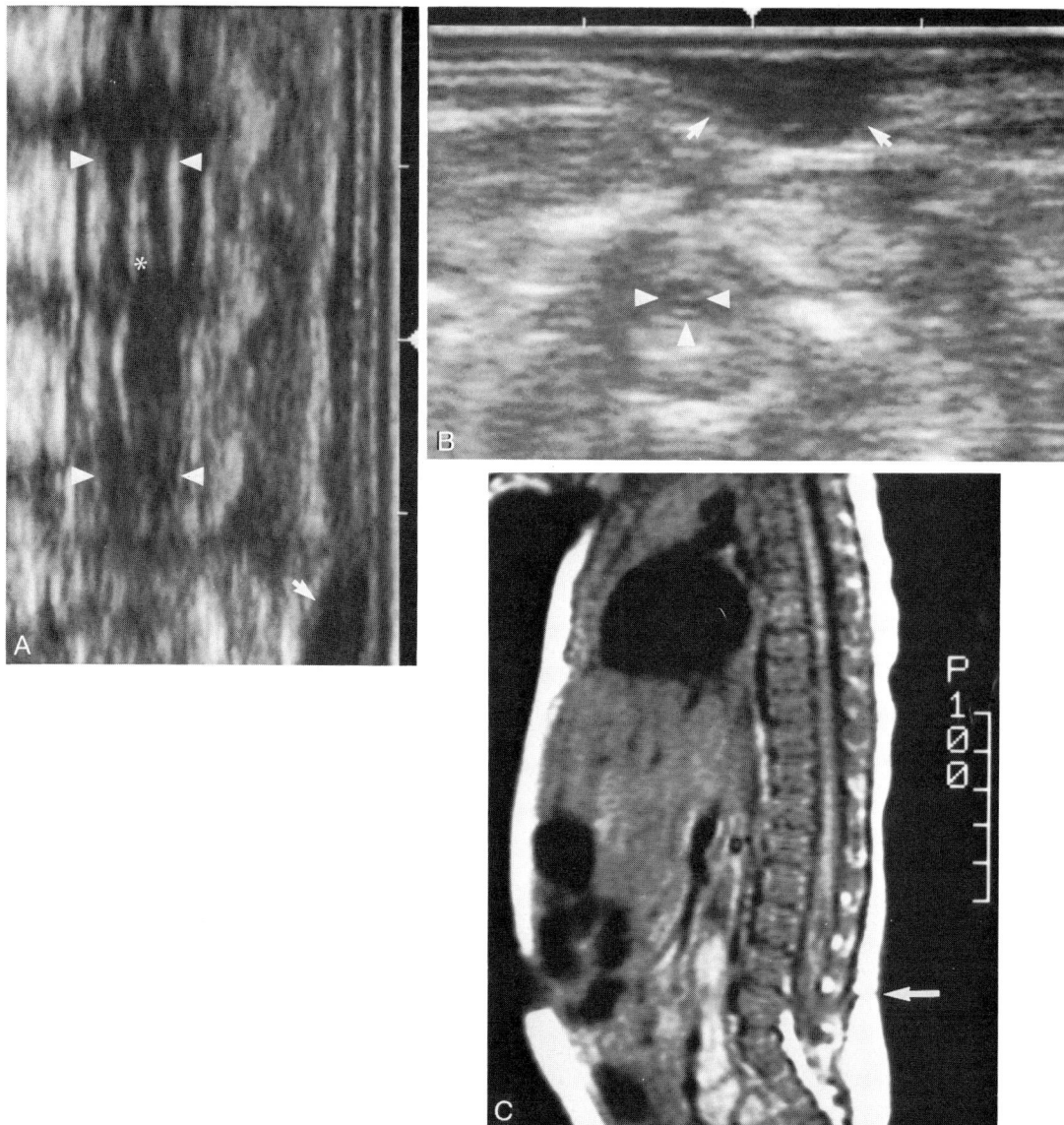

Figure 2–8. Longitudinal (**A**) and transverse (**B**) scans of this 1-day-old were performed when a fluid-filled soft tissue mass (arrows) was evident over the lower lumbar spine. The cord (arrowheads) ended at the level of L5 just proximal to the soft tissue mass. A central syrinx (asterisk) was apparent. The transverse scan (**B**) shows the slight eccentricity of the meningocele (arrows) in relation to the canal. The end of the cord (arrowheads) with its syrinx is surrounded by the cauda equina. A postoperative MRI was performed when the patient continued to have neurologic difficulties (**C**). The syrinx within the cord is apparent as a faint lucency on the sagittal scan. The low conus is again apparent. The area from prior surgery is apparent as a defect in the skin (arrow).

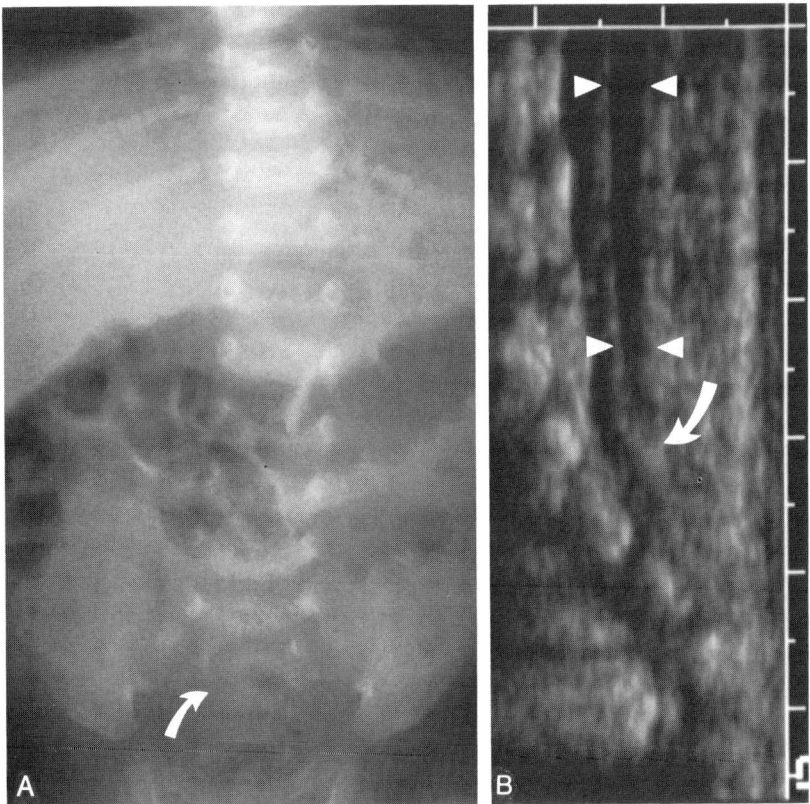

Figure 2-9. The mother of this 1-month-old boy noticed a lump between the intergluteal crease. Plain films showed anomaly of segmentation (arrow) in the upper sacrum (**A**). Sagittal ultrasonography (**B**) showed a low-lying cord (arrowheads) that was tethered posteriorly (curved arrow) and associated with fatty infiltration of the soft tissues. Lipoma with tethered cord was confirmed on MRI, and surgery was performed for its release.

Fat on the surface of the cord may be identified as a linear area of increased echogenicity or as a definite echogenic mass. When there is no bulging of meninges, when the cord is intracanalicular, and when the lipoma within the spinal canal is adherent to the cord, the term "lipomyelocele" may be used.

Abnormal Neurologic Examination

A tethered spinal cord can result in an abnormal finding on neurologic examination of a baby's lower extremities, but more commonly it is not suspected until the child is older. Sonographic features as listed by Zieger and associates (1988) include low position of the conus, an atypically shaped ("dumpy") conus, a thickened echogenic filum, dorsal placement of the spinal cord within the spinal canal, and absent movement of the spinal cord as shown with M-mode. This syndrome is at the mild end of the spectrum of dysraphic anomalies and, correspondingly, bony anomalies are minimal or absent. Hemangioma or abnormal pigmentation over the lower spine is a clue to the underlying anomaly.

Abnormal Rectum

Babies who have imperforate anus, rectal stenosis, or cloacal anomalies are at risk for associated anomalies of the lumbosacral canal and of neural elements (Figs. 2-12, 2-13; Karrer et al., 1988). We now include screening spinal ultrasonography in the initial evaluation of these babies, who usually are referred in order to rule in or out coexistent renal anomaly. Neurosurgical intervention typically follows creation of a colostomy and

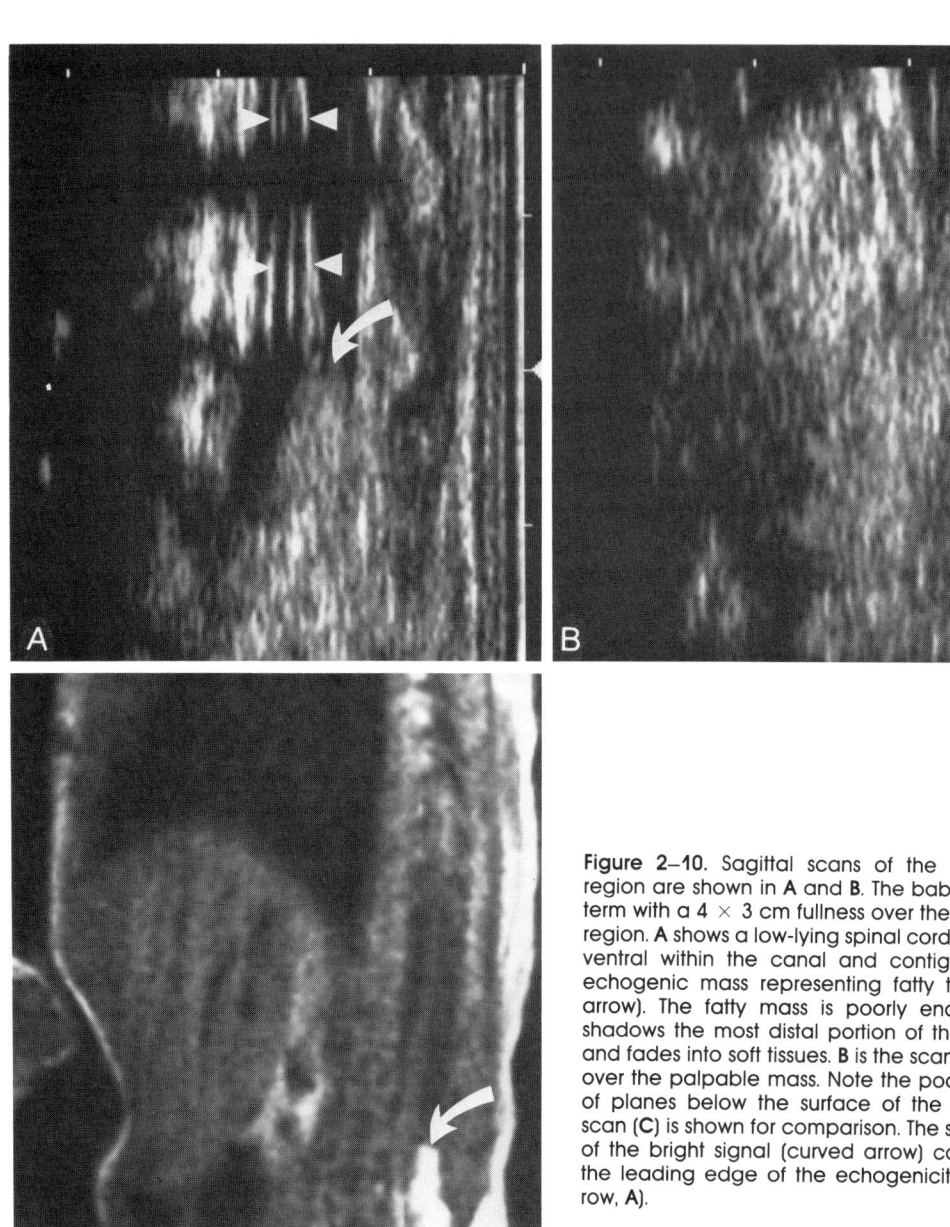

Figure 2–10. Sagittal scans of the lower lumbar region are shown in **A** and **B**. The baby was born at term with a 4 × 3 cm fullness over the lower lumbar region. **A** shows a low-lying spinal cord (arrowheads) ventral within the canal and contiguous with an echogenic mass representing fatty tissue (curved arrow). The fatty mass is poorly encapsulated. It shadows the most distal portion of the spinal cord and fades into soft tissues. **B** is the scan immediately over the palpable mass. Note the poor delineation of planes below the surface of the skin. The MRI scan (**C**) is shown for comparison. The superior edge of the bright signal (curved arrow) corresponds to the leading edge of the echogenicity (curved arrow, **A**).

Figure 2-11. This longitudinal view of the spinal canal (A) is actually coronal in its orientation. Scans immediately over the lumbar soft tissue mass, which was this child's presenting abnormality, were difficult to obtain because of the localized bulge; this bulge was shown best on the MRI scan, which is in a sagittal projection (B). The coronal ultrasonogram (A) shows splaying of the cord (arrowheads) just superior to the point at which it herniates through the spinal defect into the soft tissues of the back. When the soft tissue mass is locally protuberant, as in this baby, a thick cushion of gel or the use of standoff material above and below the mass can help in creating a more horizontal surface for the linear array transducer.

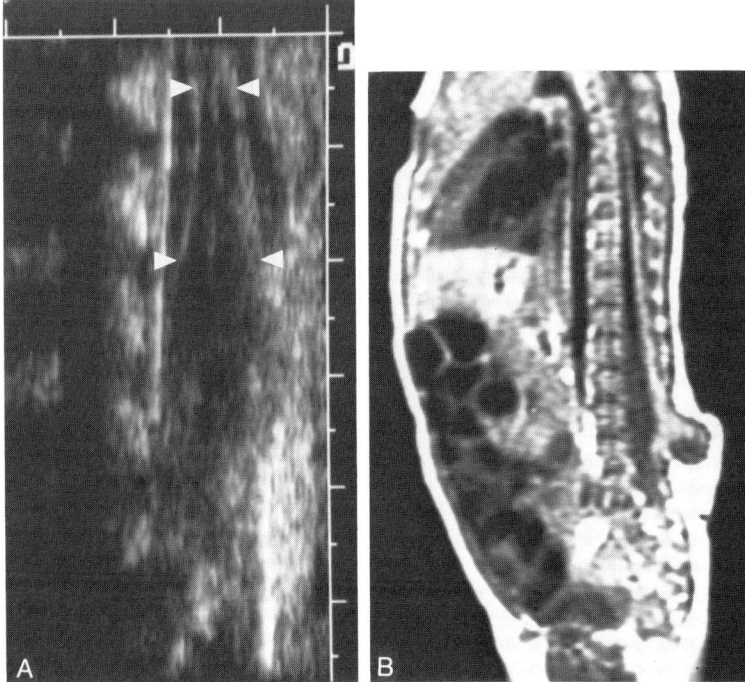

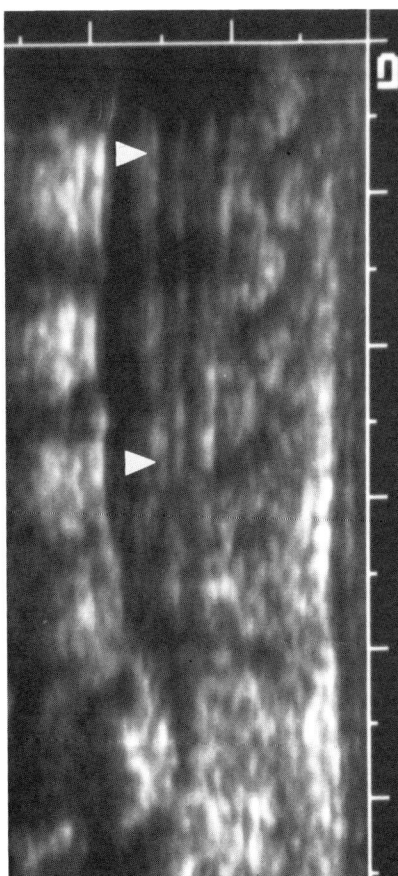

Figure 2-12. The posteriorly tethered cord (arrowheads) in this baby was associated with rectal stenosis and penile-scrotal hypoplasia. He had a normal left kidney and a right pelvic kidney.

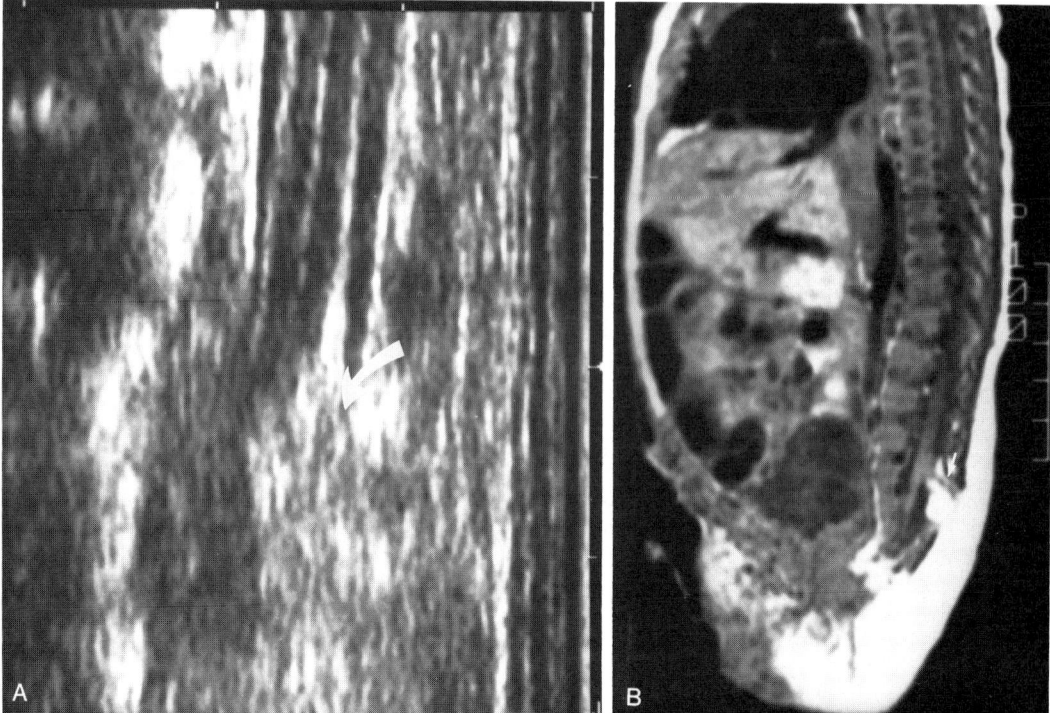

Figure 2–13. This baby was diagnosed at birth as having cloacal exstrophy. Ultrasonography included evaluation of the kidneys, spine, and hips. The sagittal sonogram of the spine (**A**) showed a low-lying spinal cord, which was tethered posteriorly in association with an ill-defined echogenic mass (arrow). The subsequent MRI scan (**B**) confirmed the low-lying tethered spinal cord, which appeared to be associated with a fibrous tract (arrow). Fatty tissue, shown on the MRI scan as a bright white signal, extended from subcutaneous tissues into the canal.

urologic repair in babies who have cloacal exstrophy. If ultrasonography can be performed before *any* surgical intervention, the problem of difficult access is avoided. Previous abdominal surgery limits positioning the baby in the prone position for spinal sonography because the baby must lie supine with hips in flexion in order that the anterior closure heal.

Sacrococcygeal Teratoma

Teratomas in the sacrococcygeal region can be huge masses with retrorectal extension into the pelvis, or they can be small masses, palpable only on careful rectal examination. They rarely extend into the spinal canal. They are variably cystic and solid in texture and have to be removed immediately upon discovery because their potential for becoming malignant increases the longer they remain in situ. (See section on pelvic masses in Chapter 8.)

INTRAMEDULLARY AND EXTRAMEDULLARY TUMORS

Most case reports of spinal tumors refer to their intraoperative localization rather than their primary diagnosis. Ultrasonography falls short of CT and MRI in its delineation of these tumors, which only rarely affect the baby or the young child. We have been interested, however, in evaluating the spinal canal in babies with paraspinal neuroblastoma (Fig. 2–14; Garcia & Keller, 1990). Intraspinal extension is marked by bony destruction, displacement of the spinal cord, and a mass in the subarachnoid space (Zieger et al., 1988). An obviously abnormal scan mandates neurosurgical consultation and further imaging before the intra-abdominal or intrathoracic component of the neuroblastoma is approached. Ultrasonography can be used after laminectomy in children with an earlier diagnosis of spinal tumor. We followed one girl who presented with neurologic decom-

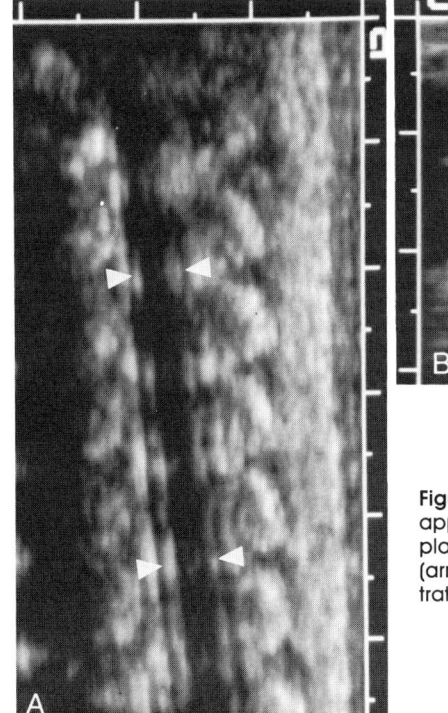
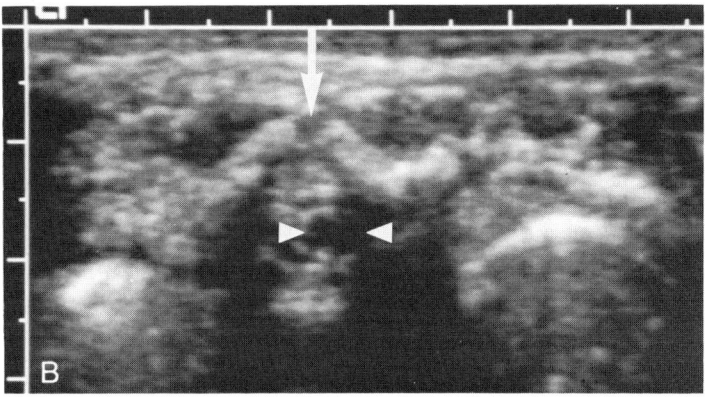

Figure 2–14. This sagittal scan of the thoracic spine (A) shows an apparently normal cord (arrowheads). However, on scans in transverse plane (B), the spinal cord (arrowheads) is shifted to the left of midline (arrow). This baby had right-sided paraspinal neuroblastoma that infiltrated the thecal sac.

pensation some years after surgery and radiotherapy for a tumor. The scans showed atrophy with syrinx, and not recurrent mass, as the source of the neurologic signs. There is no question, however, that the distortion of landmarks and the fibrosis from a scar make ultrasonographic evaluation less than ideal in postoperative patients, especially those who are older.

INTRAOPERATIVE NEUROSONOGRAPHY

There are four areas in which intraoperative use of ultrasonography has been most helpful: (1) in localizing a cerebral tumor for biopsy or removal when there is no external sign of the tumor, (2) in placing ventricular shunts, (3) in localizing bony fragments in the spinal canal during surgery for traumatic injuries, and (4) in localizing an intramedullary tumor or a syrinx within the spinal cord.

Because the access to the brain or spinal canal is limited—typically through a window less than 4 cm in diameter—we use small transducers 5 MHz or higher in frequency. One should beware of having too narrow a field of view because this limits everyone's ability to evaluate the local geography of the lesion.

On arrival in the operating room, the equipment must be plugged in with appropriate grounding (usually through adaptors on hand in the operating suite). The transducer and cord are washed first with a bactericidal agent and then with sterile saline, and then they are placed into a commercially available plastic sleeve into which sterile aqueous gel has been squeezed. Some transducers can be sterilized by gas before a procedure, but many of our patients are semi-emergent and require equipment that is in use in the department. Sterile saline is used as a coupling agent between brain and transducer. Often a surgical assistant has to use a syringe to wash over the operative field with saline if the contour is not horizontal. Before any scanning is performed, the surgeon has to be oriented to the view on the viewing screen. The easiest way is for the surgeon to move a gloved finger across the face of the transducer while watching the screen, thereby establishing right to left or top to bottom. The ultrasonographer *has* to know the positioning of the patient; it sounds easy,

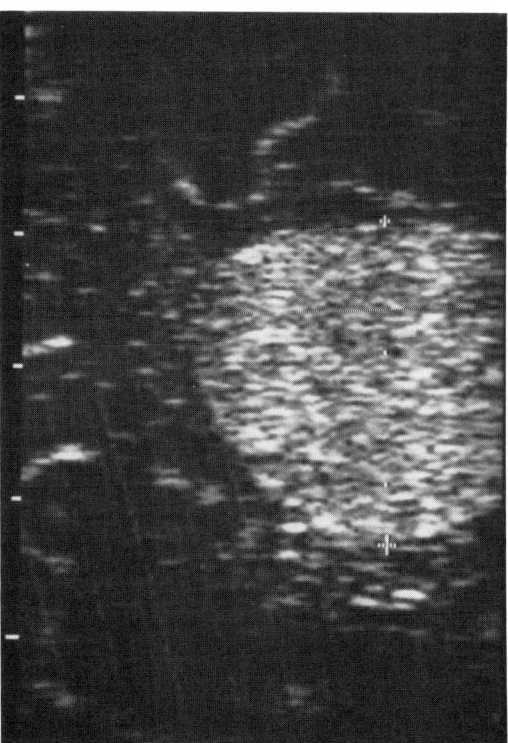

Figure 2–15. Intraoperative ultrasonography was requested when this 13-year-old, who had neurofibromatosis, was being operated on for a known left parietal tumor. After the craniotomy was performed, no parenchymal distortion was evident. Scans were performed to determine the tumor's location more precisely. This was a grade 3 astrocytoma and is shown here as an echogenic mass measuring 2.5 cm in diameter in the left parietal area. The transducer was directly on the surface of the brain; the lesion was 2 cm below the surface.

but 4 cm² of cerebral cortex surrounded by green draping gives little indication of which way the patient's nose is pointing. Ambient light in the operating room should be limited as much as possible. As the neurosurgeon places the transducer over the area of interest, the ultrasonographer changes gain settings and magnification and orients the surgeon to the anatomy. In order to identify the center of a lesion, scanning is performed in two planes, perpendicular to each other. Needle biopsy or localization is performed while the transducer is held slightly to the side of the lesion and angled to pick up the echo from the exploring needle, or the biopsy guide, previously sterilized, is attached to the transducer for use. There is often a halo effect around the primary mass. This is surrounding edema, and care must be taken to identify the nidus of the mass in order not to biopsy adjacent edematous brain (Quencer and Montalvo, 1986). Because the screen shows a minified or magnified image, markers to show the distance between surface and lesion are mandatory (Fig. 2–15). A common mistake during intraoperative procedures is the failure to document images on hard copy. The temptation is to take a look, then get on with the surgery. After biopsy is successful, the site is rescanned to show the presence or absence of hematoma (Fig. 2–16). The needle track is often evident as a linear interface because of bleeding along its path. Evolution into expanding hematoma requires its decompression before closure.

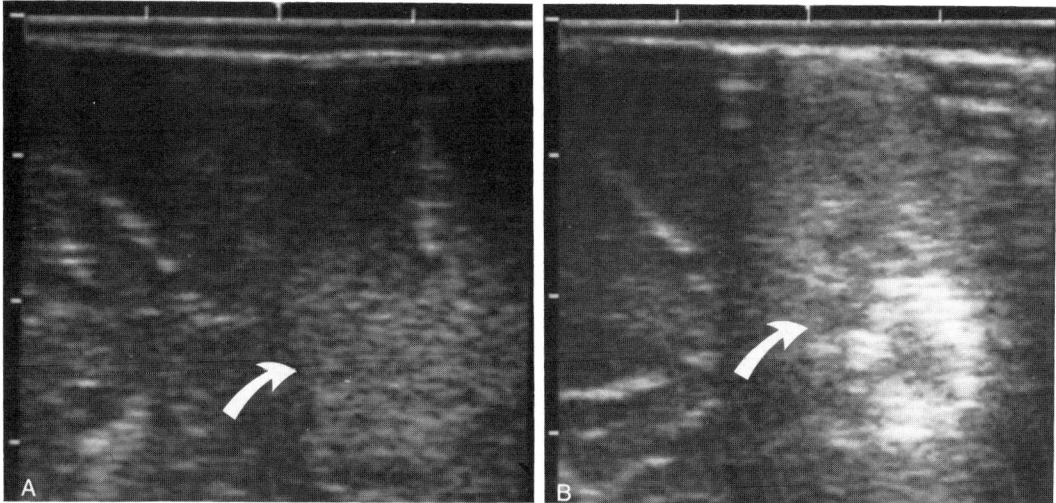

Figure 2–16. Scans before (**A**) and after (**B**) biopsy of an intracerebral mass show the mildly echogenic lesion (arrow) becoming more echogenic as bleeding occurs within it. A hamartoma was diagnosed from the histologic findings.

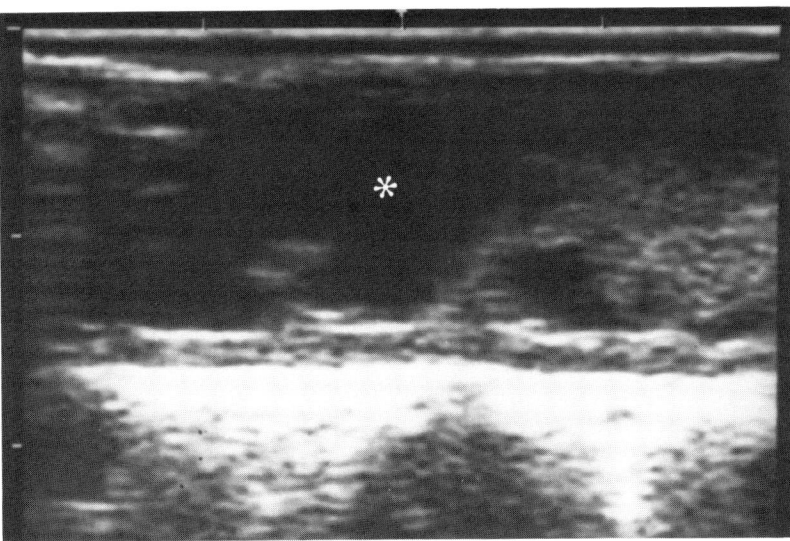

Figure 2–17. Intraoperative scans were achieved in this particular case by means of orienting the 7.5 MHz linear array transducer along the cord. The patient had an intramedullary cervicothoracic tumor that was partly cystic (asterisk). The surgeons were interested in identifying the cystic and solid components of the tumor before its resection.

During ultrasonographic localization for placement of shunts in neonates, the window to the ventricular system is the anterior fontanelle. Before the neurosurgical procedure, draping must be done in such a way that there is access to the anterior fontanelle without contamination of the surgical field. Scanning before introduction of the shunt orients the surgeons to the anatomy. The view through the transducer is generally not as familiar to them as that of the axial CT scan. Steep coronal scanning can usually show the site of entrance of the shunt into the lateral ventricle. The transducer is then turned 90 degrees to show the entire length of the tubing in the lateral ventricle. The anterior tip should lie anterior to the foramen of Monro to avoid its clogging by the choroid plexus. Bleeding during the procedure will shower the ventricle with echoes, as will introduction of air.

Intraoperative scans of the spinal cord are relatively easy because the canal is exposed by laminectomy, and there is normally a fluid bath of CSF supplemented by saline. A small linear array transducer provides the best images in this situation. Again, north–south/right–left orientation is crucial. Spicules of bone in the canal declare their presence by shadowing. Ventral compression of the cord by vertebral fracture or dislocation, or both, can be appreciated with sagittal views. Localization of small masses, syrinx, and localized hydromyelia is easily achieved (Figs. 2–17, 2–18). The same reminders as for intra-

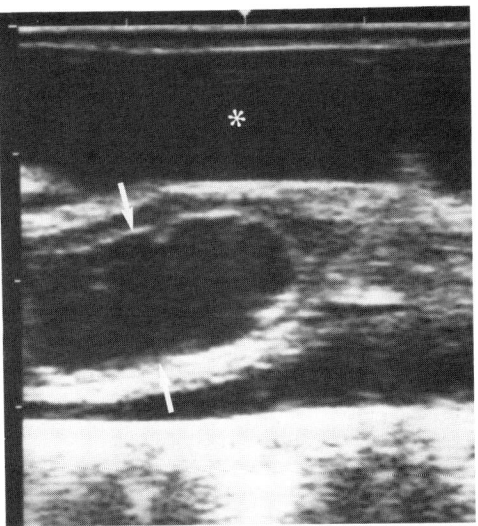

Figure 2–18. History of progressive weakness of the lower extremities resulted in this 7-year-old girl's being evaluated with MRI. Syringomyelia unassociated with any other anomaly or tumor was diagnosed, and the patient was taken to the operating room for shunting of this syrinx. Scans were performed in the operating room in order to identify the thinnest portion of the cord through which the shunt tubing could be inserted. The diameter of the syrinx is marked by arrows. In order to perform the scan, the spinal canal was filled with saline so as to have a water path (asterisk) through which to scan.

cranial work apply: use centimeter markers to emphasize true distances and obtain hard copy of views for documentation.

REFERENCES

Spine

Anderson FM: Occult spinal dysraphism: Diagnosis and management. J Pediatr 1968; 73:163–177.

Balasubramaniam C, Laurent JP, McCluggage C, et al: Tethered-cord syndrome after repair of meningomyelocele. Childs Nerv Syst 1990; 6:208–211.

Garcia CJ, Keller MS: Intraspinal extension of paraspinal masses in infants: Detection by sonography. Pediatr Radiol 1990; 20:437–439.

Glasier CM, Chadduck WM, Leithiser RE Jr, et al: Screening spinal ultrasound in newborns with neural tube defects. J Ultrasound Med 1990; 9:339–343.

Gusnard DA, Naidich TP, Yousefzadeh DK, et al: Ultrasonic anatomy of the normal neonatal and infant spine: Correlation with cryomicrotome sections and CT. Neuroradiology 1986; 28:493–511.

Holtzman RNN, Stein BM (eds): The Tethered Spinal Cord. New York: Thieme-Stratton, 1985.

Kangarloo H, Gold RH, Diament MJ, et al: High-resolution spinal sonography in infants. AJR 1984; 142:1243–1247.

Karrer FM, Flannery AM, Nelson MD Jr, et al: Anorectal malformations: Evaluation of associated spinal dysraphic syndromes. J Pediatr Surg 1988; 23:45–48.

Kawahara H, Andou Y, Takashima S, et al: Normal development of the spinal cord in neonates and infants seen on ultrasonography. Neuroradiology 1987; 29:50–52.

Kirks DR, Merten DF, Filston HC, et al: The Currarino triad: Complex of anorectal malformation, sacral bony abnormality, and presacral mass. Pediatr Radiol 1984; 14:220–225.

Naidich TP, Fernbach SK, McLone DG, et al: Sonography of the caudal spine and back: Congenital anomalies in children. AJR 1984; 142:1229–1242.

Naidich TP, Radkowski MA, Britton J: Real-time sonographic display of caudal spine anomalies. Neuroradiology 1986; 28:512–527.

Nelson MD Jr, Sedler JA, Gilles FH: Spinal cord central echo complex: Histoanatomic correlation. Radiology 1989; 170:479–481.

Raghavendra BN, Epstein FJ: Sonography of the spine and spinal cord. Radiol Clin North Am 1985; 23:91–105.

Raghavendra BN, Epstein FJ, Pinto RS, et al: The tethered spinal cord: Diagnosis by high-resolution real-time ultrasound. Radiology 1983; 149:123–128.

Raghavendra BN, Epstein FJ, Pinto RS, et al: Sonographic diagnosis of diastematomyelia. J Ultrasound Med 1988; 7:111–113.

Sarwar M: Imaging of the pediatric spine and its contents. J Child Neurol 1990; 5:3–18.

Schlessinger AE, Naidich TP, Quencer RM: Concurrent hydromyelia and diastematomyelia. AJNR 1986; 7:473–477.

Wilson DA, Prince JR: MR imaging determination of the location of the conus medullaris in normal children and in children with the tethered cord syndrome (Abstract). Pediatr Radiol 1988; 18:441.

Wright RL: Congenital dermal sinuses. Prog Neurol Surg 1971; 4:175–191.

Zieger M, Dörr U: Pediatric spinal sonography. Part I: Anatomy and examination technique. Pediatr Radiol 1988; 18:9–13.

Zieger M, Dörr U, Schulz RD: Pediatric spinal sonography. Part II: Malformations and mass lesions. Pediatr Radiol 1988; 18:105–111.

Intraoperative Cranial and Spinal Ultrasonography

Mirvis SE, Geisler FH: Intraoperative sonography of cervical spinal cord injury: Results in 30 patients. AJR 1990; 155:603–609.

Montalvo BM, Quencer RM: Intraoperative sonography in spinal surgery: Current state of the art. Neuroradiology 1986; 28:551–590.

Platt JF, Rubin JM, Chandler WF, et al: Intraoperative spinal sonography in the evaluation of intramedullary tumors. J Ultrasound Med 1988; 7:317–325.

Post MJ, Quencer RM, Montalvo BM, et al: Spinal infection: Evaluation with MR imaging and intraoperative US. Radiology 1988; 169:765–771.

Quencer RM, Montalvo BM: Intraoperative cranial sonography. Neuroradiology 1986; 28:528–550.

Rubin JM, DiPietro MA, Chandler WF, et al: Spinal ultrasonography: Intraoperative and pediatric applications. Radiol Clin North Am 1988; 26:1–27.

CHAPTER 3

THE FACE AND NECK

The written requisition for a patient who is having ultrasonography of the face or neck is typically quite focused. Most questions relate to a visible or palpable mass. This chapter is divided into discussions of masses and other abnormalities of (1) nodes (adenopathy), (2) salivary glands and sinuses, (3) thyroid and parathyroid glands, (4) vessels, and (5) connective tissues.

Technique

Children should be positioned supine with a rolled towel or sponge under the upper back so as to allow extension of the neck. Transducers of high frequency with fine resolution in the near field, preferably linear array, are needed for good examinations. Masses, if inflammatory, are typically very painful; the weight of the tissue-equivalent standoff material may be intolerable, and a thick sandwich of cold gel between skin and transducer is the only technique that these patients can tolerate. Warm gel tends to run off the skin. Because there is no fixed anatomic point of reference on transverse sections, except for midline trachea and the vessels laterally, labeling on hard copy must be explicit, and comparable right and left views must be obtained. After transverse scans, the normal side is examined in sagittal or coronal planes, or both, so that the ultrasonographer will have the normal anatomy in mind before tackling the pathologic anatomy. Because most scans are requested for a child who has a mass, the study is directed toward identifying the mass and its organ of origin, documenting its size and consistency, and showing its effect, if any, on adjacent structures. In general, the position of the mass on clinical examination, the child's history and presentation, and ancillary laboratory data (e.g., tests of thyroid function) narrow the differential diagnosis considerably.

ADENOPATHY

Cervical lymph nodes act as traps for infections of the upper respiratory tract, the teeth, the soft tissues of the face, and the scalp. The size of the glands reflects degree of edema, infiltration by leukocytes, and formation of microabscesses or necrosis. Rapid onset of purulent adenopathy generally results from staphylococcal or streptococcal infection. Facial trauma or impetigo may have been the triggering insult. An indolent onset of unilateral nodal swelling is characteristic of mycobacterial, fungal, and cat-scratch infections. Mycobacterial infection, if present, is generally atypical, and causative organisms are *M. avium-intracellulare* or *M. scrofulaceum* (Fig. 3–1). Infection with *Mycobacterium tuberculosis* is usually accompanied by a positive skin test and abnormal radiographs of the chest. Virus-related adenopathy tends to ap-

74 / THE FACE AND NECK

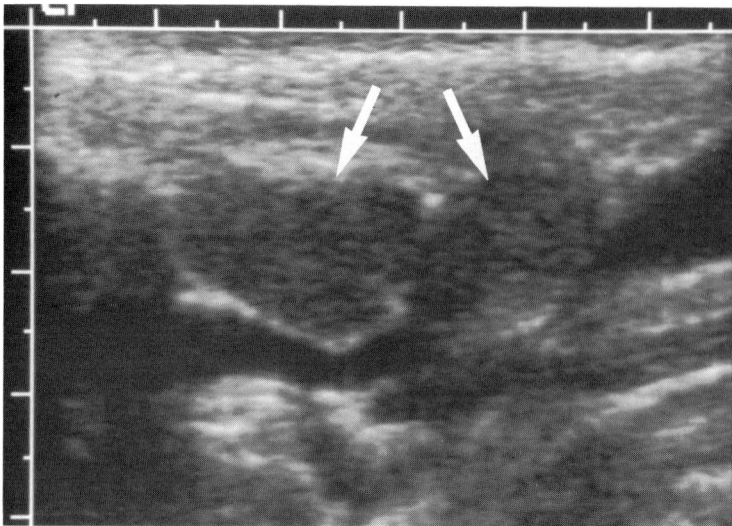

Figure 3–1. This 1½-year-old baby girl had had swelling of the neck for 4 weeks. It had not responded to antibiotics and was nontender. This longitudinal scan shows homogeneous echogenicity in two large lymph nodes (arrows) anterior to the jugular vein. These were removed, and their enlargement was proved to be secondary to infection with *Mycobacterium scrofulaceum*.

pear and resolve quickly. Although it is probably more common than bacterial adenopathy, it is encountered less often by the ultrasonographer because it is evanescent. Epstein-Barr virus, herpes simplex, cytomegalovirus, and human immunodeficiency virus have all been associated with cervical adenopathy (Brook, 1988). Determining the infectious agent in cases of cervical adenitis is the task of the clinician. Early initiation of treatment usually halts the progression of infection, and the nodes shrink (Fig. 3–2). Lack of clinical improvement after the patient has received 36 to 48 hours of empiric antimicrobial treatment indicates a need to reassess therapy. Typically, the ultrasonographer is then asked to identify those nodes that are liquefying so that needle aspiration for diagnosis or incision with drainage for therapy can be instituted (Fig. 3–3). Inflammatory and neoplastic adenopathy share the same ultrasonic appearance of uniformly enlarged, relatively echopoor, spherical or oval masses (Fig. 3–4). Neoplastic cervical adenopathy, however, usually is not tender. Hodgkin disease localized solely to cervical nodes is uncommon in childhood. In any child with de novo cervical adenopathy, radiographs of the chest should be the first imaging performed in order to rule in or out thoracic adenopathy and pulmonary disease. When suppuration occurs in an infection, the center of one or more nodes becomes more echolucent, and a shell begins to develop around it. Aspiration of a node can be done in the ultrasound room. After the skin is cleaned and anesthetized over a fluctuant node, an 18- or 20-gauge needle, which is attached to a 10-ml syringe, is passed into the node to the depth previously measured on the viewing screen. If no liquid material is obtained, 1 ml of sterile saline should be injected slowly and reaspirated. Cultures for aerobic and anaerobic bacteria, fungus, and *Mycobacterium*, as well as Gram stain and acid-fast stain of the aspirate, are requested. Incision and drainage of nodes are to be avoided for cat-scratch and atypical mycobacterial infections. Surgical removal of nodes is the therapy of choice for adenopathy secondary to atypical mycobacterial infection.

Masses that are closely related to the mandible and may be mistaken for cervical adenopathy are listed in Table 3–1. Many are associated with osteolysis or periosteal reaction of the mandible (Fig. 3–5). Bony change may actually be appreciated on ultrasonography as a change in the cortical interface of the mandible, but radiographic Panorex views are the best initial imaging for these types of masses.

Table 3–1. CAUSES OF LUMPY JAW

Actinomycosis	Ameloblastoma
Nocardiosis	Fibroma
Tuberculosis	Cementoma
Blastomycosis	Sarcoma
Pyogenic osteomyelitis	Neurofibroma
Botryomycosis	Giant cell reparative granuloma
Periapical abscess	
Eosinophilic granuloma	Caffey disease
Plasmacytoma	Cherubism

From Lerner PI: The lumpy jaw: Cervicofacial actinomycosis. Infect Dis Clin North Am 1988; 2:203–220.

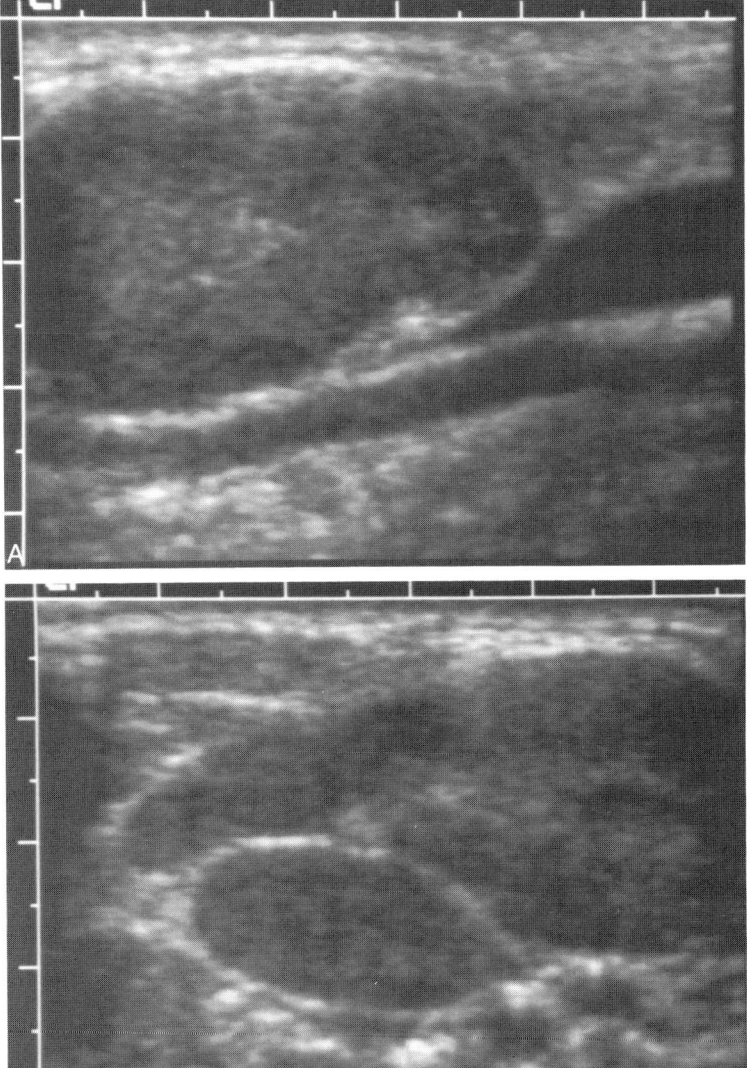

Figure 3–2. When this 17-year-old presented with swelling in the neck, which was otherwise asymptomatic, we were concerned that he might have Hodgkin lymphoma. Bilateral adenopathy is shown in these two views: longitudinal of the right side of the neck (**A**) and transverse of the left side of the neck (**B**). Chest radiographs were normal, and the adenopathy resolved when the patient was treated empirically with antibiotics. We have no proof as to whether this adenitis was staphylococcal, streptococcal, or conceivably viral in etiology.

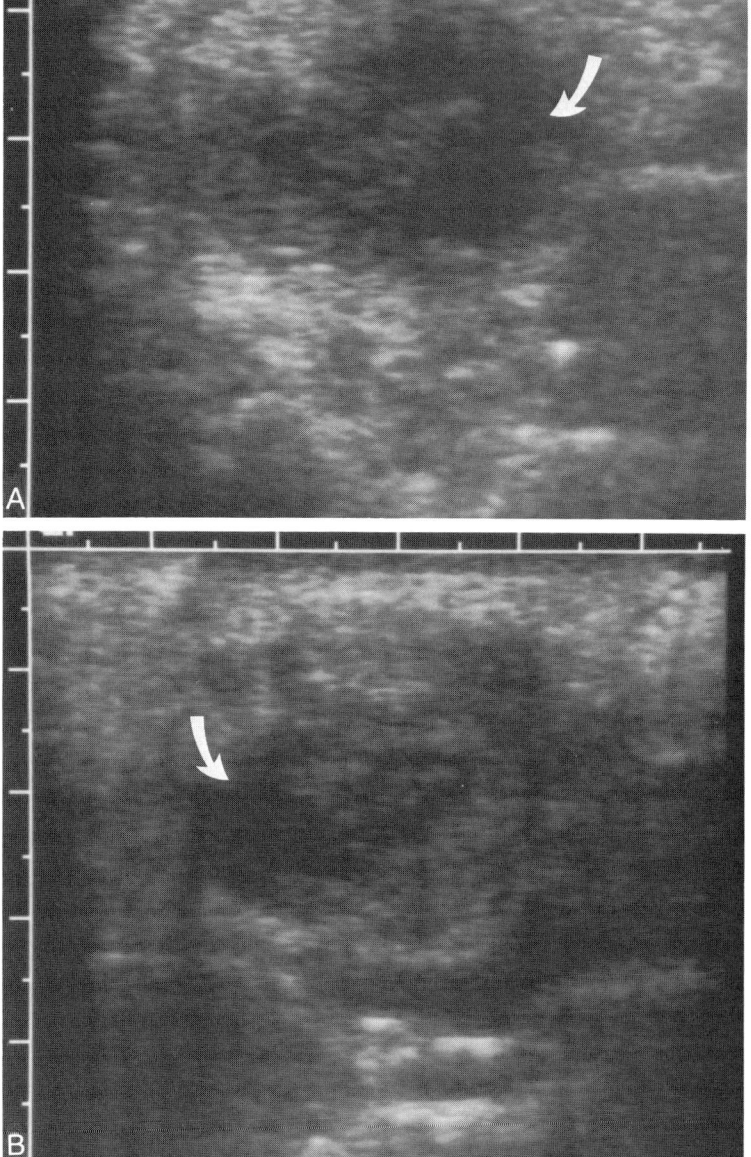

Figure 3–3. Transverse (A) and longitudinal (B) views of the swollen right neck in a 3-month-old baby, who had been cranky for 3 to 5 days, show irregular mass representing suppurating cervical adenitis. Note the irregular lucency in the center (arrow), which represents pus. *Staphylococcus aureus* was aspirated from the nodes.

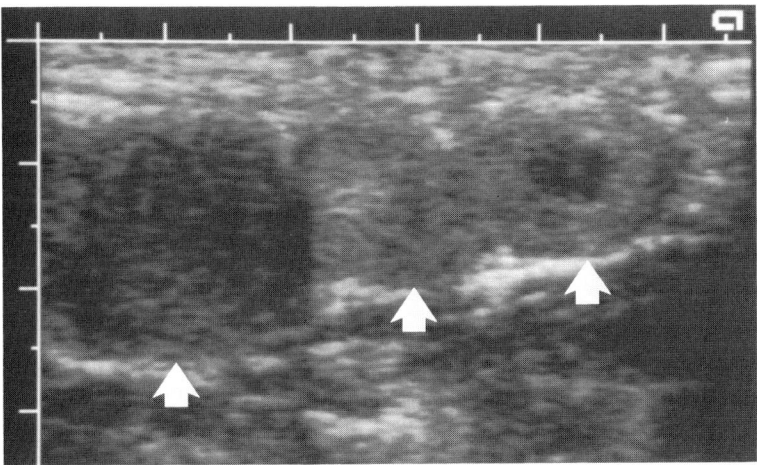

Figure 3–4. At 8 years of age, this little girl had presented with a mass in the right neck and adenopathy. Evaluation at that time revealed papillary carcinoma of the right lobe of the thyroid, and she was treated with total thyroidectomy and lymphadenectomy. Four months later, she was readmitted because of recurrent swelling in the neck. This longitudinal scan of the neck shows three lymph nodes (arrows), all involved with papillary carcinoma. It is interesting that each node shows a different ultrasonic pattern. The most superior is relatively lucent, the middle node is uniformly echogenic, and the most inferior of the nodes has a lucent center. We have no explanation for this appearance, as the histologic examinations of all the nodes were similar.

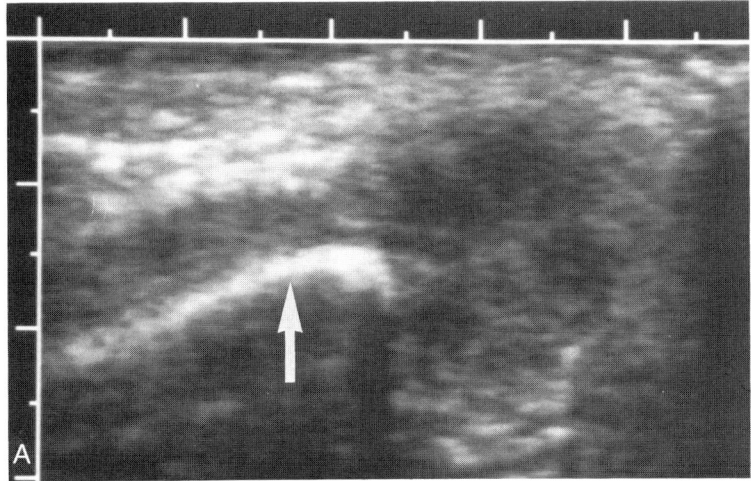

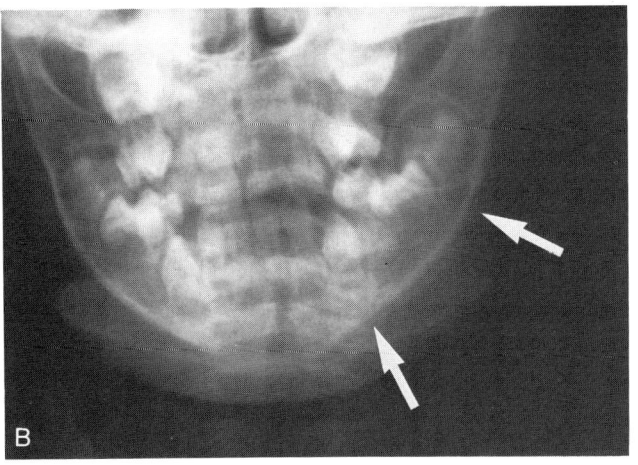

Figure 3–5. Before her admission with an enlarging right neck mass, this 17-month-old girl had fever, an upper respiratory infection, and right otitis media. Radiographs were obtained after a sonogram (**A**) showed a mass of mixed echogenicity immediately adjacent to the mandible (arrow). The radiograph (**B**) shows periosteal reaction (arrows) along the border of the mandible. Aspiration of the mass revealed *S. aureus*. The abscess may have arisen from the submandibular gland or may have been related to cervical adenitis adjacent to the mandible.

SALIVARY GLANDS AND SINUSES

Although in published articles authors have discussed ultrasonography of the salivary glands and masses related to them, imaging with computed tomography (CT; preferably with antecedent sialography) or magnetic resonance imaging (MRI) allows finer detail of the ductal anatomy, the position of the mass in relation to the facial nerve, and the delineation and characterization of the mass. However, if one is stuck on a desert island with nothing but an ultrasonographic machine, it helps if that machine is equipped with a transducer of high frequency and with linear array. Seibert and Seibert (1986, 1988) have written elegant articles on the techniques required for ultrasonographic evaluation of the parotid gland. Transverse views, perpendicular to the patient's ear, rely on two posterior and two anterior landmarks: a muscle and a shadowing bone. The anterior landmarks are the masseter muscle and the mandible; the posterior landmarks are the sternocleidomastoid muscle and the tip of the mastoid. Coronal scans are oriented parallel to the mandibular ramus, just anterior to the external ear. Normal parotid tissue is coarsely echogenic, appearing similar to normal pancreatic tissue (Fig. 3–6). Enlarged intraparotid lymph nodes present as lucent masses within the substance of the gland. A parotid abscess may occur as the lymph node suppurates (Fig. 3–7). Chronic parotitis is usually associated with sialectasis. The ultrasonic appearance is usually of multiple interfaces within the gland and thus an echogenic pattern that is coarser than normal (Lewis et al., 1989), although hypoechogenicity has also been described (Rubaltelli et al., 1987). Parotid masses are extremely rare in children. The most common is probably hemangioma, which has a variable degree of vascularity (color plate III). Angiomatous malformations are more likely to have large supplying and draining vessels and to be associated with flow rates of high velocity. Malformations rarely involute, whereas the typical hemangioma, after an initial increase in size, gradually regresses as the child ages. Stones in the salivary ducts are unusual in children, but if they do occur, they tend to be in the submaxillary duct of Wharton. Ultrasonography has been used to diagnose calculi in this location (Grünebaum et al., 1985).

The current status of ultrasonography vis-à-vis the diagnosis of sinus disease is controversial, to say the least. Our review of the literature suggests that ultrasonography is as unreliable as plain radiography (Reilly et al., 1989; Revonta and Kuuliala, 1989; Trigaux et

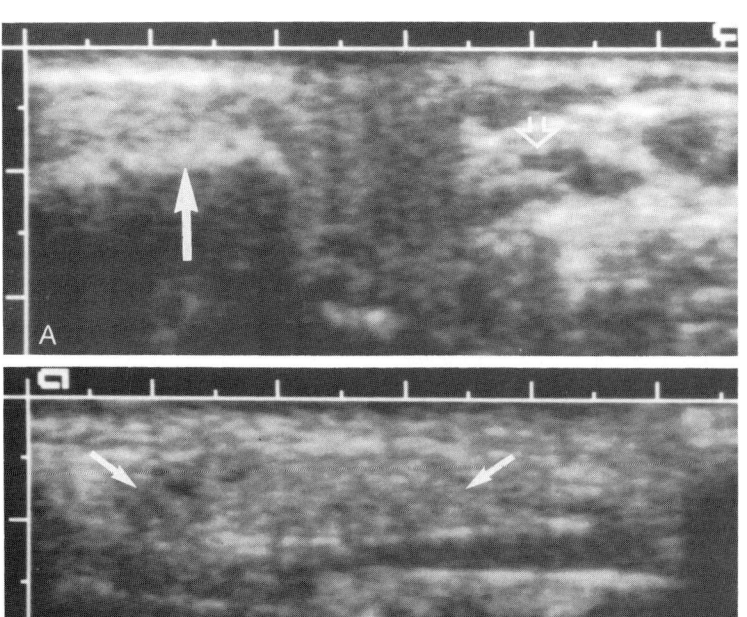

Figure 3–6. This transverse scan (A) of the normal parotid gland shows the parotid tissue as mildly echogenic in between the mandible anteriorly (arrow) and the sternocleidomastoid muscle and the tip of the mastoid posteriorly (open arrow). The coronal scan (B) shows the parotid gland as an oval mass (arrows) anterior to the masseter muscle.

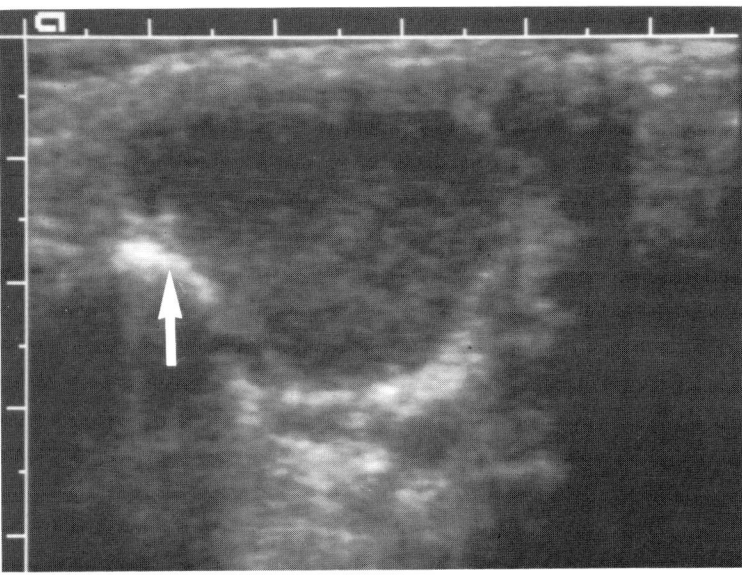

Figure 3–7. Transverse view of the parotid gland in this 9-year-old boy, who contracted infection with the human immunodeficiency virus (HIV) from his mother, shows no normal parotid glandular tissue. Arrow points to the mandible. He had had intermittent episodes of parotitis over the past 2 years. Before admission, he had developed increased swelling and pain. On clinical examination, the parotid gland was found to be fluctuant. He was treated with antibiotics without improvement. Ten cubic centimeters of brown serous fluid was aspirated from this parotid abscess, but cultures yielded no growth, probably because of earlier therapy with antibiotics.

al., 1988; Wald, 1988). A drawback to many of the studies is their comparison of ultrasonographic findings with the radiographic findings and not with sinuscopy or aspiration. We have yet to be convinced that ultrasonographic study of the sinuses is worthwhile.

THYROID AND PARATHYROID

In 1983, Bachrach and colleagues reported the ultrasonographic findings in 55 children who had thyroid disease. No recent developments have altered their conclusions, which, paraphrased, were as follows:

1. For some hypothyroid patients, thyroid tissue is poorly detected on radionuclide scans. Ultrasonography establishes the presence or absence of glandular tissue.
2. Ultrasonography is of limited usefulness in evaluating diffuse disease of the thyroid, such as Hashimoto thyroiditis and Grave disease.
3. Purely cystic masses are almost always benign. Needle aspiration with cytologic examination of the aspirate, with hormonal suppression, and with clinical follow-up is appropriate therapy.
4. Complex or solid nodules may be malignant. The likelihood of malignancy varies with the incidence of previous radiotherapy in the population of patients who are referred.

We add two further comments to this list:

5. Correlation with nuclear medicine scans is useful. Most malignant masses are cold or faintly warm on radionuclide study. Only a few cases of hot carcinoma have been reported (Fisher, 1976).
6. Family history of thyroid tumor and unusual appearance of the patient (marfanoid habitus; neuromas on the tongue, lips, and eyelids) are signs of multiple endocrine neoplasia (MEN), type III. Medullary carcinoma is associated with this syndrome. Parathyroid hyperplasia (and pheochromocytoma) is associated with medullary carcinoma in MEN, type II (Kaufman et al., 1982; McKusick, 1983).

The anatomy of a child's thyroid gland, with its relationships to great vessels, superficial musculature, and the trachea, is no different from an adult's. A baby's neck is more difficult to scan because it is short. Transverse scans from the suprasternal notch to the hyoid bone are followed by longitudinal scans of each lobe. A mass is identified as intrathyroidal or extrathyroidal, is measured, and is then classified as cystic, solid, or mixed.

A true simple cyst of the thyroid is quite rare. A cyst in the isthmus or pyramidal lobe may be a cyst of the thyroglossal duct. Ninety percent of these cysts are at or below the hyoid bone, and they present in the midline or slightly to the left of the midline. The thyroglossal tract passes from the foramen caecum in the back of the tongue to the left-sided pyramidal lobe, which itself is a remnant of the tract. In a large study of 300 children, median age at diagnosis was 5½ years, most lesions were 1 to 3 cm in diameter, and 45 percent of the cysts were inflamed at the time of surgery (Solomon and Rangecroft, 1984). Ultrasonography of a thyroglossal cyst shows a cystic mass that contains some echoes, as the fluid characteristically resembles the white of an egg. If it is infected, a complex mass may result (Fig. 3–8).

Primary abscess of the thyroid is distinctly unusual. The clinical presentation of infective thyroiditis is of pain, tenderness, dysphagia, hoarseness, local warmth, and systemic fever. Needle aspiration, under ultrasonic guidance, as with cervical adenopathy, could be done if an area becomes fluctuant, but we have not yet encountered such a situation. Localized abscess or inflammation of the left lobe of the thyroid is more likely to be secondary to a fistula from the pyriform sinus than from a primary thyroidal infection. Radiographs taken after the patient swallows barium usually show the sinus tract extending from the lowest portion of the pyriform sinus (Miller et al., 1983).

Hemorrhagic cyst may result from bleeding into an adenoma or may be a secondary result of blunt trauma to the neck. The follicular adenoma is a benign neoplasm; however, its ultrasonic features of lower echogenicity, in comparison with the parenchyma of the thyroid, and a surrounding sonolucent halo are not always present and are not pathognomonic when they appear on the scans (Fig. 3–9; Butch et al., 1985). Degeneration of an adenoma results in a mixed solid/cystic lesion (Fig. 3–10). The ultrasonic appearance of malignant tumors is similar to that of benign masses (Figs. 3–11, 3–12). The rate of malignancy in children who have thyroidal nodules varies between 14 and 40 percent, depending on the referral center and the incidence, amount, and type of previous irradiation of the neck in the population studied (Hung et al., 1982). A mean interval of 8.5 years between radiotherapy and diagnosis of thyroidal malignancy has been calculated from pooled studies. Previously irradiated children also have an increased number of benign thyroidal tumors in comparison with normal controls (Fig. 3–9; Favus et al., 1976; Hemplemann et al., 1979).

In children, diffuse thyroidal disease such as Hashimoto thyroiditis is best diagnosed with serologic studies. Ultrasonography is relatively nonspecific and does not lead to any change in clinical management (Fig. 3–13; Bachrach et al., 1983).

Parathyroid adenomas are distinctly unusual in children but may present as palpable masses in an adolescent. Typically, however, a patient is being evaluated for symptoms such as fatigue and constipation when routine laboratory tests of calcium and phosphorus in serum direct clinical attention to the parathyroid glands. Children with chronic renal failure develop secondary hyperparathyroidism, which sometimes evolves into an autonomously functioning nodule. The mean size of normal glands is $5 \times 3 \times 1$ mm. The two superior glands (derivatives of the fourth

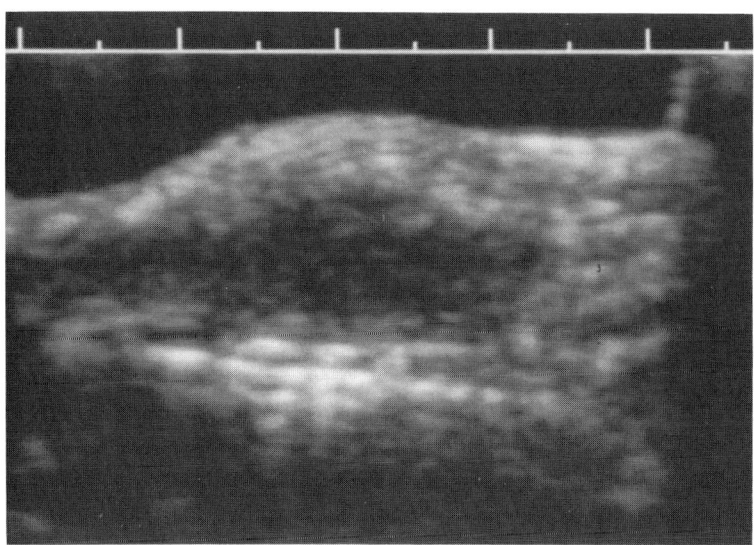

Figure 3–8. Cystic mass in the midline of the neck inferior to the hyoid is the typical presentation of a thyroglossal cyst. In this 5-year-old girl, the mass seemed to come and go, probably as the thyroglossal duct was intermittently obstructed. At surgery, an inflamed cyst of the thyroglossal duct, along with the tract that passes to the base of the tongue, was removed.

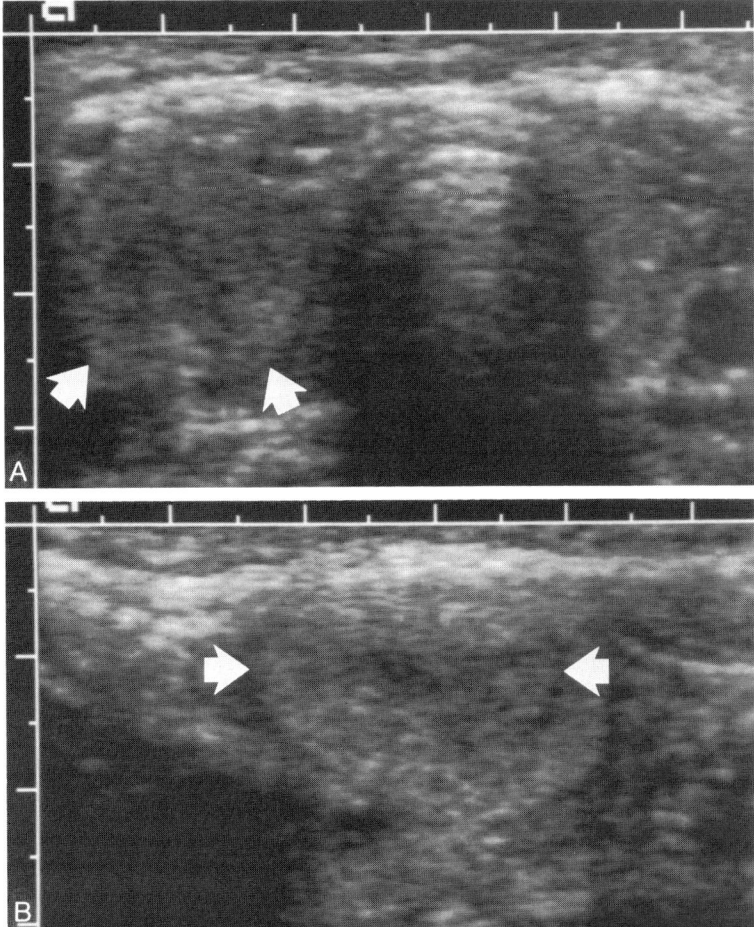

Figure 3–9. This woman had been followed at our hospital for 15 years after radiotherapy for lymphosarcoma of the neck. When she returned at age 32 with a right thyroidal mass, there was concern that this was a malignant lesion. The mass (arrows) shown on the transverse section **(A)** was in the right lobe of the thyroid. On the longitudinal section **(B)** it appeared to have a relatively lucent halo around it. Right thyroidectomy was performed, and an adenoma was removed. Both benign and malignant thyroidal masses are associated with earlier radiotherapy of the gland.

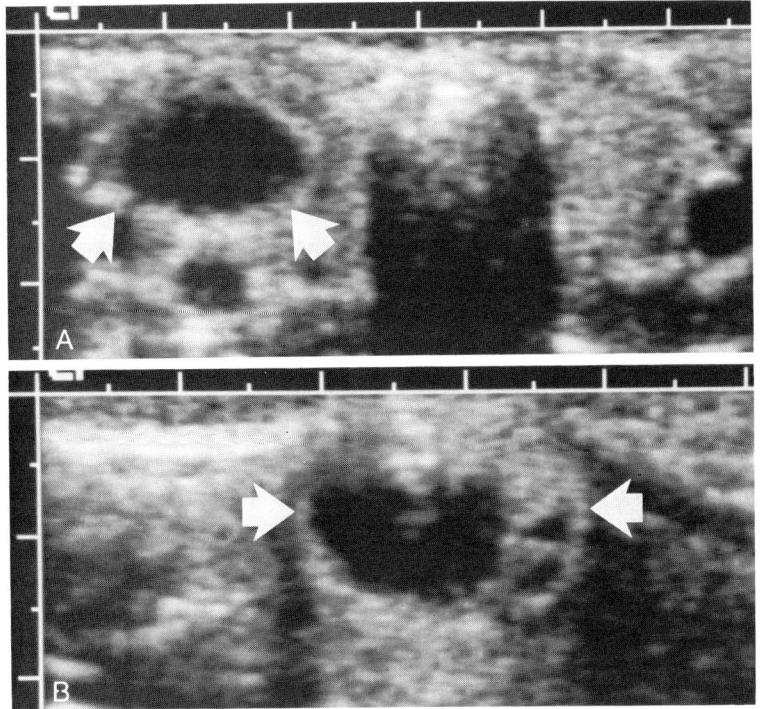

Figure 3–10. A right hemithyroidectomy was performed on this child after these scans, which showed an unusual mass in the thyroid gland. The transverse view **(A)** shows that the mass (arrows) is relatively cystic. The longitudinal view **(B)** provides more information by showing the associated solid component. Pathologic examination revealed cystic degeneration of an adenoma.

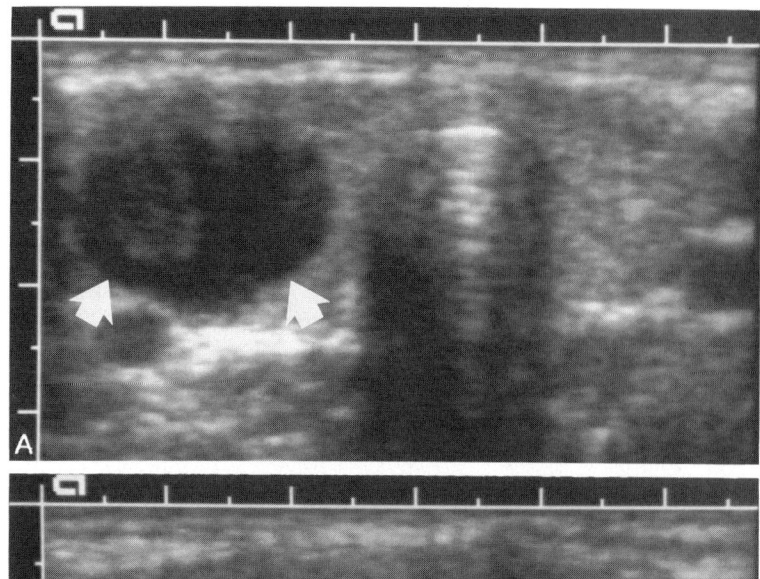

Figure 3–11. A 1-year history of a right-sided nodule that fluctuated in size was the impetus for this ultrasonogram after a radionuclide study that showed a cold area in the right lobe. The mass (arrows) on transverse (**A**) and longitudinal (**B**) scans shows a nodular mass within a cyst. Pathologic examination after its removal showed this to be a benign follicular goiter.

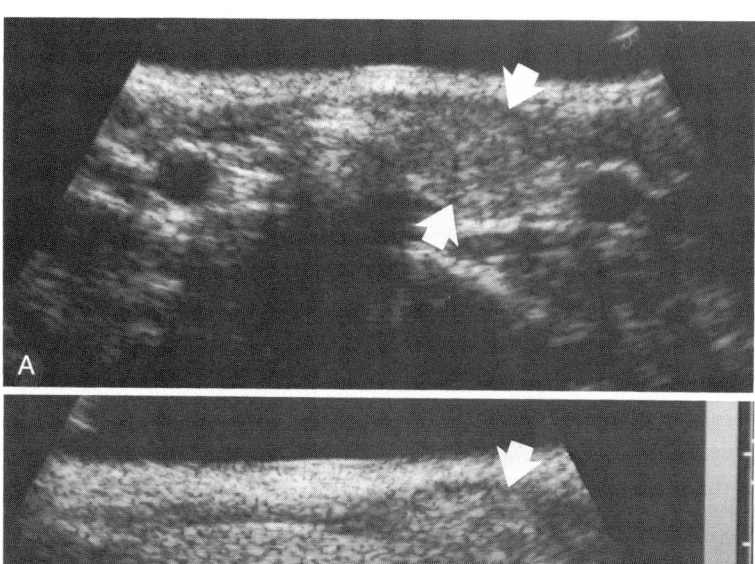

Figure 3–12. This mass (arrows), which on transverse (**A**) and longitudinal (**B**) scans extends inferiorly from the left lower edge of the thyroid gland, had been discovered during a routine school physical of this 12-year-old boy. The mass was cold on radionuclide scanning. A left-sided subtotal thyroidectomy was performed. Histologic examination revealed a mixed papillary-follicular carcinoma that was metastatic to lymph nodes.

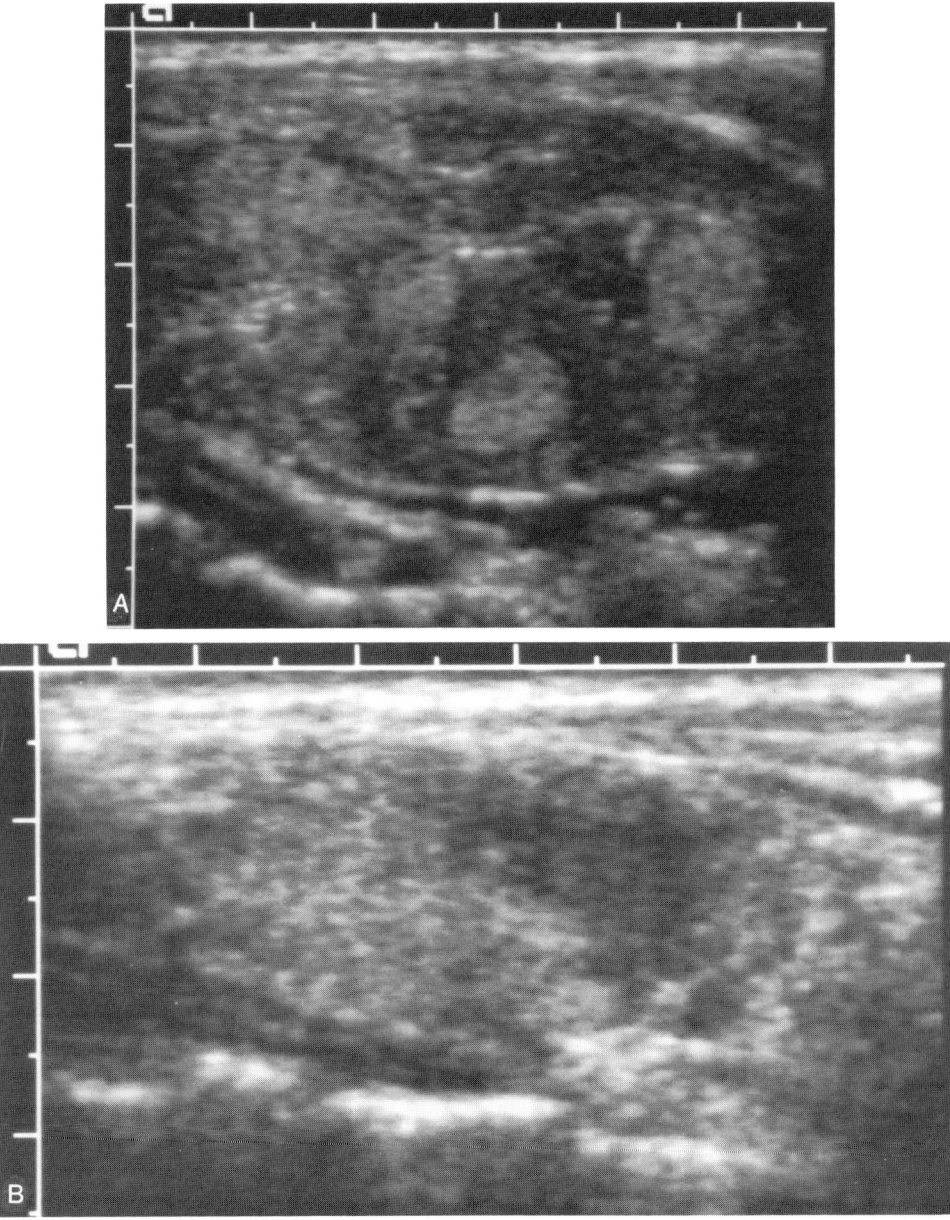

Figure 3-13. These longitudinal scans are from two patients, both of whom have diffuse disease of the thyroid. **A** is of an adolescent boy who has hyperplastic multinodular goiter. The echogenic areas represent colloid, which fills cysts. **B** is of an adolescent girl who had asymptomatic swelling and this patchy appearance of her thyroid gland on ultrasonography. She proved to have Hashimoto thyroiditis.

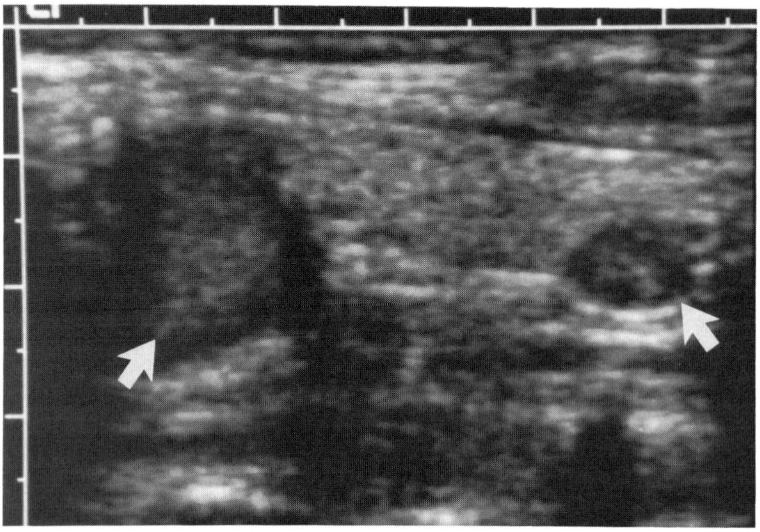

Figure 3-14. This 20-year-old male, undergoing dialysis for chronic renal failure, had clinical signs and laboratory evidence of secondary hyperparathyroidism. Longitudinal scan of the right side of the neck shows enlargement of superior and inferior parathyroid glands (arrows), which are hypoechoic in relation to the adjacent thyroidal tissue. The left-sided glands were similarly enlarged.

branchial pouch) lie in the dorsum of the upper lobes. The inferior glands are variable in location and may actually migrate into the chest with the thymus, which is derived from the third branchial pouch.

Proving that all glands are present and that they are hyperplastic (i.e., large for the child's age) is an ultrasonographic challenge indeed. Hospital centers that have large nephrology units or are scanning many adult patients are experienced in parathyroid ultrasonography and report great success rates (Fig. 3-14; Butch et al., 1985).

VESSELS

Venous aneurysm or phlebectasia of the jugular vein is characterized by a variably sized mass that changes caliber with changes in intrathoracic pressure (Hughes et al., 1988; Zohar et al., 1989; Kovanlikaya et al., 1990). Children who have this anomaly find out, very quickly, that they can amaze their classmates by doing a Valsalva maneuver, which enlarges the mass quite dramatically. Ultrasonography is an ideal method by which to show the venous nature and relationships of this type of mass, before and during a Valsalva maneuver (Fig. 3-15).

Arterial anomalies and acquired disease of carotid arteries are extremely rare (Lewis et al., 1989). We may gain more experience when more babies who have had division of the right carotid artery for extracorporeal membrane oxygenation (ECMO) come to us after surgical reconstruction of the vessel (Fig. 3-16). A few unusual children have had congenital development of a cervical, as opposed to a thoracic, aortic arch (Felson and Strife, 1989). Ultrasonography should show the arterial nature of this pulsatile mass in the base of the neck.

CONNECTIVE TISSUES

The following is an eclectic collection of masses, many of which occur only in children or tend to be diagnosed in childhood.

Cystic hygroma (termed lymphangioma or, more accurately, lymphatic malformation) is a septated cystic mass that presents anywhere in the neck but most often in the posterior triangle. Acute hemorrhage into the mass leads to an acute increase in size, which may in turn cause compromise of the airway (Fig. 3-17). The uncomplicated cystic hygroma is an infiltrative, multilocular, echolucent mass. If it is anything but superficial on ultrasonic scans, CT or MRI scan is better able to delineate its deep involvement. Unless it is completely removed, the mass regrows.

Depending on the amount of stromal tissue, hemangiomas have mixed appearances on ultrasonograms (Fig. 3-18). Flow of blood may be sluggish but occasionally can be appreciated with color Doppler scanning. CT or MRI is helpful in questionable cases.

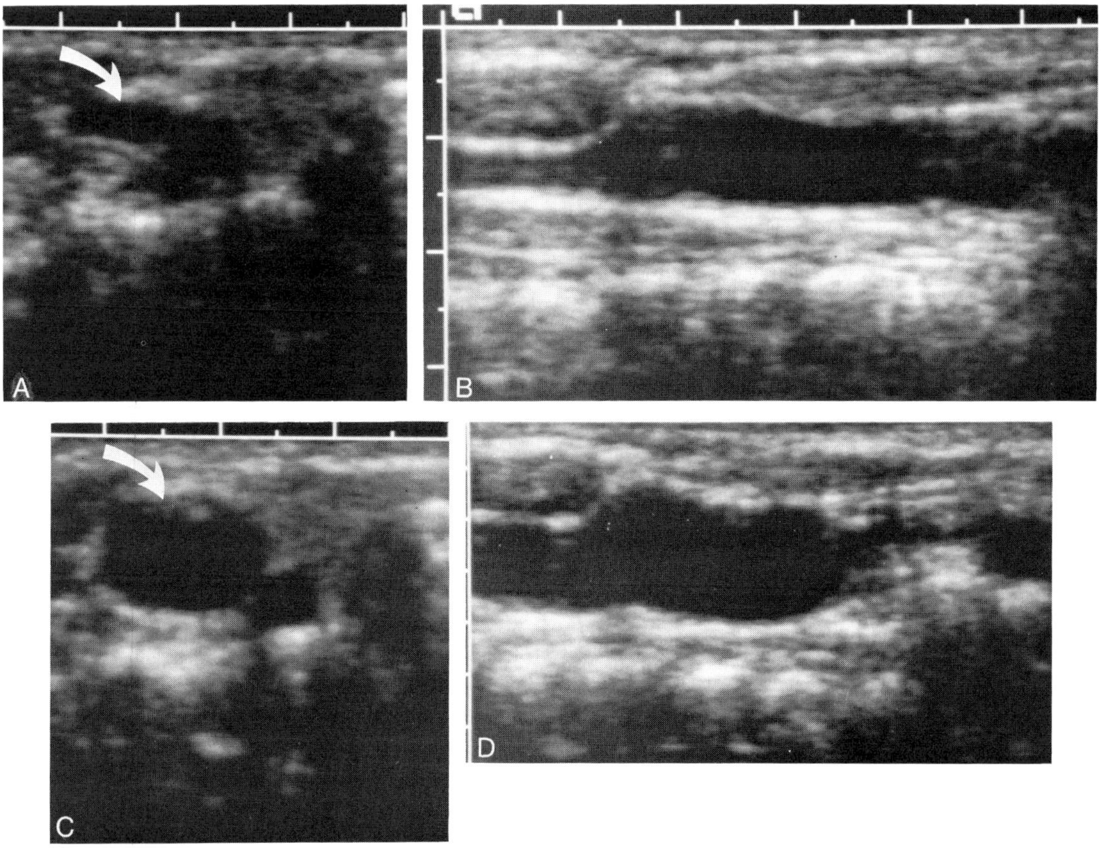

Figure 3–15. The parents of this 3-year-old boy noticed that his neck swelled dramatically when he coughed. Fluoroscopy of the neck was normal. Transverse and longitudinal scans during quiet breathing (**A** and **B**) and during cough (**C** and **D**) show that the mass was aneurysmal dilatation of the jugular vein. Arrow points to the vein on transverse scans. In general, this is otherwise asymptomatic, and removal of the phlebectasia is done only for cosmetic reasons.

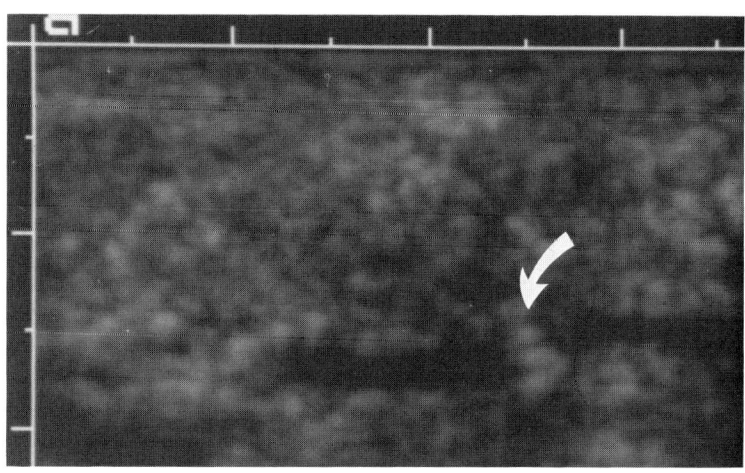

Figure 3–16. This baby girl had surgical reconstruction of the common carotid artery after extracorporeal membrane oxygenation (ECMO). The site of anastomosis is apparent as a linear interface (arrow) across the lumen on this longitudinal view of the vessel.

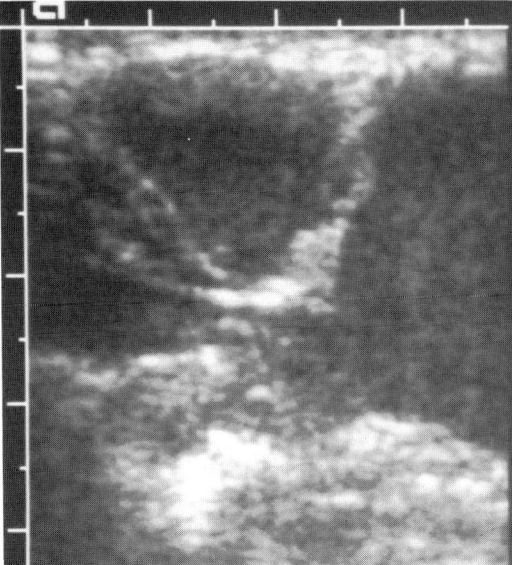

Figure 3–17. This 10-week-old boy had been diagnosed as having cystic hygroma (lymphatic malformation) of the left side of the neck. He returned to the hospital when he began to have intermittently noisy breathing. Longitudinal scan of the mass shows diffuse echogenicity, which, on real-time scans, swirled within and between the individual locules. Hemorrhage into the mass had occurred; this probably increased the size of the mass and resulted in further compression of the trachea.

Branchial cleft cysts develop from remnants of the first and second branchial clefts. A cyst from the first branchial cleft arises near the angle of the jaw and may be mistaken for a parotid mass or adenopathy. A cyst from the second branchial cleft is more common and is usually near the anterior border of the upper third of the sternocleidomastoid muscle. Cholesterol crystals in the fluid are characteristic. These may cause the cyst to appear echogenic. Infection typically brings the patient to medical attention; the mass then has the appearance of an abscess.

The thymus is derived from the third branchial pouch and occasionally may have an aberrant location, presenting as a mass in the neck (Fig. 3–19).

In contrast to a cyst of the thyroglossal duct, a dermoid cyst tends to occur above the hyoid bone. The presence of dermal appendages, fat, and keratin results in the appearance of a solid-looking mass on ultrasonography. Calcification in a solid mass suggests teratoma or neuroblastoma (Fig. 3–20). A cystic component and shardlike calcification support the diagnosis of teratoma, but in the individual case, diagnosis rests with the pathologists.

Rhabdomyosarcoma may arise in the muscles of the neck and present as a locally infiltrative mass. Calcification may be present in a necrotic center.

Fibromatosis colli is a poorly understood disorder of neonates. It is defined as fusiform swelling of the sternocleidomastoid muscle associated with torticollis. The mass is within the belly of the muscle, spindle shaped, and usually of uniformly lower echogenicity than its surroundings (Fig. 3–21; Crawford et al., 1988). Long-term follow-up of these babies vis-à-vis ultrasonograms is unreported. The major differential diagnosis is rhabdomyosarcoma or some other tumor of soft tissues, but experienced clinicians are usually able to diagnose fibromatosis colli on clinical grounds.

A laryngocele is an unusual remnant of the primitive air sac. It presents as a deflatable air-filled cyst at the side of the neck. If scanned, it would produce a confusing picture of gas artifact. Fluoroscopy of the neck is diagnostic. A pyocele results when the cyst becomes obstructed.

Ultrasonographic evaluation of the larynx is unlikely to replace laryngoscopy, but it can be a useful adjunctive study (Garel et al., 1990). A child must be able to cooperate by lying still, extending the neck, and breathing and vocalizing on command. A high-frequency linear array transducer is placed transversely across the upper neck. Use of time-equivalent material results in beautiful pictures if it can be held stationary; often a thick cushion of gel suffices. The true vocal cords form an inverted "V" with abduction (deep inspiration) and move into more parallel alignment with adduction (vocalization; Fig. 3–22). The arytenoids are small acoustic reflectors posterior to the cords. When one cord is paralyzed, there is asymmetric adduction. The paralyzed cord and the hemilarynx fail to move medially and, to some degree, anteriorly, in comparison with the normal side.

Because ultrasonography is hampered by air within the pharynx, larynx, and trachea, it is not a reliable method with which to evaluate masses related to the airway.

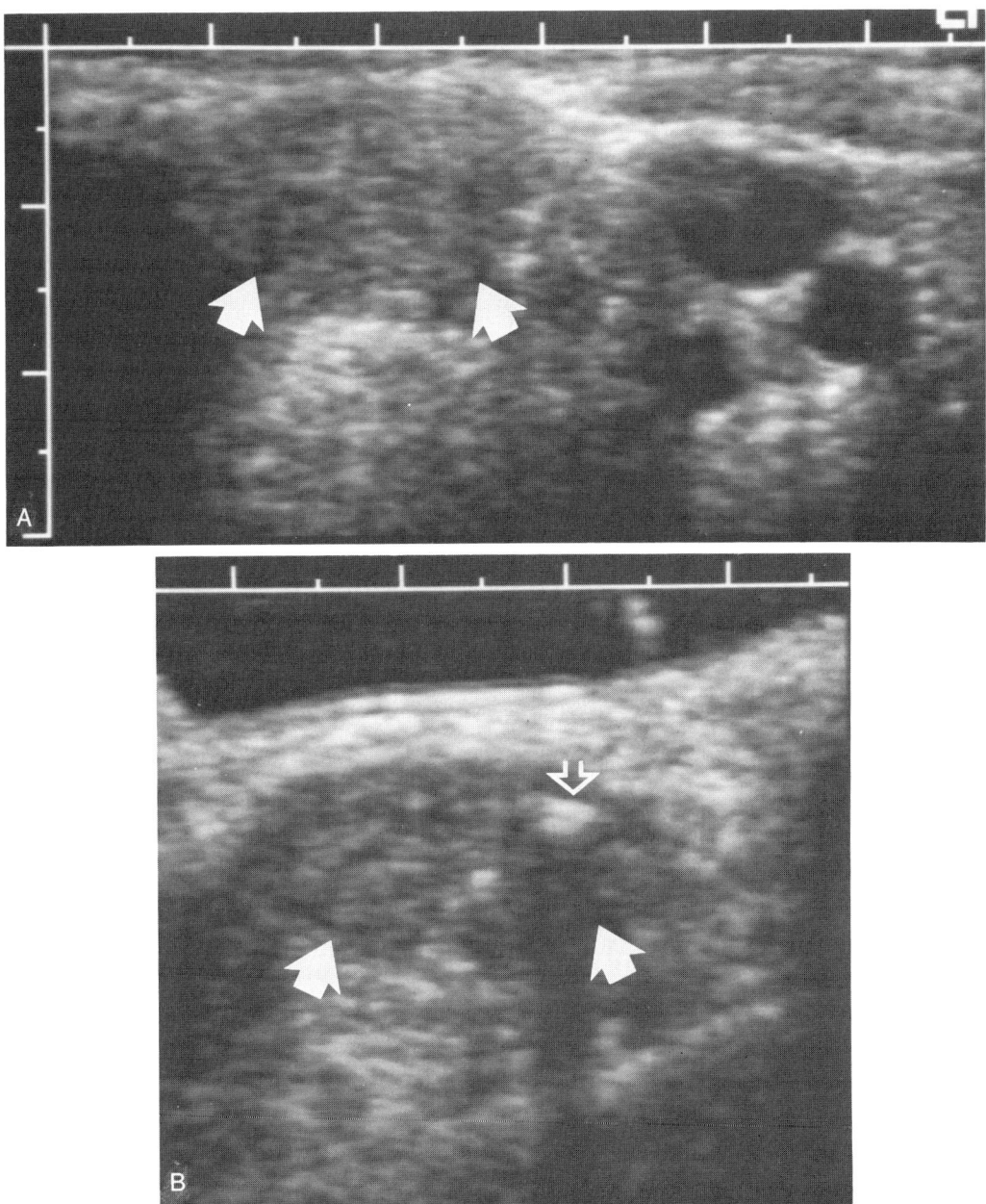

Figure 3–18. Scans shown are of a right-sided supraclavicular mass (arrows) that in most cross sections (A) has a homogeneous pattern. In one portion of the mass (B), there is a well-defined calcification (open arrow). This represents a phlebolith in this venous malformation. Flow was too sluggish to be detectable on duplex Doppler scanning.

88 / THE FACE AND NECK

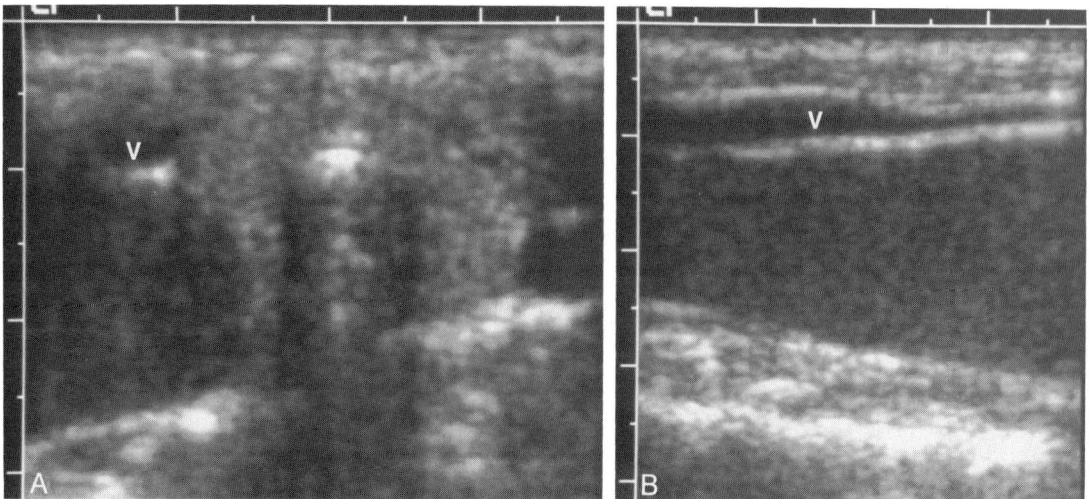

Figure 3–19. Ultrasonic pattern of a mass, shown on transverse (A) and longitudinal (B) views of the right side of the neck, is identical to that of normal thymus. In fact, this is ectopic thymus in a 7-year-old who presented with a mass in the right neck. Compression of the jugular vein (V) by the ectopic thymus had resulted in a venous hum.

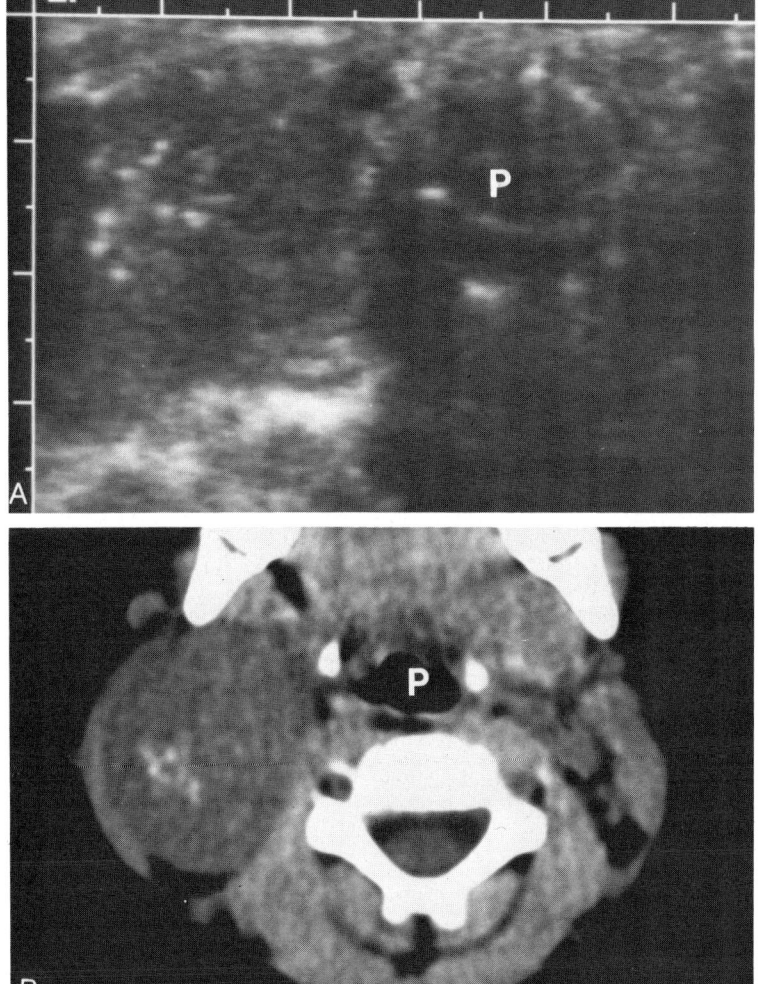

Figure 3–20. The ultrasonographic section (A) is at the same level as the subsequent CT scan (B). Both show calcification within a solid mass. This 14-month-old had presented with a 4- to 5-month history of right-sided swelling that was nontender. At surgery, neuroblastoma metastatic to one out of four lymph nodes was removed. Bone marrow was negative. Irregular calcifications within a mass usually are from teratoma or neuroblastoma. P = pharynx.

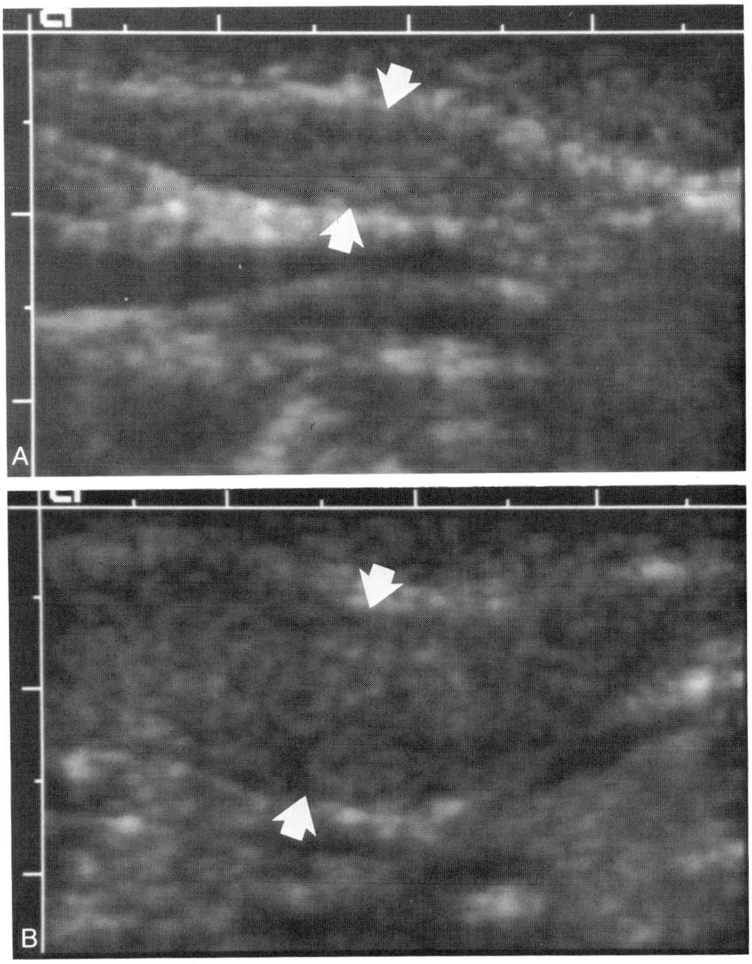

Figure 3-21. Asymptomatic swelling in the right side of the neck of this 2-week-old boy resolved spontaneously over the next few months. The ultrasonogram of the normal left side of the neck (A) shows the normal appearance of the sternocleidomastoid muscle (arrows). The longitudinal scan of the right side of the neck (B) shows the thickening of the sternocleidomastoid muscle (arrows), which is typical of fibromatosis colli.

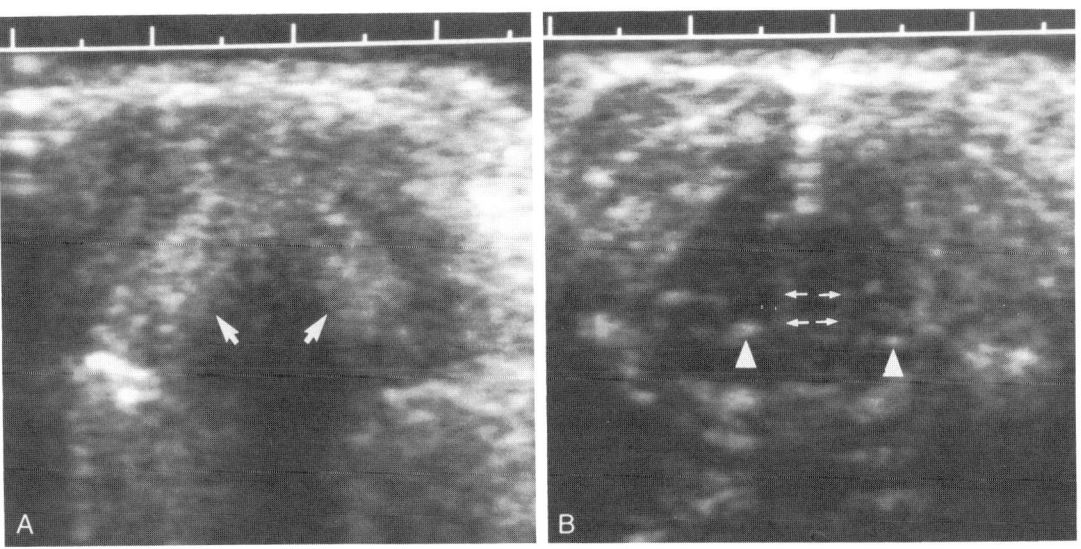

Figure 3-22. Transverse view of the larynx shows the echogenic false vocal cords (arrows, A). The true cords are less echogenic bands (arrows, B), which are slightly apart during quiet breathing. Arrowheads point to arytenoid cartilages.

REFERENCES

Salivary Glands and Sinuses

Grünebaum M, Ziv N, Mankuta DJ: Submaxillary sialadenitis with a calculus in infancy diagnosed by ultrasonography. Pediatr Radiol 1985; 15:191–192.

Hawkins DB: Advances in sinus disease in pediatrics. Otolaryngol Clin North Am 1989; 22:553–568.

Lewis GJS, Leithiser RE Jr, Glasier CM, et al: Ultrasonography of pediatric neck masses. Ultrasound Quarterly 1989; 7:315–355.

Reilly JS, Hotaling AJ, Chiponis D, et al: Use of ultrasound in detection of sinus disease in children. Int J Pediatr Otorhinolaryngol 1989; 17:225–230.

Revonta M, Kuuliala I: The diagnosis and follow-up of pediatric sinusitis: Water's view radiography versus ultrasonography. Laryngoscope 1989; 99:321–324.

Rubaltelli L, Sponga T, Candiani F, et al: Infantile recurrent sialectatic parotitis: The role of sonography and sialography in diagnosis and follow-up. Br J Radiol 1987; 60:1211–1214.

Seibert RW, Seibert JJ: High resolution ultrasonography of the parotid gland in children. Pediatr Radiol 1986; 16:374–379.

Seibert RW, Seibert JJ: High resolution ultrasonography of the parotid gland in children. Part II. Pediatr Radiol 1988; 19:13–18.

Trigaux JP, Bertrand BM, Van Beers BE: Comparison of B-mode ultrasound, radiography and sinuscopy in the diagnosis of maxillary sinusitis. Report on 177 cases. Acta Otorhinolaryngol 1988; 42:670–679.

Wald ER: Management of sinusitis in infants and children. Pediatr Infect Dis J 1988; 7:449–452.

Wittich GR, Scheible WF, Hajek PC: Ultrasonography of the salivary glands. Radiol Clin North Am 1985; 23:29–37.

Neck

Bachrach LK, Daneman D, Daneman A, et al: Use of ultrasound in childhood thyroid disorders. J Pediatr 1983; 103:547–552.

Brook I: The swollen neck. Cervical lymphadenitis, parotitis, thyroiditis and infected cysts. Infectious Dis Clin North Am 1988; 2:221–236.

Butch RJ, Simeone JF, Mueller PR: Thyroid and parathyroid ultrasonography. Radiol Clin North Am 1985; 23:57–71.

Clark OH, Stark DA, Duh QY, et al: Value of high resolution real-time ultrasonography in secondary hyperparathyroidism. Am J Surg 1985; 150:9–17.

Crawford SC, Harnsberger HR, Johnson L, et al: Fibromatosis colli of infancy: CT and sonographic findings. AJR 1988; 151:1183–1184.

Doi O, Hutson JM, Myers NA, et al: Branchial remnants: A review of 58 cases. J Pediatr Surg 1988; 23:789–792.

Favus MJ, Schneider AB, Stachura ME, et al: Thyroid cancer occurring as a late consequence of head-and-neck irradiation. Evaluation of 1056 patients. NEJM 1976; 294:1019–1025.

Felson B, Strife JL: Cervical aortic arch: A commentary. Semin Roentgenol 1989; 24:114–120.

Fisher DA: Thyroid nodules in childhood and their management. J Pediatr 1976; 89:866–868.

Friedman AP, Haller JO, Goodman JD, Nagar H: Sonographic evaluation of non-inflammatory neck masses in children. Radiology 1983; 147:693–697.

Garel C, Legrand I, Elmaleh M, et al: Laryngeal ultrasonography in infants and children: Anatomical correlation with fetal preparations. Pediatr Radiol 1990; 20:241–244.

Glasier CM, Seibert JJ, Williamson SL, et al: High resolution ultrasound characterization of soft tissue masses in children. Pediatr Radiol 1987; 17:233–237.

Hemplemann LH, Hall WJ, Phillips M, et al: Neoplasms in persons treated with x-rays in infancy: Fourth survey in 20 years. J Natl Cancer Inst 1979; 55:519–530.

Hughes PL, Qureshi SA, Galloway RW: Jugular venous aneurysm in children. Br J Radiol 1988; 61:1082–1084.

Kaufman FR, Roe TF, Isaacs H Jr, et al: Metastatic medullary thyroid carcinoma in young children with mucosal neuroma syndrome. Pediatrics 1982; 70:263–267.

Kraus R, Han BK, Babcock DS, et al: Sonography of neck masses in children. AJR 1986; 146:609–613.

Lerner PI: The lumpy jaw. Cervicofacial actinomycosis. Infectious Dis Clin North Am 1988; 2:203–220.

Lingle PA: Sonographic verification of endotracheal tube position in neonates. J Clin Ultrasound 1988; 16:605–609.

Mahoney CP: Differential diagnosis of goiter. Pediatr Clin North Am 1987; 34:891–905.

Miller D, Hill JL, Sun CC, et al: The diagnosis and management of pyriform sinus fistulae in infants and young children. J Pediatr Surg 1983; 18:377–381.

Muir A, Daneman D, Daneman A, et al: Thyroid scanning, ultrasound, and serum thyroglobulin in determining the origin of congenital hypothyroidism. Am J Dis Child 1988; 142:214–216.

Rapaport D, Ziv Y, Rubin M, et al: Primary hyperparathyroidism in children. J Pediatr Surg 1986; 21:395–397.

Salazar J, Dembrow V, Egozi I: A review of 265 cases of parathyroid explorations. Am Surg 1986; 52:174–176.

Sherman NH, Rosenberg HK, Heyman S, et al: Ultrasound evaluation of neck masses in children. J Ultrasound Med 1985; 4:127–134.

Solomon JR, Rangecroft L: Thyroglossal duct lesions in childhood. J Pediatr Surg 1984; 19:555–561.

Stewart RR, David CL, Eftekhari F, et al: Thyroid gland: US in patients with Hodgkin disease treated with radiation therapy in childhood. Radiology 1989; 172:159–163.

Zohar Y, Ben-Tovim R, Talmi YP: Phlebectasia of the jugular system. J Craniomaxillofac Surg 1989; 17:96–98.

CHAPTER 4

CHEST

The organ in the chest most amenable to ultrasonic evaluation is, of course, the heart. In most pediatric academic centers, cardiologists perform cardiac echography and integrate it with physiologic studies and angiography. In our institution, we are mindful of the cardiologists' territory, but we collaborate on research efforts and call on each other for help when ultrasonic geography is foreign. Because ultrasonography of the chest usually includes some of the heart on the edge of the films, it is worth knowing the standard four-chamber view, being able to assess the pericardial space, and being familiar with the anatomy of the great vessels (Fig. 4–1). If one recognizes that something looks truly odd, one can recommend deferring to the echocardiographer's expertise (Fig. 4–2).

Clinicians, who are looking at ultrasonic images on hard copy, have great difficulty orienting scans of the chest. After the ultrasonographer realizes the nature of the clinical problem at hand, scans should be planned so as to make each sheet of film a framed story. Some ultrasonographic units have anatomic cartoons that can be photographed with the image. Showing a normal image alongside an abnormal one is helpful. Because ultrasonography follows radiography of the chest, both sets of studies should be reviewed together to enhance the clinician's appreciation of the ultrasonic images.

Technique varies according to the clinical problem, the age of the child, and the child's ability to maintain certain positions. To gain access to pleural space and mediastinum, transducers have to fit between ribs. Normal air-filled lungs are definite walls to ultrasonic penetration. Subxiphoid, suprasternal, and parasternal windows to the mediastinum are available. Subdiaphragmatic views through liver and spleen are best for showing pleural fluid at the bases of the thorax. The larger the pleural collection is, the easier the examination. Views through inter-costal spaces from bottom to top of the chest as the child sits on the edge of the table enable one to map out the extent and character of the pleural contents. Linear array transducers and use of tissue-equivalent standoff material enhance evaluation of superficial masses of the chest wall.

PLEURAL EFFUSIONS

By far the most common reason for extracardiac ultrasonography of the chest is radiographic evidence of pleural density and the need to aspirate fluid for diagnosis. Aspiration is technically easy when the pleural collection is large and freely flowing. For small or loculated collections, ultrasonic-guided thoracentesis saves the child the pain of repeated attempts and saves the clinician

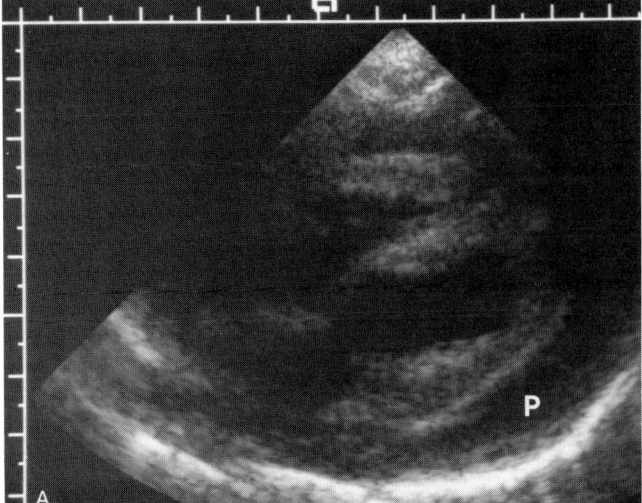
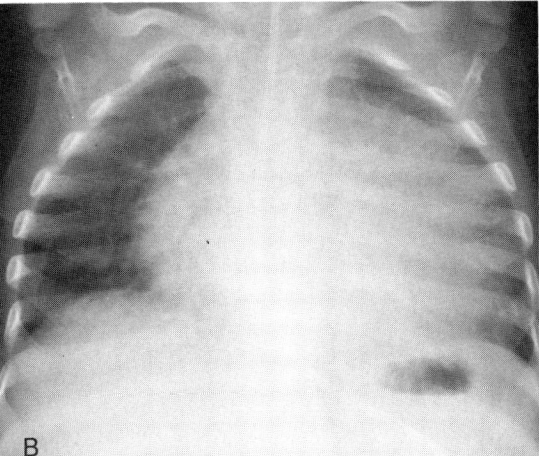
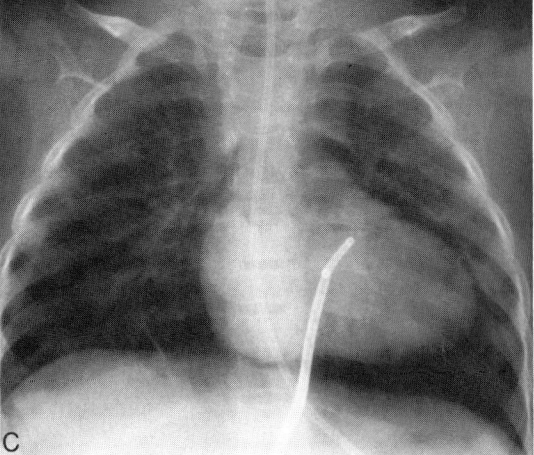

Figure 4–1. This 17-month-old boy had been followed for failure to thrive and hypothyroidism. Abnormal results from liver function tests prompted a request for abdominal ultrasonography. During this study, a large pericardial effusion (P) was noted (A). Review of the patient's chest radiograph (B) showed obvious enlargement of the cardiac silhouette, which had been attributed to simple cardiomegaly. Drainage of the pericardial effusion and instillation of air (C) was performed in an attempt to find a pericardial lesion that was causing the effusion. Follow-up testing has failed to reveal a definitive cause for this patient's pericardial fluid.

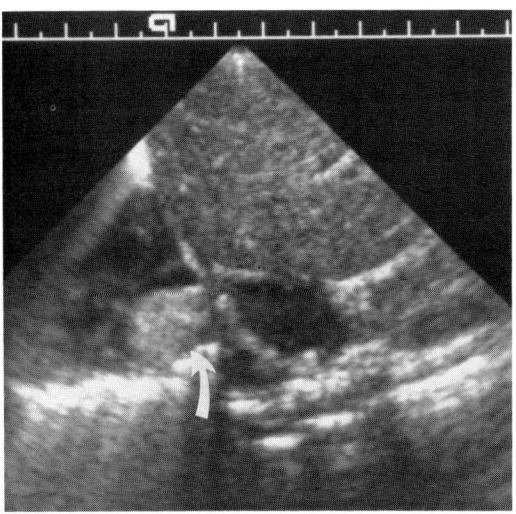

Figure 4–2. Ultrasonograms were performed on this 1-month-old after a right-sided congenital diaphragmatic hernia was repaired. During a search for subhepatic collections, the examiner noted a large echogenic focus (arrow) within the right atrium. This clot undoubtedly was caused by the venous catheter used during extracorporeal membrane oxygenation (ECMO). Further follow-up was arranged with the cardiologists. The clot decreased in size with streptokinase.

time and frustration. Fluid in the pleural space can be transudate, exudate, blood, chyle, intravenous fluid, or feedings. Review of available recent radiographs should precede ultrasonography. Tubes and catheters should be viewed with suspicion if they are on the same side of an acutely presenting pleural collection; for example, 10 premature neonates reported by Amodio and colleagues (1987) had iatrogenic collections of pleural fluid. They had hypopharyngeal perforation by feeding tube, chylothorax from superior vena caval obstruction, or hemothorax from inferior vena caval perforation, and all complications were related to catheters. We have also seen perforation of the subclavian vein and the right atrium by catheters.

Pneumonia in its early stages often causes a small pleural transudate. If antimicrobial therapy is inadequate or delayed, or if the host's defenses are compromised, the amount and content of protein in the pleural fluid (exudate) may increase, the fluid may become secondarily infected and loculated (fibrinopurulent), and then it may be invaded by fibroblasts and become a pleural rind. The ultrasonic findings parallel the pathophysiology. Questions to be answered while the scans are performed include the following: How much pleural material is present, and where is it? Is it freely flowing or loculated?

Is it clear (i.e., echofree), mildly echogenic, septated, or an echogenic rind? What is the appearance of the underlying lung vis-à-vis aeration, consolidation, abscess, or other mass (Figs. 4–3, 4–4)? Pathologists have used the term "hepatization" to describe the progression of pneumonia, and this term is also applicable to the ultrasonic picture of consolidation. Echogenic tubular structures within the consolidation are the air bronchograms of the radiographic representation of pneumonia. If the bronchi are filled with fluid, they appear as echolucent, branching tubes throughout the solid lung (Acunas et al., 1989). In order to evaluate the pleural space, good resolution in the near field is mandatory. Scans of the normal hemithorax allow one to estimate the thickness of the normal thoracic wall. Some muscular adolescents have remarkably thick soft tissues.

Bacterial infections associated with empyema, which is defined as a purulent exudate, include *Staphylococcus aureus, Haemophilus influenzae, Streptococcus pneumoniae,* microaerophilic streptococcus, and tuberculosis. Many children who have staphylococcal pneumonia have empyema, but the incidence of staphylococcal pneumonia in the U.S. has decreased dramatically. In contrast, the incidence of *H. influenzae* infections may be increasing, particularly in very young chil-

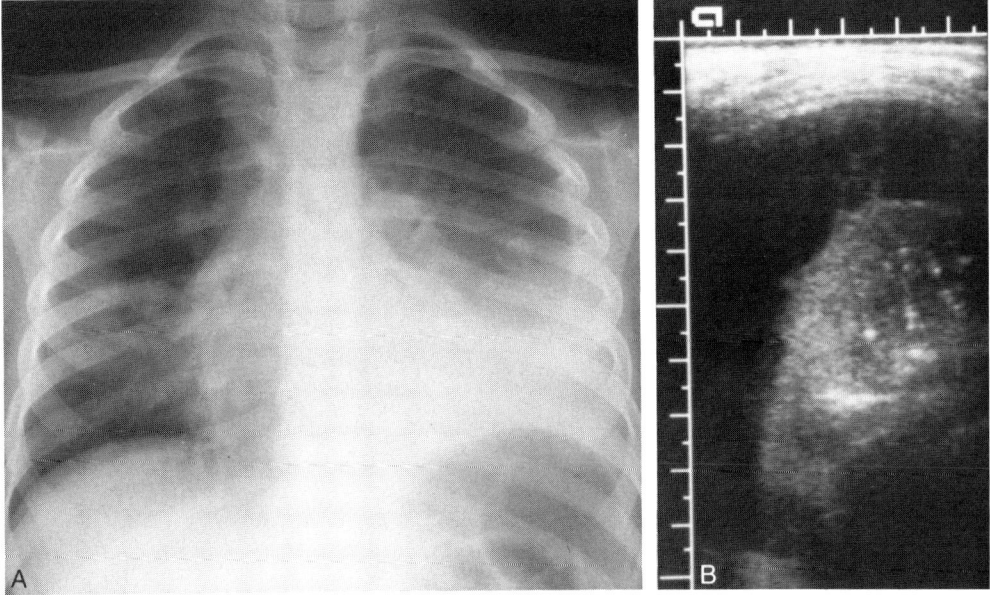

Figure 4–3. Upper respiratory infection progressed to pneumonia in this 3-year-old girl. Chest radiograph **(A)** shows the left-sided pleural effusion. This was drained, and cultures revealed *Streptococcus pneumoniae*. Treatment with antibiotics resulted in no further response. Transverse ultrasonogram **(B)** of the left lower thorax shows loculated fluid with few septi. A chest tube was placed for drainage, and the patient's symptoms resolved.

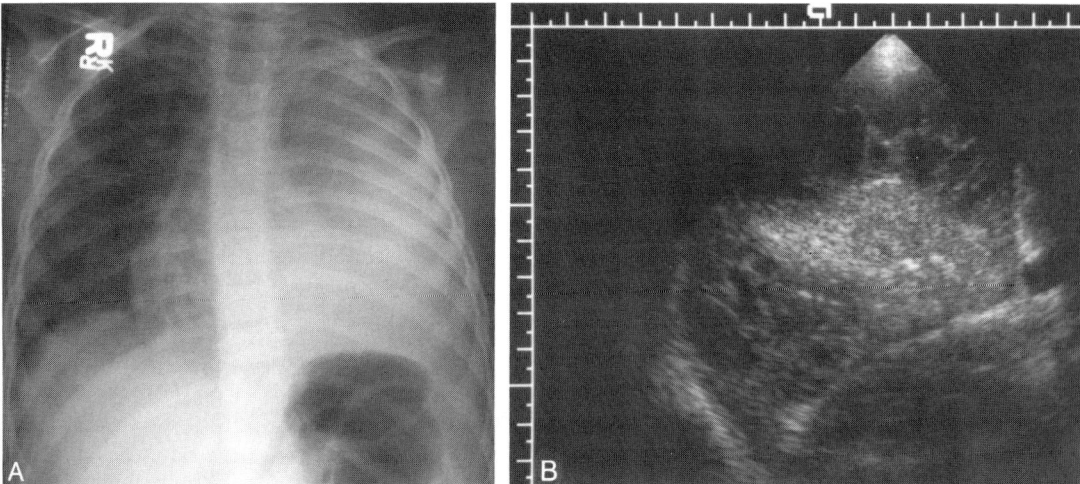

Figure 4–4. This 4-year-old boy had been given intravenous antibiotics for clinically documented pneumonia. Chest radiograph (A) shows a large left-sided effusion. Thoracentesis resulted in little fluid and no improvement of symptoms, and the patient was transferred to our hospital. Ultrasonogram (B) shows honeycomb appearance of the pleural fluid that was associated with poor aeration of the underlying lung; this appearance resembles the ultrasonographic picture of a normal liver. A chest tube was placed into the pleural space. Cultures yielded no organism in this patient.

dren. In one series, cultures of blood were positive in more than 50 percent of children with empyema, and cultures from pleural fluid were positive in almost all children with empyema (McLaughlin et al., 1984).

Transudate may be present in children with congestive heart failure, nephrotic syndrome, iatrogenic overload of fluid, and disorders of connective tissues (Figs. 4–5, 4–6). Subphrenic abscess can cause ipsilateral sympathetic pleural effusion; in rare instances, pancreatitis is associated with pleural effusion. Pulmonary or mediastinal tumor may obstruct lymphatic drainage to the hilum of the lung and result in chylous effusion. Cardiac and mediastinal surgery, which alters lymphatic drainage around the pulmonary hilum or thoracic duct, predisposes a patient to chylous effusion, which may then become superinfected (Fig. 4–7). Hemothorax results

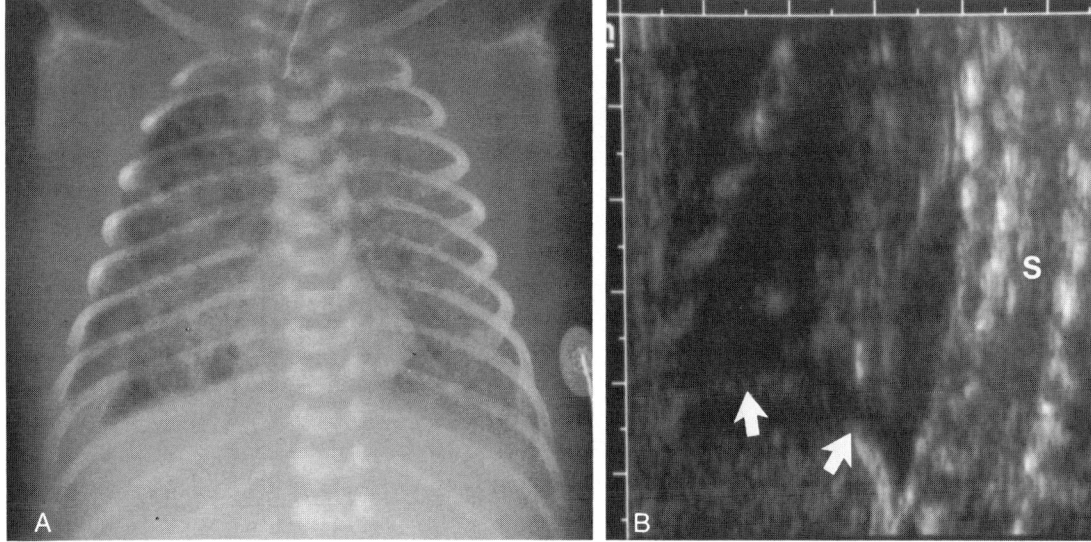

Figure 4–5. It was quite surprising to see the chest radiograph of this neonate (A) and then learn from ultransonography how much fluid was really present. The scan of the right hemithorax (B) is oriented to match the radiograph and shows pleural fluid encasing the lung. Arrows point to the diaphragm. S marks the spinal canal.

Figure 4–6. A right-sided pleural effusion was noted in this 3-year-old girl, who was undergoing abdominal ultrasonography for abdominal pain. The transverse ultrasonogram through the liver (A) shows pleural fluid at the right base. The diaphragm is marked by arrows. Note in B the thickened bowel wall (arrows) in the left flank; this thickening proved to be secondary to edema of the bowel associated with Henoch-Schönlein purpura. Vasculitis and disorders of connective tissues are associated with both pleural fluid and peritoneal fluid.

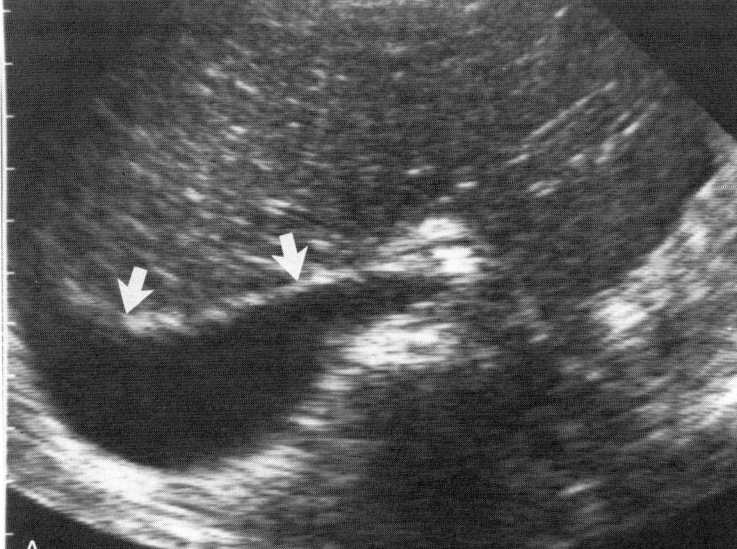

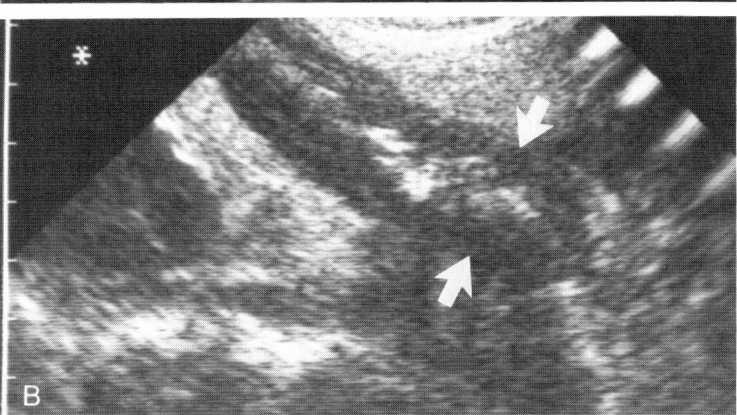

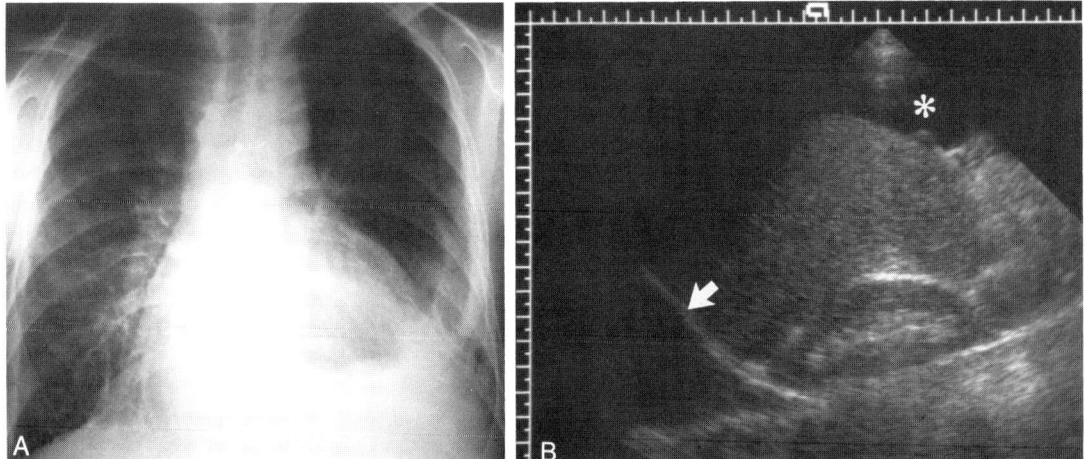

Figure 4–7. Pleural effusion is a common problem after cardiac surgery. This teenager, who had the Fontan procedure to treat single right ventricle with subaortic stenosis, has chronic pleural effusions (A). On the sagittal scan of the left upper quadrant (B), abdominal ascites is present (asterisk), as is pleural fluid. Arrow points to the diaphragm. Ascites is commonly associated with pleural effusions that follow the Fontan procedure.

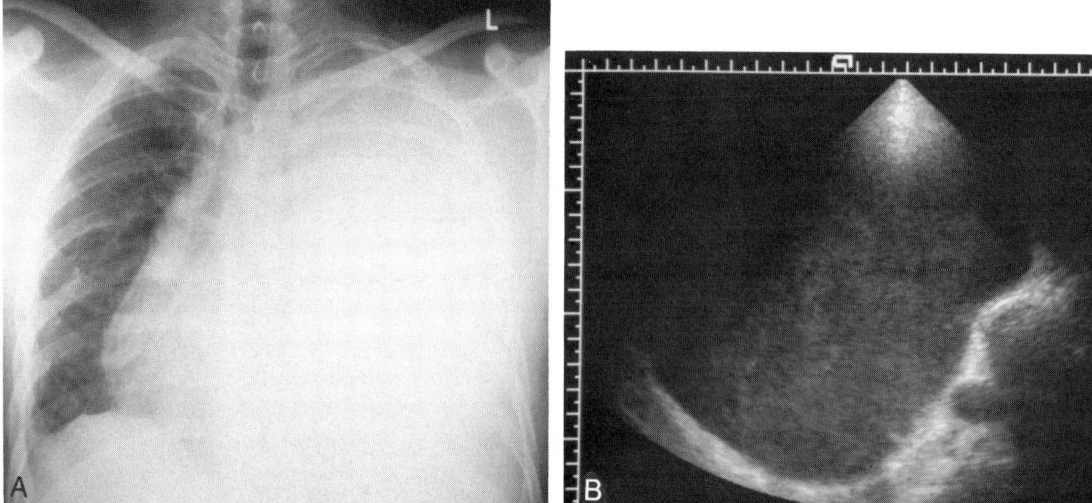

Figure 4–8. This young man had a long history of osteosarcoma, metastatic to the lung, that followed treatment for a left humeral Ewing sarcoma when he was 6. He presented with moderate dyspnea and complete opacification of the left hemithorax on the radiographs **(A)**. Ultrasonography was done immediately and showed a very echogenic collection of pleural fluid typical of hemorrhagic effusion associated with tumor **(B)**. Frankly bloody fluid was drained, and a subsequent biopsy of pleural tissue revealed, again, metastatic osteosarcoma.

from pulmonary embolus, trauma, bleeding diathesis, tumor, and occasionally infection (Fig. 4–8). Congenital thoracic cysts, bronchogenic or enteric, rarely rupture into the pleural space, but when they do, the affected child may present with a confusing clinical picture and pleural fluid.

The patient who presents with opacification of the hemithorax on initial radiographic examination is an ideal candidate for ultrasonography. Because our population of patients includes a large number of children who have a malignant condition, we have seen this situation arise when primary and, more often, secondary tumoral deposits involve most of the lung or pleura (Fig. 4–9). The scans can show whether pleural fluid is present and accessible to drainage (Fig. 4–

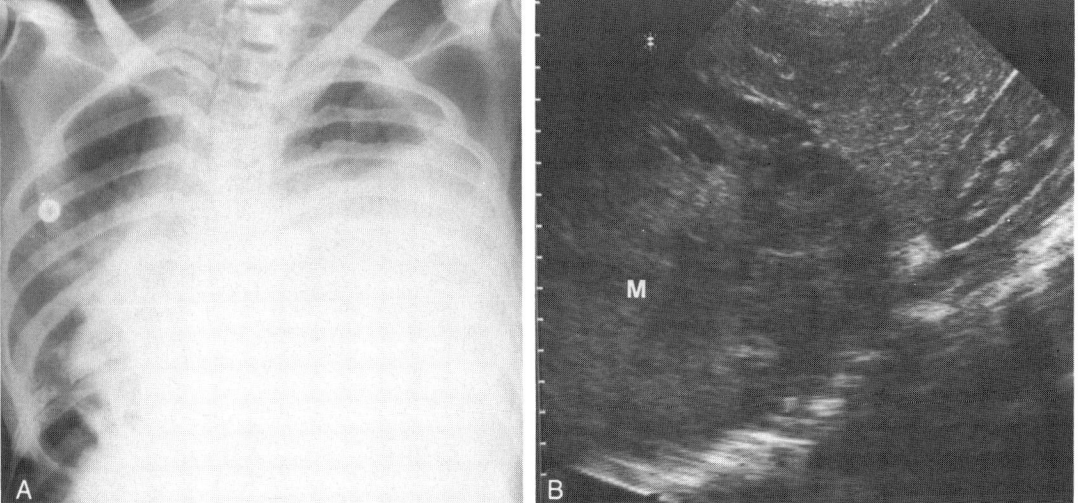

Figure 4–9. Neurofibromatosis was diagnosed in this child when she underwent resection of a right-sided Wilms tumor at age 2 years. She received chemotherapy and radiotherapy after surgery. At age 14 years, she presented with decreased appetite, weight loss, and left-sided flank pain. The radiograph of the chest **(A)** showed a large intrathoracic mass. This was confirmed with sagittal scans **(B)**, which outlined a huge, solid mass. The diaphragm and liver were depressed, and probably invaded, by what proved to be unresectable sarcoma. M = mass.

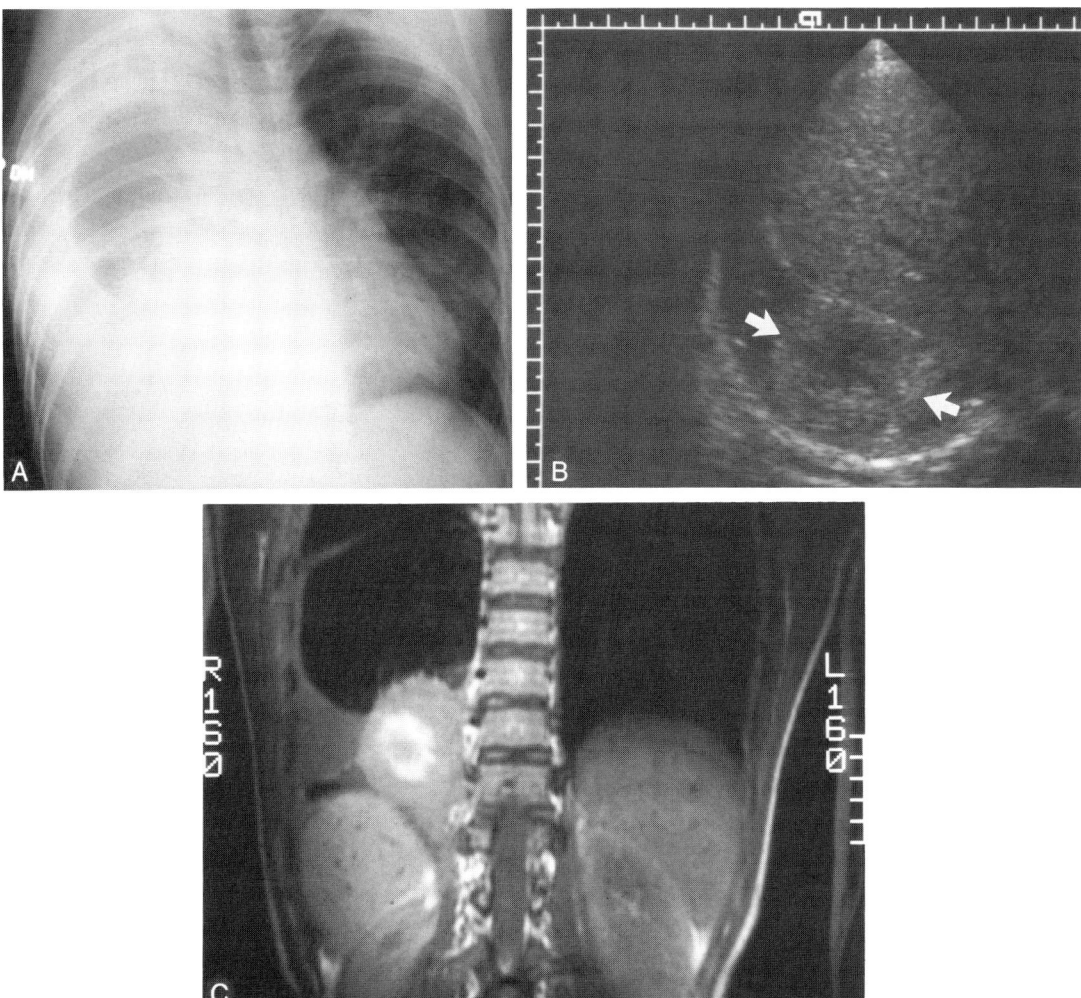

Figure 4-10. The anteroposterior radiograph of this 13-year-old girl (A) was taken as a left-side-down decubitus view of the chest. Note that the pleural density on the right does not layer. There is also a round opacity in the left upper lung, which represents a metastatic deposit. She had had a 1-month history of fatigue, dyspnea, and cough. Two days before admission she had noticed a lump posteriorly over her right lower chest. Both the transverse ultrasonogram (B) and the coronal section from magnetic resonance imaging (MRI) (C) showed a mass in the posterior costophrenic sulcus of the right hemithorax associated with pleural fluid. This proved to be a primitive neuroectodermal tumor. Arrows in B mark the mass.

10). If a biopsy for diagnosis is needed, it can be done under ultrasonic guidance. A tumor distorts the normal anatomy of the lung. Pneumonia saturates the lung with fluid and inflammatory cells, but the underlying anatomy is preserved. An air bronchogram, a fluid bronchogram, and scattered echogenic foci from residual air in the consolidated parenchyma are typical ultrasonographic features of pneumonia (Acunas et al., 1989).

Most thoracenteses are performed with patients in a sitting position. The child sits upright and hugs a pillow, thereby pulling the scapulae forward. Sagittal scans, medial to lateral across the child's back, can map the top of the pleural collection. This edge is marked on the child's back with washable ink. To establish whether there is free flow or loculation of fluid, the child is placed in a decubitus position with the abnormal side uppermost. Scans that are sagittal to the patient but now parallel to the table are repeated. If fluid is free flowing, it changes its position and layers along the mediastinum. If the fluid is loculated, the two sets of scans look similar. If preliminary radiographs show only a lateral or anterior collection of pleural fluid, loculation is virtually always present. To prove loculation at these sites, we scan the child's anterior chest while he or she is sitting upright, and then we take the same views with the child in the supine position. Subpulmonic effusions are evident as a lucent space between the inferior surface of the lower lobe of lung and the diaphragm.

If thoracentesis is deemed appropriate, it should be done immediately after ultrasonic localization. We have experienced the situation in which thoracentesis, done hours later, missed the pleural collection that had been mapped on ultrasonography and indicated on the skin by an inked cross. Changes in the child's position or a difference in the respiratory cycle may change the level of an effusion by an intercostal space or more. The aspiration can be done by a radiologist or a pediatrician. After infiltration of cleansed skin with a local anesthetic agent, a 20-gauge needle is advanced to the depth measured on the scans. The depth may be increased slightly over that suggested by the baseline scan because of the addition of local anesthesia. The biopsy transducer can be used but is rarely needed for guidance except in very small effusions or when pleural biopsy is also being performed. In cases of suspected infection, fluid acquired from aspiration must be sent for aerobic, anaerobic and mycobacterial cultures and for Gram and acid-fast stains. It is unusual for all the appropriate tubes or containers for specimens to be available in the radiology department, and we have found that the best policy is for them to arrive with the patient before the scans. The appropriate request forms can also accompany the patient. Other studies of pleural fluid that might be needed include cell count, cell block preparation, and determination of levels of protein, lactate dehydrogenase (LDH), glucose, pH, and amylase.

DIAPHRAGM

Normal excursion of the hemidiaphragms should be checked as part of any examination of the chest or abdomen. We have measured diaphragmatic excursion in normal newborns (Laing et al., 1988), but qualitative assessment is adequate in the routine clinical situation. In order to obtain maximal views of the diaphragm, sagittal scanning through the liver is the best approach on the right. A more coronal angle is needed on the left in order to use the spleen as a window. If the left lobe of the liver is large enough to act as a window, transverse scans with the transducer angled cephalad, under the xiphoid process, allow comparison of the medial portions of both hemidiaphragms (Shkolnik et al., 1982). Because the incident beam of sound is nearly perpendicular to the arching diaphragm, inspiration causes the specular diaphragmatic echo to move anteriorly; ex-

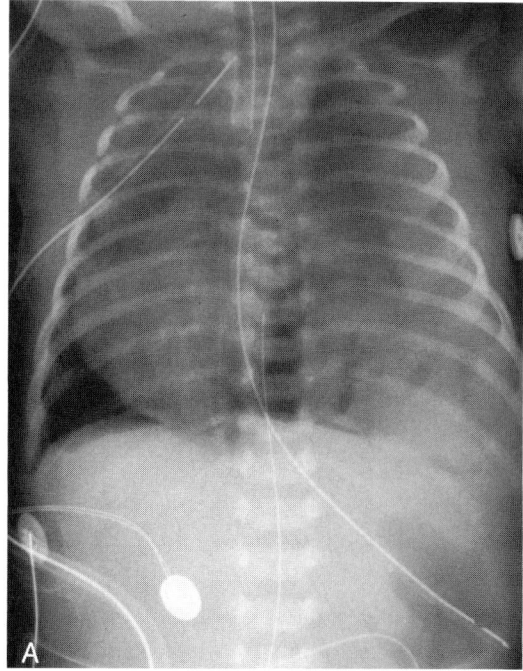
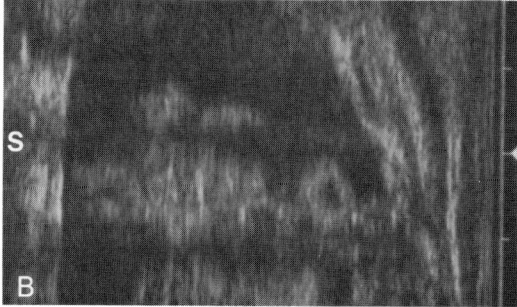

Figure 4–11. This neonate was transferred to our hospital with the diagnosis of left-sided diaphragmatic hernia. This is evident from the chest film (A), which shows a shift of the mediastinum, a hypoplastic left lung, and pleural density associated with air-filled bowel loops in the left hemithorax. A nasogastric tube in the stomach stayed within the abdominal cavity. The baby was placed on ECMO before surgical repair of the diaphragmatic hernia. The left hemithorax could be evaluated with ultrasonography (B). This left coronal scan is oriented to match the radiograph. Note that there is pleural fluid in much of the left hemithorax, with bowel loops present inferiorly. S = spine.

piration pulls it posteriorly. Overt paradoxical motion occurs with unilateral diaphragmatic paralysis if the mediastinum is mobile. If the mediastinum is fixed by earlier surgical intervention, there is less but still appreciable paradoxical motion on the paretic side. Paralysis or paresis of phrenic nerve results from disease of the cervical cord (e.g., tumor, syrinx, trauma) or from peripheral injury, which can follow extensive mediastinal or cardiac surgery or, on occasion, energetic insertion of a chest tube. Inflammatory disease adjacent to either side of the diaphragm limits excursion and is a good clue to the presence of pleural inflammation or subphrenic collection.

We do not use ultrasonography to diagnose diaphragmatic hernia in neonates. Symptoms of acute respiratory distress are best evaluated with radiography. In some of the new protocols for managing the newborn who has diaphragmatic hernia and pulmonary hypoplasia, ultrasonography has been added during the course of therapy. For example, if a baby is placed on extracorporeal membrane oxygenation (ECMO) immediately after birth, the chest and abdomen both become airless on radiographs, and the size of the hernia is indeterminate. Scans of chest and abdomen show the relative size of the lung, the presence of collections of fluid, and the contents of the hernia (Fig. 4–11). The liver and the airless lung look very similar, but vascular anatomy helps one to differentiate between them, as does the observation that pulmonary tissue is generally more pulsatile than is hepatic tissue. Extralobar sequestration is an anomaly associated with diaphragmatic hernia, but it may be difficult to diagnose as such.

Small defects in the diaphragm may go undiagnosed until later in childhood when the affected child has a radiograph of the chest either for respiratory symptoms from the hernia or for an unrelated problem. There is also a group of babies in whom, after infection with beta-streptococcal disease, diaphragmatic hernia appears (Han et al., 1988). In all children for whom the diagnosis is delayed, hernia through the foramen of Bochdalek is the most common. This diaphragmatic defect is posterior; the kidney, liver, and spleen are the solid organs that may herniate into the chest. Hernia through the foramen of Morgagni presents as a mass in the anterior mediastinum. It is rarely bilateral and may first be detected by the cardiac echographer when an unusual cardiac silhouette appears on radiographs. The liver, the omentum, and occasionally the gastrointestinal tract may herniate into the anterior chest. Hiatal hernia is less common in childhood than in adulthood. In general, only the stomach herniates through this central defect (Fig. 4–12). A small diaphragmatic hernia in a hernial sac can be difficult to differentiate from localized eventration of the diaphragm. The thinned diaphragm that is eventrated is

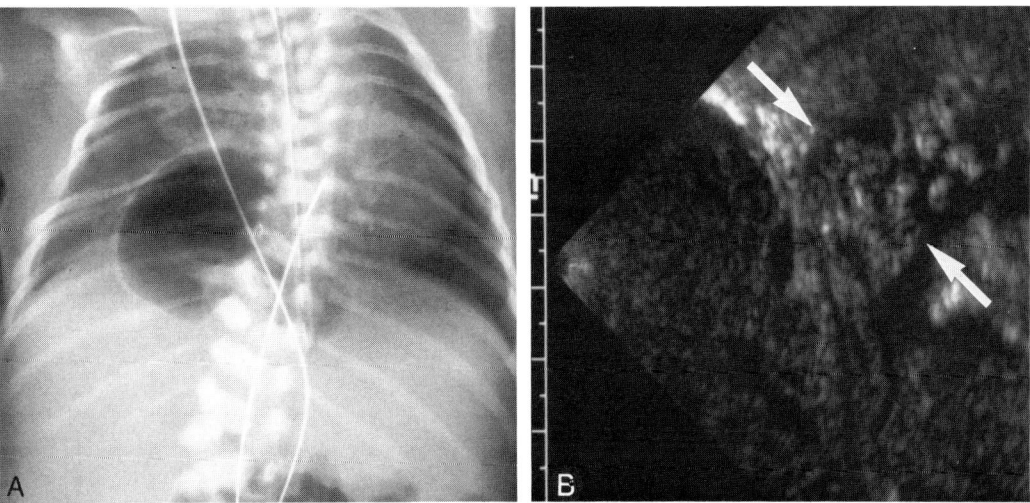

Figure 4–12. The chest and abdominal radiograph of this neonate, who had multiple anomalies, shows gas superimposed over the lower chest (A). Abdominal scans had been requested to search for renal and other anomalies. Coronal scan (B) through the right upper abdomen shows transverse position of the liver and a large mass (arrows) that represents the herniation of a twisted stomach through the hiatus of the diaphragm. The ultrasonogram is oriented to match the chest radiograph.

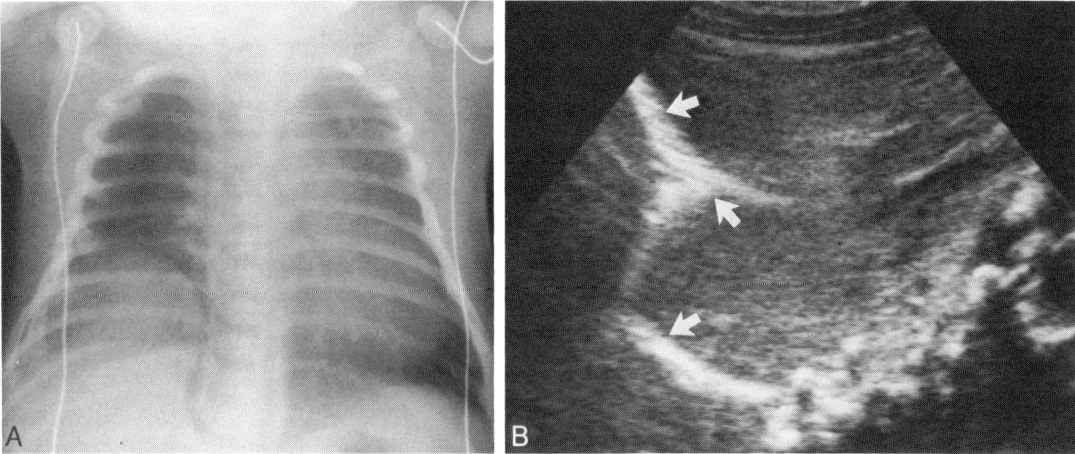

Figure 4–13. A newborn, who entered the hospital for mild respiratory distress, had an admission radiograph of the chest **(A)**, the results of which raised the possibility of eventration or right-sided herniation of the diaphragm. A sagittal, longitudinal scan of the right upper quadrant **(B)** shows a specular interface that probably represents a thinned diaphragm associated with posterior eventration. The entire specular interface moved appropriately with respiration. No further follow-up was recommended. Arrows indicate the diaphragmatic interface.

usually poorly functional, and its specular echo can be mimicked by the peritoneal/pleural interface of the hernial sac. True differentiation is possible with peritoneal insufflation of air. Coronal magnetic resonance image (MRI) scanning may be a diagnostic tool in the future, but we know of no cases to date in which it has been used as such. In practice, a smoothly contoured diaphragmatic bulge, found incidentally by radiography or ultrasonography and unassociated with respiratory distress, is considered to be eventration and is followed with radiography and no intervention (Fig. 4–13).

INTRATHORACIC MASSES

If an intrathoracic mass is juxtadiaphragmatic or abutting the pleural surface, there is no interference from the lung to prevent penetration by the ultrasonic beam. Loculated pleural fluid or a pleural rind is the most common pleural mass. Other intrathoracic masses in childhood include sequestration; congenital cystic adenomatoid malformation; lobar emphysema or bronchial atresia; expansile pneumonia; tumor (primary and metastatic); normal or abnormal thymus; pulmonary, pericardial, or bronchogenic cyst; diaphragmatic cyst; and cardiac tumor (Fig. 4–14). The origins of primary or secondary tumors of bone or cartilage should be evident from the findings on plain radiographs.

Cystic adenomatoid malformation is diagnosed in utero when a thoracic mass composed of variably sized cysts and surrounding stroma is identified. After birth, communications with the bronchi permit air to fill the cysts. Good radiographs usually allow the radiologist to make the diagnosis. Postnatal ultrasonography is hindered by the air in the malformation. In the newborn, delayed resorption of fetal fluid from a lobe supplied by an atretic bronchus or from a congenitally emphysematous lobe, usually upper or midddle, gives the appearance of a solid intrathoracic mass. Air gradually reaches the lobe through collateral pores and allows radiographic diagnosis of the anomaly.

Pulmonary sequestration is a most satisfying ultrasonographic diagnosis if one can characterize a solid mass as intrathoracic and juxtadiaphragmatic and if it is supplied by branches of the abdominal or lower thoracic aorta. Extralobar sequestration (outside visceral pleura and without bronchial communication) tends to present in infancy as a large, typically left-sided lower thoracic mass. Intralobar sequestration (inside visceral pleura and occasionally communicating with bronchi), which is six times more common, is more likely to be asymptomatic or to present with coincident or associated infection later in childhood (Mäkinen et al., 1981). Pathologists have suggested that intralobar sequestration may actually be an acquired lesion. Of 45,000 autopsies of stillborn infants and liveborn infants who died at less than 2 months of age, 12 revealed extralobar se-

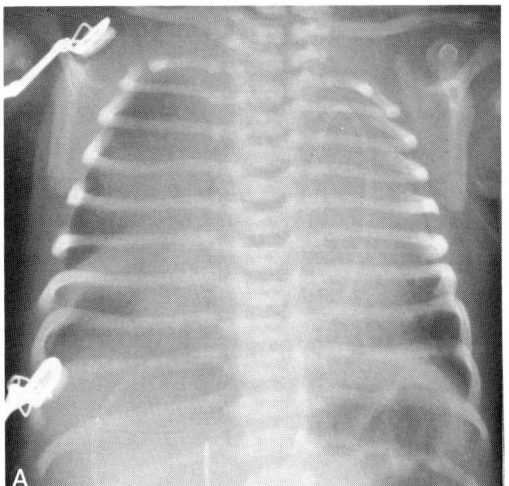 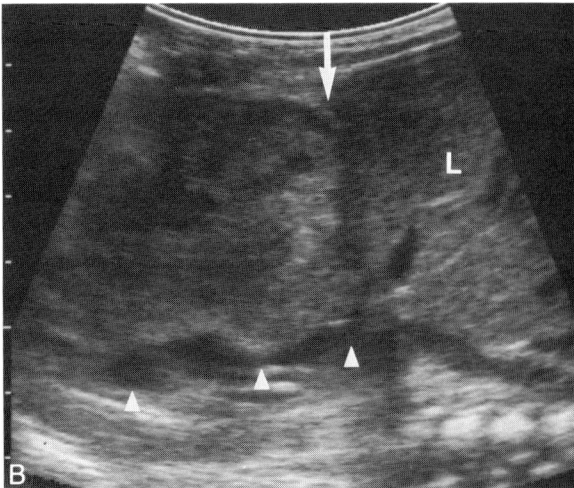

Figure 4-14. Lethargy and poor eating resulted in this baby's admission to the hospital. The radiograph of the chest was dramatically abnormal **(A)**. The cardiac silhouette could not be defined at all. Because the question of herniation of abdominal contents was raised, the abdominal ultrasonogram quickly followed. The sagittal view just to the right of the midline **(B)** shows no intrathoracic herniation but does show markedly abnormal cardiac echogenicity associated with deformity of the inferior vena cava and right atrial channel (arrowheads). Further cardiac evaluation followed, the patient was taken to the operating room, and a 5 × 6 cm sarcoma was removed from the right atrial appendage. A cardiac tumor should always raise the possibility of tuberous sclerosis, but this was not diagnosed in this particular patient. L = liver. Arrow indicates the diaphragm.

questration, but none revealed intralobar sequestration (Stocker et al., 1978). On ultrasonography, the sequestered tissue is generally more echogenic than the liver or spleen. Tubular structures within the mass should be investigated with Doppler ultrasonography to prove that they are vessels. The arterial supply to the mass may escape detection if it is from the thoracic aorta, from multiple arteries, or from vessels such as the subclavian, intercostal, or phrenic artery. Color Doppler scanning may add a significant advantage in the identification of vascular supply. The ultrasonographer should be aware that sequestration is part of the spectrum of bronchopulmonary foregut malformation (Felker and Tonkin, 1990). A sequestered lung may communicate with the esophagus. A barium swallow should be a routine examination for patients who present with possible sequestration (Fig. 4-15).

As a general rule, mediastinal masses should be evaluated with a combination of plain films, fluoroscopy with barium esophagram, and computed tomography (CT) scanning. Occasionally, this rule is broken, or ultrasonography is used as a triaging step in unusual cases (Fig. 4-16). The bronchogenic cyst—another type of bronchopulmonary foregut malformation—is typically in the middle mediastinum, smoothly walled, and intimately associated with the esophagus and tracheal bifurcation. However, it can be situated anywhere in the chest and appear noncystic on CT scans if it contains mucoid secretions. On ultrasonography, if it is accessible through the mediastinal or paraspinal window, it may contain echoes, but it transmits sound as does the typical cyst (Fig. 4-17). In contrast, a posterior mediastinal neurogenic tumor tends to be less sharply rimmed and appears as a solid mass. A neurogenic mass may be associated with an adjacent intraspinal tumor. In the newborn, intraspinal neuroblastoma can be diagnosed with ultrasonography because the posterior elements are not totally ossified. Careful scanning of the spinal canal adjacent to a thoracic or abdominal paraspinal mass is imperative. (See Chapter 2.)

Pericardial and diaphragmatic cysts, both of which are rare, may be remnants of aberrant lymphatic development. Any mass that is purely cystic is usually benign. Tumors of cardiac muscle are usually found by the cardiologist. Tuberous sclerosis is strongly associated with rhabdomyoma and rhabdomyosarcoma.

The thymus has been the unofficial symbol of pediatric radiology. One earns the title of "Pediatric Radiologist" if one can look at a radiograph and authoritatively declare that a huge anterior mediastinal mass is indeed a normal thymus—and be believed! The sono-

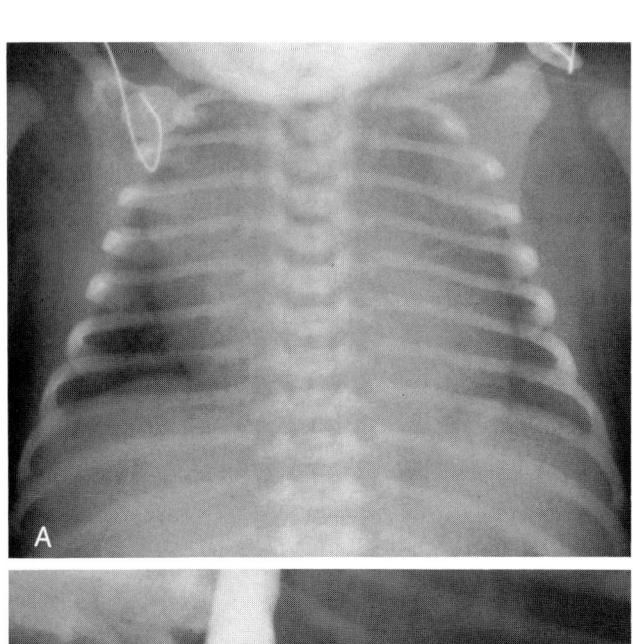
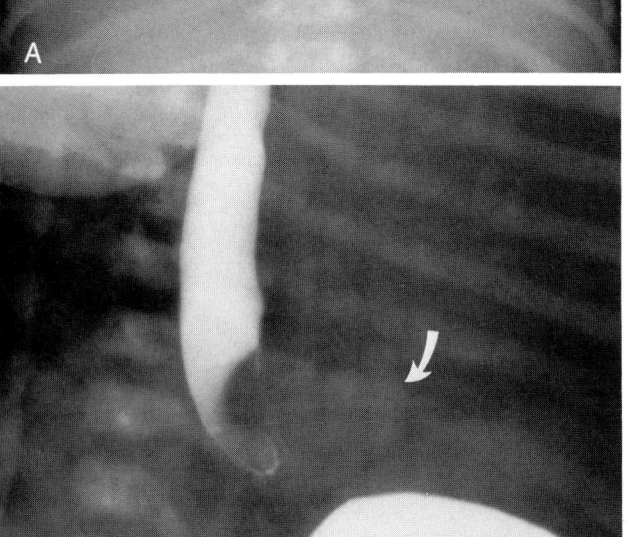
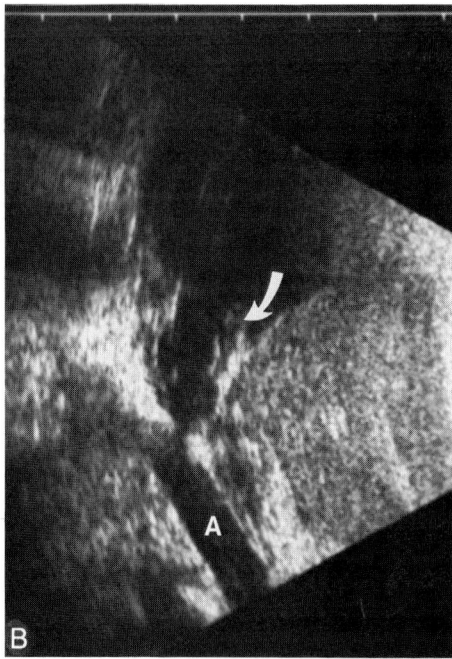

Figure 4–15. As a newborn, this baby was investigated for cyanosis. The radiograph of the chest (**A**) shows cardiomegaly, which was evaluated further with cardiac echography. This revealed an atrioventricular canal and, incidentally, a left-sided mediastinal mass. Ultrasonography (**B**) and contrast study of the esophagus (**C**) show a well-defined, cystic mass (arrow) in the costophrenic sulcus in the left hemithorax. Because of the underlying cardiac disease, this mass has never been removed. It has been diagnosed as probable cystic bronchopulmonary foregut malformation because no systemic vasculature to the area could be identified. In **B**, A = aorta.

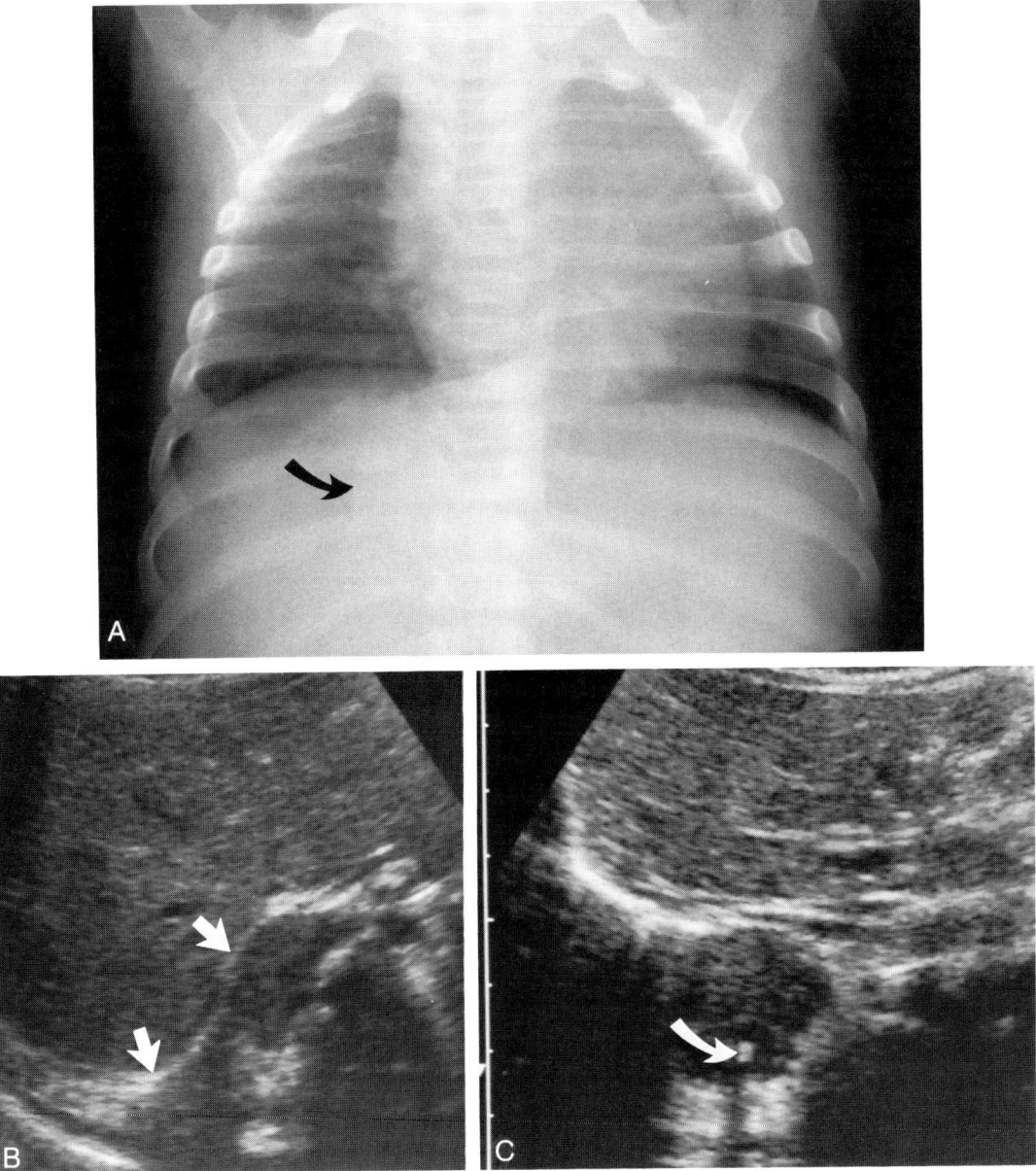

Figure 4–16. This 3½-month-old had been referred for a gastrointestinal series to evaluate causes for her repeated emesis and dehydration. The initial plain film of the chest (**A**) showed a right-sided mediastinal mass (arrow), and so the radiologist switched a cup of barium for the ultrasonic transducer. A transverse scan of the upper abdomen shows a solid mass in the right costophrenic sulcus typical of a posterior neurogenic tumor (**B**). Arrows mark the diaphragm. Note the calcification (arrow) on the sagittal ultrasonogram (**C**). During surgery, this was found to be a neuroblastoma.

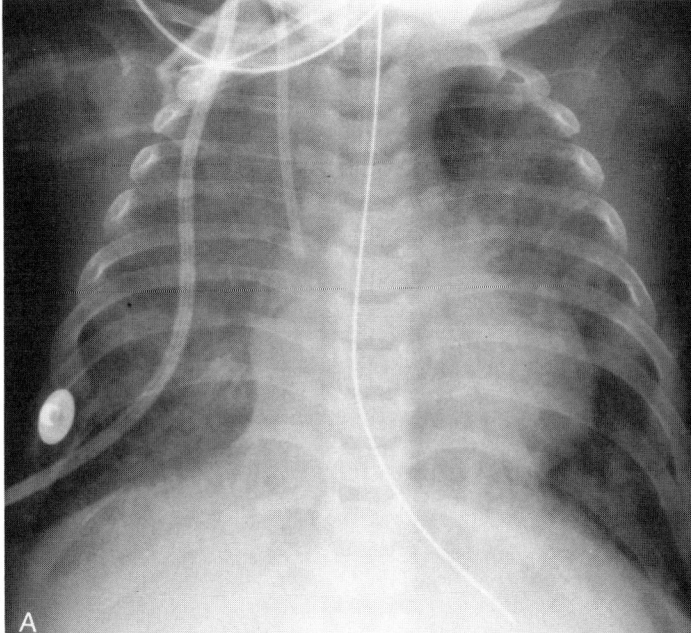
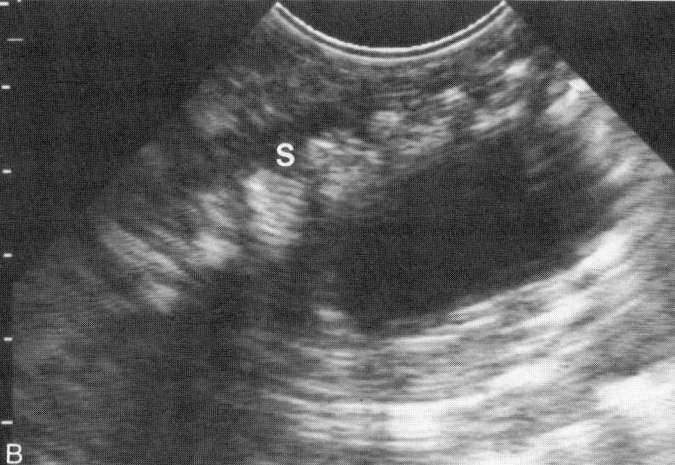

Figure 4–17. This infant with trisomy 21 had arrived at our hospital after the repair of duodenal stenosis. He also had an atrioventricular canal that had not been repaired. With his transfer note was the information that diagnosis of a right-sided intrathoracic cyst had been made on a computed tomography (CT) scan. This study was reviewed, and an apical cyst was indeed apparent. However, the current radiograph **(A)**, although showing opacity in the right upper lung, did not reveal a discrete cyst. The ultrasonogram **(B)** was requested before surgery in order to make sure that a cyst was actually still present. A well-defined 3.5-cm cyst was found immediately adjacent to the right side of the spinal canal in the upper chest. A bronchogenic cyst was removed from the posterior mediastinum during surgery. S = spine.

Figure 4–18. This split-screen view shows normal thymic tissue in comparison with normal hepatic tissue in a 6-year-old child. The thymus is homogeneous in texture and less echogenic than liver. In this sagittal view, it is immediately anterior to the main pulmonary artery. T = thymus; L = liver.

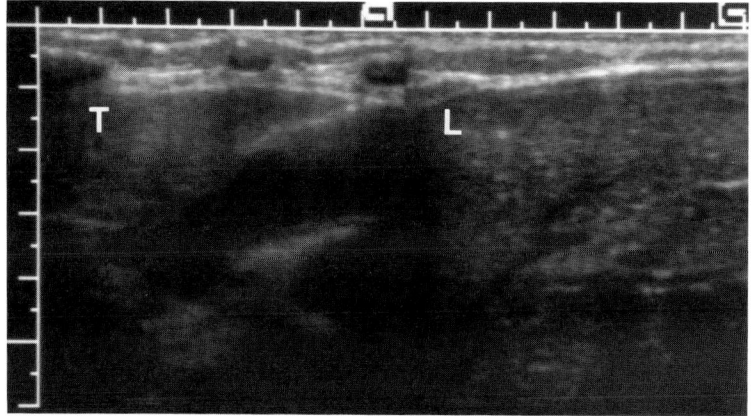

graphic characteristics of the normal thymus have been reported (Han et al., 1989). In infants, the gland has a triangular or teardrop shape on longitudinal scans. It is homogeneous in texture and less echogenic than the liver, spleen, or thyroid (Fig. 4–18). For investigating the possibly abnormal thymus, ultrasonography is less important than fluoroscopy and cross-sectional imaging. Leukemic infiltration of the thymus causes its enlargement and changes its pliability. Ultrasonography of the mediastinum can be used in addition to abdominal scans that have suggested the diagnosis of leukemia or lymphoma. It is the rare patient, however, who escapes plain radiography of the chest before ultrasonography is requested. Thymic masses also include thymic cyst, thymoma, and teratoma. Rudick and Wood (1980) reported a child who had a large multilocular thymic cyst. Cysts may result from only partial obliteration of the thymopharyngeal duct that is part of the genesis of the thymus from the ventral third branchial pouch, or they may result from degeneration of Hassall bodies. Teratoma, thymoma, and lymphoma may have a large cystic component. The presence of calcification helps confirm the diagnosis of teratoma, but CT is more sensitive in this regard.

SUPERFICIAL MASSES OF THE CHEST

Most noninflammatory masses of the chest wall are mesodermal in origin and are lipomas, hemangiomas, cystic hygromas, fibromas, neurofibromas, or tumors of muscle, bone, or cartilage. When a mass is fixed to the thoracic cage, the true extent and degree of bony involvement, if present, cannot be demonstrated nearly as well with ultrasonography as with CT scanning or MRI (Fig. 4–19). Most small, freely movable masses are simply removed without preoperative evaluation. Thus the role of ultrasonography is quite limited and frequently a stopgap measure only. Most reports of ultrasonography of superficial thoracic masses are included as parts of a larger series of reports on masses of soft tissue (Glasier et al., 1989) or as part of reviews of thoracic ultrasonography (Rosenberg, 1986). If one examines a child with a mass in the soft tissues of the chest, one should review any available radiographs and then establish the location, size, and consistency of the mass and characterize the tissue planes around the mass as displaced, altered, or invaded. For example, a very small palpable lump may be the tip of a very large infiltrating cystic hygroma (Figs. 4–20, 4–21). Bleeding into this mass produces a mixed, as opposed to septated, echolucent pattern. For masses that overlie ribs or a scapula, one occasionally can make the diagnosis of an underlying bony abnormality if the contour of the bone is changed by erosion or if the periosteum is elevated. Pathologic diagnosis is not possible with ultrasonography alone. Calcification in a mass, especially if the mass arises from skeletal muscle, should alert the examiner to the possibility of malignancy—specifically, rhabdomyosarcoma.

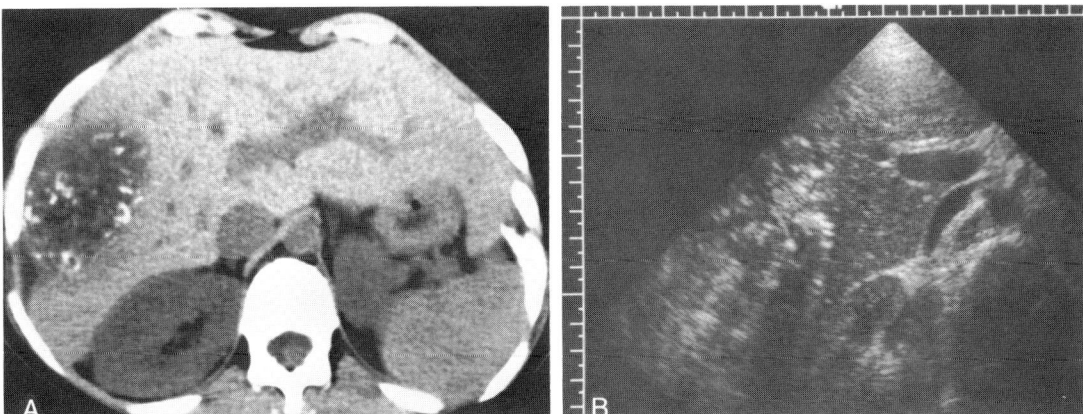

Figure 4–19. CT scan **(A)** had already shown the degree of bony and cartilaginous involvement from osteochondromas of the ribs in this adolescent girl. The ultrasonogram **(B)** was requested only to assess whether the liver was fixed by the adjacent mass. Real-time ultrasonography showed normal motion of the liver during breathing, and, therefore, lack of fixation. Surgical resection of osteochondromas followed.

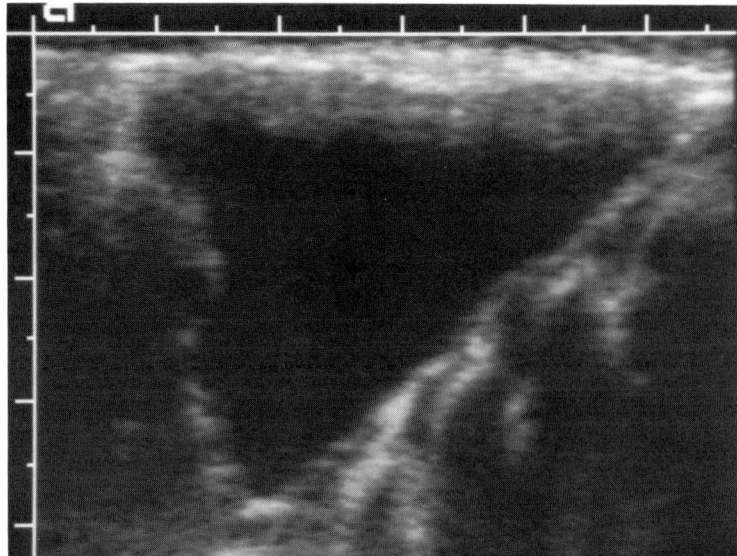

Figure 4–20. A rather small lump was felt in the axilla of this 11-week-old. Ultrasonography showed this to be a well-defined unilocular cyst, which was subsequently removed and proved to be cystic hygroma. Contrast this case with that shown in Figure 4–21.

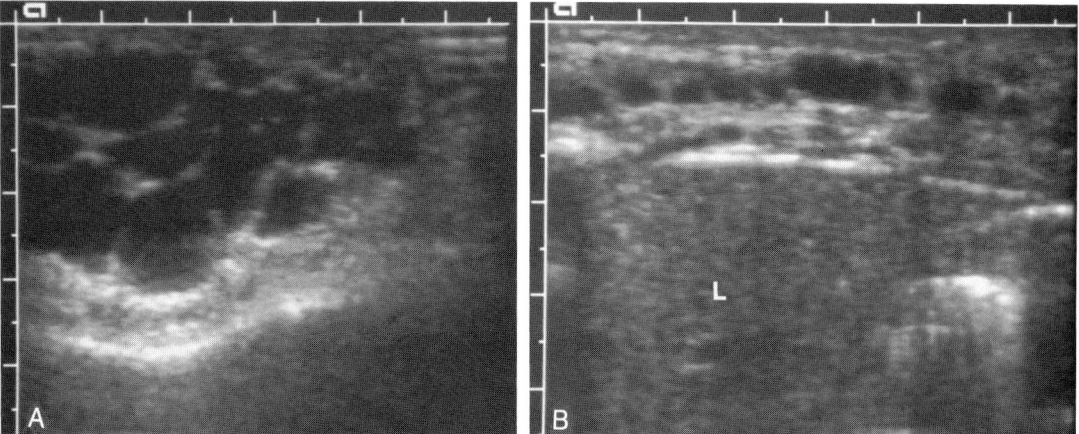

Figure 4–21. This 1-month-old girl had a palpable mass over the lower right chest **(A)**. This was a very extensive cystic hygroma extending along the abdominal wall into the upper abdomen but was separate from all intra-abdominal organs **(B)**. L = liver.

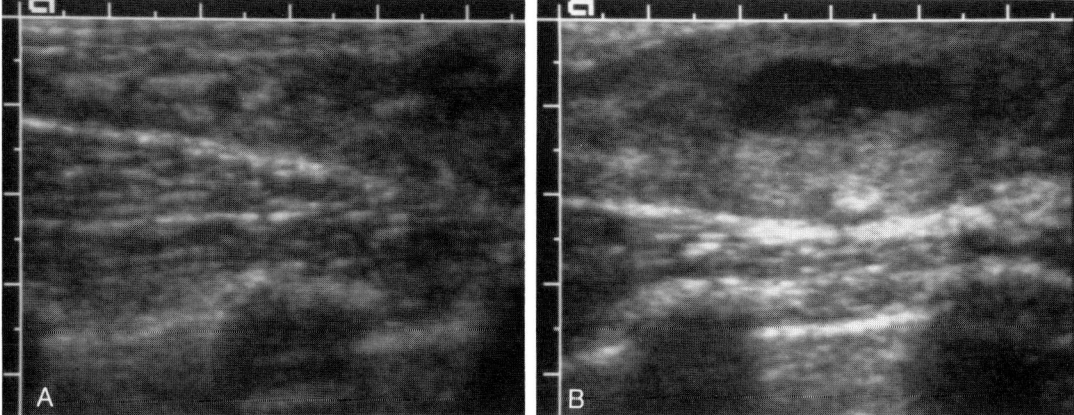

Figure 4–22. Pain in the left breast associated with 2 days of swelling brought this 15-year-old to medical attention. She was treated with antibiotics without improvement. Scans of the breast were then requested. The normal right breast **(A)** shows the typical appearance of glandular tissue over the muscles of the chest wall. Contrast this with the swollen breast **(B)** in which an abscess, associated with increased transmission of sound, is present. This abscess was drained percutaneously. Cultures were negative, probably because of the earlier therapy with antibiotics.

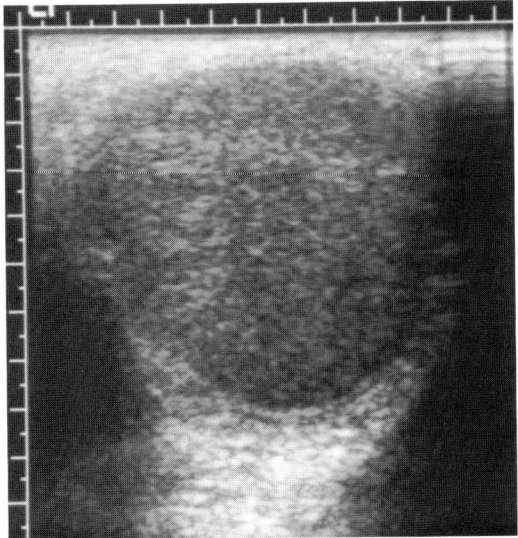

Figure 4–23. Of interest, when this 11-year-old presented with a large mass in the right breast, was the information that her mother had had a fibroadenoma removed at age 17. This transverse scan shows the typical homogeneous texture of a fibroadenoma, proved surgically.

There is little experience with ultrasonography of the breast in adolescence and childhood because the prevalence of any type of breast disease is very low. Mastitis can progress to abscess, and localization for incision and drainage is aided by preoperative ultrasonography (Fig. 4–22). Fibroadenoma is the most common neoplastic mass in adolescents. It is a benign, solid tumor managed by simple excision. Ultrasonography shows the typical fibroadenoma to be hypoechoic and homogeneous in texture (Fig. 4–23; Fornage et al., 1989). Cystosarcoma phylloides has a malignant label, but in adolescents its histologic and biologic behavior are usually benign. Clinical features typical of this mass include fast rate of growth and large size at presentation (Mollitt et al., 1987). There is a report of sarcoma of the breast induced by radiation (Squire et al., 1988). Thus a history of irradiation for malignancy is important when a patient is being evaluated for a mass in the breast.

REFERENCES

General and Pleural Disease

Ablin DS, Newell JD 2d: Diagnostic imaging for evaluation of the pediatric chest. Clin Chest Med 1987; 8:641–660.
Acunas B, Celik L, Acunas A: Chest sonography: Differentiation of pulmonary consolidation from pleural disease. Acta Radiol 1989; 30:273–275.
Amodio J, Abramson S, Berdon W, et al: Iatrogenic causes of large pleural fluid collections in the premature infant: Ultrasonic and radiographic findings. Pediatr Radiol 1987; 17:104–108.
Carey BM, Williams CE, Arthur RJ: Ultrasound demonstration of pericardial empyema in an infant with pyrexia of undetermined origin. Pediatr Radiol 1988; 18:349–350.
Cleveland RH, Foglia RP: CT in the evaluation of pleural versus pulmonary disease in children. Pediatr Radiol 1988; 18:14–19.
Glasier CM, Leithiser RE Jr, Williamson SL, et al: Extracardiac chest ultrasonography in infants and children: Radiographic and clinical implications. J Pediatr 1989; 114:540–544.
Haller JO, Schneider M, Kassner EG, et al: Sonographic evaluation of the chest in infants and children. AJR 1980; 134:1019–1027.
Hunnam GR, Flower CD: Radiologically-guided percutaneous catheter drainage of empyemas. Clin Radiol 1988; 39:121–126.
McLauglin FJ, Goldmann DA, Rosenbaum DM, et al: Empyema in children: Clinical course and long-term follow up. Pediatrics 1984; 73:587–593.
Rosenberg HK: The complementary roles of ultrasound and plain film radiography in differentiating pediatric chest abnormalities. Radiographics 1986; 6:427–445.

Diaphragm

Han BK, Towbin RB, Ball WS Jr: Pediatric case of the day. Delayed right diaphragmatic hernia following group B streptococcal infection. Radiographics 1988; 8:354–357.
Laing IA, Teele RL, Stark AR: Diaphragmatic movement in newborn infants. J Pediatr 1988; 112:638–643.
Moccia WA, Kaude JV, Felman AH: Congenital eventration of the diaphragm: Diagnosis by ultrasound. Pediatr Radiol 1981; 10:197–200.
Nussbaum A, Ben-Ami T, Treves S, et al: Diagnosis of delayed onset right-sided congenital diaphragmatic hernia using ultrasonic and radionuclide imaging. Ped Surg Int 1987; 2:149–156.
Robinson AE, Gooneratne NS, Blackburn WR, et al: Bilateral anteromedial defect of the diaphragm in children. AJR 1980; 135:301–306.
Shkolnik A, Foley MJ, Riggs TW, et al: New applications of real time ultrasound in pediatrics. Radiographics 1982; 2:422–436.

Intrathoracic Masses

Sequestration

Felker RE, Tonkin ILD: Imaging of pulmonary sequestration. AJR 1990; 154:241–249.
Fowler CL, Pokorny WJ, Wagner ML, et al: Review of bronchopulmonary foregut malformations. J Pediatr Surg 1988; 23:793–797.
Jaffe MH, Bank ER, Silver TM, et al: Pulmonary sequestration: Ultrasonic appearance. JCU 1982; 10:294–296.
Kaude JV, Laurin S: Ultrasonographic demonstration of systemic artery feeding extrapulmonary sequestration. Pediatr Radiol 1984; 14:226–227.
Mäkinen EO, Merikanto J, Rikalainen H, et al: Intralobar pulmonary sequestration occuring without alteration of pulmonary parenchyma. Pediatr Radiol 1981; 10:237–240.

Morin C, Filiatrault D, Russo P: Pulmonary sequestration with histologic changes of cystic adenomatoid malformation. 1989; 19:130–132.

Stanley P, Vachon L, Gilsanz V: Pulmonary sequestration with congenital gastroesophageal communication. Report of two cases. Pediatr Radiol 1985; 15:343–345.

Stocker JT, Drake RM, Madewell JE: Cystic and congenital lung disease in the newborn. Perspectives in Pediatric Pathology 1978; 4:93–154.

West MS, Donaldson JS, Shkolnik A: Pulmonary sequestration. Diagnosis by ultrasound. J Ultrasound Med 1989; 8:125–129.

Other Intrathoracic Masses

Ganick DJ, Kodroff MB, Marrow HG, et al: Thoracic neuroblastoma presenting as a cystic hygroma. Arch Dis Child 1988; 63:1270–1271.

Han BK, Babcock DS, Oestreich AE: Normal thymus in infancy: Sonographic characteristics. Radiology 1989; 170:471–474.

Hendry PJ, Hendry GMA: Ultrasonic diagnosis of a bronchogenic cyst in a child with persistent stridor. Pediatr Radiol 1988; 18:338.

King RM, Telander RL, Smithson WA, et al: Primary mediastinal tumors in children. J Pediatr Surg 1982; 17:512–520.

Lemaitre L, Leclerc F, Dubos JP, et al: Thymic hemorrhage: A cause of acute symptomatic mediastinal widening in an infant with late haemorrhagic disease. Sonographic findings. Pediatr Radiol 1989; 19:128–129.

Liu P, Daneman A, Stringer DA: Real-time sonography of mediastinal and juxtamediastinal masses in infants and children. J Can Assoc Radiol 1988; 39:198–203.

Nogués A, Tovar JA, Suñol M, et al: Hodgkin's disease of the thymus: A rare mediastinal cystic mass. J Pediatr Surg 1987; 22:996–997.

O'Laughlin MP, Huhta JC, Murphy DJ Jr: Ultrasound examination of extracardiac chest masses in children. Doppler diagnosis of vascular etiology. J Ultrasound Med 1987; 6:151–157.

Rudick MG, Wood BP: The use of ultrasound in the diagnosis of a large thymic cyst. Pediatr Radiol 1980; 10:113–115.

Sumner TE, Volberg FM, Kiser PE, et al: Mediastinal cystic hygroma in children. Pediatr Radiol 1981; 11:160–162.

Chest Wall and Breast

Fornage BD, Lorigan JG, Andry E: Fibroadenoma of the breast: Sonographic appearance. Radiology 1989; 172:671–675.

Glasier CM, Leithiser RE Jr, Williamson SL, et al: Extracardiac chest ultrasonography in infants and children: Radiographic and clinical implications. J Pediatr 1989; 114:540–544.

Harris VJ, Jackson VP: Indications for breast imaging in women under age 35 years. Radiology 1989; 172:445–448.

Mollitt DL, Golladay ES, Gloster ES, et al: Cystosarcoma phylloides in the adolescent female. J. Pediatr Surg 1987; 22:907–910.

Rosenberg HK: The complementary roles of ultrasound and plain film radiography in differentiating pediatric chest abnormalities. Radiographics 1986; 6:427–445.

Saito R, Kobayashi H, Kitamura S: Ultrasonographic approach to diagnosing chest wall tumors. Chest 1988; 94:1271–1275.

Scanlon EF: Benign diseases of the breast. In McKenna RJ, Murphy GP (eds): Fundamentals of Surgical Oncology. New York: Macmillan 1986; 548–556.

Squire R, Bianchi A, Jakate SM: Radiation-induced sarcoma of the breast in a female adolescent. Case report with histologic and therapeutic considerations. Cancer 1988; 61:2444–2447.

Miscellaneous

Katz R, Landman J, Dulitzky F, et al: Fracture of the clavicle in the newborn: An ultrasound diagnosis. J Ultrasound Med 1988; 7:21–23.

Shackelford GD: The pediatric airway: Radiology and new imaging. Int Anesthesiol Clin 1988; 26:3–5.

CHAPTER 5

THE EXTREMITIES

If we had written this book 5 years ago, there would have been no chapter on ultrasonography of the extremities. Rather, the few cases we had collected would have been grouped together as "miscellaneous" problems.

The proliferation of articles describing orthopedic applications of ultrasonography has coincided with an upsurge of interest in sports medicine, the development of transducers that provide good resolution in the near field, and the simple fact that musculoskeletal scanning was the last major frontier in ultrasonography. When one examines an abnormal arm or leg, one usually can view normal anatomy by scanning the opposite extremity. Because ultrasonographic views tend to be "nonstandard" in orientation, the constant comparison between normal and abnormal sides is most helpful.

In general, we rely on transducers that are configured in linear array and 5 to 7.5 MHz in frequency. The child has to be positioned in order that symmetric views of both legs or both arms can be obtained. Because internal movement is not a problem (in contrast to abdominal organs, which are affected by respiration), slow frame rate allows better resolution of anatomy without artifact of motion. Scans of the normal side provide the baseline anatomy. The split-screen function on many ultrasonographic units is ideal for comparison between extremities. The normal cross-sectional view of soft tissue consists of images of skin (which is not imaged in its entirety unless a standoff pad is employed), subcutaneous fat, muscles that are separated by echogenic fascial planes, and periosteum and bone, which together cause distal shadowing. In babies, if the section is near the joint, articular cartilage presents as a lucent shell around the stippled epiphyseal cartilage. (For those who like sweets, this looks like an image of coated candy!) The muscles are relatively lucent with echogenic streaks that parallel the long axis of each muscle. These streaks represent the connective tissues that loosely bind bundles of muscle cells. In cross-section images, the muscle appears flecked by its partitions of connective tissue and its blood vessels. (Fig. 5–1).

Ultrasonography can be used for measurements of subcutaneous fat. Nutritionists and endocrinologists have traditionally used calipers to measure the combined thickness of skin and subcutaneous fat. With its direct visualization of soft tissues, ultrasonography is an ideal substitute for the less sensitive calipers (Weiss and Clark, 1987). Pitfalls of the ultrasonic examination include the use of transducers that have poor definition in the nearfield; compression of the subcutaneous fat with the transducer, thereby producing falsely low measurement; and failure to standardize the examination so that the same site is not compared on follow-up studies. The thickness of subcutaneous fat varies dramat-

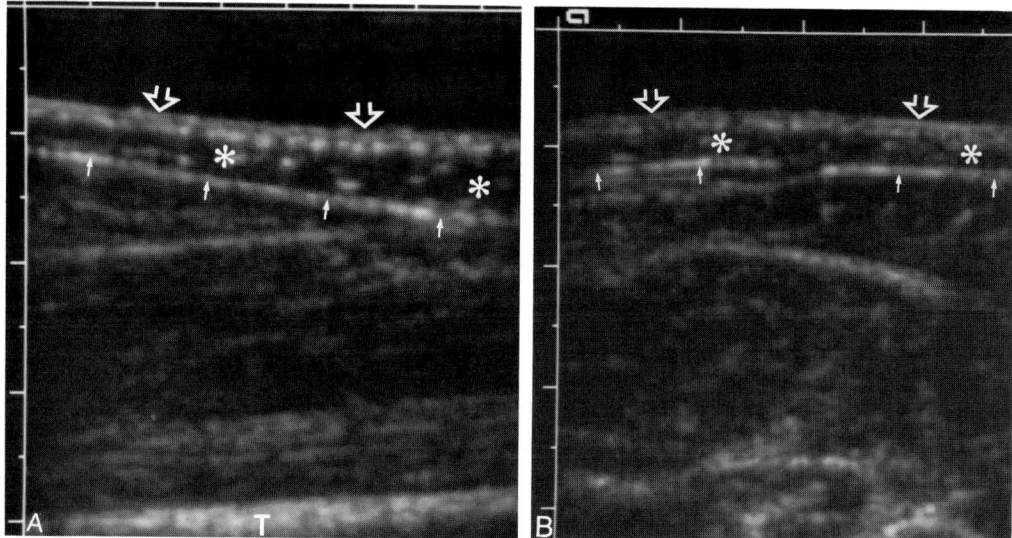

Figure 5–1. Longitudinal (A) and transverse (B) scans of the calf, for which a pad of tissue-equivalent material was used, show the typical appearance of skin (open arrows), the layer of subcutaneous fat (asterisks) above the fascial plane (small arrows), and normal muscle in this 8-year-old boy. The muscle is of low echogenicity; the linear interfaces are from connective tissue and vessels. In the axial cross-section, the muscle has a speckled pattern. In A, T = tibia.

ically between anatomic locations; we have found it almost impossible to measure its thickness in the subscapular area of most children. Scans over the triceps and the anterior thigh are most reliable and reproducible (Fig. 5–2).

Measurements of thickness and appearance of muscle are obtained for populations of children with neuromuscular diseases when research protocols are in place (Fischer and Stephens, 1988; Heckmatt et al., 1988; Lamminen et al., 1988). Muscular dystrophy appears to increase the speckled pattern of muscle. Dermatomyositis produces similar changes. Children with hypotonia of central origin or from other causes are reported as having normal scans (Heckmatt et al., 1988). Our expectation is that further experience will show that abnormal echogenicity of muscle is a nonspecific feature of primary muscular pathology that will have to be interpreted in association with the biopsy.

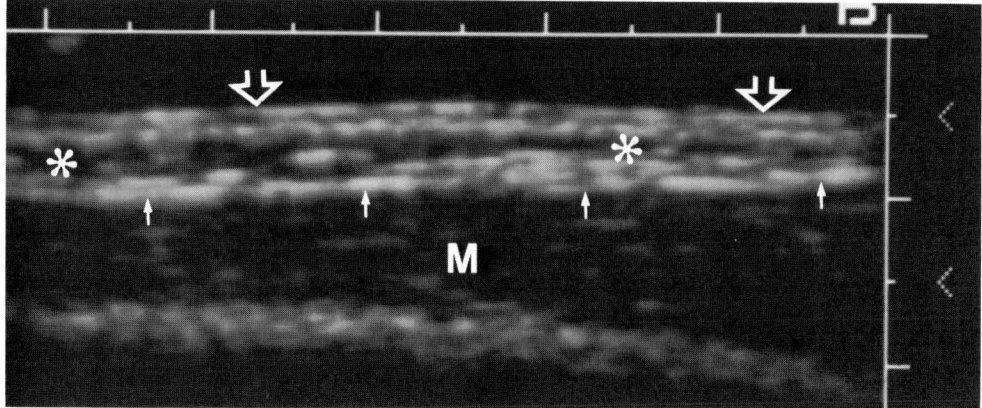

Figure 5–2. Longitudinal scan of the upper arm, with the standoff pad in place, demonstrates the layers of skin (open arrows), the subcutaneous fat (asterisks) above the fascial plane (small arrows), and the muscle (M). The standoff material allows excellent resolution of all planes, but its weight decreases the thickness of the fat and results in a falsely low measurement. A thick cushion of gel on the skin and a lightly applied transducer allow accurate and reproducible measurements.

MASSES

The most useful information from ultrasonography is the identification of a mass as (1) purely cystic or solid and (2) overtly vascular or nonvascular in origin. Vascular masses are discussed later in the sections on congenital and acquired vascular abnormalities. The overlap in appearance between benign and malignant lesions and the inadequate demonstration of bony involvement makes computed tomography (CT) scanning or magnetic resonance imaging (MRI) the study of choice for a child, otherwise asymptomatic, who presents with a palpable mass in the muscles of the extremities (Fig. 5–3).

We emphasize that all neoplasms of soft tissues are very rare in children, but of the primary malignant neoplasms, rhabdomyosarcoma is the most common. Fibrosarcoma, angiosarcoma, synovial sarcoma, and malignant schwannoma are, in decreasing order, the next most frequent (Neifeld et al., 1985). As a rule, the more poorly defined and infiltrative a solid lesion is, the more likely it is to be malignant. Lymphoma, which involves peripheral nodes, tends to present as echolucent, well-defined masses. Hemorrhage throughout a muscle from acute trauma causes diffuse, irregularly echogenic enlargement of the muscle. It is difficult to prove that an underlying lesion is present or absent in such cases. For most patients who have a history of severe trauma, conservative therapy is appropriate. Imaging is reserved for those who have a persistent mass that does not have typical features of calcifying traumatic myositis on follow-up plain radiographs (Fig. 5–4).

A mass associated with fever and tenderness can be localized to a muscle or perimuscular fascia, and ultrasonograms can guide further therapy. Although pyomyositis is uncommon in children, its ultrasonographic appearance has been reported (Yagupsky et al., 1988). Acute inflammation results in increased lucency of the muscle, and the complication of abscess can be diagnosed when obvious heterogeneity develops, if a fluid-debris level is evident or if gas accumulates. Percutaneous aspiration and drainage can follow in such cases (Fig. 5–5).

The popliteal cyst is a common orthopedic problem of childhood, typically occurring in preadolescent boys. This cyst is a thin-walled, echofree mass, which usually represents distention, with fluid, of the bursa of the gastrocnemius/semitendinous muscles or a herniation of the synovium of the joint itself. The term "Baker cyst" has been ap-

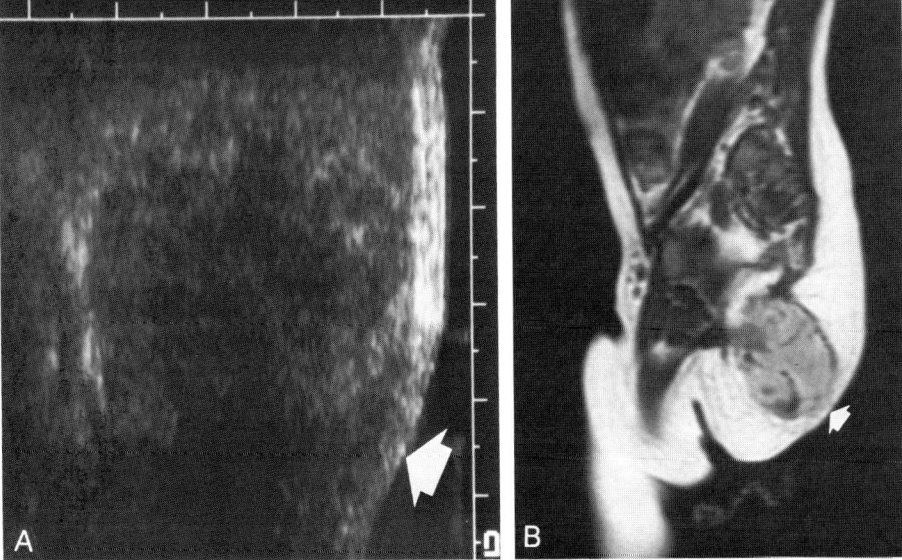

Figure 5–3. This 16-month-old presented with a gluteal mass that had been present for the preceding 2 months. The question of an abscess was raised, and ultrasonography was requested. The longitudinal scan (A) is oriented to match the subsequent magnetic resonance imaging (MRI) scan. (B). Arrow marks equivalent surface; images are of different magnification. Ultrasonography could identify the mass only as solid and atypical for abscess. MRI showed the extent and consistency of the mass, which pathologic examination showed to be benign lipoblastoma.

112 / THE EXTREMITIES

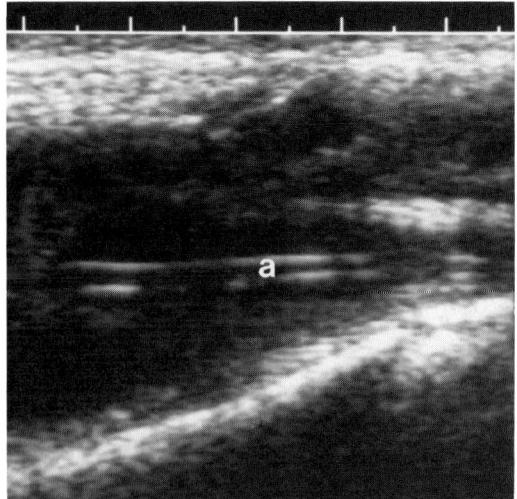

Figure 5–4. This 8-year-old boy fell into a wading pool and presented with swelling of the calf. His history was remarkable because 2 years earlier he had undergone transplantation of bone marrow after chemotherapy for acute myelogenous leukemia. Hematoma of the calf seemed a likely diagnosis after a longitudinal scan showed an ill-defined intramuscular mass surrounding an artery (a). However, the mass seems, in retrospect, unusually lucent. It increased in size over the next month, and biopsy revealed it to be a chloroma (a localized collection of leukemic cells in soft tissues). It signaled relapse of the acute myelogenous leukemia.

plied indiscriminately to popliteal cysts of all etiologies. In adults, a Baker cyst is often associated with rheumatoid arthritis or other intra-articular disease. This is not true for children who usually have no associated abnormalities. After diagnosis of popliteal cyst is confirmed by ultrasonography, conservative therapy is the rule inasmuch as the cyst usually disappears spontaneously (Fig. 5–6; Toolanen et al., 1988; Renshaw, 1986, pp. 111 to 112).

PENETRATING INJURIES OF SOFT TISSUES

Non–radio-opaque foreign bodies are typically slivers of wood or plastic. Metal and glass are virtually always radiopaque and detected on plain radiographs. Although reports indicate that ultrasonography is an ideal method for identifying splinters, a foreign body deep in the hand between metacarpals or in the foot between metatarsals can be very hard to pick out on scans. Splinters in the thenar soft tissues are easier to find, as are those in the heel pad (Fig. 5–7). Again, scans of the contralateral extremity, which provide a normal baseline, should be the first views obtained, and use of a standoff

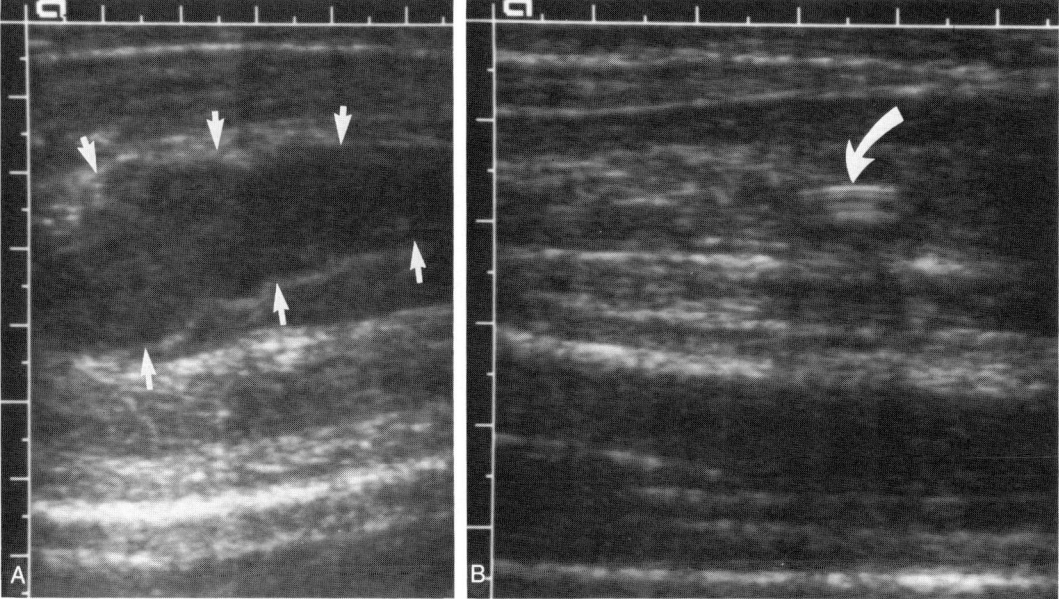

Figure 5–5. A 1-week history of pain in the left calf associated with pain and fever brought this 4½-year-old girl to the emergency room. Longitudinal scan of the calf (A) showed a heterogeneous mass (arrows) that represented an abscess in the gastrocnemius muscle. Thirty milliliters of pus was aspirated. This specimen later grew pure *Staphylococcus aureus* in culture. A catheter was left in place for drainage, and a follow-up study 3 days later (B) shows no residual locules of pus around the catheter (arrow).

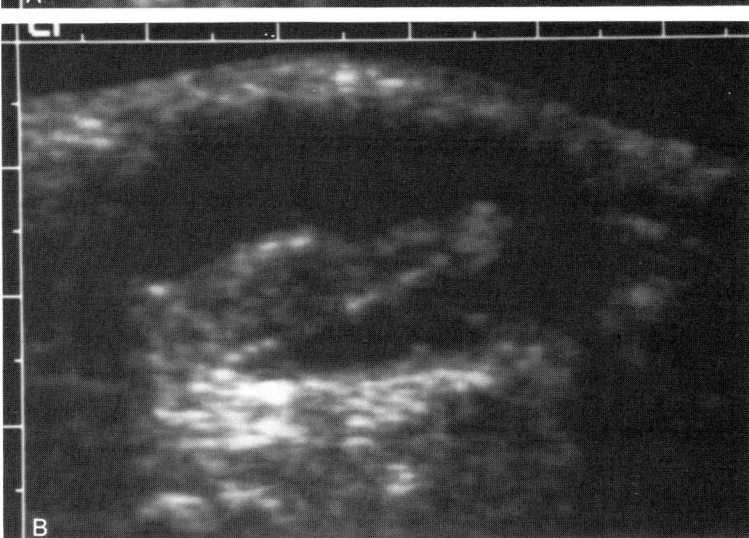

Figure 5–6. This 10-year-old boy had an asymptomatic swelling in the popliteal fossa; results of ultrasonic scans were typical of popliteal cyst. Although it appears that there are two cysts (arrows) in the longitudinal view (A), the transverse section (B) shows a single cyst that is shaped like a lobster claw. T = tibial epiphysis.

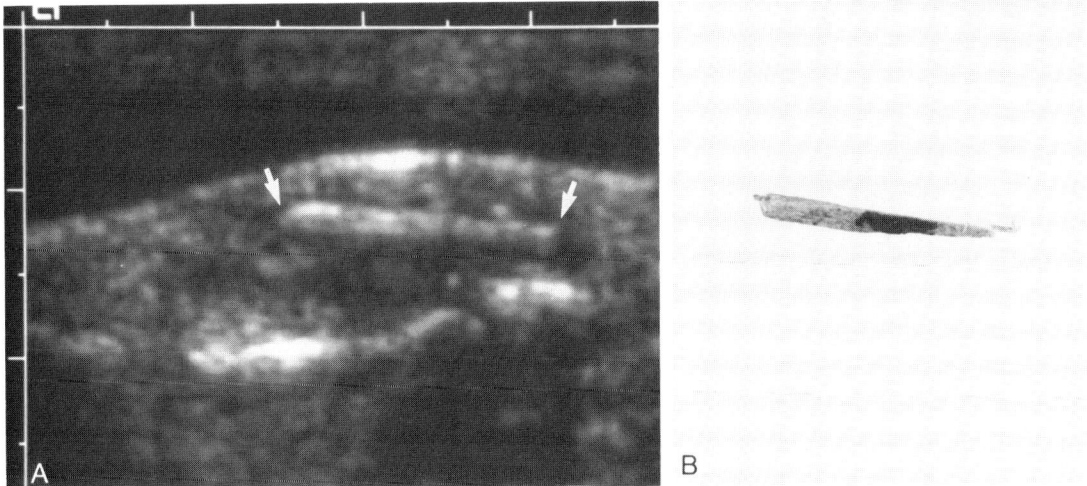

Figure 5–7. When this adolescent girl presented with a swollen thumb, radiographs showed thickening of the soft tissues but no radiopaque foreign body. In fact, she had no recollection of any traumatic episode. Longitudinal scan over the ventral portion of the interphalangeal joint (A) showed a well-defined density (arrows) in the soft tissues of the thumb. The splinter that was subsequently removed (B) is shown in the same orientation as the scan. (Courtesy of Dr. C. Hergreuter, Department of Plastic Surgery, Children's Hospital, Boston.)

pad is ideal. The foreign body produces an echogenic focus in the affected hand or foot (Fornage and Schernberg, 1986; Gooding et al., 1987; Shiels et al., 1990). The shape of the foreign body can be outlined when sequential scans are at right angles to each other, but its thickness may be underestimated. Its depth is easily measured for ease in surgical removal.

INJURIES OF TENDONS, LIGAMENTS, AND JOINTS

Experience has accumulated from ultrasonography of jumper's knee (patellar tendinitis) and a ruptured Achilles tendon (Fritschy and de Gautard, 1988; King et al., 1990; Mathieson et al., 1988). Adolescents and adults who are involved in athletic activities constitute the major group at risk for these traumatic injuries. In patients who have been reported, thickening or swelling of the tendon, in comparison with normal, was present in most symptomatic patients. Heterogeneity of the tendon was evident in many of those with patellar tendinitis or partial rupture of an Achilles tendon. In young children who have chronic tendinitis, fragmentation of the inferior edge of the patella or the tibial tuberosity may also be evident on longitudinal scans of the tendon. If the patient is able to flex and extend the extremity distal to an injury, the movement shown on real-time ultrasonography allows clearer definition of ligamentous boundaries that otherwise are obscured by adjacent edema.

The most popular use of ultrasonography in evaluating ligaments and tendons has been for injuries of the rotator cuff (Collins et al., 1987; Mack et al., 1985; Soble et al., 1989). Advocates of this technique pronounce it more accurate than arthrography. When used by experienced clinicians, this may well be true, but in our pediatric practice, injuries to the rotator cuff are few and far between. We suggest that only clinicians who are experienced in the technique and perform many studies should rely heavily on ultrasonography for diagnosis. The patient is scanned while sitting upright, with forearms resting on thighs and with humeri adducted. The biceps tendon is traced cephalad within its groove, the supraspinatus tendon is just

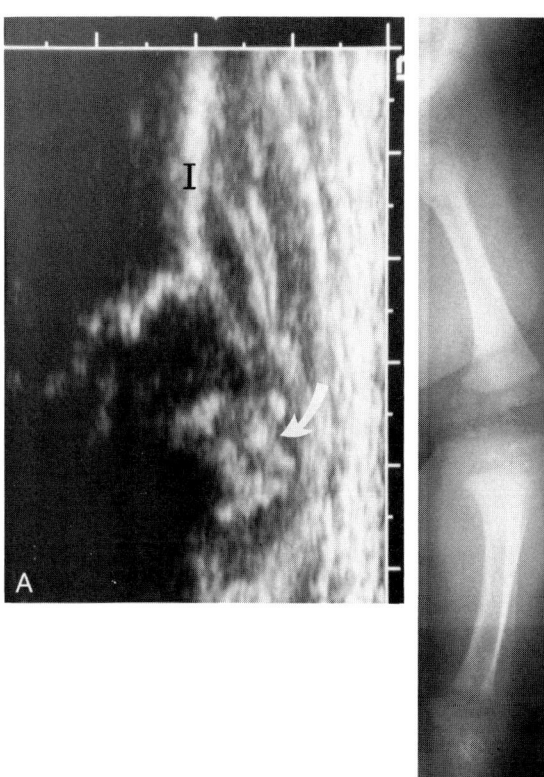

Figure 5–8. Scans of this baby's hip were remarkable for showing an unusual cluster of calcification in the region of the greater trochanter (arrow, **A**). Subsequent film of the lower extremity (**B**) does not show the greater trochanter to great advantage but does show the punctate calcifications of the tibial epiphysis and the stippled appearance of the tarsal bones in the baby, who had chondrodysplasia punctata. I = ilium. The ultrasonogram is oriented to match the radiograph.

posterolateral to the biceps tendon, and infraspinatus tendon is even more posterolateral (Mack et al., 1985). Asymmetry in these views, when one compares right and left shoulder, indicates an abnormality. Focal hyperechogenicity occurs in both partial and complete tears; discontinuity of the tendon occurs only in complete tears.

In children, cartilage and bone are much easier to scan than are their small tendons and ligaments. The normal cartilage of epiphysis and apophysis is relatively lucent. The columns of cartilage cells are represented by an irregularly regular pattern of linear echoes. Disorders of cartilage, such as chondrodysplasia punctata, result in a disorganized pattern that is detectable within the epiphyses or apophyses. (Fig. 5–8). The articular cartilage is a lucent rim, normally uniform in thickness but irregular or thinned in children with arthritis (Harcke et al., 1988). Articular cartilage of the knee is examined as the patient holds the knee in as flexed a position as possible, and the transducer is aimed into the intercondylar notch from a point just above the patella. Osteochondritis dissecans results in fragmentation of the cartilage and the subchondral bone; the osteochondral fragment can be identified on ultrasonography with transducers of high frequency (Gregersen and Rasmussen, 1989)

EFFUSION AND INFECTION

Periosteal elevation adjacent to a metaphysis can be present when osteomyelitis has resulted in subperiosteal abscess. In most clinical situations, however, the concern is proving the presence or absence of fluid within a joint. The two joints most accessible to ultrasonography are the hip and the knee. The knee is examined with the patient's leg extended and the transducer oriented longitudinally over the suprapatellar bursa. The joint may have to be squeezed in order to push a small amount of fluid into the bursa. Effusion is so readily diagnosed, clinically or with good lateral radiographs, that ultrasonography is seldom needed (Fig 5–9).

Because the coronal approach to the hip is shadowed by an overlapping acetabulum and capital femoral epiphysis in children older than 1 or 2 years, the transducer is angled along the neck of the femur through an anterior approach when their joints need

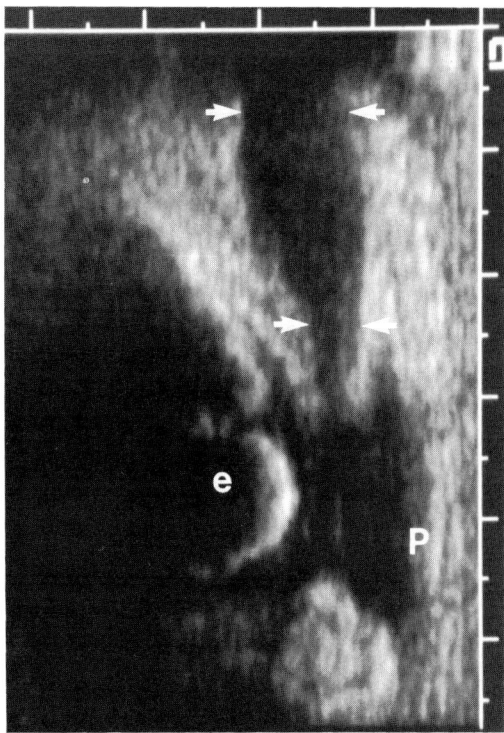

Figure 5–9. Longitudinal ultrasonogram of the left knee is oriented as a lateral radiograph. The suprapatellar bursa (arrows) is distended by echogenic fluid. This baby presented with a severely swollen knee; Haemophilus influenzae was aspirated from the joint. P = unossified patella. e = femoral epiphysis.

evaluation. Their hips must be symmetrically positioned. First the normal, and then the abnormal sides are scanned, so as to include the acetabular lip, the epiphysis, the physeal plate, and the femoral shaft. The psoas muscle is separated from the hip by the echogenic interface of the capsule. The outer boundary of articular cartilage of the femoral head is more evident if the hip is gently rotated during real-time scanning. Widening of the inferior recess of the capsule of the hip indicates that fluid is present (Fig. 5–10). Aspiration of fluid can be achieved under ultrasonic guidance, if necessary. Differentiation of blood, pus, and sterile effusion has not been possible with ultrasonography alone (Miralles et al., 1989). Ultrasonographic detection of intracapsular fluid has been far more sensitive than plain radiography; radiographs, however, provide much more information about the bones (Alexander et al., 1988). In a child who is clinically suspected of having a bacterial infection of a bone or a joint, radionuclide examination should fol-

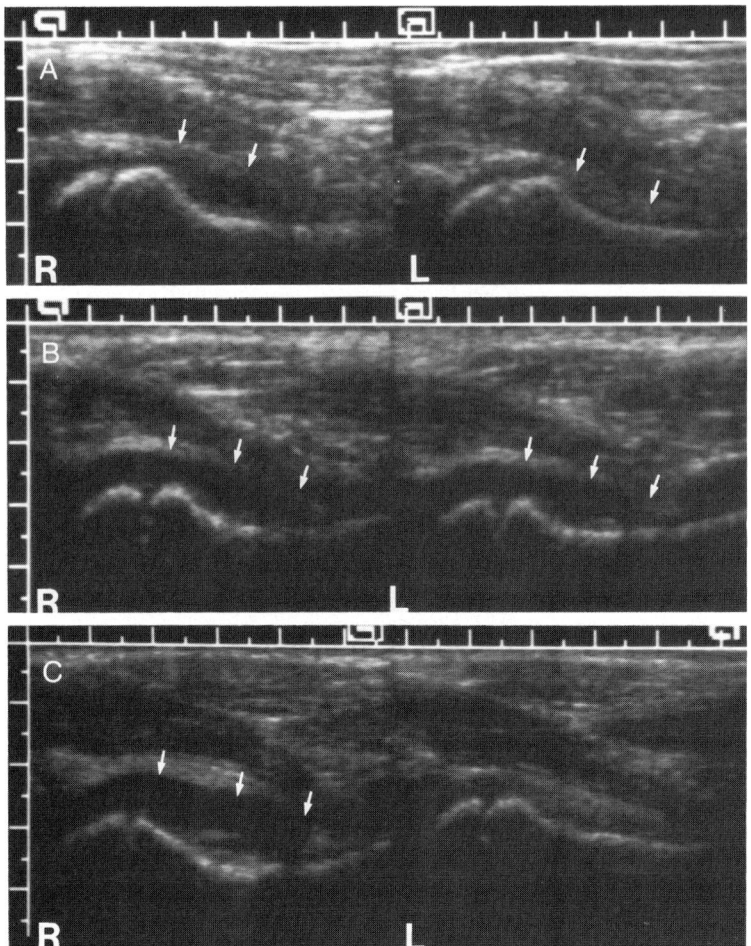

Figure 5–10. We often use the split-screen function (R = right, L = left) on the ultrasonic units in order to compare one hip with the other for a child in whom signs and symptoms suggest that fluid is present. **A** shows fluid within the right hip, lifting the anterior capsule (arrows). Compare this with the capsule (arrows) of the normal left hip. We aspirated the fluid in the right hip through the anterior soft tissues after the fluid was located with ultrasonography. The aspirate was pure pus, and the child was taken to the operating room for open drainage of septic arthritis secondary to *H. influenzae*. **B** shows bilateral effusions of the hips (arrows) in a 5-year-old with Kawasaki disease. **C** shows a very large right-sided effusion (arrows) in a 6-year-old who had a 2-day history of hip pain. The left hip is normal. Note how clear the fluid appears on this view. The pus, drained from the hip, grew *S. aureus*. Discrimination among transudate, exudate, and hemarthrosis cannot be made with ultrasonography alone.

low negative results of radiographic and ultrasonographic studies.

FRACTURE AND DEFORMITY

Other interesting uses of ultrasonography include the diagnosis of fracture (Fig. 5–11). Detection of clavicular fracture in the neonate (Katz et al., 1988) and separation of distal humeral epiphysis (Dias et al., 1988) and of proximal humeral epiphysis (Broker and Burbach, 1990) have been reported. It is worthwhile to scan neonates who have had septic arthritis of the hip, shoulder, or knee if there is concern regarding physeal separation of the epiphysis from the shaft because plain radiographs are unrevealing if the epiphysis is not ossified. Discontinuity at the physis should be evident on ultrasonography, as should an abnormal epiphysis.

Attempts to measure the degree of tibial torsion by scanning the posterior tibia proximally and distally and measuring the horizontal planes are subject to great inter- and intraobserver error, especially if the child is small. In addition, a published study describes such a large range of values for normal children that differentiation between normal and abnormal is possible only in the most exaggerated cases (Joseph et al., 1987).

VASCULAR ABNORMALITIES OF THE EXTREMITIES

In children these can be grouped into four major categories: congenital abnormalities of arteries and veins, venous thrombosis, pseudoaneurysms resulting from trauma or previous angiography, and complications of surgically created vascular shunts.

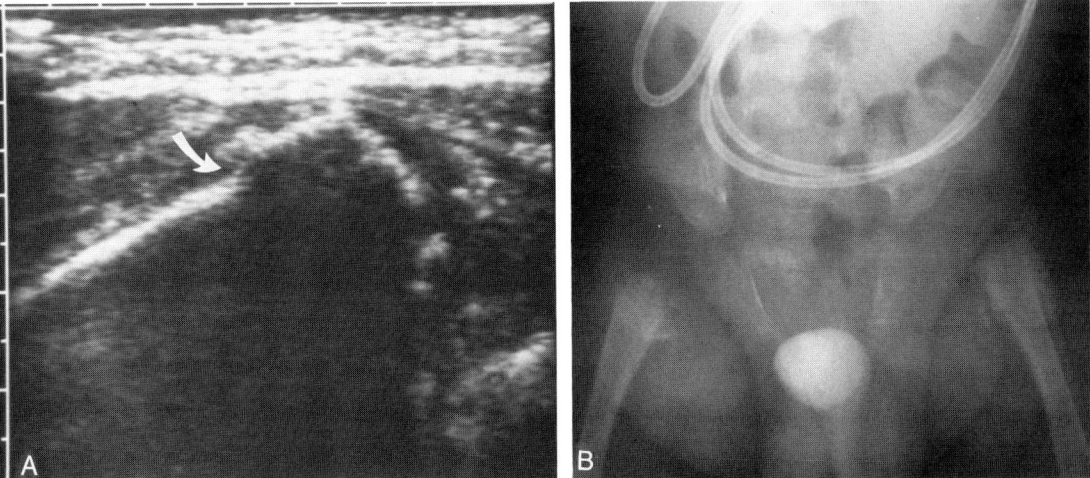

Figure 5-11. During scanning of the hips (A), requested because the baby had a meningomyelocele, an obvious stepoff in the cortex of the left femur (arrow) was apparent. The left hip was also completely dislocated. Radiography performed the same day (B) showed bilateral proximal femoral fractures with periosteal reaction and dislocated hips. The tube that is superimposed over lower abdomen is from a ventriculoperitoneal shunt. Fractures resulted from overly enthusiastic physical therapy.

Congenital Abnormalities of Vessels

Mulliken and Young (1988) have encouraged us to use their classification of vascular birthmarks as either hemangiomas or vascular malformations. Hemangiomas are characterized by a plump endothelium that has an accelerated rate of turnover, rapid postnatal proliferation, and gradual involution. Malformations may be capillary, arterial, venous, lymphatic, or mixed. Their endothelium is flat, its turnover time is slow, and growth of the lesion is usually commensurate with growth of the patient. Trauma, infection, and hormonal stimulation may increase the rate of growth. Hemangiomas may proliferate so quickly that they conscript nutritive and draining vessels, but the vessels are rarely as large as those associated with true malformations (Fig. 5-12). Doppler ultrasonography is an ideal method with which to evaluate malformations of the extremities inasmuch as one can easily correlate the characteristics of flow through the lesion with the clinical presentation. Purely lymphatic malformation (cystic hygroma) should be silent on Doppler images. The blood flow through venous malformations may be so slow that they are also "silent," but with careful technique and exercise of the extremity prior to ultrasonographic scanning, one may be able to hear the low venous hum with Doppler scanning. Arteriovenous malformation, because of the shunting, may have a palpable thrill; blood flow is quite obvious on Doppler images.

Deep Venous Thrombosis

This common affliction of adults is uncommon in children. We only occasionally see children who are referred because of a swollen leg, tenderness in the calf, or previous episode of pulmonary emboli. Predisposing factors to venous thrombosis in children include hypercoagulable state, polycythemia, previous injury to the leg, and previous injury to the veins (including earlier use of veins as an access to cardiac catheterization). We have borrowed techniques from the literature on adults to diagnose venous thrombosis, and our anecdotal experience suggests that ultrasonography is a useful first study (Plate IV).

The patient is placed supine on the examining table, and the venous system is scanned from the top down. The inferior vena cava is viewed in sagittal and transverse planes as far inferiorly as possible. In some patients—younger children and adolescents whose livers have a long right lobe—the cava can often be viewed down to its bifurcation in the coronal plane. It is difficult to scan the iliac veins, but a full bladder can make scanning easier. Doppler imaging of the iliac veins is hindered because the beam intersects the vessel in a perpendicular fashion. It has to be angled at less than 60° with the vessel in order to get a reasonable signal. Examination of the femoral veins at the groin is much easier. We use a linear array transducer of 5 MHz or greater, begin with the patient's normal leg, and adjust gain settings in order that the lumen of femoral vein is clear of

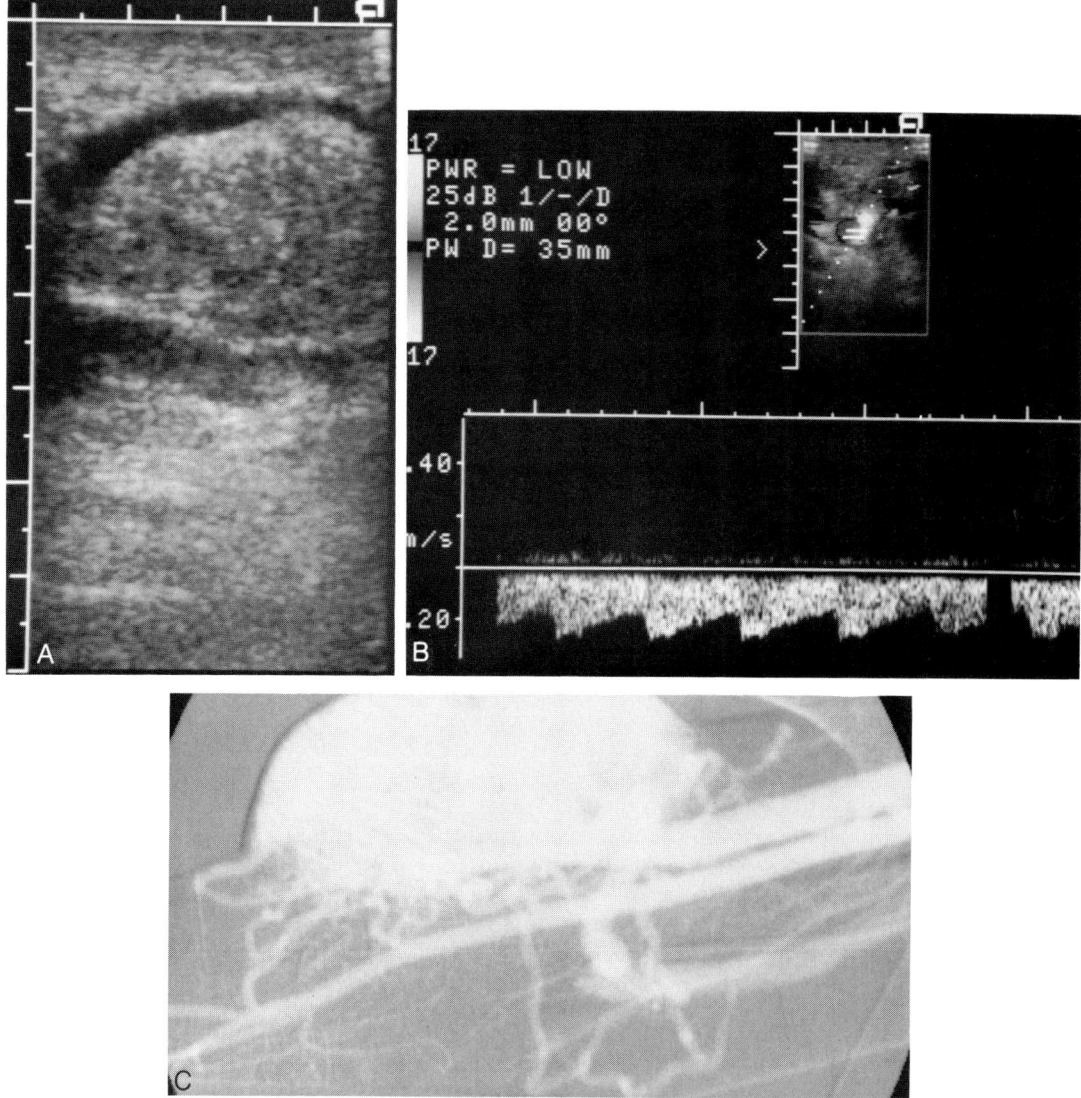

Figure 5–12. This lesion (A) was a large lump on a boy's upper arm. Veins and arteries throughout the mass were easily traced with Doppler ultrasonography (B) and angiography (C) and confirmed the vascular nature of the lesion. Although our studies indicated that this was an arteriovenous malformation, the histologic examinations of the mass revealed hemangioma, and its resection seems to have been curative; that is, there has been no recurrence. This case points out the difficulties of differentiating between an arteriovenous malformation and hemangioma.

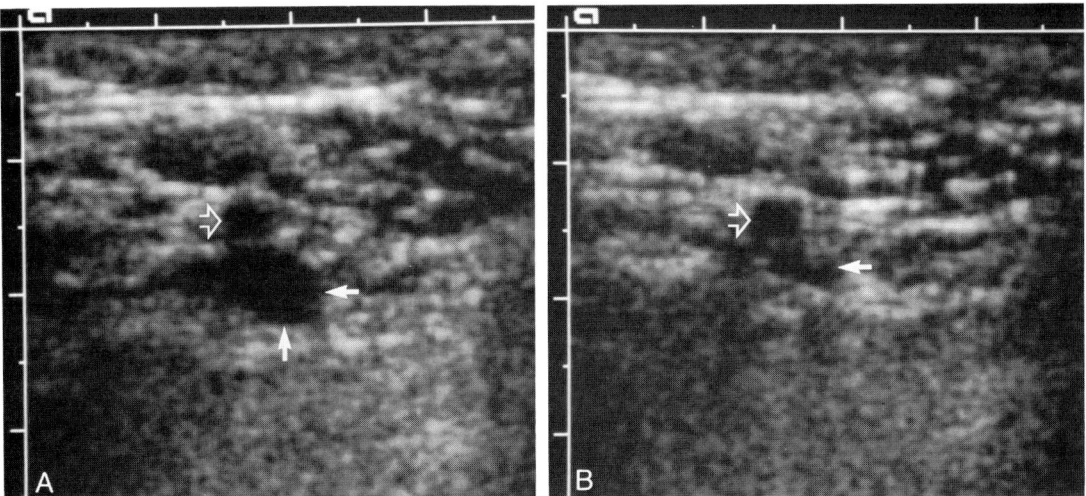

Figure 5–13. These are normal transverse views of the femoral vein (solid arrows) without (A) and with (B) compression. The artery (open arrow) is just anterior to the vein. The vein should collapse completely with compression.

artifactual echoes on the scans. After transverse and longitudinal views of the normal femoral vein, we obtain a compression view. This is done with the transducer transverse to the vein (Fig. 5–13). Longitudinal compression is not reliable because the vein may slip sideways rather than being compressed (Vogel et al., 1987). The same routine is then used to scan the symptomatic leg. Noncompressibility of the lumen implies that a clot is present. Although a clot may be faintly or obviously echogenic, some are surprisingly echolucent and are easily missed if compression of the vein is not performed (Cronan et al., 1987; Figs. 5–14, 5–15).

The common and superficial femoral veins are examined as far inferiorly as possible; images on hard copy are obtained when any abnormality is noted. A markedly diminished response of the common femoral vein to the Valsalva maneuver (i.e., less than a 10 percent increase in diameter) is useful for suggesting a thrombus in an iliac vein or the common femoral vein above the site of scanning. Children are not always able to perform the Valsalva maneuver properly, and a dampened response (10 to 50 percent increase) is neither sensitive nor specific for thrombosis (Vogel et al., 1987). Isolated iliac venous thrombosis is rare in adults and probably more unusual in children. The maneuver is worth attempting with compliant children and when a pelvic cause for thrombosis (e.g., previous surgery, infection) is strongly suspected.

The patient is turned prone for examination of popliteal areas. Distention of the popliteal veins is aided by tilting of the table, with the patient's feet downwards. The routine is similar to that used for femoral veins: transverse and longitudinal views followed by compression, first on the normal leg and then on the abnormal leg. The popliteal vein is followed inferiorly to its branching veins, but we have been unable to document the

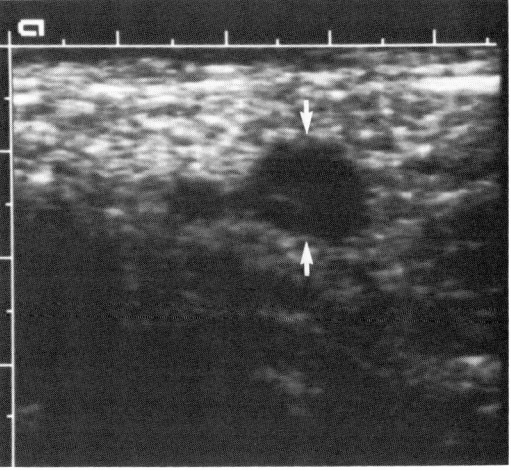

Figure 5–14. This 9-year-old boy with Down syndrome had disseminated varicella. A right femoral catheter had been placed but was removed when the leg became swollen. Ultrasonography showed, on transverse scan, a noncompressible femoral vein (arrows). This was filled with a lucent clot. Doppler scans showed no blood flow within the vein.

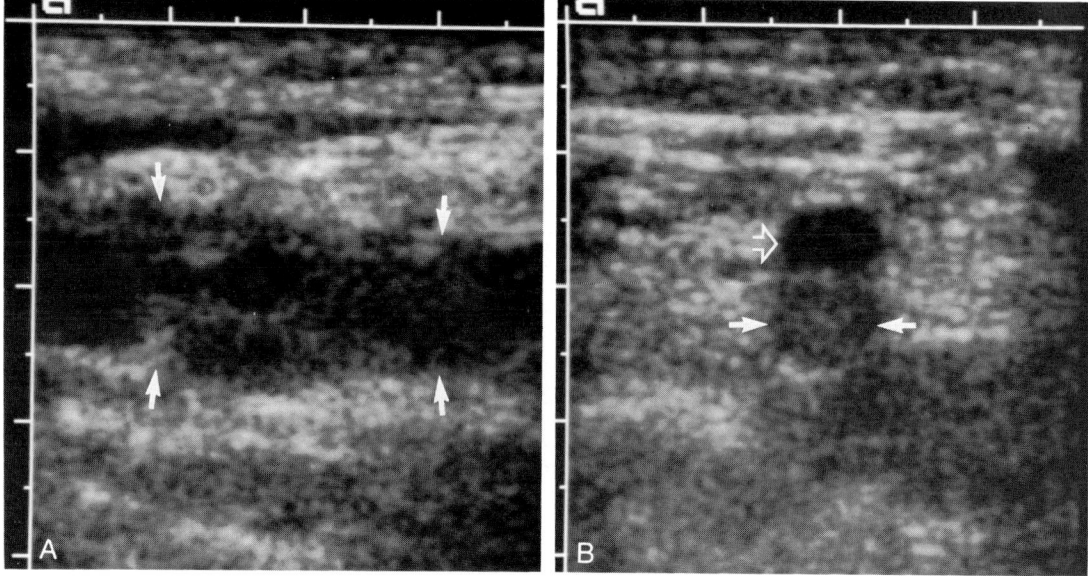

Figure 5–15. Longitudinal scan (**A**) of the femoral vein (arrows) shows that it is widened and contains an echogenic clot. Transverse view (**B**) with compression shows the femoral artery (open arrow) immediately anterior to the vein. A clot (arrows) fills the femoral vein.

presence or absence of clot in the veins of the calf. This is also the experience of others and is the major limitation of the procedure (Cronan et al., 1987, Appelman et al., 1987, Vogel et al., 1987)

Doppler imaging of the vessels can be achieved simultaneously with real-time imaging, but its use is not mandatory. Lack of Doppler ultrasonographic capability should not deter use of ultrasonography in the diagnosis of venous thrombosis (Cronan et al., 1988). Doppler imaging can be used to show a signal of higher velocity in the popliteal vein immediately after the calf is squeezed, which forces an abruptly increased volume of blood through the vein (Fig. 5–16). This Doppler response, however, is a poorly sensitive test of venous thrombosis because it would be absent only if most or all of the deep veins of the calf were clotted.

If results of the venous study are normal

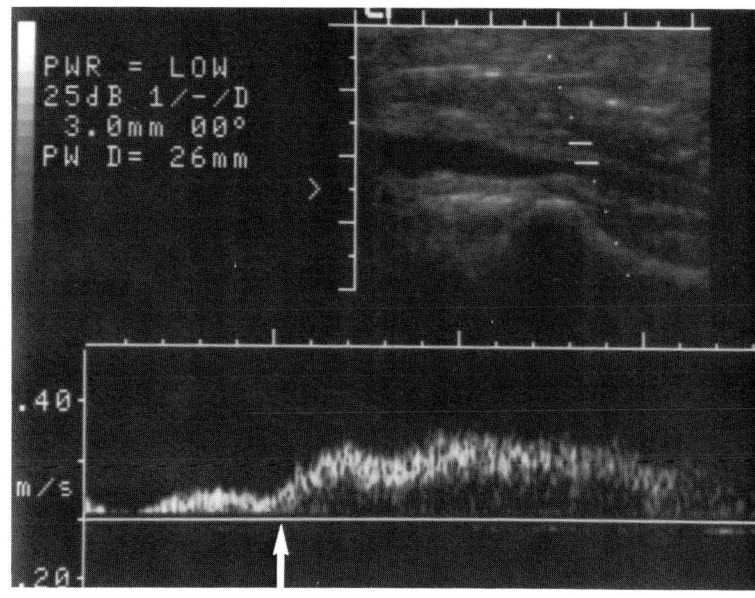

Figure 5–16. Compression of the calf (starting at arrow) results in blood flow of higher velocity through the popliteal vein when it is unobstructed by a clot.

to this point, we also scan for other causes of the clinical symptoms (soft tissue mass, hematoma, and so forth). Depending on the clinical situation and the level of suspicion of deep venous thrombosis, we advocate further evaluation for patients with negative results of ultrasonography. Scanning with I-125 labeled fibrinogen is quite sensitive for detecting thrombi in the calf and is another alternative to phlebography in this situation. The clinical significance of underdiagnosing clots in the calf veins of the adult patient is controversial. Some clinicians do not recommend use of anticoagulants unless the clot extends into the popliteal vein; others do (Salzman, 1986).

In children, however, the diagnosis of deep venous thrombosis is so unusual that documentation of venous normalcy or abnormalcy is important in both short-term and long-term management. Some children have congenital angiodysplasia of the superficial or deep venous systems, or both. These malformations are structural anomalies and present as spongy masses with a port-wine stain resulting from capillary dilation or, in extreme cases, with a swollen, painful extremity (Gorenstein et al., 1988). Children with these malformations and other children with congenital angiodysplasias are best evaluated with static and functional venography or arteriography.

Venous thrombosis associated with previous placement of intravenous catheters can be evaluated with ultrasonography. A clot in a subclavian vein can be visualized with scans along, and angling under, the clavicle. If a clot is lucent, it may be difficult to diagnose because compression of the vein is hampered by its location. The Valsalva maneuver normally increases the diameter of the vein, and cooperative older children should be asked to perform this maneuver during the study. The clot may be present and nonobstructing; it may become more evident as an intraluminal echogenicity when liquid blood outlines it during the Valsalva maneuver. Doppler imaging of the lumen of the subclavian vein is very helpful in establishing the presence of blood flow and in differentiating the vein from the adjacent artery. Color Doppler imaging is ideal in allowing quick localization of the vessels. The confluence of the internal jugular vein and the subclavian vein as they form the brachiocephalic vein can be visualized in the coronal view from the supraclavicular fossa (Falk and Smith, 1987). Normally, there is a valve in the distal section of both vessels before they join. This intraluminal echogenic structure should not be mistaken for a clot. The internal jugular vein also increases in diameter during the Valsalva maneuver. Its location allows compression in order to identify a hypoechoic intraluminal clot (Figs. 5-17, 5-18).

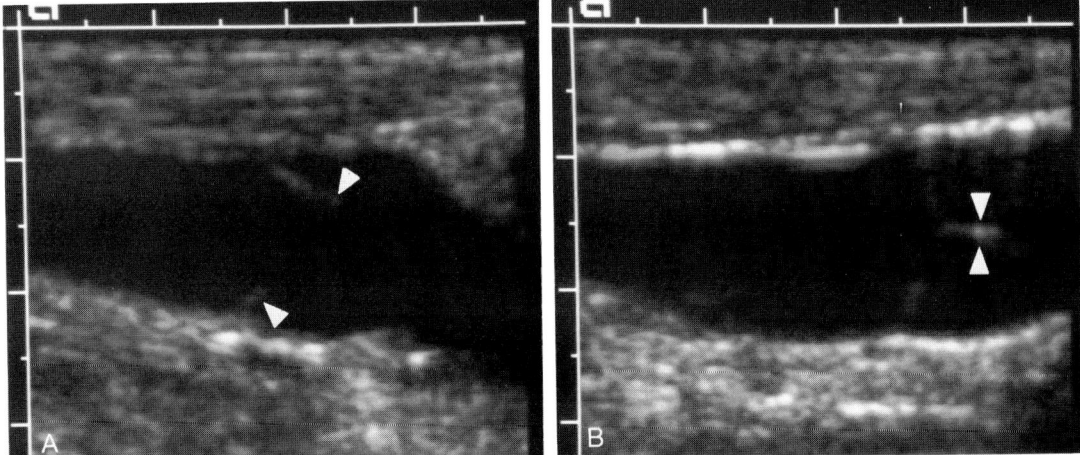

Figure 5-17. Longitudinal scans of the internal jugular vein show bicuspid valve (arrowheads), which is located 1 cm proximal to the junction of the internal jugular vein with the subclavian vein. This normally occurring structure should not be confused with an intraluminal clot. Slight dilatation of the vein distal to the valve is a normal finding. (**A**, valve open; **B**, valve closed.)

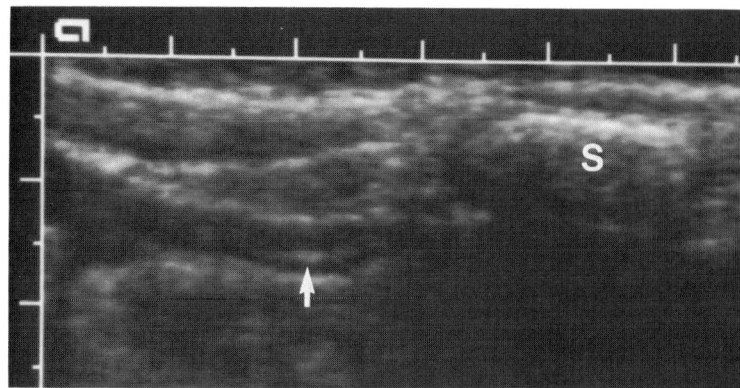

Figure 5-18. A catheter had been removed from the right subclavian vein of this patient, who had spiking temperatures. A residual clot (arrow) is still apparent within the vein. S = sternum.

Vascular Shunts and Pseudoaneurysms

Children who have vascular anastomoses that were created for hemodialysis can be evaluated with ultrasonography if they develop swelling, pain, or other symptoms referable to the surgical site. Usually, however, complications require intervention and both diagnostic and therapeutic goals are achieved by angiography (Hoffer, 1986).

There are many choices of devices or techniques for achieving vascular access (May and Andus, 1985). Most centers have favored using direct arteriovenous anastomoses to avoid the complications of infection associated with the plastic external device of the Scribner shunt. The typical locations for surgical arteriovenous communication are the wrist, the elbow, and the knee. Acute complications of the procedure include perivenous hematoma, which obstructs blood flow, as do twists or kinks in the vein. Failure of a fistula after it has been used for some time is most commonly due to venous stenosis, especially when a segment of vein has been interposed between the main artery and the vein. The stenosis typically occurs at the venovenous anastomosis or at the junction of prosthetic material with the vein.

The ultrasonographic examination should be guided by knowledge of the previous surgical procedure (Fig. 5-19). The shunted artery should show an arterial signal proximal to the anastomosis with the vein or venous segment. The anastomosis should be widely patent. The vein is usually dilated beyond the site of the anastomosis, but a hugely aneurysmic vein is abnormal and indicates that most arterial blood flow is entering the shunt. Distal ischemia of the limb may result if the shunt is too large. The vein should be traced proximally to identify stenoses that may be present. A clot in the fistula is quite evident clinically because the palpable thrill and audible bruit disappear. The extent of the clot can be diagnosed with ultrasonography before catheterization and thrombolytic therapy.

Pseudoaneurysm or arteriovenous fistula are complications of penetrating wounds of the extremities and previous catheterization

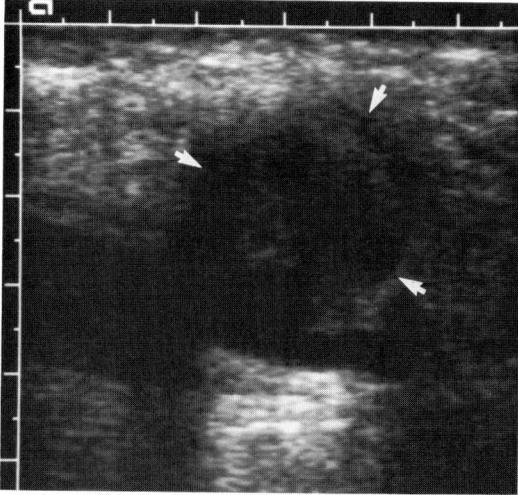

Figure 5-19. This 21-year-old patient, who had a history of chronic renal failure, presented with pain and a mass in the right thigh. His history was important, for he had previously undergone surgical creation of an arteriovenous fistula in the right leg. The mass (arrows) that was apparent on the ultrasonogram arose from the anterior surface of the right femoral artery. The Doppler scan showed no apparent blood flow within the mass. In the operating room, a clotted aneurysm, which extended from the femoral artery, appeared to be the residual blind end of a saphenous vein graft, part of the arteriovenous fistula that had since been ligated.

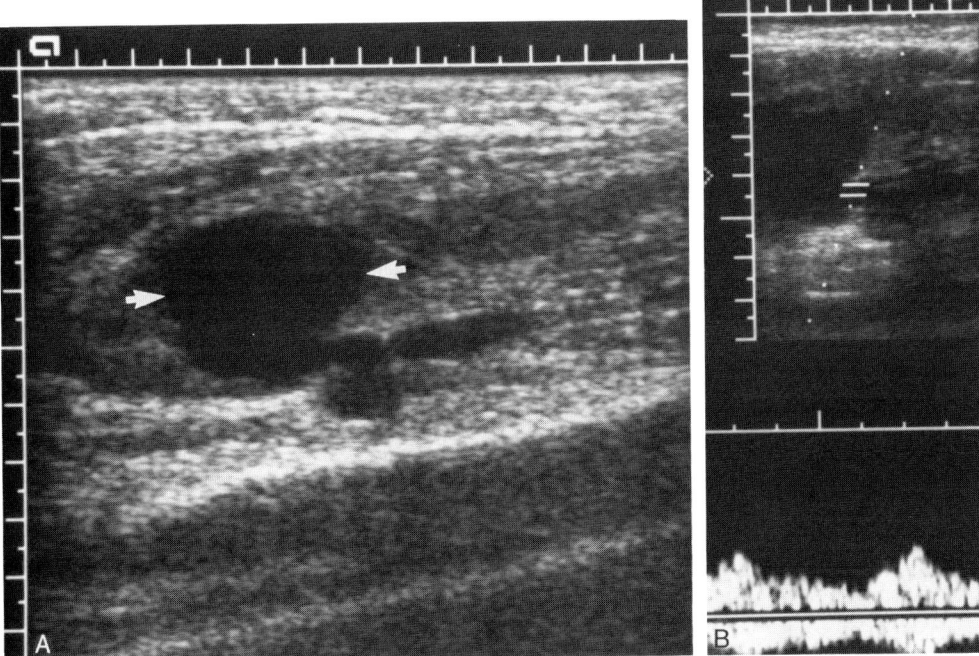

Figure 5–20. Scans of the calf were performed 1 week after this 11-year-old girl sustained a stab wound to the leg. She presented with increasing swelling of the calf. The longitudinal scan (**A**) showed a lucent mass (arrows) obviously related to vessels within the calf. Doppler ultrasonogram (**B**) showed both arterial and venous flow, depending on the site of sampling. Angiography confirmed pseudoaneurysm of the posterior tibial artery with arteriovenous communication.

of femoral arteries (Fig. 5–20). The differential diagnosis of perivascular swelling is usually between hematoma and pseudoaneurysm. Pseudoaneurysm is defined as a contained collection of blood that maintains continuity with the arterial lumen (Plate V). Complications of pseudoaneurysm include rupture, compression of neighboring structures, and retrograde propagation of thrombus.

The child who presents with acute symptoms immediately after arterial injury is evaluated with real-time imaging and Doppler scanning. The swelling may be extensive and hinder examination, as may the child's reluctance to cooperate with a study that requires a transducer on a very sore leg or arm. The aims of the study are to trace the artery through the area of injury, to document blood flow in its lumen, and to search for a localized outpouching of the vessel. If blood flow is documented within the outpouching, continuity with arterial lumen is documented, and the lesion is a pseudoaneurysm. Lack of blood flow within a collection adherent to a vessel may make differentiation between hematoma and thrombosed pseudoaneurysm impossible. Conservative therapy and follow-up scans can be done with the full realization that arteriography may be needed if there is any change in the results of the child's clinical examination. There have also been reports of spontaneous thrombosis and resolution of pseudoaneurysms (Fig. 5–21; Kotval et al., 1990).

Arterial occlusion may result from previous cardiac catheterization through the femoral artery, especially if the affected child was young at the time of initial investigation and if the catheters that were used were large in caliber. In one study, arterial occlusion was diagnosed in one third of patients who had had previous diagnostic femoral arterial catheterization before they reached their 5th birthdays (Taylor et al., 1990).

CONGENITAL DYSPLASIA OF THE HIP

Congenital dysplasia of the hip (CDH) is a continuum of anomalies referable to the hip, from slightly shallow acetabulum to irreducible dislocation. CDH does not always mean

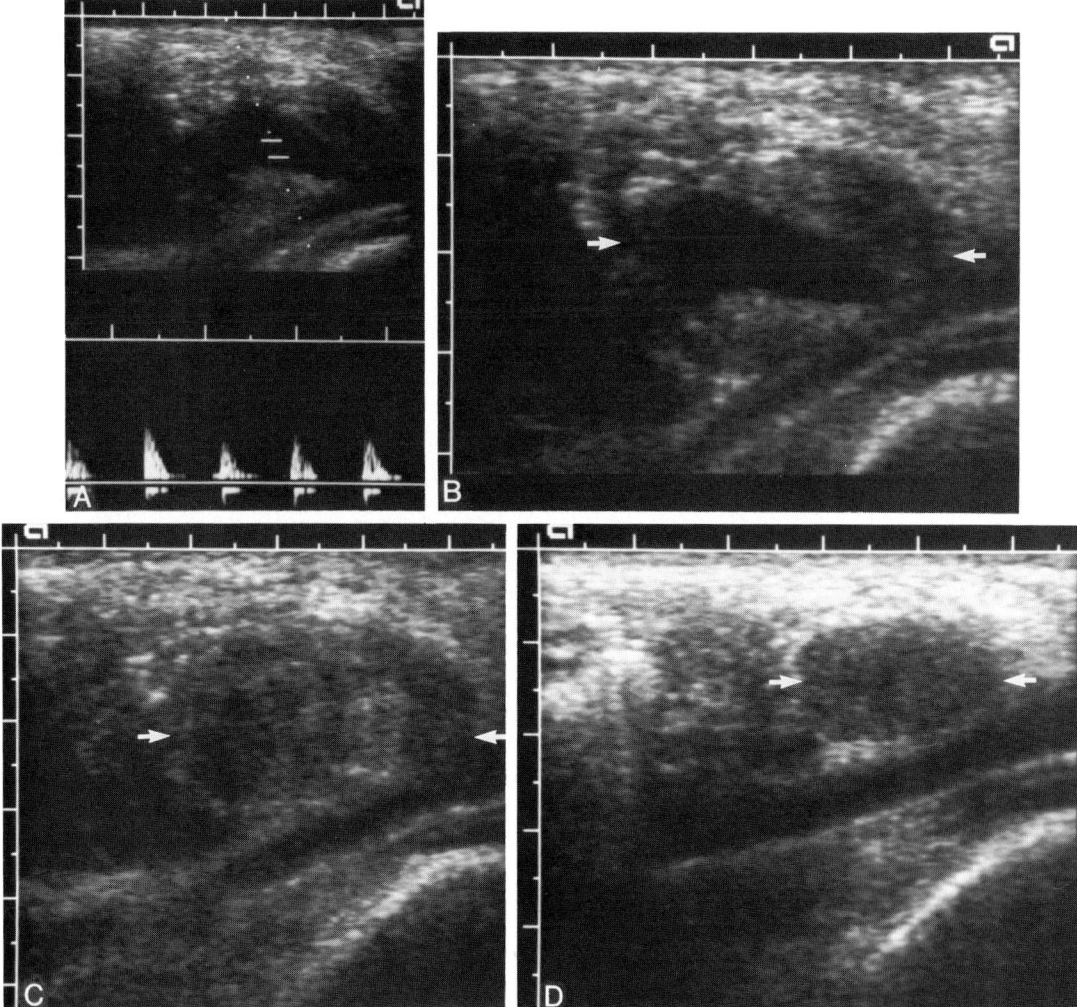

Figure 5-21. This 21-year-old had complicated congenital heart disease, which had been partially treated. He required another catheterization through a femoral arterial approach. One day after the catheterization, he complained of left-sided groin pain. The initial ultrasonogram showed a large hematoma around the left iliac artery. Hematocrit dropped from 43 to 30. Ten days later, a pulsatile mass was detected in the groin. The next ultrasonogram showed a pseudoaneurysm of the left femoral artery (**A**). Over the next month and a half, the pseudoaneurysm (arrows) gradually clotted and became smaller (**B, C,** and **D**). Surgical intervention was not performed.

congenital *dislocation* of the hip. We believe that of all ultrasonographic studies in babies, evaluation of the hip is the most difficult for the novice. It requires reacquaintance with the clinical examination of the neonatal hip and careful review of the anatomy before one approaches the baby with a transducer.

Although recognized in the writings of Hippocrates, CDH has been diagnosed, with reliability, in neonates, only since 1937, when Marino Ortolani described the maneuver that bears his name. Ortolani was a young pediatrician in Ferrara, Italy, when a mother brought her 5-month-old-baby, who had Cooley's anemia, to him for treatment. She showed him what she had noticed when washing the child's perineum: that there was a clunking as the hip was abducted and adducted. Recognizing after a radiograph was taken that the hip was dislocated, Ortolani began to examine other babies by using the same maneuver. Because he was in an area with a high incidence of CDH, he gained a considerable experience over a short time (Stanisavljevic, 1976). There are two morals of this story: fortune favors the prepared mind, and when in doubt, listen to the child's parent! Barlow (1962) reported his method

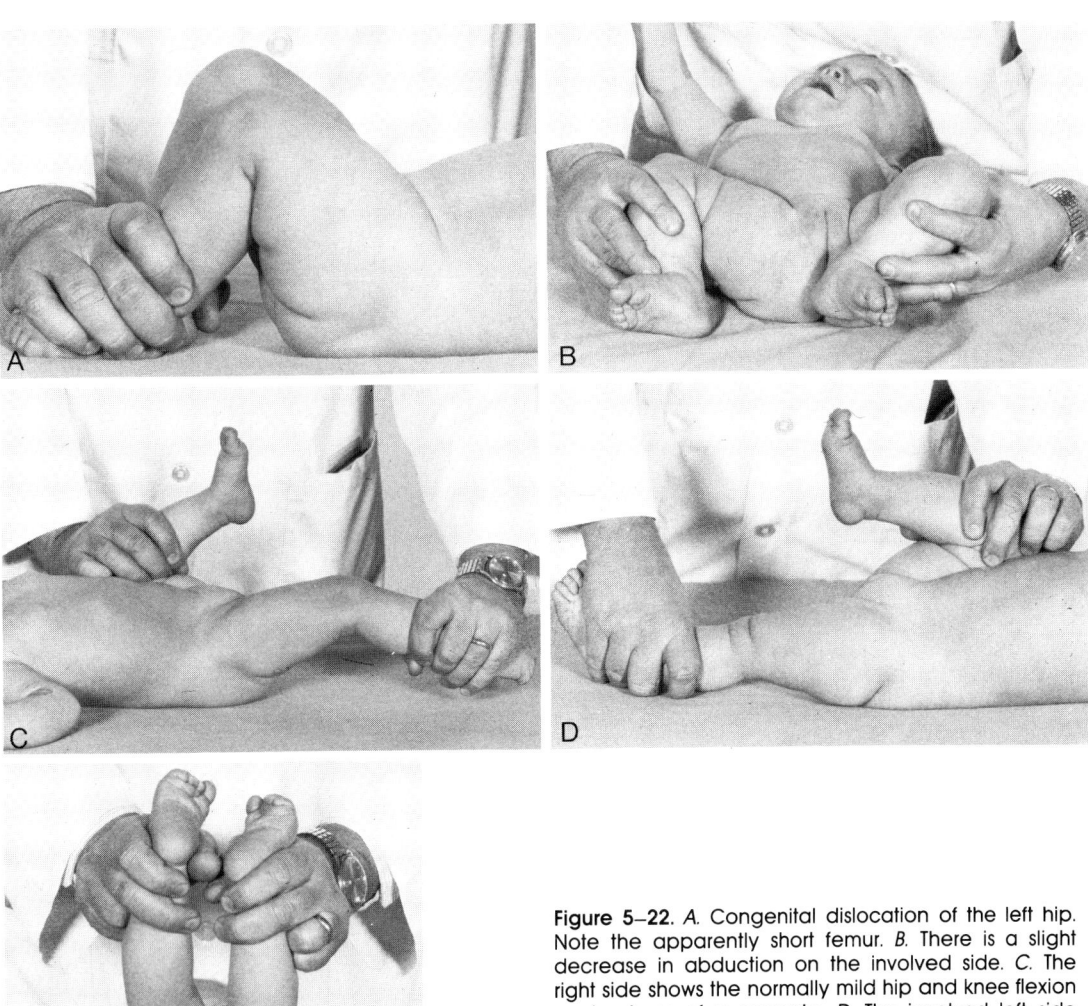

Figure 5–22. *A.* Congenital dislocation of the left hip. Note the apparently short femur. *B.* There is a slight decrease in abduction on the involved side. *C.* The right side shows the normally mild hip and knee flexion contractures of a neonate. *D.* The involved left side shows loss of the hip and knee flexion contractures. *E.* An apparently short left femur and asymmetric skin folds. (From Renshaw TS: Pediatric Orthopaedics. Philadelphia: WB Saunders, 1986.)

of clinical assessment and the results of early treatment of congenital dislocation. Clinical examination of the baby in the first 6 weeks after birth usually is characterized by the presence or absence of positive findings referable to Ortolani's and Barlow's maneuvers. The Italian orthopedist Riccardo Galeazzi contributed his sign for CDH: apparent shortening of the femur on the involved side. Two other important signs are (1) limitation of abduction when the hip is in flexion and (2) the mobility triad: loss of the normal mild (20° to 40°) adduction contracture of the newborn's hip that is related to the knee-to-chest position in utero (Fig. 5–22; Renshaw, 1986). Hip clicks alone are usually benign and probably ligamentous in origin, resulting either from the fascia lata's passing over the greater trochanter or from the psoas ligament's crossing the capsule (Chung, 1986). Asymmetric skin folds around the upper thighs are present in 30 percent of the normal population.

These findings, therefore, are not by themselves signs of CDH.

An experienced clinician can make the clinical diagnosis of CDH quite reliably, but there are still babies who are found to be affected late in infancy or in childhood, despite previous normal results of examinations. The factors contributing to CDH include a familial (presumably genetic) tendency, lack of acetabular depth, ligamentous laxity, previous abnormal position in the uterus, and swaddling practices in the neonatal period. In Japan, after the institution of a national program to discourage the traditional swaddling of babies with their hips extended, the incidence of CDH dropped to 0.2 percent from a previous high of 3.5 percent (Yamamuro and Ishida, 1984). The Navaho Indians, who used a similar position for holding babies on cradle boards, had a 6 percent incidence of CDH. In large studies, the incidence is between 1 and 2 percent of a white population, and the incidence in groups of black Africans that have been studied is virtually zero; in black Americans, the incidence is intermediate between the two, which possibly reflects genetic heterogeneity (Burke et al., 1985).

In white populations, complete dislocation of the hip at birth, called "teratologic dislocation," occurs in 1 of 500 newborns. Although the general incidence of breech presentation is 3 percent of pregnancies, 17 percent of CDH occurs in breech presentations. Of girls born from breech presentation, 7 percent have an unstable hip, and in the total population of babies with CDH, girls outnumber boys 6:1. The first-born is at greater risk than subsequent siblings. Bilateral instability is more common than unilateral instability. Interestingly, the overall incidence of CDH is higher in winter births than in summer births by 1.5:1 (Renshaw, 1986).

Radiography of CDH in the neonatal period has been notoriously unreliable except in babies with flagrant dislocation. Ultrasonography has filled the "imaging gap" with its demonstration of the cartilaginous portions of the joint. It can be repeated, when needed, to follow the results of treatment. In the last 5 years there has been a dramatic increase in the number of ultrasonic studies and in the number of journal articles reporting this experience. Some authors recommend screening all neonates with ultrasonography (Szöke et al., 1988). However, reports of long-term follow-up of large numbers of children, prospectively screened, are scanty. There is also the concern that with universal screening, overtreatment may occur. Abduction splints and harnesses are not without complications. The femoral head becomes ischemic if its blood supply via ligamentum teres is compromised. We are currently limiting our examinations to those babies whose clinical examination is abnormal and infants who have a strong family history of CDH or who are born from breech presentation. Babies who have significant abnormalities of the knee or foot, congenital torticollis, or high meningomyelocele are included in the group of infants whose clinical examination is abnormal. To handle the total neonatal population born at the adjacent obstetrical hospital alone, we would be doing 40 studies daily. Such numbers of studies also imply a hefty economic investment.

When clinicians discuss CDH, they tend to classify abnormal hips into three groups: (1) *teratologic*, the established intrauterine dislocation; (2) the *dislocatable* hip, in which the acetabulum is normally formed but the hip can be easily dislocated with the Barlow maneuver (flexion and adduction of the hip and posterior axial pressure on the thigh) and for which ligamentous laxity appears to play a major etiologic role; and (3) the *subluxable* hip, in which the acetabulum is more saucer-like than cuplike and instability varies from minor to gross; primary acetabular dysplasia is the most prominent feature in this type (Renshaw, 1986).

Babies with teratologic dislocation may have underlying musculoskeletal anomalies (e.g., arthrogryposis) or neurologic abnormalities. We often include scans of the spinal canal in such infants to rule in or out unsuspected tethering of the spinal cord or other anomalies.

Ultrasonography of the unstressed *dislocatable* hip shows normal anatomy and normal acetabular cupping. Stress views show the degree of dislocation. The *subluxable* hip appears anatomically abnormal on scans. The acetabulum appears more like the cross-section of a golf tee than that of an egg cup. Stress views will show varying degrees of mobility of the femoral head.

There have been attempts to quantify the degree of laxity of the hip by measuring differences between the femoral head and acetabular landmarks before and during the Barlow maneuver. One report suggested that laxity of 5 mm or more is present in the pathologic hip (Saies et al., 1988). Different examiners with different equipment (i.e., linear array or sector scanner) and with more or less energy or enthusiasm might not be able to duplicate these absolute numbers. The Barlow maneuver should be done with only gentle posterior pressure. When we measured the amount of force (by scientifically using a telephone receiver, to simulate a baby's femur, pushed against a kitchen scale!), we generated 5 to 8 lbs of pressure, as did the orthopedic surgeons. Too great a posterior force applied to the hip may be harmful. It should be emphasized that ligamentous laxity is common immediately after birth because the infant has been experiencing the same surge of hormones—notably, relaxin—as has the mother. It is our experience that hips seem to "tighten up" over the first 2 weeks after birth. Therefore, to avoid "falsely positive" studies, we prefer to perform ultrasonography when the baby is more than 2 weeks of age.

After this long introduction to CDH, it is time to discuss ultrasonographic technique. The initial studies reported by investigators on both sides of the Atlantic were static only. Coronal views of the femoral head and its relationship to the acetabulum were advocated by Graf (1987). Measurements of angles describing this relationship in the midiliac plane were established for normal and dysplastic hips. In the U.S., Novick and colleagues (1983) described transverse views of the hip. Harcke and associates (1984, 1990), Keller and colleagues (1986), and Boal and Schwenkter (1985), also in the U.S., were early advocates of dynamic scanning: evaluating the relationship of the femoral head to the acetabulum through the full range of motion as well as with posteriorly directed stress.

The initial scans that we take are coronal views of each hip (Fig. 5–23). The baby is placed in the decubitus or partial decubitus position with the upper leg partially extended. Some babies are so chubby that it is difficult to align the transducer properly if they lie completely supine. The transducer, preferably linear array, is placed on the skin with its long axis in line with the ilium, femoral head, and femoral shaft. The transducer is moved "through" the femoral head from anterior to posterior in order to judge its coverage by the acetabular roof. The maximal diameter of the femoral head, which

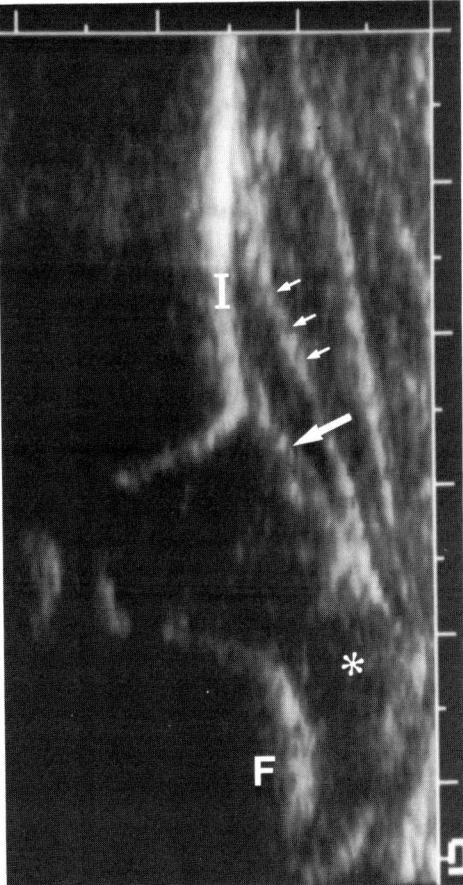

Figure 5–23. The optimal coronal scan in the midplane of the acetabulum cuts the ilium (I) in its straightest vertical portion and the spherical capital femoral epiphysis through its widest diameter. Other landmarks are the labrum acetabulare (large arrow); the fascial plane between the gluteus minimus and gluteus medius (small arrows), which insert into the greater trochanter of the femur (asterisk); and the femoral shaft (F). In this and all subsequent coronal scans, the image is oriented as an anteroposterior radiograph of the hip.

Keller (1986) termed the "equator," should be covered to at least half its width by the bony acetabular roof. The acetabulum is a composite cup formed by the ilium, the ischium, and the pubis. The Y-shaped triradiate cartilage, which lines the borders of the abutting bones, allows sound to pass through it. Far anterior, sound passes through cartilage between the ilium and the pubis; in mid-acetabulum, the stalk of the "Y" (triradiate cartilage) separates the pubis and the ischium; far posterior, the ilium abuts the ischium. There is, therefore, always a cartilaginous band that provides a visible edge to

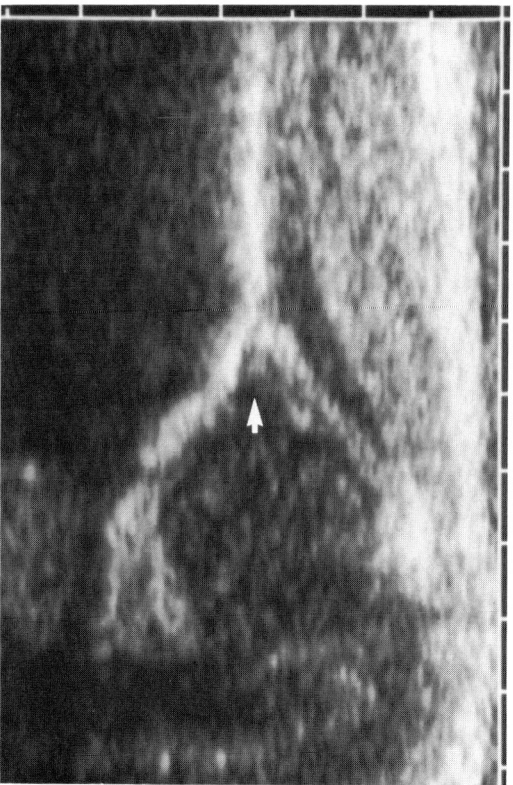

Figure 5–24. This baby has a slightly shallow acetabular roof whose edge is poorly ossified (arrow) so that the corner is not sharply defined.

the ischial acetabular roof. Every child has slightly different anatomy, and slight angulation of the transducer, in a perpendicular plane relative to the skin, is therefore needed to demonstrate these relationships for each hip examined. The capital femoral epiphysis should always be spherical and have an orderly stippled appearance from columns of cartilage. Lateral to the femoral head is the acetabular labrum and joint capsule. The tip of the labrum (also called the "limbus") is usually apparent as the tip of an echogenic "V" extending from the acetabular corner. This corner is normally sharply turned. Zieger and Schulz (1987) found a correlation between poor or delayed ossification of this corner and clinical instability (Fig. 5–24). The joint capsule continues as an echogenic interface from the labrum to the femoral neck. The gluteal muscles, medius and minimus, which are separated by a plane of connective tissue, coalesce into ligaments and insert onto the greater trochanter. Because it is apophyseal cartilage, the greater trochanter is similar in appearance to the capital femoral epiphysis. The ossified shaft of the femur gives a definite echogenic interface to sound. Interestingly, one can visualize the area of the physis; either sound finds interfaces along the physeal plate or it skims the zone

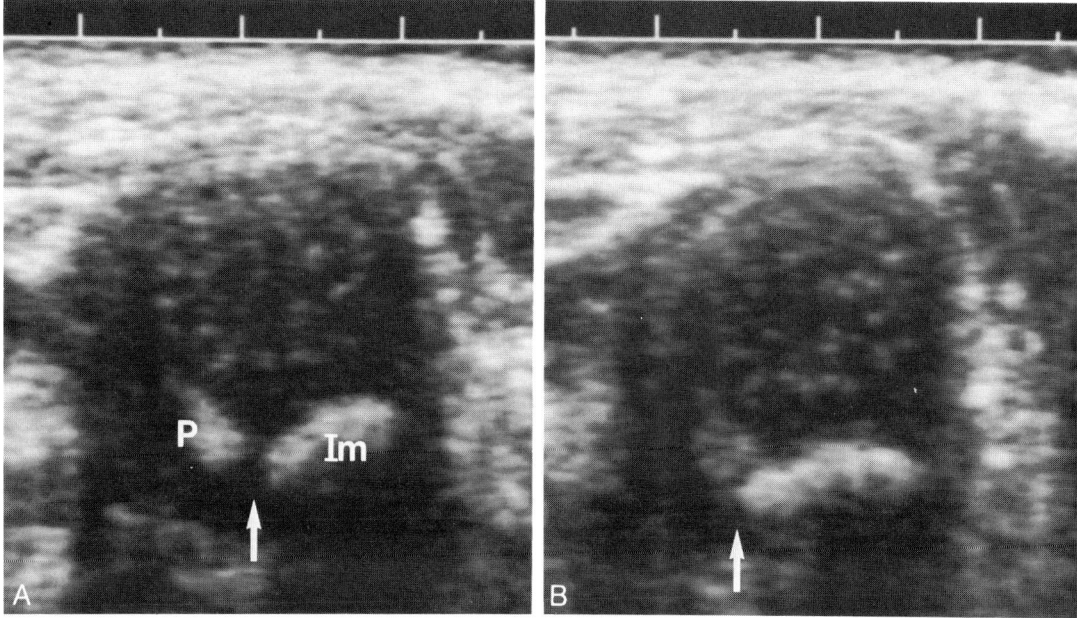

Figure 5–25. Axial view, with the hip in neutral position (A), shows the femoral epiphysis sitting in the V-shaped cup formed by the pubis (P) anteriorly and the ischium (Im) posteriorly. Arrow marks triradiate cartilage. If a hip is subluxable, the epiphysis rides over the ischium (B) when force is applied to the femur after the hip has been flexed.

of provisional calcification adjacent to it (Fig. 5–23).

After static images of each hip are obtained, the hip is viewed in the coronal plane as the femur is moved through its full range of motion. The femur can be positioned in 90° of flexion and stress applied in order to evaluate subluxation. We have found it most useful to assess the effect of anteroposterior force applied to the femoral head either by scanning at right angles to the coronal plane or by scanning along the axis of the femoral shaft while the hip is in 90° of flexion. In the first of these transverse views, the transducer is oriented so that it is scanning through the femoral head and acetabulum in the axial plane. The stalk of the triradiate cartilage allows a narrow band of sound to pass into the pelvis. The anterior bony interface is provided by the pubis, and the posterior interface by the ischium (Fig. 5–25A). When the transducer is aligned with the shaft of the flexed femur, the resulting view of the femoral head in the acetabulum looks like a scoop of ice cream in a cone (Fig. 5–26A). One can use either of these transverse views to assess the effect of force applied to the femoral head in a direction from anterior to posterior. The capital femoral epiphysis slides posteriorly over the lip of the bony ischium in both dislocatable and subluxable hips (Figs. 5–25B, 5–26B). This stress view takes a lot of practice. It is not always easy to keep the transducer appropriately oriented while stressing the hip. We have found that one also relies on the tactile stimulus as well as the visual in judging mobility because, in fact, this is a modified Barlow maneuver. It is better to do stress views at the completion of an examination because most babies, used to gentler treatment, take umbrage at being pushed and pulled. Furthermore, the pumping may increase the vacuum in the joint and create a row of gas bubbles, which blur the landmarks and result in fuzzy scans. An echogenic area in the superomedial joint

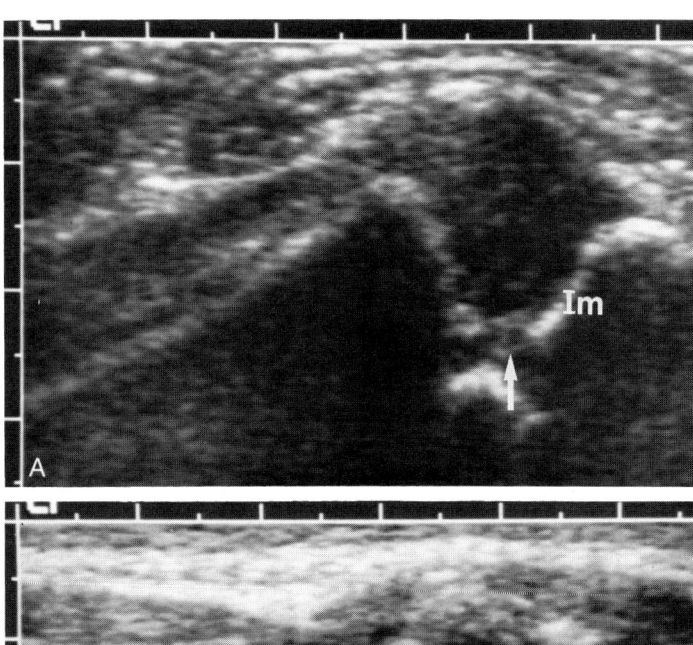

Figure 5–26. Axial view of the acetabulum, with the hip flexed and with the transducer aligned with the shaft of the femur (A), shows the normal relationship of the epiphysis with the ischium (IM) and triradiate cartilage (arrow). When stress is applied to the subluxable hip, the epiphysis slides over the ischium (B).

space is a normal finding. It represents the ligamentum teres, which carries the blood supply to the femoral head (Fig. 5–27).

The European literature—specifically that of Graf (1987), Zieger and colleagues (1986, 1987)—places great reliance on measured angles. These are very useful as a quantitative assessment of acetabular development. However, unless done with the most precise technique, there is substantial intraobserver and interobserver error. The angles are calculated from coronal scans that intersect the ilium in its midplane. The iliac interface must be perfectly straight, with no flare at its inferior edge, and the transducer is oriented so as to scan, simultaneously, the femoral head through its maximal diameter (Fig. 5–28). Criteria for normal, borderline, and dysplastic hips have been generated from these measurements (Graf, 1987). If the technique is faultless and the same landmarks are identical, these measurements are particularly useful to compare follow-up scans of individual babies undergoing treatment (Fig. 5–29). After a baby reaches 2 weeks of age, we accept an alpha angle of 60° as normal. Dictations of hip ultrasonography should include a quantitative or qualitative description of the acetabular cup, the percentage of coverage of the femoral head by the acetabular roof, the appearance of the femoral head, the position of the femoral head if dislocated, and a description of stress tests and their results.

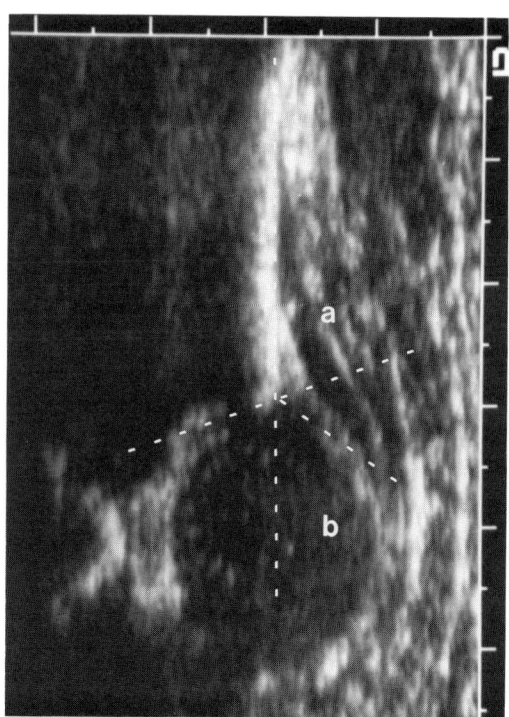

Figure 5–28. The alpha angle (a) is measured between the baseline along the ilium and the line along the ossified roof of the acetabulum. The beta angle (b) is between the labrum acetabulare and baseline.

If the clinical diagnosis of CDH has been delayed, secondary adaptive changes occur in the dysplastic hip. The acetabulum fails to deepen without the stimulus of a constantly located femoral head. The subluxing head stretches the capsular tissues, and the acetabulum tends to fill in with soft tissue (pulvinar) and redundant ligamentum teres (Fig. 5–30). The labrum may become distorted or inverted (Fig. 5–31). The femoral head loses its spherical shape and becomes oval, and the appearance of the ossification center is delayed (Fig. 5–32). Typically, ossification in normal infants appears between the ages of 3 and 6 months and is symmetric. By 8 months of age, the ossific nucleus is quite well developed and hinders ultrasonograms by shadowing the medial portion of acetabulum and the triradiate cartilage (Fig. 5–33).

If studies are being performed on children in a harness or abductor splint, they are performed without changing the position or undoing the orthosis. Scans in coronal and transverse planes show the position of the femoral head in relation to the acetabulum

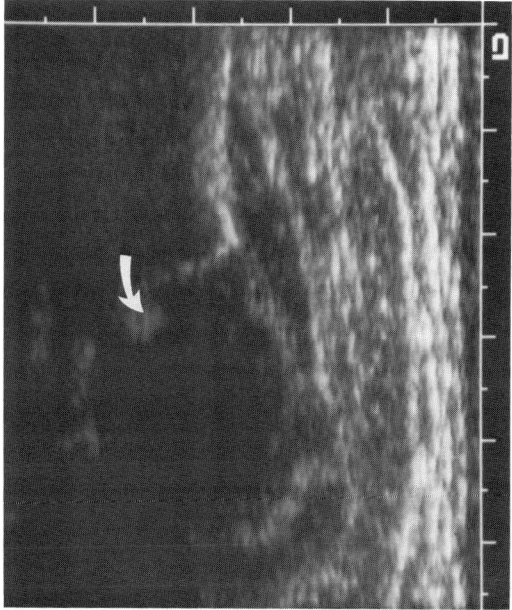

Figure 5–27. The ligamentum teres may appear as an echogenic area (arrow) in the joint space.

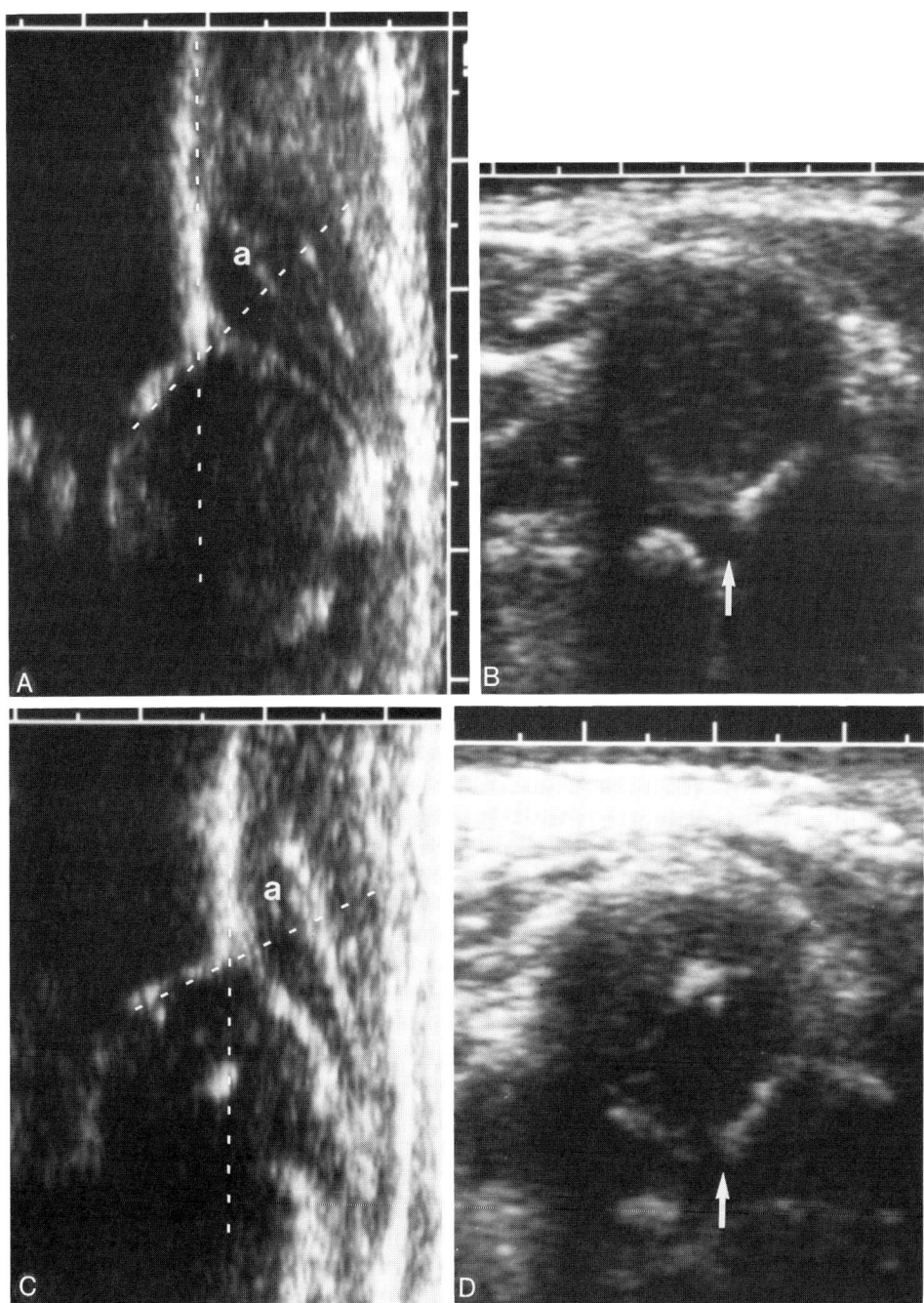

Figure 5–29. One can appreciate the maturation of this mildly abnormal hip between initial coronal (**A**) and transverse (**B**) scans and scans done 2 months later (**C** and **D**) after the baby had been placed in Pavlik harness. The alpha angle (a), marked by dotted lines, increases over time; coverage of the epiphysis increases from less than 50 percent to more than 50 percent of its diameter; and the ossification center becomes apparent. On transverse, neutral views (**B** and **D**), the femoral epiphysis becomes firmly seated in the acetabular cup. Arrow marks triradiate cartilage.

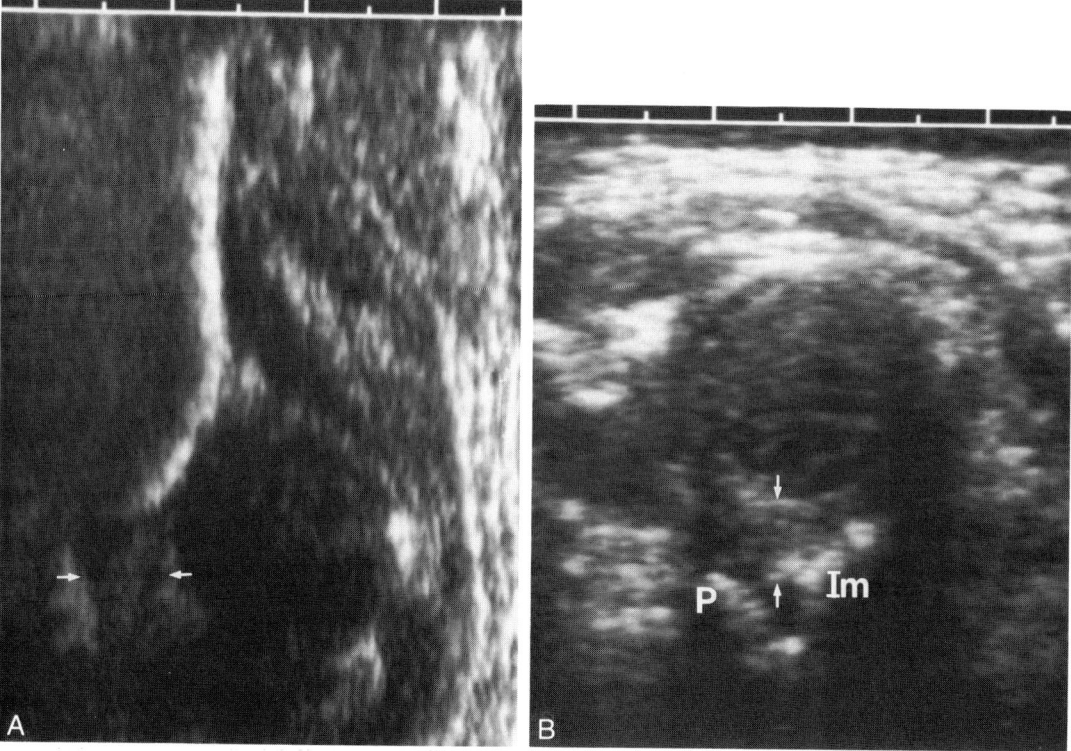

Figure 5–30. Views of the hip show a shallow acetabular roof and poor coverage of the capital femoral epiphysis on coronal scan (A) and widening of the joint space (arrows) on both coronal (A) and transverse (B) scans. P = pubis. Im = ischium.

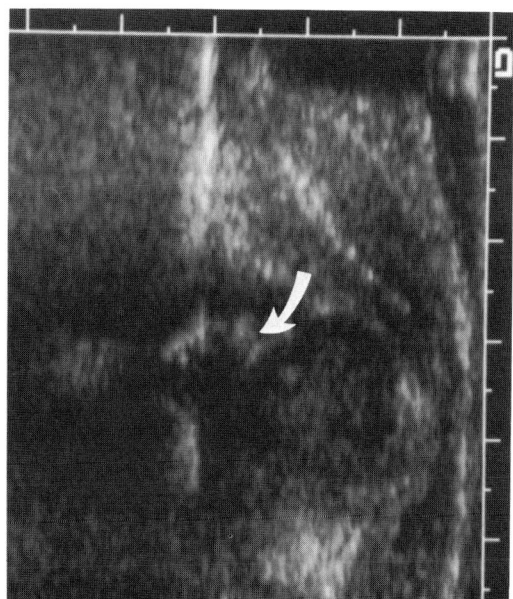

Figure 5–31. Lack of treatment for a dislocated hip resulted in the labrum's (arrow) losing its sharp, V-shaped contour.

and document its appropriate or inappropriate location. Children undergoing treatment are closely followed by the clinicians, and on follow-up ultrasonography we refrain from performing the same stress testing as used in the clinical examination unless we are specifically asked to do so. There is no certainty that repeated clinical examination is harmful, but some physicians are concerned that it may not be as benign as we consider it to be (Dickson, 1989).

Babies with dysplasia severe enough to warrant treatment in a plaster or plastic cast, either after prolonged traction or after open reduction, can be scanned by a medial or lateral transverse approach if a window is left in the cast for access to skin. The posterolateral lip of the acetabulum should be adjacent to the femoral head in the far part of the scan on the medial transverse view. These scans, however, are technically difficult to perform, and significantly more information is acquired from a few well-planned scans with CT or MRI rather than from a

THE EXTREMITIES / 133

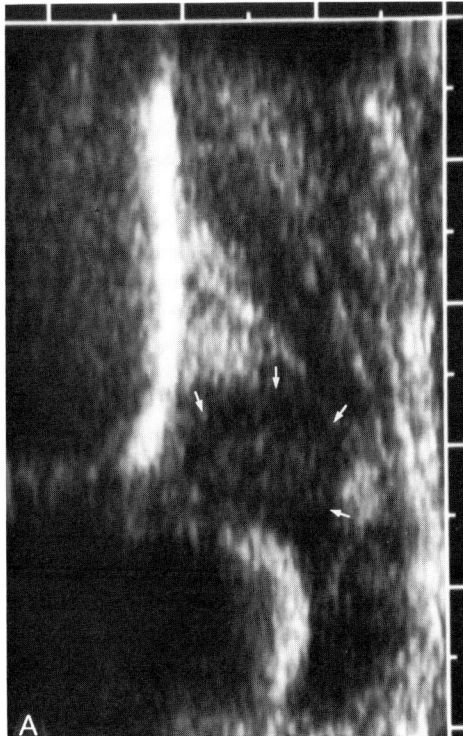

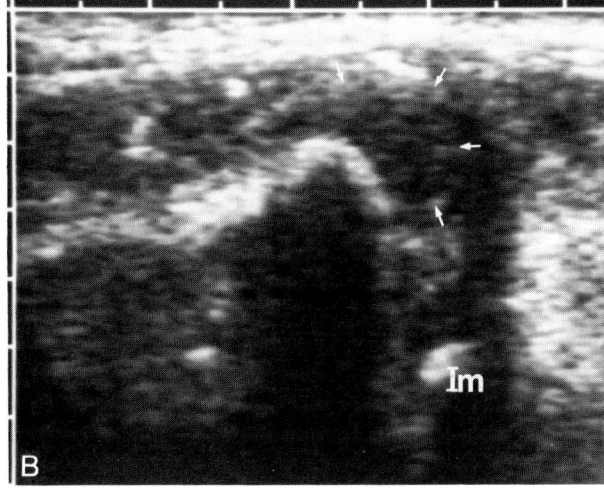

Figure 5–32. Coronal (A) and transverse (B) scans of a chronically dislocated hip in a 4-month-old girl show a small, oval capital femoral epiphysis (arrows). Im = ischium.

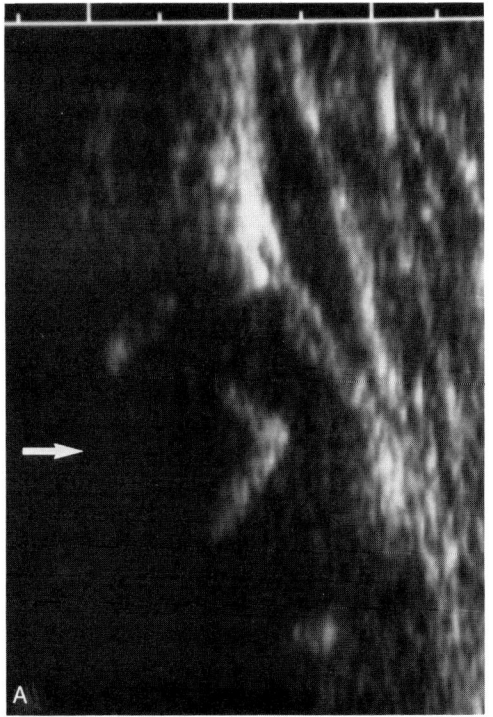

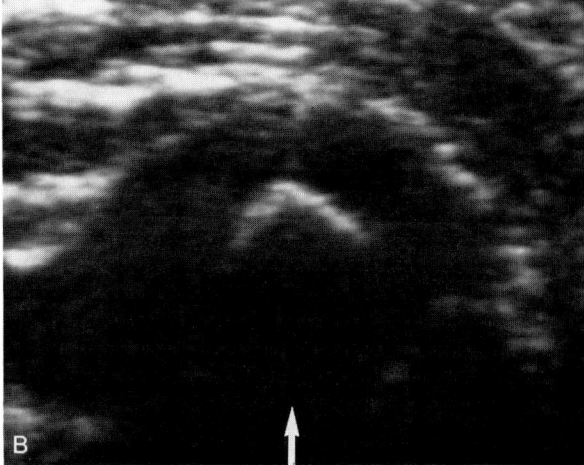

Figure 5–33. The ossification center in the capital femoral epiphysis of a 9-month-old boy shadows the triradiate cartilage (arrow) and its adjacent bony rim on coronal (A) and transverse (B) scans. The hip is normal; the capital femoral epiphysis is well seated and covered by a deep bony acetabular roof.

very limited ultrasonographic study. We have used ultrasonography in the operating room to check the appearance of a baby's hips between cast changes.

The number of initial screening studies and follow-up examinations with ultrasonography is based on the population being served, the clinical expertise in the area, the availability of technically good ultrasonography, the economic constraints, consumer demand, and governmental policy in countries with socialized medicine. As mentioned in the introduction to this section, opinions vary as to how much of a role ultrasonography should play in diagnosis. We are concerned that heavy reliance on the ultrasonographic technique, which is only as good as the examiners themselves, may lead to a gradual loss of those clinical skills that in fact are an integral part of the ultrasonographic examination.

In summary, we scan babies referred because of an abnormal clinical examination, a strong family history (particularly if the baby is a girl), prenatal history of breech presentation, and neuromuscular problems in which dysplasia is known to be frequently associated. Follow-up is individually arranged, depending on the degree of abnormality, the concerns of the orthopedic surgeon or pediatrician, and the mode of therapy.

REFERENCES

General

Fischer AQ, Stephens S: Computerized real-time neuromuscular sonography: A new application, techniques and methods. J Child Neurol 1988; 3:69–74.

Fornage BD, Eftekhari F: Sonographic diagnosis of myositis ossificans. J Ultrasound Med 1989; 8:463–466.

Harcke HT, Grissom LE, Finkelstein MS: Evaluation of the musculoskeletal system with sonography. AJR 1988; 150:1253–1261.

Heckmatt JZ, Pier N, Dubowitz V: Real-time ultrasound imaging of muscles. Muscle Nerve 1988; 11:56–65.

Heckmatt J, Rodillo E, Doherty M, et al: Quantitative sonography of muscle. J Child Neurol 1989; 4(Suppl): S101–S106.

Lamminen A, Jääskeläinen J, Rapola J, et al: High-frequency ultrasonography of skeletal muscle in children with neuromuscular disease. J Ultrasound Med 1988; 7:505–509.

Weiss LW, Clark FC: Subcutaneous fat measurements of the leg using three protocols. J Sports Med Phys Fitness 1987; 27:437–442.

Masses

Neifeld JP, Godwin D, Berg JW, et al: Prognostic features of pediatric soft-tissue sarcomas. Surgery 1985; 98:93–97.

Renshaw TS: Pediatric Orthopedics. Philadelphia: WB Saunders, 1986.

Toolanen G, Lorentzon R, Friberg S, et al: Sonography of popliteal masses. Acta Orthop Scand 1988; 59:294–296.

Yagupsky P, Shahak E, Barki Y: Non-invasive diagnosis of pyomyositis. Clin Pediatr 1988; 27:299–301.

Yamaguchi M, Takeuchi S, Matsuo S: Ultrasonic evaluation of pediatric superficial masses. JCU 1987; 15:107–113.

Penetrating Injuries of Soft Tissues

Fornage BD, Schernberg FL: Sonographic diagnosis of foreign bodies of the distal extremities. AJR 1986; 147:567–569.

Gilbert FJ, Campbell RS, Bayliss AP: The role of ultrasound in the detection of non-radiopaque foreign bodies. Clin Radiol 1990; 41:109–112.

Gooding GAW, Hardiman DPM, Sumers DPM: Sonography of the hand and foot in foreign body detection. J Ultrasound Med 1987; 6:441–447.

Hansson G, Beebe AC, Carroll NC, et al: A piece of wood in the hand diagnosed by ultrasonography. Acta Orthop Scand 1988; 59:459–460.

Shiels WE 2d, Babcock DS, Wilson JL, Burch RA: Localization and guided removal of soft-tissue foreign bodies with sonography. AJR 1990; 155:1277–1281.

Injuries of Tendons, Ligaments, and Joints

Collins RA, Gristina AG, Carter RE: Ultrasonography of the shoulder. Static and dynamic imaging. Orthop Clin North Am 1987; 18:351–360.

De Flaviis L, Nessi R, Scaglione P, et al: Ultrasonic diagnosis of Osgood-Schlatter and Sinding-Larsen-Johansson diseases of the knee. Skeletal Radiol 1989; 18:193–197.

Fritschy D, de Gautard R: Jumper's knee and ultrasonography. Am J Sports Med 1988; 16:637–640.

Gregersen HE, Rasmussen OS: Ultrasonography of osteochondritis dissecans of the knee: A preliminary report. Acta Radiol 1989; 30:552–554.

Harcke HT, Grissom LE, Finkelstein MS: Evaluation of the musculoskeletal system with sonography. AJR 1988; 150:1253–1260.

Kainberger FM, Engel A, Barton P, et al: Injury of the Achilles tendon: Diagnosis with sonography. AJR 1990; 155:1031–1036.

King JB, Perry DJ, Mourad K, et al: Lesions of the patellar ligament. J Bone Joint Surg (Br) 1990; 72:46–48.

Mack LA, Matson FA III, Kilcoyne RF, et al: US evaluation of the rotator cuff. Radiology 1985; 157:205–209.

Mathieson JR, Connell DG, Cooperberg PL, et al: Sonography of the Achilles tendon and adjacent bursae. AJR 1988; 151:127–131.

Mourad K, King J, Guggiana P: Computed tomography and ultrasound imaging of jumper's knee-patellar tendinitis. Clin Radiol 1988; 39:162–165.

Myllymäki T, Bondestam S, Suramo I, et al: Ultrasonography of jumper's knee. Acta Radiol 1990; 31:147–149.

Soble MG, Kaye AD, Guay RC: Rotator cuff tear: Clinical experience with sonographic detection. Radiology 1989; 173:319–321.

Effusion and Infection

Abiri MM, Kirpekar M, Ablow RC: Osteomyelitis: Detection with US. Radiology 1989; 172:509–511.

Alexander JE, Seibert JJ, Aronson J, et al: A protocol of plain radiographs, hip ultrasound, and triple phase bone scans in the evaluation of the painful pediatric hip. Clin Pediatr 1988; 27:175–181.

Alexander JE, Seibert JJ, Glasier CM, et al: High-resolution hip ultrasound in the limping child. JCU 1989; 17:19–24.

Dias JJ, Lamont AC, Jones JM: Ultrasonic diagnosis of neonatal separation of the distal humeral epiphysis. J Bone Joint Surg [Br] 1988; 70:825–828.

Dörr U, Zieger M, Hauke H: Ultrasonography of the painful hip. Prospective studies in 204 patients. Pediatr Radiol 1988; 19:36–40.

Egund N, Wingstrand H: Pitfalls in ultrasonography of hip joint synovitis in the child. Acta Radiol 1989; 30:375–379.

Hill SA, Maclarnon JC, Nag D: Ultrasound-guided aspiration for transient synovitis of the hip. J Bone Joint Surg (Br) 1990; 72:852–853.

Marchal GJ, Van Holsbeeck MT, Raes M, et al: Transient synovitis of the hip in children: Role of US. Radiology 1987; 162:825–828.

McGoldrick F, Bourke T, Blake N, et al: Accuracy of sonography in transient synovitis. J Pediatr Orthop 1990; 10:501–503.

Miralles M, Gonzalez G, Pulpeiro JR, et al: Sonography of the painful hip in children: 500 consecutive cases. AJR 1989; 152:579–582.

Yagupsky P, Shahak E, Barki Y: Non-invasive diagnosis of pyomyositis. Clin Pediatr 1988; 27:299–301.

Zieger MM, Dörr U, Schulz RD: Ultrasonography of hip joint effusions. Skeletal Radiol 1987; 16:607–611.

Fracture and Deformity

Broker FH, Burbach T: Ultrasonic diagnosis of separation of the proximal humeral epiphysis in the newborn. J Bone Joint Surg (Am) 1990; 72:187–191.

Clementz BG, Magnusson A: Fluoroscopic measurement of tibial torsion in adults. A comparison of three methods. Arch Orthop Trauma Surg 1989; 108:150–153.

Dias JJ, Lamont AC, Jones JM: Ultrasonic diagnosis of neonatal separation of the distal humeral epiphysis. J Bone Joint Surg (Br) 1988; 70:825–828.

Joseph B, Carver RA, Bell MJ, et al: Measurement of tibial torsion by ultrasound. J Pediatr Orthop 1987; 7:317–323.

Katz R, Landman J, Dulitzky F, et al: Fracture of the clavicle in the newborn. An ultrasound diagnosis. J Ultrasound Med 1988; 7:21–23.

Vascular Abnormalities

Congenital

Gorenstein A, Katz S, Schiller M: Congenital angiodysplasia of the superficial venous system of the lower extremities in children. Ann Surg 1988; 207:213–218.

Juul S, Ledbetter D, Wight TN, et al: New insights into idiopathic infantile arterial calcinosis. Three patient reports. Am J Dis Child 1990; 144:229–233.

Mulliken JB, Young AE: Vascular Birthmarks: Hemangiomas and Malformations. Philadelphia: WB Saunders, 1988.

Venous Thrombosis

Appelman PT, De Jong TE, Lampmann LE: Deep venous thrombosis of the leg: US findings. Radiology 1987; 163:743–746.

Cronan JJ, Dorfman GS, Scola FH, et al: Deep venous thrombosis: US assessment using vein compression. Radiology 1987; 162:191–194.

Cronan JJ, Dorfman GS, Grusmark J: Lower-extremity deep venous thrombosis: Further experience with and refinements of US assessment. Radiology 1988; 68:101–107.

Falk RL, Smith DF: Thrombosis of upper extremity thoracic inlet veins: Diagnosis with duplex Doppler sonography. AJR 1987; 149:677–682.

Lensing AW, Levi MM, Büller HR, et al: Diagnosis of deep-vein thrombosis using an objective Doppler method. Ann Intern Med 1990; 113:9–13.

Salzman EW: Venous thrombosis made easy. N Engl J Med 1986; 314:847–848.

Vogel P, Laing FC, Jeffrey RB Jr, et al: Deep venous thrombosis of the lower extremity: US evaluation. Radiology 1987; 163:747–751.

Vascular Shunts and Pseudoaneurysms

Coughlin BF, Paushter DM: Peripheral pseudoaneurysms: Evaluation with duplex US. Radiology 1988; 168:339–342.

Hoffer FA, Wyly JB, Fellow KE, et al: Maintenance of vascular access patency in pediatrics. Pediatr Radiol 1986; 16(6):456–460.

Kotval PS, Khoury A, Shah PM, et al: Doppler sonographic demonstration of the progressive spontaneous thrombosis of pseudoaneurysms. J Ultrasound Med 1990; 9:185–190.

May AC, Andus CH: Vascular access. In Rob and Smith's Operative Surgery (4th ed). London: Butterworths, 1985, 435–447.

Taylor LM Jr, Troutman R, Feliciano P, et al: Late complications after femoral artery catheterization in children less than five years of age. J Vasc Surg 1990; 11:297–304.

Vasli LR: Diagnosis of vascular injury in children with supracondylar fractures of the humerus. Injury 1988; 19:11–13.

Congenital Dysplasia of the Hip

Ando M, Gotoh E: Significance of inguinal folds for diagnosis of congenital dislocation of the hip in infants aged three to four months. J Pediatr Orthop 1990; 10:331–334.

Asher MA: Screening for scoliosis, congenital dislocation of the hip, and other abnormalities affecting the musculoskeletal system. Pediatr Clin North Am 1986; 33:1335–1353.

Barlow TG: Early diagnosis and treatment of congenital dislocation of the hip. J Bone Joint Surg (Br) 1962; 44:292–301.

Bialik V, Pery M, Kaftori JK, Fishman J: The use of ultrasound screening in the management of developmental disorders of the hip. Int Orthop 1988; 12:75–78.

Bialik V, Reuvent A, Pery M, et al: Ultrasonography in developmental displacement of the hip: A critical analysis of our results. J Pediatr Orthop 1989; 9:154–156.

Boal DKB, Schwenkter EP: The infant hip: Assessment with real-time US. Radiology 1985; 157:667–672.

Burke SW, Macey TI, Roberts JM, et al: Congenital dislocation of the hip in the American black. Clin Orthop 1985; 192:120–123.

Castelein RM, Sauter AJ: Ultrasound screening for congenital dysplasia of the hip in newborns: Its value. J Pediatr Orthop 1988; 8:666–670.

Chung SMK: Diseases of the developing hip joint. Pediatr Clin North Am 1986; 33:1457–1473.

Clarke NM, Clegg J, Al-Chalabi AN: Ultrasound screening of hips at risk for CDH. Failure to reduce the incidence of late cases. J Bone Joint Surg (Br) 1989; 71:9–12.

Dahlström H, Friberg S, Oberg L: Stabilisation and development of the hip after closed reduction of late CDH. J Bone Joint Surg (Br) 1990;72:186–189.

Dickson N: Congenital dislocation of the hip—Have we been doing harm? [abstract] N Z Med J 1989; 102:196.

Engesaeter LB, Wilson DJ, Nag D, et al: Ultrasound and congenital dislocation of the hip: The importance of dynamic assessment. J Bone Joint Surg (Br) 1990; 72:197–201.

Exner GU: Ultrasound screening for hip dysplasia in neonates. J Pediatr Orthop 1988; 8:656–660.

Faure C, Schmit P, Salvat D: Cost–benefit evaluation of systematic radiological diagnosis of congenital dislocated hip. Pediatr Radiol 1984; 14:407–412.

Fulton MJ, Barer ML: Screening for congenital dislocation of the hip: An economic appraisal. Can Med Assoc J 1984; 130:1149–1151.

Gomes A, Menanteau B, Motte J, Robiliard P: Sonography of the neonatal hip: A dynamic approach. Ann Radiol 1987; 30:503–510.

Graf R: Guide to Sonography of the Infant Hip. New York: Thieme, 1987.

Grissom LE, Harcke HT, Kumar SJ, et al: Ultrasound evaluation of hip position in the Pavlik harness. J Ultrasound Med 1988; 7:1–6.

Hampton S, Read B, Nixon W: Diagnosis of congenital dislocated hips (CDH). Radiol Technol 1988; 59:211–220.

Harcke HT, Clarke NMP, Lee MS, et al: Examination of the infant hip with real-time ultrasonography. J Ultrasound Med 1984; 3:131–137.

Harcke HT, Grissom LE: Performing dynamic sonography of the infant hip. AJR 1990; 155:837–844.

Jones DA, Powell N: Ultrasound and neonatal hip screening. A prospective study of "high risk" babies. J Bone Joint Surg (Br) 1990; 72:457–459.

Langer R, Kaufmann HJ: Ultrasound screening of the hip in newborns for the diagnosis of congenital hip dysplasia. J Belge Radiol 1987; 70:411–417.

Keller MS, Chawla HS, Weiss AA: Real-time sonography of infant hip dislocation. Radiographics 1986; 6:447–456.

Keller MS: Infant hip. Clin Diagn Ultrasound 1989; 24:217–236.

MacEwen GD, Mason B: Evaluation and treatment of congenital dislocation of the hip in infants. Orthop Clin North Am 1988; 19:815–820.

Morin C, Harcke HT, MacEwen GD: The infant hip: Real time US assessment of acetabular development. Radiology 1985; 157:673–677.

Novick GS, Ghelman B, Schneider M: Sonography of the neonatal and infant hip. AJR 1983; 141:639–645.

Novick GS: Sonography in pediatric hip disorders. Radiol Clin North Am 1988; 26:29–53.

Ortolani M: The classic: Congenital hip dysplasia in the light of early and very early diagnosis. Clin Orthop 1976; 119:6–10.

Renshaw TS: Pediatric Orthopedics. Philadelphia: WB Saunders, 1986.

Saies AD, Foster BK, Lequesne GW: The value of a new ultrasound stress test in assessment and treatment of clinically detected hip instability. J Pediatr Orthop 1988; 8:436–441.

Stanisavljevic S: Tribute to Marino Ortolani. Clin Orthop 1976; 119:4–5.

Szöke N, Kühl L, Heinrichs J: Ultrasound examination in the diagnosis of congenital hip dysplasia of newborns. J Pediatr Orthop 1988; 8:12–16.

Tönnis D, Storch K, Ulbrich H: Results of newborn screening for CDH with and without sonography and correlation of risk factors. J Pediatr Orthop 1990; 10:145–152.

Yamamuro T, Ishida K: Recent advances in the prevention, early diagnosis, and treatment of congenital dislocation of the hip in Japan. Clin Orthop 1984; 184:34–40.

Yousefzadeh DK, Ramilo JL: Normal hip in children: Correlation of US with anatomic and cryomicrotome sections. Radiology 1987; 165:647–655.

Zieger M: Ultrasound of the infant hip. Part 2. Validity of the method. Pediatr Radiol 1986; 16:488–492.

Zieger M, Hilpert S: Ultrasonography of the infant hip. Part IV: Normal development in the newborn and preterm neonate. Pediatr Radiol 1987; 17:470–473.

Zieger M, Hilpert S, Schulz RD: Ultrasound of the infant hip. Part I. Basic principles. Pediatr Radiol 1986; 16:483–487.

Zieger M, Schulz RD: Ultrasonography of the infant hip. Part III: Clinical application. Pediatr Radiol 1987; 17:226–232.

CHAPTER 6

RENAL SCREENING

In this chapter we discuss the reasons for using renal ultrasonography as a screening procedure (Table 6–1). Ideally, in order to capture all renal anomalies or abnormalities in a population at risk, a screening procedure should yield no false-negative results. Furthermore, there should be few false-positive results, so that additional, more invasive investigations are reserved for patients who actually need them. Unfortunately, renal ultrasonography is not the perfect screening tool; the errors tend to be false negative rather than false positive. However, with an appreciation of its limitations in certain diagnostic areas, one can decide for the individual patient what additional studies, if any, should be done.

THE NORMAL KIDNEYS

These paired, bean-shaped organs are easy to scan and, when normal, provide beautiful ultrasonic correlates of gross anatomy (Fig. 6–1). If the patient is a baby, we tend to begin an examination with the patient held supine. We try to get scans of the bladder first, before it empties in response to the baby's clothing being stripped off. The right kidney can often be viewed in its entire longitudinal axis through the liver. On the left, the upper pole, at least, can be viewed

Table 6–1. REASONS FOR ULTRASONOGRAPHIC RENAL SCREENING

Problem	Reasons
Rule out anomaly or cystic disease	• Patient has known syndrome and predisposition • Family has renal disease • Congenital scoliosis with vertebral anomaly • Abnormal prenatal scans
Rule out Wilms tumor	• Hemihypertrophy • Sporadic aniridia • Beckwith-Wiedemann syndrome • Drash syndrome • 13p chromosomal deletion • Cerebral gigantism • Neurofibromatosis
Abdominal pain	• Occasionally structural renal anomaly responsible for abdominal pain
Hypertension	• Need to screen for anomaly, tumor, reflux nephropathy, or vascular abnormality
Painless hematuria	• Need to rule out occult hydronephrosis, tumor
Myelodysplasia or spinal injury	• Need to rule out development of hydronephrosis, stones • Can assess function of bladder by pre-/postvoid scans
Postoperative genitourinary surgery	• Need to check for complications without continued use of ionizing radiation

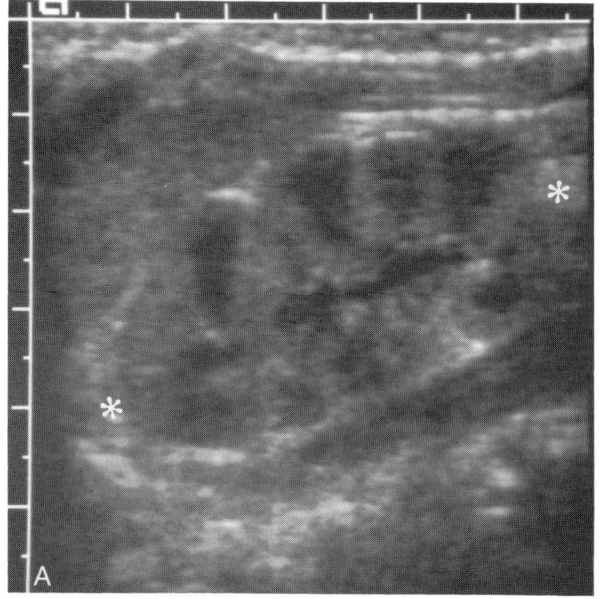
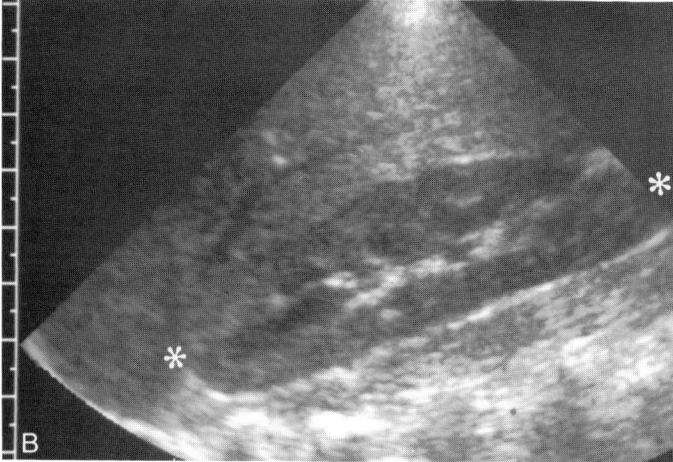

Figure 6–1. Coronal scan of the right kidney (A) in a 3-week-old shows prominent lucent medullary pyramids surrounded by echogenic cortex. The contour of the kidney is mildly lobulated at this age. Longitudinal scan of the right kidney through the liver (B) in a prepubertal girl shows the normal long oval shape of the kidney. The central echogenicity is the renal sinus composed of the collecting system fat and vessels. Medullary pyramids are lucent in relation to the cortex. The cortex is less echogenic than the adjacent liver. (In this figure, as in others throughout this chapter, asterisks outline the kidney.)

through the spleen. The wall of the bladder is normally 4 mm or less in thickness (Jequier and Rousseau, 1987), but it may appear thicker when the bladder is minimally distended. Cystic masses may simulate a bladder. In our experience, cystic teratoma, simple ovarian cyst, diverticulum of the bladder, ureterocele, and urinoma have all masqueraded as the bladder. Methods of avoiding this pitfall include critical evaluation of the shape of the "cyst." The transverse cross-sectional shape of the normal bladder is not a circle but a rounded-off square. The wall of most cysts is thinner than that of the normal bladder. In girls of all ages, the uterus should indent the posterior wall of the bladder (Fig. 6–2). Throughout an examination, the bladder should increase in size as it fills with urine, and all urine should disappear when the patient voids. A diverticulum of the bladder may fill with urine as the patient voids. Its cross-sectional shape is oval or circular, and its relationship to the bladder is usually evident when the bladder fills with more urine. A small, lentiform mass, just anterior to the bladder, may be apparent on routine scans and represents the remnant of the urachus (Cacciarelli et al., 1990; Fig. 6–2B, 6–2C).

The ureters may be seen intermittently as they conduct a bolus of urine to the bladder, but ureters of normal caliber are not consistently identifiable on scans. Mild ureteral distention may occur in the normal child who has a very full bladder and in a child who is undergoing diuresis from any cause.

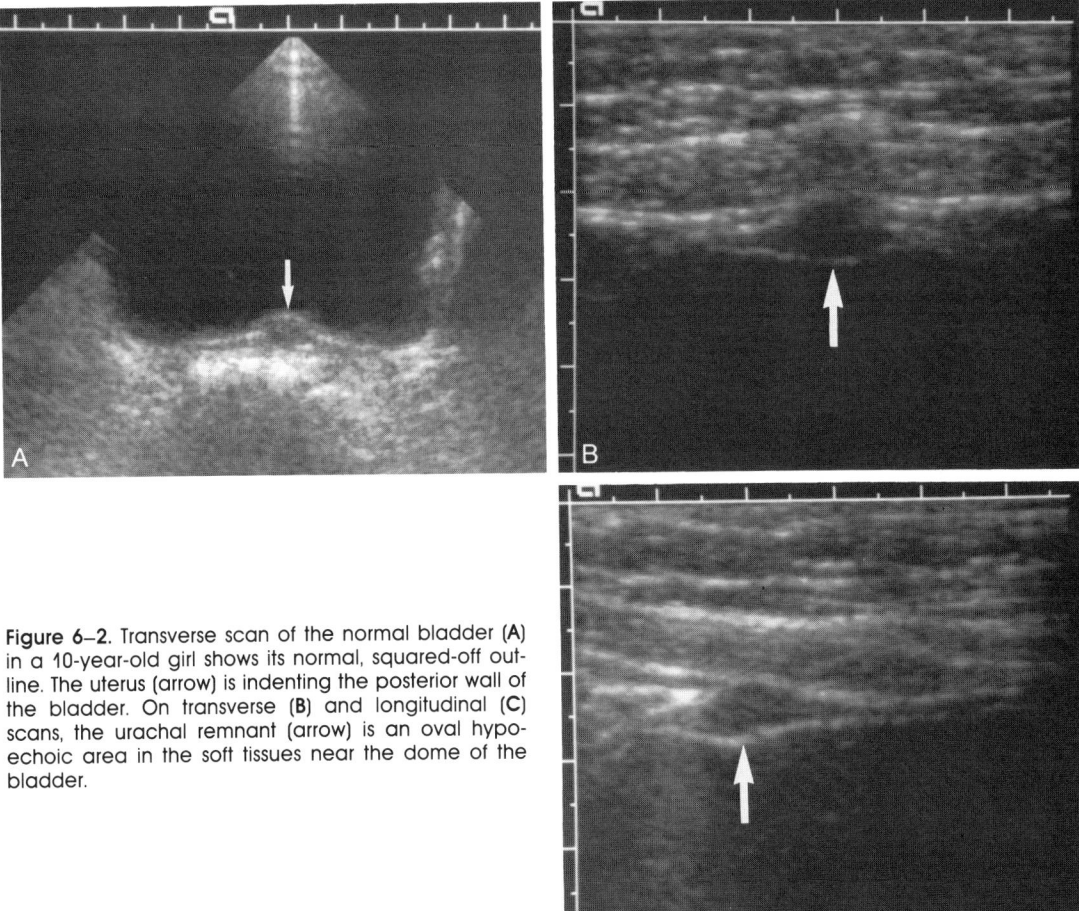

Figure 6–2. Transverse scan of the normal bladder (A) in a 10-year-old girl shows its normal, squared-off outline. The uterus (arrow) is indenting the posterior wall of the bladder. On transverse (B) and longitudinal (C) scans, the urachal remnant (arrow) is an oval hypoechoic area in the soft tissues near the dome of the bladder.

Transverse, coronal, and sagittal scanning of kidneys is recommended in order to simulate a three-dimensional view of the renal parenchyma and the collecting system. The collecting system is part of the central renal echogenicity that is created by pelvic and infundibular walls, vessels, lymphatics, nerves, and fat. Children usually have less fat, both within and around the kidney, than do adults. Babies have a barely perceptible central sinus. If the system is duplex, coronal scanning may hint at splitting of the echoes from the central sinus as the pelves exit medially at the renal hilum (Fig. 6–3).

The walls of the renal pelvis are separated by urine, especially if the pelvis is extrarenal. A normal extrarenal pelvis may look quite large on coronal scans, but its anteroposterior width may appear narrow on transverse sections. There is no absolute measurement to separate normal distention from that present with hydronephrosis, but a pelvic diameter of greater than 1 cm causes us to look more closely at the scans. Dilation that extends into infundibula and calices cannot be considered normal. Because of the iatrogenic diuresis, scans that follow intravenous urography with ionic contrast show more dilation of the renal pelvis than do scans performed before the radiographic procedure. The arcuate arteries of the kidney often show up as double tracks or echogenic points between the cortex and the medulla (Fig. 6–4). Magnification views and Doppler imaging allow differentiation of normal vessels from other echogenic interfaces. The renal veins are not as obvious until they coalesce near the hilum. Coronal or sagittal scanning across the renal vein may show what looks like a small parapelvic cyst. A cyst, however, should not appear cylindrical on a transverse view; that shape is what characterizes the renal vein as

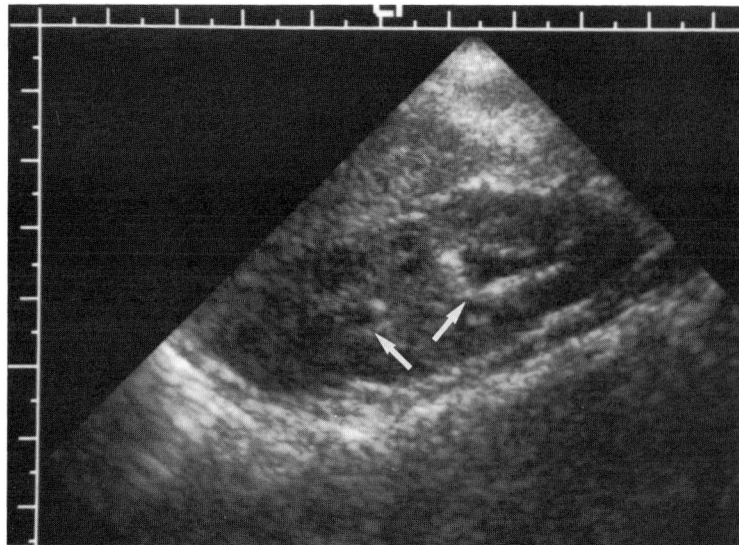

Figure 6–3. This is a longitudinal scan of a duplex kidney. The kidney was longer than normal for age, and the collecting system echoes (arrows) were split by a thick column of cortex.

it drains into the inferior vena cava. The parenchyma of the kidney is divided into the medulla and the cortex. The normal medulla is more lucent than the cortex in all age groups. Increased cortical echogenicity in babies, from birth to approximately 6 months of age, has been attributed to glomeruli occupying 18 percent of the volume of cortex and to the presence of up to 20 percent of loops of Henle in the cortex, in comparison with 8.6 percent in the adult (Hricak et al., 1983). The medulla of the neonate is relatively larger in volume (in comparison with the cortex) than the medulla of the adult. Its apparent increased lucency may be a result of its size or a result of an absolute increase in its content of water (Fig. 6–5). In older babies, toddlers, and children, the cortex is less echogenic than the adjacent normal liver. The medulla, particularly in the polar regions of the kidney, may simulate a lucent mass if a composite papilla is associated with a compound calix. Most medullary areas are triangular in cross-section, but the composite papilla is quite large and lumpy and may simulate a mass (Fig. 6–6). The arcuate artery marking the boundary of the papilla from the adjacent cortex and the lack of any dis-

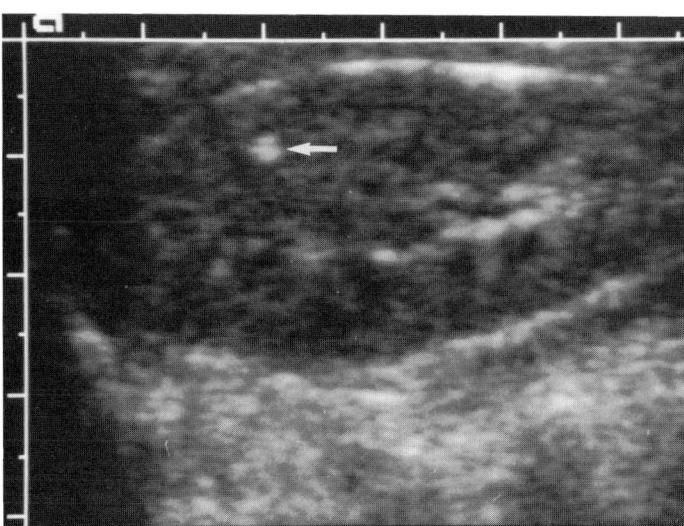

Figure 6–4. Longitudinal view of the right kidney in this baby shows echogenic double track (arrow), which represents the two walls of a renal artery. It is not unusual to see very prominent echogenic vascular walls, especially in very young babies. Color or pulsed Doppler ultrasonography can be used to verify their vascular nature.

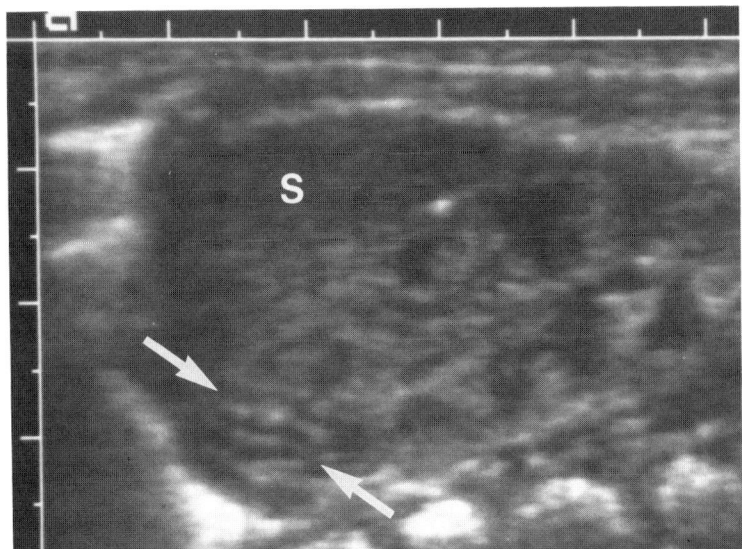

Figure 6–5. This is a normal neonatal kidney. Note the adrenal gland superior to it (arrows). The medullae are quite lucent and relatively prominent. The cortex is echogenic in relation to the adjacent spleen (S).

tortion of renal contour are clues to its normalcy. Neonatal kidneys retain variable amounts of fetal lobulation for some weeks after birth (Fig. 6–7). The interrenicular plane between the upper and middle kidney results in an oblique echogenic interface on parasagittal scans or a triangular defect on transverse views (Fig. 6–8; Hoffer et al., 1985). Cortical infoldings or columns of Bertin are common and usually detected in midsections of kidneys on transverse sections (Fig. 6–9).

In a child, the kidneys lie parallel to the long axis of the spine. As the child grows into adolescence, the lower poles deviate laterally and the psoas muscles increase in size. The left kidney is generally a little higher than the right, and the left often has a more tapered upper pole and bulbous midsection than the right, which is more properly bean-shaped (Fig. 6–10).

Renal length may be underestimated (1) if sector scans, which truncate the upper margins, are used; (2) if scans are oblique to the axis of the kidney; and (3) if the longest axis is not chosen. We think, although it is difficult to prove, that scans in suspended deep inspiration may show a slight decrease in renal length, in comparison with scans in full expiration, in which the kidney is not as squashed in a superoinferior direction. There

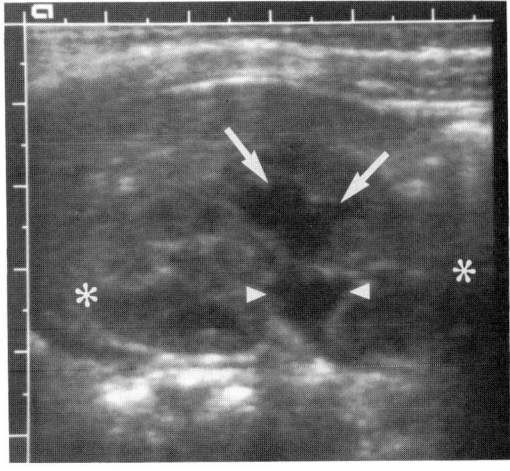

Figure 6–6. This baby had been referred because previous ultrasonography had suggested the presence of a renal cyst. The coronal view of the left kidney shows that the "cyst" is actually a lucent composite papilla (arrows) in the midportion of the kidney. The mild prominence of the renal pelvis (arrowheads) is within normal range.

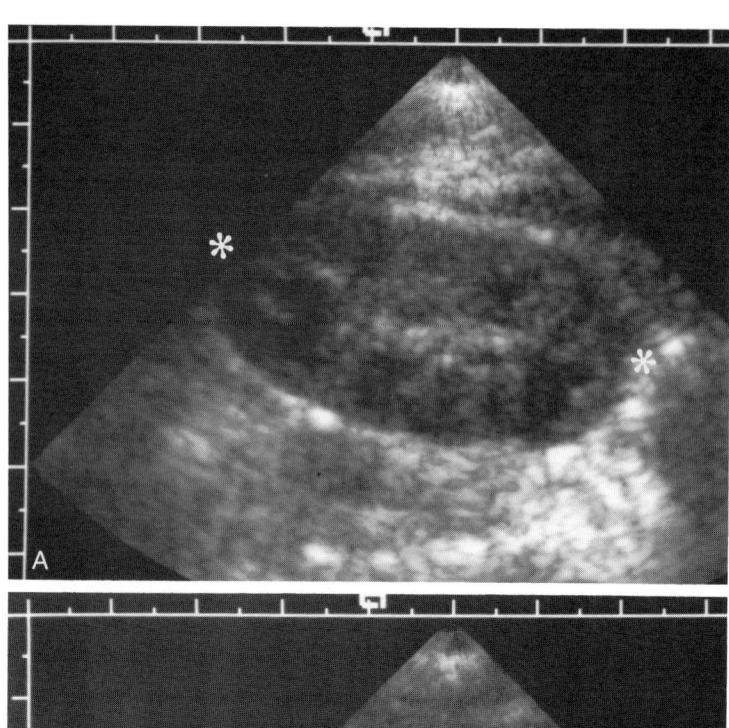

Figure 6–7. The right kidney of this baby is relatively smooth in contour (**A**). The outline of the left kidney is quite lobular (**B**).

can be a difference between measurements acquired from mechanical sector scanners and those from phased linear array scanners (Fig. 6–11). When scanning children in follow-up studies, we try to use the same transducer and ultrasonic unit that was used for their baseline scans.

Measurements of renal length and charts of renal length and volume in comparison with age, height, weight, and body surface area have been published and are listed in the references. We recommend that the reader select one chart that is easy to use, is based on a population of patients similar to the reader's, and involves the use of equipment similar to that available. The most important feature of normal renal growth in a child is sustained growth along the same curve. To establish this, one needs good scans, similar techniques, and the same method of measurement and charting. Ultrasonography, in comparison with intravenous urography, shows a kidney that is approximately 1 cm "shorter" because of lack of swelling (from ionic contrast media) and lack of radiographic magnification.

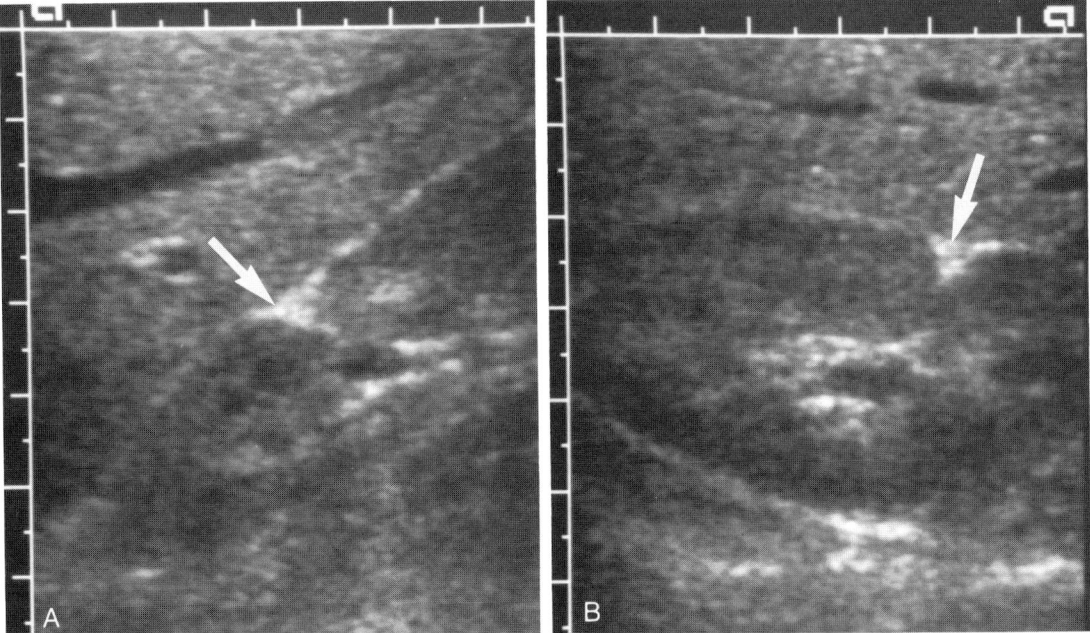

Figure 6–8. Longitudinal (A) and transverse (B) scans show the normal indentation (arrow) in the kidney from a plane of connective tissue that separates the kidney into two reniculi.

RULING OUT RENAL ABNORMALITY

A patient may be sent for ultrasonography because of a known, named syndrome, because of dysmorphism, or because relatives have renal disease. The ultrasonographer must know what question is being asked when a patient arrives for a screening study. The necessity for screening renal ultrasonography is controversial in some situations. Although a single umbilical artery is associated with malformations, these malformations are typically lethal or multiple, or both, and evident by birth if the fetus survives. Results from studies of babies who have presented with a single umbilical artery as their only abnormality have not supported an increased incidence of renal anomalies (Leung and Robson, 1989). However, very large numbers of babies would have to be screened in order to find a small increase over the normal "background" incidence of renal anomalies. The fact that in babies with the VATER association (vertebral defects, imperforate anus, tracheoesophageal fistula, and radial and renal dysplasia) there is a high incidence of single umbilical artery also makes us suspect that there is more of a spectrum than has been proved to date. Supernumerary nipples, unless associated with other obvious anomalies, are not indicative of renal anomaly. "Funny ears" without other abnormality are not a problem worthy of renal ultrasonography! Simple hypospadias is unassociated with anomalies, as is undescended testis in most cases. However, in one study of 144 asymptomatic boys with cryptorchidism, major anomalies were detected in 8 (5.5 percent) on intravenous urography (Pappis et al., 1988). Six of these 8 had an intra-abdominal or canalicular testis, and bilateral undescended testes were more than twice as likely to be associated with a major anomaly. If it is assumed that 1 to 2 percent of the population has a major renal anomaly, this study's findings represent a threefold increase. Babies who have congenital heart disease are more likely than the normal population to have renal anomalies. In babies with congenital heart disease, the presence of additional anomalies increases the incidence of renal anomaly from 5 to 39 percent (Murugasu et al., 1990). Many babies with multiple anomalies are among those with the VATER association.

The syndromes associated with renal tu-

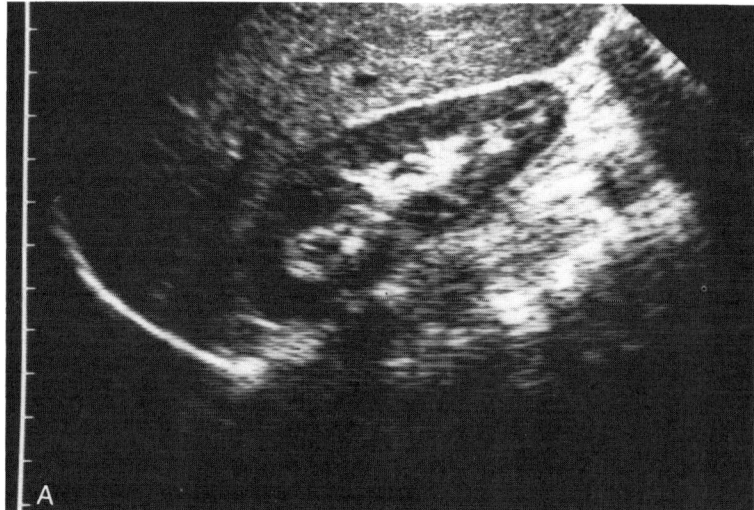

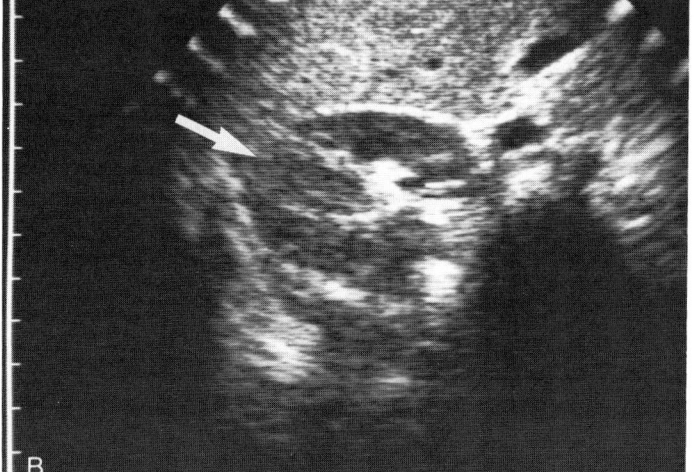

Figure 6–9. Longitudinal scan of the right kidney through the liver (**A**) shows the normal relationship of the collecting system to the parenchyma. The transverse scan through the midportion of kidney (**B**) shows a column of Bertin (arrow). This should not be mistaken for an intrarenal mass.

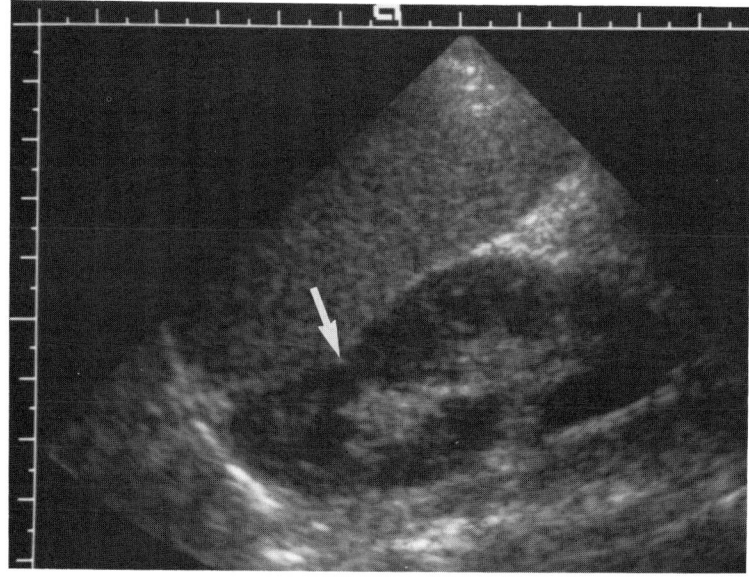

Figure 6–10. Coronal view of the left kidney in a normal 3-year-old shows apparent narrowing of the parenchyma (arrow) in the upper portion of the kidney. This is normal tapering associated with the spleen and the interrenicular junction. It should not be mistaken for scarring.

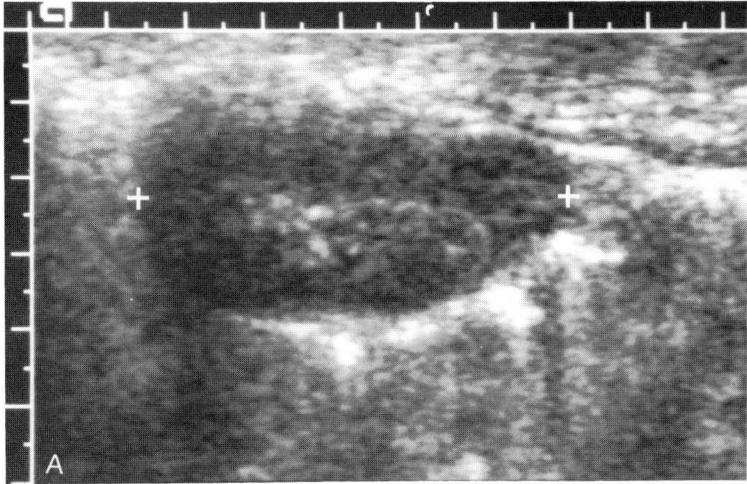
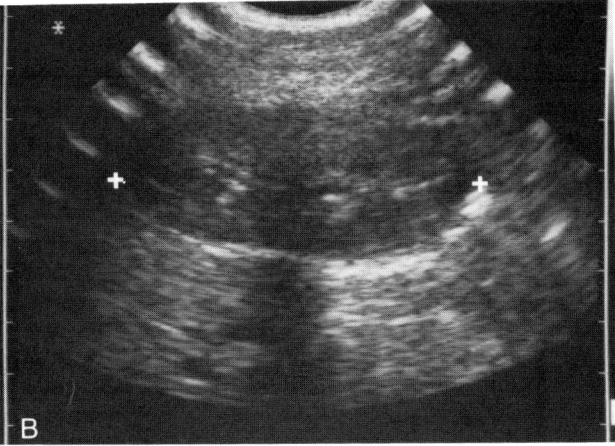
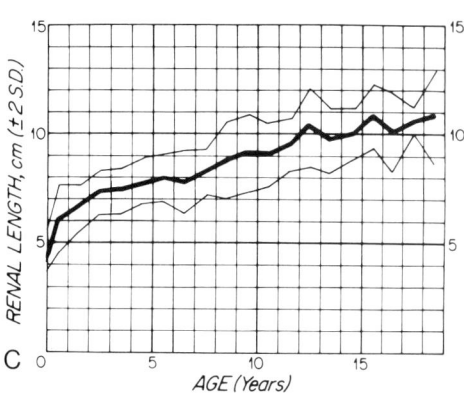

Figure 6–11. Note the difference in measured renal lengths, which depends on the transducer used. These two scans (**A** and **B**) were performed on the same day on the same patient with different transducers, and there is a difference of 1 cm in the lengths measured. Change in length (i.e., growth) is important in following children who have reflux and other renal problems. We always try to use the same equipment as that used for the patients' baseline studies. Plus signs in **A** and **B** mark edges of the kidney. **C**. Renal length charted against age in years. (From Rosenbaum DM, et al: Sonographic assessment of renal length in normal children. AJR 1984; 142:467–469.)

mors are included in Table 6–1. Those syndromes commonly associated with renal anomaly or abnormality are listed in Table 6–2. Various types of renal cystic disease and associations are included in Table 6–3. The tables include only the most common syndromes and associations, and it is apparent that some syndromes are associated with both renal anomaly and cystic disease. An easily accessible reference is *Radiology of Syndromes, Metabolic Disorders and Skeletal Dysplasia* by H. Taybi and R. S. Lachman. For unusual cases, we recommend use of the computer programs available through departments of genetics (e.g., POSSUM) or a literature search of the references in the U.S. National Library of Medicine.

The examiner should realize that the parents, and the child if old enough, are usually aware of the primary diagnosis and ramifications for the child if scans are abnormal. This situation can be difficult for all concerned, especially when disease known to be genetic in origin is being evaluated. There is always a measure of guilt, anger, and depression in the families of affected children, and the last thing they need is "variable input" from several sources. The best person to discuss the ultrasonographic findings with a family is the physician who has prime responsibility for their care. If possible, that person should be available soon after the study is completed so that implications of abnormal studies can be discussed.

RENAL ANOMALIES

The reported prevalence of renal anomalies in a defined population varies, depending on the extent of investigation. In large clinical studies reported before ultrasonography was available or applied to unselected populations, renal anomalies were detected by pal-

Table 6–2. COMMON SYNDROMES ASSOCIATED WITH RENAL ABNORMALITY

Syndrome	Type of Renal Abnormality
VATER complex	45% to 60% with anomaly, usually single kidney
Imperforate anus	4% (low imperforate anus), >37% (high imperforate anus) with anomaly, usually single kidney
Vertebral anomaly/congenital scoliosis	16% with anomaly, usually single kidney; also duplex, hydronephrosis
Müllerian duct aplasia, renal aplasia, cervical somite dysplasia (MURCS)	Single kidney
Fanconi anemia	Single kidney
Brachio-oto-renal syndrome	Renal agenesis/hypoplasia
Cloacal exstrophy	Pelvic or subdiaphragmatic kidney
Prune-belly syndrome	Varying degrees of hydronephrosis, hydroureter, and renal hypoplasia
Nail-patella syndrome (Fong)	Nephropathy: small kidneys with interstitial fibrosis, tubular dilatation, glomerular atrophy
Alport syndrome (congenital cataracts, deafness)	Nephropathy
Drash syndrome (glomerulopathy, male pseudohermaphroditism)	Chronic glomerulonephropathy (predisposition for Wilms tumor)
Cockayne syndrome (deafness, dwarfism, retinal atrophy)	Glomerular dysplasia
Trisomy 21 (Down)	Microscopic renal dysplasia with or without cysts
Trisomy 13 (Patau)	Renocortical cysts, hydronephrosis/hydroureter
Trisomy 18 (Edwards)	Hydronephrosis/hydroureter ectopic, horseshoe kidney
Triploidy (dispermy, diandry, or digyny)	Hydronephrosis, renal dysplasia
Turner syndrome (45,X)	50% with anomaly: horseshoe, agenesis, or hypoplasia; hydronephrosis; retrocaval ureter (Mosaics and variants have lower incidence of anomaly)

pation at a rate of 0.6 percent (Museles et al., 1971). In large ultrasonographic studies now being reported, it appears that significant renal anomalies (all types) can occur in more than 1 percent of the liveborn population (Steinhart et al., 1988).

Renal Agenesis

Renal agenesis results from failure of the ureteric bud, which arises from the wolffian duct, to make contact with nephrogenic blastema at the proper time (6 weeks after conception). If the entire urogenital ridge has failed to form on one side, there will be ipsilateral absence of the genital and upper urinary tracts (including the trigone). The ipsilateral adrenal gland will fail to develop, as will the gonad. Gray and Skandalakis (1972) noted that the adrenal gland is absent in only 10 percent of cases of renal agenesis. If the urogenital ridge has formed but the wolffian duct fails to produce a ureteric bud, or if the developing ureter fails to reach the nephrogenic blastema, renal agenesis will result, but the ipsilateral gonad and adrenal gland will be present. Renal agenesis allows the adrenal gland (if present), the spleen, and the colon (on the left) to fill the renal fossa. In the neonate who has renal agenesis, the adrenal gland appears larger than usual and assumes an oval rather than lambdoid shape (Fig. 6–12).

Renal agenesis is associated with many of the named syndromes and with the VATER complex. One can readily realize that any insult to the embryo early in its development might affect the development of multiple organ systems.

Because urinary and genital tracts share ductal systems and geography, renal agenesis is strongly associated with gynecologic anomalies in girls and, to a lesser extent, genital anomalies in boys. It has been estimated that 70 percent of girls with renal agenesis have a gynecologic anomaly (Wiersma et al., 1976). This percentage may be misleading and may be an underestimate of the association between true renal agenesis and genital malformation. Early studies usually relied heavily on intravenous urography for the diagnosis of renal agenesis. Unilateral nonfunction with compensatory hypertrophy of the other kidney was often interpreted as agenesis. However, a nubbin of renal tissue from an involuted, multicystic, dysplastic kidney and a kidney that is nonfunctional as a result of a neonatal vascular accident can masquerade as agenesis (Fig. 6–13). They are not, however, the sequelae of embryologic accidents during the first 6 weeks of gestation. In boys and men, cyst of the seminal

Table 6–3. CYSTIC DISEASES

Syndrome	Inheritance if Known	Type of Involvement
Autosomal dominant ("adult" type) polycystic kidney disease	AD	Macroscopic cysts that usually connect to some part of nephron or collecting duct
Autosomal recessive ("infantile" type) polycystic kidney disease	AR	Microscopic cysts that represent marked ectasia of collecting ducts
Familial juvenile nephronophthisis	AR	Normal-sized to small kidneys, small or microscopic medullary and cortical cysts
Medullary cystic disease	AD	Same as above
Renal-retinal dysplasia	AR	Same as above
Mainzer-Saldino syndrome (cerebellar ataxia, skeletal dysplasia, and renal-retinal dysplasia)		
Medullary sponge kidney	AD and sporadic	Dilated medullary collecting tubules with or without calcifications
Glomerulocystic kidney disease	AD or sporadic	Infants: glomerular cysts, large kidneys (simulates AR polycystic kidney disease); older children: smaller kidneys, macroscopic cysts develop
Tuberous sclerosis	AD	Noncommunicating macroscopic cysts, angiomyolipomas, renal artery aneurysms
von Hippel-Lindau disease (cerebelloretinal angiomatosis)	AD	Variably sized renal cysts (also renal cell carcinoma)
Beckwith-Wiedemann syndrome (exomphalos-macroglossia-gigantism)		Cystic medullary-cortical dysplasia; pyelocaliceal diverticula
Laurence-Moon-Biedl syndrome (obesity, polydactyly, mental retardation, retinitis pigmentosa, hypogenitalism)	AR	Small kidneys, clubbed calices, microcystic dysplasia of cortex and medulla
Ehlers-Danlos syndrome (hyperelastica)	AD	Variable renal involvement: from normal to cortical microcysts to "polycystic"
Apert syndrome (acrocephalosyndactyly)	AD	Microcystic renal dysplasia
Jeune syndrome (asphyxiating thoracic dystrophy)	AR	Spectrum of cystic dysplasia
Zellweger syndrome (cerebrohepatorenal syndrome)	AR	Glomerulocystic involvement with or without cortical cysts
Goldston syndrome (Dandy-Walker malformation and cystic kidneys)	AR	Cystic renal dysplasia
Meckel-Gruber syndrome (polydactyly, cystic renal dysplasia, encephalocele or other cranial anomalies)	AR	Cystic renal dysplasia
Oral-facial-digital syndrome, type I (Gorlin)	X-linked	Macroscopic cysts (similar to AD polycystic kidney disease)
Trisomy 13		30% glomerulocystic or cystic dysplasia
Trisomy 18		<10% glomerulocystic or cystic dysplasia
Triploidy		Cystic dysplasia, microcystic dysplasia
Trisomy 21		Microscopic cysts occasionally present
Partial chromosome 19 translocation		Cystic renal dysplasia

Note: AD = autosomal dominant; AR = autosomal recessive.

vesicle ipsilateral to renal agenesis has been described (Denes et al., 1986). Absence of derivatives of the wolffian duct (epididymis, ductus deferens, and seminal vesicle) associated with ipsilateral renal agenesis may well be clinically silent, and therefore their incidence may be underestimated.

For all children in whom only one kidney is apparent, it is important to use the bladder as a scanning window to search both for a pelvic kidney and for associated genital anomalies. In prepubertal girls in whom the uterus and related structures are small, an anomaly, even if present, may not be apparent on ultrasonography. Pubertal growth with its hormonal stimulation usually reveals duplication with or without obstruction on the side of the renal agenesis (see Chapter 8).

The absence of one kidney results, over time, in hypertrophy of the remaining kidney. In the neonate, whose excretory function has been managed by the mother for 9 months, absence of one kidney does not

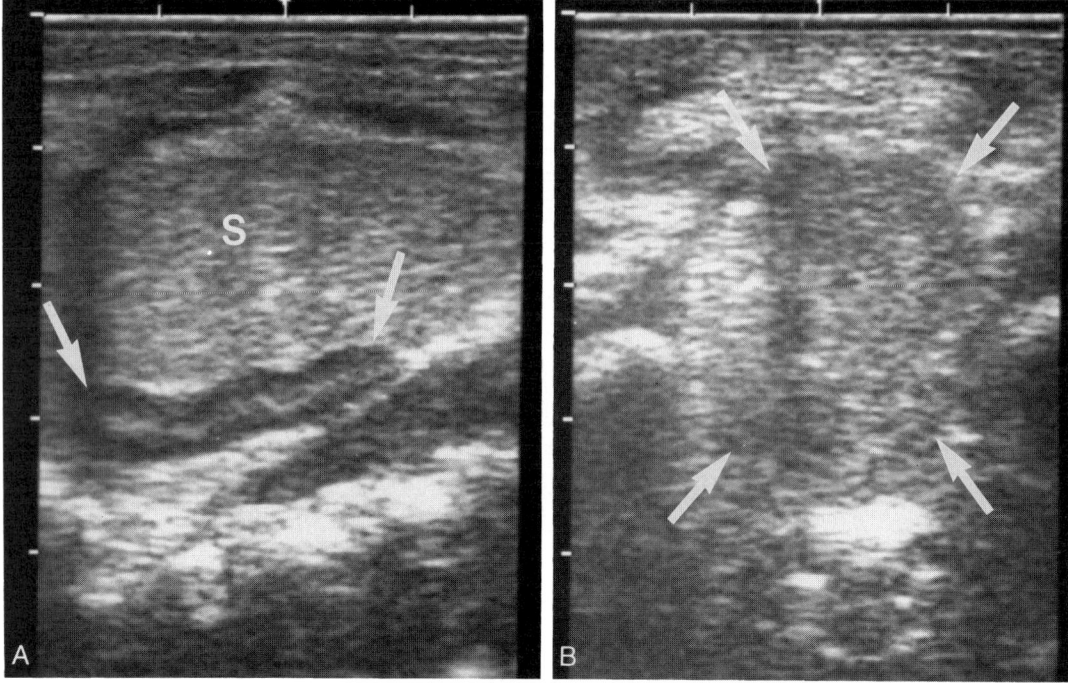

Figure 6–12. This newborn boy was scanned emergently when he presented with bilateral pneumothoraces, club feet, and Potter facies. Scans of each renal fossa were similar. No kidney was identified. On the longitudinal scan of the left renal fossa (**A**), the adrenal gland (arrows) has slipped into the space normally occupied by the kidney. It has assumed an oval appearance. The spleen (S) is also more posterior because the kidney is absent. The transverse scan of the pelvis (**B**) shows a mass 2.5 cm in diameter that represents the contracted, unused bladder (arrows).

result in obvious hypertrophy of the other until some weeks have passed. In a child, if one renal fossa is empty, the other kidney, if solitary, should be large. However, a dysplastic kidney, hidden in the retroperitoneum or the pelvis, may be functioning so poorly that the remaining kidney still hypertrophies (Fig. 6–14). Dysplastic kidneys are difficult to identify with ultrasonography because they blend with surrounding connective tissue in the retroperitoneum or are obscured by the bowel in the pelvis (Fig. 6–15). A plain radiograph that documents normal position of the splenic flexure of the colon, rather than a posteromedial position, suggests that renal tissue is present in the left renal fossa. There is no reliably comparable sign for the right side. Unless the child carries the diagnosis of a syndrome that has a known association with agenesis, we extend the diagnostic evaluation of presumed solitary kidney by performing radionuclide studies to localize a small kidney that has some function.

A number of published articles have established the familial nature of renal agenesis and dysgenesis. An ultrasonographic study of the first-degree relatives of babies with agenesis or dysgenesis (unassociated with any obvious syndrome) showed a 9 percent incidence of asymptomatic renal disease. Of all these relatives, 4.5 percent had renal agenesis, whereas the incidence in the control population was 0.3 percent (Roodhooft et al., 1984). In the absence of economic or other constraints, it is reasonable to screen siblings and parents of children found to have renal agenesis because the solitary kidney does appear to be more prone to complications than are two kidneys. It certainly is more exposed to the effects of abdominal trauma.

"Acquired" single kidney may result from surgical removal, previous arterial occlusion (e.g., trauma, insertion of a catheter during a stay in the neonatal nursery), and, less commonly, previous venous occlusion of a kidney. Venous occlusion probably results in hypoplasia of the kidney more often than in its complete disappearance. A multicystic, dysplastic kidney may evolve from the cystic

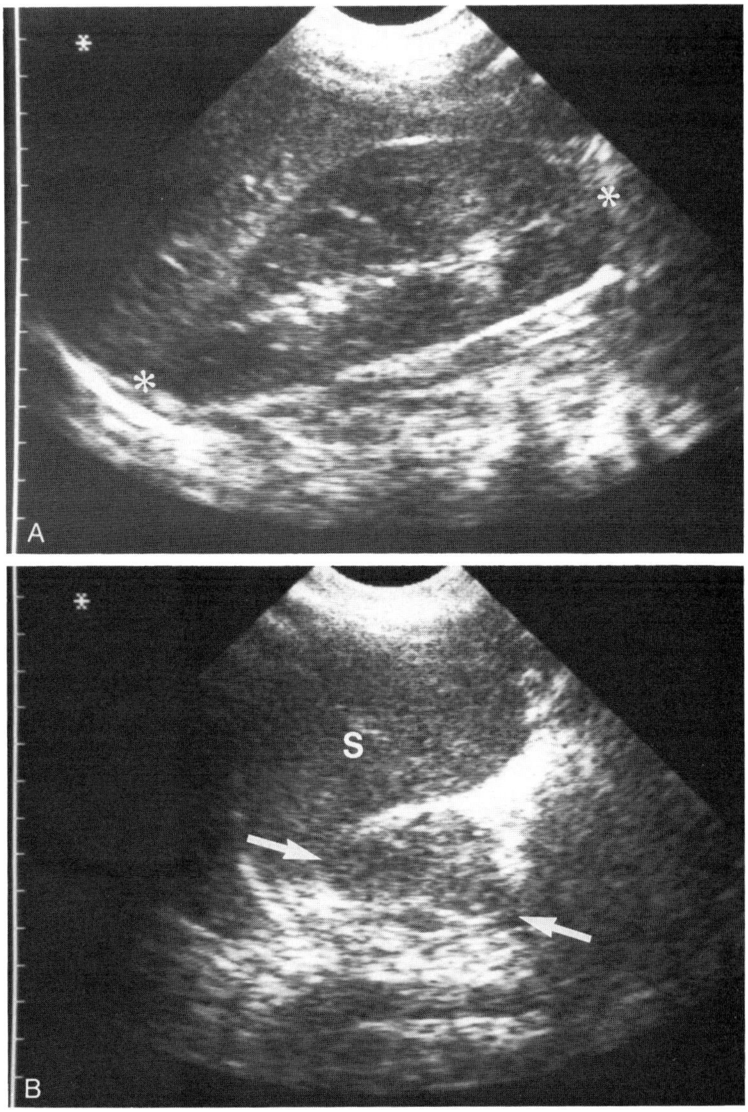

Figure 6–13. The hypertrophied single kidney on the right (**A**) was an incidental finding in this teenage girl, who had no symptoms referable to the genitourinary tract. She had no pelvic abnormality. Scan of the left renal fossa (**B**) shows the spleen (S) and an indistinct echogenic mass (arrows) in the left renal fossa. This had no function on subsequent radionuclide studies. Whether this represents a nubbin of renal tissue from multicystic dysplasia or an earlier vascular accident is unknown. The colon was in normal position in this patient. Renal agenesis on the left allows the left colon to fall into the left renal fossa. Occasionally, the stool-filled left colon masquerades as a kidney or a mass.

stage to a completely dysplastic nubbin and disappear into retroperitoneal connective tissue (Avni, 1987).

Renal Ectopia

"Renal ectopia" is a kidney that is fixed in position outside its renal fossa. If a kidney is simply mobile, one may ultrasonographically demonstrate its change in position with the patient prone, supine, and then upright. Most low kidneys are pelvic and fixed and diagnosed as part of an evaluation for urinary tract infection, pelvic mass, pelvic pain, or unusual pelvic symptoms (Fig. 6–16).

Failure of a kidney to ascend normally at 6 to 7 weeks' conceptual age results in its being ectopic. A pelvic kidney may be difficult to evaluate thoroughly with ultrasonography. Viewed anteriorly, the kidney is usually partially hidden by loops of bowel. The iliac crest and spine shield it from posterior viewing. Scanning through a very full bladder may suffice if the kidney is low in the pelvis. The collecting system of this anomalous kidney tends to be predominantly extrarenal, and the central oval-shaped collection

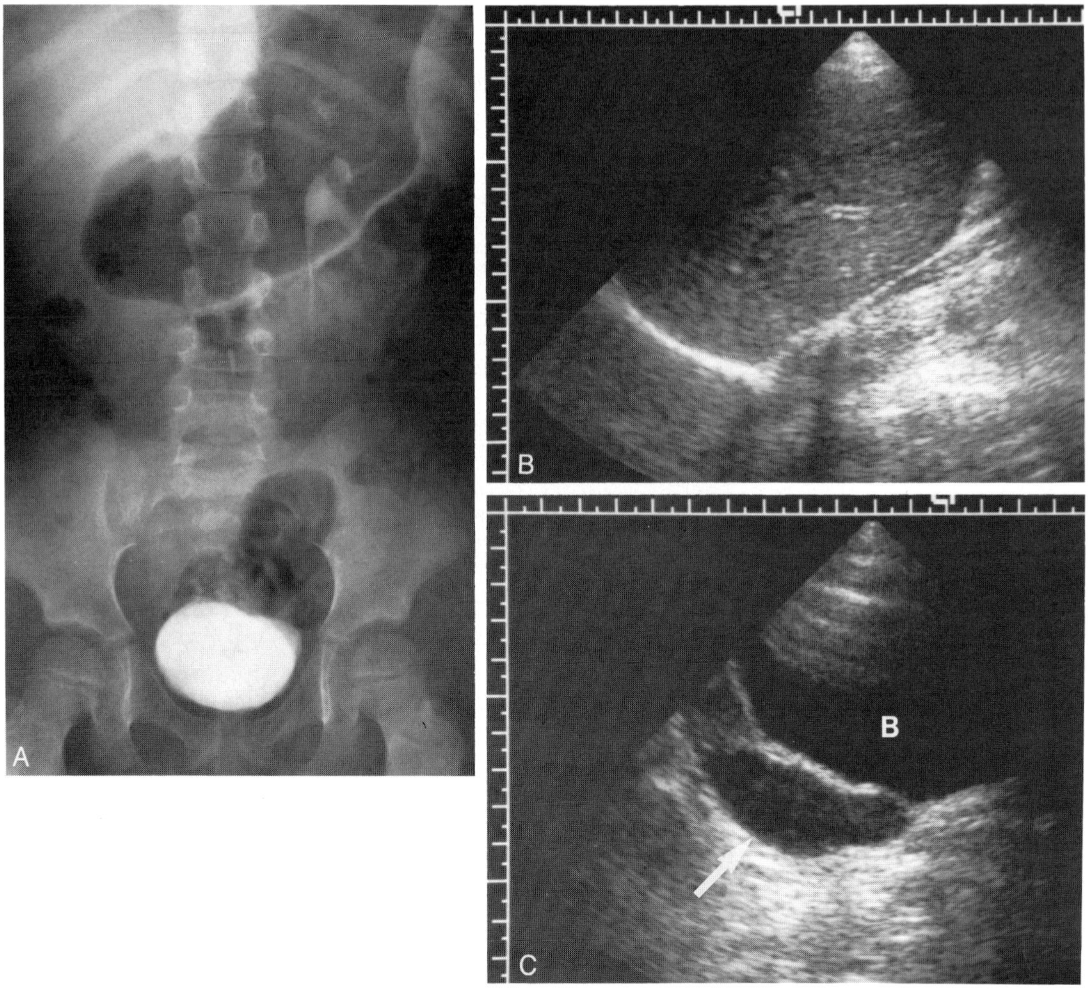

Figure 6–14. This 12-year-old girl had been constantly wet, day and night, since birth. She had been evaluated with multiple previous studies, which resulted in a diagnosis of solitary kidney and presumed neurogenic bladder. Intravenous urogram is shown in **A**. The bladder seems normal in contour. The left kidney is hypertrophied. Longitudinal scan of the right renal fossa (**B**) shows the liver occupying the space normally taken by the kidney. Longitudinal scan of the right pelvis (**C**), however, shows a cylindrical lucency (arrow) behind the bladder, which is typical of an obstructed ureter. This patient had a dysplastic right pelvic kidney associated with ectopic insertion of its ureter into vagina. When this renal unit was removed, the patient's wetting vanished. B = bladder.

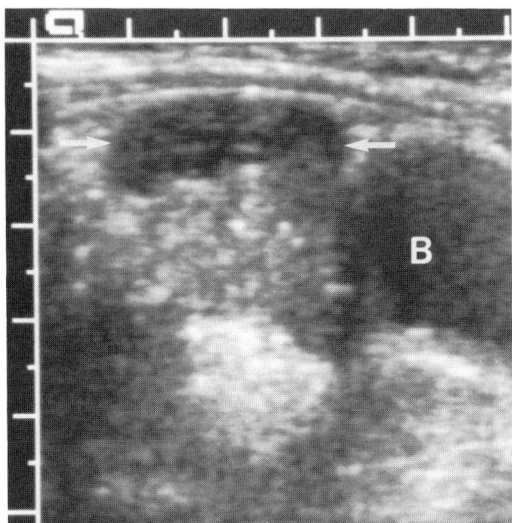

Figure 6–15. This 2.5 cm dysplastic pelvic kidney (arrows) was responsible for bloody vaginal discharge. Its ureter drained into a paravaginal cyst, which was assumed to communicate intermittently with the vagina. The baby also had uterine duplication, which could not be recognized during ultrasonography. The dysplastic pelvic kidney was removed, and the patient had no further symptoms. B = bladder.

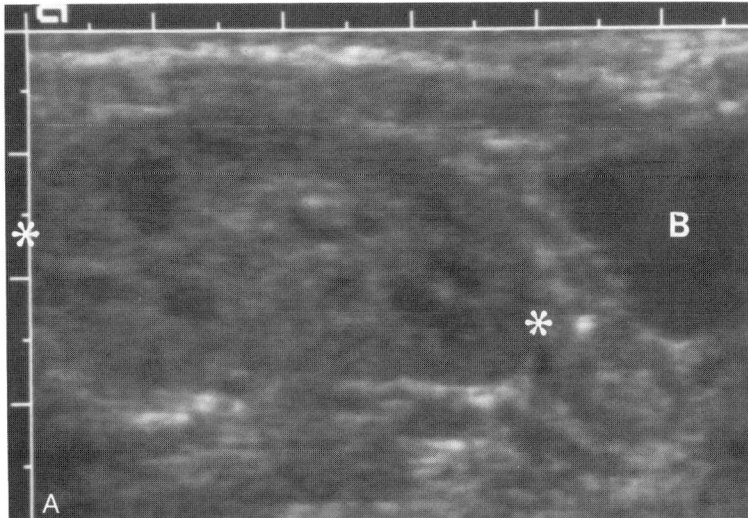

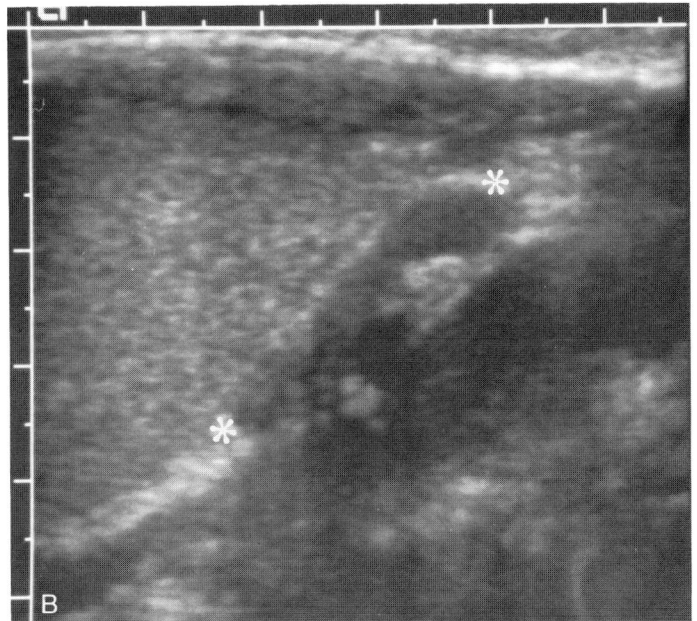

Figure 6–16. Prenatal ultrasonography had revealed a pelvic kidney in this baby. The postnatal follow-up study shows pelvic kidney immediately superior to the bladder (A). B = bladder. Longitudinal scan of the right renal fossa (B) demonstrated a dysplastic kidney. The left renal fossa was empty.

of echoes seen in the normal kidney may be completely missing. Intravenous urography with tomography or radionuclide imaging, or both, is usually needed in such cases to delineate both anatomy and function.

Among children who have cloacal exstrophy, there is a high incidence of pelvic kidney (Herman et al., 1986). Absence of normally pelvic organs, such as bladder and lower gut, may allow kidneys to stay in the pelvis rather than be forced to ascend. Could girls with Turner syndrome have a similar embryologic history, with partial failure of ascent (horseshoe kidney), because genital structures are absent or hypoplastic? A single kidney in an ectopic location, typically the pelvis, is a rare anomaly and should not be evaluated with ultrasonography alone. This type of kidney has also been called "lump," "cake," or "discoid" kidney. It likely results from fusion of the metanephric stroma, associated with failure of ascent, that occurs earlier than that blamed for producing horseshoe kidney. The orientation and number of pelves and calices are unusual, and we recommend good radiologic baseline studies because these kidneys are prone to formation of calculi and may have a higher rate of infection.

When renal ascent has been not only in-

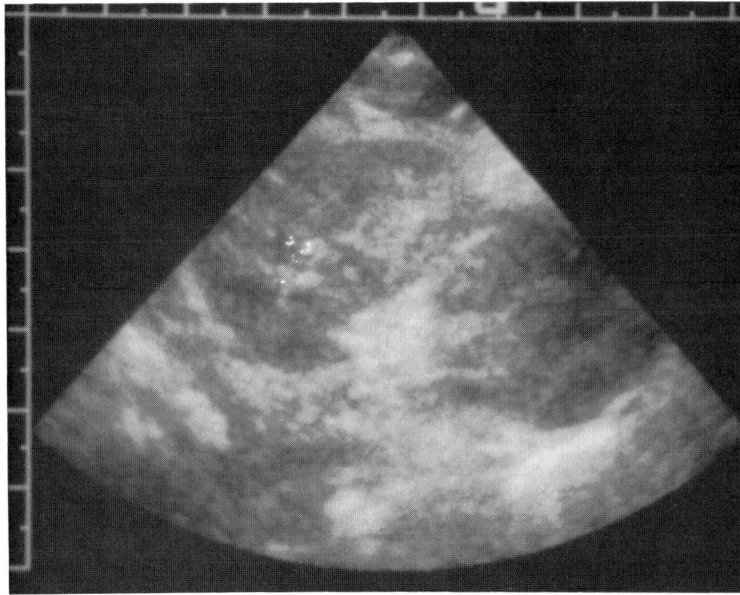

Figure 6–17. Postnatal scan of this baby was to follow up a prenatal diagnosis of cross-fused renal ectopia. This oblique scan is actually a transverse view of each kidney, both of which lie to the right of the spine. Interestingly, this patient had a single umbilical artery.

complete but confused, both kidneys may lie separately on the same side (crossed renal ectopia), or they may be a conglomerate mass (cross-fused renal ectopia; Fig. 6–17). Fusion is 10 times more common than nonfusion (Perlmutter et al., 1986). In many situations of renal ectopia, other imaging such as intravenous urography or scintigraphy is needed to sort out the anatomy and physiology, as these kidneys seem to be predisposed to other anomalies such as multicystic dysplasia and obstruction (Fig. 6–18; Lubat et al., 1989).

Horseshoe kidney results from partial failure of renal ascent and variable fusion of renal tissue anterior to the spine. The kidneys are lower than normal in position, they lie on a vertical axis (although in normal children kidneys tend to lie parallel to spine, anyway, until psoas muscles enlarge in early puberty), the collecting systems exit anteriorly, and there is usually a bridge of renal tissue that connects the lower poles (Figs. 6–19, 6–20). In rare instances, renal tissue fuses between upper poles. Even more rare is fusion between both upper and lower poles that results in a "doughnut" kidney. If only sagittal scans are done, the horseshoe kidney can be completely missed. Coronal views are best for showing the bridge of renal tissue, if it is present. Turner syndrome has a well-known association with this anomaly.

In the embryo, after ascent at 6 to 7 weeks after conception the kidneys normally make a 90° medial turn; as a result, the ureters exit the renal pelves in the same coronal plane as the great vessels. A malrotated kidney has a collecting system that exits anteriorly or (much less commonly) posteriorly, rather than medially (Fig. 6–21). Malrotation appears to have no clinical significance except that we suspect that some cases of obstruction at the ureteropelvic junction might be secondary to vessels crossing an abnormally rotated pelvis. Recognition of a malrotated kidney is important in order to avoid assigning some other, less benign diagnosis to the anomaly. In the malrotated kidneys that we have examined, the collecting system echoes tend to be more extrarenal.

A high, medial position of both kidneys is typical in children who have undergone previous repair of an omphalocele, especially those in whom a large portion of the liver was in the sac. The kidneys, allowed some freedom of movement, appear to favor the superior position in the abdomen. After repair of an omphalocele, replacement of abdominal contents under pressure may obstruct the ureters, especially on the right. Eventration of the diaphragm or previous diaphragmatic hernia may be associated with a very high placement of the kidney on the side of the diaphragmatic anomaly (Fig. 6–22).

Anomalies of Duplication

A duplex kidney is not difficult to diagnose when there is obstruction of, or reflux to,

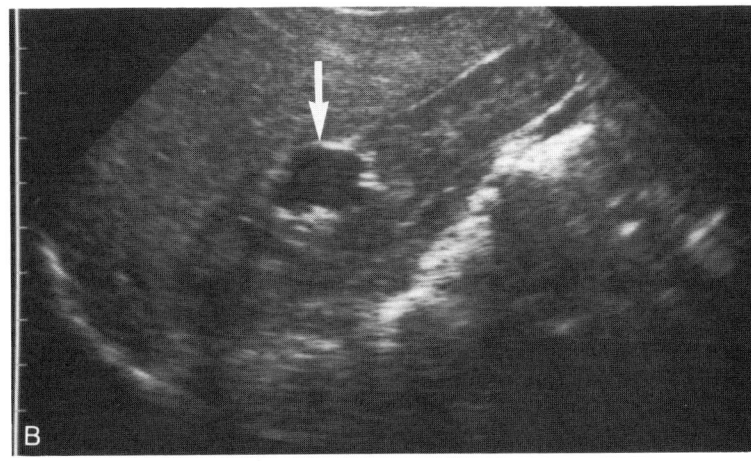

Figure 6–18. Transverse scan of the upper abdomen was performed as a screening study for this little boy, who had multiple segmentation anomalies of the thoracic spine. He also had hemifacial microsomia. The transverse scan (A) shows a mantle of renal tissue, representing cross-fused ectopia, to the right of the spine. S = spine. G = gallbladder. B is an oblique view along the long axis of the fused kidneys. There is prominence of the renal pelvis (arrow), which is related to the upper renal unit. Radionuclide studies with furosemide (lasix) showed no significant obstruction.

one of its components (Fig. 6–23). If reflux into the lower pole of a duplex kidney has resulted in scarring, there will be an obvious difference in the parenchymal cushion of upper and lower poles. Obstruction of the upper unit is typically associated with an ectopic ureter and a ureterocele (see section on hydronephrosis, Chapter 8). A duplex system may be difficult to diagnose with ultrasonography when it is uncomplicated. Because the central collection of echoes in the kidney is representative not just of the collecting system but of fat, blood vessels, and lymphatics, it is not absolutely reliable for distinguishing single from duplex systems. A discrepancy of more than 1 cm in size between kidneys is an inconstant clue to the presence of a duplex kidney. Careful coronal scanning can, at times, allow delineation of superior and inferior pelves, but these may join out of ultrasonic view and be a bifid rather than completely duplex system. There are two situations in which clinicians should be aware of the difficulty in diagnosing duplex kidney: (1) during pelvic surgery

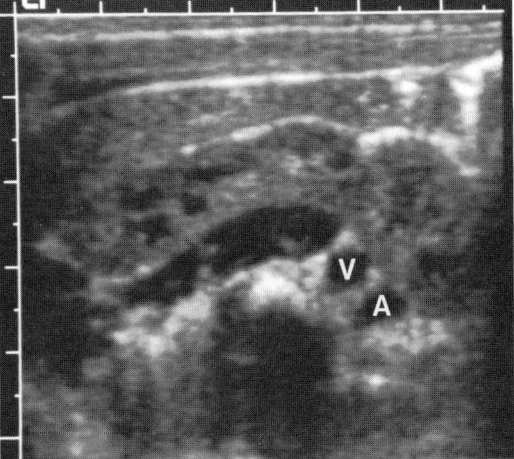

Figure 6–19. Horseshoe kidney was an incidental finding in this baby, who was being scanned for question of pyloric stenosis. This is an axial view through the right side of the abdomen. There is a bridge of renal tissue anterior to the great vessels. The psoas muscle on the right presents as a lucent pad posterior to the right kidney. A = aorta. V = inferior vena cava.

154 / RENAL SCREENING

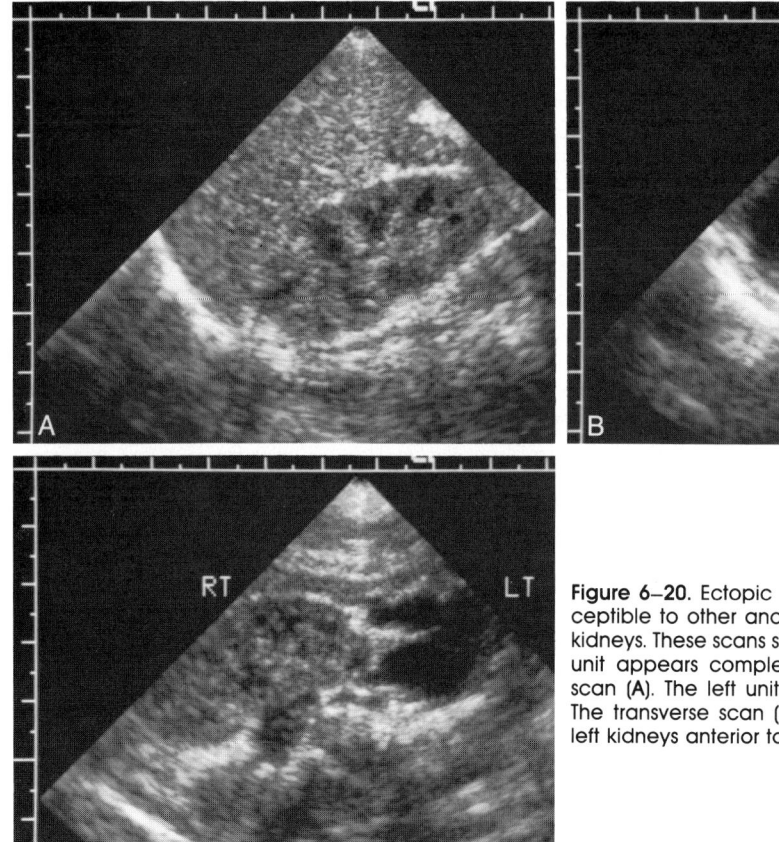

Figure 6–20. Ectopic kidneys appear to be more susceptible to other anomalies than do normally placed kidneys. These scans show a horseshoe kidney; the right unit appears completely normal on the longitudinal scan (A). The left unit is multicystic and dysplastic (B). The transverse scan (C) shows the fusion of right and left kidneys anterior to the spine.

in which a previous "normal" renal ultrasonogram does not rule out the possibility of there being two ureters on one or both sides, and (2) the existence of an unobstructed ectopic ureter. For a girl experiencing chronic wetting (not enuresis or occasional incontinence), investigation should be targeted at finding an ectopic ureter draining into the vagina or urethra from the upper pole of a duplex kidney. A normal ultrasonogram, in this clinical situation, is not enough. A small dysplastic upper pole of a duplex system may not be detected, even with careful scanning and when its presence is certain (Fig. 6–24).

A supernumerary kidney is the most extravagant form of duplex kidney and is very rare. Duplication of the collecting system is explained by aberrant ureteral budding from the wolffian duct at 5 weeks after conception. If the tip of the bud bifurcates before invading the metanephric stroma, a bifid pelvis results. If bifurcation from the wolffian duct is more proximal but the resultant ureters stay close together, the collecting system is duplex. If duplicated or even triplicated ureters diverge, the metanephric tissue becomes separated into clumps, and a supernumerary kidney results. The inferior kidney tends to be the smaller of the two and may be hypoplastic.

RENAL SCREENING

Ruling Out Tumor

Babies and children with known predisposition to Wilms tumor (Table 6–1) present the problem of how often to screen them. We saw one child in whom a second Wilms tumor developed in the remaining kidney, which had been thought normal according to radiologic, ultrasonographic, and surgical examination only 6 weeks previously. Semiannual or annual screening is helpful only when it happens to coincide with the onset of neoplasia (Fig. 6–25; Azouz et al., 1990).

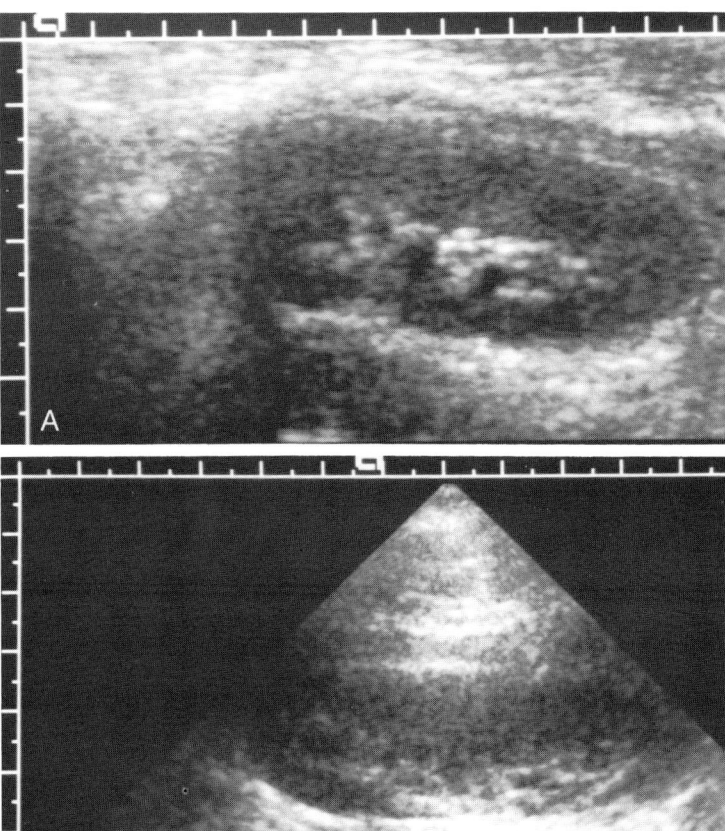

Figure 6-21. Longitudinal scan of the right kidney, performed while the patient was prone, shows the normal relationship of the collecting system echoes to renal parenchyma (A). The collecting system of the left kidney exits anteriorly (arrow, B). This normal variant should not be mistaken for scarring.

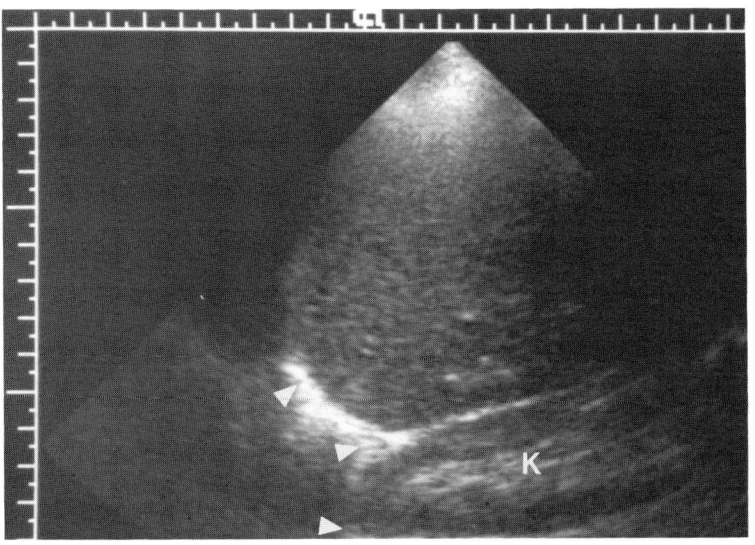

Figure 6-22. The high position of the right kidney (K) in this patient is related to previous congenital diaphragmatic hernia on that side. This scan is a longitudinal view of the right upper quadrant. Arrowheads mark reconstructed diaphragm.

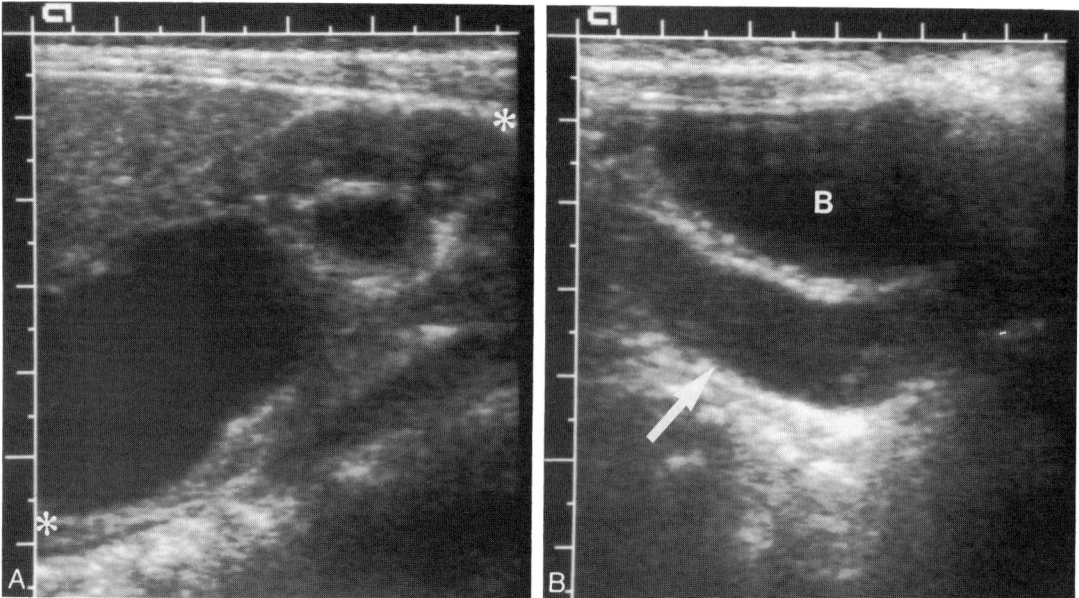

Figure 6–23. Prenatal diagnosis of hydronephrosis was confirmed on these postnatal scans. Longitudinal view of the right kidney **(A)** shows obstruction of the upper pole of a duplex kidney. Dilation of the collecting system in the lower pole was secondary to reflux. Longitudinal scan of the bladder **(B)** shows the ureter (arrow), whose dilation and ectopia were associated with the upper-pole moiety. There was no associated ureterocele. The baby underwent common sheath reimplantation after plication of the dilated ureter. B = bladder.

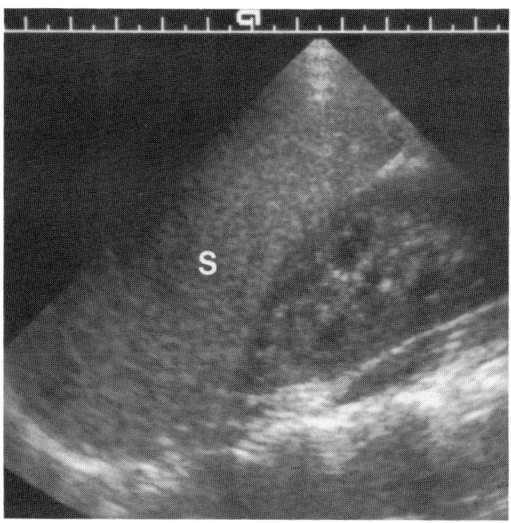

Figure 6–24. The coronal scan of the left kidney showed no obvious abnormality, but this patient was chronically wet, and the orifice of an ectopic ureter, which entered the vagina, had been visualized during a cystoscopy. The small dysplastic nubbin of the upper pole, which was connected to the ectopic ureter, could not be identified even with careful scanning. S = spleen.

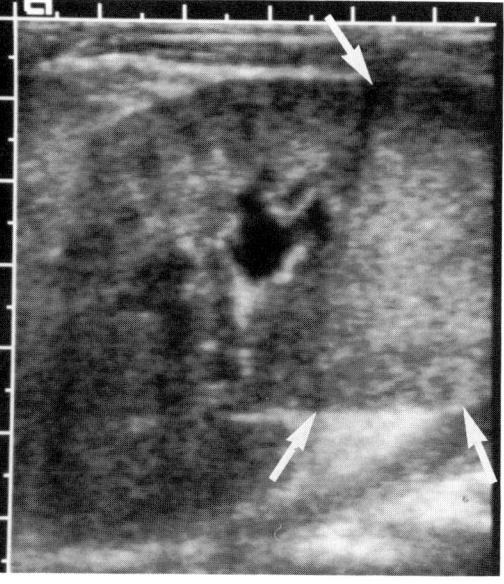

Figure 6–25. At birth, this girl was diagnosed as possibly having Beckwith-Weidemann syndrome. The neonatal scan was normal. At 7 months of age she returned for routine evaluation and at this time had a poorly defined mass in the lower pole of the left kidney (arrows). She came to surgery, at which time a Wilms tumor of the lower pole of the kidney was resected. This mass was barely palpable in the clinical examination, and it was fortunate that she had returned for screening when she did.

Also, the presence of nephroblastomatosis is frequently underestimated on ultrasonography (Fernbach et al., 1988). In spite of reservations in this regard, our practice with children who are considered at risk is to screen them semiannually until the age of 6 years and annually thereafter until age 12 or at any time when new clinical findings arise. At each session we obtain views by which to judge renal size and to evaluate growth, and we always look at renal veins and the inferior vena cava, although we have not seen involvement of vessels with tumor in the absence of a sizable renal mass.

Of patients with aniridia, 33 percent develop Wilms tumors, whereas of those with hemihypertrophy alone, only 3 percent develop the tumor. Hereditary and bilateral cases of Wilms tumor occur earlier (at a mean age of 2.5 years) than sporadic cases (at a mean age of 3.5 years; Mesrobian, 1988). A horseshoe kidney entails an increased risk of Wilms tumor (approximately 1 in 25,000); its occurrence in the general population is 7.8 per 1 million children (Beseghi et al., 1988). For children with Beckwith-Wiedemann syndrome, who have a predisposition to other tumors, we also scan the liver and the entire retroperitoneum (Fig. 6–26). (See Chapter 8 for further discussion of Wilms tumor.)

Abdominal Pain

For patients with chronic recurrent abdominal pain that is renal in origin, there are usually some corroborative clinical or laboratory data (e.g., abnormal urinalysis results, a flank mass) that also point to the urinary tract. However, as part of our evaluation for diffuse abdominal pain, we always include views of each kidney (see Chapter 10). A small number of children with pain have a renal anomaly that is difficult to diagnose. Scans may be falsely "negative" between painful episodes caused by intermittent obstruction of the ureteropelvic junction by a crossing vessel or a retroperitoneal band. Perlmutter and colleagues (1986) stated that 60 percent of kidneys have extra vessels to the lower pole that could act as obstructing bands. We have seen several children in whom overt hydronephrosis—shown by ultrasonography or intravenous urography—is evident only during their episodes of pain; at other times the affected kidney has looked normal. In retrospect, the redundant, collapsed walls of a previously dilated pelvis and calices have provided more interfaces and thus a more prominent cluster of central echoes than has the contralateral kidney. The patient's history is helpful in these cases: pain can usually be localized to the flank and tends to have an abrupt onset and just as abrupt a cessation. The child may be pale, anorexic, or nauseated. Strong suspicion of hydronephrosis and the use of imaging during the episode of pain can confirm the diagnosis. Pain related to intermittent obstruction of a pelvic kidney may occur in a similar fashion. The substitution of nonionic for ionic contrast media in urography will probably make the diagnosis of intermittent obstruction at the ureteropelvic junction even more occult as the diuretic effect from the injection of ionic contrast media is lost. Diuresis from any cause may uncover an otherwise silent partial obstruction at the ureteropelvic or ureterovesical junction (Fig. 6–27).

Hypertension

The children who are referred to our hospital for evaluation of hypertension are likely

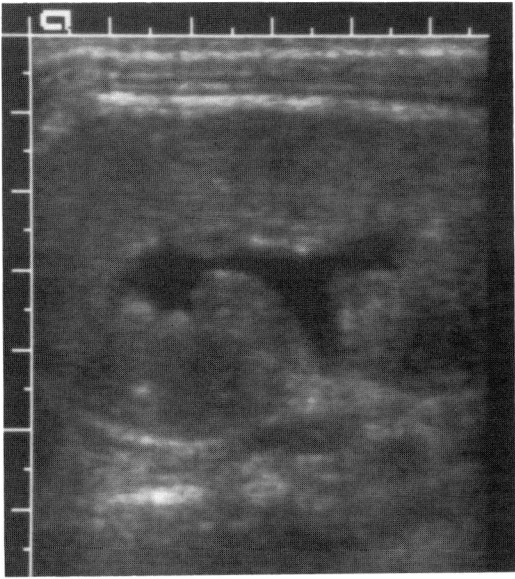

Figure 6–26. This is a longitudinal scan of the left kidney in a baby with Beckwith-Weidemann syndrome. Both kidneys were large for the patient's chronologic age of 3 months. Organomegaly is commonly associated with this syndrome. This baby did not develop a Wilms tumor or other intra-abdominal malignancy.

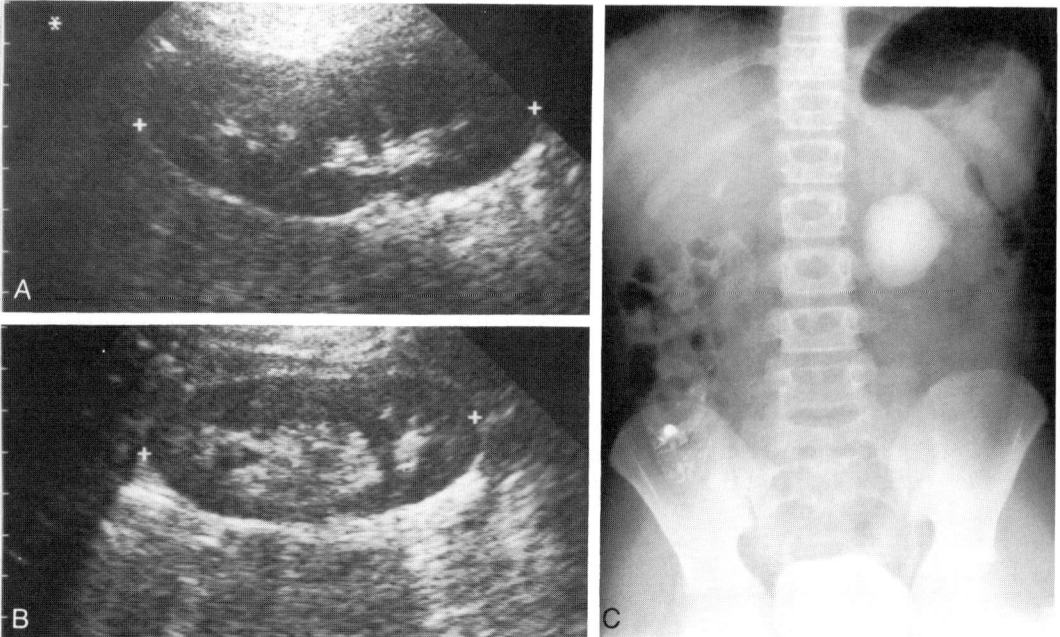

Figure 6–27. The normal right kidney (A) has less central echogenicity than the otherwise normal left kidney (B). Because of intermittent obstruction of the ureteropelvic junction by a crossing vessel, the surface area of the collecting system is greater on the left. An intravenous urogram, performed when the patient was in pain, shows the obstruction (C).

only a fraction of the pediatric population with elevated blood pressure. Measurements of blood pressure are not routinely performed for children, even on annual visits for physical examinations. Measurements are often in error in the infant and toddler population if the size of the cuff is incorrect, and there is a tendency to compare the measurements with adult norms rather than with age-adjusted or height/weight-adjusted normative values. Thus the last Task Force on Blood Pressure Control in Children (1987) began its report by encouraging routine measurement of blood pressure once yearly in healthy children 3 years of age and older, explaining the mechanics of appropriate measurement, and setting out normative data derived from published studies. In brief, the following values were provided in the tables supplied in the report: in the first month of age, systolic blood pressure higher than 100 mm of mercury is abnormal; systolic and diastolic pressures increase with age; 115/75 borders on hypertension for a 5-year-old; and 135/85 is at the top of the normal range for a 12-year-old.

The true incidence of hypertension in children is unknown; neither are there adequate data to determine what proportion of hypertension is primary (i.e., essential) and what is secondary. Reports published in the literature reflect the interests and patients of the physician-authors. In primary clinics, essential hypertension has been estimated as present in 93 percent of the hypertensive population. This proportion is completely reversed in selected referral populations, in which secondary hypertension can account for 65 to 85 percent of diagnoses. In a study from our institution, which offers primary and referral care of patients, 16 percent of hypertensive children who were referred for nuclear renograms had an identifiable cause of the hypertension (Rosen et al., 1985).

The report of the task force spells out in some detail the specific criteria for the investigation of a child, otherwise healthy, who is judged to be hypertensive. Diagnostic imaging is recommended for very few patients and only after careful review of family history and the patient's history, a thorough physical examination, and results of basic laboratory studies support a secondary cause.

Because most secondary hypertension is associated with renal problems, we combine the anatomic information from renal ultrasonography with the physiologic results from radionuclide scanning. In general, we start

Table 6–4. ABDOMINAL CAUSES OF HYPERTENSION IN CHILDREN

Congenital renal malformation
Renal parenchymal diseases
    Scarring after infection
    Nephritis
    Polycystic disease
    Tumor
    Collagen vascular disease
Perinephric/intrarenal hematoma
Renal arterial thrombosis
Renal arterial stenosis
Aortic coarctation
Aortic/renal aneurysm
Adrenal neoplasm

with ultrasonography because finding an obvious structural abnormality, such as obstructive hydronephrosis, is helpful to specialists in nuclear medicine. In Table 6–4 we list the problems associated with secondary hypertension that may be diagnosed with ultrasonography.

In the neonatal nursery, we commonly are asked to perform abdominal and renal ultrasonography for babies who are hypertensive. Indwelling umbilical arterial catheters are a major cause of vascular complications. A catheter can generate clots that become renal emboli or can induce spasm of renal arteries. The aorta can be imaged in coronal planes through the liver or spleen, usually from diaphragm to bifurcation. Sagittal and transverse views are too often limited to the upper aorta because gas in the bowel obscures the great vessels below the superior mesenteric artery. If the catheter has been removed, any echogenicity within the lumen of the aorta is abnormal and usually represents a clot or an elevated flap of intima (Fig. 6–28). When a high umbilical arterial catheter is in place, flat clots adherent to the tubing may not be visible. Usually, the renal arteries can be seen quite well on scans, although evidence of blood flow can be proved only with Doppler imaging. With duplex Doppler imaging it is impossible to know whether every branch of renal arterial vasculature has been examined. In fact, we are pleased when we can obtain a signal showing arterial and venous blood flow at the hilum of each kidney. Coronal scanning is best because blood flow is almost parallel to the transducer in this plane. Color Doppler imaging has been superb in demonstrating blood flow to and from the kidney (Plate VI). A kidney with an acutely obstructed main renal artery can at first look normal on routine scanning, but then the normal differentiation of medulla and cortex is lost and the kidney gradually shrinks, becoming more echodense with time (Fig. 6–29). We have noted relatively silent arterial occlusion in a few babies. Undoubtedly some children who are diagnosed as having renal agenesis or dysplasia when older actually lost a kidney to ischemia in the neonatal period.

We have emphasized renal arterial obstruction as a cause of hypertension, but ischemia secondary to renal venous obstruction may also cause hypertension in the neonate. The diagnosis of renal venous thrombosis is made when (1) the kidney is large, (2) the medullary-cortical differentiation is disorganized, or (3) a clot or absence of blood flow is documented in the renal vein (Plate VII). Adrenal hemorrhage rupturing into the retroperitoneum around the kidney has also been associated with hypertension in a neonate (Starinsky et al., 1986).

For children and adolescents who are hypertensive, the renal examination consists of (1) identifying each kidney; (2) evaluating the size, the collecting system, and the parenchymal pattern; (3) carefully searching for scars to diagnose reflux nephropathy; (4) scanning the bladder, specifically in those with reflux nephropathy; (5) scanning renal arteries and the aorta; and (6) viewing each adrenal area.

Of 18 hypertensive children who were reported by Diament and coauthors (1986), 5 had renal parenchymal disease of various types, 6 had neoplasms of the endocrine system, and 6 had renovascular disease. We emphasize that this study represents findings from a selected population. In an unselected hypertensive population, most have normal scans. "Positive" diagnostic imaging is more likely to be present in the young, symptomatic patient with moderate to severe elevation of blood pressure and retinopathy or left ventricular hypertrophy (Fig. 6–30). The diagnosis of pheochromocytoma is usually suspected on the basis of clinical and laboratory data (Fig. 6–31). Because these children tend to be older (aged 8 to 13 years in Farrelly et al.'s 1984 study), computed tomography (CT) scanning is preferable to ultrasonography in their evaluation. In addition, 30 percent of pheochromocytomas may be extra-adrenal or multiple, or both, a problem that is much better tackled with CT than with ultrasonography. A family history of

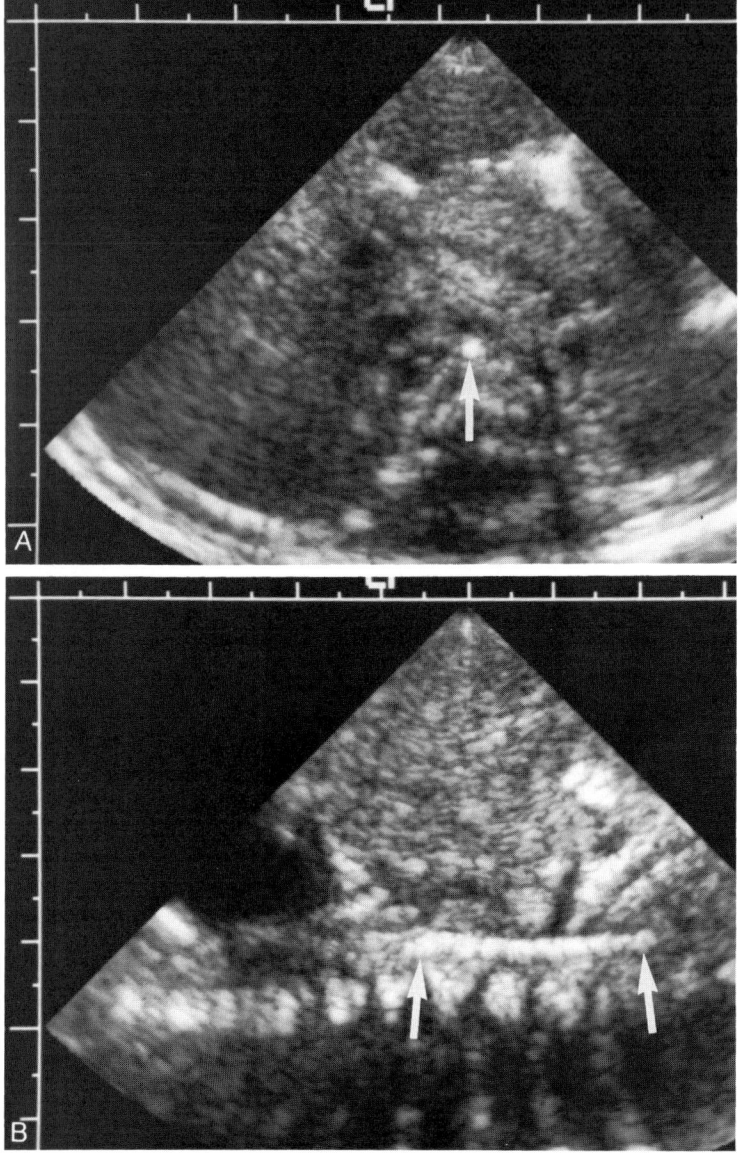

Figure 6–28. Transverse (A) and longitudinal (B) scans of the upper abdomen in a baby who was born at 26 weeks of gestational age and weighed 870 g show echogenic focus from clot within the aorta (arrows). An umbilical artery catheter had been placed for monitoring but was removed before these scans. The baby had both hypertension and hematuria.

endocrinopathy or neurofibromatosis is associated with pheochromocytoma.

Our ability to recognize renovascular hypertension with ultrasonography alone has not been good, but the diagnosis in these cases is supported by abnormal scintigraphy or evidence of elevated levels of plasma renin that encourage further evaluation with angiography. Doppler imaging of renal arteries, in an attempt to identify children with primary renovascular disease, has not been reported in any large study to date. Renovascular disease in 40 patients, reported by Stanley and Fry in 1981, was associated with an abnormal previous intravenous urogram in only 27 percent. Ultrasonography was not mentioned. Of importance is that 25 percent of patients had neurofibromatosis, and most of these patients had extrarenal vascular disease. Any child with neurofibromatosis who comes to ultrasonography for any reason should undergo complete renal, adrenal, and aortic scanning.

If we find renal parenchymal disease on ultrasonography, it is usually reflux nephropathy. Participants at the 1983 Symposium on Reflux Nephropathy estimated that 10 percent of patients with reflux nephropathy

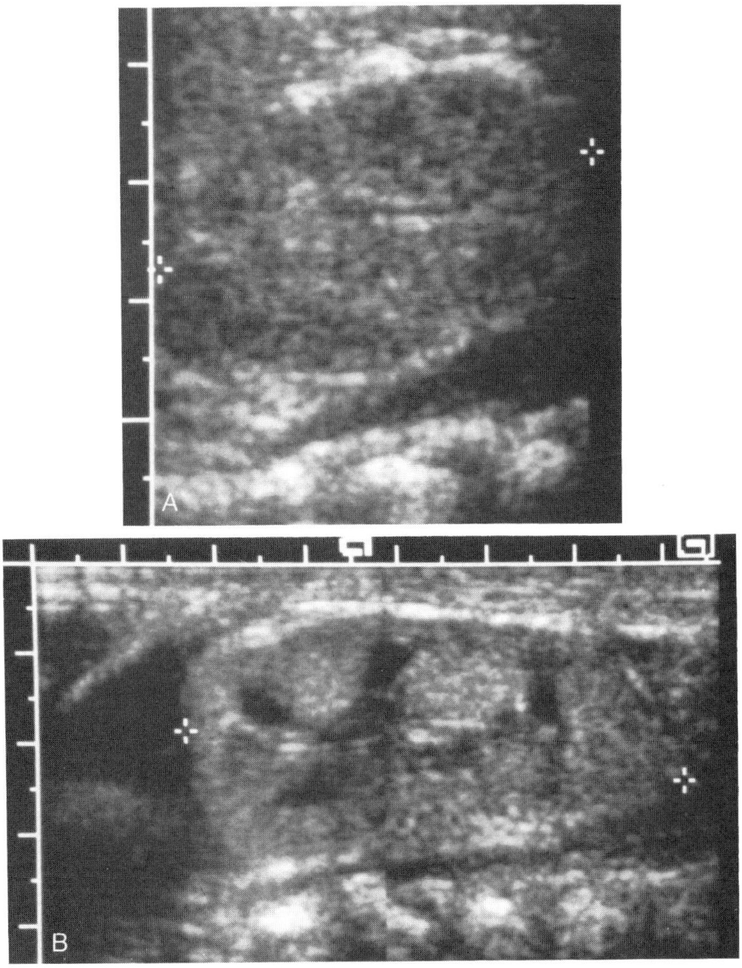

Figure 6–29. Complete obstruction of the right renal artery by aortic clot resulted in a right kidney (**A**) that was smaller than the normally perfused left kidney (**B**). Medullary-cortical differentiation is poor on the right; examination with color Doppler ultrasonography revealed no blood flow to that kidney.

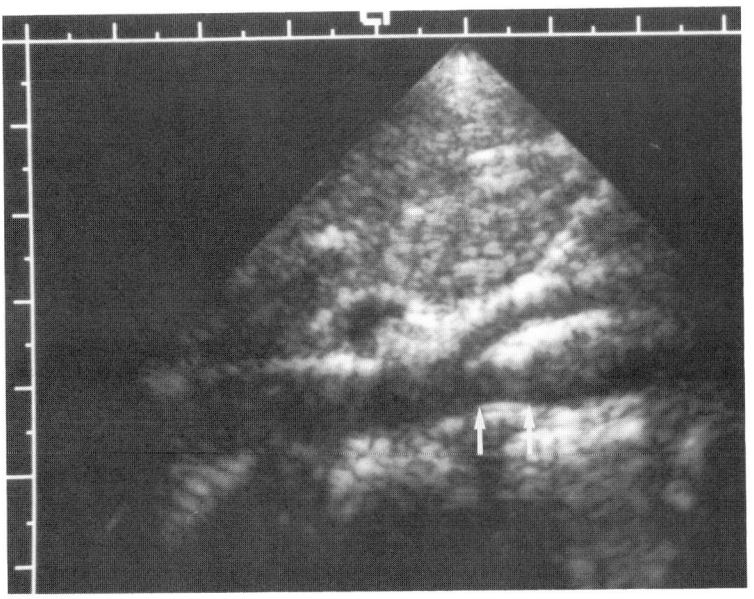

Figure 6–30. Screening ultrasonography was performed on this 6-year-old, who had a blood pressure of 140/80 and an abdominal bruit, both noted during a routine physical examination. The longitudinal scan of the aorta revealed a discrete area of narrowing (arrows) just distal to the superior mesenteric artery. Angiography confirmed this localized narrowing, which extended into the orifice of the right renal artery. The patient is being managed medically at present. He has no stigmata of neurofibromatosis.

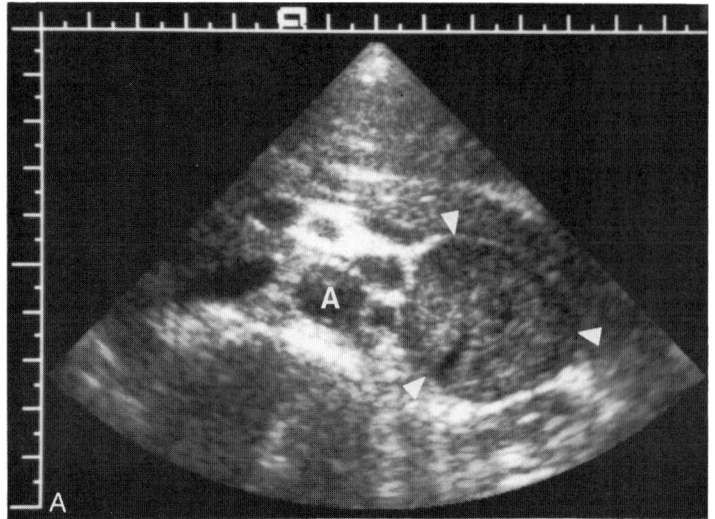

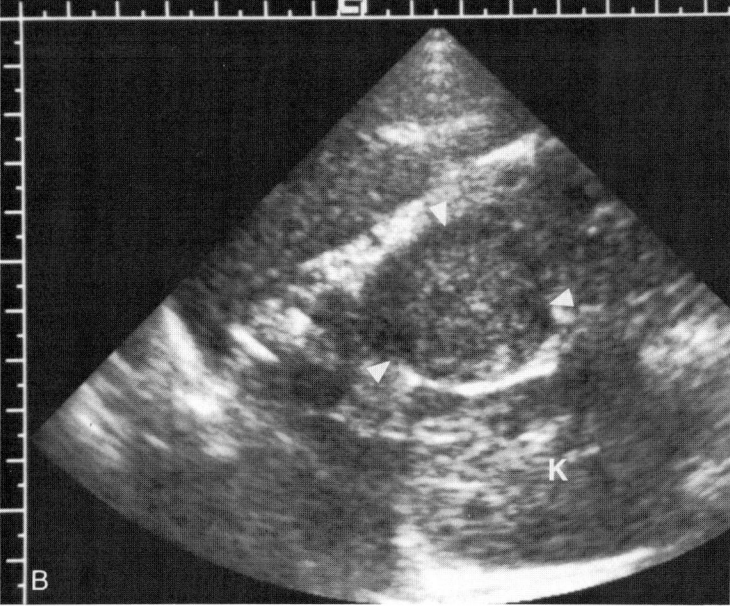

Figure 6–31. The results of laboratory studies were not available when this 11-year-old boy was referred for ultrasonograms after his blood pressure was found to be 150/100. A well-defined mass (arrowheads) was evident anterior to the left kidney (K) on transverse (A) and longitudinal scans (B). This was a pheochromocytoma of the left adrenal medulla. Note how medial and anterior the location of the left adrenal is in relation to the kidney. Levels in serum of norepinephrine, epinephrine, and vanillylmandelic acid were all elevated. A = aorta.

would be hypertensive (Hodson et al., 1984). This opinion, however, is likely an overestimate, as it was derived from results of intravenous urography in selected groups of patients. On ultrasonography, scars are generally polar but can be quite subtle. Loss of medullary-cortical differentiation, thinning of parenchyma, and ectasia of adjacent calix are all signs of reflux nephropathy. Scintigraphy with ^{99m}Tc DMSA or some other cortical labeling agent appears to be the most sensitive technique with which to diagnose scars and can be used as part of the scintigraphic evaluation to confirm their presence in suspicious cases (see Chapter 7).

Other types of renal parenchymal disease are usually accompanied by abnormal results of urinalysis and abnormalities in renal function that are evident in the initial screening of a hypertensive patient. Changes in renal echogenicity and size are characteristic of renal parenchymal disease (see Chapter 19.) Wilms tumor rarely presents with hypertension as its only sign. Renal anomalies assumed to be causally related to hypertension are infrequent but can occur. In our experience, a multicystic, dysplastic kidney and obstruction at the ureteropelvic junction have been associated with hypertension. One little girl, whom we followed before and after renal transplantation, had had unrecognized hypertension from severe unilateral obstruction. Nephrosclerosis destroyed her other kidney before the hypertension was diagnosed.

Hematuria

Hematuria is usually classified as gross when urine is visibly red and as microscopic when it is discovered only on urinalysis (>5 red blood cells per high-power field). Surveys of prevalence have shown microscopic hematuria to be present in 0.05 to 2 percent of the pediatric population. Gross hematuria usually results in the child's or family's seeking medical attention. In one large survey, 1.3 per 1000 visits to an outpatient emergency room were for gross hematuria (Ingelfinger et al., 1977). Physicians who perform imaging are likely to see a selected group of children who present with hematuria. Many patients receive a diagnosis (e.g., acute infection) after physical examination or basic laboratory examinations and are not investigated further. A list of conditions causing hematuria is included in Table 6–5. "Idiopathic" hematuria accounts for an estimated 40 percent of the total population with hematuria (Stapleton et al., 1984). The type and degree of diagnostic evaluation depends greatly on the referring physician. The surgeon is interested in the plumbing; the physician tends to think along metabolic or immunologic lines. Both are concerned with ruling out renal neoplasm as a cause for hematuria. Our evaluation for those with asymptomatic hematuria consists of ultrasonography of the kidneys, bladder, and renal vasculature. A stone in the bladder or diverticulum or evidence of cystitis has occasionally been identified as a cause of hematuria (Fig. 6–32). On rare occasion, a tumor or a polyp has been identified in the bladder or the urethra. Obstruction at any level can be associated with hematuria, and hydronephrosis does not always present with a mass, pain, or infection (Fig. 6–33). Because of the prevalence of glomerulonephritis in the pediatric population, we are very interested in the appearance of renal parenchyma (see Chapter 19). The patient who has polycystic disease of the kidneys may present with hematuria. Although we always look for vascular abnormalities, it is rare for a vascular malformation to cause hematuria in a child (Fig. 6–34).

Table 6–5. CAUSES OF HEMATURIA

Acute Glomerulonephritis
Immunologic Injury
   Subacute and chronic glomerulonephritis
   Henoch-Schönlein purpura
   Collagen vascular disease
   Subacute bacterial endocarditis
   Goodpasture syndrome
   Hemolytic uremic syndrome
Infection of Urinary Tract
Familial and Congenital
   Alport syndrome
   Benign familial
   Polycystic disease
   Congenital anomalies
Bleeding and Vascular Disorders
   Coagulation and platelet deficiencies
   Hemoglobinopathies
   Hemangiomas
   Renal venous thrombosis
   Varices
   Neoplasm
   Trauma
   Direct (including child abuse)
   Shock/anoxia
   Renal stones, foreign body, excoriation of skin
   Meatal stenosis with ulcer
   Drug or chemically induced
Miscellaneous
   Exercise
   Munchausen or Munchausen syndrome by proxy
   Recurrent, benign

Adapted from Northway JD: Hematuria in children. J Pediatr 1971; 78:381–396.

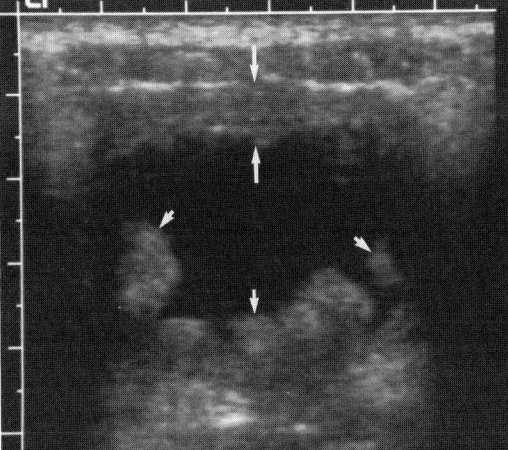

Figure 6–32. Ultrasonography confirmed the clinical impression that cystitis caused by cyclophosphamide (cytoxan) given to treat Burkitt lymphoma was the cause of this patient's hematuria. The transverse ultrasonogram shows marked mucosal thickening (arrows) that was secondary to cystitis.

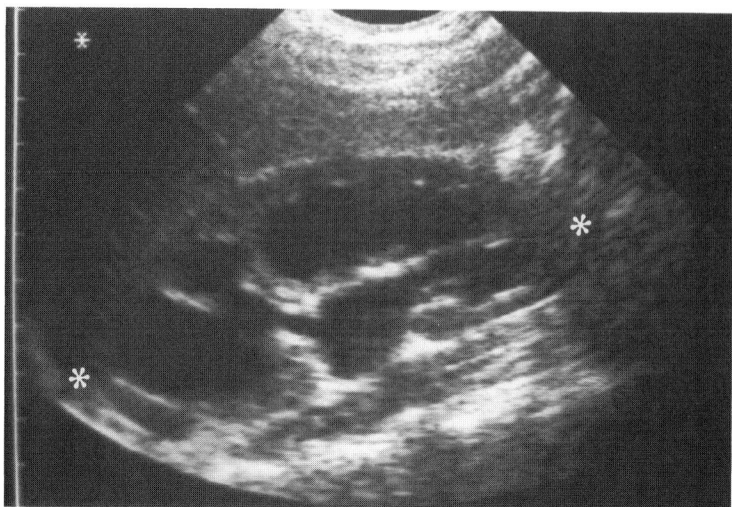

Figure 6–33. Recurrent gross hematuria was the only sign of hydronephrosis secondary to obstruction at the ureteropelvic junction in this 7-year-old boy. Scan is a coronal view of the right kidney.

Urolithiasis

Documentation of hypercalciuria in 25 percent of a large group of children with unexplained gross hematuria (Stapleton et al., 1984) suggests that a state of "prelithiasis" in childhood may be more common than realized to date. The hypothesis is that deposition of calcium occurs in medullary pyramids if the load of calcium in the interstitium exceeds renal lymphatic capacity. As calcium aggregates at the tips and margins of the pyramids, it appears to fuse into plaques and migrates toward uroepithelium (Patriquin and Robitaille, 1986). Epithelial erosion by small calculi is blamed for hematuria.

Microscopic hematuria is virtually always present in patients with bona fide urolithiasis. Fever and mass are other, less common presentations (Sinno et al., 1979). In general, one can divide children with urinary stones into four major groups: those with anatomic abnormalities or infection, or both, of the urinary tract; those with metabolic disorders; those on medications that change normal renal homeostasis; and those who have idiopathic lithiasis. Depending on the population served by a hospital or clinic, the absolute numbers of patients in these groups will vary. Appropriate, early intervention to treat malformations of the urinary tract should decrease the proportion of patients who have

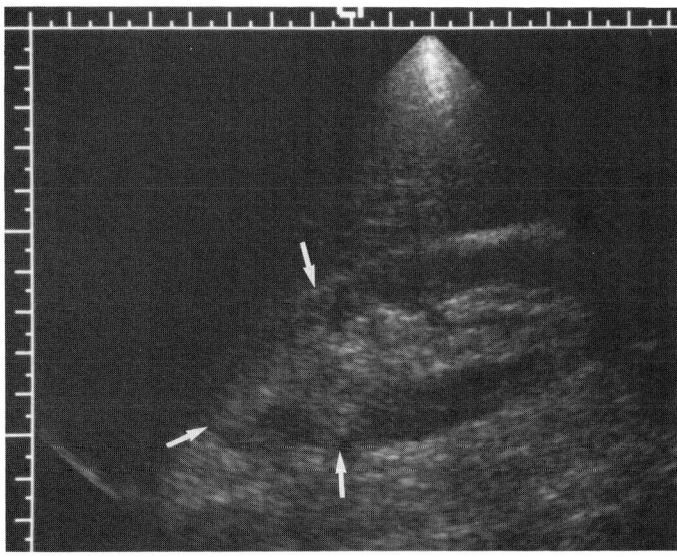

Figure 6–34. Longitudinal scan of the right kidney is of a teenage boy who had multiple episodes of gross hematuria. The ill-defined echogenicity in the upper pole (arrows) did not change over several examinations. Preoperative diagnosis was that of possible angiomyolipoma, but an arteriovenous malformation was diagnosed and removed at surgery.

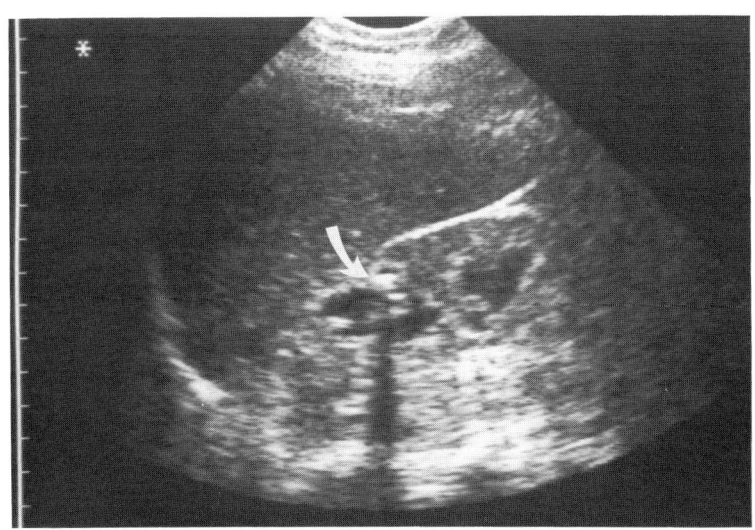

Figure 6-35. This boy had had a complex urologic history consisting of transurethral resection of posterior urethral valve, urethroplasty to treat subsequent stricture, and bilateral ureteral reimplantation. He developed nephrogenic diabetes insipidus with distal renal tubular acidosis. This longitudinal scan of the right kidney shows a well-defined shadowing focus (arrow) as well as parenchymal scarring and calicectasis.

lithiasis secondary to stasis of urine (Figs. 6-35, 6-36, 6-37). Infection of urine with *Proteus mirabilis* is commonly associated with urinary stones and, in our experience, is a problem particularly for patients with myelodysplasia who have poorly functioning urinary tracts. Involuntary immobilization, which is a common fate of patients with neurologic dysfunction, is known to encourage the development of renal lithiasis, and infection only complicates matters.

High doses of furosemide given to premature neonates during treatment of cardiac failure and bronchopulmonary dysplasia cause hypercalciuria and deposition of calcium in the medullary pyramids (Fig. 6-38; Myracle et al., 1986; Jacinto et al., 1988).

Forty to 60 percent of children with apparent idiopathic renal stones have a family history of this disorder (Sinno et al., 1979; Churchill et al., 1980). As noted earlier, sophisticated studies of calcium balance indicate that these children likely have a defect in absorption or excretion of calcium and that their disease can be classified as metabolic (Stapleton et al., 1984). Other unusual met-

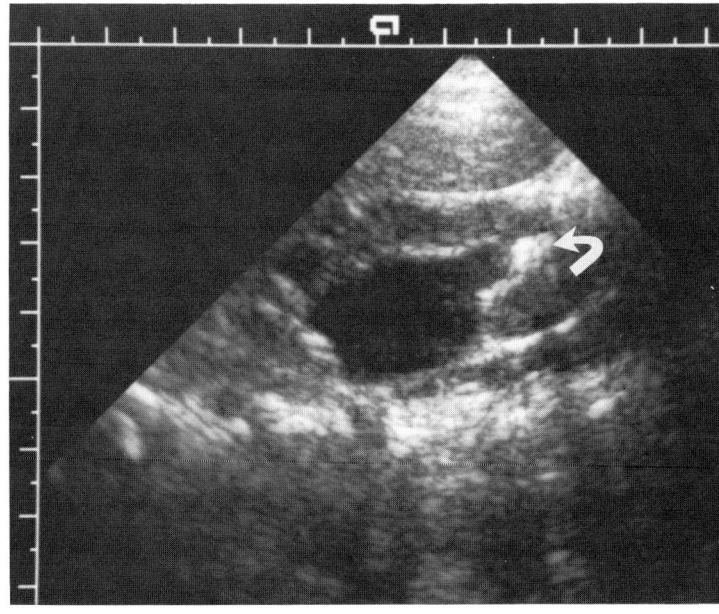

Figure 6-36. This baby reached 22 months of age before the diagnosis of a right-sided obstruction at the ureteropelvic junction was made. He had had two well-documented urinary tract infections with *Escherichia coli*. A stone was present in the collecting system of the lower pole (arrow). He underwent right pyelolithotomy and pyeloplasty.

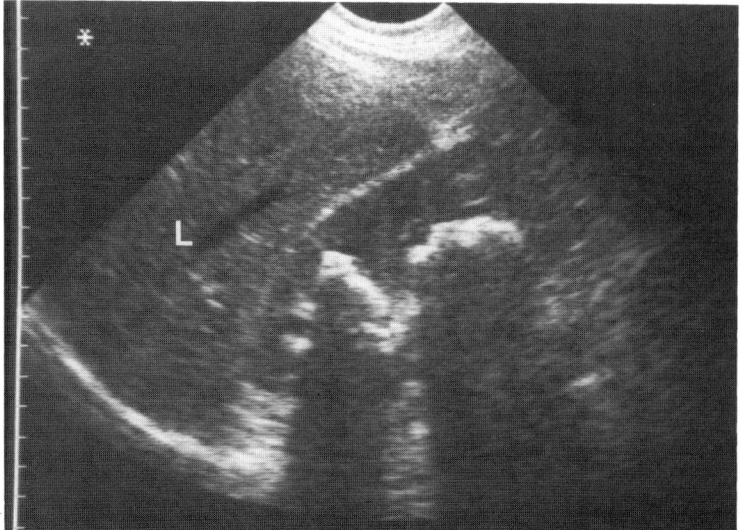

Figure 6–37. Hypoperistalsis associated with prune belly syndrome probably contributed to this patient's nephrolithiasis. This longitudinal scan of the right kidney through the liver (L) shows dense echogenic foci representing multiple stones in an ectatic collecting system.

abolic diseases or situations that cause urolithiasis are listed in Table 6–6 (Figs. 6–39, 6–40).

Urinary stones may be appreciated on plain radiographs, but their variable content of calcium, their typically small size, and an observer's low level of suspicion of stones in

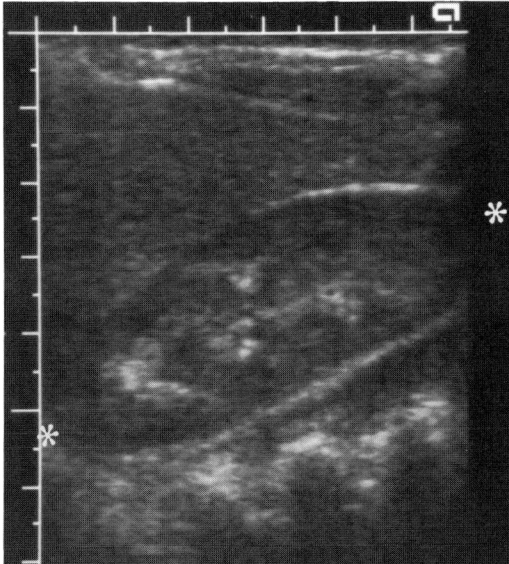

Figure 6–38. This 5-month-old baby was a graduate of the Neonatal Intensive Care Unit, where he had been since his early delivery at 28 weeks of gestational age. He had been receiving chronic therapy with furosemide. Scan of the right kidney shows echogenic foci within medullary pyramids secondary to deposition of calcium. The left kidney had a similar appearance.

Table 6–6. UROLITHIASIS IN CHILDREN

Renal Tubular Diseases
 *Renal tubular acidosis (distal tubule)
 Carbonic anhydrase inhibitors (acetazolamide)
 *Cystinuria
 Glycinuria (oxalate urolithiasis, rare)
Enzyme Disorders
 *Primary hyperoxaluria
 Xanthinuria
Hypercalciuric States
 Furosemide
 Primary hyperparathyroidism
 Sarcoidosis
 Hypervitaminosis D
 Milk-alkali syndrome (milk, antacids)
 Neoplasm
 Exogenous or endogenous steroids
 Hyperthyroidism
 Infantile hypercalcemia (Williams syndrome)
 Immobilization
Uric Acid Lithiasis
 Increased purine metabolism (tumor breakdown)
 Idiopathic uric acid lithiasis
 Lesch-Nyhan syndrome
Associated Intestinal Disease
 Acquired hyperoxaluria (inflammatory bowel disease)
Renal Malformations
 Horseshoe kidney
 Obstruction at ureteropelvic junction, ureterovesical junction
*Infected Urolithiasis and Urinary Stasis (e.g., Myelodysplasia)
*Idiopathic Urolithiasis
*Endemic Calculi in Developing Countries

Adapted from Kelalis PP, King LR, Belman AB: Clinical Pediatric Urology, 2nd ed. Philadelphia: WB Saunders, 1985.
*Most common.

RENAL SCREENING / 167

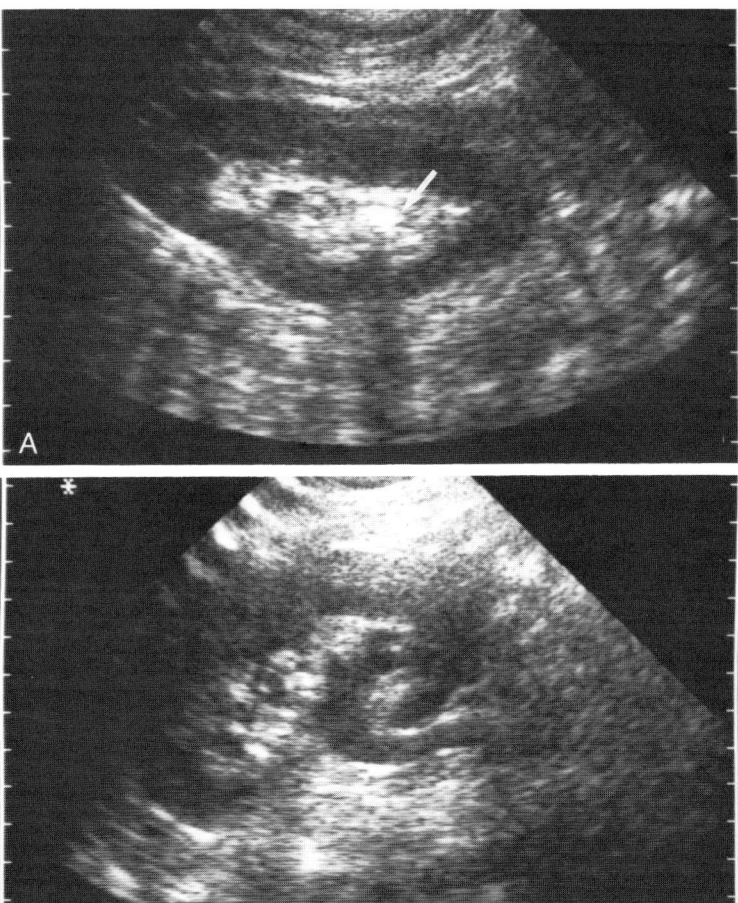

Figure 6–39. Recurrent oxalate stones (arrow, **A**) are a problem for this patient, who has cystic fibrosis and malabsorption. Intermittently, she has renal colic and dilation of the collecting system (**B**) when a stone obstructs the ureter.

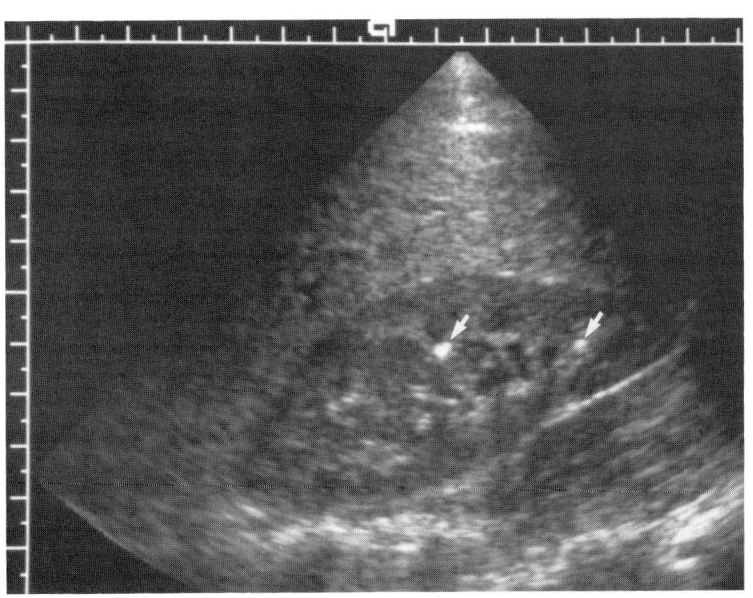

Figure 6–40. Urate stones cause small shadowing foci (arrows) in this boy, who has Lesch-Nyhan syndrome.

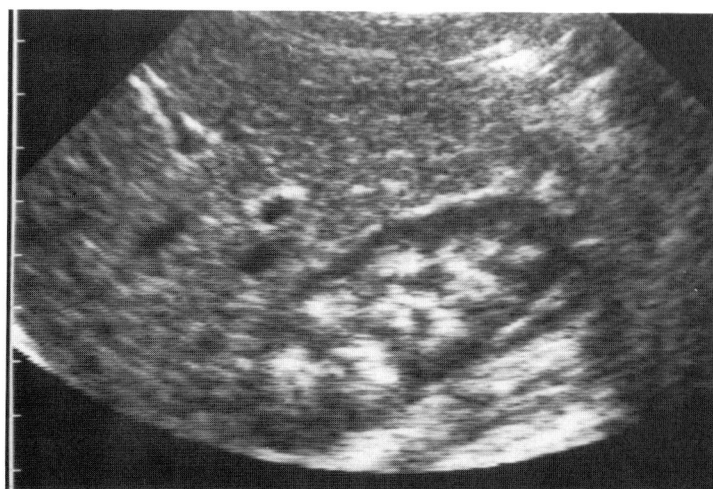

Figure 6–41. Longitudinal scan of the right kidney shows medullary calcinosis in this child, who has X-linked hypophosphatemic rickets. She has been treated with high doses of vitamin D and supplemental calcium, as well as phosphorus.

a child makes diagnosis from plain films unusual. Intravenous urography is the study most frequently, and appropriately, requested when lithiasis is suspected by the clinicians. The stone or stones may be apparent on closer inspection or tomography, differences in renal function and the obstruction caused by a stone are obvious on the urogram, and the diuresis caused by intravenous injection of contrast may be therapeutic. Acute, total obstruction by a ureteral stone may result in very little dilation of the renal collecting system. Therefore, a normal ultrasonogram may be falsely reassuring.

Children undergoing screening ultrasonography for hematuria should be studied with a view toward identifying medullary calcinosis if it is present. Calcification tends to outline the pyramidal shape or to conglomerate at the tips of the pyramids (Fig. 6–41; Patriquin and Robitaille, 1986). Only when there is a dense focus will the calcification shadow. Shadowing from stones does not imply that calcium is present, but most stones do contain calcium. Most stones, of all types, that are in the collecting system are difficult to identify if small and unassociated with hydronephrosis. They get lost among the echogenicity of fat and vessels in renal sinus. Conversely, intrarenal vessels in babies and small children should not be mistaken for stones. The walls of the arteries can be very reflective and may even cast a shadow. The vessel, however, usually has the appearance of a double track and if the baby is cooperative, Doppler imaging can show it to have arterial blood flow. Bubbles of gas in the collecting system of the kidney can produce reflective interfaces and simulate stones. Vesicoureteral reflux of air that has been introduced by catheter, reflux of gas into ureters from an ileal loop, or incompetent ureterosigmoid anastomosis following ureterosigmoidostomy are all causes of intrarenal gas (Fig. 6–42).

It is always a surprise, when performing ultrasonography, to be the first to find urolithiasis as a cause for a child's hematuria or pain (Fig. 6–43). Such patients have usually had undiagnosed metabolic disease or have been given large doses of calcium or vitamin D without the referring physician's knowl-

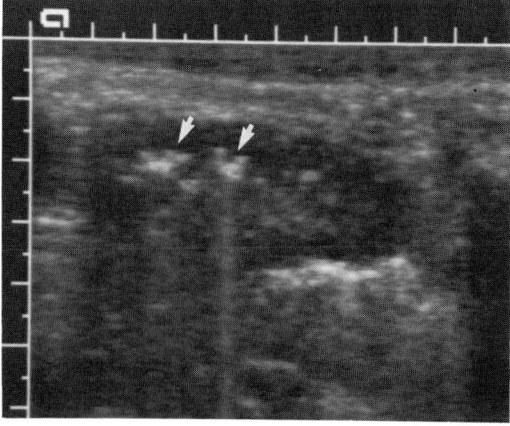

Figure 6–42. Echogenic foci (arrows) in the upper pole of the left kidney were caused by vesicoureteral reflux of air mixed with urine and contrast material after catheterization for voiding cystourethrography. Air in the collecting system blocks transmission of sound. It may be present in patients who have refluxing ileal loop or ureterosigmoidostomy.

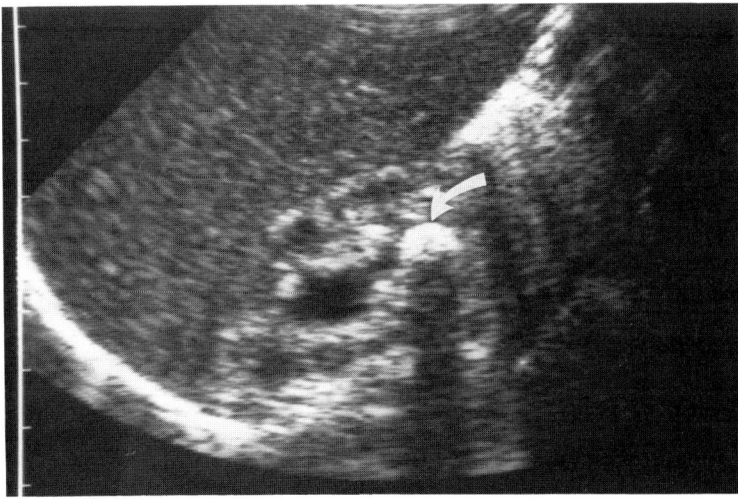

Figure 6–43. At 4 years of age, this patient was scanned because of asymptomatic hematuria. The patient had William syndrome, which is associated with hypercalcemia. The longitudinal scan of the right kidney shows a well-defined stone (arrow) within the collecting system. It casts a distinct shadow. This stone was removed percutaneously.

edge. When stones are found in the upper tract, it is important to search for ureteral and vesical stones, and in order to do this, the bladder must be distended with urine.

Myelodysplasia or Other Cause for Neurogenic Injury

The baby born with a neurogenic bladder should have a baseline ultrasonographic study of the urinary tract, another study at 6 months of age, and a periodic yearly study until at least 6 years of age. Scans performed every 2 to 3 years through puberty are sufficient unless an abnormality develops. Baseline urodynamic evaluation, shortly after birth, characterizes function of the bladder.

In a study from our hospital (Bauer et al., 1984), 18 of 36 babies with meningomyelocele had incoordination of the detrusor with the external urethral sphincter (dyssynergia). Of these 18 patients, 13 (72 percent) developed early onset of hydroureteronephrosis, reflux, or vesiculomegaly, requiring cutaneous vesicotomy or a program of intermittent catheterization. Dyssynergia impairs emptying of the bladder and causes elevation of intravesical pressure during voiding. Decompensation of the upper tracts results because of physiologic obstruction or reflux. Babies with complete denervation of the external urethral sphincter are unlikely to have any problem with upper tracts unless a urinary tract infection (UTI) intervenes.

If a baby has a large amount of residual urine after voiding, if sphincteric dyssynergia is identified with urodynamic testing, or if a UTI is found, a voiding cystourethrogram (VCUG) is performed, predominantly to rule in or out vesicoureteral reflux. A normal ultrasonographic study cannot rule out the presence of significant reflux. Presence of reflux is a contraindication to Credé voiding. Reflux associated with outlet obstruction and with UTI is more likely to lead to reflux nephropathy (Hodson et al., 1984).

In the population of older children with myelodysplasia, renal scanning is hampered by anatomic deformities (scoliosis and kyphosis) that have developed, by gaseous distention of the bowel resulting from previous neurosurgery or orthopedic surgery on the back, and by abnormal connective tissues, especially fat, that attenuate the ultrasonic beam. To put it frankly, the periodic renal scans of older children and adolescents who have had high meningomyelocele usually look dreadful (Fig. 6–44). We cannot reliably measure renal size and rule out scars, but we can document the presence of hydronephrosis. Onset of dilation usually indicates occult physiologic or anatomic obstruction or reflux. Further radiologic evaluation must follow.

In all patients with a neurogenic bladder who come for screening ultrasonography, we inquire as to how the bladder is emptied and perform a study only if emptying has occurred in the past hour. A full bladder causes relative obstruction to ureteral flow even in normal persons and can produce a picture of

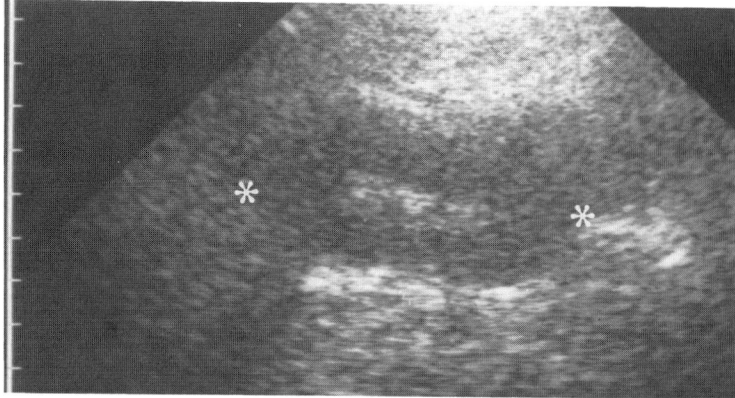

Figure 6–44. Not all renal scans of patients who have myelodysplasia are this poor, but many are. The abnormal soft tissues of the back prevent good transmission of sound, and anatomic deformity from scoliosis or kyphosis prevents good "access" to the kidneys.

hydronephrosis (Fig. 6–45). After spontaneous voiding, catheterization as part of an established regimen, or the Credé maneuver, we scan the bladder to evaluate the amount of residual urine. There are formulas for measuring this quantitatively (Bis and Slovis, 1990), but the categories "no residual," "small," "moderate" and "large" are easily assigned. As part of a training program in the use of the Credé maneuver or catheterization, the ultrasonic scans are ideal for showing parents, children, or nurses how well or how poorly the bladder is emptied by the procedure. Renal scans are directed at identifying hydronephrosis, parenchymal scars, and stones (Fig. 6–46). Renal stones, unless associated with hydronephrosis, can be missed on ultrasonography. Unexplained hematuria, pain, and repeated infection (especially with organisms other than *Escherichia*

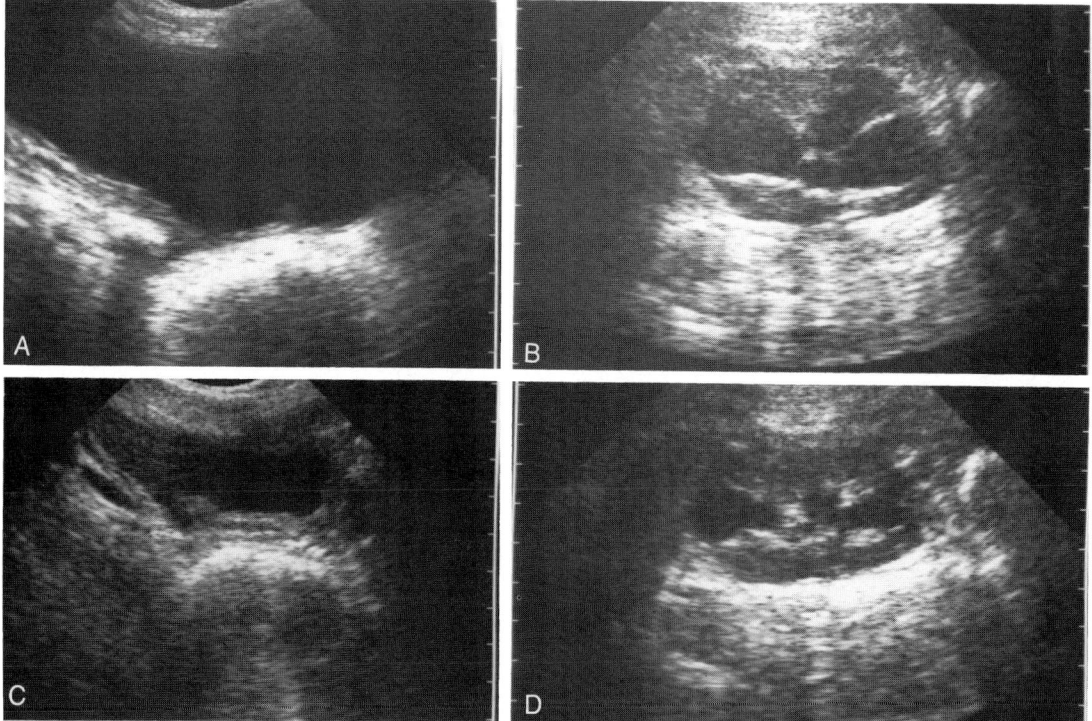

Figure 6–45. A full urinary bladder (A) in this patient, who has a meningomyelocele, is associated with dilation of a right renal collecting system in a scarred kidney (B). After catheterization of the bladder, residual urine is small in amount (C). Decompression of the intrarenal collecting system (D) occurs when the bladder is emptied.

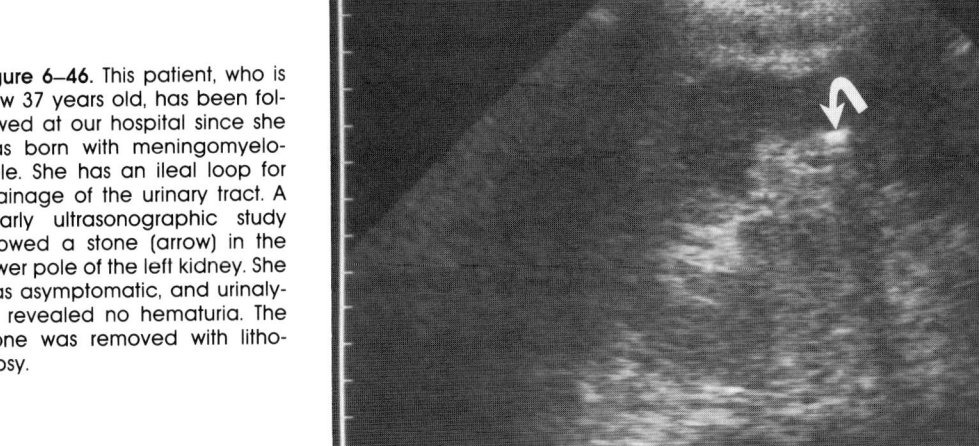

Figure 6–46. This patient, who is now 37 years old, has been followed at our hospital since she was born with meningomyelocele. She has an ileal loop for drainage of the urinary tract. A yearly ultrasonographic study showed a stone (arrow) in the lower pole of the left kidney. She was asymptomatic, and urinalysis revealed no hematuria. The stone was removed with lithotripsy.

coli) mandate more extensive evaluation. Thin-section CT for these patients, who typically have a great deal of perinephric and retroperitoneal fat, is ideal for identifying renal stones. Intravenous urography, preceded by plain radiographs, and linear tomography are not as reliable as CT in the diagnosis of stones.

It is worthwhile to quickly scan the gallbladder in older patients who have myelodysplasia. Their histories usually include extensive orthopedic surgery; ileal loops may have been constructed for urinary diversion, and their mobility is generally limited. This combination is conducive to the development of gallstones (see Chapter 17). Causes of neurogenic bladder other than myelodysplasia include caudal regression syndrome, tethered spinal cord, previous spinal injury, tumor within the spinal canal, and previous irradiation of the cord. There is also a small number of children who have "nonneurogenic neurogenic" bladder. For all intents and purposes, they have typical urodynamic features of a neurogenic bladder but have no identifiable primary reason for their neurologic deficit.

Occasionally, the diagnosis of neurogenic bladder is first made during ultrasonography (Fig. 6–47). A child may present with a pelvic mass that is in fact a bladder distended because of sphincteric dysfunction, or the wall of the bladder may be obviously thickened or trabeculated because of chronic obstruction. Further investigation of these children requires voiding cystourethrography to rule out anatomic obstruction and urodynamic testing to define the physiologic problem.

EVALUATION OF THE POSTOPERATIVE PATIENT

Reimplantation of the ureter, because there is either an obstruction at the ureterovesical junction or gross vesicoureteral reflux, is a common pediatric urologic procedure in our hospital. Reimplantation, with the creation

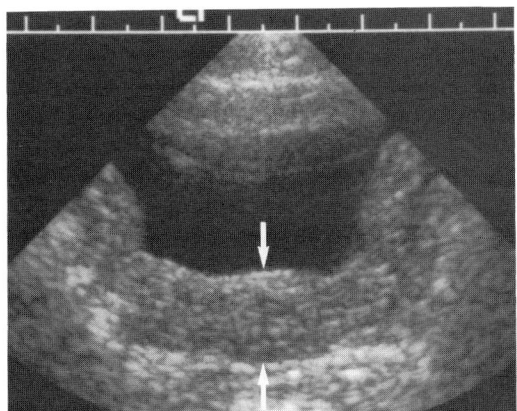

Figure 6–47. This child had presented with urinary tract infection, and on scans of the pelvis, it was apparent that the wall of the bladder was markedly thickened (between arrows). Urodynamic study showed that she had uninhibited contractions of the bladder. Her neurologic examination was otherwise completely normal.

of a long submucosal tunnel to prevent reflux, is usually done in an extraperitoneal approach. The new ureteral tunnel may be ipsilateral (Leadbetter-Politano technique) or supratrigonal and crossing to the other side (Cohen technique). Within 1 month of surgery the child has an intravenous urogram, which consists of a single radiograph that is obtained 15 minutes after injection of contrast. The dilation of the collecting system on this postoperative study should not exceed that shown by reflux on the preoperative VCUG; otherwise we infer significant obstruction at the ureterovesical junction. If the postoperative course is uncomplicated, further follow-up is performed with ultrasonography. Immediate postoperative ultrasonography cannot replace urography because it cannot show function. We have encountered the situation in which complete obstruction to urinary flow at the site of reimplantation was unassociated with an appreciable increase in dilation, and the severity of the problem was recognized only with urography. One could argue that radionuclide scanning with diethylenetriaminepenta-acetic acid (DTPA) could be used instead of the radiographic urogram, but a single urographic film provides all the necessary information with little irradiation and can be compared with the preoperative cystogram. Timing of ultrasonographic follow-up is at the discretion of the urologist. We generally scan the kidneys, looking for hydronephrosis, scars, or growth 18 months, 3 years, and 5 years after surgery. These children typically have a history of UTI; many are subjects of the International Study on Reflux and, therefore, are followed very closely. We scan the bladder at each follow-up study. The creation of a submucosal tunnel may produce a tubular ridge of the mucosal surface of the bladder and should be recognized as the normal postoperative appearance (Fig. 6–48; Mezzacappa et al., 1987). Complications associated with reimplantation include granuloma or abscess around a stitch, ureteral stone, inflammatory epithelial polyp, and ischemic stricture, but these are all quite rare. If hydroureteronephrosis is found in the postoperative study, it is important to trace the dilation to its end (Fig. 6–49). Ischemic damage to a long segment of distal ureter may occur if there has been ureteral tapering before reimplantation. Occasionally, a ureter is brought through the mesentery of sigmoid colon, and obstruction occurs at that level: generally between the lower third and the proximal two thirds of the ureter. The specific details of the surgery should be known to the clinicians performing the postoperative evaluation. To avoid dilation of the upper tracts that is secondary to a full bladder (pseudohydronephrosis), we usually perform postoperative scans after the bladder has been emptied. However, if hydronephrosis is present, the patient has to wait until the bladder is full so that ancillary scans of the pelvis can be performed and the region of ureteral reimplantation viewed.

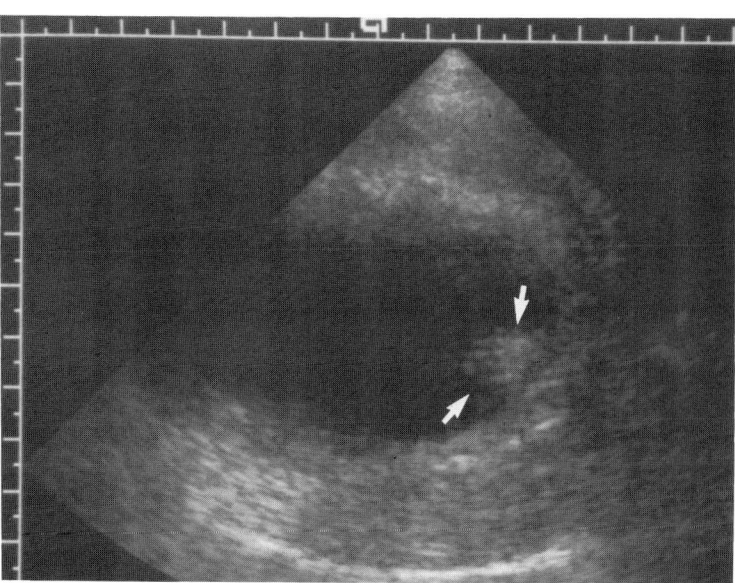

Figure 6–48. This transverse view of the bladder was taken a few days after left-sided ureteroreimplantation. Edema at the site of reimplantation of the left ureter created a soft tissue mass within the bladder (arrows). Six months later, routine follow-up revealed that the contour of the bladder was completely smooth.

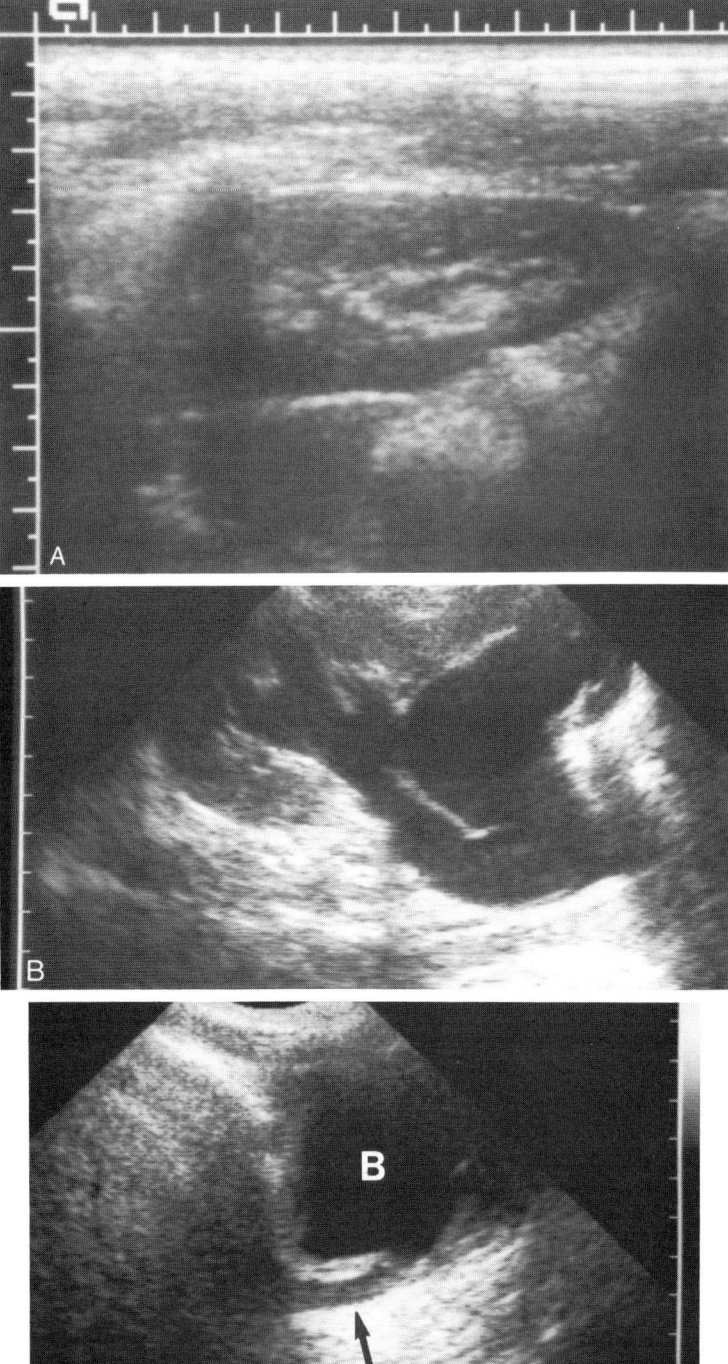

Figure 6–49. Longitudinal scan of the left kidney before surgery for reimplantation of the left distal ureter shows no dilation of the intrarenal collecting system (**A**). One month after surgery, the patient presented with an episode of acute left-sided flank pain. Obstruction of the distal left ureter from scarring at the site of reimplantation caused significant hydronephrosis of the left kidney (**B**). Dilation of the ureter (arrow, **C**) could be traced to the bladder. Nephrostomy was placed to decompress the collecting system, and reimplantation of the ureter followed. B = bladder.

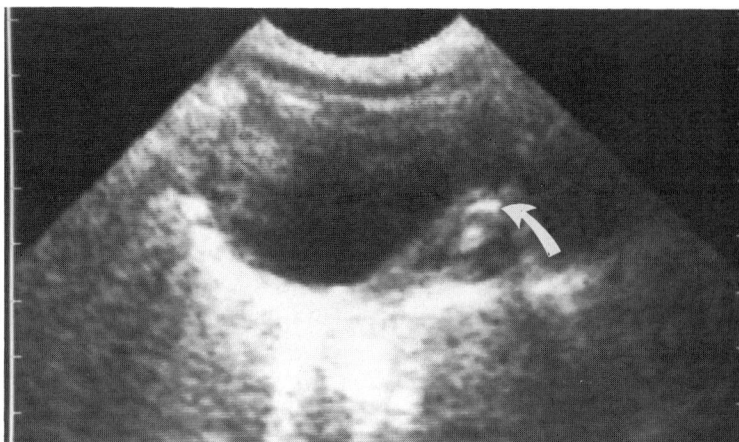

Figure 6–50. Intramural injection of Teflon causes an echogenic focus (arrow) within the wall of the bladder.

A relatively new technique, intramural injection of Teflon, is being used in some hospitals for treatment of vesicoureteral reflux (Mann et al., 1988; Gore et al., 1989; Giuliano et al., 1990; Blake and O'Connell, 1989). Under cystoscopic visualization, 0.2 to 0.4 ml of Teflon paste is injected intramurally, inferior to the ureteral orifice, with the purpose of increasing the length of the intravesical submucosal ureteral tunnel and preventing reflux. The subsequent ultrasonograms show a shadowing, hyperechogenic mass within the wall of the bladder (Fig. 6–50; Mann et al., 1988). The mass, which initially measures approximately 0.5 cm in diameter, may shrink with time as the glycerine carrier is absorbed. Extravesical extravasation of the Teflon, and complications such as obstruction, can be shown with ultrasonography.

The population of pediatric patients who have an ileal conduit is rapidly shrinking. Intermittent catheterization and the use of artificial sphincters have limited the need for ileal conduits. Many of those who have undergone ileal conduit are being "dediverted" with reconstructions of their urinary tract. For those who have ileal conduit, yearly ultrasonographic scans are combined with liberal use of plain or tomographic radiographs or CT to uncover complications of infection, hydronephrosis, and renal stones. If ultrasonography shows new, or an increase in, hydronephrosis from baseline, loopogram follows.

For that small proportion of patients who have undergone ureterosigmoidostomies, hydronephrosis may develop from a stricture at the site of ureteral implantation in the colon, from incompetent ureterocolonic tunneling, from reflux and infection, or from colonic tumor. Adenocarcinoma is a well-recognized complication of ureterosigmoidostomy, and this fact has led to the decline in popularity of the procedure.

In some patients who have had urinary diversion, the bladder is left in place. Pyocystis may develop if there is an obstruction to the outlet of the bladder; in men, if ejaculation is retrograde, spermatocystis may result.

Reconstruction of the urinary tract in those with no or an inadequate bladder has led to appropriation of pieces of the gastrointestinal tract for augmentation of the bladder. There

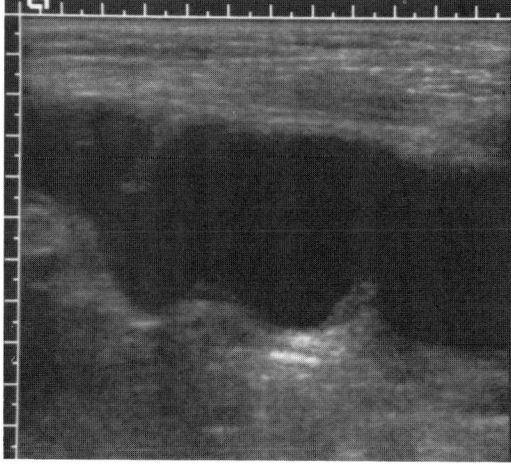

Figure 6–51. Longitudinal view of the bladder is unusually serpentine because of its augmentation with ileum.

is nothing as helpful as good surgical history for performing follow-up scans for these patients. Hertzberg and colleagues (1987) described the types of surgical procedures in detail. Since then, the stomach has been added to the list of organs available for bladder augmentation. The newly constructed bladder can appear most bizarre on ultrasonograms (Fig. 6–51). Its shape depends on the type of augmentation. If the ileum has been intussuscepted into the cecal reservoir or the ileal pouch, then a cylindrical mass will bulge into the urine-filled neobladder. Because stapling is required to maintain the intussusception, echogenic shadowing foci may be present. Unfortunately, the staples appear to encourage formation of stones, and deciding from ultrasonograms which reflector is stone and which might be staple is generally futile (Figs. 6–52, 6–53). Stones are generated partly because of mucus in the urine. The intestinal mucosa sheds both cells and mucus, creating a turbid urine, often with strands and debris that shift with changes in the patient's position. The haustra from the colon or valvulae from the small bowel are typically evident as pseudomasses in the wall of the neobladder. In unusually shaped bladders, comparison with cystography is most helpful in visualizing the anatomy. Augmented bladders are susceptible to spontaneous or catheter-associated perforation (Elder et al., 1988). High pressures within a full bladder that is being poorly emptied have resulted in perforation through the intestinal augmentation. Free fluid within the abdomen may be a clue to

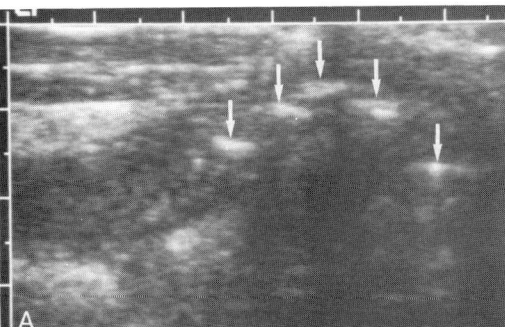
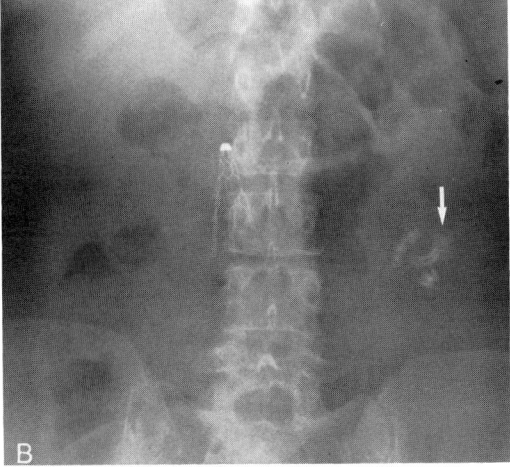

Figure 6–52. A continent ileal pouch was created for the diversion of this young woman's urine. Multiple echogenic foci (arrows) within the pouch were present (A). These were a combination of staples and stones forming on the staples. The plain film (B) shows the metallic staples to the left of the midline. The hazy opacity is a stone (arrow). The patient also has a vena caval umbrella because of previous pulmonary emboli.

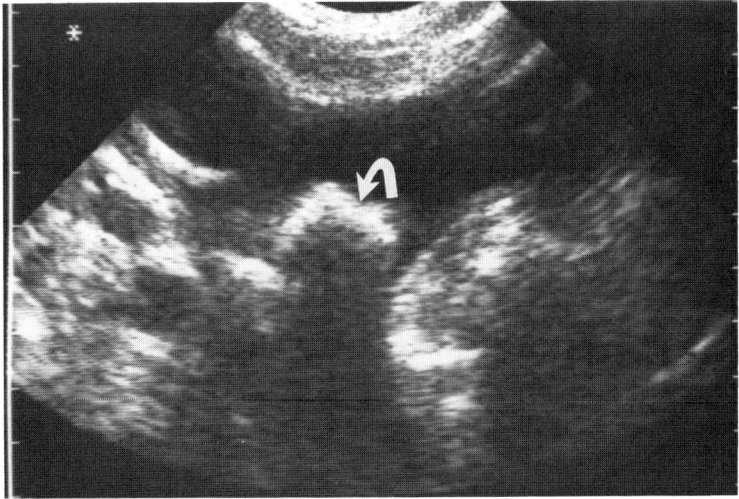

Figure 6–53. An augmented bladder that is partially filled with urine shows a well-defined echogenic focus (arrow), which is shadowing. This focus changed when the patient changed position, which thereby proved that it was a stone within the bladder.

this occurrence on ultrasonography, but many of the same patients have fluid from ventriculoperitoneal shunting of cerebrospinal fluid. Cystography is recommended as an emergent procedure for patients suspected of perforation.

The common type of prosthetic urinary sphincter in current use has a spherical, fluid-filled reservoir, that is subcutaneous. This should not be mistaken for a cystic mass (Fig. 6–54). Functional studies of the sphincter are usually done with fluoroscopy, but ultrasonography can be used for simple assessments of residual urine in the bladder after the sphincter is opened to permit its emptying.

RENAL CYSTIC DISEASE

Before discussing each type of renal cystic disease in depth, we have several comments regarding ultrasonography in this area.

1. The presence of multiple cysts does not necessarily connote "polycystic" disease—that is, disease associated with a specific syndrome. Cysts are associated with renal dysplasia with or without obstruction. Multicystic dysplastic kidney (MDK) specifically is discussed in Chapter 8 (Fig. 6–55).

2. Paradoxically, a kidney that is echogenic may be cystic. Microscopic cystic renal dis-

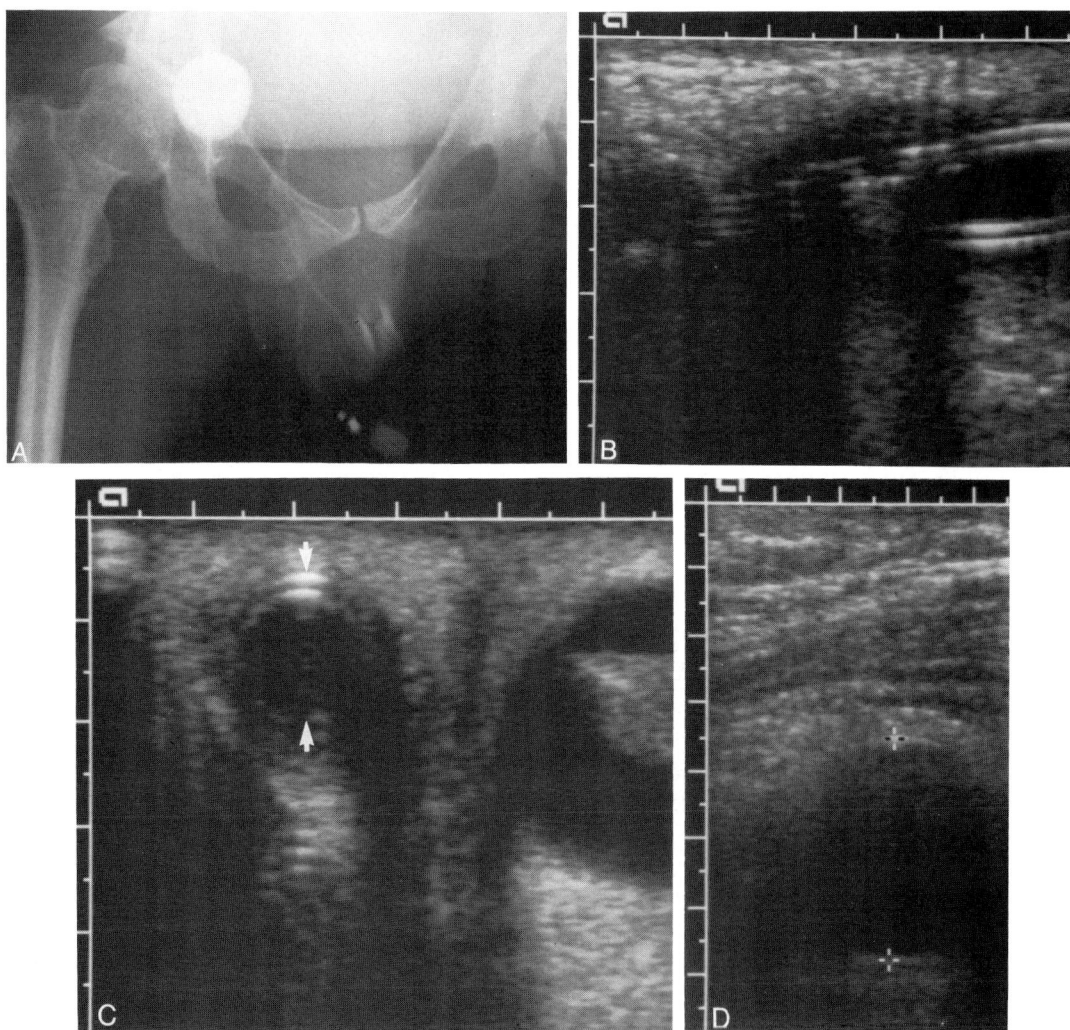

Figure 6–54. An artificial sphincter, filled with contrast material, is shown on plain radiograph of the pelvis (**A**). The catheters, outlined by fluid—possibly cerebrospinal fluid (CSF) from the ventriculoperitoneal shunt—are shown in a longitudinal scan of the right groin (**B**). The pump mechanism that lies in the right scrotal sac is shown in cross-section (arrows) in **C**. The reservoir is shown in cross-section in **D**. This fluid-filled chamber, which may be placed anywhere in the lower abdomen, should not be mistaken for a mass.

ease results in hyperechogenicity of the involved parenchyma because the multiple interfaces provide thousands of reflecting surfaces to the ultrasonic beam.

3. Renal cystic disease has as many classifications as ultrasonography has decibels. Several recent reviews of renal cystic disease are listed in the references. Information from morphologic study of affected kidneys has probably served its usefulness in these schemata. The more precise relationship between different types of cysts awaits identification by geneticists of chromosomal markers for certain diseases.

4. A specific diagnosis of the type of cystic disease may be impossible from ultrasonography alone. A label should not be attached unless the diagnosis is certain. Genetic considerations for the family may change with the label.

Single Cyst

The term "simple renal cyst" is an oxymoron in pediatric practice. It is a diagnosis of exclusion, which is frequently more complicated a process than we would like. Most simple renal cysts appear to be, like wrinkles and gray hair, another sign of aging. In an ultrasonographic survey of asymptomatic patients by Yamagishi and associates (1988), no cysts could be found in anyone younger than 23 years of age. How does one explain pe-

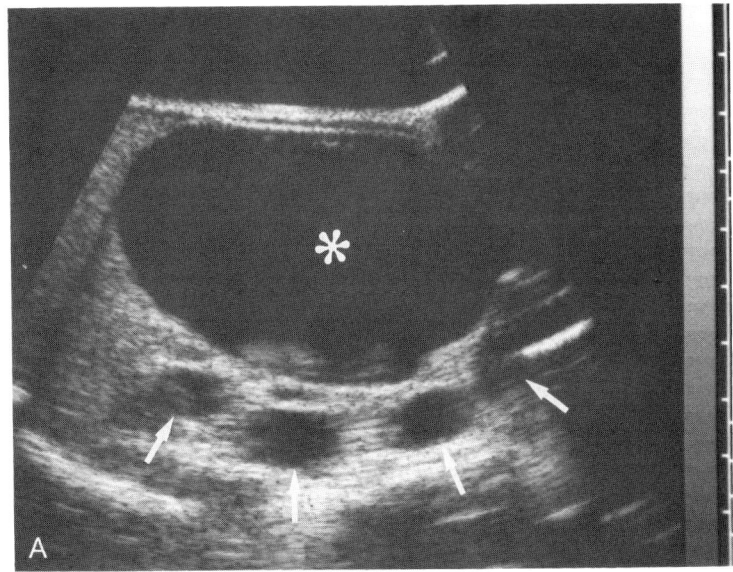
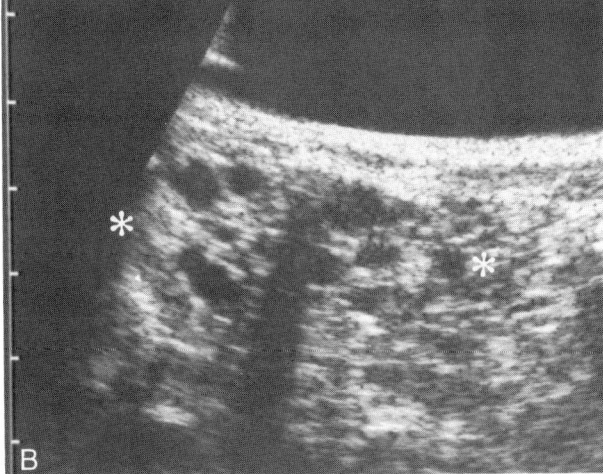

Figure 6–55. Bilateral renal cysts do not necessarily mean polycystic disease. Occasionally, a baby with bilateral multicystic dysplasia can survive. This child was admitted at 3 weeks of age for metabolic acidosis, weight loss, and a mass in the right upper quadrant. The right kidney (A) had been replaced by one large central cyst (asterisk) and several peripheral cysts (arrows). The left kidney (B), although containing several cysts, was distinctly smaller and indistinguishable from surrounding retroperitoneal tissue. Radionuclide scanning revealed virtually no function in the right kidney. There was poor function on the left. Bilateral multicystic dysplasia was diagnosed when both kidneys were removed before renal transplantation when the baby was 10 months old.

diatric studies that report a 5 percent incidence of simple cysts (Mir et al., 1983)? These are studies selected from autopsy material, not from a general pediatric population. Extrapolating their data to the general population, one would expect to find a simple renal cyst in fewer than 0.1 percent of patients examined. The reports of simple renal cyst that have been published in urologic and radiologic literature generally lack pathologic proof or long-term follow-up of a child. Any child with an apparent single cyst should be followed carefully for possible polycystic disease, particularly if the kidneys are large for the patient's size and age and if the parenchyma is more echogenic than usual. A "cyst" may also be a caliceal diverticulum, localized obstructive hydronephrosis (particularly in the upper pole, where the cyst may represent the obstructed unit of a duplex kidney), an ectatic calix, a liquefied hematoma, or, in rare instances, a renal artery aneurysm or venous malformation (Fig. 6–56).

A pyelocaliceal diverticulum presenting as a cyst may be more common than realized to date (Fig. 6–57). The incidence in children has been cited as 3.3 diagnosed per 1000 intravenous urograms (Wulfsohn, 1980), but these instances represent diverticula that communicate with the collecting system during the time of the radiographic study. We have seen children who have shown, on intravenous urography, communication on one occasion and not on another. The ultrasonograms have shown "classic" features of a simple cyst with sharply defined walls, clear fluid, and posterior enhancement. Aspiration of the cyst is frequently associated with reaccumulation of fluid. Pyelocaliceal diverticula are commonly polar in location, although they may be peripelvic and central; they are likely formed from aberrant budding of the ureteral nubbin that invades the metanephros. Infection of a pyelocaliceal diverticulum may occur, as may formation of renal stones or milk of calcium. An increased incidence with vesicoureteral reflux has been reported, but this may be a sampling, rather than a causal, relationship. Posttraumatic cyst may account for some simple cysts, and we are willing to admit that some "true" simple cysts likely occur in pediatric patients (Fig. 6–58).

Usually, a single cyst is identified incidentally during evaluation for UTI or other problem. It is our policy to obtain both urography and ultrasonography in such a case and to rescan the patient, assuming no clinical problems arise, in 6 months. One of our patients had hypertension associated with a single cyst. The hypertension resolved after aspiration of the cyst and recurred with reaccumulation of fluid. Failure of sclerosis of the cyst led to surgical unroofing of the cyst and a return to normotensive pressures. Of interest is that this patient was concurrently diagnosed as having basal cell nevus syndrome (Fig. 6–59). We do not think that aspiration of a benign-appearing cyst is warranted unless there are mitigating circumstances, as noted in the case just mentioned. If scans during the 6-month follow-up are unchanged, further care is discussed with the referring physician and family. In our view, it is best to rescan such a patient at puberty to determine whether other cysts have developed (Fig. 6–60).

Multiple Renal Cysts

Renal cysts are a definite component of renal dysplasia (Fig. 6–61). In this context, the terms "multiple cysts" and "multicystic" are appropriate. "Polycystic disease" implies syndromic disease. Although obstruction of

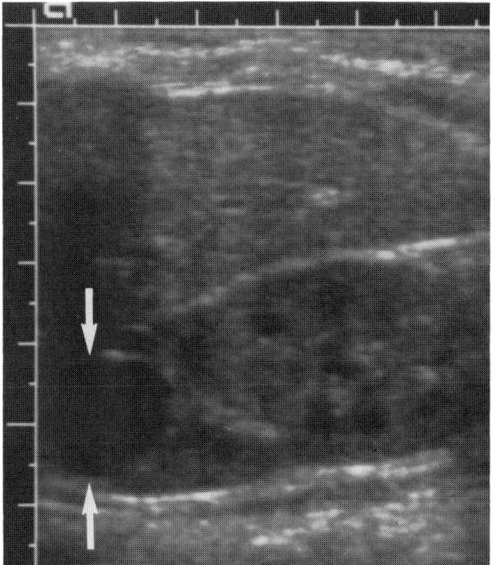

Figure 6–56. Longitudinal scan of the right kidney in this baby shows a "cyst" (arrows) in the upper pole. This is the dilated, obstructed collecting system of the upper pole of a duplex kidney. There was enough function, according to radionuclide study, to allow common sheath reimplantation of the ureters on the right.

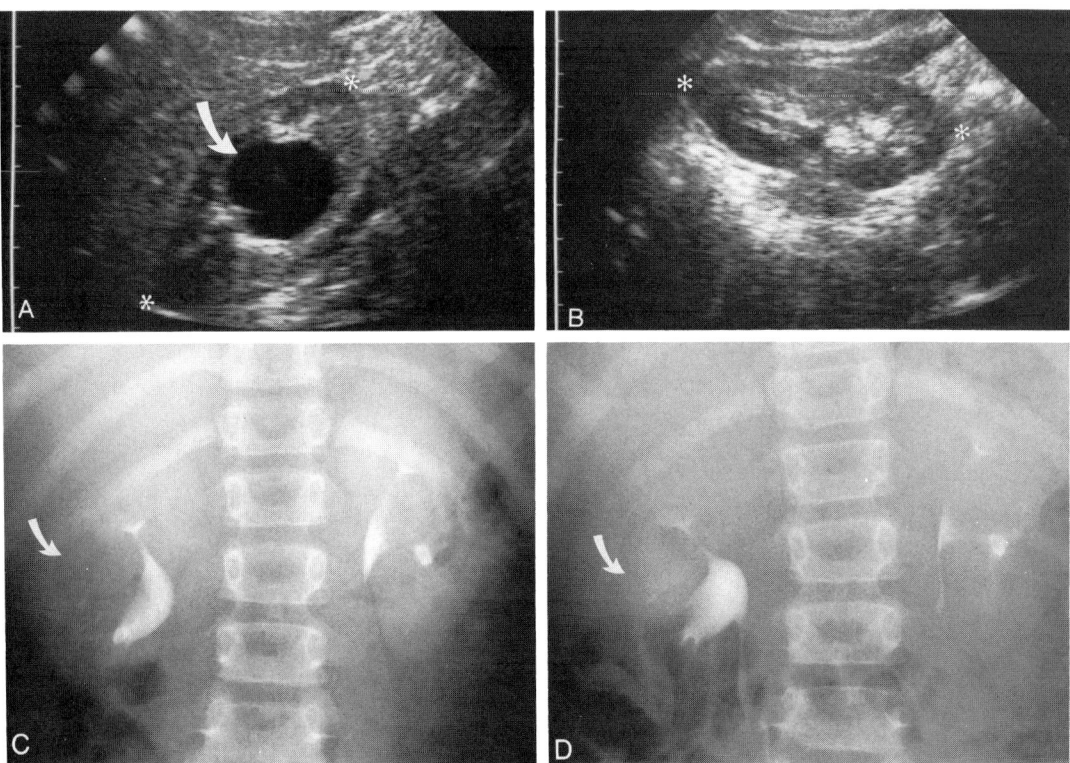

Figure 6–57. This 8-year-old girl had had a single infection of the urinary tract, and findings of a preceding vesicoureterogram were normal. Routine ultrasonography (A) showed a large cyst in the right kidney (arrow). Compare the right kidney with the normal left kidney (B). The intravenous urogram showed, on initial films (C), a nonopaque mass (arrow) in the center of the right kidney. Note the appearance of the left kidney. A column of Bertin separates the upper and lower parts of the collecting system. Delayed film (D) shows contrast material accumulating in the cyst (arrow), indicating that this is a diverticulum from the collecting system. No treatment was initiated because she had no further infection. She is being followed with yearly ultrasonograms.

the urinary tract in utero is a major associated finding in patients with cystic dysplasia, it is not always present. In general, the more proximal the obstruction is (at the proximal ureter or pelvis), the larger are the cysts. Patients with a distal ureteral or urethral obstruction tend to have small kidneys with small cysts (Sanders et al., 1988). In babies with bilateral involvement, previous abnormal intrauterine ultrasonograms, failure to thrive, and abnormal results from tests of urinary function are the usual reasons for referral. Careful scanning with transducers of high resolution often allows discrimination

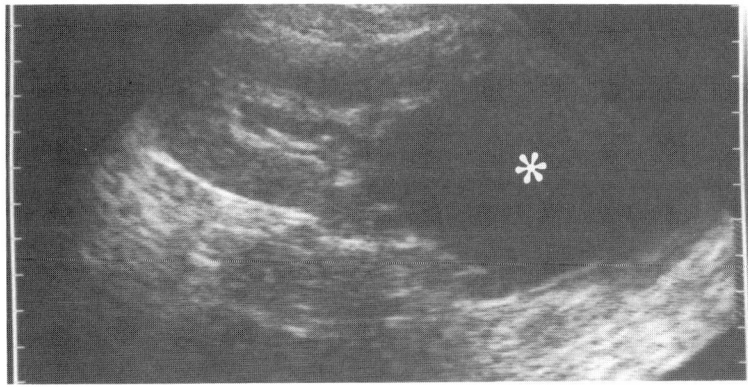

Figure 6–58. This large cyst (asterisk) in the lower pole of the left kidney was found incidentally during evaluation for presumed cystitis. At the time of the study, the patient was 18 years old. There was no family history of cystic disease. The cyst was aspirated; it contained clear fluid, and cytologic results were normal. We have no proof that this is a simple cyst, but that is its label for lack of any other diagnosis.

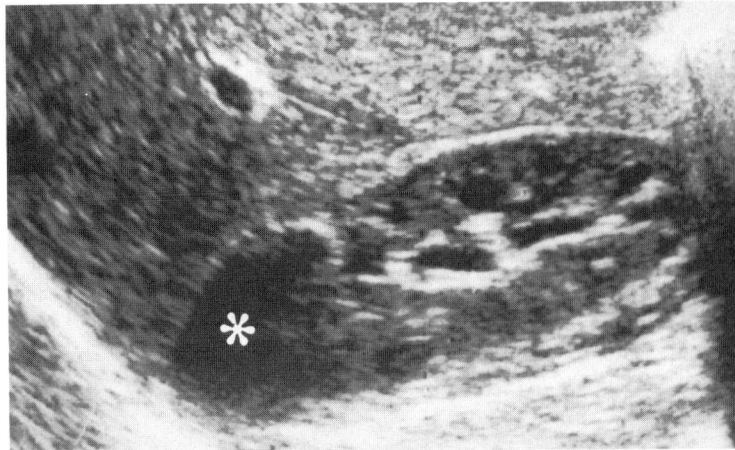

Figure 6–59. Although we have termed this a simple cyst (asterisk) of the upper pole, it may be a component of this patient's basal cell nevus syndrome.

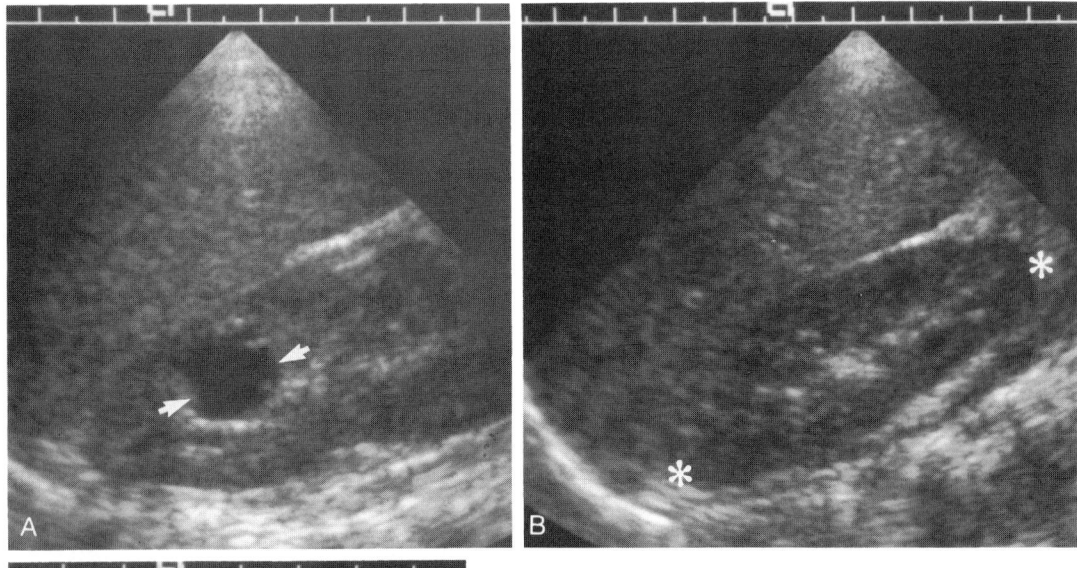

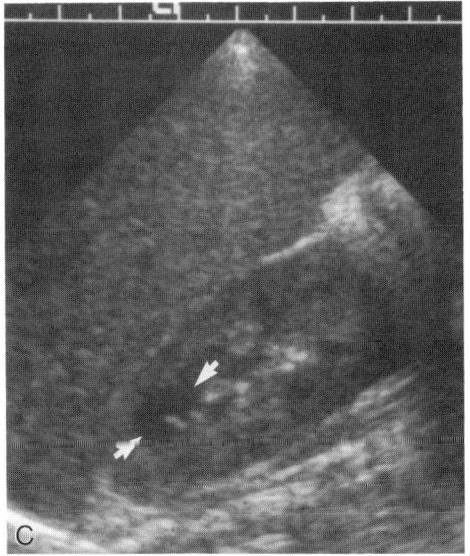

Figure 6–60. A 3-year-old boy was referred for ultrasonography to confirm the clinical impression of hepatosplenomegaly. The liver and spleen were normal, but a cyst in the upper pole of the left kidney (arrows, **A**) was apparent. In the initial study, scans of the right kidney (**B**) showed no overt abnormality. Six months later, a cyst in the right kidney had appeared (arrows, **C**). When dealing with small children who have only a single cyst found on initial ultrasonographic study, we are always concerned about the possibility of autosomal dominant polycystic renal disease, because its presentation may be unilateral, as in this patient.

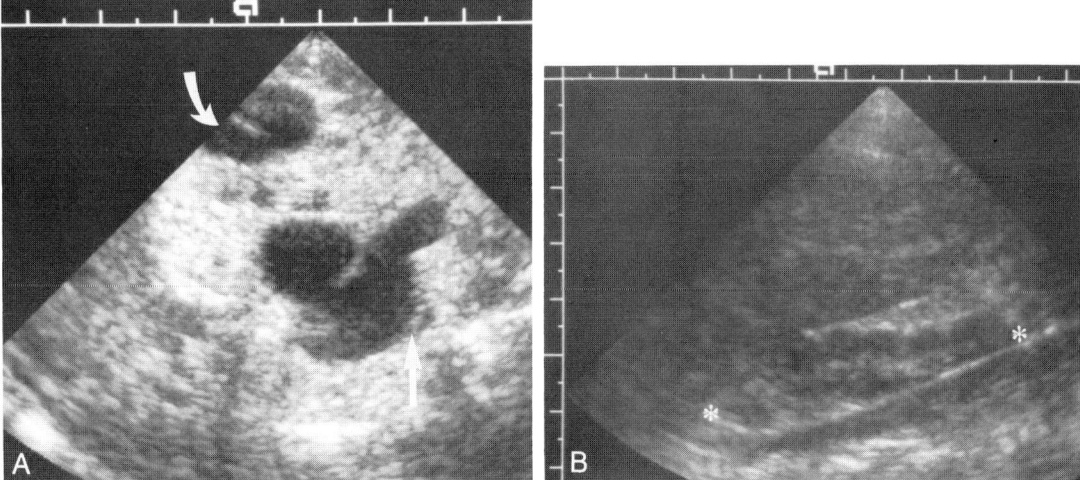

Figure 6–61. Cystic dysplasia of the right kidney with one large cyst predominating (curved arrow) was associated with obstruction at the ureteropelvic junction (straight arrow) on coronal scan (**A**). Repair of the obstruction was performed because some function was present on the right side. Postoperative scan (**B**) shows resolution of the cystic change and decrease in parenchymal echogenicity after pyeloplasty.

of small cysts. The cortex and medulla are poorly differentiated, and overall echogenicity of the dysplastic kidney is higher than in normal kidneys. A voiding cystourethrogram is an adjunctive study for two reasons: massive reflux may be present intermittently and may be missed on ultrasonography, but it may be the likely cause of renal maldevelopment. Also, minor degrees of reflux may outline the caliceal system and show it to be spindly or rudimentary, thereby corroborating a diagnosis of dysplasia.

Polycystic Kidney Disease (PKD)

Most patients with autosomal dominant polycystic kidney disease (ADPD) have a strong family history of the disorder, but occasional sporadic cases do occur. The estimated frequency of disease is 1 per 1000 children. It is now recognized that renal cysts, formerly called "adult-type" polycystic disease, may be present in childhood, although the syndrome is fully developed only in adulthood. The kidneys are usually enlarged, although they may be normal in size; macroscopic cysts are characteristic; and the renal parenchyma is often slightly more echogenic than expected (Fig. 6–62). Occasionally, the cystic kidneys are quite asymmetric in size. Cysts of the liver, pancreas, and spleen are rare in childhood but can be identified in some adolescents with the ADPD syndrome (Fig. 6–63). Complications of ADPD disease include hemorrhage into a cyst, which may be recognized on ultrasonography as a change from a baseline scan (Fig. 6–64). Infection of a polycystic kidney is very difficult to diagnose with routine methods of imaging.

When should offspring of an affected parent be scanned? Unless the family is part of a longitudinal study of polycystic kidney disease, the decision to scan children is made on an individual basis. Finding no overt abnormality on ultrasonograms of a baby or a small child does not rule out later development of renal cysts. Finding one or more cysts in a small child does not change the course of the disease and may change the psychosocial milieu within a family. Any offspring in a family at risk should be followed clinically with periodic measurements of blood pressure and renal function, whether they have abnormal scans early in life or not. There is good reason to scan adolescents before they begin childbearing so that genetic counseling can be initiated. Perhaps geneticists will make things easier or perhaps more complicated: prenatal diagnosis has been made with a deoxyribonucleic acid (DNA) probe genetically linked to the locus of ADPD on the short arm of chromosome 16 (Reeders, 1986).

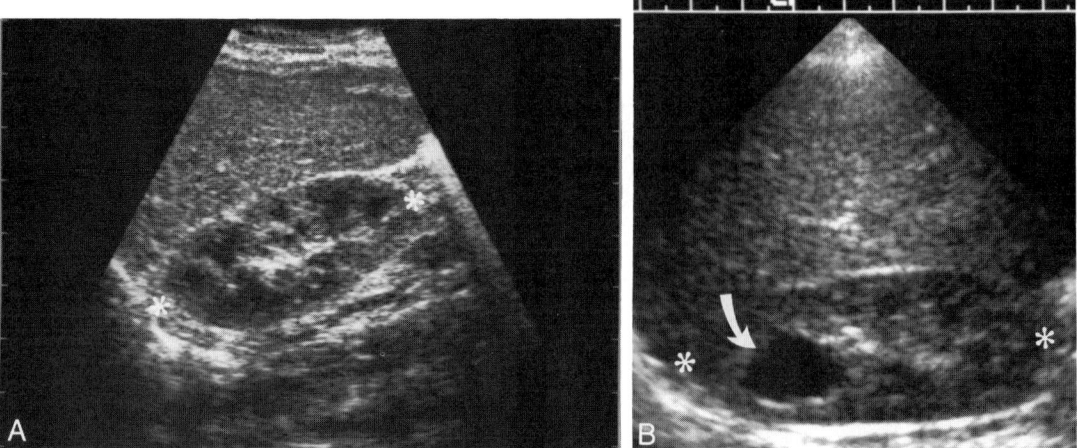

Figure 6–62. Autosomal dominant disease had been diagnosed in the sibling of this 3-year-old boy. Initial scans were done when this boy was 2 months old, and the results were normal (A). When he was 3 years old, another ultrasonogram showed a macroscopic cyst (arrow, B) in the upper pole of the right kidney. Renal screening of babies and children who have a family history of autosomal dominant disease and a normal initial scan does not rule out the possibility that cysts will develop later in life. We do not advocate routine screening of babies and children. Documentation of cystic disease does not change the clinical care of these patients. All such decisions, however, have to be made in concert with the pediatrician and the affected family.

Autosomal recessive polycystic kidney disease (ARPD) was previously termed "infantile" polycystic kidney disease, but this term has lost favor because the disease can manifest in toddlers and older children (Fig. 6–65). Because the syndrome is expressed only in homozygotes, a family history of the disease frequently is lacking. In the newborn, the kidneys tend to be large and increased in echogenicity in relation to hepatic and splenic parenchyma (Fig. 6–66). The "cysts" are actually dilated collecting tubules. The dilation results in multiple interfaces on ultrasonography and prolonged radial streaking of contrast media on intravenous urography. If the dilated tubules do not extend to the surface of the kidney, the compressed renal cortex provides a rim of relative sonolucency (Hayden et al., 1986; Premkumar et al., 1988). If the baby survives, macroscopic cysts may develop, although they are not as numerous or generally as large as those found in ADPD. Associated with ARPD disease is congenital hepatic fibrosis and biliary ectasia (Fig. 6–65; Boal and Teele, 1980; Premkumar et al., 1988). The ectasia of intrahepatic ducts is also termed Caroli's disease when the dilations are macroscopic (Davies et al., 1985). The spectrum of hepatic abnormalities may be subtle in the newborn, but if the baby survives, the hepatic disease comes to clinical attention. The periportal areas are echogenic from fibrosis and proliferation of biliary ducts; lucencies in the liver, if present, represent communicating biliary cysts, a lollipop appearance of the biliary tree. Portal hypertension results in spleno-

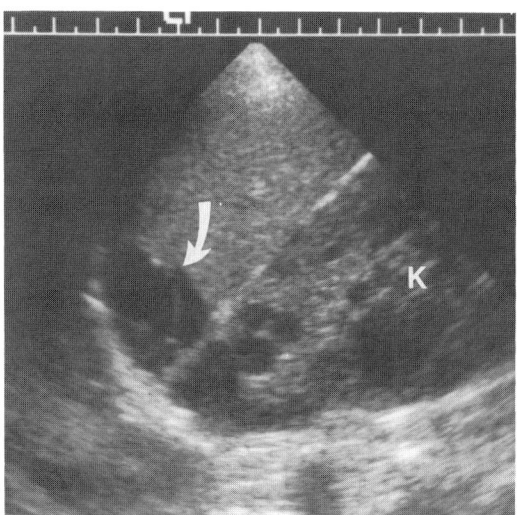

Figure 6–63. Autosomal dominant polycystic renal disease was diagnosed in this 17-year-old girl when her physician felt an abdominal mass during a routine physical examination. The patient has a splenic cyst (arrow), shown on this coronal scan of both the spleen and the polycystic left kidney (K). We assume that this is related to her renal disease, but it could have been posttraumatic, inasmuch as the patient is a competitive athlete. Splenic and hepatic cysts in autosomal dominant renal disease are an unusual occurrence before affected patients reach adulthood.

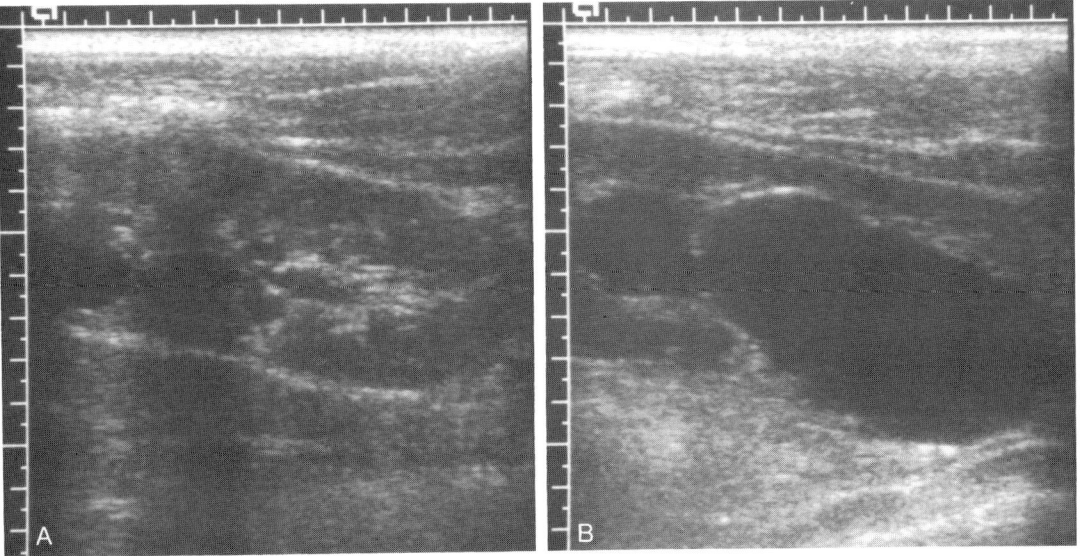

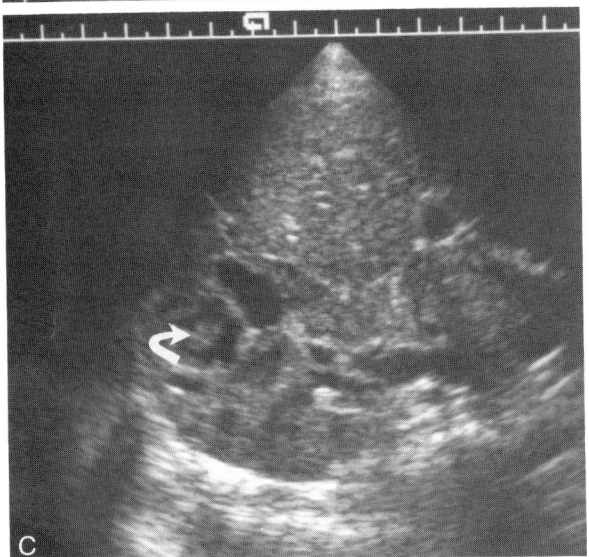

Figure 6–64. Diagnosis of autosomal dominant polycystic disease had been made previously in this adolescent girl. Note the asymmetry of involvement in comparisons of the longitudinal scan of the right kidney (A) with that of the left kidney (B). The cysts on the left are much larger. The patient was admitted to the hospital when she complained of severe flank pain and had symptoms of hematuria. A clot in one of the cysts (arrow) was apparent on careful scanning of the right kidney, as shown on this transverse scan (C).

megaly in some patients. In any baby or child with ultrasonographic features of polycystic renal disease, investigation of the liver and spleen should be included in the examination.

Some conditions masquerade as ARPD. Stapleton and coauthors (1981) reported transient nephromegaly, which resulted possibly from intrarenal tubular obstruction from Tamm-Horsfall mucoprotein or some other precipitating protein, as mimicking ARPD. Glomerulocystic kidney disease (GKD) in the neonate may be indistinguishable from classic ARPD and from some cases of ADPD (Fig. 6–67). Some early reports of "atypical" ARPD, for which biopsies were unavailable, may in fact have been describing cases of GKD. Cystic dilation of the Bowman space around glomeruli is the hallmark of this cystic disease. Although cysts occur in all parts of the nephron in ADPD, the predominance of glomerular cysts characterizes GKD (Worthington et al., 1988). Hepatic lesions have been reported with GKD, and so involvement of the liver is not a differentiating feature of the disease. For a child reported by Fitch and Stapleton (1986), the initial diagnosis of ARPD was changed to one of GKD as the kidneys decreased in size over 15 months, becoming small with macrocysts. Renal function did not deteriorate, and the diagnosis of GKD was made after biopsy.

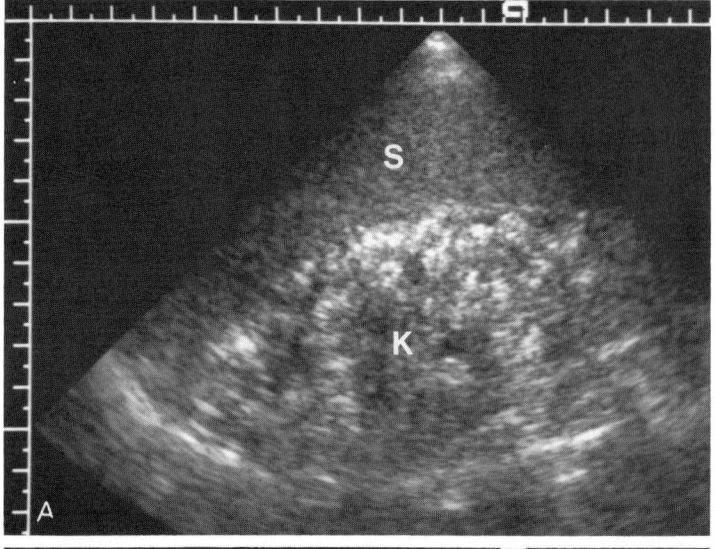

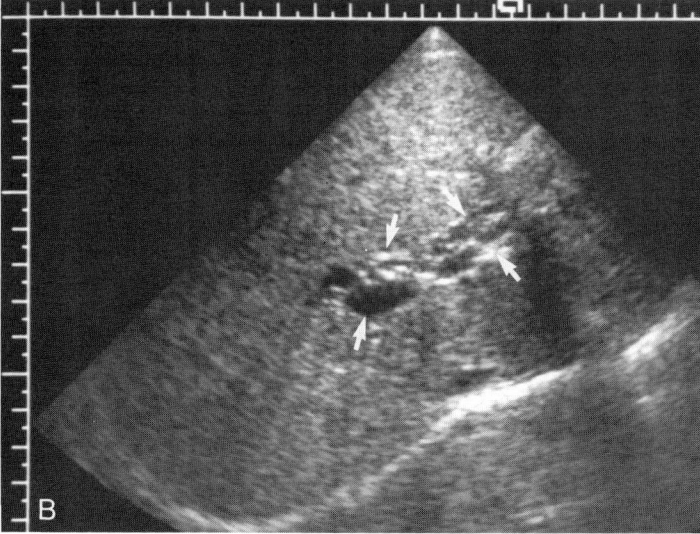

Figure 6–65. This 8-year-old girl presented with splenomegaly. Coronal scan of the left flank (A) showed enlargement of the spleen (S). The adjacent diffuse echogenicity of the kidney (K) is typical of autosomal recessive polycystic disease. The multiple small cystic interfaces cause its diffuse echogenicity on ultrasonography. In all patients who have renal cystic disease, the liver and spleen should be carefully scanned. The transverse view of the liver (B) shows saccular dilation of the biliary tree manifested by too many lucencies within portal triads (arrows).

Sporadic cases seem to be the norm; determination of genetic transmission of GKD has not been well established to date.

The conclusions and recommendations from a review article on polycystic kidney disease in infants (Worthington et al., 1988) are worth citing (with some additions).

1. Variable clinical and sonographic features occur with all types of polycystic kidney disease.
2. Macrocysts in infants are less common in ARPD, but not invariably absent.
3. Absence of macrocysts does not rule out a diagnosis of ADPD or of GKD.
4. GKD may be indistinguishable from either ADPD or ARPD on ultrasonography.
5. Family history is of utmost importance in diagnosis. Genetic markers, when developed fully, will be invaluable.

As a practical matter, renal and hepatic biopsies are indicated for babies and children with atypical cystic renal disease primarily for the genetic counseling of parents who wish to have more children (Fig. 6–68). Management of the individual patient is based on symptoms and generally is not altered by the pathologic findings.

GKD is a feature of several syndromes that are associated with renal cystic disease and are listed in Table 6–3. Cortical cysts and cystic distention of the Bowman space usually result in mild to moderate renal enlargement. As a general rule, any baby shown on screening renal ultrasonography to have cys-

RENAL SCREENING / 185

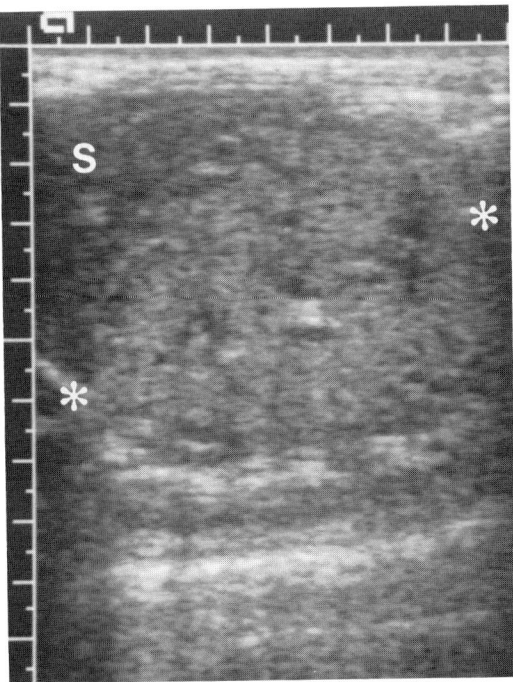

Figure 6–66. Longitudinal scan of the left kidney was similar to scans of the right kidney in this baby, who had autosomal recessive kidney disease. The spleen (S) is adjacent to the kidney. The renal outline is poorly defined. Multiple small cysts create multiple interfaces within the kidney.

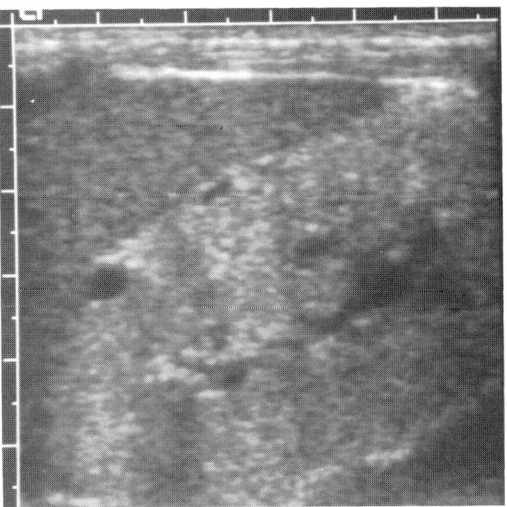

Figure 6–68. Renal and hepatic biopsies were performed on this baby after he presented with an asymptomatic abdominal mass. Both kidneys were involved in a similar fashion. A longitudinal scan of the right kidney is shown. There were peripheral macrocysts and diffuse echogenicity throughout the rest of the kidney. The central renal collecting system is mildly prominent. There was no family history of cystic renal disease, and both parents were scanned and shown to have kidneys that appeared normal. The final pathologic diagnosis for this baby was of dominant polycystic kidney disease. It is obvious, from these and other pathologic reports, that there is overlap between the cystic diseases even at the cellular level. We believe that investigations of genetic material will provide the final answer to the puzzle of polycystic diseases of the kidney.

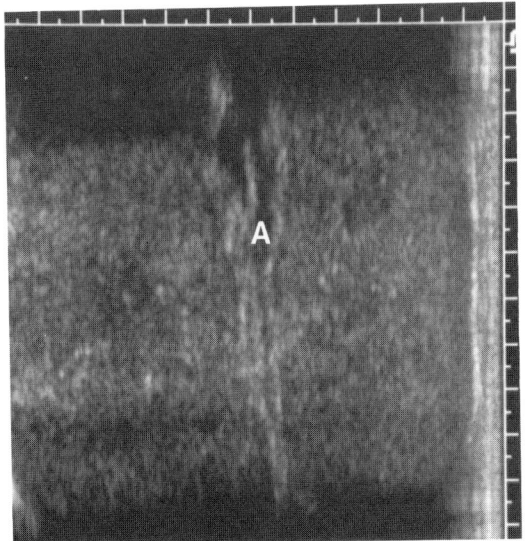

Figure 6–67. Left coronal scan of the kidneys, oriented as an anteroposterior radiograph, shows huge kidneys filling the abdomen. This baby was admitted to the hospital because of renal insufficiency and hypertension. A biopsy was performed and reviewed by several pathologists. Final diagnosis was probable glomerulocystic disease. A = aorta.

tic kidneys should have cranial ultrasonography. In a baby whom we scanned and who received a diagnosis of polycystic kidney disease, occult Dandy-Walker malformation was discovered on cranial ultrasonography at a later date. Meckel-Gruber syndrome is more frequently associated with cystic kidneys than with occipital encephalocele. Other anomalies of the brain that are commonly present can be diagnosed on ultrasonography (Fig. 6–69). The macrocysts associated with tuberous sclerosis resemble ADPD, but scans of the brain may reveal the disorder if calcified tubers of the walls of lateral ventricles are present (see last section for more discussion of tuberous sclerosis).

Juvenile Nephronophthisis: Renal Medullary Cystic Disease

Idiopathic renal failure in adolescents is most often caused by this disease (Glassberg

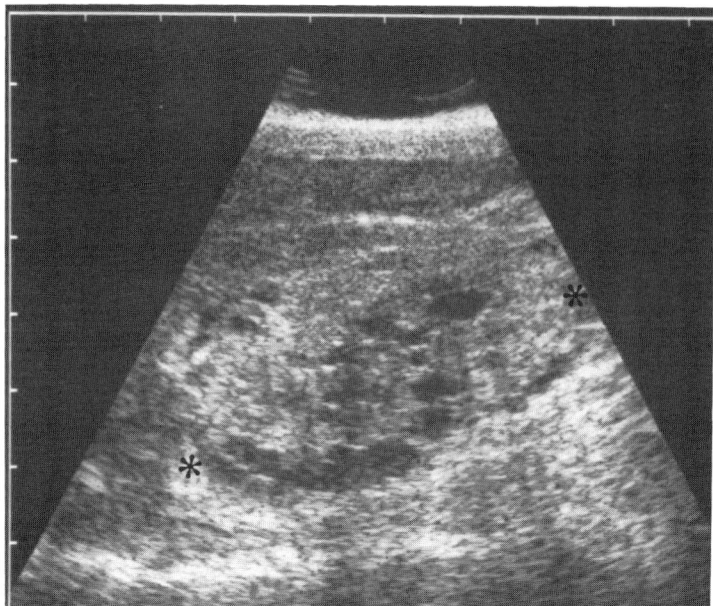

Figure 6-69. Longitudinal scan of the right kidney shows irregular lucencies associated with generalized diffuse increase in parenchymal echogenicity of the kidney. This baby had polydactyly and multiple intracranial anomalies consisting of lissencephaly and cerebellar hypoplasia. Although encephalocele was not present, this constellation of anomalies is typical of Meckel-Gruber syndrome.

et al., 1987). Medullary cysts associated with chronic tubulointerstitial nephritis is the pathologic hallmark, although the cysts are not always obvious on ultrasonography. The kidneys tend to be small and diffusely echogenic, with a variable number of small cysts (Figs. 6-70, 6-71; Garel et al., 1984c). The terms "juvenile nephronophthisis" and "renal medullary cystic disease" refer to the same pathologic renal abnormality but to different modes of inheritance. Autosomal recessive inheritance is associated with juvenile nephronophthisis; autosomal dominant inheritance, with medullary cystic disease. Retinitis pigmentosa (renal-retinal dysplasia) and cone-shaped epiphyses (Mainzer-Saldino syndrome) can be associated with this renal abnormality.

Medullary sponge kidney is characterized by cystic dilation of the collecting ducts and is therefore a medullary, rather than cortical, disease. Its inheritance is uncertain, and it is

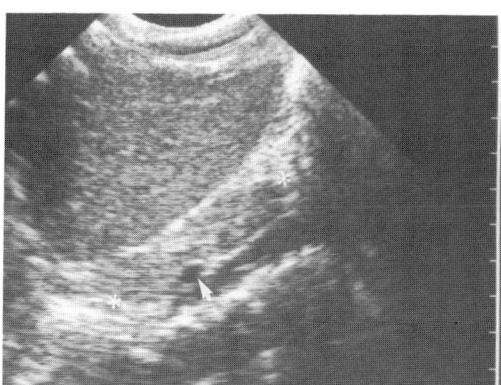

Figure 6-70. The diagnosis of nephronophthisis was made when this patient presented at 12 years of age with short stature, elevated creatinine levels, and hypertension. Both kidneys were small and echogenic. A small cyst was present (arrow) on the left kidney.

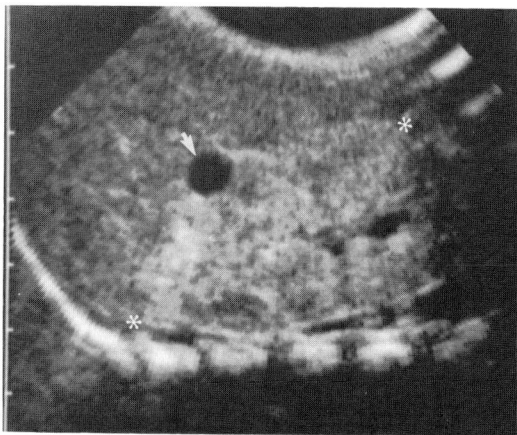

Figure 6-71. Nephronophthisis was diagnosed in another child at age 2½ years. Note the presence of a cortical cyst (arrow) in association with echogenic renal parenchyma. Both kidneys were removed at the time of renal transplantation. There was no family history of renal disease.

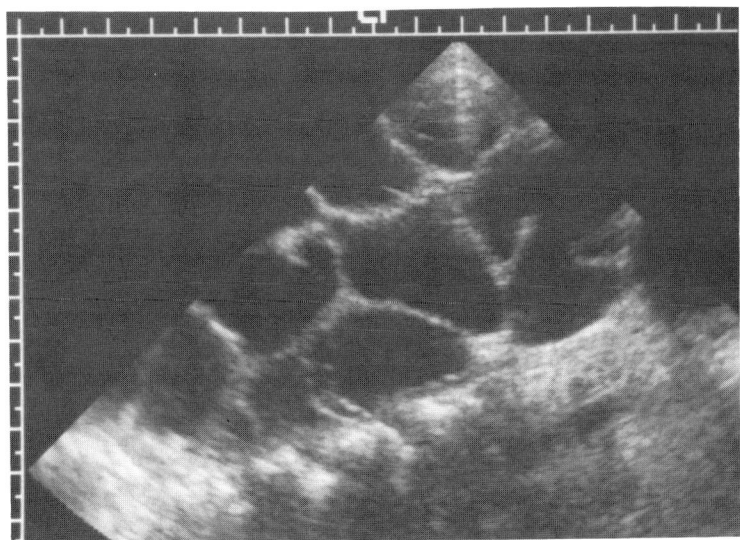

Figure 6–72. At 12 months of age, this baby was noted to have a blood pressure of 190/108 during a routine physical examination. His mother had also been concerned that his belly was protuberant. Scans show replacement of renal tissue by macrocysts. View is of the right kidney. The left kidney was similar in appearance. Scans of the brain done at the same time showed shadowing foci that were adjacent to the ventricular system and that represented calcified tubers of tuberous sclerosis.

unassociated with other anomalies. Hyperechogenicity of the renal pyramids seen on ultrasonograms of children who have this disease is probably from calcium in dilated ducts (Patriquin and O'Regan, 1985). Medullary sponge kidney is usually diagnosed after childhood. Children may present with hematuria from frank calculi or UTI that may be incidental to the disease. The major differential diagnosis on ultrasonography is renal tubular acidosis with secondary deposition of calcium in the medulla.

Miscellaneous

The syndromes known to be associated with chromosomal abnormalities are commonly also associated with renal cysts, dysplasia, and anomalies. They are listed in Table 6–2. "Renal nephropathy" is an all-encompassing term, indicating poorly functioning kidneys, and the disorder occurs in association with several named syndromes. The most common are also listed in Table 6–2. Prune-belly syndrome is discussed in the section on hydronephrosis in Chapter 8.

Tuberous sclerosis is inherited as an autosomal dominant syndrome, but a family history of the syndrome is lacking for 50 percent of the patients. The affected newborn may present with macroscopic cystic disease that resembles ADPD (Fig. 6–72). Usually, however, renal involvement with cysts and angiomyolipomas increases with age (Figs. 6–73, 6–74; Narla et al., 1988). The angiomyolipomata are echogenic and may be quite large, 5 to 6 cm in diameter. Renal cysts are usually less than 2 cm in diameter. Distortion of the renal architecture by the masses makes comparison of scans, on follow-up ultrasonographic studies, quite difficult. In contrast to an angiomyolipoma, acute hemorrhage into a cyst tends not to shadow, but the differentiation may not be possible except through CT. Renal aneurysm is an associated anomaly, and on static scans it may simulate a

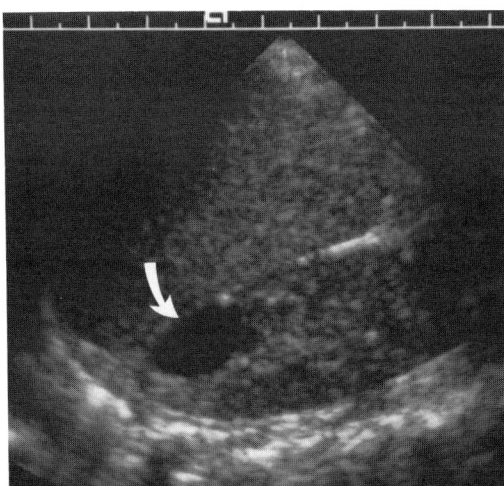

Figure 6–73. A single renal cyst (arrow) in the upper pole of the left kidney was found in this patient, newly diagnosed with seizures. Diagnosis of tuberous sclerosis was subsequently made.

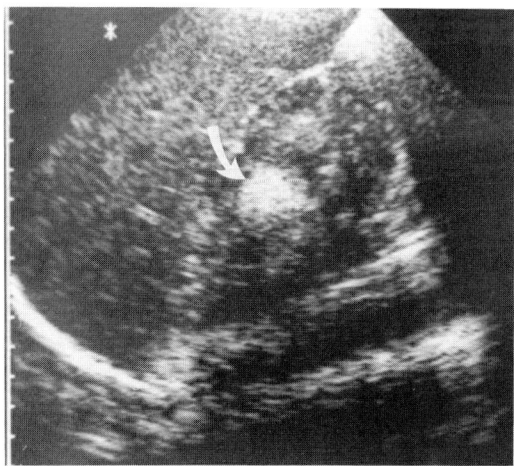

Figure 6–74. Angiomyolipoma of the upper pole of the right kidney is an echogenic focus (arrow) in this 13-year-old boy, who has tuberous sclerosis.

cyst. Doppler imaging of suspicious masses will discriminate between vascular and nonvascular lesions.

REFERENCES

Normal Renal Ultrasonography

Bis KG, Slovis TL: Accuracy of ultrasonic bladder volume measurement in children. Pediatr Radiol 1990; 20:457–460.

Blane CE, Bookstein FL, DiPietro MA, et al: Sonographic standards for normal infant kidney length. AJR 1985; 145:1289–1291.

Cacciarelli AA, Kass EJ, Yang SS, et al: Urachal remnants: Sonographic demonstration in children. Radiology 1990; 174:473–475.

Chiara A, Chirico G, Barbarini, M: Ultrasonic evaluation of kidney length in term and preterm infants. Eur J Pediatr 1989; 149:94–95.

DeVries L, Levene MI: Measurement of renal size in preterm and term infants by real-time ultrasound. Arch Dis Child 1983; 58:145–147.

Dinkel E, Ertel M, Dittrich M, et al: Kidney size in childhood. Sonographical growth charts for kidney length and volume. Pediatr Radiol 1985; 15:38–43.

Dremsek PA, Kritscher H, Böhm G, et al: Kidney dimensions in ultrasound compared to somatometric parameters in normal children. Pediatr Radiol 1987; 17:285–290.

Erasmie U, Lidefelt KJ: Accuracy of ultrasonic assessment of residual urine in children. Pediatr Radiol 1989; 19:388–390.

Fendel H, Schneider K, Bakowski C, et al: Common use of diagnostic imaging for childhood wetting (enuresis): A survey of practicing paediatricians in the Federal Republic of Germany and West Berlin. Ann Radiol 1987; 30:473–477.

Haller JO, Berdon WE, Friedman AP: Increased renal cortical echogenicity: A normal finding in neonates and infants. Radiology 1982; 142:173–174.

Han BK, Babcock DS: Sonographic measurements and appearance of normal kidneys in children. AJR 1985; 145:611–616.

Hoffer FA, Hanabergh AM, Teele RL: The interrenicular junction: A mimic of renal scarring on normal pediatric sonograms. AJR 1985; 145:1075–1078.

Horgan JG, Rosenfield NS, Weiss RM, et al: Is renal ultrasound a reliable indicator of a nonobstructed duplication anomaly? Pediatr Radiol 1984; 14:388–391.

Hricak H, Slovis TL, Callen CW, et al: Neonatal kidneys: Sonographic anatomic correlation. Radiology 1983; 147:699–702.

Jequier S, Rousseau O: Sonographic measurements of the normal bladder wall in children. AJR 1987; 149:563–566.

Rosenbaum DM, Korngold E, Teele RL: Sonographic assessment of renal length in normal children. AJR 1984; 142:467–469.

Steinhart JM, Kuhn JP, Eisenberg B, et al: Ultrasound screening of healthy infants for urinary tract abnormalities. Pediatrics 1988; 82:609–614.

Troell S, Berg U, Johansson B, et al: Renal parenchymal volume in children. Normal values assessed by ultrasonography. Acta Radiol 1988; 29:127–130.

Williot P, McLorie GA, Gilmour RF, et al: Accuracy of bladder volume determination in children using a suprapubic ultrasonic bi-polar technique. J Urol 1989; 141:900–902.

Syndromes

Azouz EM, Larson EJ, Patel J, Gyepes MT: Beckwith-Wiedemann syndrome: Development of nephroblastoma during the surveillance period. Pediatr Radiol 1990; 20:550–552.

Baker D: Turner's syndrome and pseudo-Turner's syndrome. Am J Roentgenol 1967; 100:40–47.

Bronk JB, Parker BR: Pyelocalyceal diverticula in the Beckwith-Wiedemann syndrome. Pediatr Radiol 1987; 17:80–81.

Cramer B, Green J, Harnett J et al: Sonographic and urographic correlation in Bardet-Biedl syndrome (formerly Laurence-Moon-Biedl syndrome). Urol Radiol 1988; 10:176–180.

Darlington D, Hawkins CF: Nail-patella syndrome with iliac horns and hereditary nephropathy. Necropsy report and anatomical dissection. J Bone Joint Surg 1967; 49B:164–174.

Ferguson AC, Rance CP: Hereditary nephropathy with nerve deafness (Alport's Syndrome). Am J Dis Child 1972; 124:84–88.

Greenberg CR, Trevenen CL, Evans JA: The BOR syndrome and renal agenesis—prenatal diagnosis and further clinical delineation. Prenat Diagn 1988; 8:103–108.

Hegde HR, Leung AK: Aplasia of pectoralis major muscle and renal anomalies. Am J Genet 1989; 32:109–111.

Jennings CM, Gaines PA: The abdominal manifestation of von Hippel-Lindau disease and a radiological screening protocol for an affected family. Clin Radiol 1988; 39:363–367.

Linné T, Wikstad I, Zetterström R: Renal involvement in the Laurence-Moon-Biedl Syndrome. Functional and radiological studies. Acta Pediatr Scand 1986; 75:240–244.

Lippe B, Geffner ME, Dietrich RB, et al: Renal malformations in patients with Turner syndrome: Imaging in 141 patients. Pediatrics 1988; 82:852–856.

Luisiri A, Sotelo-Avila C, Silberstein MJ, et al: Sonog-

raphy of the Zellweger syndrome. J Ultrasound Med 1988; 7:169–173.
Mainzer F, Saldino RM, Ozonoff MB, et al: Familial nephropathy associated with retinitis pigmentosa, cerebellar ataxia and skeletal abnormalities. Am J Med 1970; 49:556–562.
Miller WB Jr, Boal DK, Teele RL: Neurofibromatosis of the bladder: Sonographic findings. JCU 1983; 11:460–462.
Shah KJ: Beckwith-Weidemann syndrome: Role of ultrasound in its management. Clin Radiol 1983; 34:313–319.
Taybi H, Lachman RS: Radiology of Syndromes, Metabolic Disorders and Skeletal Dysplasias, 3rd ed. Chicago: Year Book Medical Publishers, 1990.
Weese-Mayer DE, Smith KM, Reddy JK, et al: Computerized tomography and ultrasound in the diagnosis of cerebro-hepato-renal syndrome of Zellweger. Pediatr Radiol 1987; 17:170–172.

Screening to Rule Out Renal Anomaly

Avni EF, Thoua Y, Lalmand B, et al: Multicystic dysplastic kidney: Natural history from in utero diagnosis and postnatal followup. J Urol 1987; 138:1420–1424.
Bourne GL, Benirschke K: Absent umbilical artery. A review of 113 cases. Arch Dis Child 1960; 35:534–543.
Denes FT, Montellato NID, Lopes RN, et al: Seminal vesicle cyst and ipsilateral renal agenesis. Urology 1986; 28:313–315.
Eisenberg D, Luis-Jorge JC, Himmelfarb EH, et al: Sonographic diagnosis of seminal vesicle cysts. JCU 1986; 14:213–215.
Emanuel B, Nachman R, Aronson N, et al: Congenital solitary kidney: A review of 74 cases. Am J Dis Child 1974; 127:17–19.
Escobar LF, Weaver DD, Bixler D, et al: Urorectal septum malformation sequence. Am J Dis Child 1987; 141:1021–1024.
Fendel H, Schneider K, Bakowski C, et al: Common use of diagnostic imaging for childhood wetting (enuresis): A survey of practicing pediatricians in the Federal Republic of Germany and West Berlin. Ann Radiol 1987; 30:473–477.
Fernbach SK, Glass RBJ: The expanded spectrum of limb anomalies in the Vater association. Pediatr Radiol 1988; 18:215–220.
Gordon AC, Thomas DF, Arthur RJ, et al: Prenatally diagnosed reflux: A follow-up study. Br J Urol 1990; 65:407–412.
Gray SW, Skandalakis JE: Embryology for Surgeons. Philadelphia: WB Saunders, 1972.
Greig JD, Raine PA, Young DG, et al: Value of antenatal diagnosis of abnormalities of the urinary tract. Br Med J 1989; 298:1417–1419.
Heifetz SA: Single umbilical artery: A statistical analysis of 237 autopsy cases and review of the literature. Perspect Pediatr Pathol 1984; 8:345–378.
Herman TE, Cleveland RH, Kushner DC: Pelvic kidney in cloacal extrophy. Pediatr Radiol 1986; 16:306–308.
Herrmann UJ Jr, Sidiropoulos D: Single umbilical artery: prenatal findings. Prenat Diagn 1988; 8:275–280.
Kenny RD, Flippo JL, Black EB: Supernumerary nipples and renal anomalies in neonates. Am J Dis Child 1987; 141:987–988.
Knight PJ, Clatworthy HW: Screening for latent malformations: Cost effectiveness in neonates with correctable anomalies. J Pediatr Surg 1982; 17:123–129.
Kohn G, Borns PF: The association of bilateral and unilateral renal aplasia in the same family. J Pediatr 1973; 83:95–97.
Leung AKC, Robson WLM: Single umbilical artery: A report of 159 cases. Am J Dis Child 1989; 143:108–111.
Liddell RM, Rosenbaum DM, Blumhagen JD: Delayed radiologic appearance of bilateral thoracic ectopic kidneys. AJR 1989; 152:120–122.
Livera LN, Brookfield DS, Egginton JA, Hawnaur JM: Antenatal ultrasonography to detect fetal renal abnormalities: A prospective screening programme. Br Med J 1989; 298:1421–1423.
Lubat E, Hernanz-Schulman M, Genieser NB, et al: Sonography of the simple and complicated ipsilateral fused kidney. J Ultrasound Med 1989; 8:109–114.
McArdle R, Lebowitz RL: Uncomplicated hypospadias and anomalies of upper urinary tract. Need for screening? Urology 1975; 5:712–716.
Meglin AJ, Balotin RJ, Jelinek JS, et al: Cloacal exstrophy: Radiologic findings in 13 patients. AJR 1990; 155:1267–1272.
Muller P: Association of genital and urinary malformations in women. Gynecology 1968; 165:285–294.
Murugasu B, Yip WC, Tay JS et al: Sonographic screening for renal tract anomalies associated with congenital heart disease. JCU 1990; 18:79–83.
Museles M, Gaudry CL, Bason WM: Renal anomalies in the newborn found by deep palpation. Pediatrics 1971; 47:97–100.
Najmaldin A, Burge DM, Atwell JD: Fetal vesicoureteric reflux. Br J Urol 1990; 65:403–406.
Pappis CH, Argianas SA, Bousgas D, et al: Unsuspected urological anomalies in asymptomatic cryptorchid boys. Pediatr Radiol 1988; 18:51–53.
Pavanello RdeCM, Eigier A, Otto PA: Relationship between Mayer-Rokitansky-Küster (MRK) anomaly and hereditary renal adysplasia (HRA). Am J Med Genet 1988; 29:845–849.
Perlmutter AD, Retik AB, Bauer SB: Anomalies of the upper urinary tract. In Walsh PC, Gittes RF, Perlmutter AD, Stamey TA (eds): Campbell's Urology (5th ed). Philadelphia: WB Saunders, 1986, 1665–1759.
Quan L, Smith DW: The VATER association: Vertebral defects, anal atresia, T-E fistula with esophageal atresia, radial and renal dysplasia: A spectrum of associated defects. J Pediatr 1973; 82:104–107.
Roodhooft AM, Birnholz JC, Holmes LB: Familial nature of congenital absence and severe dysgenesis of both kidneys. N Engl J Med 1984; 310:1341–1345.
Rosenstein BJ, Wheeler JS, Heid PL: Congenital renal abnormalities in infants with in utero cocaine exposure. J Urol 1990; 144:110–112.
Sheih CP, Liu MB, Hung CS, et al: Renal abnormalities in school children. Pediatrics 1989; 84:1086–1090.
Singh MP, Haddadin A, Zachary RB, et al: Renal tract disease in imperforate anus. J Pediatr Surg 1974; 9:197–202.
Steinhart JM, Kuhn JP, Eisenberg B, et al: Ultrasound screening of healthy infants for urinary tract abnormalities. Pediatrics 1988; 82:609–614.
Sumner TE, Volberg FM, Smolen PM: Intrathoracic kidney—Diagnosis by ultrasound. Pediatr Radiol 1982; 12:78–80.
Temtamy SA, Miller JD: Extending the scope of the VATER association: Definition of the VATER syndrome. J Pediatr 1974; 85:345–349.
Van den Abbeele AD, Treves ST, Lebowitz RL, et al: Vesicoureteral reflux in asymptomatic siblings of patients with known reflux: Radionuclide cystography. Pediatrics 1987; 79:147–153.

Wiersma AF, Peterson LF, Justema EJ: Uterine anomalies associated with unilateral renal agenesis. Obstet Gynecol 1976; 47:654–657.

Wilms Tumor*

Beseghi U, Del Rossi C, Cerasoli G, et al: Diagnostic problems in a Wilms' tumour of the horseshoe kidney. Z Kinderchir 1988; 43:110–111.
Boechat MI, Kangarloo H: MR imaging in Drash syndrome. J Comput Assist Tomogr 1988; 12:405–408.
Drash A, Sherman F, Hartmann WH, et al: A syndrome of pseudohermaphroditism, Wilms tumor, hypertension, and degenerative renal disease. J Pediatr 1970; 76:585–593.
Fernbach SK, Feinstein KA, Donaldson JS, et al: Nephroblastomatosis: Comparison of CT with US and urography. Radiology 1988; 166:153–156.
Friedman AL, Finlay JL: The Drash syndrome revisited: Diagnosis and follow-up. Am J Med Genet Suppl 1987; 3:293–296.
Gallo GE, Chemes HE: The association of Wilms' tumor, male pseudohermaphroditism and diffuse glomerular disease (Drash syndrome): Report of eight cases with clinical and morphologic findings and review of the literature. Pediatr Pathol 1987; 7:175–189.
Garel L, Musset D, Habib R, et al: Interest of ultrasound in Drash syndrome: A report of three cases. Ann Radiol 1984a; 27:223–227.
Mesrobian H-GJ: Wilms' tumor: Past, present, future. J Urol 1988; 140:231–238.

Hypertension

Baldwin CE, Holder TM, Ashcroft KW, et al: Neonatal renovascular hypertension—A complication of aortic monitoring catheters. J Pediatr Surg 1981; 16:820–821.
Caplan MS, Cohn RA, Langman CB, et al: Favorable outcome of neonatal aortic thrombosis and renovascular hypertension. J Pediatr 1989; 115:291–295.
Diament MJ, Stanley P, Boechat MI, et al: Pediatric hypertension: An approach to imaging. Pediatr Radiol 1986; 16:461–467.
Farrelly CA, Daneman A, Martin DJ, et al: Pheochromocytoma in childhood: The important role of computed tomography in tumour localization. Pediatr Radiol 1984; 14:210–214.
Garel LA, Pariente DM, Gubler MC, et al: The dotted corticomedullary junction: A sonographic indicator of small-vessel renal disease in hypertensive children. Radiology 1984b; 152:419–422.
Hodson CJ, Heptinstall RH, Winberg J: Reflux Nephropathy Update: 1983. New York: Karger Basel, 1984.
Loggie JMH: Evaluation and management of childhood hypertension. Surgical Clin North Am 1985; 65:1623–1649.
Martin JE Jr, Moran JF, Cook LS, et al: Neonatal aortic thrombosis complicating umbilical artery catheterization: Successful treatment with retroperitoneal aortic thrombectomy. Surgery 1989; 105:793–796.
Mentser M: Diagnosis and treatment of hypertension in children. Pediatr Clin North Am 1982; 29:933–945.
Robertson R, Murphy A, Dubbins PA: Renal artery stenosis: The use of duplex ultrasound as a screening technique. Br J Radiol 1988; 61:196–201.
Rosen PR, Treves S, Ingelfinger J: Hypertension in children. Increased efficacy of Technetium (Tc) 99m succimer in screening for renal disease. Am J Dis Child 1985; 139:173–177.
Seibert JJ, Taylor BJ, Williamson SL, et al: Sonographic detection of neonatal umbilical artery thrombosis: Clinical correlation. AJR 1987; 148:965–968.
Stanley JC, Fry WJ: Pediatric renal artery occlusive disease and renovascular hypertension: Etiology, diagnosis and operative treatment. Arch Surg 1981; 116:669–676.
Starinsky R, Manor A, Segal M: Non-functioning kidney associated with neonatal adrenal hemorrhage. Report of two cases. Pediatr Radiol 1986; 16:427–429.
Stringer DA, de Bruyn R, Dillon MJ, et al: Comparison of aortography, renal vein renin sampling, radionuclide scans, ultrasound and the IVU in the investigation of childhood renovascular hypertension. Br J Radiol 1984; 57:111–121.
Task Force on Blood Pressure Control in Children. Report of the second Task Force on Blood Pressure Control in Children—1987. Pediatrics 1987; 79:1–25.
Taylor DC, Kettler MD, Moneta GL, et al: Duplex ultrasound scanning in the diagnosis of renal artery stenosis: A prospective evaluation. J Vasc Surg 1988; 7:363–369.
Thornbury JR, Stanley JC, Fryback DG, et al: Limited use of hypertensive excretory urography. Urol Radiol 1982; 3:209–211.
Wallace DMA, Rothwell DL, Williams DI: The long-term follow-up of surgically treated vesico-ureteric reflux. Br J Urol 1978; 50:479–484.

Hematuria and Urolithiasis

Alton DJ, Gu L, Daneman A: Transient opacification of the urinary pathways by amorphous debris in children with leukemia. Pediatr Radiol 1988; 18:392–394.
Baggio B, Gambaro G, Favaro S, et al: Juvenile renal stone disease: A study of urinary promoting and inhibiting factors. J Urol 1983; 130:1133–1135.
Churchill DN, Maloney CM, Nolan R, et al: Pediatric urolithiasis in the 1970s. J Urol 1980; 123:237–238.
Diament MJ, Malekzadeh M: Ultrasound and the diagnosis of renal and ureteral calculi. J Pediatr 1986; 109:980–983.
Hymes LC, Warshaw BL: Idiopathic hypercalciuria: Renal and absorptive subtypes in children. Am J Dis Child 1984; 138:176–180.
Ingelfinger JR, Davis AE, Grupe WE: Frequency and etiology of gross hematuria in a general pediatric setting. Pediatrics 1977; 59:557–561.
Jacinto JS, Modanlou HD, Grade M, et al: Renal calcification incidence in very low birth weight infants. Pediatrics 1988; 81:31–35.
Janetschek G, Kunzel KH: Percutaneous nephrolithotomy in horseshoe kidneys: Applied anatomy and clinical experience. Br J Urol 1988; 62:117–122.
Leonard MP, Nickel JC, Morales A: Cavernous hemangiomas of the bladder in the pediatric age group. J Urol 1988; 140:1503–1504.
MacDonald I, Azmy AF: Recurrent and residual renal calculi in children. Br J Urol 1988; 61:395–398.
Myracle MR, McGahan JP, Goetzman BW, et al: Ultrasound diagnosis of renal calcification in infants on chronic furosemide therapy. JCU 1986; 14:281–287.
Northway JD: Hematuria in children. J Pediatr 1971; 78:381–396.
Patriquin H, Robitaille P: Renal calcium deposition in children: sonographic demonstration of the Anderson-Carr progression. AJR 1986; 146:1253–1256.

---

*Also see references for Chapter 8.

Shepherd P, Thomas R, Harmon EP: Urolithiasis in children: Innovations in management. J Urol 1988; 140:790–792.

Sinno K, Boyce WH, Resnick MI: Childhood urolithiasis. J Urol 1979; 121:662–664.

Stapleton FB, Roy S III, Noe HN, et al: Hypercalciuria in children with hematuria. N Engl J Med 1984; 310:1345–1348.

Williams JL, Cumming WA, Walker RD III, et al: Transitional cell papilloma of the bladder. Pediatr Radiol 1986; 16:322–323.

Woolfield N, Haslam R, LeQuesne G et al: Ultrasound diagnosis of nephrocalcinosis in preterm infants. Arch Dis Child 1988; 63:86–88.

Renal Screening in Patients Who Have Myelodysplasia or Other Neurologic Abnormality

Bauer SB, Hallett M, Khoshbin S, et al: Predictive value of urodynamic evaluation in newborns with myelodysplasia. JAMA 1984; 252:650–652.

Boling RO, Schipul AH Jr, Barnhill DR, et al: Prevalence of neural tube defects in United States Army treatment facilities, 1975–1985; cost analysis of routine screening. Milit Med 1988; 153:293–295.

Gross GW, Boal DK: Sonographic assessment of normal renal size in children with myelodysplasia. J Urol 1988; 140:784–786.

Massagli TL, Jaffe KM, Cardenas DD: Ultrasound measurement of urine volume of children with neurogenic bladder. Dev Med Child Neurol 1990; 32:314–318.

Morcos SK, Thomas DG: A comparison of real-time ultrasonography with intravenous urography in the follow-up of patients with spinal cord injury. Clin Radiol 1988; 39:49–50.

Postoperative Screening of the Urinary Tract

Amis ES Jr, Newhouse JH, Olsson CA: Continent urinary diversions: Review of current surgical procedures and radiologic imaging. Radiology 1988; 168:395–401.

Blake NS, O'Connell E: Endoscopic correction of vesicoureteric reflux by subureteric Teflon injection: Follow-up ultrasound and voiding cystography. Br J Radiol 1989; 62:443–446.

Elder JS, Snyder HM, Hulbert WC, et al: Perforation of the augmented bladder in patients undergoing clean intermittent catheterization. J Urol 1988; 140:1159–1162.

Giuliano CT, Cohen HL, Haller JO, et al: The Sting procedure and its complications: Sonographic evaluation. JCU 1990; 18:415–420.

Gore MD, Fernbach SK, Donaldson JS, et al: Radiographic evaluation of subureteric injection of teflon to correct vesicoureteral reflux. AJR 1989; 152:115–119.

Hertzberg BS, Bowie JD, King LR, et al: Augmentation and replacement cystoplasty: Sonographic findings. Radiology 1987; 165:853–856.

Kroovand RL, Chang CH, Brocker BH: Epithelial lesions of the bladder mucosa following ureteral reimplantation. J Urol 1981; 126:822–826.

Mann CI, Jequier S, Patriquin H, et al: Intramural Teflon injection of the ureter for treatment of vesicoureteral reflux: Sonographic appearance. AJR 1988; 151:543–545.

Mezzacappa PM, Price AP, Kassner EG et al: Cohen ureteral reimplantation: Sonographic appearance. Radiology 1987; 165:851–852.

Cystic Renal Disease

Boal DKB, Teele RL: Sonography of infantile polycystic renal disease. AJR 1980; 135:575–580.

Cachero S, Montgomery P, Seidel FG, et al: Glomerulocystic kidney disease: Case report. Pediatr Radiol 1990; 20:491–493.

Chilcote WA: A simple renal cyst in a child. J Canad Assoc Radiol 1982; 33:51–52.

Davies CH, Stringer DA, Whyte H, et al: Congenital hepatic fibrosis with saccular dilatation of intrahepatic bile ducts and infantile polycystic kidneys. Pediatr Radiol 1985; 16:302–305.

del Senno L, de Paoli Vitali E, Zamorani G, et al: Use of 3'HVR genomic probe for presymptomatic diagnosis of adult polycystic kidney disease in northern Italy: Comparison of DNA analysis and renal ultrasonographic data. Nephrol Dial Transplant 1988; 3:752–755.

Fitch SJ, Stapleton FB: Ultrasonographic features of glomerulocystic disease in infancy: Similarity to infantile polycystic kidney disease. Pediatr Radiol 1986; 16:400–402.

Garel LA, Habib R, Pariente D, et al: Juvenile nephronophthisis: Sonographic appearance in children with severe uremia. Radiology 1984c; 151:93–95.

Glassberg KI, Stephens FD, Lebowitz RL, et al: Renal dysgenesis and cystic disease of the kidney: A report of the committee on terminology, nomenclature and classification, Section on Urology, American Academy of Pediatrics. J Urol 1987; 138:1085–1092.

Gordon RL, Pollack HM, Popky GL, et al: Simple serous cyst of the kidney in children. Radiology 1979; 131:357–366.

Grossman H, Rosenberg ER, Bowie JD, et al: Sonographic diagnosis of renal cystic disease. AJR 1983; 140:81–85.

Hayden CK Jr, Swischuk LE, Smith TH, et al: Renal cystic disease in childhood. Radiographics 1986; 6:97–116.

Kääriäinen H, Jääskeläinen J, Kivisaari L, et al: Dominant and recessive polycystic kidney disease in children: Classification by intravenous pyelography, ultrasound and computed tomography. Pediatr Radiol 1988; 18:45–50.

Landing BH, Gwinn JL, Lieberman E: Cystic diseases of the kidney in children. In Gardner KD Jr (ed): Cystic Diseases of the Kidney. New York: J Wiley, 1976.

McAlister WH, Siegel MJ: Pediatric radiology case of the day. Congenital hepatic fibrosis with saccular dilatation of the intrahepatic bile ducts and infantile polycystic kidneys. AJR 1989; 152:1329–1330.

Melson GL, Shackelford GD, Cole BR, et al: The spectrum of sonographic findings in infantile polycystic kidney disease with urographic and clinical correlations. JCU 1985; 13:113–119.

Mir S, Rapola J, Koskimies O: Renal cysts in pediatric autopsy material. Nephron 1983; 33:189–195.

Narla LD, Slovis TL, Watts FB, et al: The renal lesions of tuberosclerosis (cysts and angiomyolipoma)— Screening with sonography and computerized tomography. Pediatr Radiol 1988; 18:205–209.

Patriquin HB, O'Regan S: Medullary sponge kidney in childhood. AJR 1985; 145:315–319.

Premkumar A, Berdon WE, Levy J, et al: The emergence of hepatic fibrosis and portal hypertension in infants and children with autosomal recessive polycystic kidney disease: Initial and follow-up sonographic and radiographic findings. Pediatr Radiol 1988; 18:123–129.

Reeders ST, Breuning MH, Corney G, et al: Two genetic markers closely linked to adult polycystic kidney disease on chromosome 16. Br Med J 1986; 292:851–853.

Sanders RC, Nussbaum AR, Solez K: Renal dysplasia: Sonographic findings. Radiology 1988; 167:623–626.

Stapleton FB, Bernstein J, Kok G, et al: Cystic kidneys in a patient with oral-facial-digital syndrome type I. Am Kidney Dis 1982; 1:288–293.

Stapleton FB, Hilton S, Wilcox J, et al: Transient nephromegaly simulating infantile polycystic disease of the kidneys. Pediatrics 1981; 67:554–559.

Strand WR, Rushton HG, Markle BM, et al: Autosomal dominant polycystic disease in infants: Asymmetric disease mimicking a unilateral renal mass. J Urol 1989; 141:1151–1153.

Watson ML, Macnicol AM, Wright AF: Adult polycystic kidney disease. Br Med J 1990; 300:62–63.

Worthington JL, Shackelford GD, Cole BR, et al: Sonographically detectable cysts in polycystic kidney disease in newborn and young infants. Pediatr Radiol 1988; 18:287–293.

Wulfsohn MA: Pyelocaliceal diverticula. J Urol 1980; 123:1–8.

Yamagishi F, Kitahara N, Mogi W, et al: Age-related occurrence of simple renal cysts studied by ultrasonography. Klin Wochenschr 1988; 66:385–387.

CHAPTER 7

INFECTION OF THE URINARY TRACT

The investigation of children with infection of the urinary tract (UTI) seems to provoke more argument than in any other subject in pediatric medicine. The type and sequence of studies considered appropriate or necessary vary among hospitals, cities, and nations. We believe that there are very good reasons for these differing points of view. In the following introduction to the subject, we hope to cover the salient points used in the clinical arguments.

The first problem, in the evaluation of any sick child who is suspected of having UTI, is in procuring a specimen of urine for culture. Plastic bags applied to the perineum are notorious for collecting urine contaminated by organisms on the perineum, from stool, or from vaginal flora. In a study of 53 premature babies who had positive cultures from bagged specimens, only 4 had a positive culture from a bladder tap (Edelmann et al., 1973). Midstream collection of urine from a toilet-trained but combative 2-year-old is subject to contamination if the perineum cannot be cleansed adequately. The reliability of clean-voided, midstream specimens increases with the age of the patient. If the sample of urine is not processed rapidly, a spuriously high number of bacterial colonies will grow; the doubling time of *Escherichia coli* in a warm environment is only 30 minutes. Determining a true infection of the urinary tract is established solely with specimens of urine obtained by suprapubic aspiration or catheterization of bladder. The presence of *any* number of bacteria in such specimens is abnormal. The radiologist has to know how rigorously the definition of UTI is applied in the community. Much of the radiologic literature concerning evaluation of UTI is flawed because of its reliance on data from populations for whom infection has been poorly documented.

E. coli is the pathogen most frequently implicated in UTI, causing 90 percent of acute infections in preschool and school-aged children. *Proteus* and *Pseudomonas* species are responsible for many infections acquired in hospitals. *Proteus* is also associated with urinary stones. Staphylococcal infections appear to reach the kidney through the hematogenous route. The presence of adhesins on the bacteria's surface allows certain serogroups of *E. coli* to attach to mucosal cells; the virulence of *E. coli* is enhanced by its elaboration of toxins. The response of the host at a cellular level also dictates whether a given bacterium will cause disease or will be challenged by the host's immune response and be rendered impotent (Winberg et al., 1982;

Lebowitz and Mandell, 1987). Bacterial virulence and the response of the host may vary among communities and populations.

The practice of circumcision varies in frequency among communities. UTI is more prevalent among uncircumcised baby boys than among circumcised boys (Wiswell et al., 1987). Of 100 infants hospitalized for acute UTI and reported in 1982 by Ginsburg and McCracken (pediatricians), 75 were boys, 95 percent of whom were uncircumcised. Abnormal radiographic studies were found in only 4 of 55 boys studied. In contrast, of 83 boys with UTI reported 2 years later by Burbige and colleagues (pediatric urologists), only 8 (10 percent) were reported to be uncircumcised. Abnormal radiographic results were found for 7 of the 17 boys less than 1 year old. The latter study is from a surgical unit in our teaching hospital. Statistics reflect the type of hospital practice from which patients are drawn and the specific interests of the authors.

The objective of early diagnosis and treatment of UTI is prevention of destruction and subsequent scarring of renal parenchyma. The younger the child is, the greater is the risk of renal scarring with infection. If there is an underlying anatomic abnormality of the urinary tract, the child is at even greater risk of parenchymal damage. No one would argue that obstruction should not be surgically relieved if it is severe and associated with urinary infection. The arguments revolve around the uncertainty of how to treat vesicoureteral reflux if it is diagnosed. Children tend to outgrow vesicoureteral reflux as they enter puberty. This phenomenon is supported by several studies, including that of Skoog and coworkers (1987), who showed gradual resolution of reflux in a population of 545 children who were managed without intervention. Reflux of low grade took 20 months, on average, to resolve; reflux of high grades took 24 to 43 months to resolve.

Reflux is dependent on the structure of the ureterovesical junction and the competency of the ureterovesical tunnel. Although reflux is probably not caused by infection, clinical and experimental evidence suggests that ongoing infection affects ureteral peristalsis and prevents resolution of high grades of reflux (Roberts et al., 1988). When, therefore, is reflux a surgical problem, and how much imaging should be mobilized to identify this elusive percentage and the population it represents? The International Vesicoureteral Reflux Study Group was established in 1980 to follow children with moderately severe reflux who were randomly assigned to medical or surgical treatment. Its findings are expected to parallel those of the Birmingham Reflux Study Group (1983), which found no differences, as measured by multiple variables of outcome, between surgically treated and untreated groups.

Depending on where in the world one lives, reflux may or may not be a problem at all. For those of us who see the world from a North American vantage point, it is important to remember that the prevalence of vesicoureteral reflux varies with race; for example, in black children, reflux associated with UTI is distinctly uncommon (Askari and Belman, 1982).

Reflux nephropathy is the scarring and caliceal clubbing that results from waves of bacteria-laden urine reaching the kidneys on the tides of reflux. However, some authors have expressed the opinion that infection is not always necessary for reflux nephropathy to occur (Shindo et al., 1983). They believe that reflux under high pressure (typically that found with distal obstruction) can cause scarring in the absence of infection. However, scars may take months or years to develop. Thus their exact genesis, whether from infected or sterile urine, may never be known.

The demands on imaging depend, to some extent, on the referring physicians. The interests of the pediatrician are not necessarily those of the urologic surgeon. Imaging is invasive. A voiding study, whether done with fluoroscopy or with scanning after the instillation of radionuclide, requires catheterization or suprapubic puncture. Voiding cystourethrography and intravenous urography rely on ionizing radiation. Because the gonads are close neighbors of the urinary tract, the irradiation is regarded with more concern, certainly by the parents, than is irradiation of other parts of the body. We do not perform ultrasonographic evaluation to diagnose reflux, although it has its advocates (Schneider et al., 1984; Kessler and Altman, 1982). (See section on hydronephrosis in Chapter 8 for further discussion.) Intravenous urography depends on injection of contrast material with its rare but known hazards. Imaging is inconsistently available; for example, facilities for performing good radionuclide voiding studies in children may or may not be available in the community. Ultrasonography is only as good as the equipment and operator, and in a cost-conscious environment, there is no doubt that comprehensive imaging is very costly.

Our practice at present is to evaluate, with an initial radiographic cystogram, each child who is 5 years of age or younger and who has had well-documented UTI. Otherwise, the evaluation and sequence of studies vary, depending on clinical evaluation and age of the patient. We try to tailor the examinations in order to avoid duplication, to minimize invasiveness, and to maximize information gained. Our policies are based on our experience in a pediatric hospital in the northeastern U.S. that serves as both a referral center and a primary care facility. There are currently five genitourinary surgeons on the staff, and this group has been particularly interested in UTI. The institution is participating in the International Vesicoureteral Reflux Study. There is access to all modalities of imaging within the department of radiology. We are lucky to be surrounded by modern technology, interested clinicians, an expert uroradiologist, and excellent technologists. Much of the world is not as luxuriously endowed.

The baby aged 1 year or younger who presents with acute UTI usually has nonspecific signs: fever, irritability, and perhaps

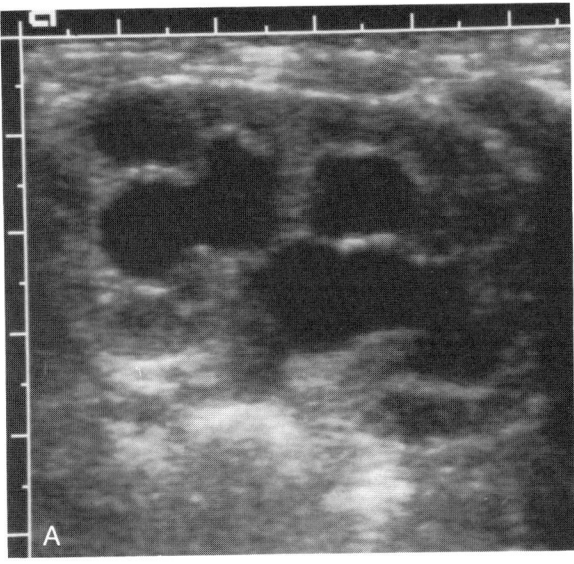
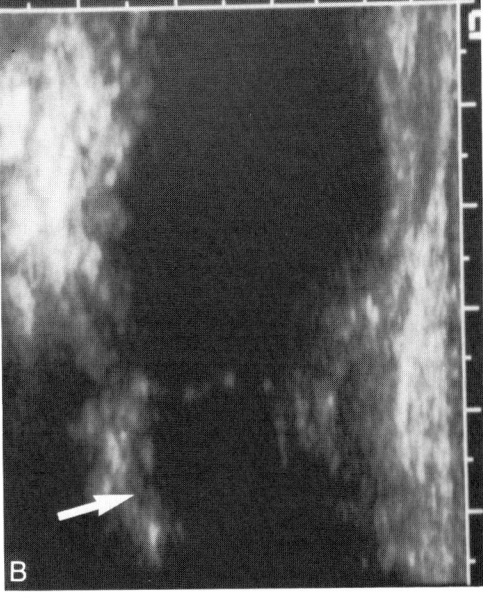
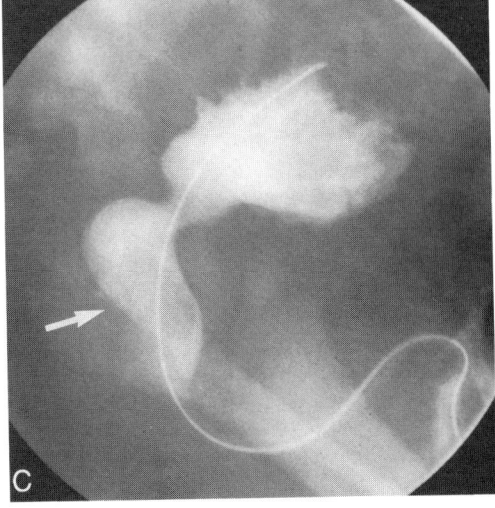

Figure 7–1. Ultrasonography was performed when this 2-week-old boy was admitted to hospital for vomiting, dehydration, and a temperature of 39.8°C. Urine sent for culture grew more than 100,000 colonies of *Escherichia coli*. Longitudinal scans of each kidney were similar: each showed a hydronephrotic kidney (**A**). Scans of the bladder were unusual: the bladder was not grossly distended but had an irregular wall, and this irregularity was associated with dilation of the posterior urethra (arrow) extending below the symphysis pubis on the longitudinal scan (**B**). (**B** is oriented to match **C**.) The baby was immediately studied with voiding cystourography. This lateral view (**C**) shows the obstruction to be from posterior urethral valve. There was no reflux. When bilateral hydronephrosis is diagnosed in a boy, the possibility of posterior urethral valve should always be considered.

vomiting. Often, no single finding differentiates upper from lower tract infections. The first imaging performed in this acute situation is ultrasonography. Scans are used to evaluate renal size; parenchymal appearance; degree of caliceal, pelvic, and ureteral dilation; size and configuration of bladder; and thickness of vesical wall. The scan serves to triage patients, identifying those who need immediate radiologic evaluation and surgical attention (Fig. 7–1). Congenital obstruction at the ureteropelvic, ureterovesical, or urethral levels is usually easily detected because not only has obstruction been chronic, since at least the last trimester in utero, but infection tends to render the urinary tract aperistaltic. Dilation may also result from severe vesicoureteral reflux. Clues to its presence in infants include a small kidney on the side of the reflux, poor delineation of the medullary-cortical interface, and variability in the size of the ureter and renal pelvis during scanning (Figs. 7–2, 7–3, 7–4). Occasionally, a reversal of ureteric peristalsis or a patulous ureterovesical junction may be detected. If the ultrasonograms are normal, voiding cystourethrography is delayed for 4 to 6 weeks. This is no magical interval of time; rather, it allows

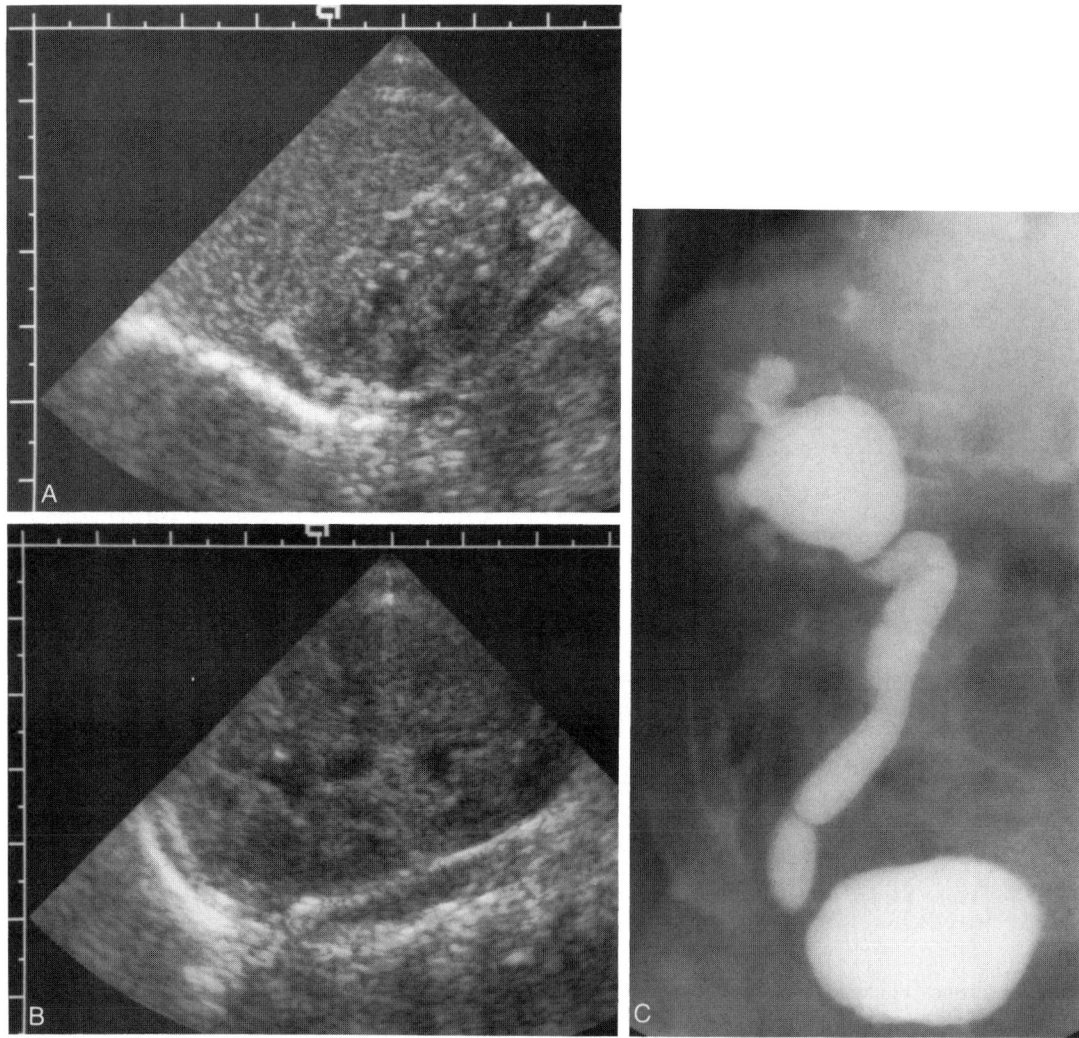

Figure 7–2. Prenatal ultrasonography had revealed right-sided hydronephrosis in this baby. Postnatal scan showed, not hydronephrosis, but an obvious discrepancy in the size of the two kidneys. Note the smaller right kidney on this longitudinal scan (A) in comparison with the large, plump left-sided kidney (B). Voiding cystourethrography (C) shows grade 4 to 5 reflux into the right kidney. Reimplantation of the right ureter followed.

the baby to recover and also allows the urinary tract, if it has been paralyzed to any extent by bacterial endotoxins, to return to its usual state. A sample of urine cultured at the time of catheterization for voiding cystourethrography provides the clinician with bacteriologic follow-up. Smellie and associates (1985) recommended that antimicrobial therapy be extended for all patients with UTI until radiographic studies of the urinary tract were done. This recommendation was based on a study of 69 patients who developed renal scars; 68 were shown to have vesicoureteral reflux when studied.

Radionuclide, rather than radiographic, cystography may be more sensitive to the presence or absence of reflux. However, its lack of anatomic detail of the posterior urethra and bladder, and the lack of standardization in grading reflux, makes it less than ideal for this young age group.

For the 1- to 5-year-old child who has UTI that responds quickly to antimicrobial therapy, and for older children with clinical pyelonephritis that responds within 2 or 3 days to treatment, the first study is a radiographic voiding cystourethrogram. This is performed when the child is asymptomatic, has completed a course of treatment, and is continuing to receive prophylaxis. Reflux is graded I through V according to the international system that was created in 1980 as part of the collaborative study of reflux (Fig. 7–5). If reflux is severe (i.e., grade III to V), the catheter is left in place to drain the bladder during excretory urography. In this situation, reflux cannot occur and therefore cannot mimic urinary function. If reflux is minor or absent, the child comes to ultrasonography for assessment of renal size, parenchymal pattern, and caliceal abnormalities. In spite of previous normal cystography, we always look at the bladder with ultrasonography. Usually there is nothing abnormal to be seen, but occasionally we find distal ureteric dilation from primary megaureter, discover a ureterocele that was inapparent, show that vaginal reflux has occurred, or even spot a calculus that was invisible on cystography (Fig. 7–6). Infection of the lower tract is commonly accompanied by mild thickening of the wall of the bladder (Fig. 7–7).

In any child at any age, renal scarring from an acute episode of pyelonephritis takes weeks to months to develop. We certainly do not see many children with a renal scar from a recent infection at the 4- to 6-week follow-up. Ultrasonography during the acute episode may show a localized area of parenchymal abnormality within the kidney—hyperechogenic or hypoechogenic—that represents an area of acute inflammation, so-called

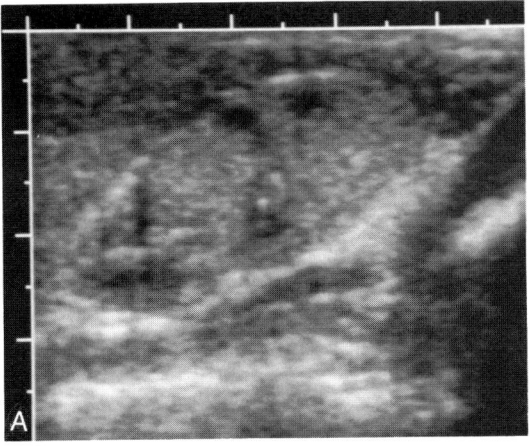
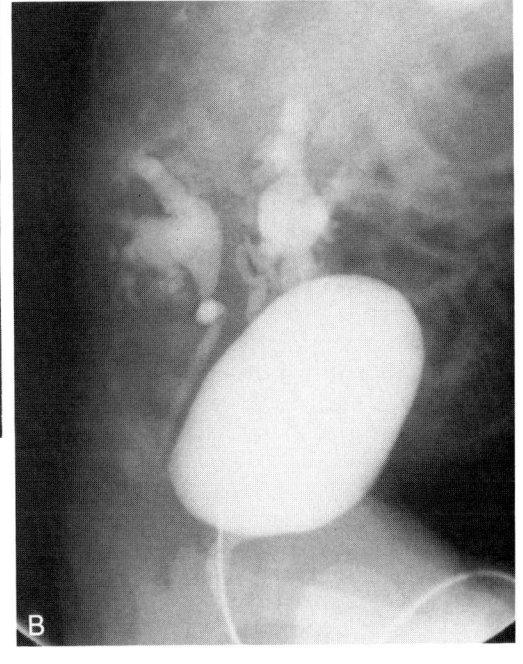

Figure 7–3. Poor delineation of medullary-cortical interface may result from dysplasia associated with reflux. This is a longitudinal scan of the right kidney (A) in a two-month-old. Note the small size of the kidney. The left kidney was similar in its appearance. Voiding cystourethrogram (B) showed bilateral grade 4, and intrarenal, reflux.

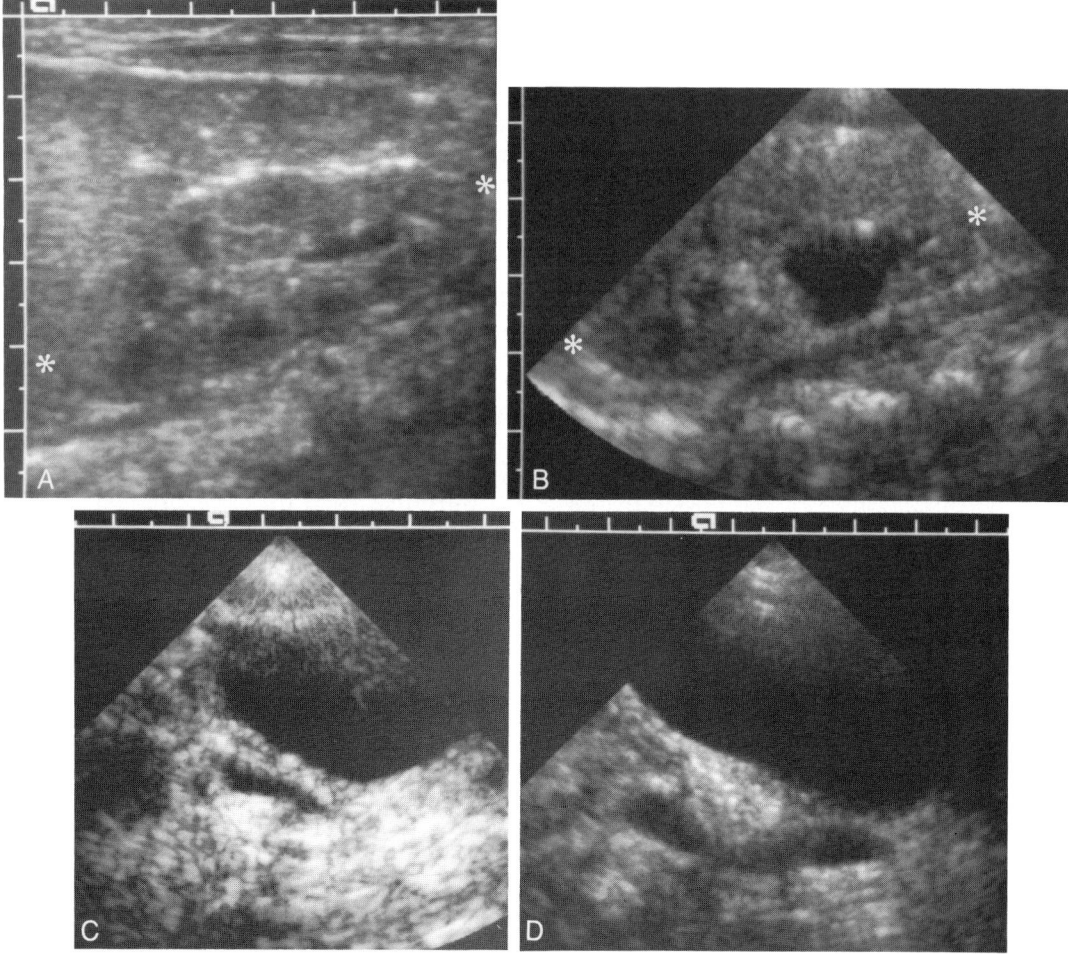

Figure 7–4. Ultrasonography was performed for this 7-week-old girl after sepsis from infection of the urinary tract was diagnosed. On the scan, it was apparent that the pelvis of the lower pole of a duplex left kidney was changing in size (**A** and **B**). When the bladder was scanned, it was also apparent that a ureter on the left side was variable in size (**C** and **D**). The ultrasonographic study was followed by a voiding cystourethrogram, which showed grade 4 reflux into the lower pole of the duplex kidney on the left side. There was also grade II reflux on the right side, which we had not detected on ultrasonography.

lobar nephronia (Fig. 7–8). Localized medullary echogenicity may represent areas affected by intrarenal reflux (Diard et al., 1987), although there is rarely ultrasonographic evidence of this phenomenon. There is no question that ultrasonography is less sensitive in identifying focal inflammation than are radionuclide scans in which a cortical labeling agent, Tc99m glucoheptonate or dimercaptosuccinate (DMSA), is used (Traisman et al., 1986; Verber et al., 1988). To prove acute renal parenchymal involvement, such studies have to be done. We see our role in ultrasonography as identifying children who have had scarring from previous, unrecognized UTI and who therefore may be at greater risk for sustained damage to their kidneys and as finding the children with underlying anatomic abnormality. We assume that any child who has documented UTI will be carefully followed with cultures of urine when the course of antimicrobial therapy is over.

Older children (generally girls between 5 and 10 years of age) who have signs of infection of only the lower urinary tract are investigated with nuclear cystography. If the results are normal, ultrasonography follows to assess renal size, the parenchymal pattern, and collecting systems. Intravenous urography (IVU) follows if there is evidence of underlying structural anomaly. This group may be equally well served by "indirect"

INFECTION OF THE URINARY TRACT / 199

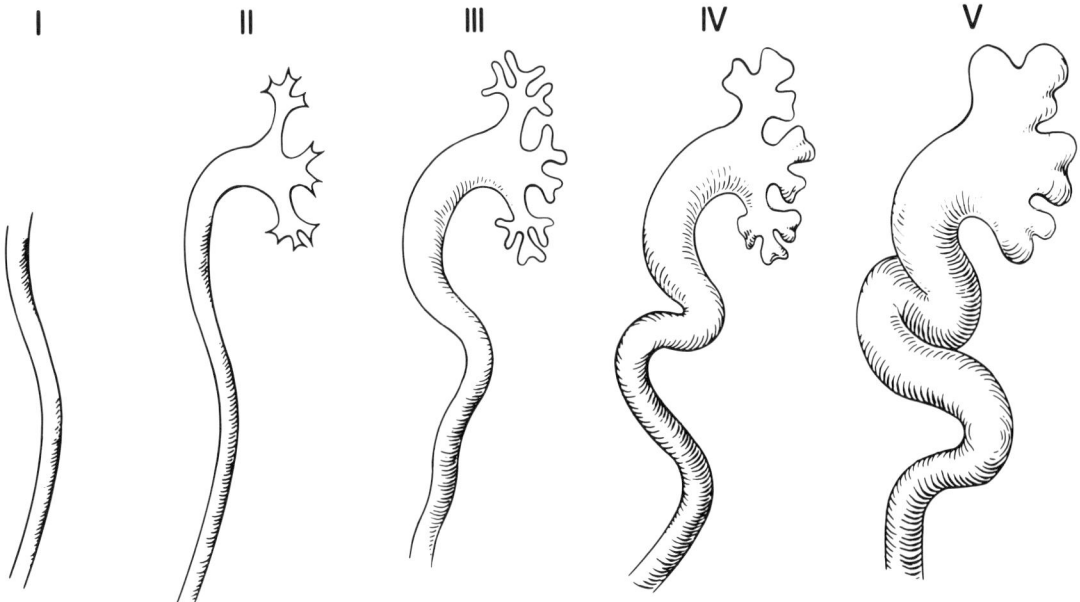

Figure 7–5. Grading I to V of vesicoureteral reflux was established for the International Reflux Study. (Photograph courtesy of Dr. Robert Lebowitz, Department of Radiology, Children's Hospital, Boston.)

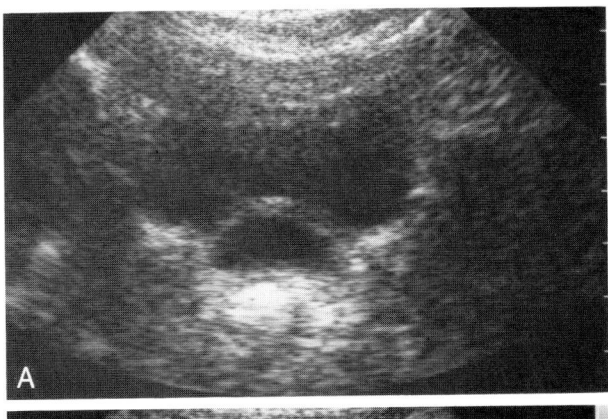
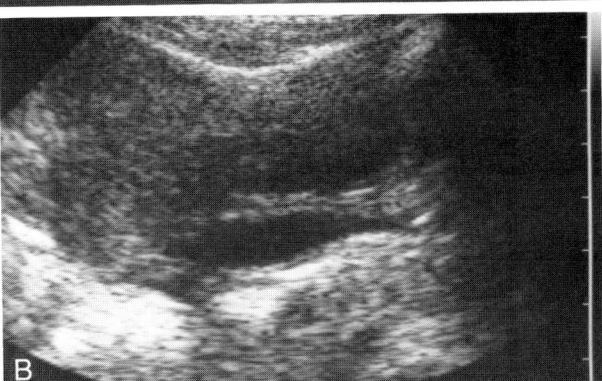
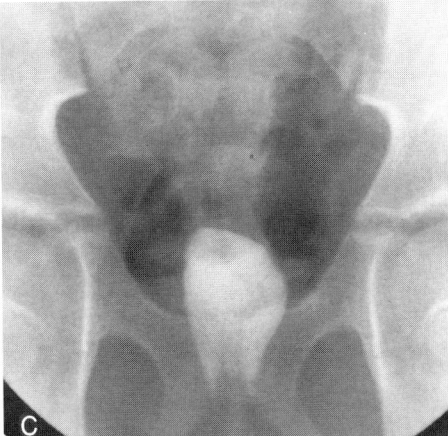

Figure 7–6. Vaginal reflux of urine may present a puzzling ultrasonographic picture to people who are not aware that it occurs in girls. Transverse (A) and longitudinal (B) scans of the pelvis show a lucent mass immediately posterior to the bladder. A view of the pelvis taken after a voiding cystourethrogram and after the bladder is completely emptied is shown for reference. The contrast is in the vagina (C).

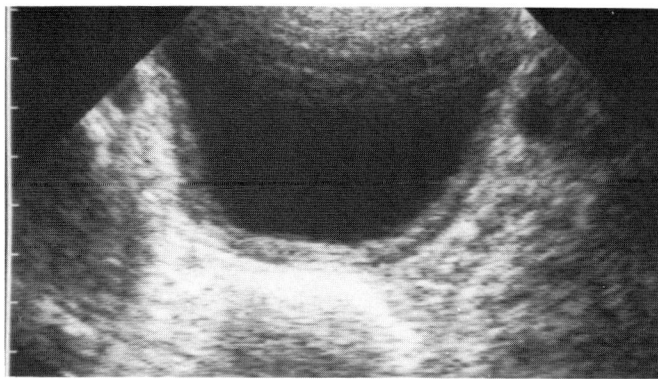

Figure 7-7. Slight thickening of the bladder wall is often associated with cystitis, as in this boy who presented with his first documented urinary tract infection *(E. coli)*. He had frequency, dysuria, and hematuria. A voiding cystourethrogram showed no reflux.

cystography (Chapman et al., 1988). This procedure involves intravenous injection of ^{99m}Tc diethylenetriamine penta-acetic acid (DTPA), measurement of split renal function, diuresis induced by ingested fluid, and then scanning during voiding. Other researchers feel that there are too many false-negative results for this technique to replace standard radionuclide cystography (Conway, 1983, cited by Hodson et al., 1984), but this procedure warrants further study because it avoids catheterization, which many patients and parents find objectionable.

The oldest children and adolescents who present with their first UTI are scanned with ultrasonography. Any abnormality that is discovered is further evaluated. We have seen the rare patient who presents at this age with severe reflux nephropathy. Careful review of the patient's history usually reveals evidence of earlier UTI that was overlooked or masked by antibiotics given for other illness (Fig. 7-9).

These protocols for older children are based on the facts that (1) incidence of reflux decreases in the population of children as they age, (2) scarring with reflux and infection generally affects children younger than 5 years, and (3) children older than 5 years are generally able to distinguish symptoms of infection in the lower tract from those in the upper tract.

It is important to emphasize that in any age group, neither normal results of ultraso-

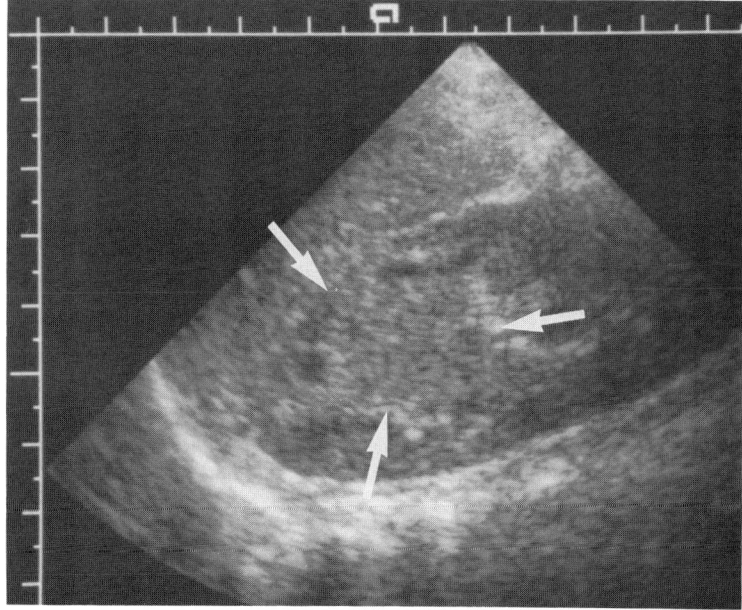

Figure 7-8. *Escherichia coli* was grown from cultures of blood and of urine from this 2-year-old girl, who was admitted to the hospital for fever, vomiting, and a white blood cell count of 21,900. An echogenic focus in the upper pole of the right kidney (arrows) shown on this longitudinal scan represented focal infection in the kidney. Treatment was instituted immediately, and follow-up scans 8 days later showed resolution of the infection.

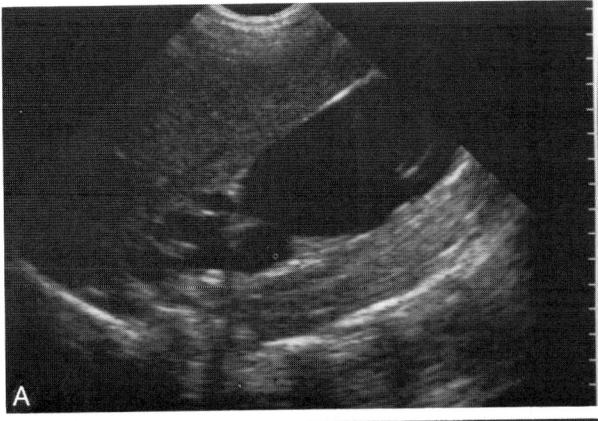
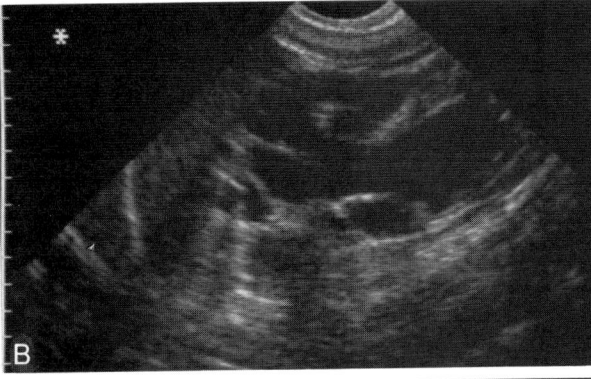
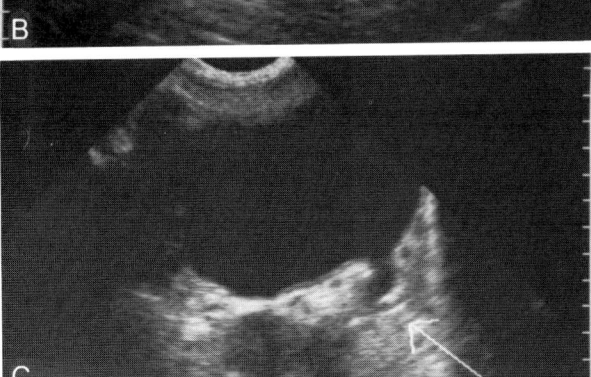
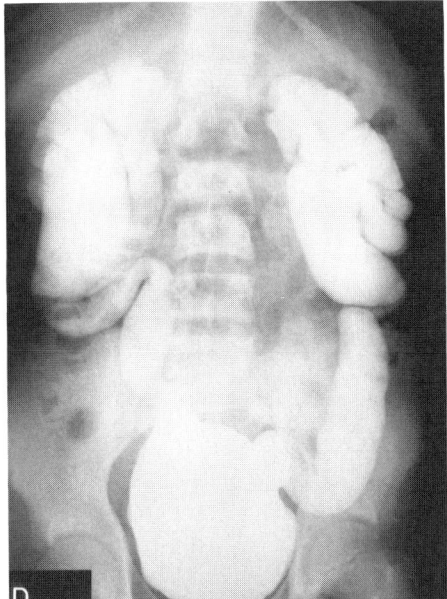

Figure 7–9. End-stage renal disease that is secondary to reflux and infection is usually diagnosed before adolescence. This adolescent, who presented with urinary tract infection, had a creatinine level of 7. Ultrasonography showed severe scarring of right (A) and left (B) kidneys that was associated with massive dilation of the collecting systems. Transverse scan of the bladder (C) showed a patulous ureterovesical junction on the left (arrow). A voiding cystourethrogram was done immediately, and bilateral reflux was shown to be the cause of the patient's renal failure (D).

nography nor normal results of excretory urography rule out the possibility of significant reflux. Of 133 patients with reflux who were studied at our institution, half (14) of those with grade III reflux (28) and more than a third (4) with grade IV reflux (11) had normal excretory findings on urography (Fig. 7–10; Blickman et al., 1985).

Although some authors have advocated ultrasonography as a means of diagnosing vesicoureteral reflux (Kessler and Altman, 1982; Schneider et al., 1984), we believe it to be unreliable, especially for the younger age groups. It is an invasive procedure because catheterization is needed (see the section on hydronephrosis in Chapter 8 for further discussion).

Ultrasonography should be available for any child of any age who is ill with acute UTI and not responding as expected to clinical management. Although acute pyelonephritis may not always be revealed ultrasonographically as a parenchymal abnormality, there are other clues to its presence: (1) the kidney does not move well with respiration; (2) the perinephric outline is indistinct, and perinephric tissues are thickened; (3) the affected kidney appears swollen

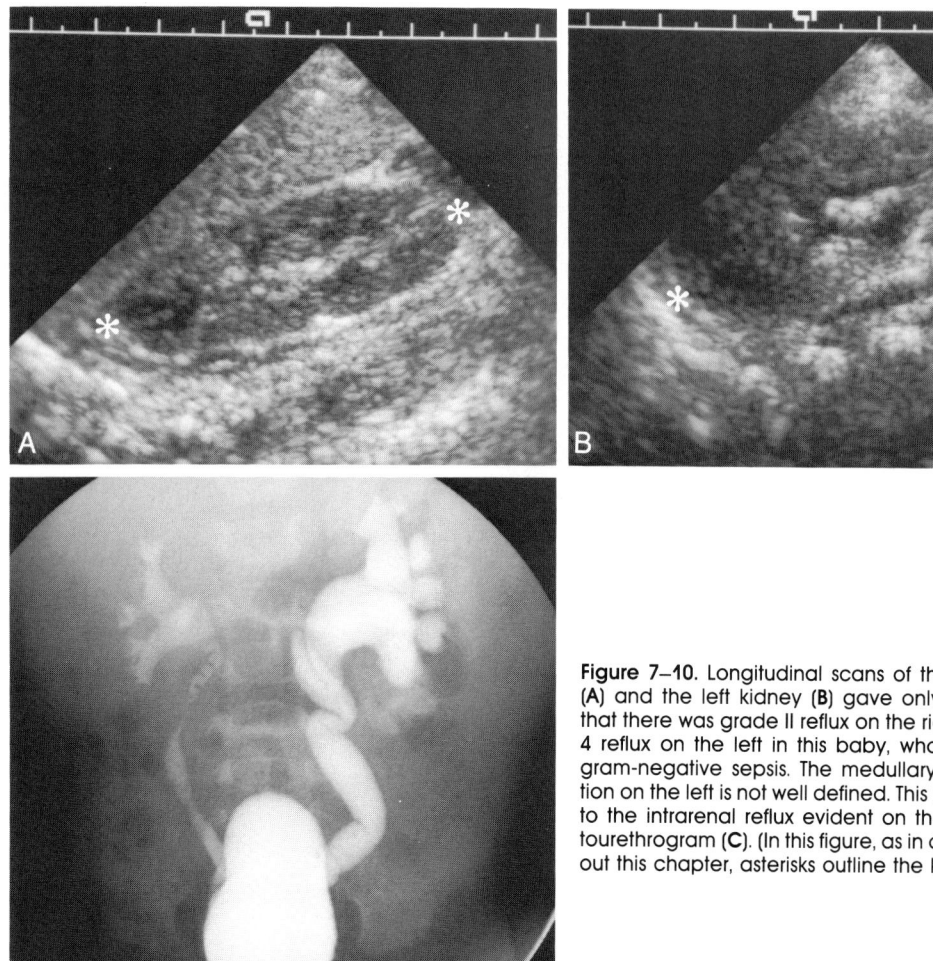

Figure 7-10. Longitudinal scans of the right kidney (A) and the left kidney (B) gave only a subtle hint that there was grade II reflux on the right and grade 4 reflux on the left in this baby, who presented in gram-negative sepsis. The medullary-cortical junction on the left is not well defined. This is likely related to the intrarenal reflux evident on the voiding cystourethrogram (C). (In this figure, as in others throughout this chapter, asterisks outline the kidney.)

in comparison with its mate; and (4) thickening of ureteric and renal pelvic wall from edema may occur (Fig. 7-11; Avni et al., 1988). Complications of pyelonephritis include (1) renal carbuncle, (2) perinephric abscess, and (3) pyonephrosis. Renal carbuncle or abscess in its early stages may be difficult to differentiate from lobar nephronia because it is a continuation of the infective process (Fig. 7-12). In later stages, the abscess is a more spherical, rimmed mass (Fig. 7-13). If the bacterial pathogen is known from cultures of urine, antimicrobial therapy at high dosages is usually curative. If bacterial proof of infection is lacking, or if the abscess is not resolving with antibiotic therapy, the cavity can be drained percutaneously. This achieves diagnostic and therapeutic goals. A small pigtail catheter is left in place if the cavity is large; complete aspiration typically is curative. A Wilms tumor may occasionally mimic a renal abscess, and vice versa. Actually, Wilms tumor is a more common cause of intrarenal mass than is an abscess. The ultrasonographer should be aware of this differential diagnosis and discuss the clinical context with the physicians involved. Percutaneous manipulation of a Wilms tumor is contraindicated because the staging of the tumor may be increased with transgression of the pseudocapsule.

Pyonephrosis is pus in an obstructed system. In our experience, it is more common a presentation in babies than in older children

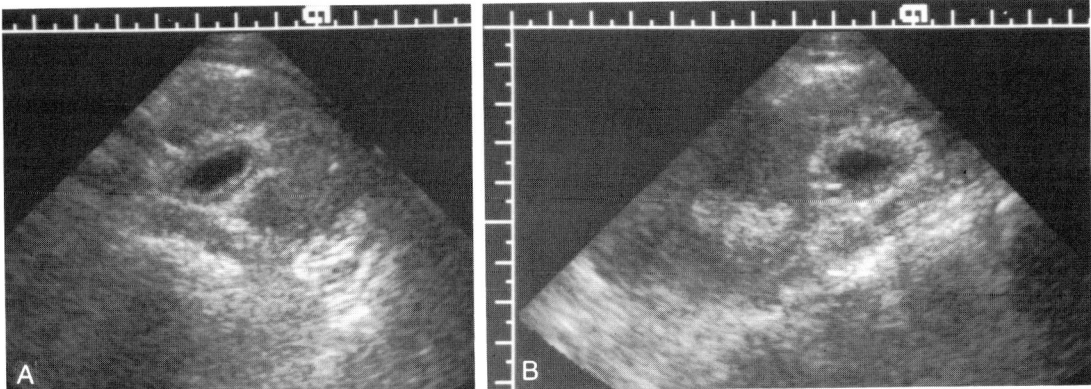

Figure 7–11. Transverse (A) and longitudinal (B) ultrasonograms show submucosal edema of the renal pelvis of the lower pole of this left kidney. Symptoms were certainly consistent with a urinary tract infection, but cultures grew no bacteria, probably because this child had earlier received antibiotic therapy.

(Fig. 7–14). The cellular debris may completely fill a hydronephrotic system or may layer, creating a fluid/sludge level. Echogenic debris from desquamated cells and crystalline material may be present in an obstructed system that is not infected. Children who have pyonephrosis are usually quite ill with high fever and neutrophilia, and Gram stains of spun urine are positive for bacteria. If there is no immediate response to aggressive treatment with appropriate antibiotics, drainage of the obstructed system through percu-

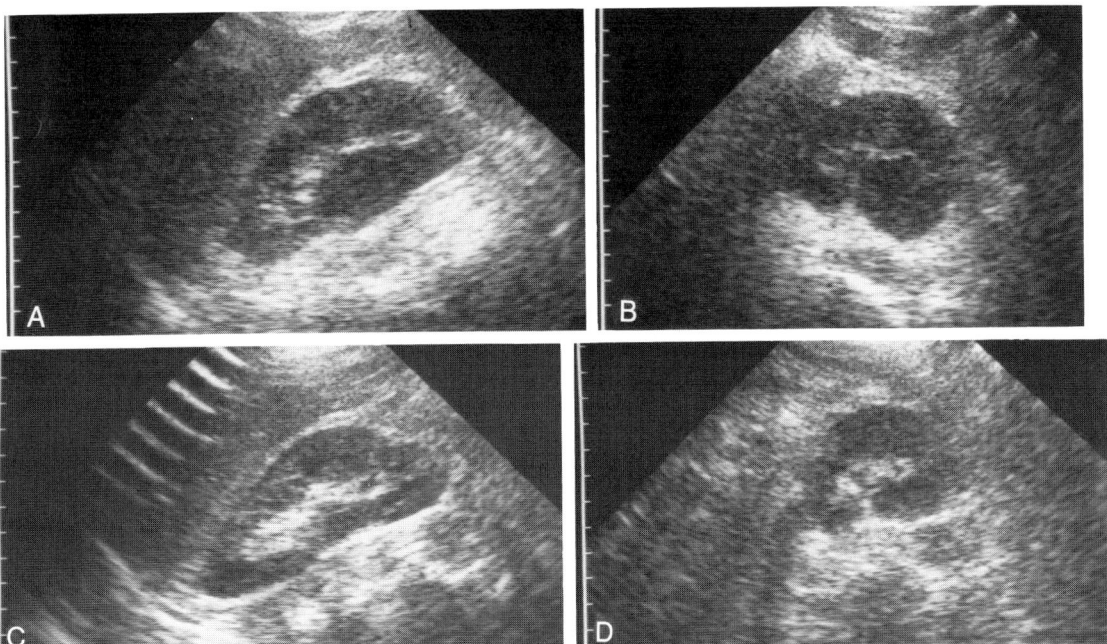

Figure 7–12. Renal abscess may simulate intrarenal tumor in some patients. This 8-year-old girl had had a documented urinary tract infection about 5 weeks before admission to the hospital. One day before admission, she had recurrent left-sided flank pain, which had increased in severity. Her white blood cell count was 19,000, and she was admitted to the hospital after this ultrasonographic study, which shows a mass in the left kidney on both coronal (A) and transverse (B) scans. Evaluation included radionuclide and computed tomography (CT) scans, which supported the diagnosis of abscess. One milliliter of pus was aspirated from the kidney and grew *E. coli*. Intensive antibiotic therapy was instituted, and 1 month later a normal kidney was shown on coronal (C) and transverse (D) scans.

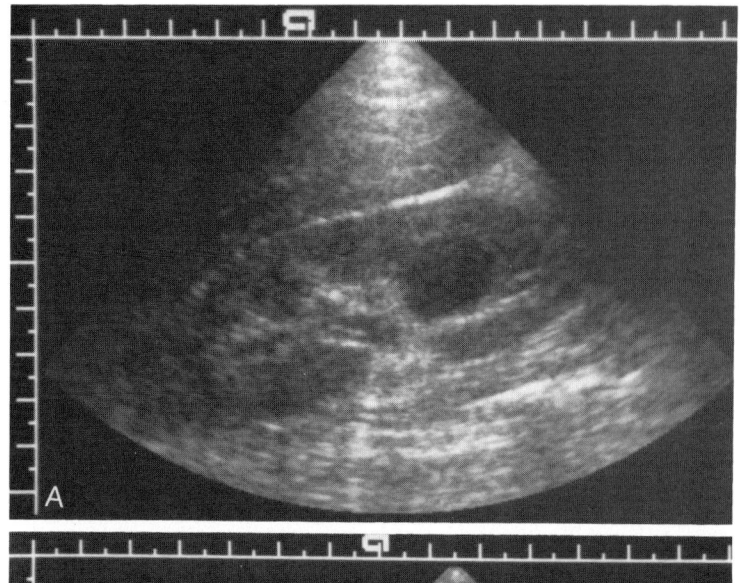

Figure 7–13. Established renal abscess is usually well defined, as in this patient, who presented only with fever without source. The coronal scan of the left kidney (**A**) shows an abscess in the lower pole. Follow-up scans 1 month later (**B**) show no residual abscess after treatment with antibiotics.

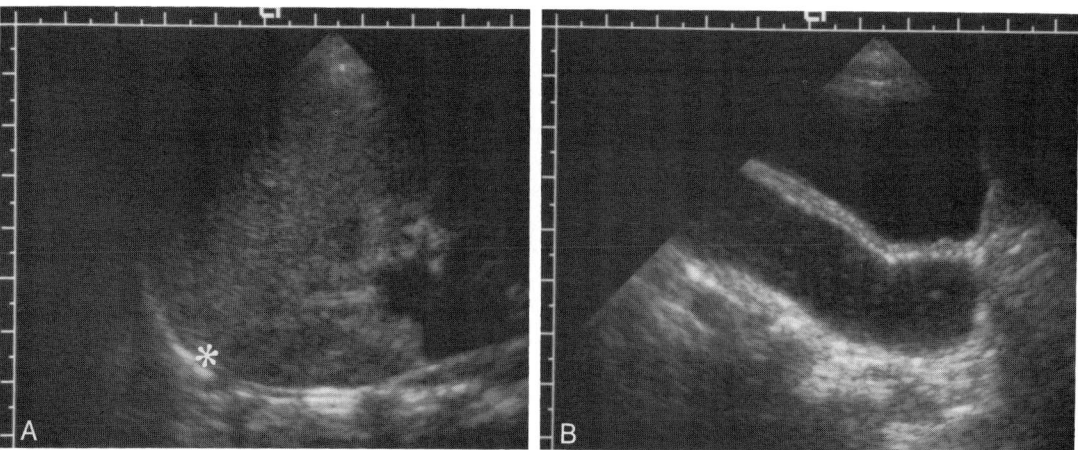

Figure 7–14. Although the renal pelvis was relatively echo free, as seen on the coronal view of the left kidney (**A**), the dilated ureter, which extended along the posterior wall of the bladder, was filled with debris (**B**). These scans were obtained for a 16-month-old boy who presented to the emergency room with a 24-hour history of shaking, chills, temperatures up to 40.5°C, and a white blood cell count of 28,000. Cultures of urine and blood grew *E. coli*. The baby responded to intensive antibiotic therapy and did not require percutaneous drainage of the obstructed system. Repair of the primary megaureter was achieved when the infection had cleared.

taneous catheter achieves clearance of the infection. Surgery is performed when cultures of urine are sterile (Fig. 7–15).

When a kidney has been damaged by pyelonephritis, whether reflux is associated or not, scarring occurs. There is evidence to suggest that rapid institution of antimicrobial therapy at the onset of disease may prevent such damage. Therapeutic delay is rarely addressed in papers on the sequelae of urinary infection (Winberg et al., 1982). Over time—and this may be months to years—focal thinning of the cortex in the region of previous infection may occur (Fig. 7–16).

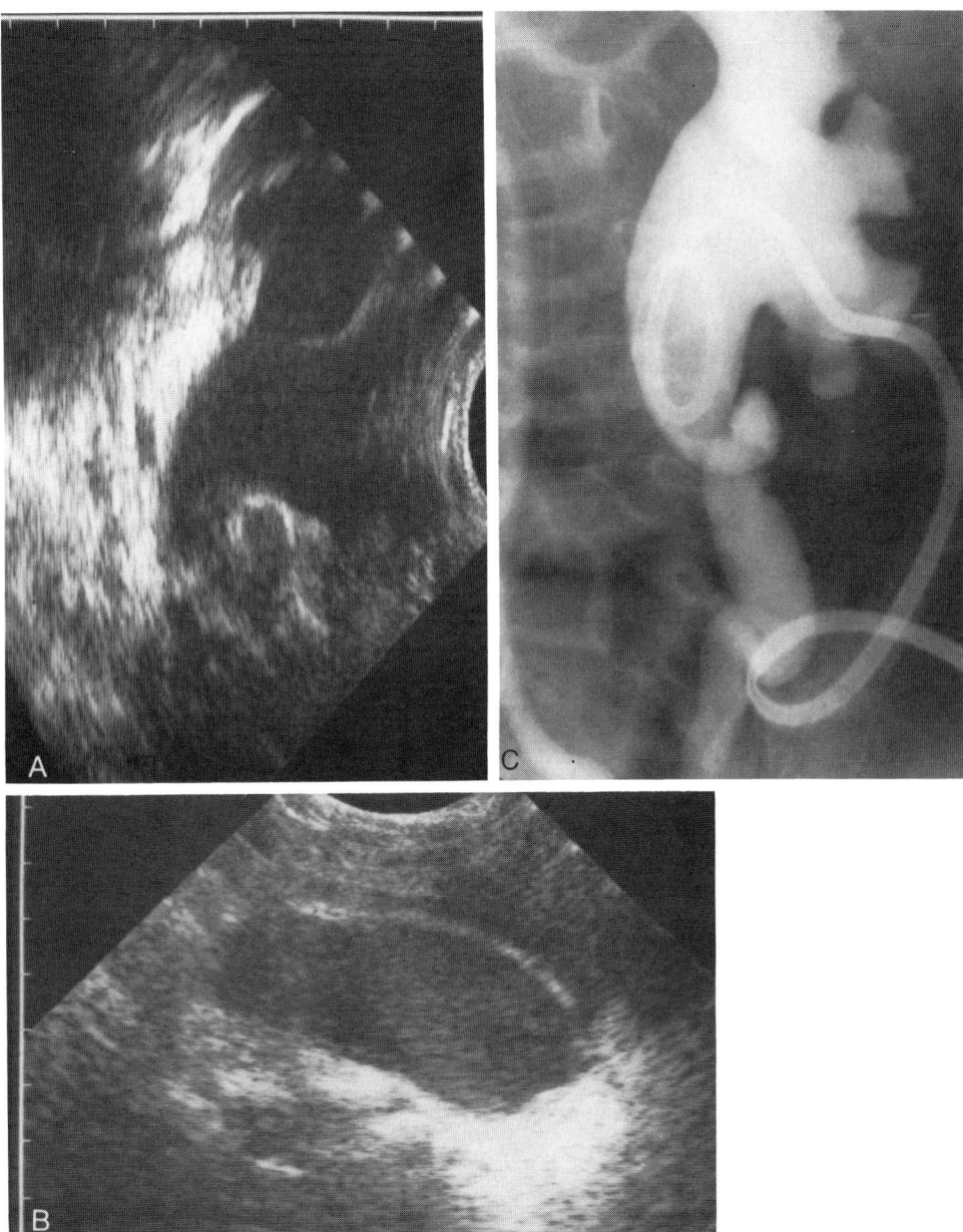

Figure 7–15. Left-sided hydroureteronephrosis in this 13-month-old boy was secondary to primary megaureter. He presented with urinary infection secondary to *Proteus mirabilis*. Prompt response to antibiotics did not occur, and he underwent drainage through percutaneous nephrostomy. Note the debris throughout the dilated renal collecting system on the coronal scan (A). Debris in the distal dilated ureter is evident on a longitudinal scan of the pelvis (B). Study with contrast (C) followed percutaneous nephrostomy by several days. Ultrasonogram (A) is oriented to match radiograph (C).

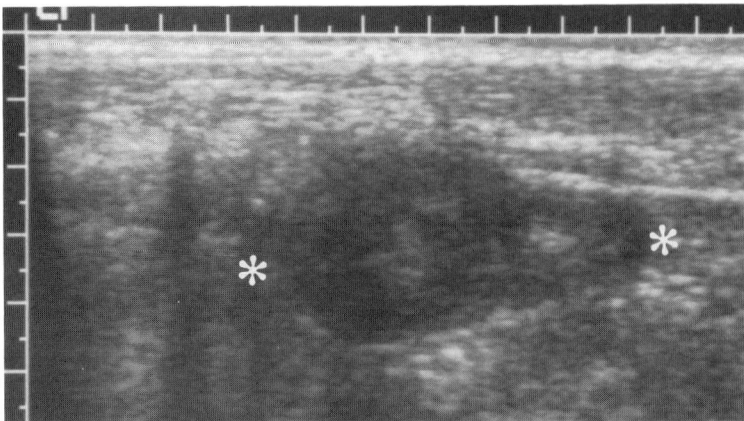

Figure 7–16. Longitudinal scan of the right kidney shows parenchymal thinning of the lower pole of a duplex system. The scan is of a 5-year-old who had a long history of multiple urinary tract infections. She had undergone bilateral reimplantation of the ureters 1 year before this ultrasonographic study.

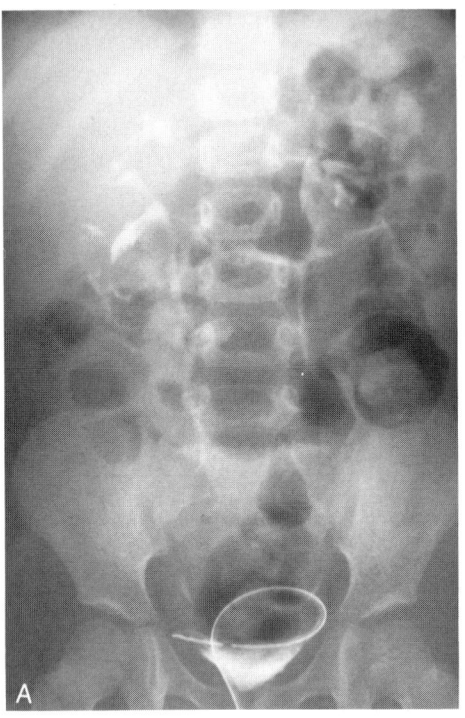
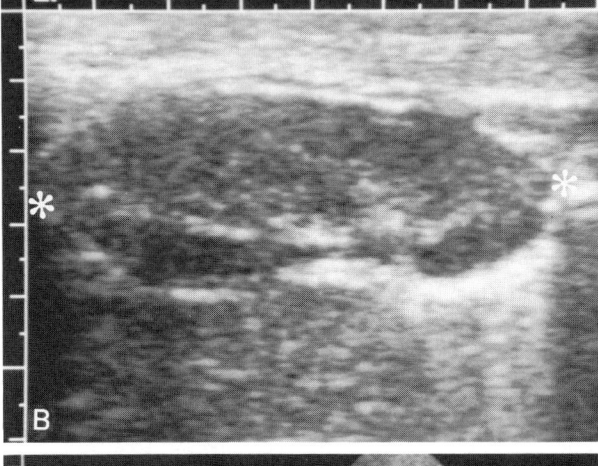
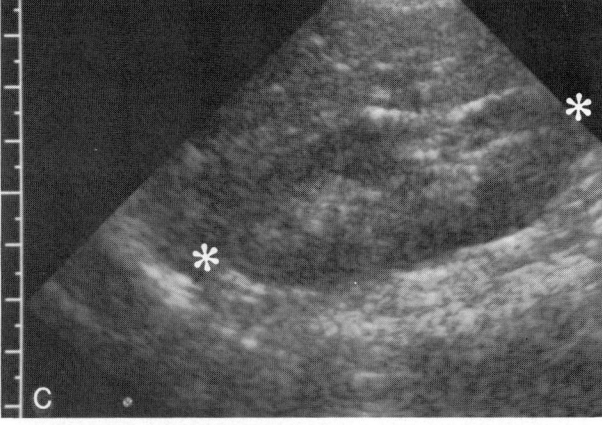
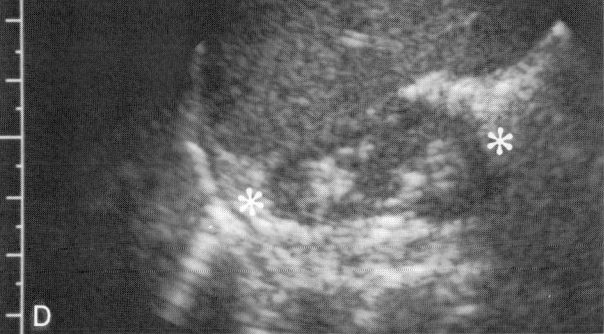

Figure 7–17. This 3½-year-old girl had had two documented episodes of urinary tract infection when she was evaluated with voiding cystourethrography. This showed bilateral grade III to IV reflux. Prophylactic therapy with antibiotics failed to suppress the infection, and she underwent bilateral cross-trigonal ureteral reimplantation. Follow-up intravenous urogram (**A**) shows bilaterally scarred kidneys. Note how scarring is manifest on ultrasonograms as focal parenchymal thinning. The prone longitudinal scan of the right kidney (**B**) shows the echoes of the collecting system closer than normal to the anterior edge of the kidney. The supine longitudinal scan (**C**) also shows the anterior thinning. The obviously small left kidney (**D**) has suffered global parenchymal loss.

There has been great debate over which method of imaging is best for detecting scars. Monsour and colleagues (1987) reiterated what others had previously stated: radionuclide scans with DMSA, especially in children aged 0 to 2 years, are more sensitive than other methods of detecting scarring. If therapy and follow-up are driven by the presence of scars, one can make the argument that every child younger than 5 years who presents with a UTI should have a DMSA scan. If therapy and follow-up are not dependent on the presence of scarring alone, one can use IVU or ultrasonography, which are less sensitive to scarring but provide more information regarding anatomy and, with IVU, physiology of the renal tract. One should remember that all the vast literature on pediatric urinary infection before about 1978 relied on IVU for data concerning the prevalence of scarring. Current literature should be viewed with the realization that the prevalence of scarring may change, not as a result of the disease necessarily, but as a result of the techniques used to measure it.

To evaluate the kidneys for scarring, ultrasonic scanning must be done in at least two planes; three—sagittal, coronal, and transverse—are ideal (Fig. 7–17). The upper pole of the left kidney is the most difficult to assess properly. The left upper pole is often unusual in shape and is tucked behind a variable splenic window, behind an artifact-producing stomach, and between ticklish ribs (Fig. 7–18). The unusual conglomerate lucency, produced by fusion of the medullary pyramids, which is associated with a complex papilla and which typically is polar, should not be mistaken for abnormal renal parenchyma (Fig. 7–19). A linear interface on sagittal or coronal scans of the medial portions of kidney represents a plane of connective tissue between the inferior and superior reniculi. On transverse sections this presents as a V-shaped defect (a junctional parenchymal defect) in the anteromedial aspect of the kidney. This normal finding should not be

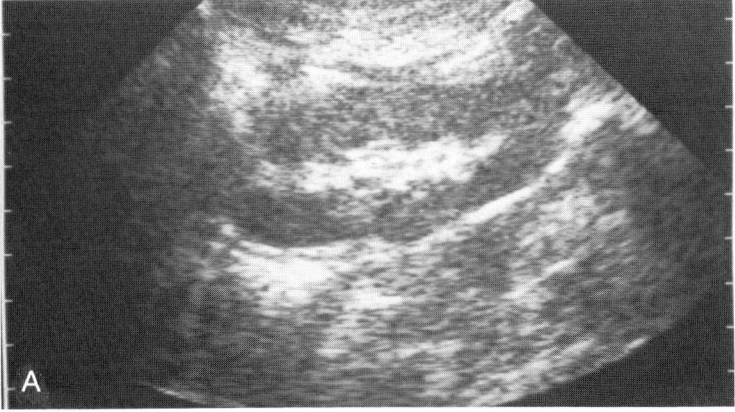
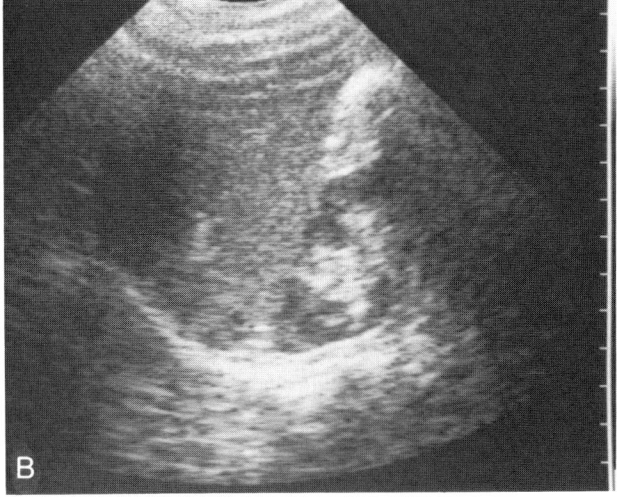

Figure 7–18. Prone longitudinal scan of the left kidney (A) shows the echoes from the collecting system extending toward the edge of the parenchyma in the upper pole. However, artifact from the overlying ribs makes identification of the true renal edge difficult on prone views. To evaluate the upper pole more completely, we rely on coronal views through the spleen (B). The echoes from the collecting system are obviously abutting the edge of the renal outline on this view. This represents severe scarring in the left upper pole.

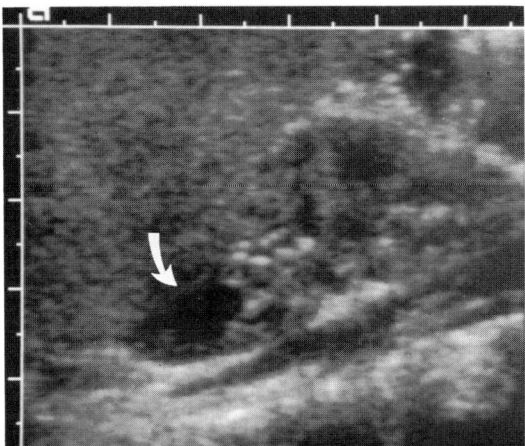

Figure 7–19. Compound pyramid in the upper pole of the kidney should not be mistaken for abnormal parenchyma or even a renal cyst. This 2½-month-old has a normal left kidney with a very prominent, lucent, compound pyramid (arrow).

mistaken for a scar (Fig. 7–20; Hoffer et al., 1985). Caliectasis is frequently associated with focal parenchymal thinning on urography because ionic contrast media provides a diuretic load to the kidney that distends the collecting system. Unless there is ongoing reflux or obstruction, the calices generally are collapsed during ultrasonography, and caliectasis is covert (Fig. 7–21). Comparison of renal volume is the most reliable method by which to assess renal growth over time but only if carefully performed. Renal length is a more gross measure of renal growth but is more easily reproduced. There are charts that provide the range of normal measurements based on age, height and weight, or body surface area (see Chapter 6). These charts are useful if precise measurements can be obtained and if follow-up scans are performed with the same equipment, which is accurately calibrated. Linear array and mechanical sector scanners used to measure the same organ do not always give the same result. For purposes of measurement, the entire kidney should be included on the field of view of the scan. A typical routine for ultrasonography of the kidneys after a normal voiding cystourethrogram (VCUG) is (1) prone sagittal views of each kidney for measurements, (2) prone transverse views of each kidney, (3) supine coronal views with special attention to the upper renal poles, and (4) views of the bladder in transverse and longitudinal planes. Scans of the bladder are left

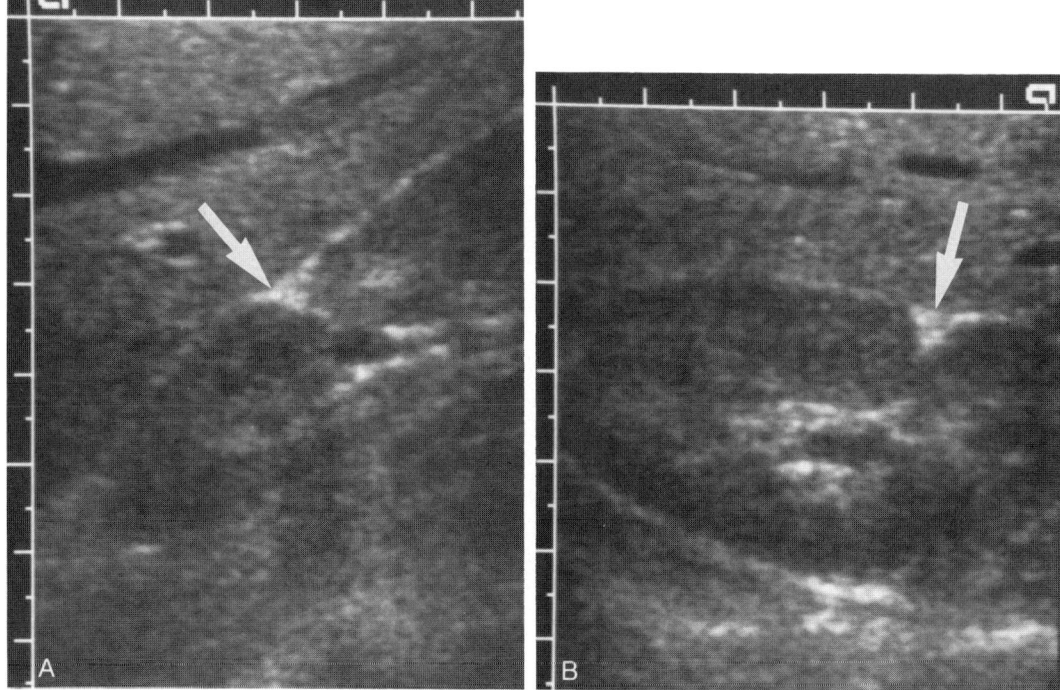

Figure 7–20. A plane of connective tissue between inferior and superior reniculi is a normal finding. It presents as a linear interface (arrow) on the coronal scan (**A**). On the transverse scan, it is a V-shaped defect (arrow, **B**).

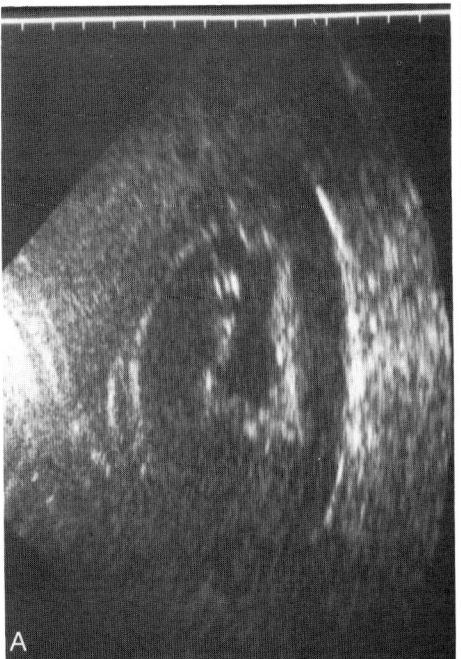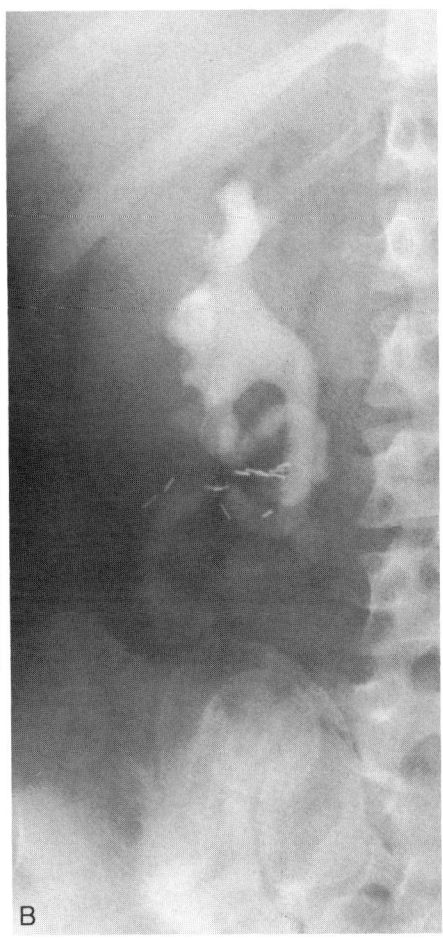

Figure 7–21. Caliectasis usually is not detected on ultrasonography, but in this patient, who has a single kidney handling all her urinary flow, the collecting system is always full. Caliectasis associated with focal parenchymal scarring of the upper pole can be seen on the ultrasonogram (**A**), which is oriented to match the intravenous urogram (**B**).

until the end of the study in order that some urine will have partially filled it after the VCUG. Also, beginning a pelvic scan immediately after a VCUG is guaranteed to convince the child that a repeat catheterization is next!

Xanthogranulomatous pyelonephritis is a rarity in children (Yazaki et al., 1982; Braun et al., 1985; Kierce et al., 1985). It is less consistently associated with obstruction from renal stones in children than it is in adults. The chronic infective process is characterized by destruction of renal parenchyma and its replacement by sheets of macrophages filled with lipids. It may be diffuse (in about 75 percent of cases) or segmental. Ultrasonography shows irregular or sometimes nodular echogenicity replacing normal architecture. The outline of the kidney may be indistinct from adjacent inflammation of soft tissues. One of our patients had an associated perinephric abscess. Scans have to be correlated with other imaging such as radionuclide or radiographic studies, which will show the involved segment of kidney to be nonfunctioning (Fig. 7–22). A gallium scan yields positive findings in xanthogranulomatous pyelonephritis. Differentiation from a tumor may be difficult, but there is less of a mass effect with this disease, and there is usually other clinical evidence of an inflammatory etiology.

Candidal infection of the urinary tract usually affects premature, and occasionally full-term, babies who have been receiving chronic antimicrobial therapy for bacterial infections. Patients who have received organ transplants, are immunosuppressed, and are taking antibiotics are also at risk. Renal involvement results from hematogenous dissemination of the fungus. There is one case report of a baby who possibly had ascending renal infection, or at least exacerbation of underlying infection, from vesicoureteral re-

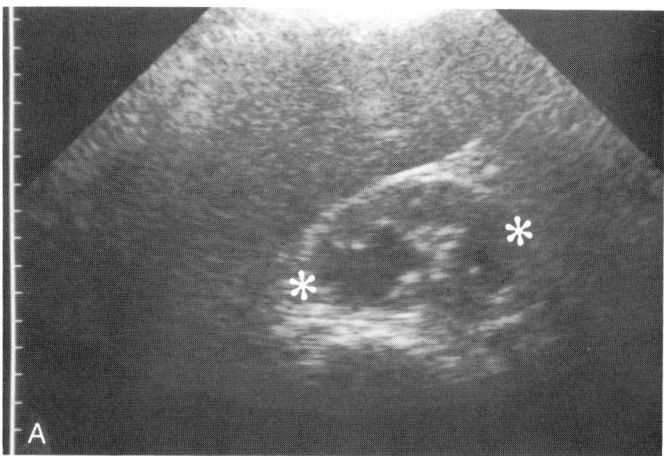

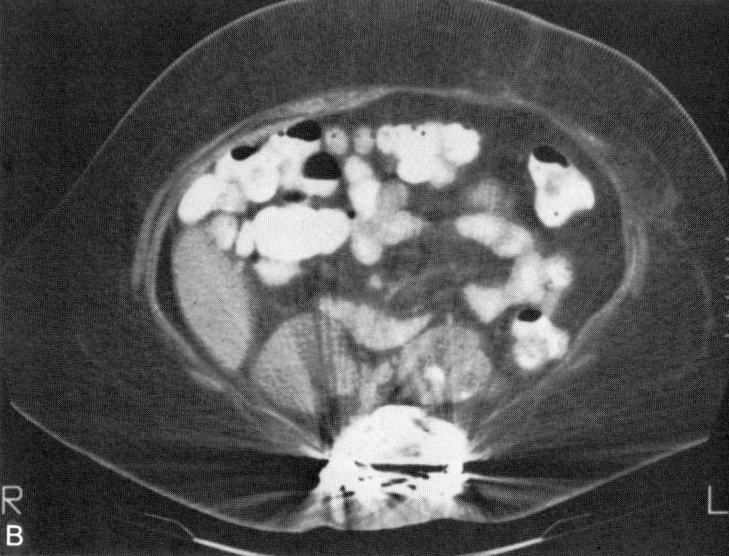

Figure 7–22. This patient, who had myelodysplasia and many of the urinary and orthopedic complications associated with it, presented at the hospital with temperatures up to 40°C. Ultrasonography had always been difficult to perform for this patient because of her size and because of the previous surgery on her back. The right kidney seemed stable in its appearance with focal ectasia of the upper collecting system (A). The other kidney looked similar in appearance. Because of persisting evidence of infection and poor response to antibiotics, CT scan was requested to identify stones, which were indeed present in the left kidney (B). Tc99m dimethyl captosuccinate (DMSA) scan that finally followed showed complete nonfunction of the right kidney. Nephrostomy of the right kidney revealed pyonephrosis. The kidney failed to regain any function and was removed. Xanthogranulomatous pyelonephritis was diagnosed on histologic examination of the renal parenchyma. It is important to remember that routine ultrasonography cannot provide information regarding function of the kidney. In addition, in patients for whom scanning is difficult (such as those with myelodysplasia), stones may be missed. Ultrasonographic scans have to be correlated with other imaging when clinical signs and symptoms are present but unexplained.

flux of contaminated urine (Sirinelli et al., 1987). The usual pathogenesis of infection is parenchymal seeding, cortical abscesses, and then extension into tubules and the collecting system with formation of mycotic conglomerates. The ultrasonic correlates are enlargement and diffuse echogenicity of renal parenchyma, followed by nonshadowing echogenicity in the collecting system (Fig. 7–23). If the kidney is hydronephrotic from congenital obstruction, reflux, or obstruction secondary to the fungus itself, the fungal balls are outlined by urine and are much easier to diagnose. Blood clots in the collecting system may appear identical to fungus balls, and results of urinalysis differentiate the two problems. Increased parenchymal echogenicity is a nonspecific sign. Nephrotoxic antibiotics, cyclosporine, and acute tubular necrosis can cause this appearance. The brain is often affected simultaneously with metastatic candidiasis and should be scanned if the fontanelle is patent (Kirpekar et al., 1986).

The incidence of bacterial urinary infection in children pales beside reported incidence of infection with *Schistosoma haematobium* in many parts of the world. In one area in Kenya, 69 percent of all children examined were infected (King et al., 1988). In Africa and the Middle East, an estimated 80 million people have this disease. The parasite burrows into the mucosa of the bladder and lays its ova. Both pathologically and ultrasonographically, thickening of the wall of the bladder, polypoid hyperplasia of mucosa, calcifications around dead ova, and obstruction of the upper urinary tract by acute and

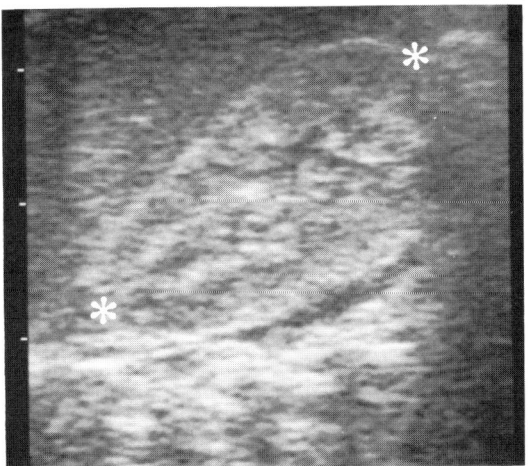

Figure 7-23. This longitudinal scan is of a premature baby in the intensive care unit whose urine cultures were growing *Candida*. Both kidneys appeared similar, with diffusely echogenic renal parenchyma bilaterally and poor differentiation between cortex and medulla.

chronic distal ureteral and vesical inflammation are characteristic of this infection (Fig. 7–24). In an ultrasonographic survey done in an endemic area in the Democratic Republic of the Congo, abnormalities were apparent in 93 to 98 percent of people with moderate to heavy urinary excretion of ova (Dittrich and Doehring, 1986). Reversal of obstruction to the upper urinary tract can be achieved if specific treatment is instituted in the young.

Renal tuberculosis in children is uncommon even in developing countries. In only 6 of 12 children reported from South Africa was there radiologic evidence of pulmonary disease (Cremin, 1987). Miliary spread of the bacillus carries it to the renal arteriole, from which it may pass to the papilla through the nephron. Destruction of the papilla, followed by more extensive cavitation, may be focal or result in granulomatous autonephrectomy. Infection of the ureter and bladder results in a poorly distensible bladder, gaping ureteral orifices, and mucosal irregularity. Depending on the stage and extent of renal involvement, scans may show abnormalities of medullary pyramids, focal caseation, or complete destruction of normal anatomy by relatively echofree nodular caseation. The bladder, when affected, is more spherical than normal on transverse views, and the ureteral junctions may be patulous.

REFERENCES

Alon U, Berant M, Pery M: Intravenous pyelography in children with urinary tract infection and vesicoureteral reflux. Pediatrics 1989; 83:332–336.

Aronson AS, Gustafson B, Srenningsen NW: Combined suprapubic aspiration and clean-voided urine examination in infants and children. Acta Paediatr Scand 1973; 62:396–400.

Askari A, Belman AB: Vesicoureteral reflux in black girls. J Urol 1982; 127:747–748.

Avni EF, Van Gansbeke D, Thoua Y, et al: US demonstration of pyelitis and ureteritis in children. Pediatr Radiol 1988; 18:134–139.

Baetz-Greenwalt B, Debaz B, Kumar ML: Bladder fungus ball: A reversible cause of neonatal obstructive uropathy. Pediatrics 1988; 81:826–829.

Baley JE, Kliegman RM, Fanaroff AA: Disseminated fungal infections in very low-birth weight infants: Clinical manifestations and epidemiology. Pediatrics 1984; 73:144-152.

Ben-Ami T, Rozin M, Hertz M: Imaging of children with urinary tract infection: A tailored approach. Clin Radiol 1989; 40:64–67.

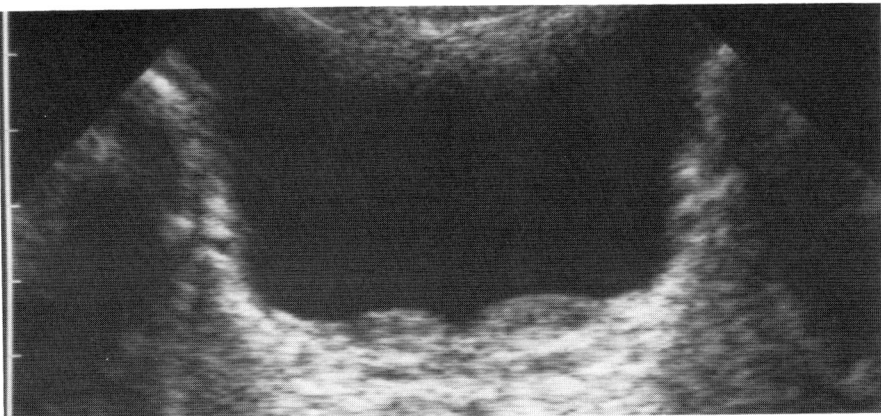

Figure 7–24. Mild symmetric thickening of the posterior wall of the bladder was the result of schistosomal infection in this 10-year-old girl, who had been living in Africa. The ova of *Schistosoma haematobium* were recovered from the urine.

Bergius AR, Niskanen K, Kekomäki M: Detection of significant vesico-ureteric reflux by ultrasound in infants and children. Z Kinderchir 1990; 45:144–145.

Berman LH, Stringer DA, St. Onge O, et al: An assessment of sonography in the diagnosis and management of neonatal candidiasis. Clin Radiol 1989; 40:577–581.

Birmingham Reflux Study Group: Prospective trial of operative versus non-operative treatment of severe vesico-ureteric reflux: Two years' observation in 96 children. Br Med J 1983; 287:171–174.

Blickman JG, Taylor GA, Lebowitz RL: Voiding cystourethrography: The initial radiologic study in children with urinary tract infection. Radiology 1985; 156:659–662.

Braun G, Moussali L, Balanzar JL: Xanthogranulomatous pyelonephritis in children. J Urol 1985; 133:236–239.

Burbige KA, Retik AB, Colodny AH, et al: Urinary tract infection in boys. J Urol 1984; 132:541–542.

Burns MW, Burns JL, Krieger JN: Pediatric urinary tract infection. Diagnosis, classification and significance. Pediatr Clin North Am 1987; 34:1111–1120.

Chapman SJ, Chantler C, Haycock GB, et al: Radionuclide cystography in vesicoureteric reflux. Arch Dis Child 1988; 63:650–651.

Cremin BJ: Radiological imaging of urogenital tuberculosis in children with emphasis on ultrasound. Pediatr Radiol 1987; 17:34–38.

Diament MJ: Is ultrasound screening for urinary tract infection "cost effective"? Pediatr Radiol 1988; 18:157–159.

Diard F, Nicolau A, Bernard S: Intra-renal reflux: A new cause of medullary hyperechogenicity? Pediatr Radiol 1987; 17:154–155.

Dinkel E, Orth S, Dittrich M: Renal sonography in the differentiation of upper from lower urinary tract infection. AJR 1986; 146:775–780.

Dittrich M, Doehring E: Ultrasonographical aspects of urinary schistosomiasis: Assessment of morphological lesions in the upper and lower urinary tract. Pediatr Radiol 1986; 16:225–230.

Edelmann CM, Ogwo JE, Fine BP, Martinez AB: The prevalence of bacteriuria in full-term and premature newborn infants. J Pediatr 1973; 82:125–132.

Ehrlich RM: Vesicoureteral reflux: A surgeon's perspective. Ped Clin North Am 1982; 29:827–834.

Faix RG: Systemic candida infections in infants in intensive care nurseries: high incidence of central nervous system involvement. J Pediatr 1984; 105:616–622.

Ginsburg CM, McCracken GH: Urinary tract infections in young infants. Pediatrics 1982; 69:409–412.

Gordon I: Urinary tract infection in paediatrics: The role of diagnostic imaging. Br J Radiol 1990; 63:507–511.

Hanbury DC, Coulden RA, Farman P, et al: Ultrasound cystography in the diagnosis of vesicoureteric reflux. Br J Urol 1990; 65:250–233.

Hatz C, Mayombana C, de Savigny D, et al: Ultrasound scanning for detecting morbidity due to *Schistosoma haematobium* and its resolution following treatment with different doses of praziquantel. Trans R Soc Trop Med Hyg 1990; 84:84–88.

Hayden CK Jr, Swischuk LE, Fawcett HD, et al: Urinary tract infections in childhood: A current imaging approach. Radiographics 1986; 6:1023–1038.

Hodson CJ: Reflux nephropathy: A personal historical review. Neuhauser lecture. AJR 1981; 137:451–462.

Hodson CJ, Heptinstall RH, Winberg J: Reflux Nephropathy Update: 1983. New York: Karger Basel, 1984.

Hoffer FA, Hanabergh AM, Teele RL: The interrenicular junction: A mimic of renal scarring on normal pediatric sonograms. AJR 1985; 145:1075–1078.

Hughes PM, Gupta SC, Thomas NB: Xanthogranulomatous pyelonephritis in childhood. Clin Radiol 1990; 41:360–362.

Irving HC, Arthur RJ, Thomas DFM: Percutaneous nephrostomy in paediatrics. Clinical Radiology 1987; 38:245–248.

Jequier S, Paltiel H, Lafortune M: Ureterovesical jets in infants and children: Duplex and color Doppler US studies. Radiology 1990; 175:349–353.

Johansson B, Troell S, Berg U: Renal parenchymal volume during and after acute pyelonephritis measured by ultrasonography. Arch Dis Child 1988; 63:1309–1314.

Kenda R, Kenig T, Silc M, et al: Renal ultrasound and excretory urography in infants and young children with urinary tract infection. Pediatr Radiol 1989; 19:299–301.

Kessler RM, Altman DH: Real-time sonographic detection of vesicoureteral reflux in children. AJR 1982; 138:1033–1036.

Kierce F, Carroll R, Guiney EJ: Xanthogranulomatous pyelonephritis in childhood. Br J Urol 1985; 57:261–263.

King CH, Lombardi G, Lombardi C, et al: Chemotherapy-based control of schistosomiasis haematobia. I. Metrifonate versus praziquantel in control of intensity and prevalence of infection. Am J Trop Med Hyg 1988; 39:295–305.

Kirpekar M, Abini MM, Hilfer C, Emerson R: Ultrasound in the diagnosis of systemic candidiasis (renal and cranial) in very low birth weight premature infants. Pediatr Radiol 1986; 16:17–20.

Lebowitz RL, Mandell J: Urinary tract infection in children: Putting radiology in its place. Radiology 1987; 165:1–9.

Lebowitz RL, Olbing H, Parkkulainen KV, et al: International system of radiographic grading of vesicoureteric reflux. Pediatr Radiol 1985; 15:105–109.

Lich R Jr, Howerton LW Jr, Goode LS, et al: The ureterovesical junction of the newborn. J Urol 1964; 92:436–438.

Marshall JL, Johnson ND, DeCampo MP: Vesicoureteric reflux in children: Prediction with color Doppler imaging. Work in progress. Radiology 1990; 175:355–358.

Monsour M, Azmy AF, MacKenzie JR: Renal scarring secondary to vesicoureteric reflux. Critical assessment and new grading. Br J Urol 1987; 70:320–324.

Nosher JL, Tamminen JL, Amorosa JK, et al: Acute focal bacterial nephritis. Am J Kidney Dis 1988; 11:36–42.

Ogra PL, Faden HS: Urinary tract infections in childhood: An update. J Pediatr 1985; 106:1023–1029.

Peters PC, Johnson DE, Jackson JH Jr: The incidence of vesicoureteral reflux in the premature child. J Urol 1967; 97:259–260.

Reid BS, Bender TM: Radiographic evaluation of children with urinary tract infections. Radiol Clin North Am 1988; 26:393–407.

Roberts JA, Kaack MB, Morvant AB: Vesicoureteral reflux in the primate. IV. Infection as a cause of prolonged high-grade reflux. Pediatrics 1988; 82:91–95.

Schneider K, Helmig FJ, Eife R, et al: Pyonephrosis in childhood—Is ultrasound sufficient for diagnosis? Pediatr Radiol 1989; 19:302–307.

Schneider K, Jablonski C, Wiessner M, et al: Screening for vesicoureteral reflux in children using real-time sonography. Pediatr Radiol 1984; 14:400–403.

Shindo S, Bernstein J, Arant BS: Evolution of renal segmental atrophy (Ask-Upmark kidney) in children with vesicoureteric reflux: Radiographic and morphologic studies. J Pediatr 1983; 102:847–854.

Sirinelli D, Biniotti V, Schmit P, et al: Urinoma and

arterial hypertension complicating neonatal renal candidiasis. Pediatr Radiol 1987; 17:156–158.

Skoog SJ, Belman AB, Majd M: A nonsurgical approach to the management of primary vesicoureteral reflux. J Urol 1987; 138:941–946.

Smellie JM, Ransley PG, Normand ICS, et al: Development of new renal scars: A collaborative study. Br Med J 1985; 290:1957–1960.

Strife JL, Bisset GS 3d, Kirks DR, et al: Nuclear cystography and renal sonography: Findings in girls with urinary tract infection. AJR 1989; 153:115–119.

Sty Jr, Wells RG, Starshak RJ: Imaging in acute renal infection in children. AJR 1987; 148:471–477.

Traisman ES, Conway JJ, Traisman HS, et al: The localization of urinary tract infection with 99m Tc glucoheptonate scintigraphy. Pediatr Radiol 1986; 16:403–406.

Troell S, Berg U, Johansson B, et al : Renal parenchymal volume in children. Normal values assessed by ultrasonography. Acta Radiol 1988; 29:127–130.

Verber IG, Strudley MR, Meller ST: 99m Tc dimercaptosuccinic acid (DMSA) scan as first investigation of urinary tract infection. Arch Dis Child 1988; 63:1320–1325.

Verboven M, Ingels M, Delree M, Piepsz A: 99mTc-DMSA scintigraphy in acute urinary tract infection in children. Pediatr Radiol 1990; 20:540–542.

Whyte KM, Abbott GD, Kennedy JC, et al: A protocol for the investigation of infants and children with urinary tract infection. Clinical Radiology 1988; 39:278–280.

Winberg J, Bollgren I, Källenius G, et al: Clinical pyelonephritis and focal renal scarring. Ped Clin North Am 1982; 29:801–814.

Wiswell TE, Enzenauer RW, Cornish JD et al: Declining frequency of circumcision. Implications for changes in the absolute incidence and male to female sex ratio of urinary tract infections in early infancy. Pediatrics 1987; 79:338–342.

Yadin O, Gradus Ben-Ezer D, Golan A, et al: Survival of a premature neonate with obstructive anuria due to *Candida*: The role of early sonographic diagnosis and antimycotic treatment. Eur J Pediatr 1988; 147:653–655.

Yazaki T, Ishikawa S, Ogawa Y, et al: Xanthogranulomatous pyelonephritis in childhood: Case report and review of English and Japanese literature. J Urol 1982; 127:80–83.

CHAPTER 8

EVALUATING AN ABDOMINAL MASS

APPROACH TO THE INFANT

A baby who has an abdominal mass typically comes to ultrasonography with a pair of distressed parents and a covey of concerned doctors. All want the diagnosis the second the transducer touches the abdomen. If we have learned anything through experience, it is the practice of performing an examination carefully and thoroughly. We always regret the rushed or incomplete study.

The widespread use of ultrasonography during pregnancy has led to an increase in detection of abdominal masses in fetuses. This development has several implications: (1) the parents have been under stress for a while; (2) the referral may be through the obstetric rather than pediatric service, and clinical examination of the baby may be bypassed; (3) a baby may be delivered early because of a mass and have problems of immaturity superimposed on those of the mass; (4) because cystic masses are easier to spot in utero than are solid masses, more cases of hydronephrosis are identified early, and more and earlier genitourinary surgery will likely be performed; (5) an otherwise silent mass, which might have regressed spontaneously without any intervention, may end up as a surgical specimen; (6) on the other hand, covert renal obstruction and subsequent renal failure in childhood may decrease in incidence because obstructive uropathy is diagnosed early.

Infants also come to ultrasonography when the examining clinician has palpated a mass or when other studies have indicated that a mass might be present. In Japan, for example, screening levels of urinary vanillylmandelic acid are obtained from neonates. Those who have elevated levels are referred for ultrasonograms to search for neuroblastoma (Fujioka et al., 1988).

Earlier published studies of babies with abdominal masses tended to be "clinically" biased. Current and future series will describe a mixed population, diagnosed either prenatally or postnatally.

Plain radiographs of the abdomen and chest and results from a good clinical examination should accompany the baby to ultrasonography. It has been our observation that with the current reliance on imaging, thorough clinical examination seems to be an endangered art form. Plain radiographs and clinical concerns help in orienting the ultrasonographic study; furthermore, the information gathered from each source has to be consolidated before a decision regarding management of the baby is made. For example, skeletal anomalies may signal a renal anomaly; peritoneal calcification occurs when a viscus is perforated in utero, which results in meconium peritonitis. The gas pattern in the intestines may hint or reveal that intestinal obstruction is present. Gas-filled loops may be distorted over or around a soft tissue mass. Cardiomegaly and hepatic mass point to one or more shunting vascular tumors of the liver. Pulmonary hypoplasia often coexists with renomegaly when polycystic renal disease is present.

Babies, particularly premature neonates, have to be kept warm in the examining room. Infrared heaters are ideal because they do not cast the bright light of warming lamps. Covering the baby's head reduces radiant loss of heat. Warm gel for acoustic coupling is preferable to cold gel for obvious reasons. Transducers have to be washed, as do the examiner's hands. Transducers should be high in frequency but also allow good penetration and a large field of view. "Keyhole" views should be saved until the end of the examination, after the nature of the abnormality has been uncovered.

The baby is placed supine on the examining table and, if restless, is offered a pacifier or parental finger to suck. Most will stop crying and remain quiet during an examination if the room is darkened and quiet. Sustained light pressure from the transducer is less stimulating than irregular contact; therefore, we tend to hold the transducer on the baby's abdomen even when films are being changed and labeling is done.

EVALUATION OF AN ABDOMINAL MASS (ALL AGES)

Ultrasonography of an abdominal mass should include the following tasks:

1. Determination of the organ of origin: most abdominal masses are retroperitoneal, and most of those are renal; sometimes, the larger the mass is, the more difficult it is to identify its source.

2. Assessing the size of the mass: good measurements, done in a plane that can be reproduced, provide a baseline for follow-up studies if the mass is not removed surgically.

3. Defining the character of the mass (i.e., solid, cystic, mixed): as a rule, a purely cystic mass is benign.

4. Establishing the relationship of the mass to contiguous organs and blood vessels: as mentioned earlier, a very large mass may distort adjacent organs to the extent that its origin is indeterminate; with smaller masses, relationships are easier to judge. For example, a right-sided retroperitoneal mass will lift the inferior vena cava anteriorly; a fixed pelvic mass may cause ipsilateral hydronephrosis; a mass in the right upper abdomen can be shown as separate from the liver on real-time scanning if the liver glides over the mass during respiration.

5. Documentation of adenopathy or metastases: adjacent lymphadenopathy may be appreciated at the hilum in some patients with renal tumor. Non-Hodgkin lymphoma, particularly Burkitt lymphoma, may present with extranodal mass or widespread or localized adenopathy, or both. Metastatic disease in the abdomen is unusual except in the case of neuroblastoma, which may involve nodes and the liver.

6. Determination of vascularity: if color or pulsed Doppler scanning is available, it should be used to assess the vascularity of a lesion. Doppler scanning is particularly helpful in assessing unusual cystic masses and proving or disproving their vascular nature (Plate VIII).

RETROPERITONEAL MASSES: HYDRONEPHROSIS

INTRODUCTION TO HYDRONEPHROSIS AND RELATED CONDITIONS

"Hydronephrosis" simply means dilatation of the renal collecting system. Although most hydronephrosis in children is obstructive, there are other reasons for its presence: vesicoureteral reflux, primary megacalices, prune-belly syndrome, occasional dilatation from sepsis, and vigorous diuresis. Hydronephrosis associated with a palpable kidney is usually obstructive in nature.

Obstruction at the ureteropelvic junction (UPJ) is typically from congenital stenosis and occasionally from a crossing vessel or extrinsic band. Ureteral valves have been described as a rare cause of ureteral obstruction (Reinberg et al., 1987; Mandell et al., 1988). Obstruction at the ureterovesical level can be caused by an aperistaltic segment of the ureter (primary megaureter), ureteral stenosis, a polyp, or a stone. The latter two causes are rare in all pediatric age groups.

Obstruction by urethral valve occurs in boys. The degree of hydronephrosis depends on the severity of obstruction, the competence of the ureterovesical junctions, and the presence of decompressive urinoma or urinary ascites. Urethral obstruction in girls may occur with cyst or inflammation of the Cowper gland. Abnormal sphincteric function, a prolapsed ureterocele, and, in rare instances, a polyp of the urethra may cause obstruction in both sexes.

An ectopic ureterocele of a single drainage system is far less common than an ectopic ureterocele that is associated with the obstructed upper unit of a duplex system. Hydronephrosis of the lower unit of a duplex kidney may result from vesicoureteral reflux, from obstruction at its ureteropelvic junction, or from extrinsic pressure of its distal ureter by an adjacent ureterocele.

Multicystic dysplastic kidney (MDK) is discussed in this section because it is likely the result of chronic, severe obstruction in utero (Griscom et al., 1975; Felson and Cussen, 1975). On occasion, severe obstruction at the ureteropelvic junction simulates MDK, and vice versa. Functional studies can usually differentiate between the two.

ULTRASONOGRAPHY OF HYDRONEPHROSIS AND RELATED CONDITIONS

If a newborn has had a prenatal diagnosis of unilateral hydronephrosis and if the clinical condition is good and urinary function seems normal, we delay follow-up ultrasonography for 7 to 10 days. This enables the baby to go home and have a scheduled examination under controlled conditions. More important, on scans performed too soon after birth, we have the problem of missing significant hydronephrosis from obstruction at the UPJ (Fig. 8–1). Laing and associates (1984) suggested that scans are falsely normal because of relative oliguria in the few days after birth. It should be emphasized that a normal postnatal scan at any time does not rule out the possibility that intermittent vesicoureteral reflux was responsible for earlier, prenatal dilatation. The incidence of vesicoureteral reflux in the general population of normal newborns is unknown. Cystograms have been performed for premature babies (Peters et al., 1967); it appears, however, that most of those studied were black. This group is recognized as having a lower rate of vesi-

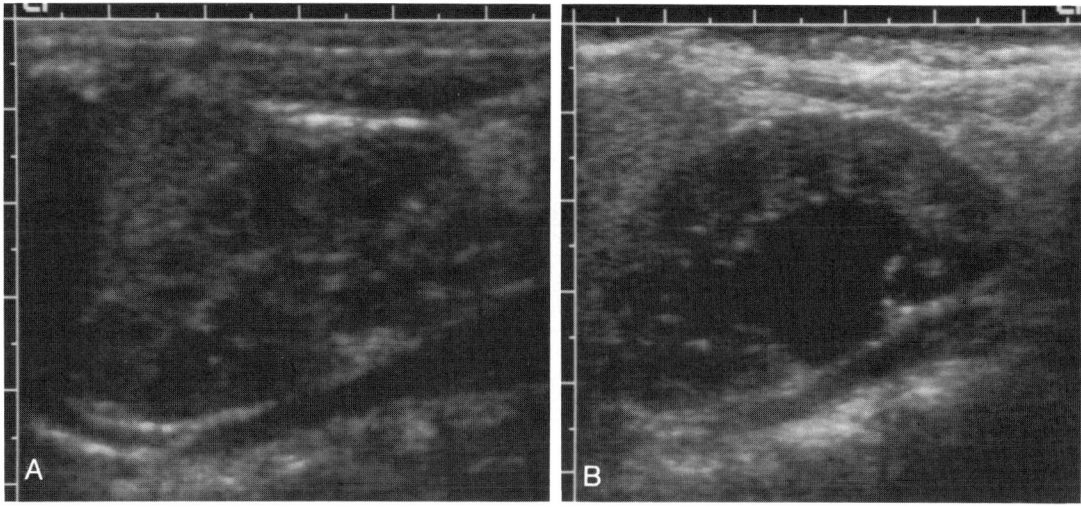

Figure 8–1. Prenatal ultrasonography had shown dilatation of the left renal collecting system. When this baby was 2 days old, the left kidney was completely normal (A). When the baby was 1 month old, dilatation of the renal collecting system secondary to narrowing at the ureteropelvic junction was evident (B).

coureteral reflux than do whites. A published but unattributed comment in a symposium on reflux nephropathy mentioned that 10 percent of a group of normal babies studied had reflux (Hodson et al., 1984). Because we know that older children outgrow reflux, it is tempting to believe that there is a continuum of maturation of the ureterovesical tunnel that bridges prenatal and postnatal existence and that some normal babies may have reflux. If postnatal scans show no dilatation, if renal size and parenchyma are normal, and if the baby is asymptomatic, we do not perform voiding cystourethrography unless prenatal scans have shown striking dilatation. If, however, the kidneys are asymmetric in size or show a change from the normal parenchymal pattern, or if there is urinary symptomatology, we pursue a radiographic evaluation with voiding cystourethrography. Sterile reflux, grades 3 to 5, has been associated with ipsilateral hypoplasia, and possibly dysplasia, in several neonates whom we have examined (Fig. 8–2).

For babies with a prenatal diagnosis of *bilateral* hydronephrosis, we are more concerned (Reznik et al., 1988). If dilatation has been moderate to severe, we rescan the baby soon after delivery. If dilatation has been mild to moderate, if urinary output seems normal, and if the kidneys and bladder are not palpable, we defer evaluation from hours to days, depending on the level of clinical concern (Fig. 8–3). If early scans are normal, we recommend another follow-up study at 2 weeks to avoid missing covert obstruction at the UPJ. Ideally, the ultrasonographer should have the obstetric scans in hand when performing the follow-up study, but in reality we often rely on information supplied by the mother.

Series from the obstetric experience with prenatal ultrasonography suggest that 1 in 1000 liveborn infants has a urinary anomaly (Watson et al., 1988). The pediatric experience suggests that this is far too low an estimate and that 1 in 100 to 200 babies has a urinary anomaly (Steinhart et al., 1988; Sheih et al., 1989). An anomaly detected in utero is most likely one that is manifest as hydronephrosis because a dilated collecting system is easy to identify. Obstructive uropathy does appear to affect 1 or 2 per 1000 liveborn infants (Reznik et al., 1988) and thus better matches the numbers from the obstetric experience. Obstruction at the UPJ is the most common lesion, accounting for approximately 40 percent of all cases of significant hydronephrosis (Figs. 8–4, 8–5; Brown et al., 1987). It should be noted that scans performed before the affected fetus is in the last trimester of gestation may appear normal (Reznik et al., 1988).

Intervention to drain or repair the obstructed fetal urinary tract is infrequently performed. A flurry of interest in performing fetal surgery has subsided (Sholder et al., 1988), leaving us with the reminder that

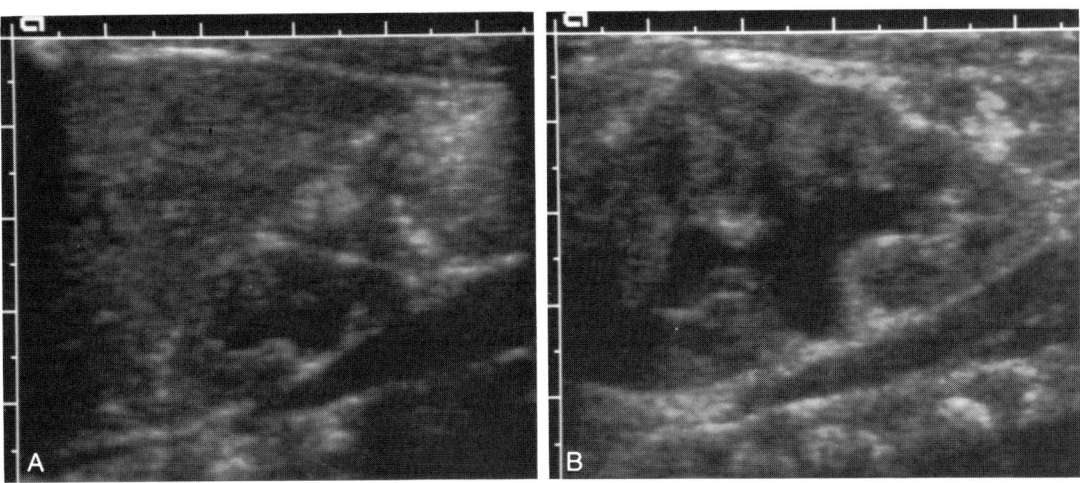

Figure 8–2. Prenatal diagnosis of a small right kidney had been made in this baby boy. Postnatal scans confirmed the small size of the right kidney (A) and showed dilatation of the left renal collecting system (B). Bilateral reflux was present on a subsequent voiding cystourethrogram: grade 4 on the right and grade 3 on the left.

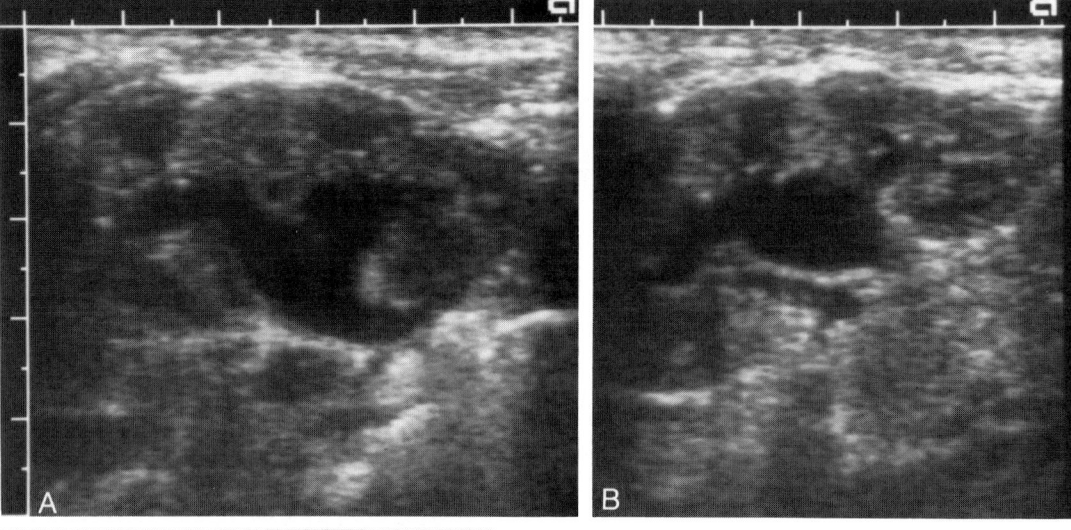
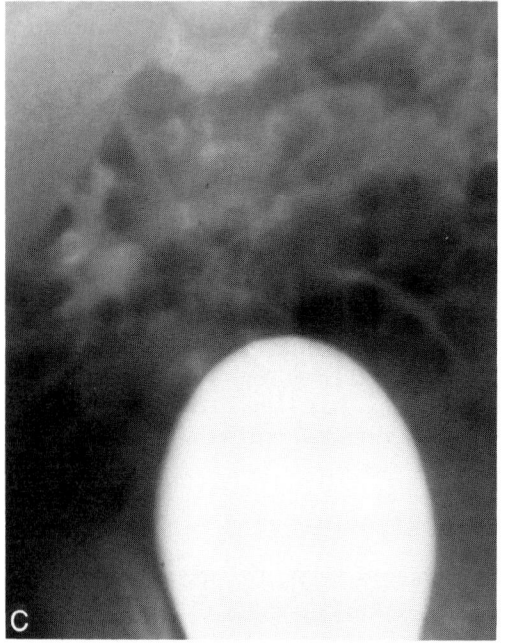

Figure 8–3. This baby boy had received a prenatal diagnosis of bilateral hydronephrosis. However, dilatation had been mild to moderate, and the bladder had been normal on all studies in utero. The baby was normal on physical examination at delivery and appeared to void normally. Postnatal scanning was therefore delayed until the baby was 2 weeks old. At that time, there was bilateral dilatation of upper tracts (**A**, right kidney; **B**, left kidney). Further radiographic work-up that included voiding cystourethrography (**C**) showed grade 2 vesicoureteral reflux on the right. Dilatation on the left was secondary to mild narrowing at the ureteropelvic junction. Both situations were managed without surgery.

although we may understand fetal anatomy, we are less informed about fetal physiology and embryology. Consequently, the ultrasonographic window on the fetus has stimulated basic research into fetal physiology, particularly that of the kidney and lung.

If hydronephrosis is apparent on follow-up postnatal scans, we follow a mental checklist in order to limit the differential diagnosis. This approach is applied to children of all ages, some of whom may have had hydronephrosis that was discovered incidentally or during the initial evaluation of hypertension, hematuria, or urinary tract infection. Therefore, the following discussion applies to older children as well as to babies.

Multicystic dysplasia of the kidney is at the far end of the spectrum of obstructive hydronephrosis. If it is the result of pelvoinfundibular atresia with associated atretic ureter, the kidney is a cluster of variably sized cysts intermixed with echogenic stroma (Fig. 8–6; Griscom et al., 1975). If the atretic process has not extended as thoroughly into the renal pelvis and infundibula, the cysts, representing dilated calices, may connect to a central pelvis (Fig. 8–7; Felson and Cussen, 1975). In each case, the parenchyma is dys-

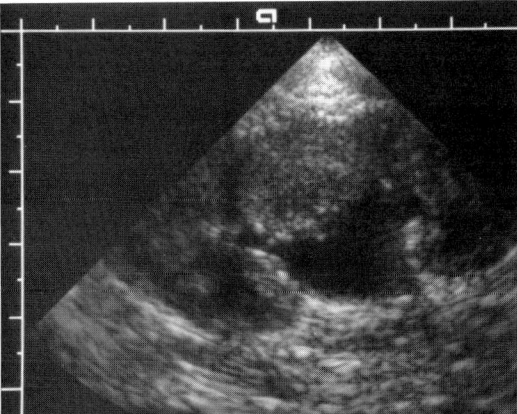

Figure 8–4. Longitudinal scan of the left kidney in a baby in whom a prenatal diagnosis of hydronephrosis was made shows typical features of mild narrowing at the ureteropelvic junction. No surgical intervention was performed.

plastic and the kidney usually lobular in contour. Scintigraphy is helpful in showing a nonfunctional kidney, although a few cases of MDK have shown enough function from a few dysplastic glomeruli to confuse matters (Carey and Howards, 1988). Percutaneous nephrostomy is also useful in doubtful situations to evaluate the quality and quantity of urine being made and to opacify the cysts (Blane et al., 1988). Noncommunication of cysts is typical of an MDK although it is not invariably present. Contralateral hydrone-

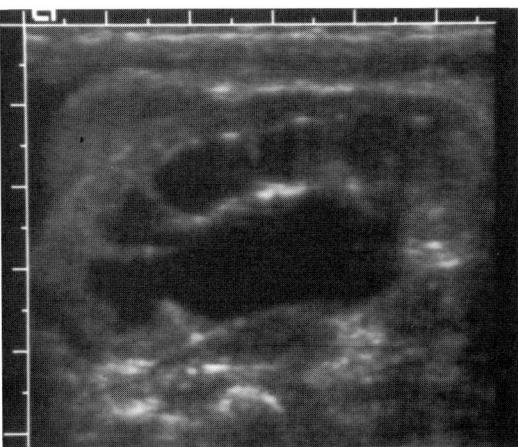

Figure 8–5. Severe narrowing at the ureteropelvic junction resulted in dilatation of the renal pelvis, infundibula, and calices in this baby, in whom a prenatal diagnosis of hydronephrosis had been made. This obstruction was surgically repaired.

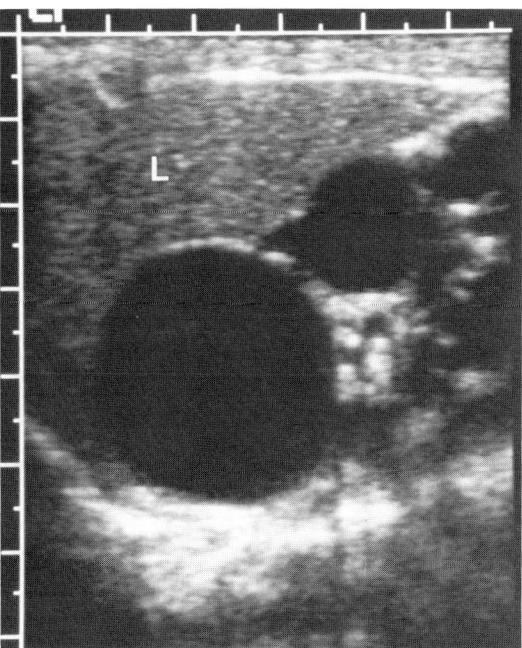

Figure 8–6. Longitudinal scan of the right kidney through the right lobe of the liver (L) shows the typical appearance of a multicystic dysplastic kidney. Cysts of varying size create a lobular renal outline.

phrosis resulting from obstruction of varying degrees at the UPJ is a common association (Kleiner et al., 1986). Bilateral multicystic dysplasia, although usually a lethal condition, may be associated with enough renal function that an affected baby can be nursed through the 1st year of life and come to renal transplantation.

Current controversies center on the management of babies who have unilateral MDK. The incidence is cited as 1 per 4300 live births, and in one series only 3 of 25 patients with an MDK had a palpable mass (Gordon et al., 1988). Prenatal ultrasonography is responsible for the apparent increase in number of cases. Those who encourage removal of an MDK cite the possibility of silent malignancy developing in the kidney or of hypertension secondary to dysplastic elements. Over 20 years there have been six reports of malignancy (two with Wilms tumor) and nine reports of concurrent hypertension. It has been our experience and others' (Avni et al., 1987, Vinocur et al., 1988) that the natural history of an MDK is regression in size and disappearance of the cysts: "dysplasia" evolves into hypoplasia. Currently, the popular recommendation is against routine re-

220 / EVALUATING AN ABDOMINAL MASS

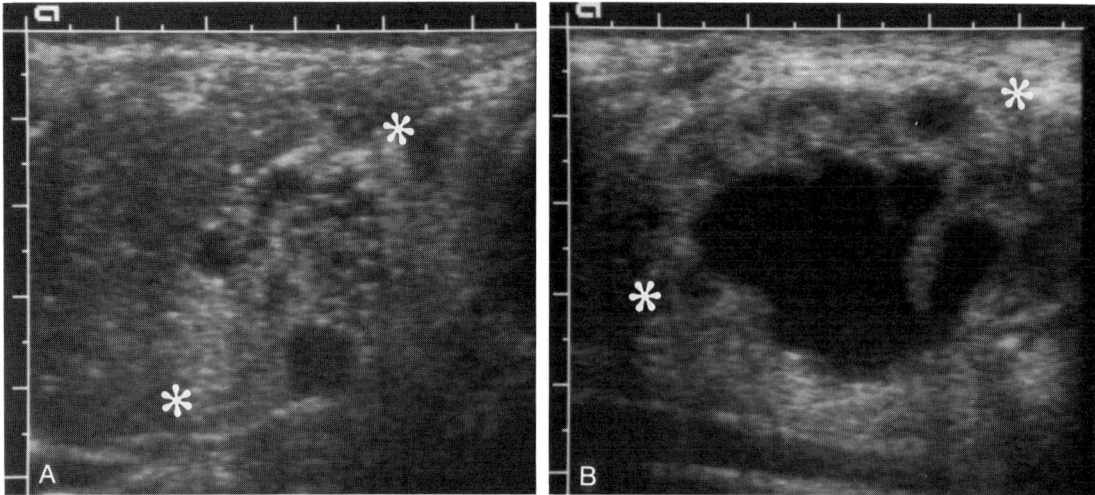

Figure 8–7. This baby was born at 37 weeks' gestational age and immediately developed bilateral pneumothoraces. The mother had had oligohydramnios during her pregnancy. Scan of the right kidney (A) shows cysts of varying size associated with an echogenic stroma. On the left (B), there is a central lucency that represents the renal pelvis. The baby had bilateral multicystic dysplasia; the left kidney had the hydronephrotic type. In an attempt to salvage some renal function, a left pyeloplasty was performed. The dysplastic kidneys were able to function well enough during the baby's 1st year of life that he could grow large enough to receive a renal transplant. (In this and other figures throughout this chapter, asterisks outline the kidneys.)

moval of the MDK (Gordon et al., 1988; Vinocur et al., 1988). We suspect, however, that any future patient who is diagnosed as having both an MDK and a tumor will re-stimulate the discussion of what represents appropriate management of an MDK.

In contrast to that of an MDK, the contour of a hydronephrotic kidney is smooth and reniform. Dilatation from obstruction affects a collecting system in a uniform manner. Presence or absence of ureteral distention distinguishes those kidneys with proximal obstruction from those with distal problems. The ureter is in the same coronal plane as the great vessels (Fig. 8–8). The relatively echolucent but more posterior psoas muscle should not be mistaken for the ureter (Fig. 8–9).

Coronal scans of patients with an obstruction at the UPJ show uniformly dilated calices emptying into a central dilated pelvis. There is no ureteral dilatation. The dilated pelvis

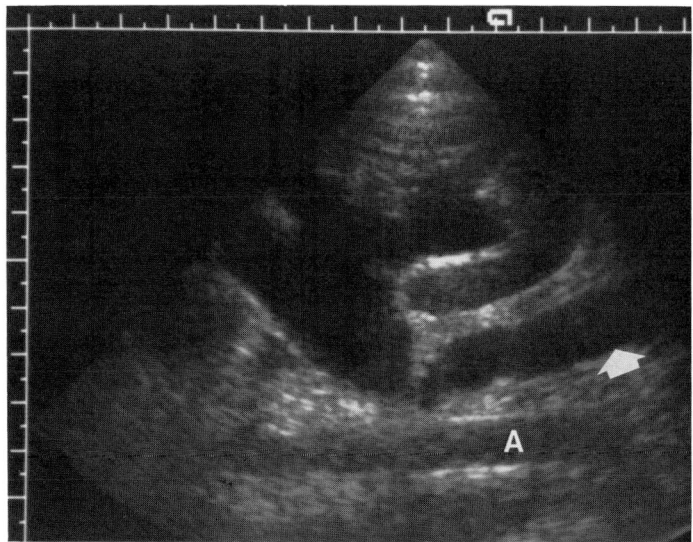

Figure 8–8. Coronal scan allows identification of the dilated ureter (arrow) in a baby who has an obstruction at the ureterovesical junction. A = aorta.

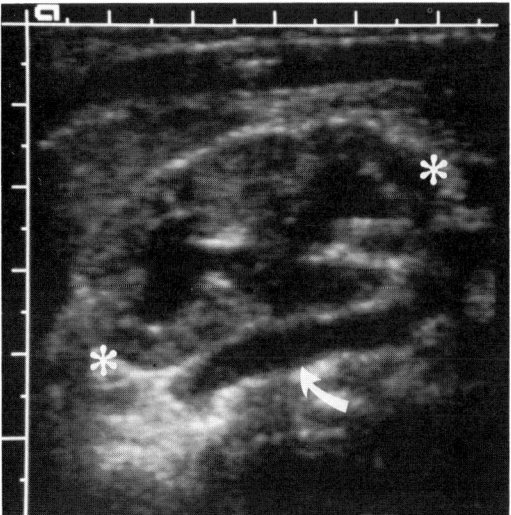

Figure 8–9. This coronal scan of the right kidney shows a moderately dilated collecting system. The psoas muscle (arrow) medial to the kidney is quite lucent. It should not be mistaken for a dilated ureter.

may be pyramidal or spherical, and in some cases, the apex of the pyramid is situated quite low in the retroperitoneum (Figs. 8–10, 8–11). A retrocaval ureter, which developmentally is actually a preureteric cava, may simulate a low, right-sided obstruction at the UPJ. Careful transverse scanning might be able to show the lateral position of the inferior vena cava and the dilated ureter passing posterior to it. A very low tapered narrowing of the upper tract should suggest some other ureteral obstruction or a long segment of an aperistaltic distal ureter (primary megaureter). Scans of the bladder show no abnormality in patients with an uncomplicated obstruction at the UPJ. A small number of children have two levels of partial obstruction: at the UPJ and the ureterovesical junction (UVJ) (McGrath et al., 1987). Occasionally, scans of these children show both distal ureteral dilatation and proximal narrowing at the UPJ (Fig. 8–12). Usually there is no way to identify the affected child, either by radiography or by ultrasonography, until surgery to relieve the proximal obstruction reveals the distal problem. A very small number of children have obstruction at the UPJ as well as vesicoureteral reflux. An ultrasonographic mismatch between the hydronephrosis affecting the renal pelvis and the degree of ureteral dilatation should raise this possibility (Fig. 8–13).

Ebel and colleagues (1988) made the point that diagnosis of obstructive UPJ may be missed if the child being examined is poorly hydrated. Furosemide can be used during ultrasonography as a renal stress test. When children are given furosemide, they have to be well hydrated and be able to maintain good input of fluids after the examination. Scanning performed 10, 20, and 30 minutes after furosemide is administered (0.3 mg/kg intravenous dose or 1 mg/kg orally) is directed at the renal pelvis. If dilatation of the pelvis increases during that time, we perform delayed scans until the pelvic diameter reaches its maximal dimensions. A normal child shows no or very minor separation of the walls of the renal pelvis. There should be minimal ureteral dilatation, if any. The bladder, when it becomes full, should be

Figure 8–10. This patient had moderate dilatation of the right renal collecting system associated with narrowing of the ureteropelvic junction, which in this patient was quite low in the retroperitoneum (arrow).

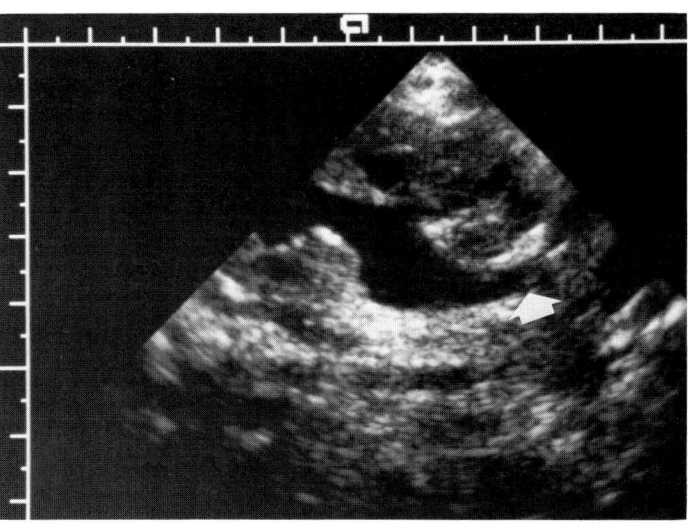

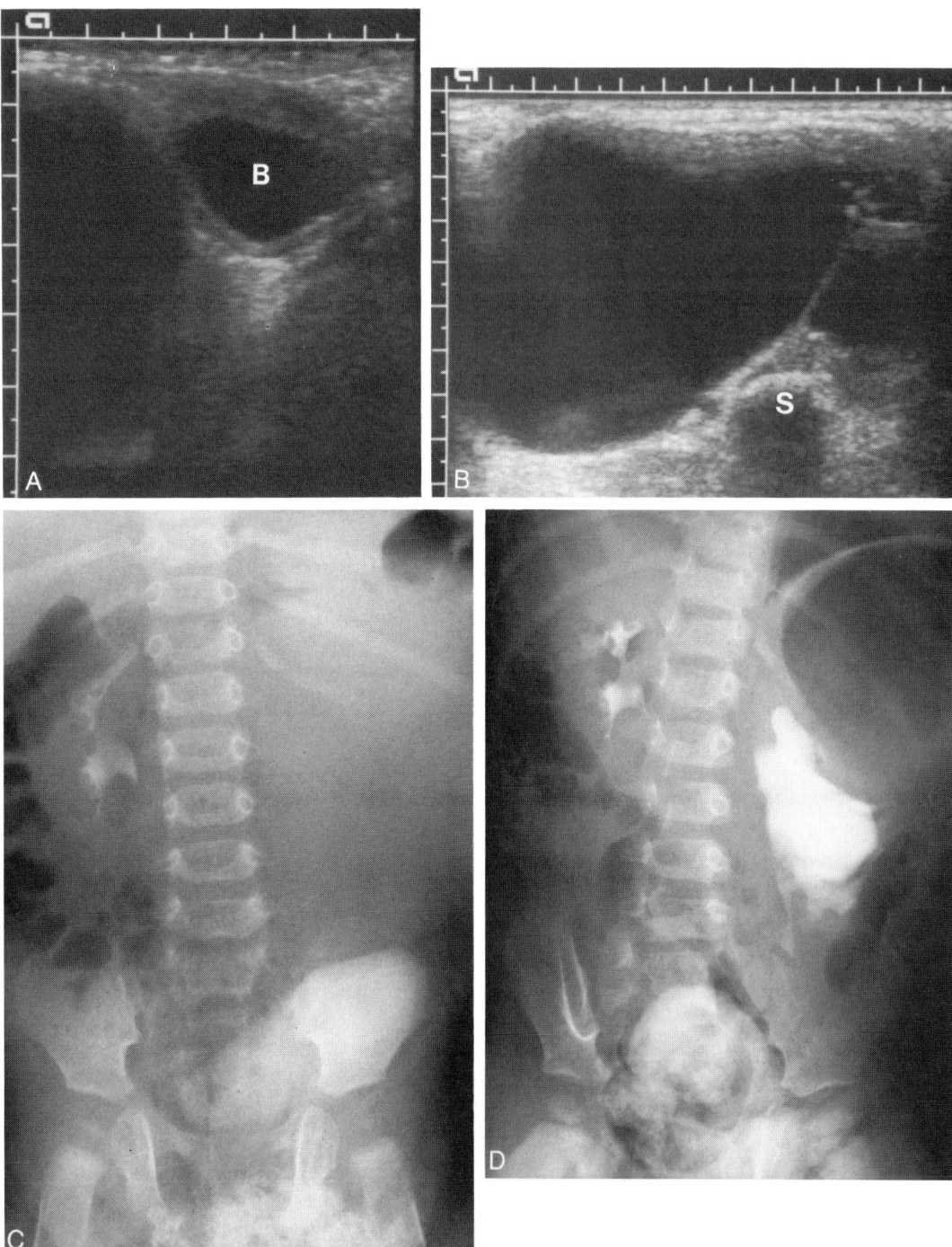

Figure 8–11. Chronic, severe obstruction at the ureteropelvic junction may result in a huge sphere of fluid representing the obstructed renal pelvis. This baby had not had prenatal scans; rather, he was sent for ultrasonography when he was 6 months old because the clinicians thought he had a distended bladder. Longitudinal scan in the midline (**A**) shows the lucent renal pelvis extending down to the level of the bladder (B). Transverse scan at the level of the umbilicus (**B**) shows the renal pelvis extending across midline. S = spine. Intravenous urography performed shortly thereafter shows normal function on the right and confirms the massive hydronephrosis on the left (**C**). Pyeloplasty was performed. Postoperative intravenous urogram (**D**) shows much improved function of the left kidney after its decompression.

emptied in order that its distention not cause pseudohydronephrosis. Diuretic-assisted renal scintigraphy better enables the clinician to quantify renal function and degree of obstruction, and in most situations it should be done instead of the ultrasonographic study. Diuretic ultrasonography is helpful for examining children who have obscure abdominal pain and whose renal pelvis appears mildly prominent on routine ultrasonography. When dilatation occurs coincidentally with reproduction of the patient's pain, intermittent obstruction to either renal pelvis or ureter is certain. If the ureter becomes obvious during the study, obstruction at the ureterovesical junction is likely (Fig. 8–14).

Narrowing at the UPJ, which causes mild to moderate dilatation of the renal pelvis but is unassociated with caliceal dilatation, does not require surgical intervention. However, we have now had experience with two asymptomatic boys in whom hydronephrosis

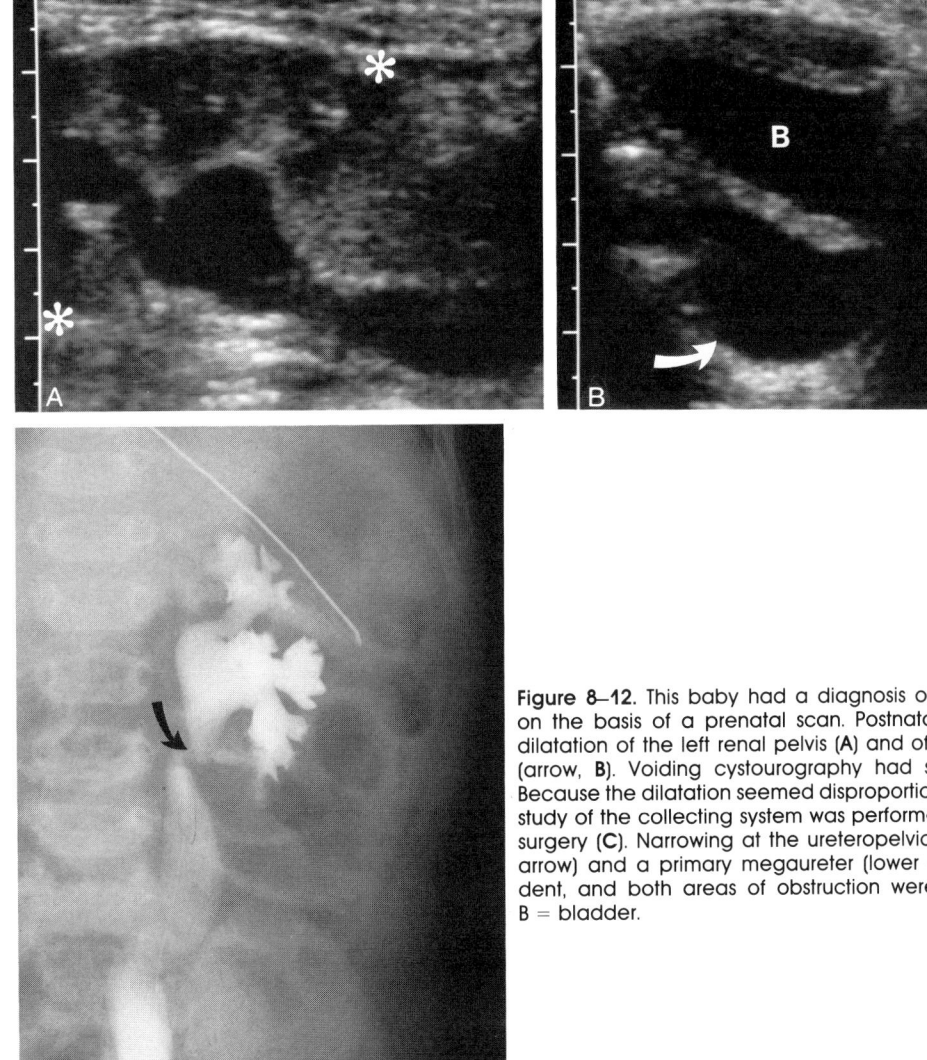

Figure 8–12. This baby had a diagnosis of hydronephrosis on the basis of a prenatal scan. Postnatal scans showed dilatation of the left renal pelvis (**A**) and of the distal ureter (arrow, **B**). Voiding cystourography had shown no reflux. Because the dilatation seemed disproportionate, retrograde study of the collecting system was performed at the time of surgery (**C**). Narrowing at the ureteropelvic junction (upper arrow) and a primary megaureter (lower arrow) were evident, and both areas of obstruction were repaired. In B, B = bladder.

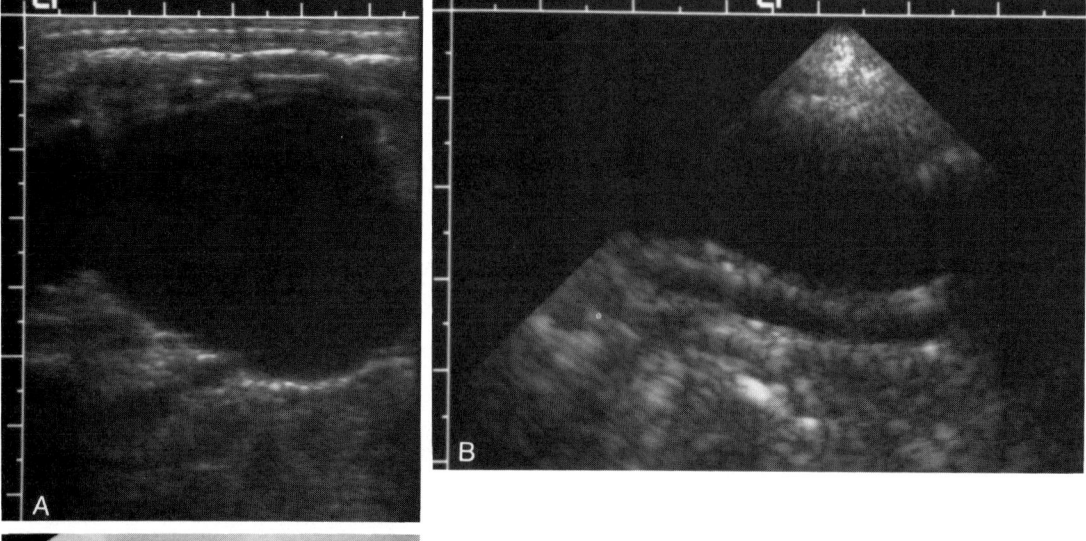

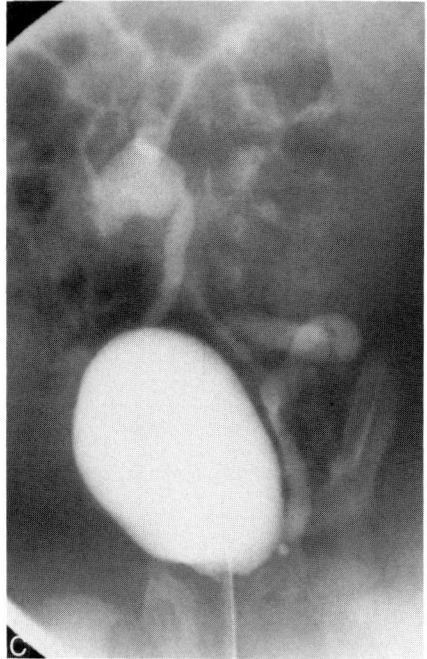

Figure 8–13. Prenatal ultrasonography had shown hydronephrosis of the left kidney. Postnatal longitudinal scan done when this girl was 7 weeks old showed huge distention of the left renal pelvis and calices with thinning of the renal cortex (**A**). Longitudinal scan of the pelvis through the partially filled bladder showed dilatation of the left distal ureter (**B**). However, the degree of dilatation of the renal pelvis was out of proportion to the ureteral dilatation. Voiding cystourethrogram followed (**C**). Bilateral reflux was present. Contrast reflux into the left ureter was stopped by the obstruction at the left ureteropelvic junction. Pyeloplasty was performed, and the child is being followed while she receives prophylactic treatment; she is expected to outgrow the reflux.

increased significantly years (4 and 5, respectively) after prenatal scans and postnatal evaluations showed mild obstruction at the UPJ. We now extend ultrasonographic follow-up of such children to at least 4 years after birth.

Primary megaureter results from aperistalsis of a variable length of the distal ureter. This functional obstruction causes variable proximal dilatation. The etiology of this anomaly is still poorly understood. Many more cases of primary megaureter have been diagnosed with prenatal scanning than were identified in children in studies that predated fetal ultrasonography (Brown et al., 1987). It is apparent that significant spontaneous regression or complete resolution of dilatation often occurs in infancy (Babut et al., 1988). Because it is difficult to predict which ureters will regress in size, surgery is now reserved for children with moderately severe obstruction, urinary infection, or some other

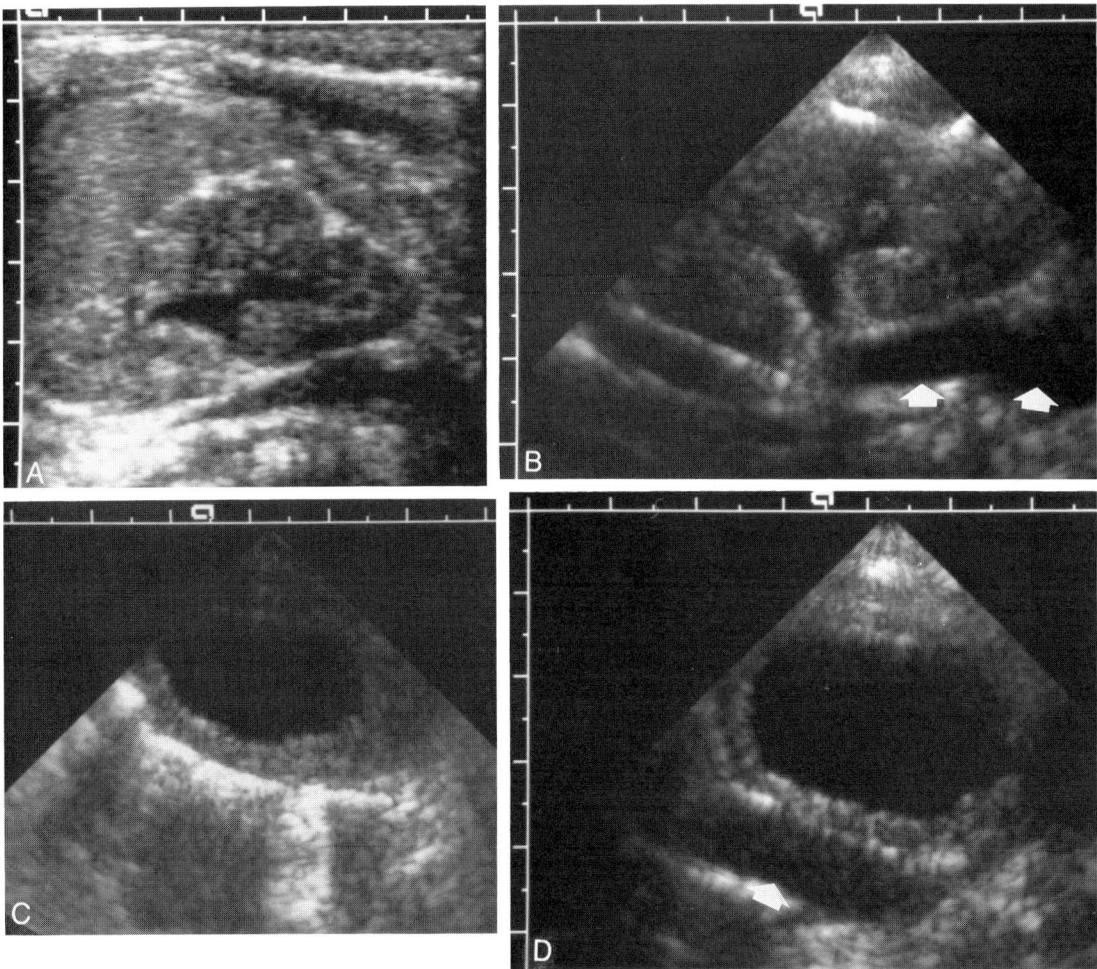

Figure 8-14. Scans were done before and after administration of furosemide. **A** shows mild dilatation of the intrarenal collecting system. After diuresis (**B**) the proximal left ureter becomes apparent (arrows). Longitudinal view of the bladder before diuresis (**C**) shows no evidence of the distal ureter. After diuresis (**D**) it becomes readily apparent (arrow) in this baby with primary megaureter.

complication such as failure to thrive or pain. Ureteral dilatation, proportionately more pronounced than ipsilateral pelvicaliceal dilatation, is typical of primary megaureter. Also characteristic is rhythmic peristalsis in the distal ureter (Fig. 8–15; Wood et al., 1985). Patience is needed in order to spot this ultrasonographic sign. The transducer has to be aligned with the long axis of the distal ureter, in either the sagittal or the coronal plane, and the ureter must be kept in view in order to appreciate the antegrade stripping of urine. If infection is present, peristalsis may be inhibited by endotoxin.

Distal ureteral obstruction can be caused by stenosis (which is rare), a primary uretero- cele (which is uncommon), an intrinsic or extrinsic mass, a stone (also uncommon), or postoperative edema or stricture (Figs. 8–16, 8–17). Distal ureteral stenosis may cause such ureteral obstruction that the dilated ureter indents the bladder and appears to be intravesical. However, the interface, composed of vesical wall and ureteral wall, is much thicker than that associated with an intravesical ureterocele. A primary ureterocele of a single collecting system can be orthotopic or ectopic. Typically the orthotopic ureterocele is associated with only mild hydronephrosis and often requires no surgical repair (Mandell et al., 1980). The simple orthotopic ureterocele appears on scans as a fluid-filled

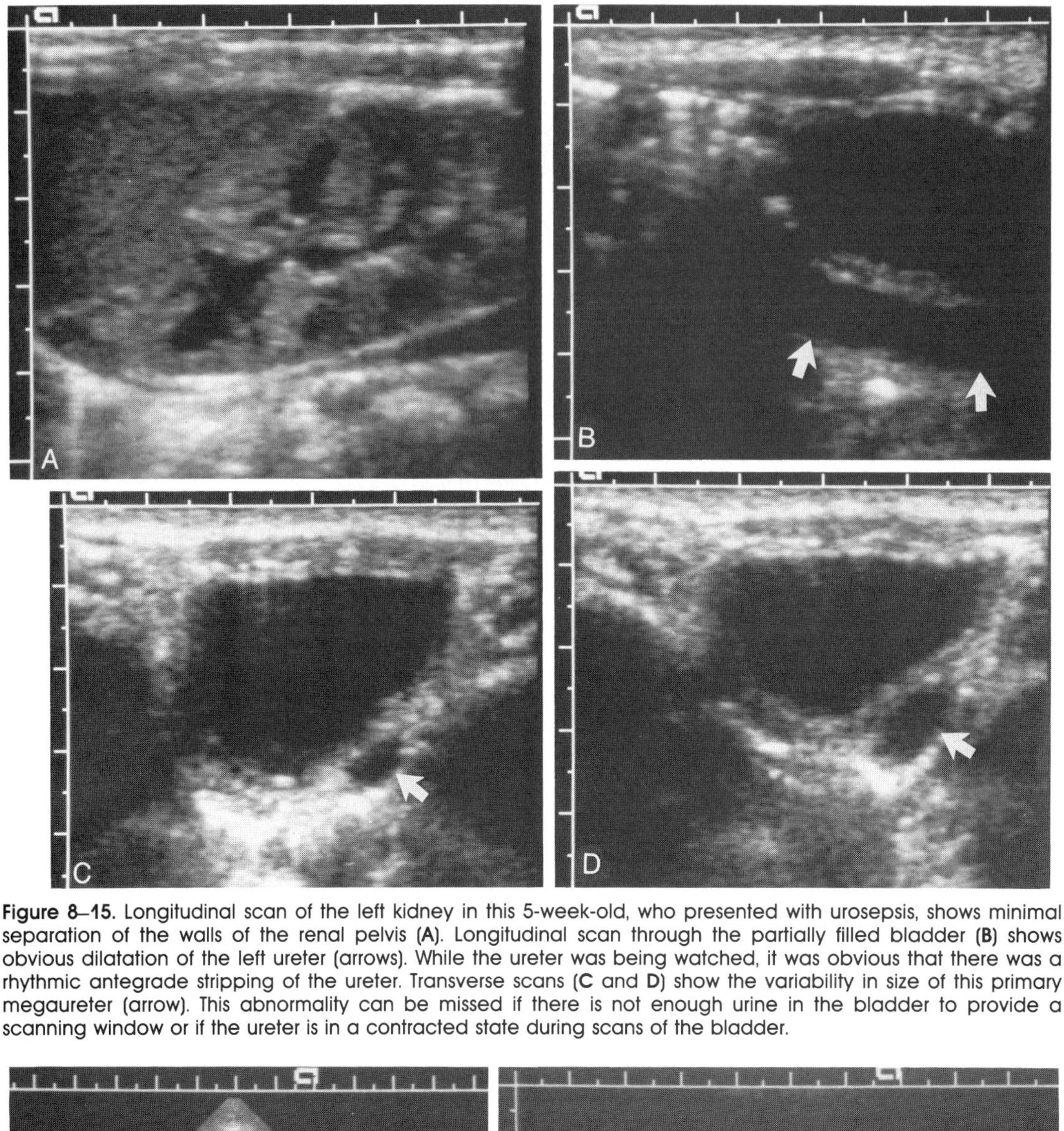

Figure 8–15. Longitudinal scan of the left kidney in this 5-week-old, who presented with urosepsis, shows minimal separation of the walls of the renal pelvis (**A**). Longitudinal scan through the partially filled bladder (**B**) shows obvious dilatation of the left ureter (arrows). While the ureter was being watched, it was obvious that there was a rhythmic antegrade stripping of the ureter. Transverse scans (**C** and **D**) show the variability in size of this primary megaureter (arrow). This abnormality can be missed if there is not enough urine in the bladder to provide a scanning window or if the ureter is in a contracted state during scans of the bladder.

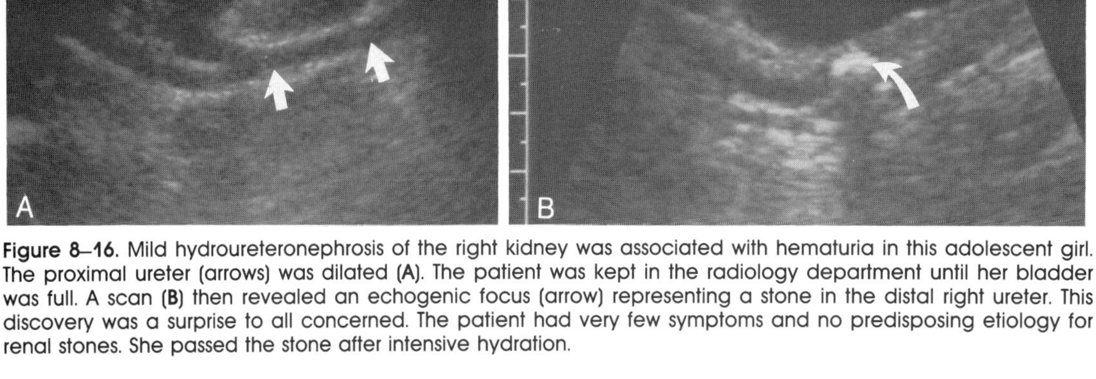

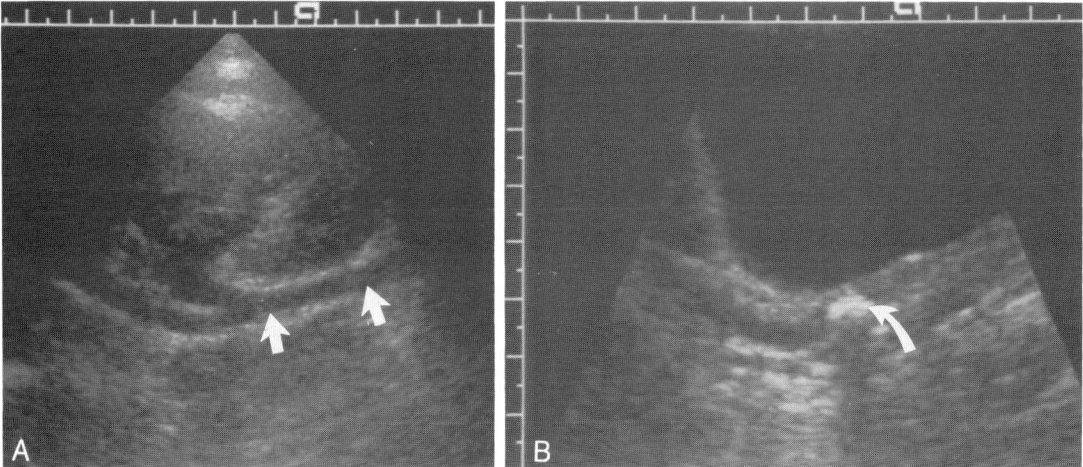

Figure 8–16. Mild hydroureteronephrosis of the right kidney was associated with hematuria in this adolescent girl. The proximal ureter (arrows) was dilated (**A**). The patient was kept in the radiology department until her bladder was full. A scan (**B**) then revealed an echogenic focus (arrow) representing a stone in the distal right ureter. This discovery was a surprise to all concerned. The patient had very few symptoms and no predisposing etiology for renal stones. She passed the stone after intensive hydration.

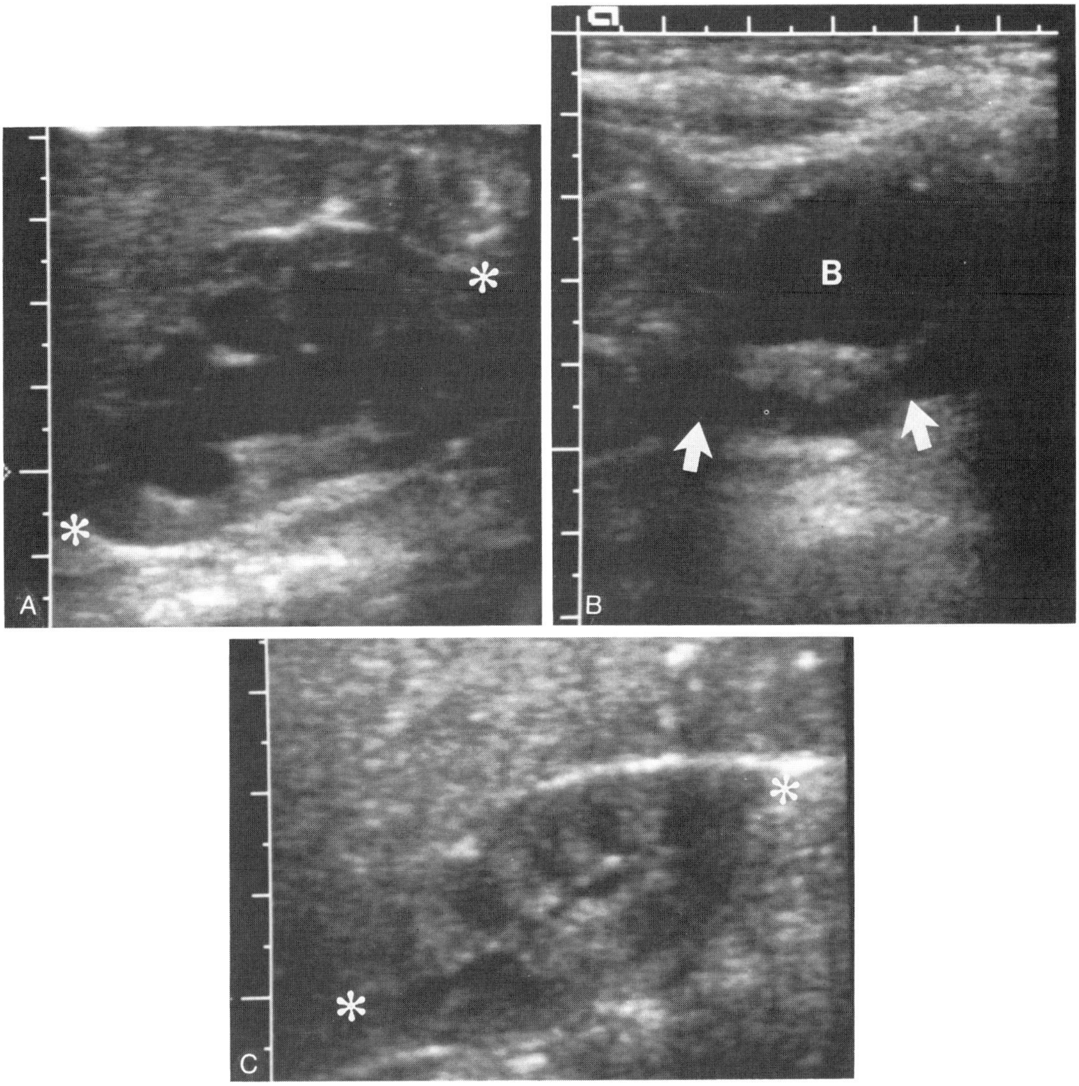

Figure 8–17. Severe postoperative edema at the site of ureteral reimplantation was the cause of this patient's hydronephrosis (**A**) and distal ureteral dilatation (arrows, **B**). B = bladder. Preoperative scan of the kidney is shown for comparison (**C**). Postoperative dilatation should not exceed the degree seen on the preoperative voiding cystourethrogram in patients who have undergone reimplantation for reflux. This child was managed conservatively, the edema subsided, and the kidney returned to normal size over the next 2 months.

intravesical blister, contiguous with its ureter (Figs. 8–18, 8–19). In contrast, the ectopic ureterocele tends to be large and draining a dysplastic or poorly functional kidney through a large ureter (Fig. 8–20). Identification of a single, rather than duplex, system should follow, as should functional studies. (See the later section on duplex kidneys.)

Although ultrasonography has been advocated as a means of documenting vesicoureteral reflux (Kessler and Altman, 1982; Schneider et al., 1984), identification and degree of reflux are better established with radiography. If the situation dictates—that is, if parents refuse any radiography and the presence of suspected gross reflux has to be established—ultrasonography can be implemented. The child is catheterized, the bladder is emptied, and scans of each kidney are done as baseline views. Normal saline is introduced into the bladder while the ureterovesical junctions are monitored with scanning.

Routine, normal ultrasonographic scans of the kidneys and bladder cannot rule out the

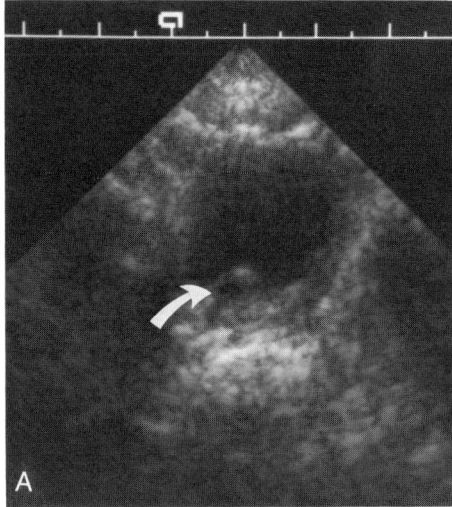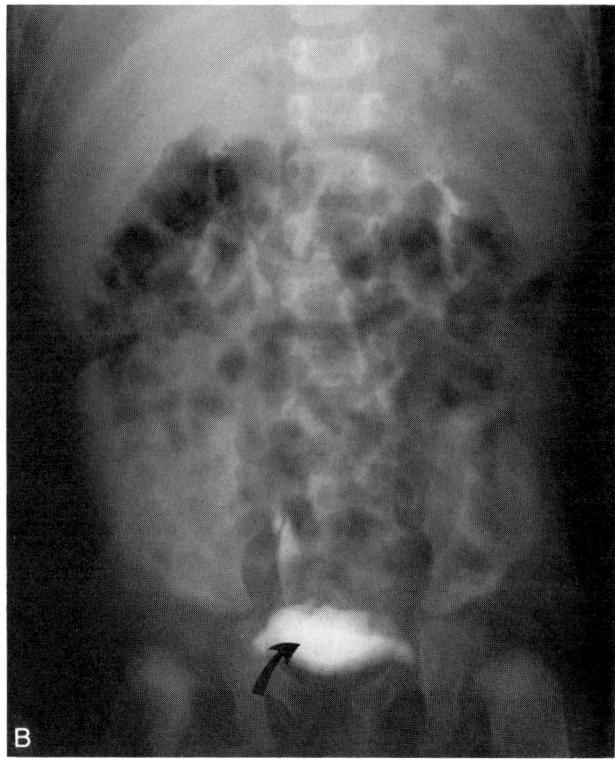

Figure 8–18. Episodic abdominal pain and fever resulted in screening ultrasonography for this 5-month-old boy. Both kidneys were normal. Scan **(A)** through a partially filled bladder showed a small intraluminal cyst typical of a simple ureterocele (arrow). Intravenous urogram **(B)** confirmed this diagnosis. There is a single collecting system on the right associated with a simple ureterocele (arrow).

presence of significant vesicoureteral reflux (Fig. 8–21). Parents should be told, and physicians reminded, of this fact, particularly when ultrasonography is performed before voiding cystourethrography in the evaluation of a child with a urinary tract infection.

On occasion, reflux is apparent on routine ultrasonography. A patulous vesicoureteral junction is present in situations of gross reflux (Fig. 8–22). Variable dilatation of the ureter and renal pelvis during an examination is characteristic of moderate reflux. Rapid refilling of the bladder with a moderate to large amount of urine immediately after voiding indicates earlier reflux: "aberrant micturition" and drainage of refluxed urine back into the bladder. A baby or child with gross reflux develops a capacious bladder, megacystis-megaureter, from this situation (Willi and Lebowitz, 1979).

A posterior urethral valve results from obstructing folds of tissue in the posterior urethra of boys. These folds, fused anteriorly, cause variable degrees of dilatation of the bladder and upper tracts by preventing normal drainage of urine from the bladder. Each affected patient has only one valve, and purists suggest that the singular rather than plural term be used (Cremin, 1986). We circumvent the argument by using the acronym PUV. The ultrasonographic findings are those of obstructive uropathy and variable degrees of renal dysplasia. Most cases of significant PUV are diagnosed during the first 2 years of life. Prenatal ultrasonography has changed the mode of presentation of PUV. A boy who has severe obstruction is diagnosed when his mother is referred for evaluation of oligohydramnios. A urinary tract infection, a lower abdominal mass representing a distended bladder, incontinence, and poor urinary stream are other clinical presentations after delivery. Exaggerated but normal folds of plicae colliculi that can be demonstrated on voiding cystourethrography in some older boys should not be mistaken for PUV.

Bilateral hydronephrosis in a boy should always make the clinician consider the diagnosis of PUV. Chronic urethral obstruction results in dilatation of the posterior urethra and utricle. The bladder enlarges, the wall of the bladder thickens, becoming trabeculated as obstruction persists, and the upper tracts

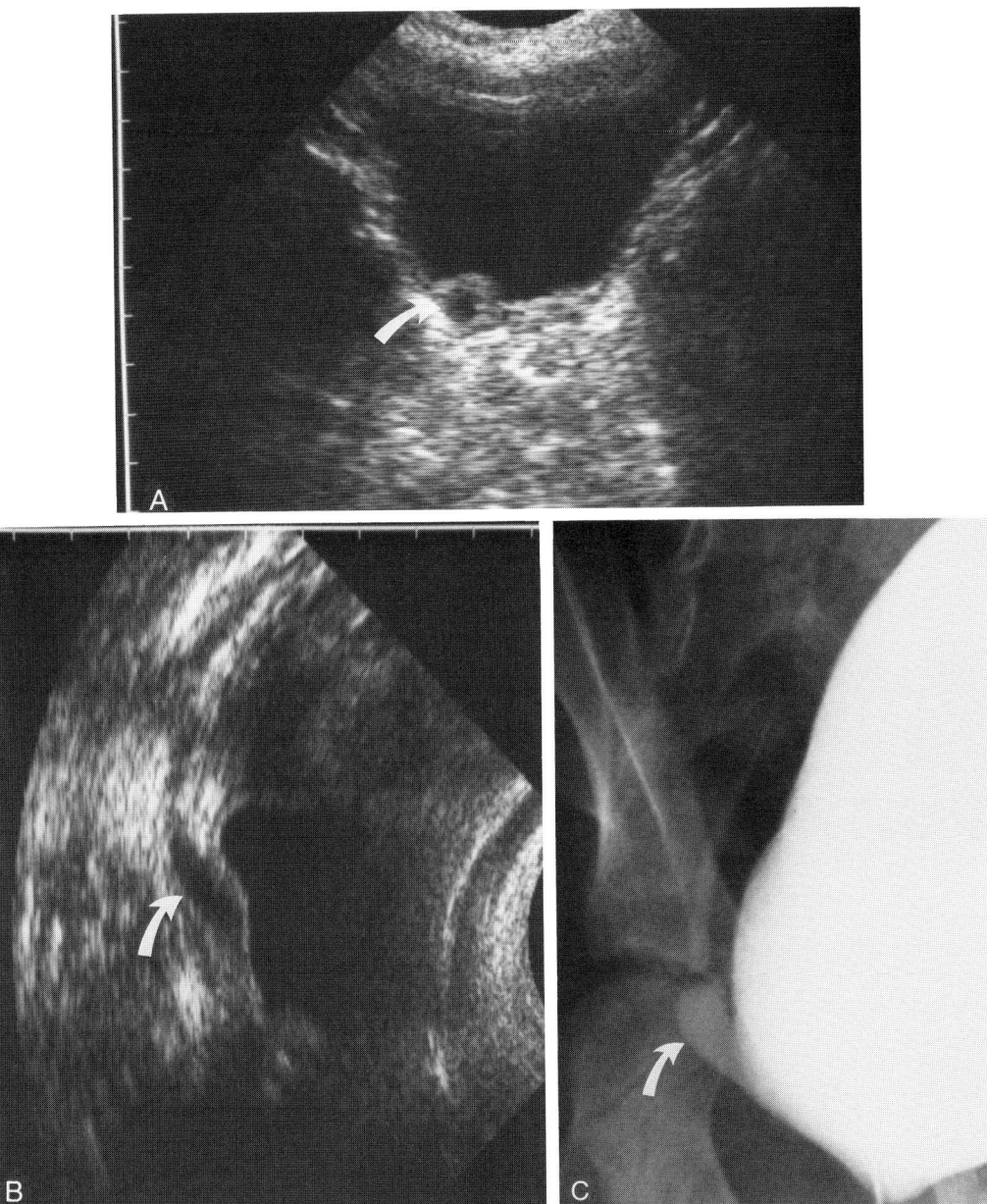

Figure 8–19. A diverticulum can simulate a ureterocele on ultrasonograms. Transverse scan of the bladder (A) suggests a ureterocele, except that the wall (arrow) appears too thick. Longitudinal view of the bladder (B) is oriented to conform to the cystogram (C). The patient has a diverticulum of the bladder (arrow) associated with reflux on the right.

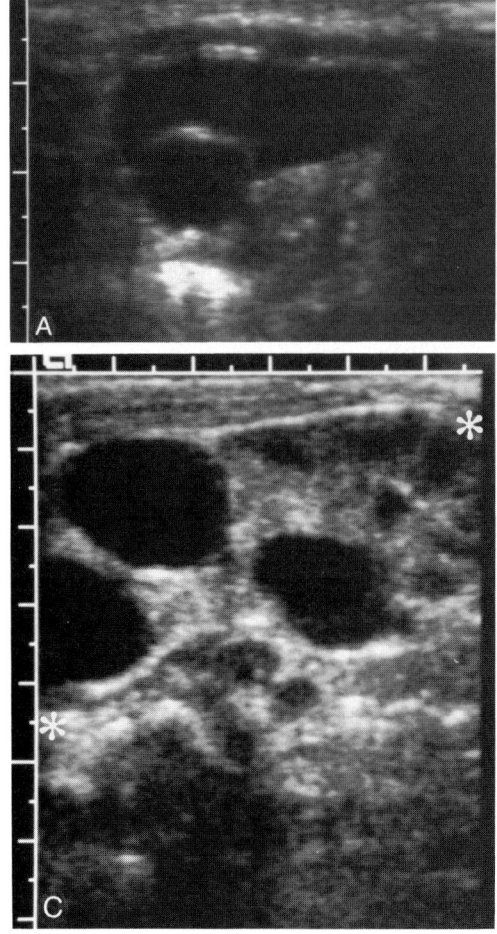
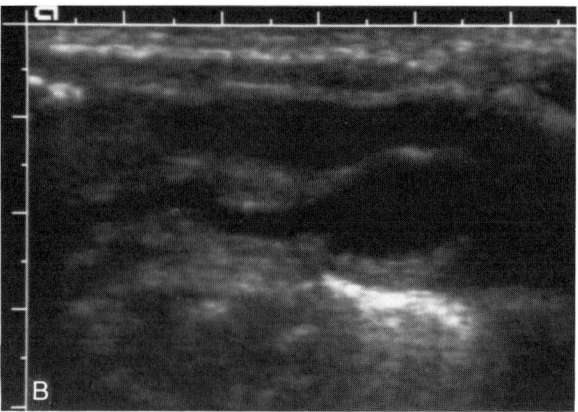

Figure 8–20. An ectopic ureterocele tends to be large, thin-walled, and associated with the upper pole of a duplex system. Transverse **(A)** and longitudinal **(B)** scans of the pelvis show the association of a ureterocele with both the bladder and its ureter. A coronal scan of the right kidney **(C)** shows multicystic dysplasia of the upper pole secondary to chronic obstruction. Heminephroureterectomy was performed.

dilate in response to the increased intravesical pressure. To complicate matters, vesicoureteral reflux supervenes or coexists in a large number of patients. Cerniglia and coworkers (1988) reported that 40 percent of their 66 patients with PUV had vesicoureteral reflux.

Decompression of the urinary tract in utero or after birth can occur as urine, under pressure, escapes from the collecting system into the retroperitoneum or the peritoneum, or both. The pathophysiology of this occurrence is hypothetical; most explanations invoke perforation of a caliceal fornix and accumulation of urine in a subcapsular or perirenal location with subsequent rupture or transudation across the peritoneum (Connor et al., 1988). In rare instances, perforation of the bladder may occur (Trulock et al., 1985). It is possible that decompression, through extravasation, allows more normal development of nephrons than is possible in the presence of chronically raised intrapelvic pressure. Renal dysplasia is associated with obstructive uropathy. Vesicoureteral reflux *plus* obstruction seems to be a combination powerful enough to prevent normal metanephric differentiation. If, however, there is a decompressive mechanism in the form of urinoma or ascites, diverticula of the bladder, or unilateral reflux with dysplasia, then renal function after ablation of the valve is better preserved (Rittenberg et al., 1988).

The ultrasonograms of patients with PUV may show any or all of the following features: a dilated posterior urethra and utricle in perineal or abdominal scanning; a large bladder with a thickened trabeculated wall; hydroureteronephrosis; a perinephric cyst representing urinoma; urinary ascites; and an abnormal renal parenchyma (Figs. 8–23, 8–24). If decompression of the system has resulted from urinoma or ascites, the bladder may be small and its wall close to normal in

EVALUATING AN ABDOMINAL MASS / 231

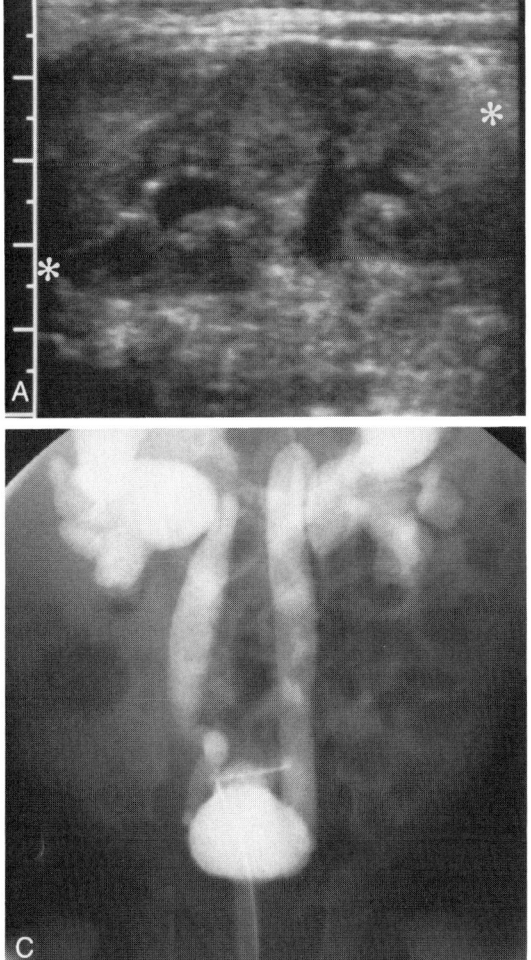

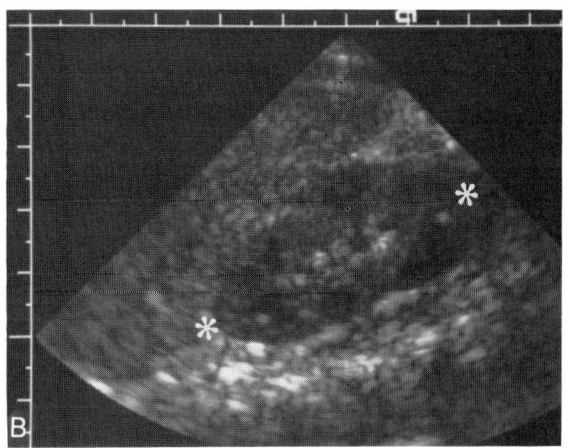

Figure 8–21. Septicemia with *Escherichia coli* was diagnosed in this 6-week-old girl. Scan of the left kidney showed mild dilatation of the intrarenal collecting system (A). Scan of the right kidney looked completely normal (B). Voiding cystourethrogram shows grade 4 bilateral reflux (C). It has been our experience that normal renal ultrasonograms cannot rule out the presence of significant vesicoureteral reflux.

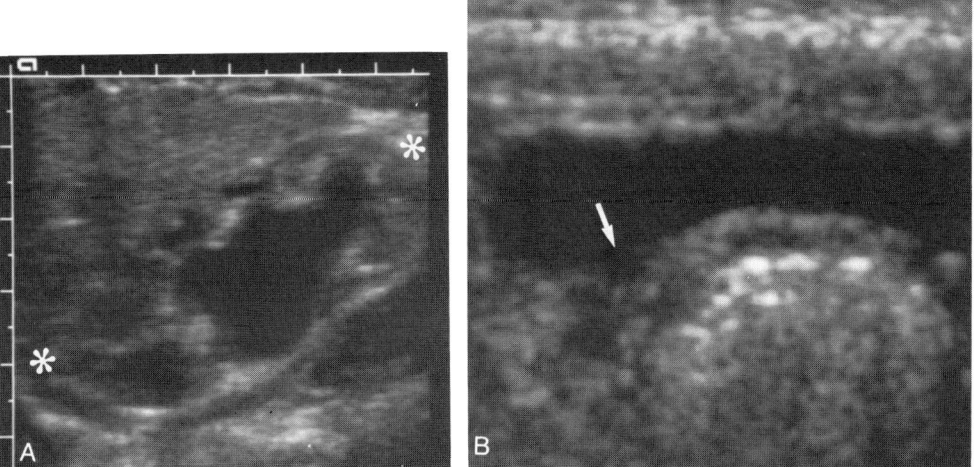

Figure 8–22. Prenatal diagnosis of hydronephrosis brought this baby to ultrasonography when she was 3 weeks old. There is hydronephrosis of the lower pole of a duplex system (A). Scans of the bladder (B) showed a patulous vesicoureteral junction (arrow) with variable dilatation of the distal ureter. Voiding cystourethrography confirmed the ultrasonographic impression of reflux into the lower pole of the duplex system.

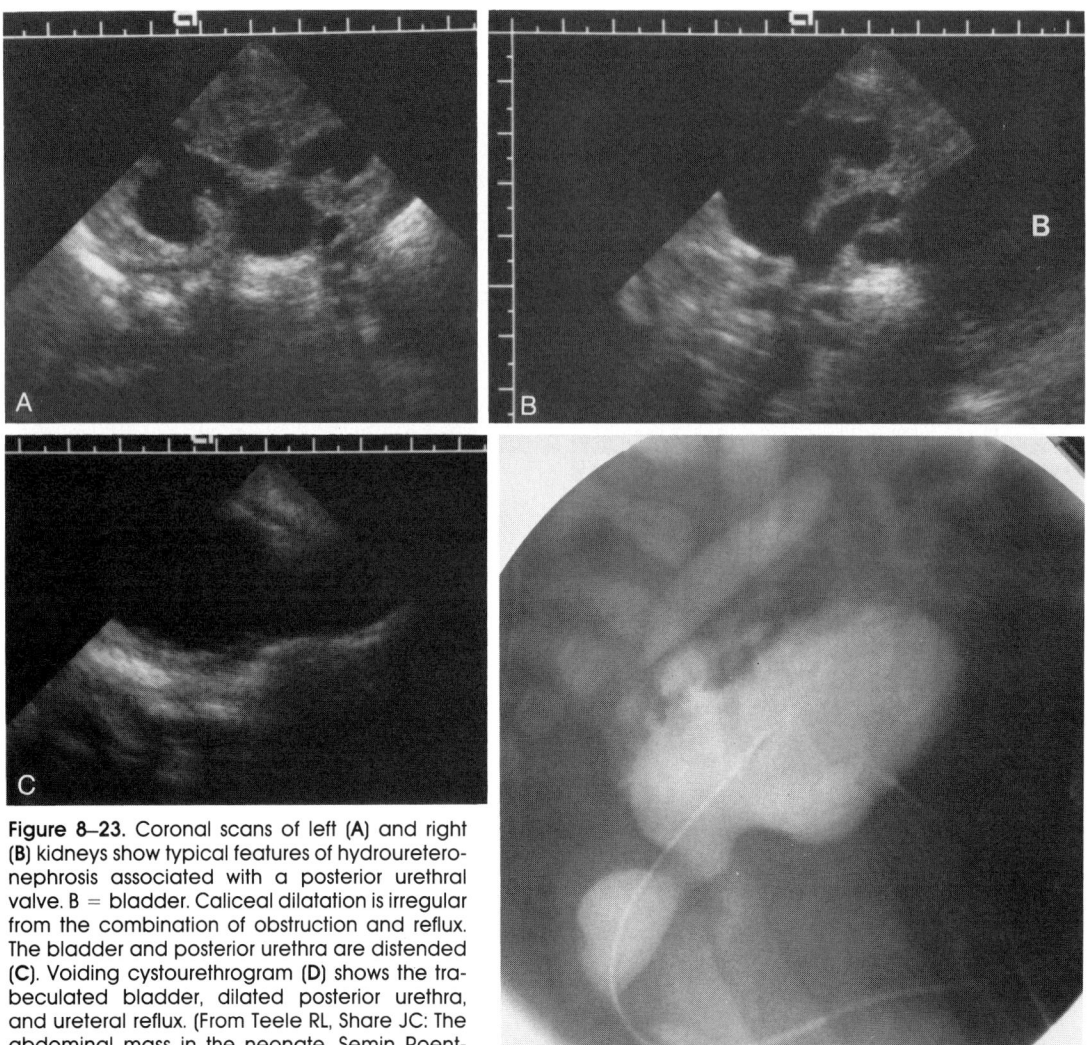

Figure 8–23. Coronal scans of left (A) and right (B) kidneys show typical features of hydroureteronephrosis associated with a posterior urethral valve. B = bladder. Caliceal dilatation is irregular from the combination of obstruction and reflux. The bladder and posterior urethra are distended (C). Voiding cystourethrogram (D) shows the trabeculated bladder, dilated posterior urethra, and ureteral reflux. (From Teele RL, Share JC: The abdominal mass in the neonate. Semin Roentgenol 1988; 23:175–184.)

thickness. The kidney ipsilateral to a urinoma may be distorted and displaced by the collection. Echogenic material within a urinoma suggests a clot or superinfection. In most cases, a urinoma gradually resorbs after the primary obstruction is relieved. Percutaneous drainage is appropriate if the mass causes respiratory compromise or if infection is present. The renal parenchyma may be quite overtly echogenic with poor medullary-cortical differentiation, and it is our impression that this appearance likely represents dysplasia in response to chronic obstruction (Fig. 8–25). Unlike the situation in which there is simple obstruction at the UPJ or the ureterovesical junction, calices are often irregularly, rather than uniformly, dilated. Coexistent reflux is possibly responsible for this appearance. Any patient in whom PUV is diagnosed on ultrasonography must have a voiding cystourethrogram in order to document the valve and to make the diagnosis of reflux if it is present. If the radiographic study cannot be done immediately, catheterization of the bladder, in order to decompress the system, is warranted.

Obstruction to the outlet of the bladder may also occur as a result of sphincteric dysfunction, a urethral stricture (postinflammatory, posttraumatic, or after instrumentation of the bladder), a polyp or tumor, and, in rare instances, a calculus (Fig. 8–26).

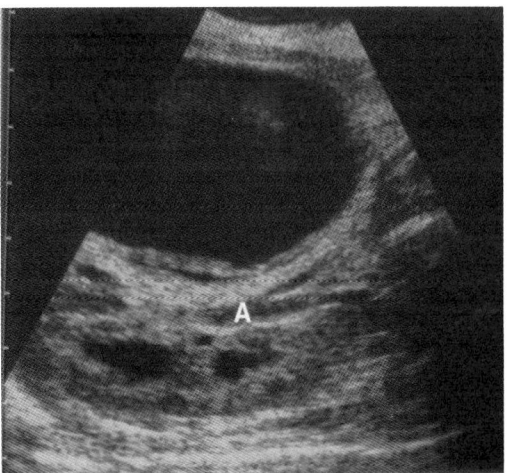

Figure 8–24. This newborn boy presented with a left-sided abdominal mass during routine physical examination. Scan through the left flank shows a large cyst representing a urinoma. The aorta (A) is bowed to the right. Residual renal tissue on the left is flattened by the urinoma. The right kidney is mildly hydronephrotic. The bladder, although decompressed at the time, had a thickened wall. Obstructed by the posterior urethral valve, it was decompressed as urine refluxed into the left kidney through a forniceal tear and into the retroperitoneum.

Duplex systems are subject to all the anatomic and physiologic vagaries that affect single systems; in addition, they have problems peculiar to duplication. Complete duplication occurs when two ureteral buds arise from the same wolffian duct early in fetal life. With caudal migration of the wolffian duct, the ureter from the lower pole is the first to become absorbed into the bladder. It therefore occupies a more cephalad and lateral position than its mate, which continues to migrate with the wolffian duct and becomes the ectopic ureter. Because of early implantation into the bladder, the ureter from the lower pole may have a short or no submucosal tunnel. This embryologic mistake in timing predisposes the ureter to vesicoureteral reflux. Reflux into the collecting system of the lower pole is cited as the most common problem seen in association with duplex systems, but its true incidence is unknown. The ureter from the upper pole may function normally or may be obstructed; reflux into the upper pole is rare. Obstruction is usually associated with an ectopic ureterocele. This submucosal ballooning of the distal ureter results in a cystic intravesical mass when the bladder is empty or partially filled with urine (Plate IX). The ureterocele may be

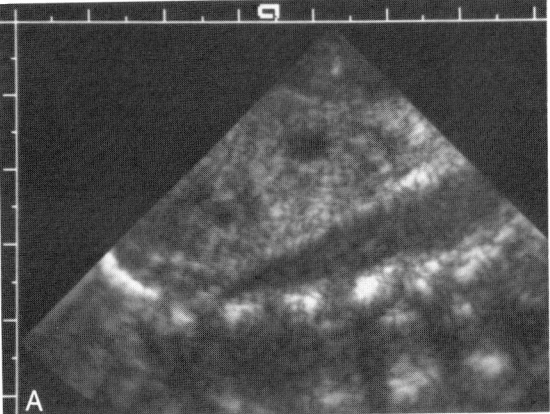
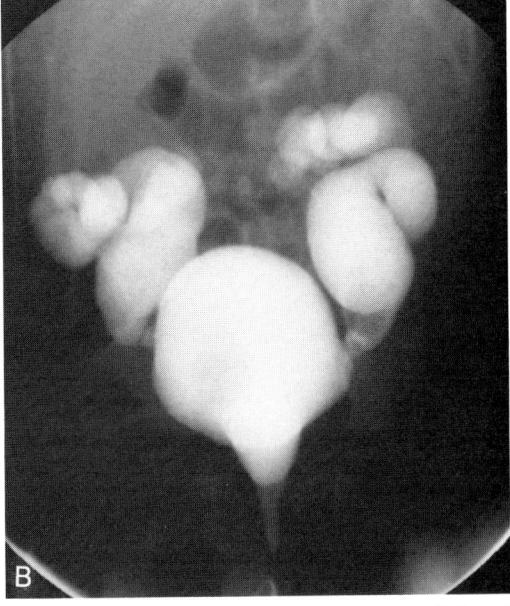

Figure 8–25. The renal outline is difficult to discern because fibrosis associated with dysplasia causes the kidney to lose its silhouette against retroperitoneal connective tissues (A). This baby had small, dysplastic kidneys secondary to posterior urethral valve with vesicoureteral reflux (B). Even though the obstruction had been relieved shortly after the infant's birth, the kidneys had been permanently damaged, and the baby was in chronic renal failure.

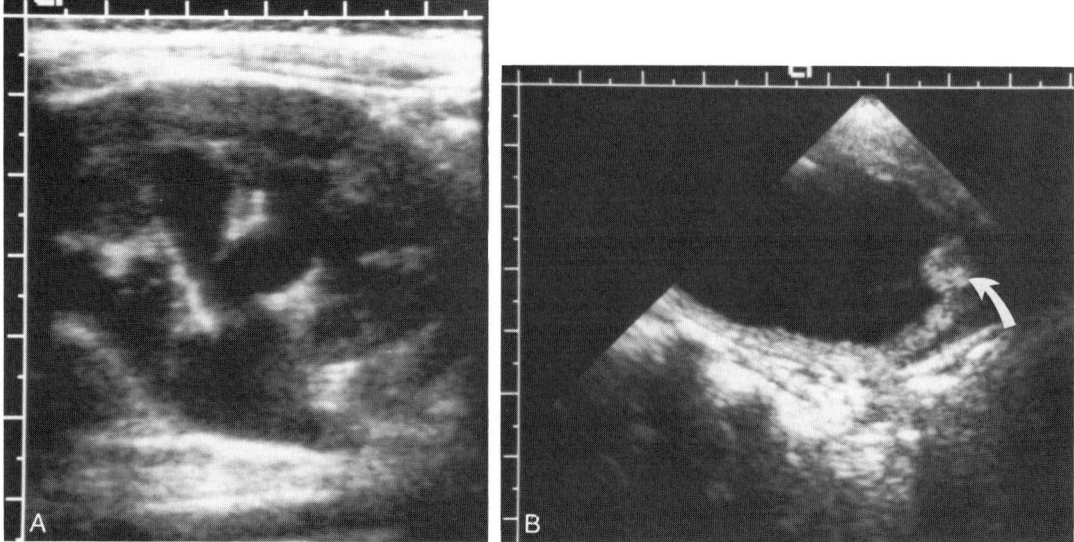

Figure 8–26. Bilateral hydronephrosis was present in this 8-month-old, who presented with irritability, decreased appetite, and temperatures up to 39°C. The creatinine level was 2.9. Longitudinal scan of the right kidney (A) was similar to that of the left. The bladder was distended (B). At the base of the bladder, a prolapsing urethral polyp (arrow) was obvious and was the cause of the baby's obstruction. Hydronephrosis resolved with resection of the polyp.

forced outside the confines of the bladder wall if the intravesical pressure is high and the musculature of the bladder is weak in that area. It may also intussuscept into its own ureter. The ureterocele may be large enough or close enough to ipsilateral or contralateral ureters that it obstructs them. If its position is low, it may cause obstruction of the outlet of the bladder. Ectopic insertion of a ureter is usually into the bladder, but because of the relationship with the wolffian duct, the ectopic ureter may be dragged as far as the urethral ejaculatory duct in boys and the vagina in girls. In rare instances the ureter remains attached to the wolffian duct and empties into a wolffian derivative (i.e., the vas deferens or the seminal vesicle). The upper pole associated with the ectopic ureter is variable both in size and in its degree of metanephric differentiation. A dysplastic nubbin of renal tissue may be all that is present. Usually the volume of the upper pole is 25 to 40 percent of the entire renal volume.

The typical ultrasonographic appearance of an uncomplicated duplex kidney is that of a large kidney with a split central sinus. (See section on renal anomalies in Chapter 6.) The *complicated* duplex kidney is affected by reflux, obstruction, or both. A disparity in degree of distention between upper and lower collecting systems is a clue to the presence of a complicated duplex kidney. Dilatation of the collecting system in the lower pole may be secondary to reflux, to obstruction at its ureteropelvic junction, or to obstruction at the ureterovesical junction from an adjacent ipsilateral or contralateral ureterocele (Figs. 8–27, 8–28). Primary megaureter is another but much rarer cause of obstruction to a lower renal unit. The collecting system of the upper pole may be normal or dilated. An unobstructed and yet ectopic ureter that drains into the vagina in a girl may be invisible on ultrasonography. Chronic wetting is the clinical presentation in most girls with this anomaly. Chronic vaginal discharge and inflammation from infected, pooled urine are other presentations. In such cases, we occasionally see fluid in the vagina trapped behind the hymen, but we emphasize that a "normal" ultrasonogram does not rule out ectopic insertion of the ureter into the vagina. We scanned at least one patient who was known to have an unobstructed ectopic ureter draining into the vagina but in whom no identifiable abnormality was visible on ultrasonography. Excretory urography should be the first study done for girls who have constant wetting and normal findings on neurologic examination. On occasion, an ectopic ureter is stenotic at

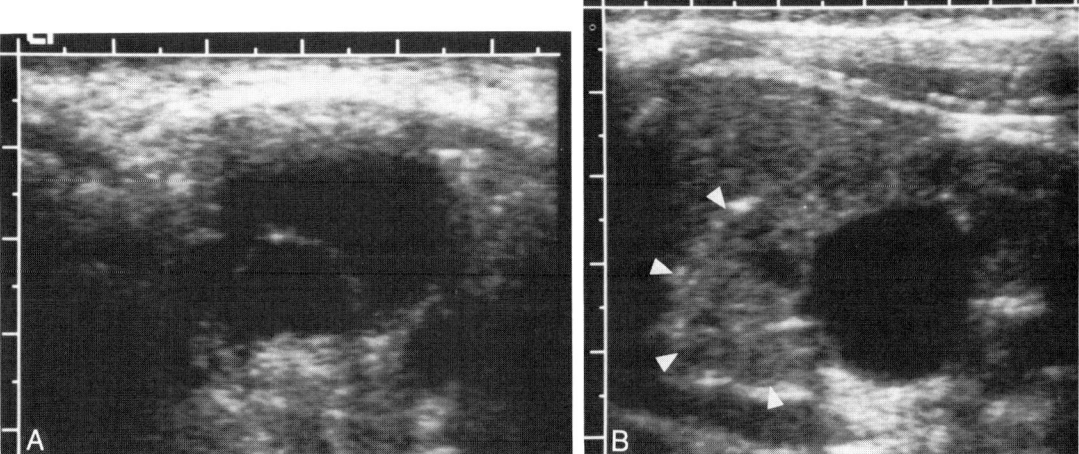

Figure 8–27. Prenatal diagnosis of a ureterocele had been made in this baby, who was referred for postnatal follow-up at 18 days of age. Transverse scan of the bladder (**A**) shows the ureterocele. No dilatation of an associated ureter was apparent. The coronal scan of the right kidney (**B**) shows an echogenic upper pole (arrowheads), which represents dysplasia. The lower pole is abnormal, with dilatation of its collecting system. A voiding cystourethrogram that followed showed grade 4 reflux into the lower pole. The dysplastic upper pole was left in place, and the ureterocele was incised.

its junction with the vagina and, being dilated, can be identified on pelvic ultrasonography as a cylindric lucent mass coursing parallel to the posterior wall of the bladder (Fig. 8–29).

An obstructed ectopic ureter usually can be traced from the upper pole to its termination (Fig. 8–30). Obstruction of the collecting system of the upper unit often appears as a central renal "cyst" on sagittal scans. Transverse and coronal scans of the kidney should reveal the ureter exiting from the upper pelvis. If obstruction has been severe and chronic, the upper pole may be a dysplastic nubbin of parenchyma and may have the same appearance as multicystic dysplasia of a single system (Nussbaum et al., 1986). Occasionally, the ureter from the upper pole resembles a string of beads (Fig. 8–31). An associated ureterocele is detected by means of scanning the bladder while angling the transducer. The wall of the ureterocele is often very thin and is imaged only when it is directly perpendicular to the beam of sound. A large ureterocele may be mistaken for the bladder, especially in small infants. As the bladder fills with urine, eversion of a ureterocele may occur, and the intraluminal cystic mass may disappear. Duplex kidneys are commonly bilateral. When both are complicated, the dilated ureters and pelvicaliceal systems may fill the abdomen (Fig. 8–32). Ultrasonography has to be used in association with radiography to sort out the anatomy in these cases. In all patients with complicated duplex systems, physiologic information from radiography or scintigraphy, or both, is necessary before surgical repair is performed.

In summary, when hydronephrosis is encountered, at any age, the ultrasonographic checklist is as follows: (1) Is this a single or duplex system? (2) Is the ureter dilated or

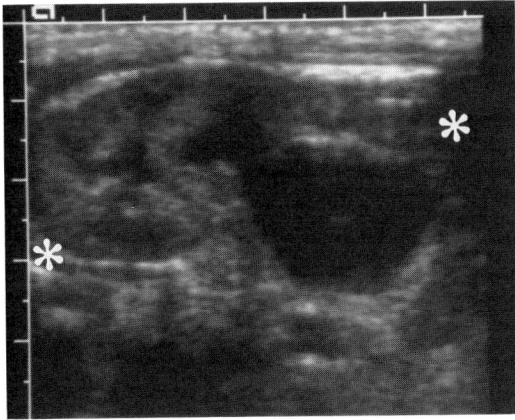

Figure 8–28. The dilatation of the collecting system of the lower pole in this duplex kidney was secondary to obstruction at the ureteropelvic junction. The upper pole was functioning normally. View shown is a coronal scan of the left kidney.

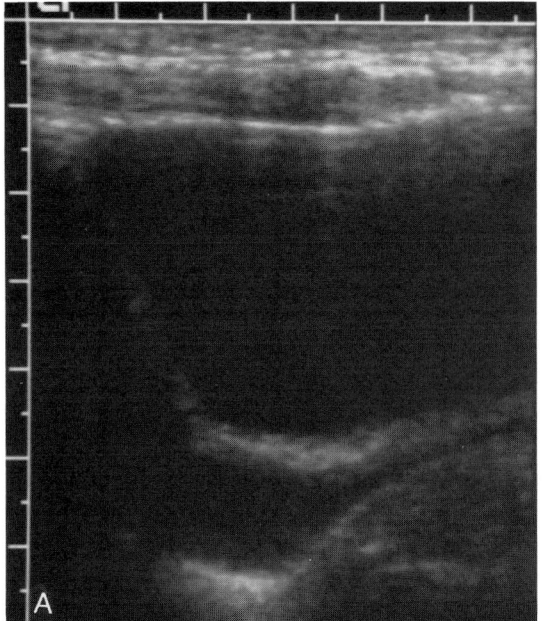
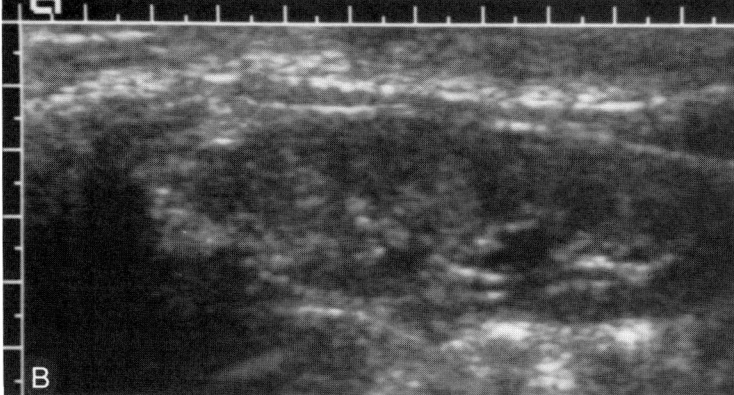

Figure 8–29. In spite of extensive earlier evaluation, no diagnosis had been made for this 8-year-old girl, whose underwear was constantly wet. Scans showed dilatation of a distal right ureter (A), although the longitudinal scan of the right kidney (B) was close to normal in appearance. These findings indicated the presence of a duplex system on the right. Right hemiureteronephrectomy was performed, and the ultrasonographic finding was confirmed. The patient's wetness persisted. Ultrasonograms were unremarkable, but careful clinical examination showed an ectopic orifice just inside the meatus on the left. Subsequent left heminephrectomy with removal of a similarly dysplastic upper pole resulted in complete eradication of her symptoms.

not? (3) Is urinary flow appreciably antegrade, retrograde, or static in a dilated ureter? (4) Is the bladder normal? (5) Is there an extrinsic retroperitoneal or pelvic mass? (6) What about the other kidney? (7) How can other imaging help?

The major differential diagnoses of obstructive hydronephrosis are a multicystic dysplastic kidney, obstruction at the ureteropelvic junction, obstruction at the vesicoureteral junction, posterior urethral valve, a neurogenic bladder, and an extrinsic pelvic mass. Rare causes of obstructive hydronephrosis include a tumor, a stone, a ureteral valve or stricture, and a urethral mass. As a general rule, voiding cystourethrography should follow ultrasonography if there is ureteral dilatation, a ureterocele, or suspicion of a posterior urethral valve. Intravenous urography or scintigraphy, or both, should follow when there is upper obstruction or a multicystic dysplastic kidney.

Not all hydronephrosis is obstructive. Vesicoureteral reflux, as discussed previously, is the most common example of nonobstructive dilatation. Prune-belly syndrome, originally named by Sir William Osler in 1901, almost always affects boys and is characterized by congenital absence or deficiency of abdominal musculature, cryptorchidism, and anomalies of the genitourinary tract (Greskovich and Nyberg, 1988). Vesicoureteral reflux is common in this syndrome, but even in patients without reflux, the ureters are dilated

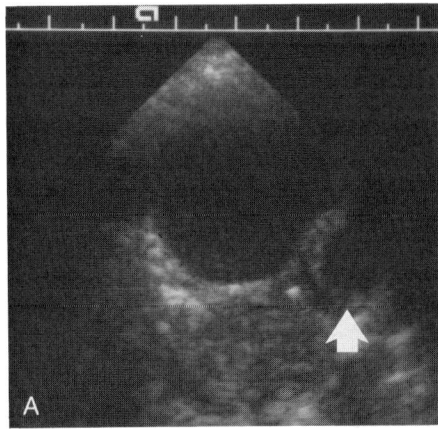

Figure 8–30. Three months before these scans, the patient had been treated for a urinary tract infection. She was admitted at 11 months of age when her mother noticed a mass in the introitus. Radiographic evaluation began with these scans. Transverse (**A**) and longitudinal (**B**) views of the bladder show a dilated left ureter (arrow, **A**). On ultrasonography, the ureter could not be traced farther distally because of the pubic symphysis. It was obvious, however, that the intralabial mass was the prolapsing ureterocele associated with this dilated ureter. Scans of the left kidney through the spleen (**C**) showed that the ureter was related to the upper pole of the duplex kidney. The patient underwent left hemiuretero-nephrectomy. In **B**, B = bladder.

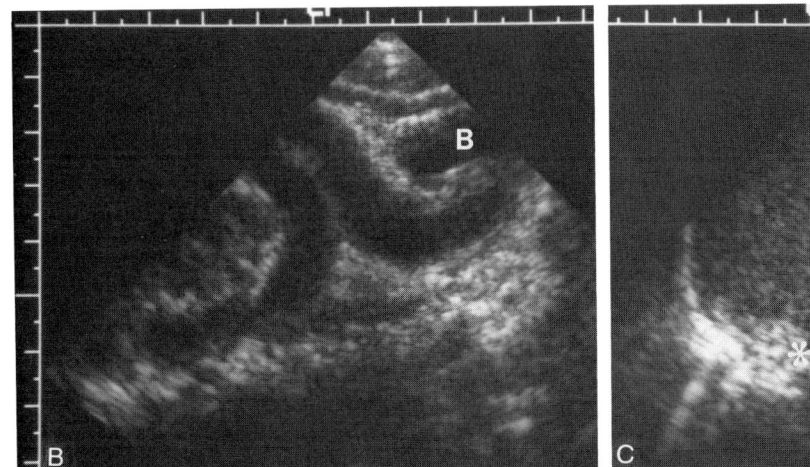

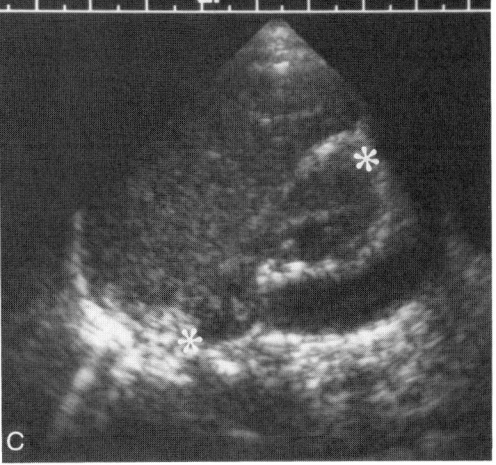

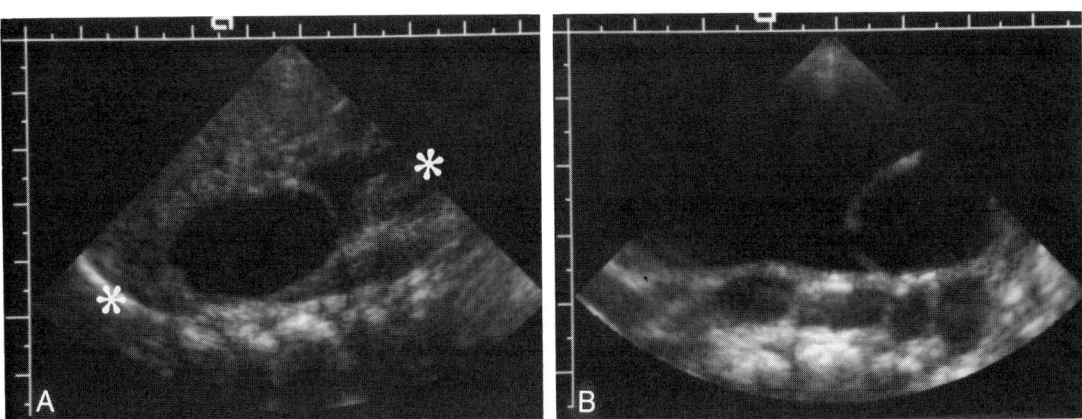

Figure 8–31. This baby had been diagnosed as having hydronephrosis in utero. Coronal scan of the right kidney (**A**) shows a duplex kidney with a central cyst in the upper pole representing an obstructed system. Its ureter could be traced to the bladder, where it entered a ureterocele (**B**). Note the beadlike appearance of the obstructed distal ureter on this longitudinal scan.

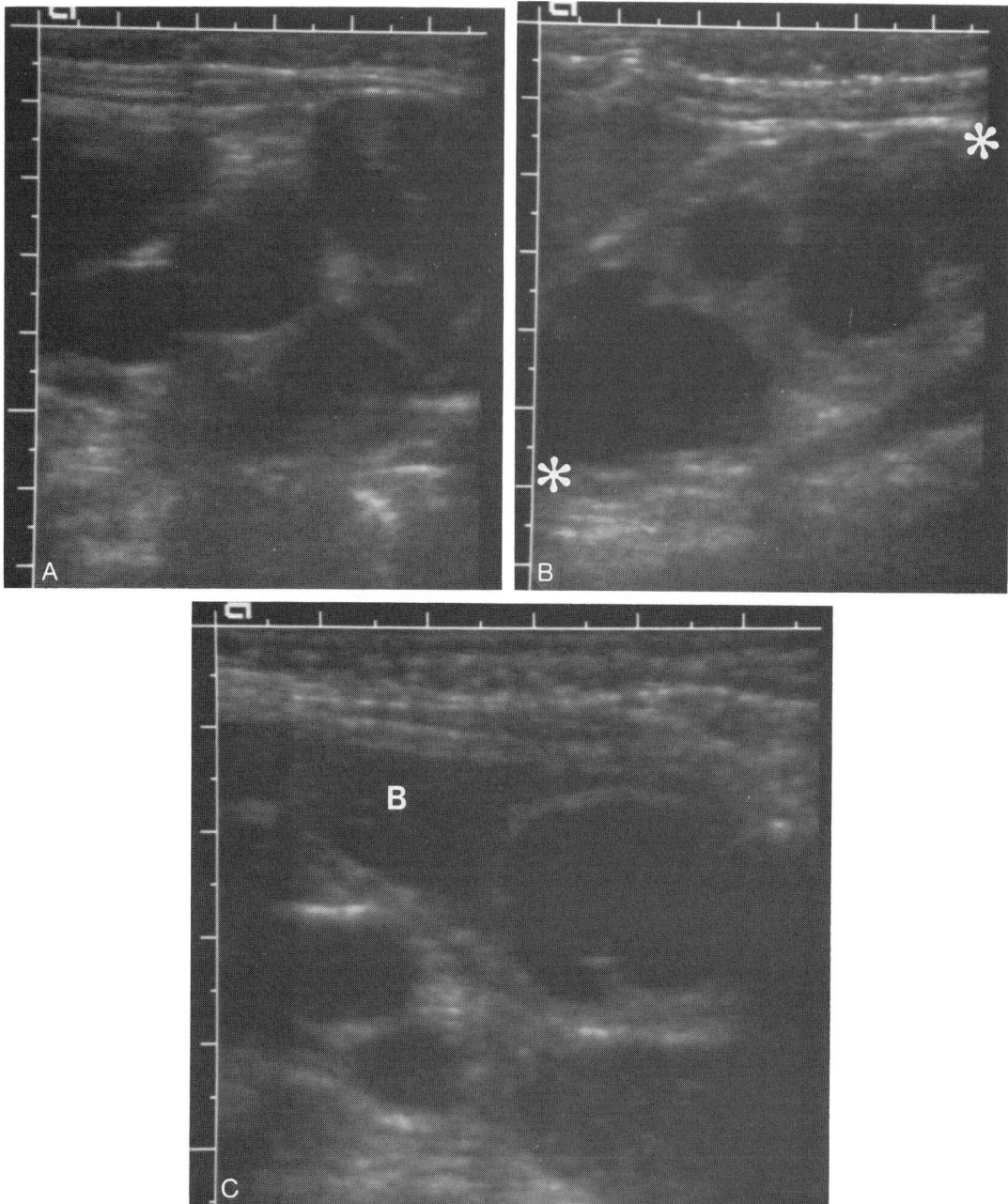

Figure 8–32. When there is severe chronic obstruction associated with duplex kidneys, the ultrasonographic anatomy can become extremely complicated. Coronal scan through the left flank (**A**) shows multiple fluid-filled structures in the abdomen of this baby girl. Coronal scan of the left kidney (**B**) shows dilatation of collecting systems to both upper and lower poles. Transverse scan of the pelvis (**C**) shows a large ureterocele in a partially filled bladder (B). A ureterocele may be mistaken for the bladder if the bladder is empty. In this patient, both left-sided ureters were dilated. The ureter from the upper pole was obstructed in association with the ureterocele, and the ureter to the lower pole was dilated because of massive reflux. Furthermore, there was right-sided hydroureteronephrosis from obstruction by the large ectopic ureterocele.

EVALUATING AN ABDOMINAL MASS / 239

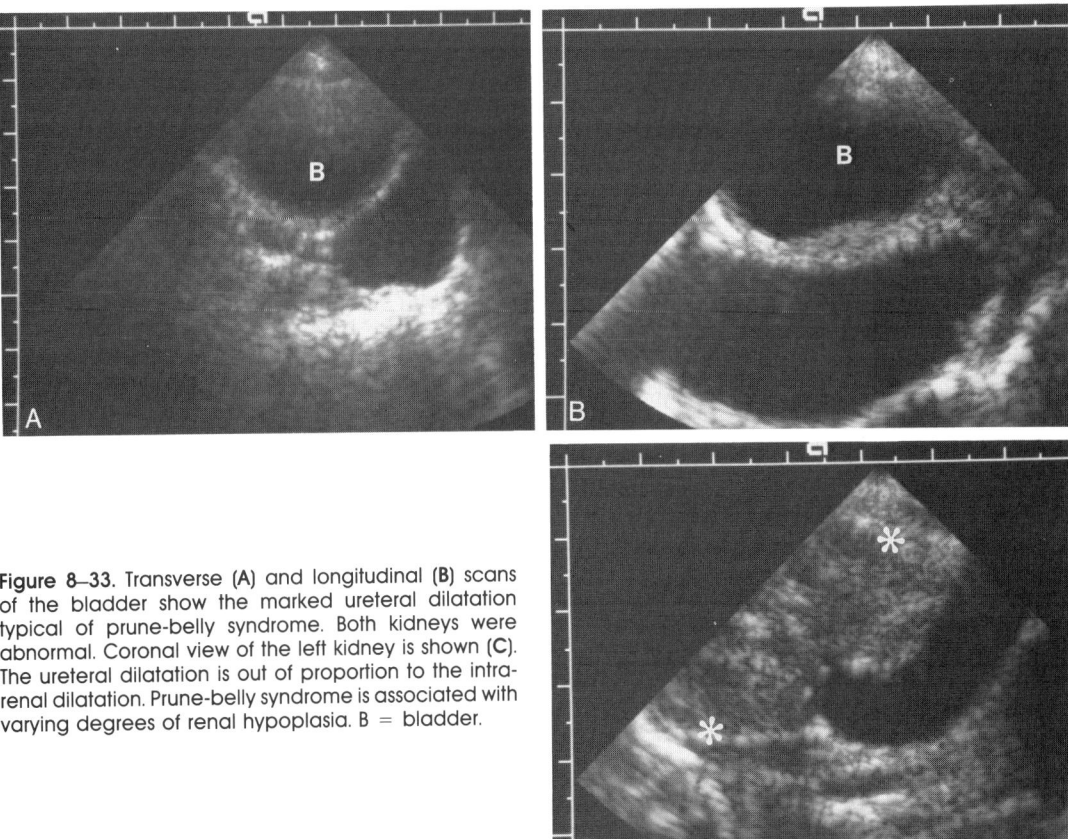

Figure 8–33. Transverse (A) and longitudinal (B) scans of the bladder show the marked ureteral dilatation typical of prune-belly syndrome. Both kidneys were abnormal. Coronal view of the left kidney is shown (C). The ureteral dilatation is out of proportion to the intra-renal dilatation. Prune-belly syndrome is associated with varying degrees of renal hypoplasia. B = bladder.

(Fig. 8–33). The bladder tends to be very large and poorly contractile. Urachal extension of the dome of the bladder is common. Hydronephrosis or renal hypoplasia is present with great variability between patients. Prenatal scans may be mistaken as being those of a baby who has a posterior urethral valve. The typical flabby appearance of the abdominal wall makes diagnosis much more obvious in the neonate.

Megacalicosis is a rare anomaly of the collecting system that also simulates obstructive hydronephrosis. Typically, the calices are large, more numerous than usual, and associated with a normal renal pelvis. The medullary-cortical ratio is 1:1 rather than the normal thickness of 3:1 (Mandell et al., 1986).

RETROPERITONEAL MASSES OTHER THAN HYDRONEPHROSIS

Some retroperitoneal masses, particularly those with a cystic component, are being discovered on prenatal ultrasonography. Most are diagnosed during clinical examination. An experienced pediatrician usually is able to localize a mass to the retroperitoneum, peritoneal cavity, pelvis, or liver. The origins of masses in the right upper quadrant are occasionally indeterminate on clinical examination alone. Most retroperitoneal masses

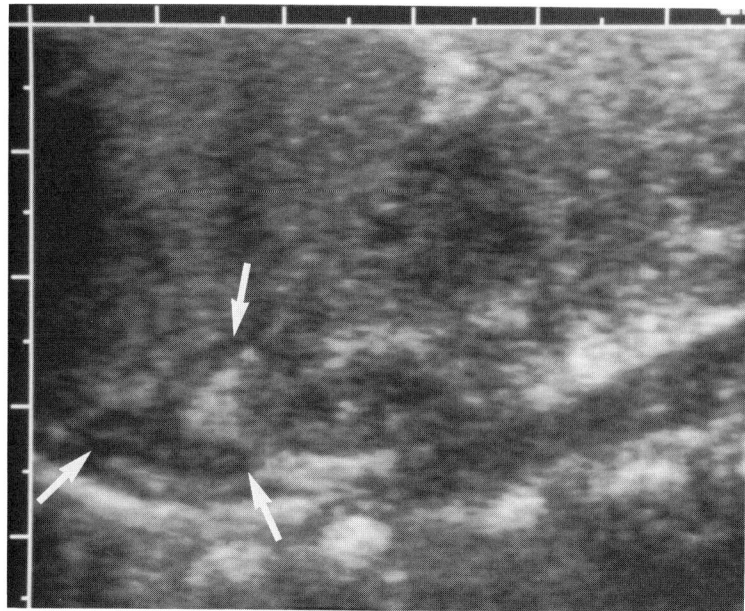

Figure 8–34. The coronal scan through the spleen of this 3-day-old baby shows the normal lambdoid appearance of the adrenal gland (arrows). In this particular case, the adrenal gland is superior to the left kidney. In many babies, the left adrenal slips medially and anteriorly.

in neonates are in the kidney or the adrenal gland. On rare occasions, such masses as teratoma, rhabdomyosarcoma, or lipoblastoma arise in this region. In older children, lymphangioma, lymphoma, pancreatic masses, and neural tumors related to sympathetic ganglia are added to the list. Ultrasonography follows plain radiographs, and the principles of examination for all children are those outlined at the beginning of this chapter.

ADRENAL MASS

Normal and Hypertrophied Adrenal Glands

To our way of thinking, a normal adrenal gland capping a normal neonatal kidney makes for one of the prettiest ultrasonograms. The normal adrenal gland makes only a brief ultrasonographic appearance; it involutes quickly after birth (Scott et al., 1990). In one study, the calculated adrenal surface area dropped by two thirds during the first postnatal week (Hata et al., 1988; Menzel and Hauffa, 1990). On coronal scans, the normal neonatal adrenal gland appears lambdoid in outline with a central linear echogenicity representing the medulla and a thicker outer coat representing the cortex (Fig. 8–34). On the right, the adrenal gland caps the kidney and is best shown on coronal views. On the left, the adrenal gland is medial and anterior to the kidney so that it is occasionally seen best on transverse rather than coronal scans. When the ipsilateral kidney is absent or ectopic, the adrenal gland slips into the renal fossa, acquires a more oval configuration,

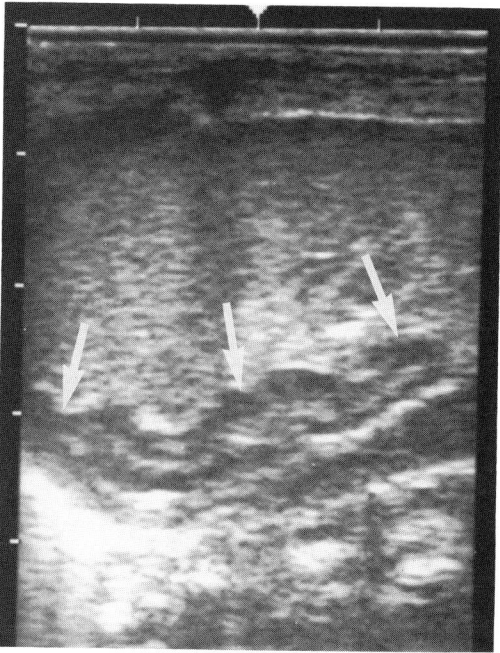

Figure 8–35. Coronal view of the left renal fossa shows the adrenal gland (arrows), which has moved into the space normally occupied by the kidney. This baby died because of bilateral renal agenesis.

and actually is larger than normal both in volume and in weight (Fig. 8–35). Absence of the adrenal gland may occur in some cases of renal agenesis, but failure to image the neonatal adrenal gland is otherwise distinctly abnormal and is diagnostic of adrenal hypoplasia.

Enlargement of the adrenal cortex occurs in many but not all babies who have congenital adrenal hyperplasia due to 21-hydroxylase deficiency (Hauffa et al., 1988). The normal cross-sectional area (about 20 percent of the normal ipsilateral kidney) increases, especially in infants with salt wasting (Fig. 8–36).

Wolman disease is also associated with adrenomegaly. This rare, lethal storage disease, which results from deficiency of the lysosomal enzyme acid lipase, appears particularly often in multiple choice questions in examinations of the American Board of Radiology! Of the approximately 40 cases that have been reported, one was published with ultrasonograms and computed tomography (CT) scans of enlarged, calcified adrenals in an affected baby girl (Dutton, 1985). Adrenal enlargement with cortical calcification is the radiologic hallmark of this disease, which is inherited in an autosomal recessive manner. Hepatosplenomegaly is usually also present.

On coronal scans of normal children older than 6 months, the adrenal area is marked only by a small triangular echogenicity. This likely represents both the adrenal gland and its surrounding fat. Large adrenal masses can be diagnosed, but small tumors in older children, especially tumors that are left-sided, are better delineated with CT.

Adrenal Hemorrhage

A large size, a difficult delivery, and perinatal asphyxia have been reported as predisposing a neonate to adrenal hemorrhage. However, a rough entry into the world is not a mandatory prerequisite, and many babies whom we have examined have presented with an asymptomatic mass or jaundice. Wright and Bear (1987) supported this statement in their review of adrenal hemorrhage. On ultrasonography, established hemorrhage can be echogenic, lucent, or mixed in appearance, depending on its age and the extent of parenchymal destruction. The adrenal gland may be discernible in part or completely obliterated. If large, the mass

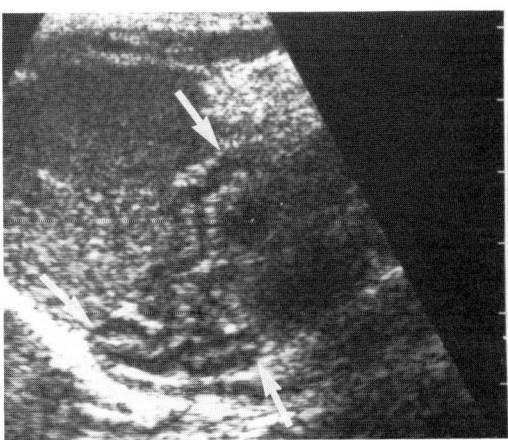

Figure 8–36. Compare the abnormal left adrenal gland (arrows) with the normal one shown in Figure 8–34. This gland is large, and the limbs have a wavy configuration. The right adrenal gland was similar in appearance. This baby had presented with ambiguous genitalia. Chromosomal analysis showed the baby to be female, and a uterus could be identified on ultrasonography. Further endocrinologic work-up revealed that the infant had 21-hydroxylase deficiency.

tends to indent the superior pole of the adjacent kidney. Sludge may be present in the gallbladder, presumably as a result of breakdown of red blood cells and production of bilirubin. The question always asked by clinicians is whether we can prove that what appears to be an adrenal hemorrhage is not neuroblastoma. Normal levels of urinary catecholamines support but do not prove the diagnosis of adrenal hemorrhage. Tincture of time is the most useful commodity available to the ultrasonographer. Hemorrhage does resorb, often slowly, but it should not increase in size nor stay completely unchanged. It also tends to assume a pyramidal, rather than spherical, shape especially as it resorbs. We routinely scan a baby with assumed adrenal hemorrhage 7 to 10 days after the first study. If the mass is shrinking or changing, we rescan after 4 weeks. By this time, the mass should have shrunk further although, on occasion, it takes 6 weeks or longer to completely resolve (Fig. 8–37). Calcification that follows hemorrhage is common and may be identified on an ultrasonogram by shadowing in the suprarenal area.

Every so often, calcification in the area of the adrenal gland is found on a plain radiograph or abdominal scans of an asymptomatic child. If it is unassociated with a mass or other abnormality, no further work-

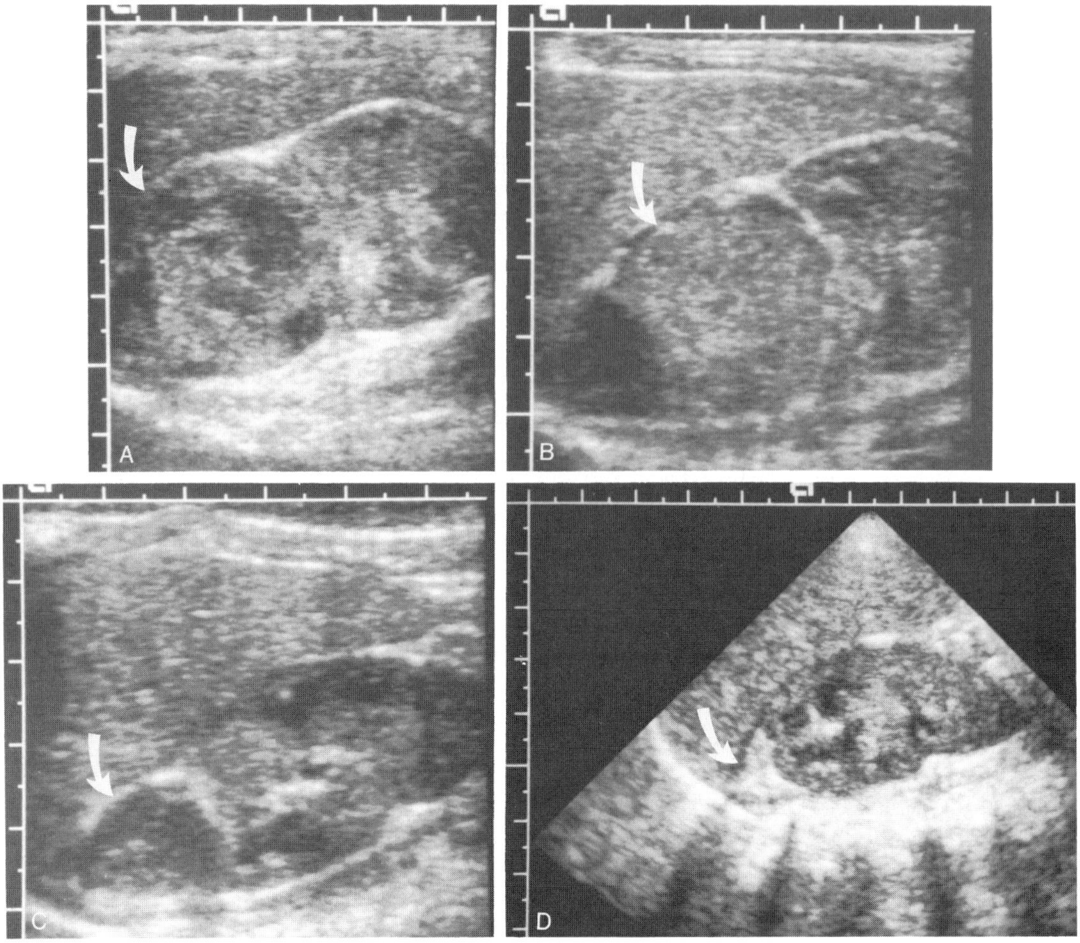

Figure 8–37. These four scans span a period of 3 months. This child was born at full term after prolonged labor and delivery with forceps. At 12 hours of age, he presented with bilious vomiting and a mass in the right flank. The first scan was performed when he was 1½ days old. The left adrenal gland (A) was hugely enlarged (arrows). Six days later (B), the pattern of echogenicity had changed slightly, but the size of the adrenal mass had not decreased. Note, however, that the mass maintained a triangular as opposed to spherical shape. One month later (C), there was a definite decrease in the size of the adrenal hemorrhage. When the child was 3 months old (D), the adrenal gland had become an echogenic triangle (arrow).

up is needed. Undoubtedly this represents a previous neonatal adrenal hemorrhage (Fig. 8–38).

Adrenal hemorrhage shown by ultrasonography has been reported in two children, 3 months and 28 months of age, who had meningococcemia (Sarnaik et al., 1988). Bacterial sepsis with any organism can produce diffuse intravascular coagulation, adrenal hemorrhage, and shock (Waterhouse-Friderichsen syndrome), but it is most commonly associated with the meningococcus. We have also seen scans of two older children whose adrenal hemorrhage followed trauma—in one case, secondary to child abuse.

Adrenal abscess is probably a complication of adrenal hemorrhage in which hematoma is seeded by bacteria during an episode of sepsis. *Escherichia coli* is the bacteria most commonly isolated in cases that have been reported (Atkinson et al., 1985). The diagnosis should be considered for a baby who has an adrenal mass associated with high fever and other systemic signs of infection.

Neuroblastoma

We have yet to be convinced that adrenal hemorrhage can occur, in utero, in a normal gland. Patients whom we have seen with a diagnosis, made in utero, of an adrenal mass

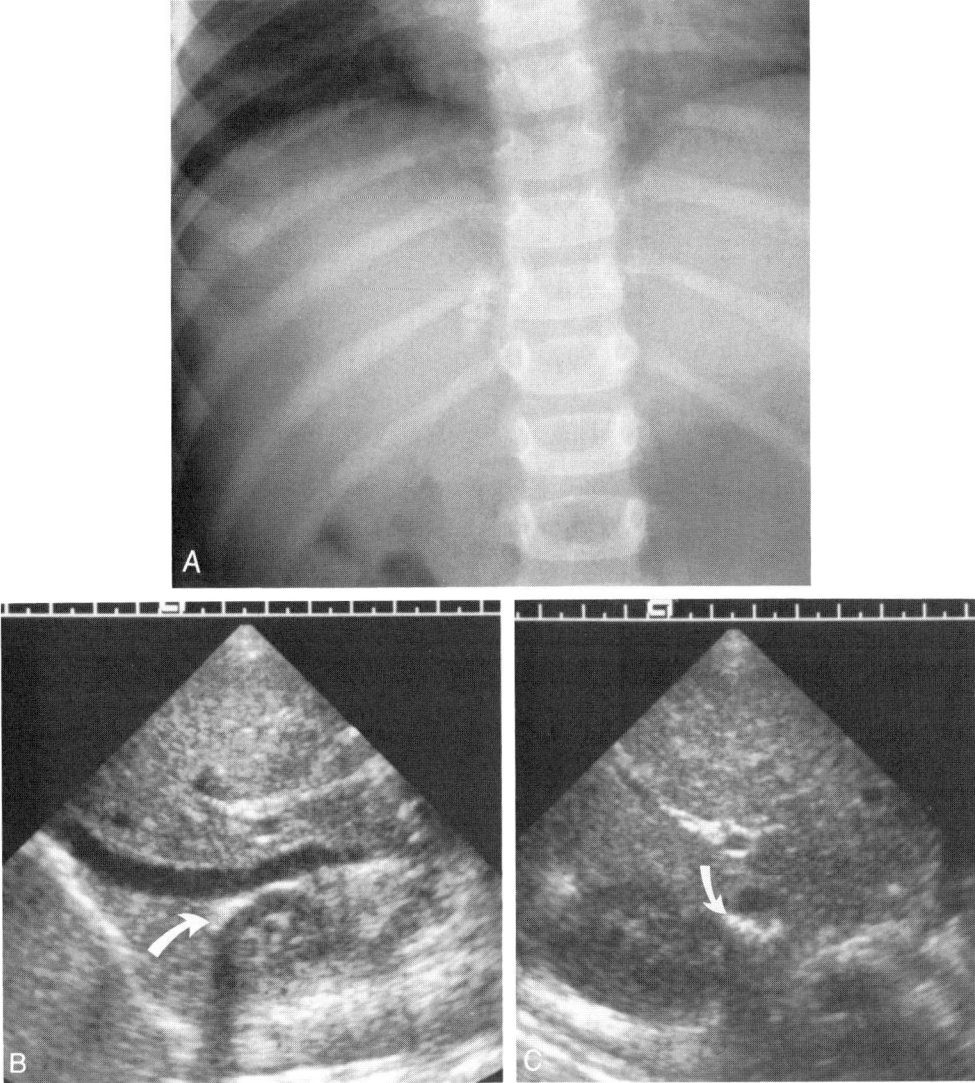

Figure 8–38. A radiograph of the abdomen was obtained because this 2-year-old child presented with crampy abdominal pain; it shows calcification in the right upper quadrant (A). Ultrasonography followed and showed a shell of calcification (arrow) on longitudinal (B) and transverse (C) scans. Past medical history was unremarkable. Because no mass effect was associated with the calcification, no further evaluation was performed. Previous adrenal hemorrhage is often detected incidentally when calcification is noted on plain radiograph or ultrasonography.

have been found, during surgery after delivery, to have neuroblastoma. There are likely some neuroblastomas that self-destruct with hemorrhage or regress spontaneously. According to autopsy studies, neuroblastoma in situ can be identified in 0.3 to 2 percent of miscarried fetuses and stillborn neonates (Beckwith and Perrin, 1963; Guin et al., 1969), although this conclusion was challenged by Ikeda and colleagues (1981). Although some neuroblastomas are detected early, most present as a mass in children who are about 2 years of age. Neuroblastoma rarely occurs in children older than 10 years. Presentation is that of an abdominal mass, failure to thrive, fever, or anemia. Two unusual paraneoplastic syndromes are associated with neuroblastoma. Myoclonic encephalopathy of infancy (opsoclonus, myoclonus, and cerebellar ataxia) is present in 2 per cent of patients with neuroblastoma (Bousvaros et al., 1986). This syndrome is thought to be secondary to antibodies to neuroblastoma that cross-react with cerebellar tissue. The reverse proportion (i.e., how many patients with the neurologic syndrome have neuroblastoma) has been the source of argument. Publication of cases is biased toward positive findings and results, and there may be less than the touted 50 percent association. Small lesions, an increased propensity for mediastinal location in comparison with other neuroblastomas, and good prognosis are characteristic of this association. For patients presenting with myoclonic encephalopathy, we recommend good chest radiography and, if the radiograph does not reveal a mediastinal tumor, abdominal CT scans. Radionuclide scans with ^{123}I-meta-iodobenzylguanidine (MIBG) may be another diagnostic tool; data from large groups of patients are not yet available. The second paraneoplastic syndrome associated with neuroblastoma is linked to excess secretion of vasoactive peptides and occurs in approximately 7 percent of children with tumors originating from the neural crest (Bousvaros et al., 1986). Watery diarrhea, hypokalemia, and hypochlorhydria are the consequences of this association.

Laboratory tests that support the diagnosis of neuroblastoma include elevation of levels of urinary vanillylmandelic acid or homovanillic acid. These levels are elevated in 80 percent of children with tumors. Plain radiographs may show the mass, often with speckled calcification (55 percent of tumors have calcification that is evident on plain films), retroperitoneal widening from nodal spread, disease metastatic to bones, or hepatomegaly from metastases. If a child presents with blatant neuroblastoma visible on plain radiographs, then CT or magnetic resonance imaging (MRI) is the most cost-effective method of confirming the diagnosis and staging the tumor (Table 8–1). Otherwise, ultrasonography is reasonable for diagnosis, less useful for staging, but very helpful in follow-up of an upper abdominal tumor while the child undergoes radiation or chemotherapy (Dershaw and Helson, 1988).

Although it is always stated in the literature that two thirds of abdominal neuroblastomas originate from the adrenal glands, 70 percent of children have disseminated disease at the time of presentation (Evans, 1980). Any retroperitoneal mass, therefore, may be a neuroblastoma. This tumor is usually echogenic, but cystic neuroblastoma in babies has been described (Atkinson et al., 1986), and we have seen such cases (Fig. 8–39). It is noteworthy that two of three cases of cystic neuroblastoma, described by Atkinson and coauthors, were identified on prenatal scans. All four patients whom we studied had had abnormal prenatal scans. Cystic masses are relatively easy to spot on prenatal ultrasonography; the solid asymptomatic tumor may be overlooked.

Table 8–1. EVANS SYSTEM OF STAGING NEUROBLASTOMA

Stage I	Tumor confined to organ or structure of origin
Stage II	Extension of tumor in continuity beyond organ or structure of origin but not across midline
Stage III	Extension of tumor in continuity across midline (includes bilateral extension of midline tumor)
Stage IV	Disseminated disease with metastases involving skeleton, soft tissues, distant lymph nodes, distant organs
Stage IV-S	Stage I or II tumor, no obvious bony metastases, and metastatic disease limited to liver, skin, or bone marrow singly or in combination

From Evans AE, D'Angio GJ, Randolph J: A proposed staging for children with neuroblastoma. Cancer 1971; 27:374–378.

Neuroblastoma is truly cancerous (i.e., crablike) when it spreads. Tentacles of the tumor encircle the great vessels and appear to infiltrate the pancreas (Fig. 8–40). Remarkably, there is usually little effect on the ductal or vascular systems of the organs encased by the tumor. On ultrasonograms, small shadowing foci within the mass represent calcification (Fig. 8–41). Although one child whom we saw had localized lymphangiectasia of bowel caused by obstruction of lymphatics at the base of the mesentery and another child had an obstruction of the common bile duct, these are extremely unusual complications (Fig. 8–42). Aggressive neuroblastoma may infiltrate the kidney and simulate a Wilms tumor (Fig. 8–43; Rosenfield et al., 1988). This is distinctly unusual behavior and is associated with a poorly differentiated tumor. In general, neuroblastoma displaces or flattens one or both kidneys (Fig. 8–44). A complete study of patients who have neuroblastoma should include the spine because intraspinal extension is reported to occur in 15 percent of such patients (Armstrong et al., 1981). In older children, this is feasible only with CT or MRI, but in babies, ultrasonography can penetrate the cartilaginous portions of posterior elements and can produce reasonable evidence of spinal involvement or the lack of it.

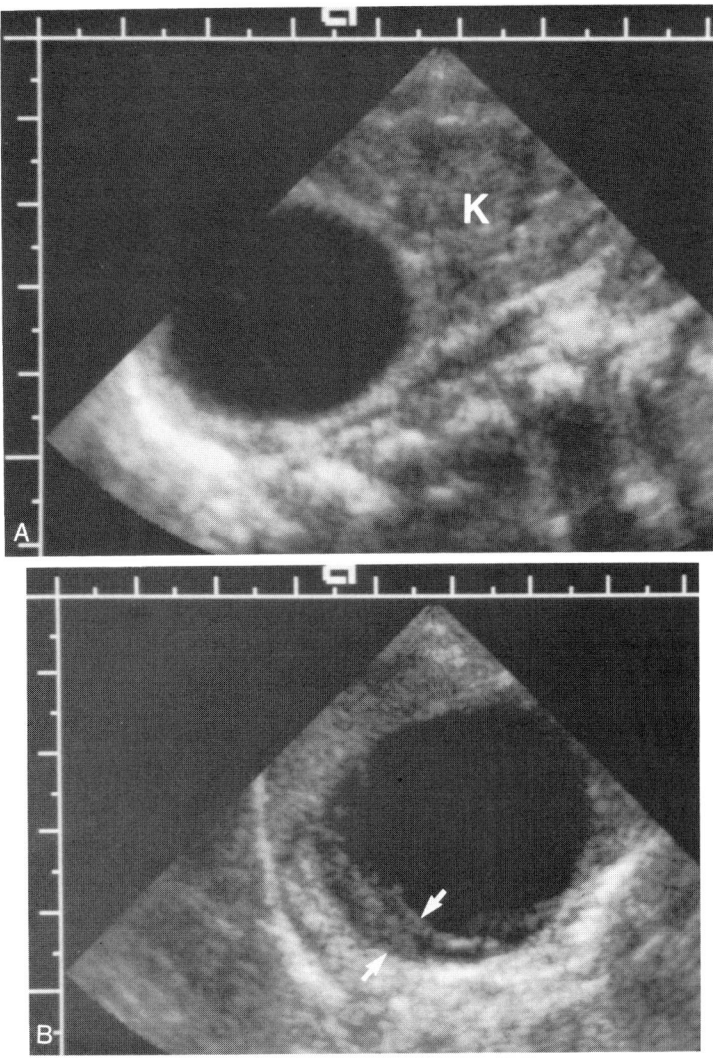

Figure 8–39. A suprarenal cyst had been diagnosed in this baby boy on prenatal ultrasonography. He presented for follow-up ultrasonography at 1 month of age. The initial coronal scan (**A**) showed what appeared to be a simple cyst in the suprarenal area. K = kidney. Closer evaluation (**B**) suggested that there was a double margin (arrows) to the medial and inferior portions of the cyst. Because the mass had not changed between prenatal and postnatal scans, this baby went to surgery, and a cystic neuroblastoma was removed. Bone marrow biopsy yielded normal results. The baby has been disease free for 1 year.

246 / EVALUATING AN ABDOMINAL MASS

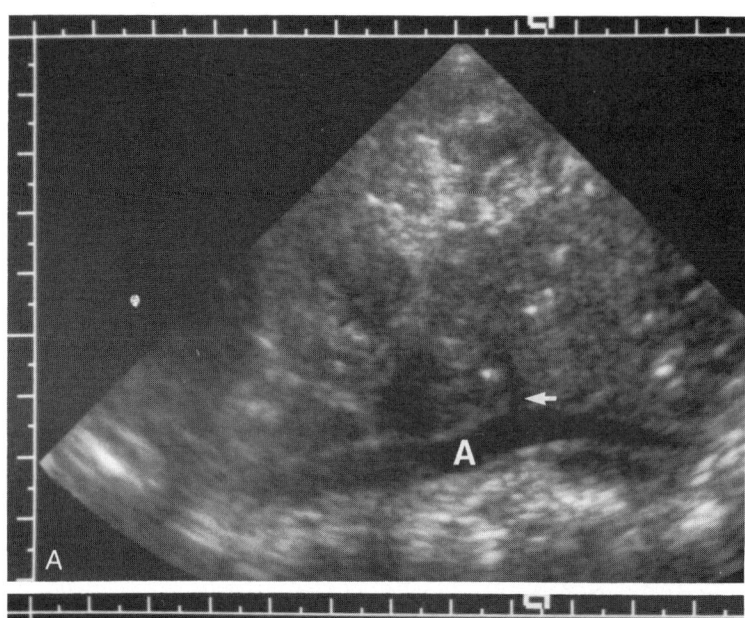

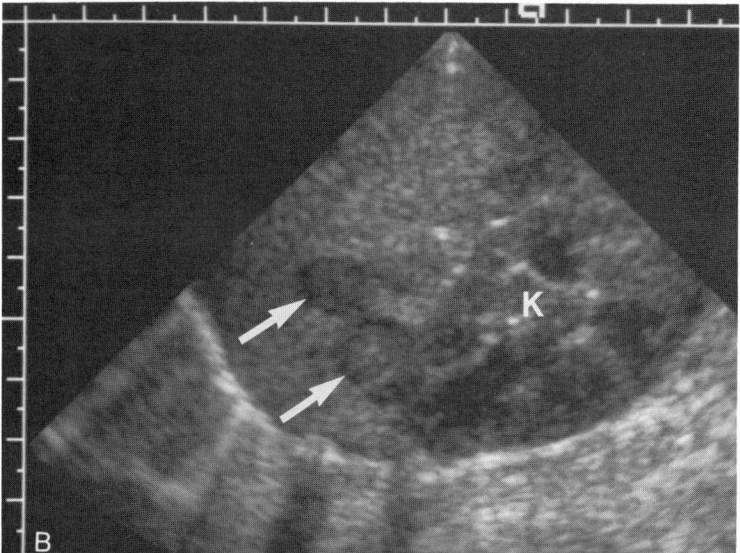

Figure 8–40. Increasing abdominal girth brought this 6½-month-old child to medical attention. Physical examination revealed a midline abdominal mass. Longitudinal scan of the aorta (**A**) shows a mass of low echogenicity anterior to the aorta and encasing the superior mesenteric artery (arrow). A = aorta. **B** shows hepatic metastases (arrows) that were present at the time of the child's evaluation. He was treated with chemotherapy for metastatic neuroblastoma. K = kidney.

Figure 8–41. The coronal scan of the left upper quadrant in this 7-year-old girl followed the discovery of a palpable mass. She had presented to her pediatrician with a chronic, low-grade fever. The mass was a neuroblastoma (arrows) in the left adrenal gland that depressed and rotated the ipsilateral kidney (K). The echogenic areas within the mass represent calcification. This is the textbook appearance of neuroblastoma as shown on ultrasonography. During surgery, the mass and the left kidney were removed in toto. Pathologic examination revealed ganglioneuroma with areas of neuroblastoma.

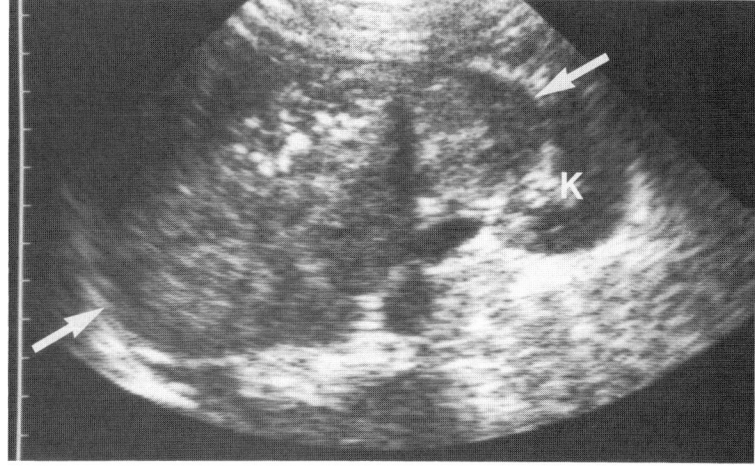

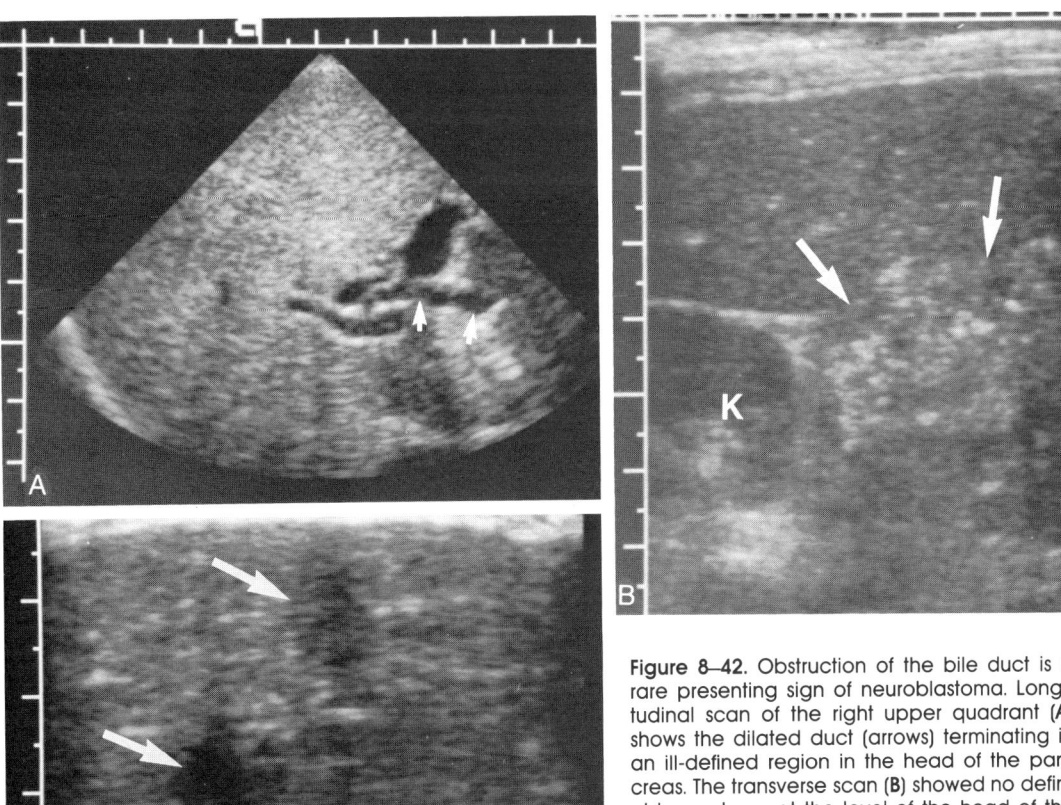

Figure 8–42. Obstruction of the bile duct is a rare presenting sign of neuroblastoma. Longitudinal scan of the right upper quadrant (**A**) shows the dilated duct (arrows) terminating in an ill-defined region in the head of the pancreas. The transverse scan (**B**) showed no definable anatomy at the level of the head of the pancreas. K = kidney. Arrows outline the irregular mass, which proved to be a neuroblastoma in the retroperitoneum obstructing the common bile duct. Closer evaluation of the liver with linear array transducer (**C**) shows two lucent areas (arrows) that represent metastatic deposits of neuroblastoma in the liver.

Figure 8–43. Prone longitudinal scan of the right kidney shows a huge, lobular mass insinuating itself into the hilum of the kidney (marked by asterisks). Occasionally, it is difficult to differentiate an aggressive neuroblastoma that is invading a kidney from an exophytic Wilms tumor. In this case, echogenic foci (arrow) throughout the mass are typical of neuroblastoma.

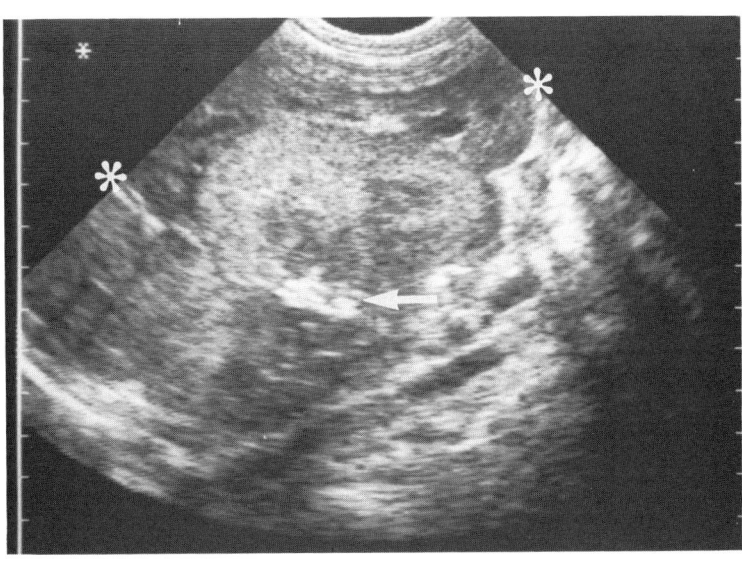

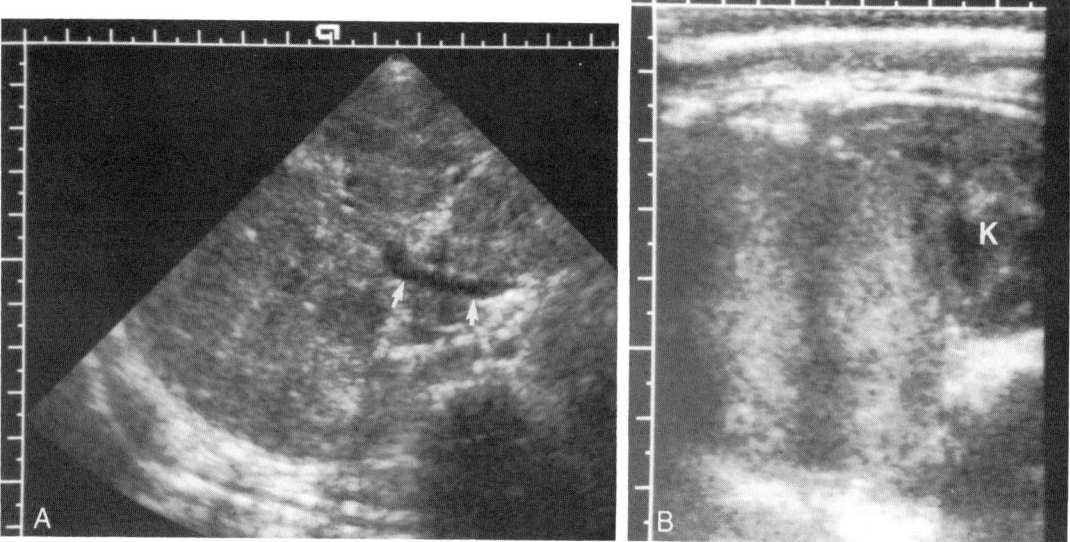

Figure 8–44. A baby who presents with hepatomegaly and patchy appearance of hepatic parenchyma, as seen on the transverse scan (A), may have metastatic neuroblastoma to the liver. Arrows mark the portal vein. The study is then expanded to look for the primary lesion. In this case, the left adrenal gland was the site of the primary tumor. Coronal scan (B) shows the mass indenting and displacing the left kidney (K).

Fine-needle biopsy of suspected neuroblastoma is reasonable when a child has inoperable disease at the outset. However, pathologists interested in refining histologic criteria so as to improve prediction of outcome may need more tissue than is available from aspiration with the fine needle alone (Shimada et al., 1984).

Follow-up with ultrasonography during therapy is appropriate if most of the tumor is in the upper abdomen and is easily visualized. Lower abdominal masses are too obscured by the bowel or pelvic bones to be adequately monitored. When no tumor or a stable one is detected on ultrasonography, CT or MRI can be used. Neuroblastoma does not melt with therapy, as does lymphoma. It often matures into ganglioneuroma or leaves behind calcified stroma, both of which persist as a residual mass (Fig. 8–45). Residual malignancy and benign residua cannot be differentiated without histopathologic study. Often, therefore, a second-look operation is performed after chemotherapy or radiotherapy.

Pheochromocytoma

This is a rare tumor in childhood and is diagnosed when abnormal levels of urinary

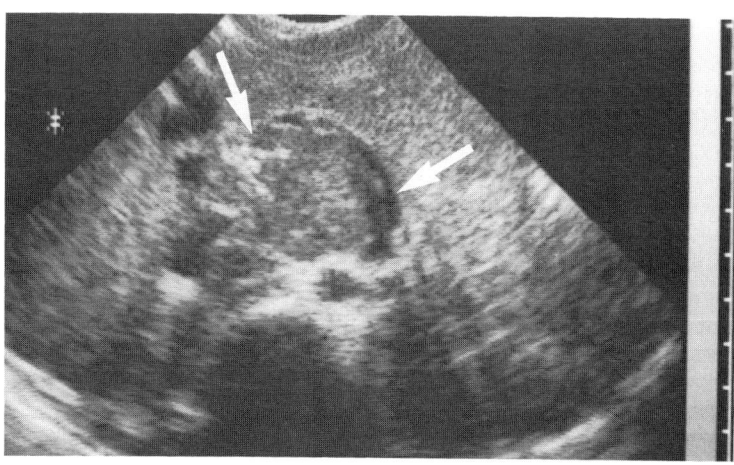

Figure 8–45. This is the transverse scan of an 8-year-old who had received treatment for neuroblastoma at age 3. The prevertebral mass (arrows), which elevated splenic vessels, was mature ganglioma, proved at second-look exploratory laparotomy.

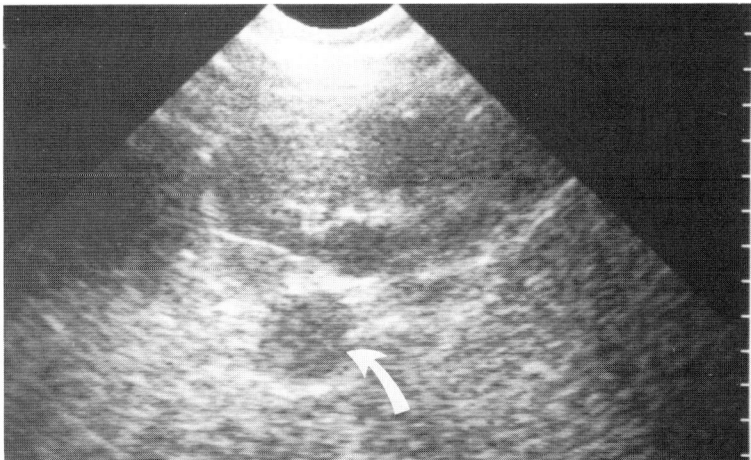

Figure 8–46. Increased blood pressure resulted in this 12-year-old boy's undergoing renal ultrasonography as a screening modality. He presented with a dull pain around the eyes and a blood pressure of 140/110. Results from laboratory studies were not back at the time of the scans, which showed a well-defined mass (arrow) anterior to the left kidney. This was confirmed on computed tomography (CT) scanning as being adrenal in origin. Note, however, how inferior and medial this adrenal gland is. Results of urine tests were positive for vanillylmandelic acid and metanorepinephrine. A left pheochromocytoma was removed during surgery, and the blood pressure fell after surgery to 110/60.

vanillylmandelic acid, catecholamines, or both are detected in a child with severe episodic or sustained hypertension (Fig. 8–46). Finding the tumor is best accomplished with CT or MRI. Ultrasonography can reveal moderately sized adrenal lesions, but multiple lesions (33 percent of cases) and extra-adrenal lesions (30 percent of cases) are more common in children than in adults. Malignancy is unusual, although Daneman (1988) mentioned malignancy in 3 of 11 children with pheochromocytoma. Associated syndromes include neurofibromatosis, von Hippel-Lindau disease, Sturge-Weber syndrome, and tuberous sclerosis, as well as the group of multiple endocrine neoplasias.

Adenoma and Carcinoma

Both adenoma and carcinoma are rare. It is difficult to differentiate one from the other,

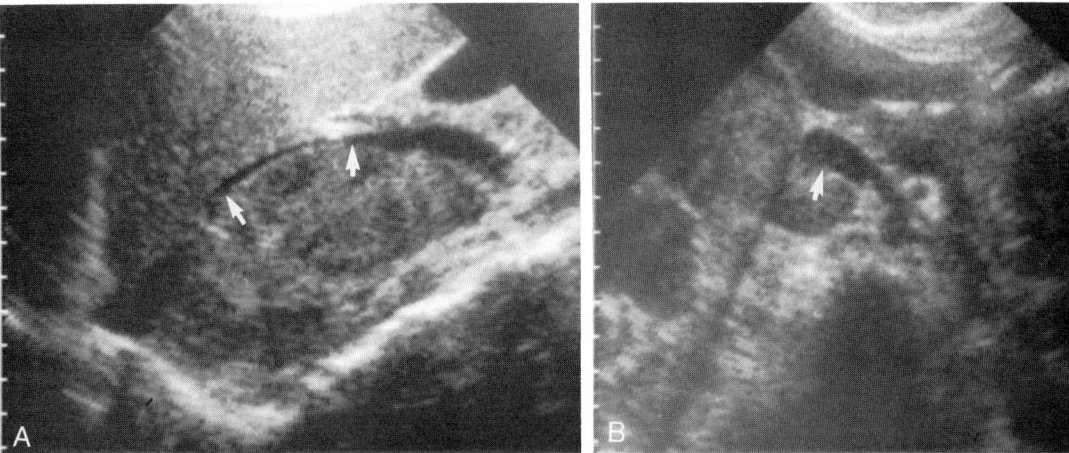

Figure 8–47. Longitudinal (A) and transverse (B) scans of the right hemiabdomen show elevation of the inferior vena cava (arrows) from a retroperitoneal mass associated with the right adrenal gland. This was a nonfunctioning adrenal carcinoma that had invaded the liver. In spite of chemotherapy, the patient died of widespread metastatic disease shortly after diagnosis.

and either from adrenal pheochromocytoma, with ultrasonography alone. An adenoma tends to be uniform in echogenicity, whereas the more rapid growth of an adrenal carcinoma produces central areas of necrosis. Calcification is more likely to occur in an adrenal carcinoma. The clinical presentation of both adenoma and carcinoma is of precocious puberty in boys and virilization in girls. Rarely is a tumor nonfunctional. An adrenal carcinoma is highly invasive locally and metastasizes to the liver and lung (Fig. 8–47). If an adrenal mass is identified during an ultrasonographic evaluation for precocious puberty or virilization, the inferior vena cava should be evaluated for possible tumor thrombus and the liver surveyed for metastatic disease. CT should follow in order to evaluate pulmonary parenchyma and to re-evaluate the abdomen.

RENAL MASS

This section includes discussion of renal neoplasms, benign and malignant, that affect infants, children, and adolescents. A tumor in the neonatal kidney is a rare occurrence. With few exceptions, a solid mass in the kidney of a neonate is a mesoblastic nephroma. Malignant rhabdoid tumor of the kidney, which fortunately is extremely rare, may present in the neonatal period. It is associated with midline intracranial tumors (Bonnin et al., 1984). For this reason, scans of the brain are a worthwhile screening procedure if a renal mass is identified in the infant. Wilms tumors occur most often between 1 and 5 years of age. The diagnosis of renal venous thrombosis in the neonate is usually suspected on clinical grounds, but the enlarged, distorted renal architecture may be mistaken on scans for a neoplasm. Ultrasonography with color Doppler imaging can be used for the immediate identification of venous obstruction (Plate VII). Renal abscesses in neonates are unusual. Abscesses in older children may be misdiagnosed as tumors, and vice versa. (Features of renal abscesses are discussed in Chapter 7.)

Because most malignant tumors are more vascular than benign tumors, and because tumor vascularity is abnormal, Doppler imaging has been used to evaluate the margins of renal masses where the feeding vessels are located (Ramos et al., 1988). The frequency shift near the tumor has to be compared with that in the ipsilateral renal artery. We recommend adding examination with Doppler imaging in the evaluation of children with intrarenal tumors so that pediatric experience can be accumulated.

Mesoblastic Nephroma

Uniform spindle-shaped cells arranged in bundles produce a yellow-gray whorled appearance when this tumor is sectioned. This benign tumor (also called "fetal renal hamartoma," "leiomyomatous hamartoma," or "mesenchymal hamartoma") is the most common neonatal renal neoplasm and almost invariably is discovered early in life as a palpable mass. On ultrasonography, the appearance of the mass is variable: uniformly to irregularly echogenic, blending with normal renal parenchyma rather than having a discrete interface (Fig. 8–48). We have noticed that the renal vein draining the involved kidney may be larger than its mate. Although the tumor itself is not hypervascular, dilated blood vessels at its periphery have been described on pathologic examination (Chan et al., 1987). The mass should be surgically removed with its kidney because there is no way, preoperatively, to prove that malignancy is not present. Atypical congenital mesoblastic nephroma, which appears to border on renal sarcoma, has been described. An atypical tumor is more cellular, locally invasive, and centrally necrotic. It may be associated with hypercalcemia (Ferraro et al., 1986).

Multilocular Cystic Nephroma

This multinamed mass (also called "cystic nephroblastoma," "immature unilateral multilocular cyst," "polycystic nephroblastoma," or "cystic partially differentiated nephroblastoma"), benign in its activity, occurs more frequently in boys than in girls. In infants the stroma may include elements of nephroblastoma, hence the incorporation of this term into some of its nomenclature. Nephrectomy is curative. Multilocular cystic nephroma appears both in gross examination and on ultrasonography as a well-defined, intrarenal, septated cystic mass, as if soap bubbles had been blown into a tennis ball

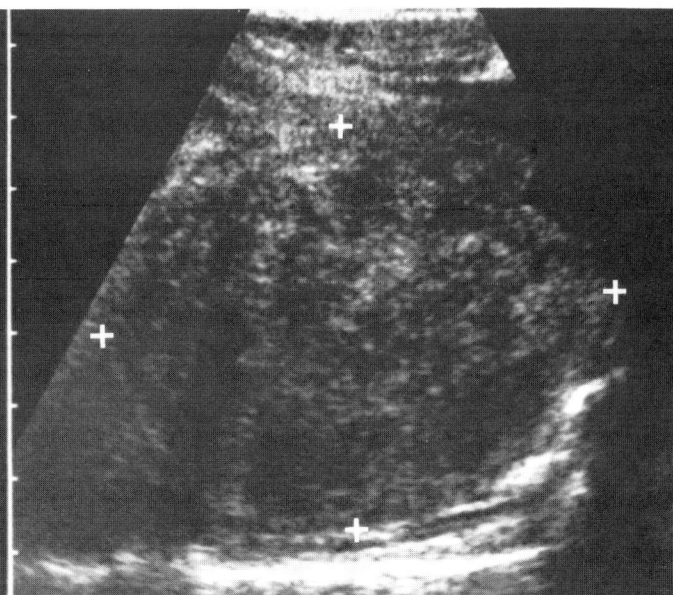

Figure 8–48. The most common solid mass of the neonate is mesoblastic nephroma. This coronal scan of the right flank, performed after the baby was found to have a right-sided mass during routine examination at 1 day of age, shows the typical appearance of mesoblastic nephroma: a hypoechoic mass occupying the right renal fossa. The mass is marked by crosses.

(Fig. 8–49). It presents as a palpable abdominal mass in a child younger than 4 years of age. Cystic Wilms tumor, which is the major differential diagnosis, tends to have spherical, as opposed to faceted, cystic spaces and has more irregular and thicker bands of stroma.

Nephroblastomatosis (Nodular Renal Blastema)

A primitive metanephric epithelium may persist in the kidney as small microscopic rests or gross nodules. It is found in nearly 1 percent of autopsies of stillborn infants and in 12 to 40 percent of kidneys resected for Wilms tumor (Davis, 1987). How a nodular renal blastema changes into a Wilms tumor is unknown, but it is generally regarded as a precursor of malignancy (Kirks et al., 1987). In current usage, "nephroblastomatosis" is defined as normal or mildly enlarged kidneys containing one or more Wilms tumors and microscopic or macroscopic nodules of pure or differentiating blastema or regressing derivatives (Bove, 1988). Multifocal nephroblastomatosis is found in 25 percent of patients

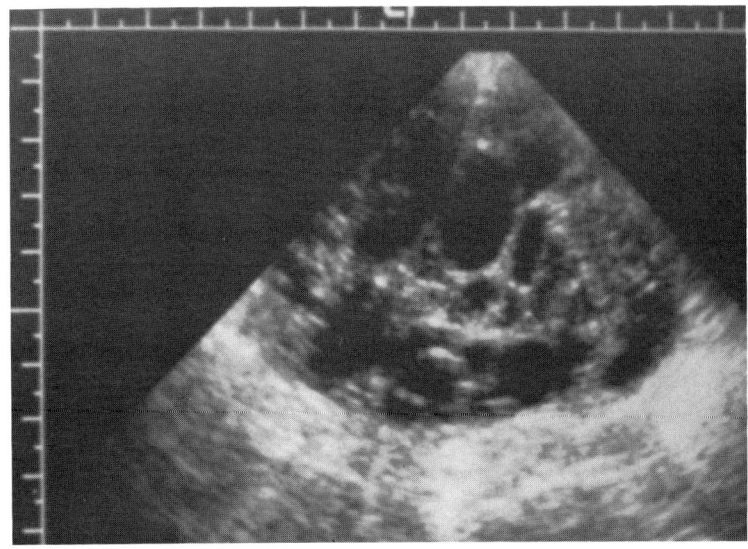

Figure 8–49. A palpable abdominal mass was found in this 2-year-old boy. The scan shows a multilocular cystic mass. This is the typical appearance of multilocular cystic nephroma. (From Teele RL, Share JC: The abdominal mass in the neonate. Semin Roentgenol 1988; 23:175–184.)

with Wilms tumors and is present in most patients with bilateral Wilms tumors. These numbers may be underestimates; the estimates are dependent on the skill and interest of the pathologist and the number of sections taken from a submitted specimen. Ultrasonography is not as sensitive as CT in detecting nephroblastomatosis (Fernbach et al., 1988). This is one reason why we use contrast-enhanced CT scanning after a Wilms tumor has been diagnosed on ultrasonography. The data from MRI are not yet available.

Wilms Tumor

Information regarding Wilms tumors is easier to retrieve than that on other tumors because the diagnosis is straightforward, because most children in the U.S. are referred for treatment to large hospitals that accumulate statistics, and because the National Wilms Tumor Study consolidates and updates much of the data from these centers. An excellent review of Wilms tumor (Mesrobian, 1988) includes the clinical, histologic, genetic, and therapeutic aspects of this specifically pediatric abdominal malignancy. Regardless of race or country, Wilms tumors affect 7.8 per 1 million children aged 0 to 15 years. Sporadic cases occur at a mean age of 3.5 years; hereditary and bilateral cases occur at a mean age of 2.5 years. Most children who have Wilms tumor have an abdominal mass on presentation. Hypertension, hematuria, and pain are less common presentations.

Table 8–2. NATIONAL WILMS TUMOR STUDY GROUPING SYSTEM

Group I	Tumor limited to kidney and completely excised (surface of capsule intact, no rupture of tumor, no residual tumor apparent)
Group II	Tumor extends beyond kidney but is completely excised (includes penetration beyond pseudocapsule or periaortic lymph node involvement; renal vessels may be infiltrated or contain thrombus; no residual tumor apparent)
Group III	Residual nonhematogenous tumor confined to abdomen (includes one or more of following: tumor biopsied or ruptured before or during surgery, implants on peritoneum, nodes involved beyond abdominal periaortic chains, tumor incompletely removed because of local infiltration into vital structures)
Group IV	Hematogenous metastases (e.g., lung, liver, bone, brain)
Group V	Bilateral renal involvement, synchronous or metachronous

Associated congenital malformations, seen in approximately 15 percent of children with Wilms tumor, include renal anomalies, hemihypertrophy, sporadic nonfamilial aniridia (33 percent develop Wilms tumor), Beckwith-Wiedemann syndrome, cerebral gigantism, pseudohermaphroditism (Drash syndrome), and neurofibromatosis (Kirks et al., 1987; see Chapter 6). Genetic research with deoxyribonucleic acid (DNA) probes is focusing on the short arm of chromosome 11, band 13. Deletions of portions of this band have been

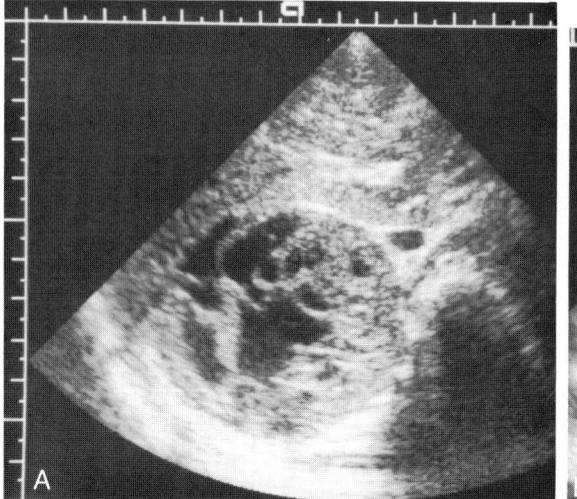 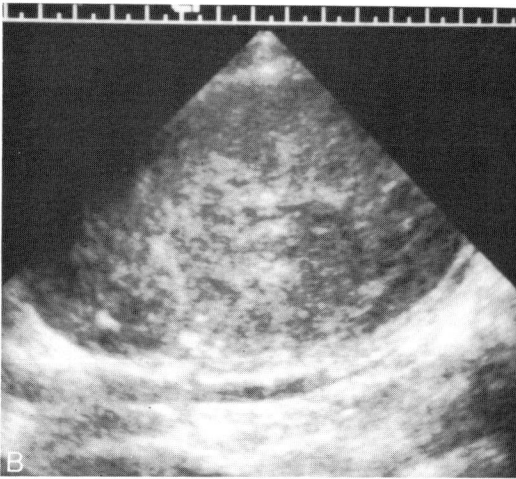

Figure 8–50. Bilateral Wilms tumor in this 4-year-old boy, who presented with hematuria, shows different pattern between right and left renal masses. On the right side (**A**), the Wilms tumor is cystic. On the left (**B**), it is purely solid.

found in one third of patients with sporadic aniridia and Wilms tumor (Mesrobian, 1988).

Bilateral tumors occur in 4.4 to 9 percent of all patients with Wilms tumor (Fig. 8–50). These children tend to be young at the time of presentation, have associated anomalies, typically or perhaps invariably have nephroblastomatosis, and rarely present with hypertension. Two thirds of bilateral tumors are synchronous; one third are metachronous. It is uncertain, however, whether patients with metachronous tumors may have had an undetected small synchronous tumor at the time of the initial diagnosis of Wilms tumor.

Survival after therapy for Wilms tumor is directly related to grouping at time of diagnosis (Table 8–2) and to the histology of the tumor, which is classified as favorable or unfavorable depending on degree of cytologic atypism and sarcomatous stroma (Fig. 8–51; Beckwith and Palmer, 1978). Those with favorable histologic findings, grouped I to III, have a 92.1 percent rate of 2-year survival. With unfavorable histologic findings, at all stages, and at stage IV with favorable histologic findings, the survival rate drops to 78.5 percent (extrapolated from D'Angio et al.'s 1984 findings). The presence of metachronous tumors cuts the survival rate in half, to 39 percent (Mesrobian, 1988).

Wilms tumors arise from any part of the kidney and, rarely, in an extrarenal location (Fig. 8–52). As Wilms tumor enlarges, its center becomes necrotic. It is prone to hemorrhage and may rupture with or without superimposed abdominal trauma. Calcification, which used to be thought rare and hence a differentiating feature between a Wilms tumor and neuroblastoma, is actually present 15 percent of the time. In 5 to 10 percent of patients, the tumor may infiltrate the renal vein to emerge in the inferior vena cava (IVC). Intracaval and atrial involvement, if recognized during imaging, does not affect survival (Ritchey et al., 1988). Infiltration of the tumor into the collecting system may obstruct the kidney in part or in toto. Nonfunction of the affected kidney occurred in 5 of 50 patients with Wilms tumor in one reported study (Nakayama et al., 1988).

Answers to the following questions are needed by the surgeon and oncologist before treatment of Wilms tumor begins: (1) Is the palpable abdominal mass an intrarenal Wilms tumor? (2) Is a congenital renal anomaly present? (3) Is there evidence of the extrarenal extent of the tumor (e.g., adjacent nodes or rupture of the pseudocapsule)? (4) Is the renal vein or the IVC, or are both, involved with tumor thrombus? (5) Is the contralateral kidney normal? (6) Is there metastatic disease? (Lungs are the most common site; the liver, bones, and central nervous system are distinctly less commonly involved.) Ultrasonography can answer most but not all of these questions. A combination of ultrasonography (as the initial diagnostic study and particularly to document patent or thrombosed cava) with contrast-enhanced CT (to assess function, allow more precise preoperative staging, diagnose nephroblastomatosis,

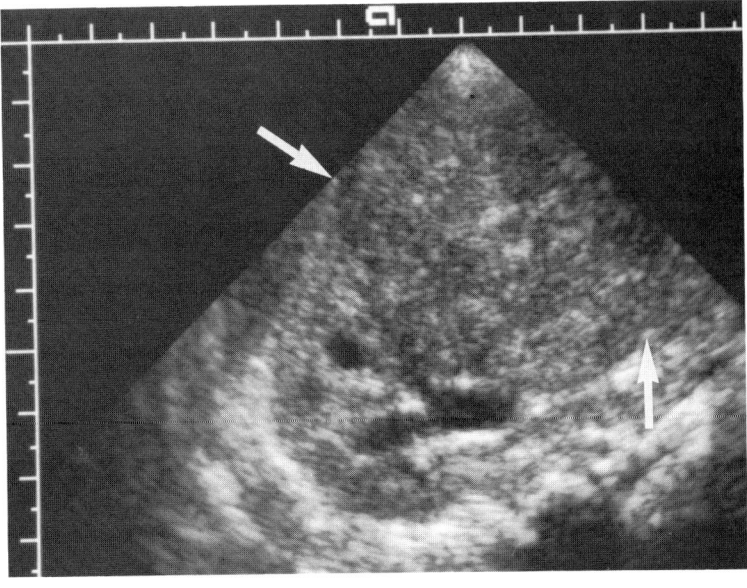

Figure 8–51. Transverse scan of the right upper quadrant shows an exophytic renal mass (arrows). Pathologic examination proved this to be a renal sarcoma with mixed histology. The baby was 7 months old at presentation. Six months later, she suffered relapse of the tumor in the abdomen and lungs and died shortly thereafter.

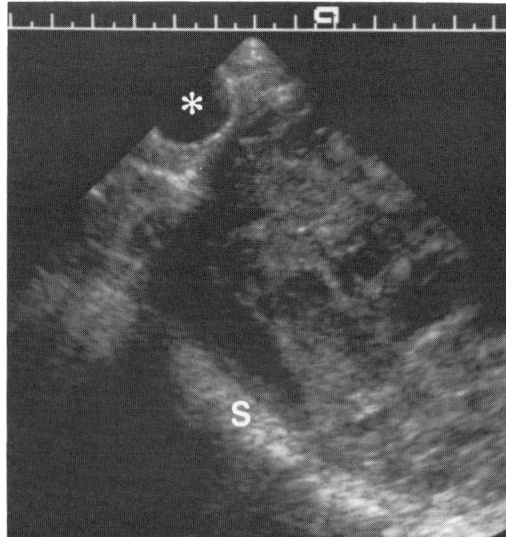

Figure 8–52. Longitudinal scan of the pelvis shows a mass arising from the pelvis. A Foley catheter (asterisk) is in the bladder, which is lifted anteriorly and superiorly. Initial diagnosis was prostatic rhabdomyosarcoma in a 5-year-old boy who had presented with acute urinary retention. However, biopsy revealed this to be an extrarenal Wilms tumor that was attached to the base of the bladder. S = sacrum.

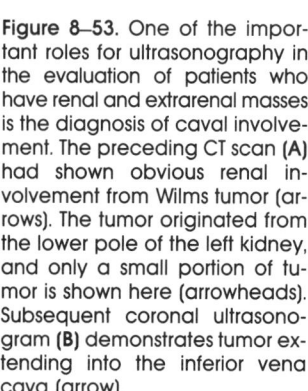

Figure 8–53. One of the important roles for ultrasonography in the evaluation of patients who have renal and extrarenal masses is the diagnosis of caval involvement. The preceding CT scan **(A)** had shown obvious renal involvement from Wilms tumor (arrows). The tumor originated from the lower pole of the left kidney, and only a small portion of tumor is shown here (arrowheads). Subsequent coronal ultrasonogram **(B)** demonstrates tumor extending into the inferior vena cava (arrow).

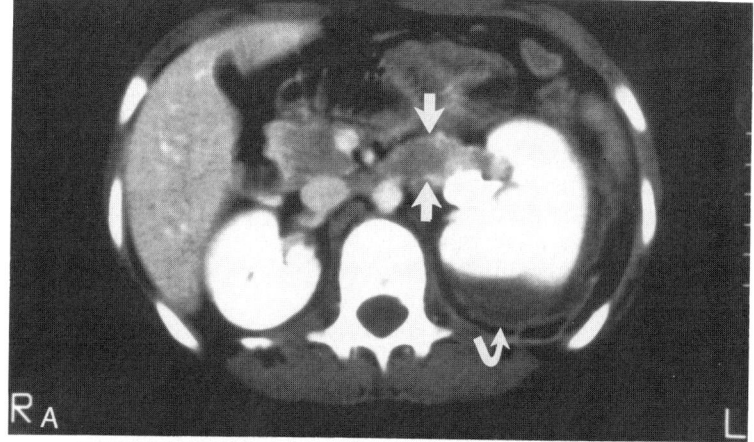

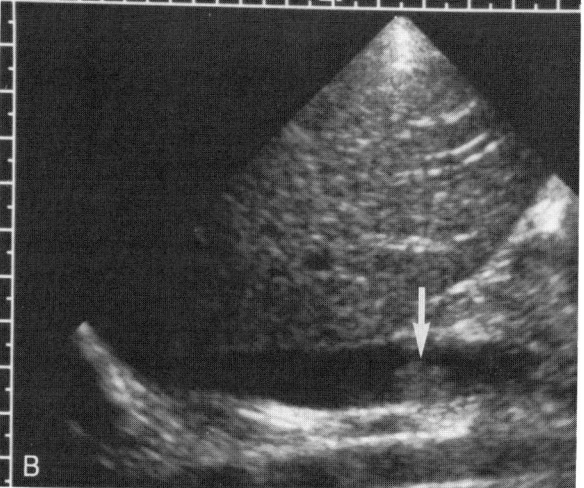

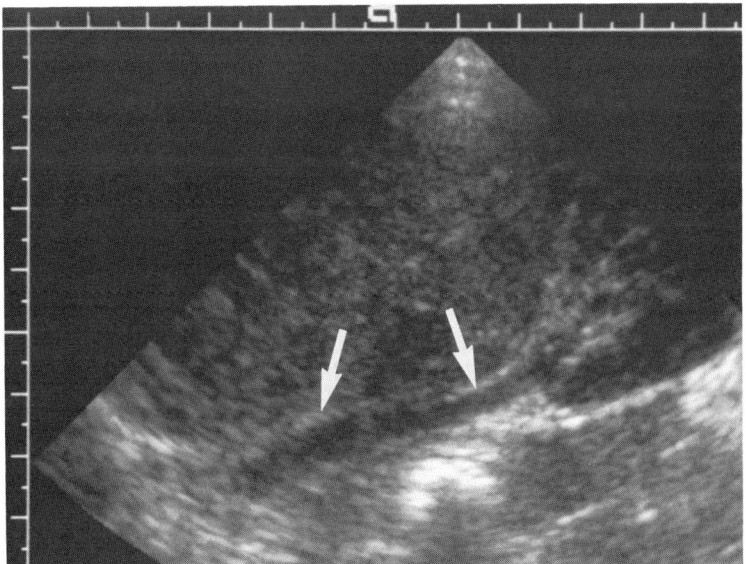

Figure 8–54. A large exophytic Wilms tumor often displaces the kidney that it is attached to. In this case, the left renal vein (arrows) is depressed by the Wilms tumor in the upper pole of the left kidney. This is a coronal view through the left flank.

and evaluate lungs) is reasonable in medical centers in which both modalities are available (Fig. 8–53). However, in spite of sophisticated preoperative diagnostic imaging, a third of bilateral tumors are detected only during exploration (Mesrobian, 1988). This statistic may change with more liberal use of MRI.

Wilms tumors vary in size among patients but typically are very large when discovered. They tend to push blood vessels and organs aside rather than encase them (Fig. 8–54). A tumor may produce any type of ultrasonographic echogenic pattern from homogeneous to blotchy and hyperechogenic with cystic areas that represent necrosis. Dilated calices in the adjacent normal renal parenchyma may be present if the tumor is compressing or infiltrating the collecting system. The presence of enlarged nodes along the IVC and aorta moves a patient beyond the classification of stage I. The IVC and renal vein must be scanned in both axial and coronal or sagittal planes. A thrombus may be adherent to the wall of either vessel and invisible on a single plane. Occasionally a right-sided tumor is so large that the IVC is completely compressed and bowed across midline. Good evaluation in this situation requires some help from gravity. Coronal scans are done with the patient upright so that the IVC is distended as much as possible. If there is any question about the patency or normalcy of the IVC, old-fashioned but simple venacavography can be done if MRI is unavailable. CT occasionally presents problems defining extrinsic from intrinsic involvement of the IVC. We ask help from our colleagues in the department of cardiology if we see, in the IVC, a tumor thrombus extending into supradiaphragmatic territory. Our cardiologists are more skilled than we at evaluating right atrial contours and contents. We always carefully scan the contralateral kidney of a patient with Wilms tumor, but on occasion we have been unable to detect a small contralateral tumor shown to be present by CT and surgery.

Follow-up of patients who have undergone nephrectomy for Wilms tumor is scheduled in collaboration with the oncologists and depends on the protocols used for treatment, the stage of the disease when diagnosed, and clinical concerns. The growth and parenchymal pattern of the remaining kidney is carefully monitored. Both chemotherapy and radiotherapy may inhibit growth. In addition, the single kidney appears susceptible to injury from hyperfiltration; increasing parenchymal echogenicity over time may be an ultrasonographic sign of this phenomenon. Views of the IVC and a survey of the liver are included in each examination.

Renal Carcinoma

A rare tumor of childhood, renal carcinoma usually presents at a later age than does Wilms tumor. In two studies, the mean ages at diagnosis were 10.5 years and 12 years, respectively (Cassady et al., 1974, Chan et al., 1983). At any given time, there are likely to be 20 patients who have Wilms tumor for every child who has renal cell carcinoma.

256 / EVALUATING AN ABDOMINAL MASS

However, the presentation is similar for each: hematuria associated with a retroperitoneal mass. The imaging is similar for each tumor as well, although carcinoma is more likely than Wilms tumor to appear calcified on CT scans (25 percent in comparison with 15 percent; Kirks et al., 1987). Disease that is already beyond the confines of the kidney when the patient presents appears to be the rule for renal carcinoma. Therefore, ultrasonograms should include a careful search for adjacent hilar or periaortic adenopathy (Fig. 8–55).

OTHER RETROPERITONEAL MASSES

Teratoma has to be included in the differential diagnosis of any mixed cystic/solid

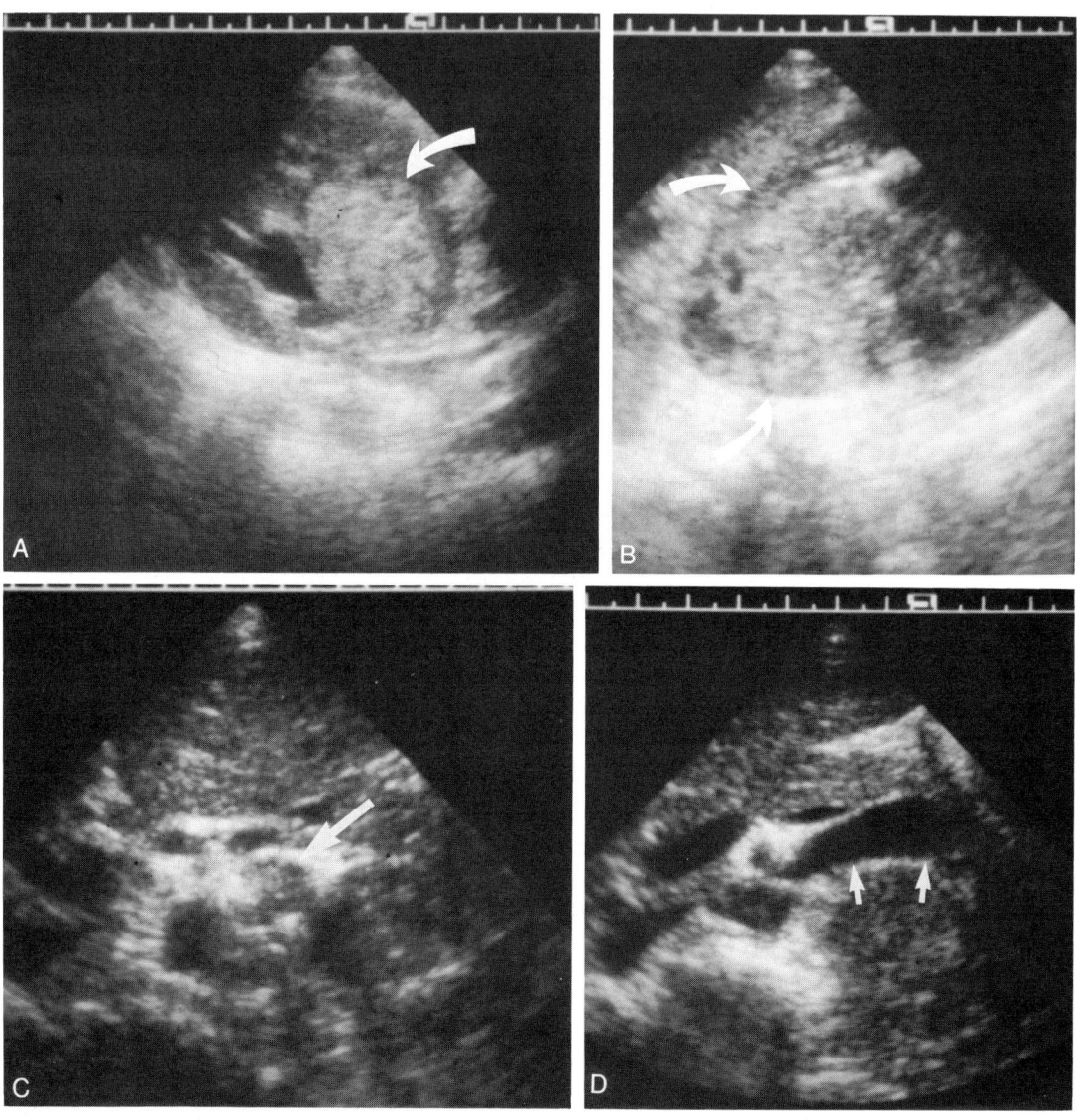

Figure 8–55. This 11-year-old girl presented with flank pain and documented infection of her urine. Presence of an intrarenal mass was an unexpected finding on ultrasonic examination. Transverse (A) and coronal (B) scans show the mass (arrows). The transverse view of the renal hilum (C) showed a pararenal node (arrow). The renal vein (arrows, D) was elevated by the intrarenal mass but not invaded. Renal cell carcinoma, metastatic to local nodes, was diagnosed on histologic examination after radical nephrectomy. The infection was probably coincidental but may have been related to partial obstruction of the collecting system by the tumor.

mass, especially those that are calcified. Diagnosis of teratoma can be made on plain radiographs when shardlike calcification is present (Schey et al., 1986). When calcification is lacking, the mass may resemble neuroblastoma or a tumor of connective tissues or muscle. It can arise from anywhere in the retroperitoneum. Fetus in fetu is likely an extremely well-differentiated, highly organized teratoma (Heifetz et al., 1988). Teratoma is the third most common tumor of the retroperitoneum; only in rare cases is it shown to be malignant on histopathologic examination.

Extensive involvement of the retroperitoneum, similar to that in some cases of neuroblastoma, is also characteristic of rhabdomyosarcoma. Luckily, this tumor is uncommon. Its resectability usually is limited, and its response to chemotherapy is poor (Ransom et al., 1980). Lipoblastoma is a benign tumor of the neonate or young child. Lipoma is a related tumor that affects older children. Both can spread through the retroperitoneum, distorting and encircling organs (Bowen et al., 1982). Both present as echogenic masses, often poorly defined, on ultrasonography. Lipoma is quite radiolucent and often betrays itself on plain films. Lipoblastoma does not have as great a content of pure fat; neither does liposarcoma, the rare malignant counterpart of lipoma.

Tumors of the psoas muscle are distinctly unusual. Rhabdomyosarcoma is the most important of any inasmuch as it may involve the entire muscle and be difficult to treat surgically. Asymmetric thickening of the psoas muscle was the ultrasonographic appearance in one such patient whom we studied years ago. Neurogenic tumors, of types other than neuroblastoma, may arise from the sympathetic chain in any part of the retroperitoneum (Fig. 8–56).

A much more common mass in the iliopsoas muscle is abscess. Primary iliopsoas abscess occurs most often in adolescence and is usually staphylococcal. Secondary abscess evolves from a perforated appendix or adjacent Crohn disease. The clinical presentation of psoas abscess is frequently that of hip or back pain. An elevated erythrocyte sedimentation rate (ESR), an increased number of white blood cells in serum, and fever are usually present. Most patients who have secondary abscess have a history of inflammatory bowel disease or intra-abdominal symptoms. Ultrasonography can demonstrate the abscess quite well unless it is low in the psoas or iliacus muscle. CT is better able to demonstrate an abscess in either of these locations, as well as provide information regarding adjacent bowel in patients with secondary abscess. Either ultrasonography or CT can be used for guided drainage of the mass (Fig. 8–57; Hoffer et al., 1987).

Bleeding into the retroperitoneum occurs after retroperitoneal surgery, after extrinsic trauma, and in patients who have an under-

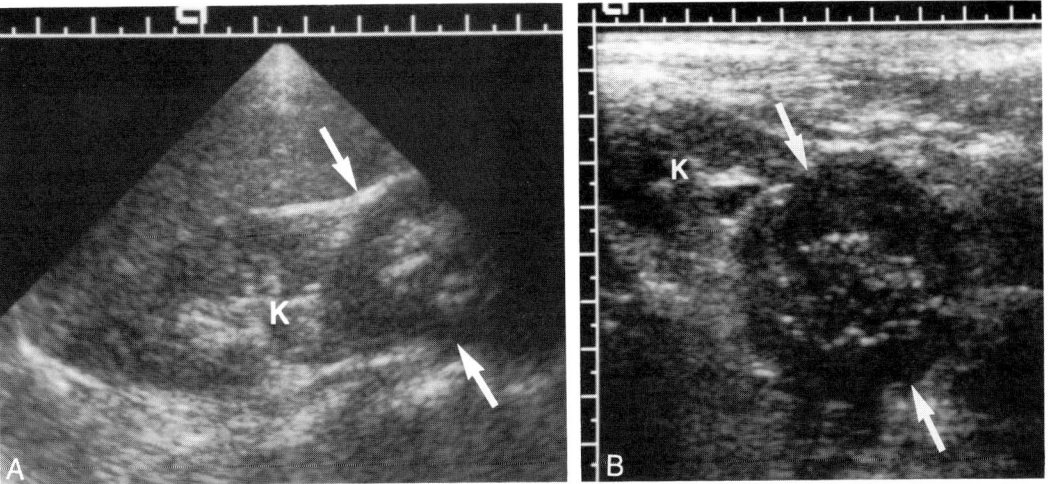

Figure 8–56. Retroperitoneal tumors are often of neurogenic origin. Longitudinal (A) and transverse (B) scans show a mass (arrows) adjacent to the lower pole of the left kidney but separate from it. Central echogenicity represents calcium. Ganglioneuroma with microfoci of neuroblasts was removed without sacrificing of the ipsilateral kidney in this 3-year-old boy. K = kidney.

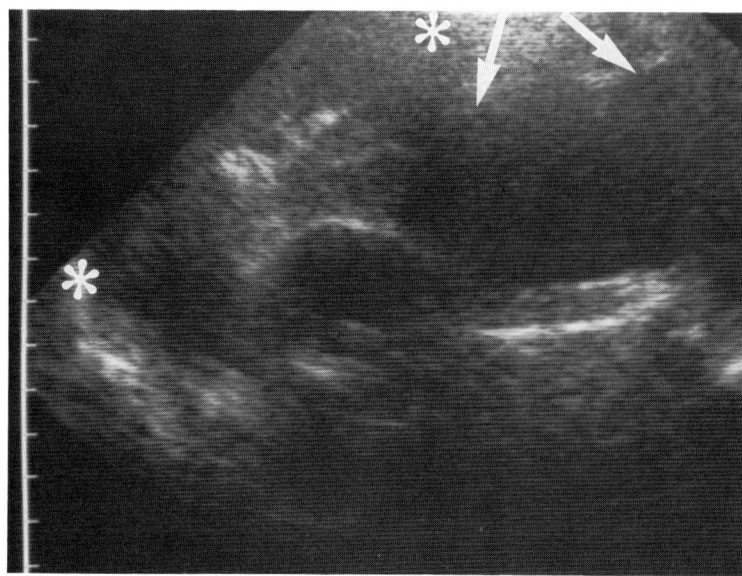

Figure 8-57. Coronal view of the left upper quadrant in this rather large 19-year-old shows the kidney (asterisks) altered in its axis by a large echolucent collection (arrows), which follows the course of the psoas muscle. This represents a large staphyloccal abscess of the psoas. It was drained percutaneously.

lying coagulopathy (Graif et al., 1987). The clinical situation is such that hematoma is rarely mistaken for a tumor or an abscess. Ill-defined margins are the norm for postsurgical hemorrhage in the retroperitoneum. Hematoma in the psoas muscle produces asymmetric thickening of the muscle and appears similar to an abscess on coronal ultrasonograms. In general, CT is better able to demonstrate the extent of the hemorrhage. Ultrasonography is often limited by the accompanying ileus.

The base of the mesentery is anchored to the retroperitoneum, and tumors at this site are usually lymphangiomas (Blumhagen et al., 1987). These multilocular cystic masses may be poorly marginated. They tend to gently displace, rather than obstruct, adjacent organs. Lymphangioma may be identified in a patient because a displaced organ is palpable or because abdominal girth is increased.

Lymphoma accounts for only 10 percent of all cancers in children but is third in frequency after the acute leukemias and brain tumors. Lymphoma is divided into two major classifications: Hodgkin disease and non-Hodgkin lymphoma. Hodgkin disease is rare in children younger than 5 years of age; when it occurs in children who are younger than 10 years of age, it is more likely to occur in boys. Whites are affected more often than other racial groups. Diagnosis is based on establishing the presence of Reed-Sternberg cells in pathologic material, which is generally obtained from enlarged lymph nodes. Lymphocytic predominance, mixed cellularity, lymphocytic depletion, and nodular sclerosis are subclassifications of the disease that are based on proportions of lymphocytes and fibrosis. In most children and adolescents who have Hodgkin disease, the disease presents above the diaphragm in supraclavicular nodes, as a mediastinal mass or a nasopharyngeal mass (Leventhal and Donaldson, 1989). Ultrasonography is not part of the routine diagnostic evaluation because it cannot provide detailed information regarding the presence or absence of abnormal nodes in the retroperitoneum and pelvis. Even CT has problems with false positives and false negatives: enlarged nodes may be reactive and not malignant; small splenic deposits are routinely missed both on imaging and at surgery. Exploratory laparotomy follows clinical and radiologic classification if the child is thought to have disease that is stage I or II. Results from nodal biopsies, wedge biopsy of liver, and splenic removal may advance the staging.

We are more likely to encounter a child with non-Hodgkin lymphoma as he or she enters ultrasonography for evaluation of a palpable abdominal mass. The classification of this malignancy seems to change each year as new methods of diagnosis, which now are reaching into the DNA of the cell, become available. Three major classifications of lymphoma are now in vogue: (1) Lymphoblastic lymphoma (derived from T cells) usually pre-

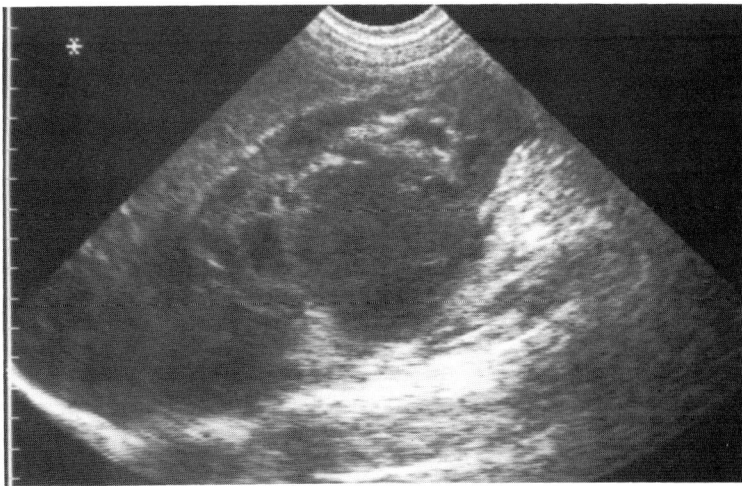

Figure 8–58. Renal involvement with lymphoma may be invisible on routine ultrasonography. However, in this patient, large lucent deposits are distorting the anatomy of the right kidney. The left kidney was similarly involved. The patient presented with central nervous system relapse of lymphoblastic lymphoma.

sents above the diaphragm with mediastinal mass, adenopathy, and pleural effusions. (2) Small, noncleaved cell lymphoma is subdivided into two groups, classic Burkitt lymphoma and non-Burkitt lymphoma. In Western countries, both tend to present as an abdominal tumor with or without pain, intussusception, nausea and vomiting, intestinal bleeding, and, rarely, perforation. The right lower quadrant is a common site of involvement. Endemic African Burkitt lymphoma, although histologically identical to sporadic Burkitt lymphoma, presents with involvement of the jaw or the orbit in 69 percent of patients. (3) Large-cell lymphoma and other unusual, poorly classified lymphomas occur in another 20 to 30 percent of patients. Large-cell lymphoma tends to favor unusual sites of origin, such as the face, lungs, and brain (Magrath, 1989).

Lymphoma causes enlargement of nodes, and typically these nodes are hypoechoic on ultrasonography. The discovery of nodal enlargement or of a large extranodal mass should provoke careful assessment of the liver, spleen, and kidneys because involvement of abdominal organs changes the classification of both Hodgkin disease and non-Hodgkin lymphoma (Figs. 8–58, 8–59). As with Hodgkin disease, ultrasonograms of solid organs may be falsely negative, and we rely on CT imaging for more accurate staging.

Tragically, we now are seeing babies and children who have abdominal masses associated with acquired immunodeficiency syndrome (AIDS). Lymphadenopathy in the abdomen is common in children who are infected with the human immunodeficiency virus (HIV) or who are immunodeficient for other reasons. Lymphocytic proliferation and infection with *Mycobacterium avium–intracellulare* are the most common etiologies of

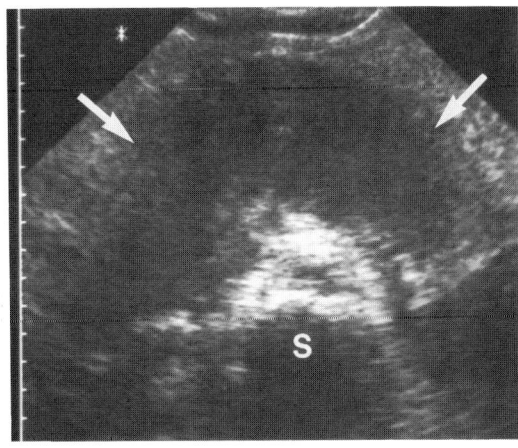

Figure 8–59. An echolucent mantle of tumor (arrows) represents abdominal and peripancreatic involvement with lymphoblastic lymphoma in this 16-year-old. S = spine.

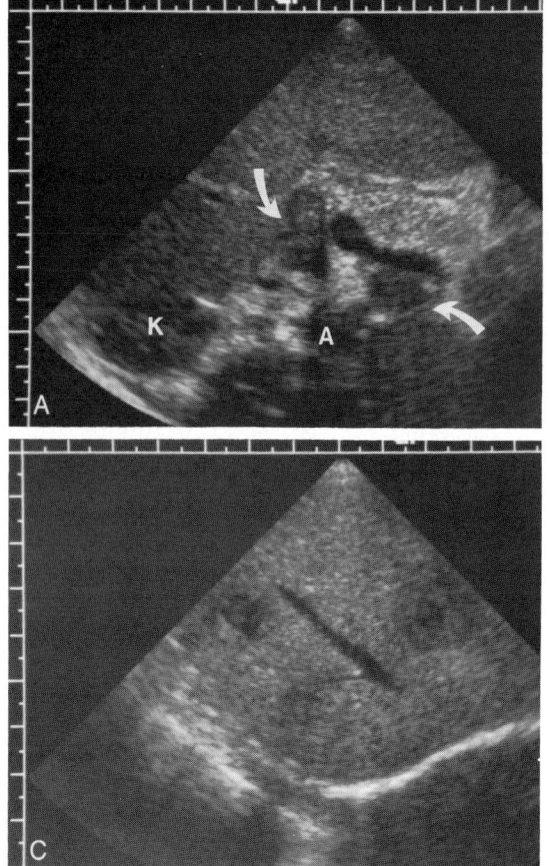
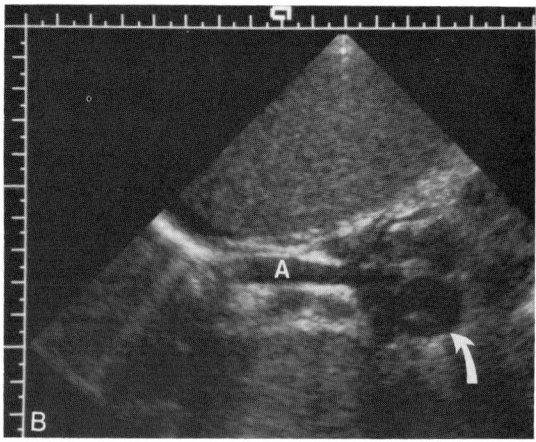

Figure 8–60. Multiple nodes (arrows) around the pancreas (A) and the aorta (B) and lucent deposits in the liver (C) were all secondary to disseminated *Mycobacterium avium–intracellulare* in this child, who had immunodeficiency unassociated with human immunodeficiency virus (HIV). K = kidney; A = aorta.

lymphadenopathy (Fig. 8–60). However, the differential diagnosis in these patients does include lymphoma (Fig. 8–61). Lymphoma can be diagnosed by biopsy if this information is needed. Nodal involvement with Kaposi sarcoma has been reported in children with AIDS (Bradford et al., 1988).

Pancreatic masses are discussed in Chapter 15.

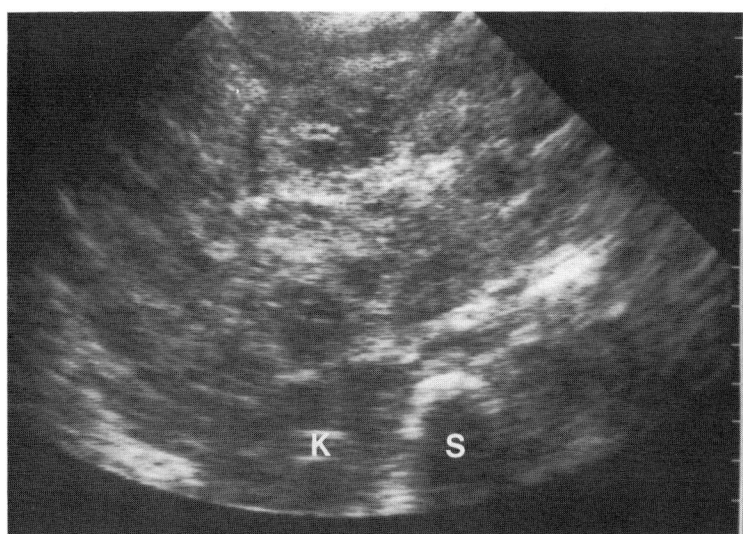

Figure 8–61. Lymphoma throughout the liver caused this diffusely abnormal parenchymal pattern on transverse scan. This child was 3 years old and had acquired immunodeficiency syndrome (AIDS). He died of rapidly proliferating lymphoma. S = spine; K = kidney.

HEPATIC MASSES

INTRODUCTION

Hepatic masses, benign and malignant, can arise from hepatocytes (epithelial tumors), from the supporting skeleton of connective tissues and blood vessels (mesenchymal tumors), or from the biliary system. Hepatic masses can also occur when tumors seed the liver through the portal system. Because primary carcinomas of the gastrointestinal tract are so rare in children, metastatic disease is less common in children than in adults. In Miller and Greenspan's (1985a) review of 40 children with hepatic malignancy, 25 malignancies were classified as "metastatic." Neuroblastoma is the major tumor of childhood to spread to the liver. Children with metastatic neuroblastoma may present only with mild hepatomegaly on clinical examination. On the other hand, we have

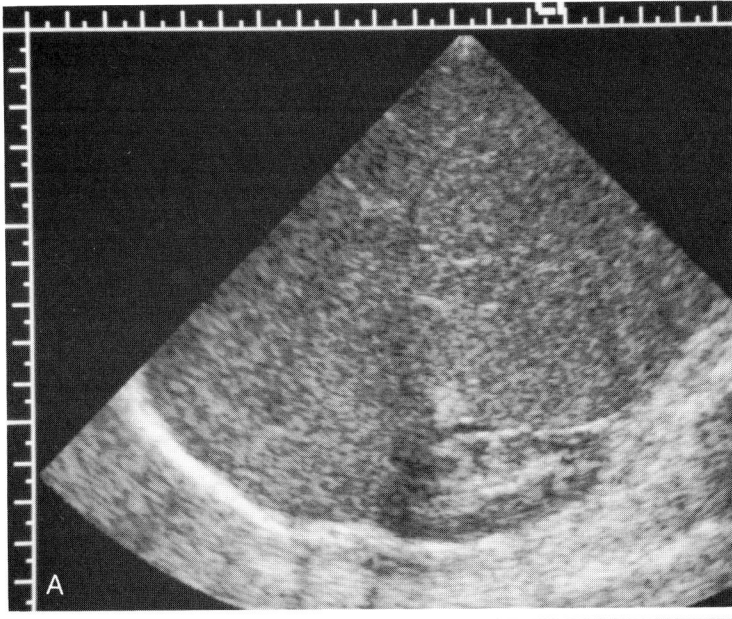

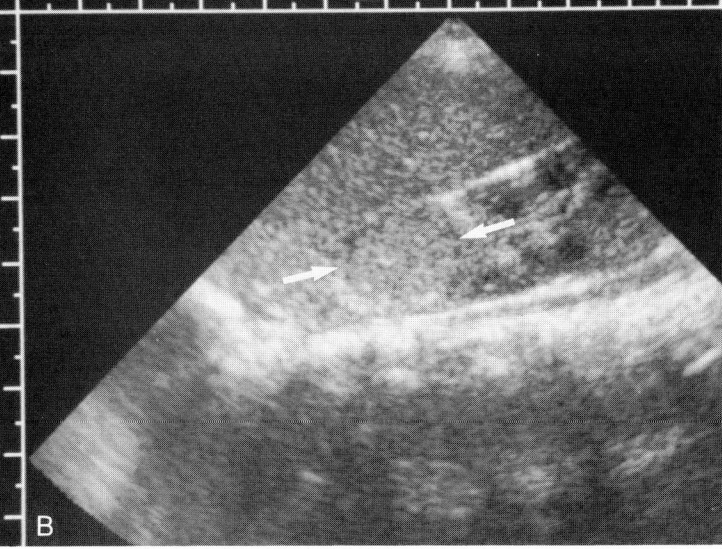

Figure 8–62. Stage IV neuroblastoma was diagnosed in this 4-month-old baby. He presented with a distended abdomen. His liver was large with relatively inhomogeneous texture on ultrasonography (**A**). Attention was directed toward finding a primary lesion. Coronal scan of the left upper quadrant (**B**) shows a solid mass in the left adrenal gland (arrows) that measured just under 2 cm in diameter. Bone marrow biopsy was normal; thus he fulfilled the criteria for stage IV-S disease.

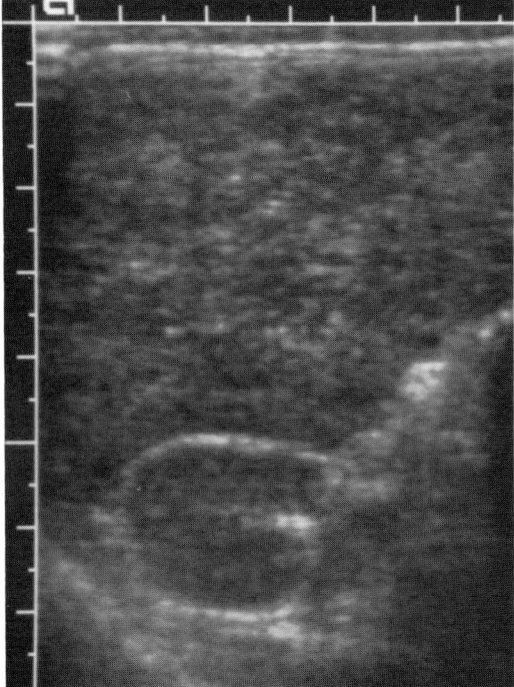

Figure 8–63. Thoracic neuroblastoma had been diagnosed prenatally in this child. The thoracic mass was resected. Because of an increase in the size of the liver 2 months after surgery, ultrasonography was performed and revealed a salt-and-pepper appearance of metastatic neuroblastoma.

seen neuroblastoma produce such massive enlargement of the liver that it caused respiratory and gastrointestinal compromise. In any baby or small child in whom a patchy or nodular pattern appears throughout the hepatic parenchyma on ultrasonography, we spend the rest of the study searching for the primary focus of neuroblastoma. It may be extra-abdominal; therefore, good radiographs of the chest should be obtained if the abdominal search is unrevealing. Children who have neuroblastoma with a small primary tumor and distant foci in the liver, skin, or bone marrow but without radiographic evidence of bony metastases are a small subset of patients with stage IV disease and have been classified as IV-S (S for special). They are usually, but not always, infants. Their prognosis is good, and many such patients have spontaneous regression of their primary tumors and metastases (Figs. 8–62, 8–63).

Lymphoma and leukemia are classified as "metastatic" when they involve the liver. Burkitt lymphoma is particularly likely to produce focal lesions, which are often very echolucent on ultrasonography. Other types of lymphoma and Hodgkin disease are usually more infiltrative. Other metastasizing tumors include rhabdomyosarcoma, teratocarcinoma, gastrointestinal tumors, and Wilms tumor (Fig. 8–64). In our experience, right-sided Wilms tumor may invade the right hepatic lobe but metastatic disease to the liver is distinctly less common than is indicated by the literature (Smith et al., 1983; Boechat et al., 1988).

Technique

In evaluating a mass in the liver, we need answers to the following questions: (1) Is the palpable mass truly part of the liver? The

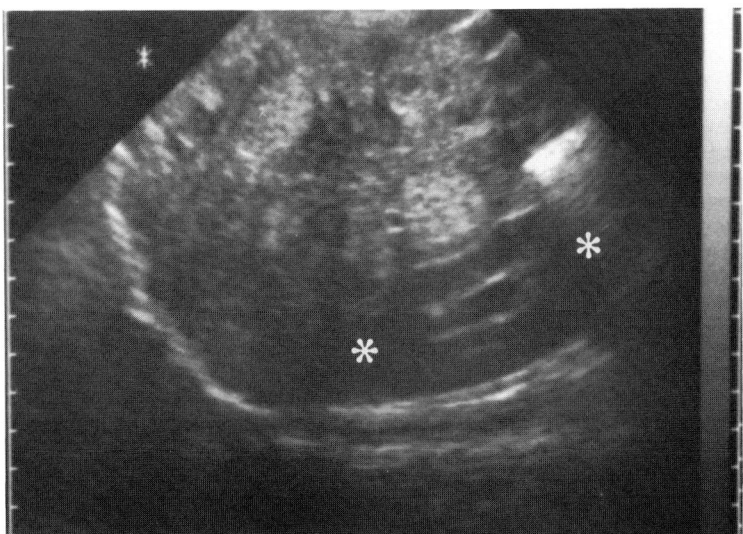

Figure 8–64. Pelvic rhabdomyosarcoma was the primary lesion in this little boy. This longitudinal scan of the liver shows obvious deposits of tumor within the hepatic parenchyma. Mild dilation of the right kidney (marked by asterisks) is from obstruction by the primary tumor.

right upper quadrant is one of the most difficult to assess when a mass is present. The clinician may mistake an exophytic Wilms tumor for a "hepatic" mass. Because the liver moves well with inspiration, a difference in response to deep breathing suggests that the liver and the mass are separate. (2) Where is the mass in relationship to hepatic venous anatomy, and are the veins normal? The draining hepatic veins—right, left, and middle—define the surgical lobar anatomy (Cosgrove et al., 1987). The patency of the vessels may be compromised by an extrinsic mass effect or an intrinsic tumor thrombus. The hepatic veins draining a vascular mass are dilated. (3) Are portal venous and hepatic arterial anatomy normal? Portal veins may be amputated from a primary hepatic malignancy (Brunelle and Chaumont, 1984). An overtly enlarged hepatic artery is probably feeding a benign vascular tumor or malformation (Abramson et al., 1982). The presence of a replaced right hepatic artery is useful information for angiographer or surgeon. (4) Is the biliary tract normal? A cystic mass may represent a normal, distended gallbladder. Obstruction to the biliary tract can be extrinsic or can be intrinsic as a result of primary rhabdomyosarcoma of the duct. (5) Is there any other abnormality in the abdomen? For example, is there a pelvic mass that could be a primary tumor? Is there ascites that could be aspirated for cytologic examination? (6) Finally, is the mass solid, cystic, or mixed? What are its size and contour? And is the remaining hepatic parenchyma normal?

Primary Hepatic Mass

Epithelial Derivatives

Ultrasonographic differential diagnosis of a primary hepatic mass is based heavily on its pattern: solid, cystic, or mixed. Most solid masses are epithelial derivatives. Fewer than one third of solid lesions are benign; therefore, any such mass has to be considered malignant until proved otherwise. In spite of all the help from the literature on imaging, we find that diagnosis of primary hepatic masses is not easy, particularly in older children.

Hepatoblastoma is more common than hepatocarcinoma in the pediatric population of the U.S. However, hepatocarcinoma is likely more prevalent in countries with a high incidence of cirrhosis in childhood (Smith et al., 1983). Hepatoblastoma arises from the primitive epithelial cells of the fetal liver. Hepatocarcinoma, also termed "hepatoma," is derived from mature hepatocytes. Clinical presentation of both types of tumor is usually of an asymptomatic mass or hepatomegaly. Hepatoblastoma typically occurs in children aged 0 to 3 years; hepatocarcinoma presents throughout childhood with two modal frequency peaks at 1 year and 13 years of age (Exelby et al., 1975). Certain clinical features help in differential diagnosis: hepatoblastoma is associated in some cases with hemihypertrophy and Beckwith-Wiedemann syndrome. In this regard, ongoing research in genetics localizes the fault or predisposition for embryonal tumors, including hepatoblastoma, to the 11p13 chromosome (Koufos et al., 1985). Also of interest is a report of hepatoblastoma associated with polyposis coli (Li et al., 1987). Some cases of hepatocellular carcinoma occur in children with preexisting cirrhosis; one third of patients with tyrosinemia develop malignancy. Elevated levels of alpha-fetoprotein in serum can occur with both hepatoblastoma and hepatocarcinoma. Multifocality is more likely with hepatocarcinoma, but because only one third of patients have multiple lesions, this is a poorly sensitive discriminatory sign. Scans of patients with either type of tumor typically show a poorly marginated echogenic mass in the hepatic parenchyma. In some tumors, microcystic degeneration is responsible for the echogenicity that is increased in comparison to normal hepatic parenchyma. Calcification is occasionally evident as a shadowing focus within a tumor. Portal venous amputation or invasion of adjacent hepatic vein supports a diagnosis of malignancy (Brunelle and Chaumont, 1984), but these signs are not always present (Figs. 8–65 to 8–68).

An unusual variant of hepatoma has been termed "fibrolamellar carcinoma." Affected patients tend to be older adolescents, the tumor rarely elevates levels in serum of alpha-fetoprotein, and its appearance simulates that of focal nodular hyperplasia (Titelbaum et al., 1988). Calcification was present in 5 of 13 cases from the Armed Forces Institute of Pathology (Friedman et al., 1985).

The benign epithelial tumors also appear as solid echogenic lesions and usually are identified as benign only in retrospect after surgical resection. The classic pathologic fea-

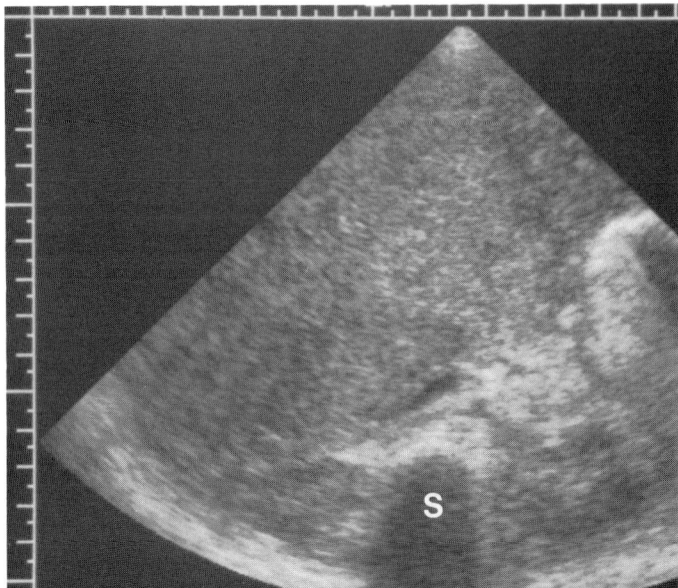

Figure 8–65. The mother of this 6½-month-old baby noticed that he had a very large liver. He had had a 1-week history of lethargy and vomiting. At the time of evaluation, his chest radiograph showed pulmonary metastases. Ultrasonography showed patchy increased echogenicity in the liver, very similar to a pattern we see with neuroblastoma. However, this was a yolk sac tumor. Alpha-fetoprotein levels were 16 times normal. The baby died of progressive disease. S = spine.

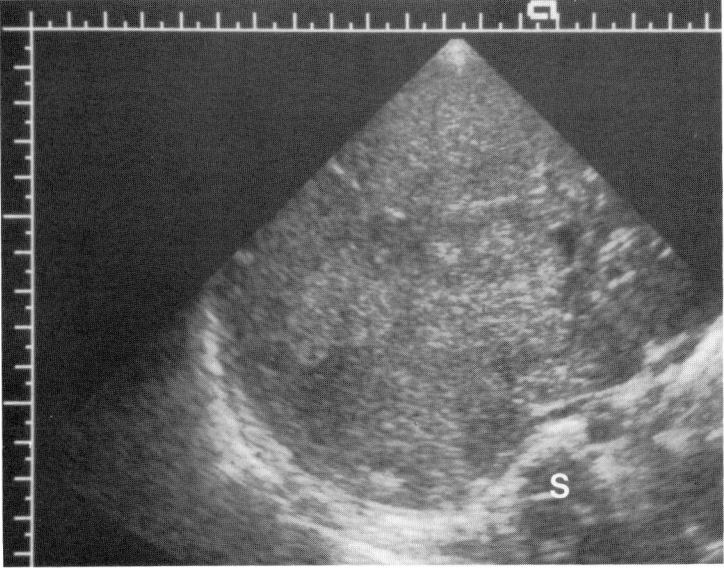

Figure 8–66. At 3½ years of age, a child presented with abdominal distention. It was apparent on clinical examination that his liver was firm and large. Multiple echogenic masses were identified in the right lobe of the liver, and on several sections, it appeared that the hepatic veins were truncated. He did not have pulmonary metastases at the time, but his multifocal hepatoblastoma was nonresectable, and he was treated with chemotherapy. S = spine.

EVALUATING AN ABDOMINAL MASS / 265

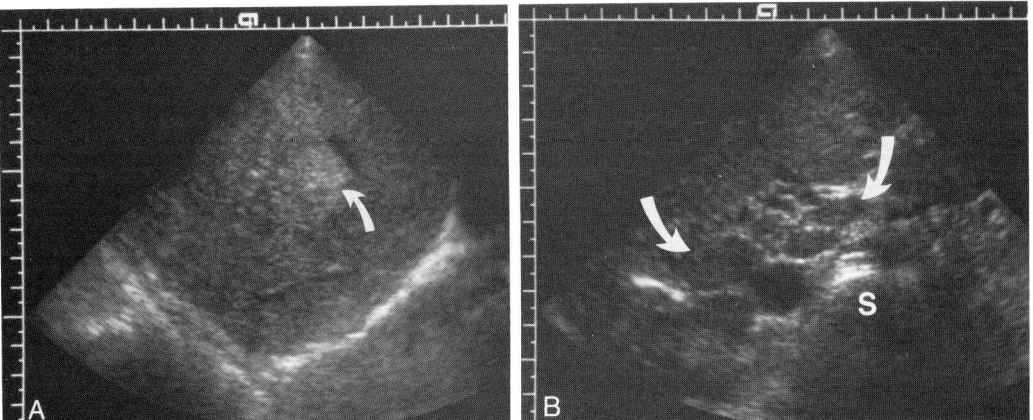

Figure 8–67. This 6-year-old had hepatocellular carcinoma. Transverse scan (**A**) high in the right lobe of the liver shows a poorly defined echogenic mass (arrow). Note the similarity to hepatoblastoma as shown in preceding figures. The child had multiple nodes around the porta hepatis (arrows, **B**). She was treated with chemotherapy. S = spine.

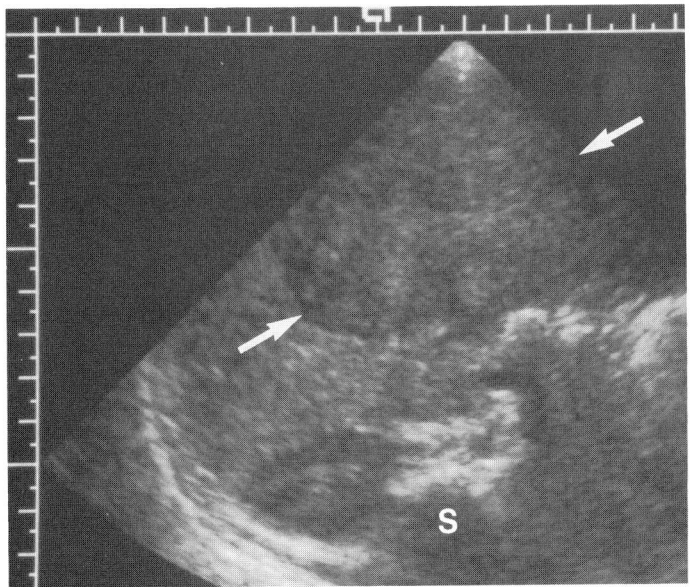

Figure 8–68. The transverse scan shown is of a 3-year-old child. Biopsy of the relatively hypoechogenic mass (arrows) showed embryonal hepatoblastoma. This is an atypical appearance for hepatoblastoma. Most are echogenic. S = spine.

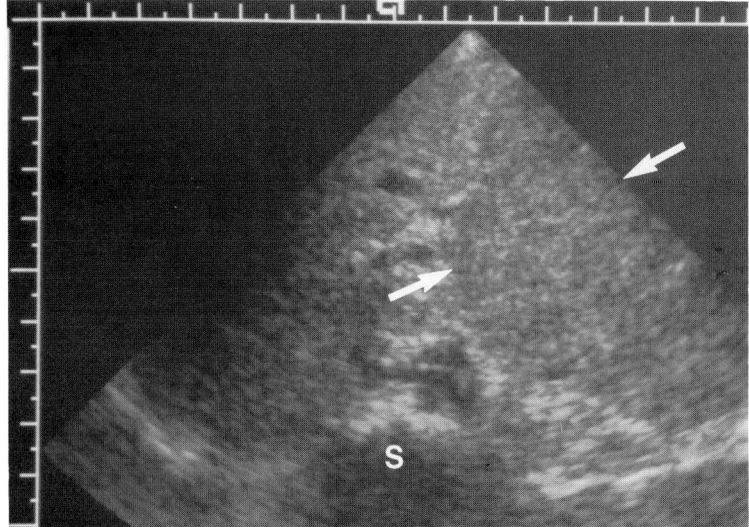

Figure 8–69. A relatively well circumscribed mass (arrows) involved most of the left lobe of the liver in this 2-year-old girl. The preoperative diagnosis was that of hepatoblastoma, but pathologic examination revealed focal nodular hyperplasia. The central scar was not apparent on any of the preoperative images. S = spine.

Figure 8–70. Transverse scans show a large mass in the lateral segment of the left lobe of the liver (A) and a small mass low in the right lobe of the liver (arrow, B). These are scans from a patient who is now 19 years old and has been followed for many years since receiving a diagnosis of glycogen storage disease, type I. The size of the lesions has stayed stable, and we assume that they represent hepatic adenomas.

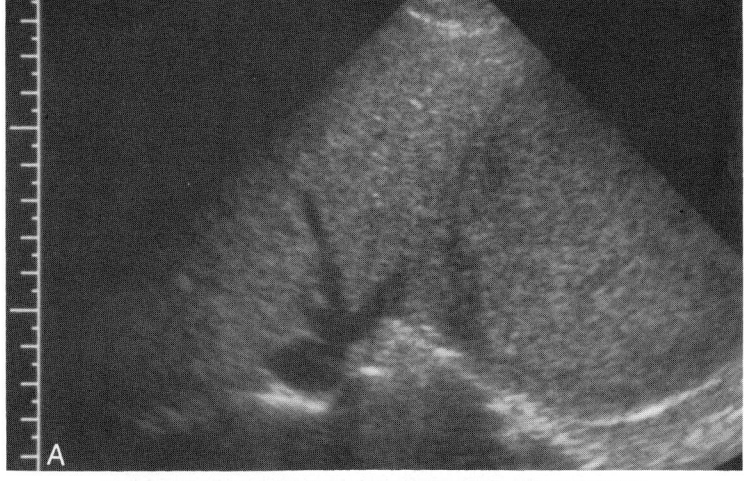
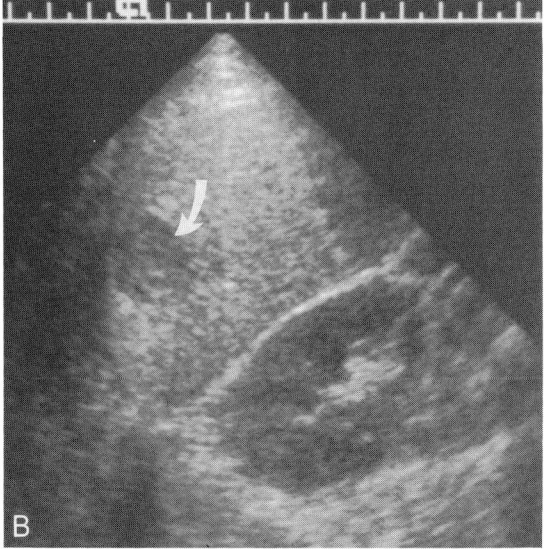

ture of focal nodular hyperplasia is a central scar, but this cannot be identified with reliability on ultrasonograms (Fig. 8–69). One third of patients with focal nodular hyperplasia show, on scintigrams, normal or increased uptake of ^{99m}Tc sulfur colloid in the mass. This is in contrast to patients with malignancy, whose scans usually show a defect. Angiography of focal nodular hyperplasia may reveal the central fibrous scar and septa as defects in the center of a sharply defined and otherwise uniformly dense blush (D'Souza et al., 1983).

Hepatic adenoma occurs in childhood, albeit uncommonly. Its association with glycogen storage disease is well known. Adenomas, when found in children with glycogen storage disease (almost invariably type I, glucose-6-phosphatase deficiency, or von Gierke disease), are usually multiple (Fig. 8–70). Their ultrasonographic appearance (hypoechogenic, isoechogenic, or hyperechogenic) can vary in the same patient. We have noted waxing and waning lesions in patients followed over months to years. There is no correlation between ultrasonographic and angiographic appearances (Brunelle et al., 1984). Malignant degeneration has been reported but is rare. Evaluation with CT or angiography follows semiannual ultrasonographic screening only if vascular changes (i.e., portal or hepatic venous) occur, if a lesion increases dramatically in size, or if alpha-fetoprotein levels in serum have increased. Hepatic adenoma may also develop in children who are receiving androgenic

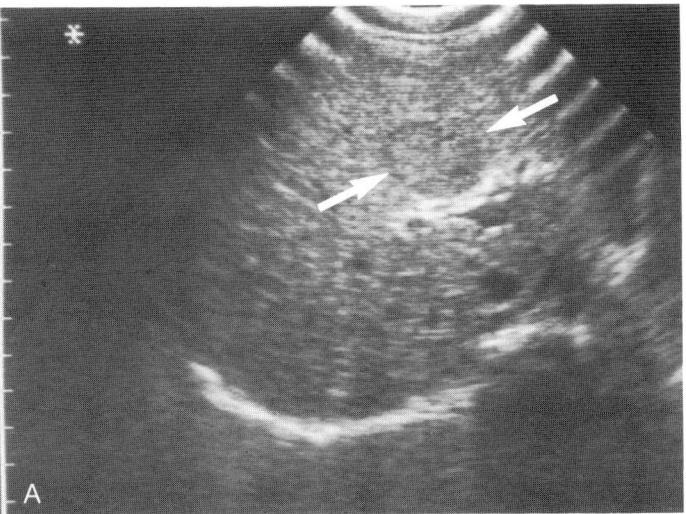

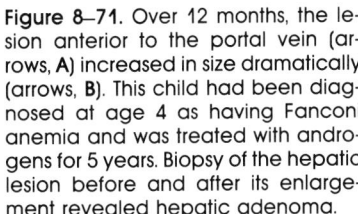

Figure 8–71. Over 12 months, the lesion anterior to the portal vein (arrows, **A**) increased in size dramatically (arrows, **B**). This child had been diagnosed at age 4 as having Fanconi anemia and was treated with androgens for 5 years. Biopsy of the hepatic lesion before and after its enlargement revealed hepatic adenoma.

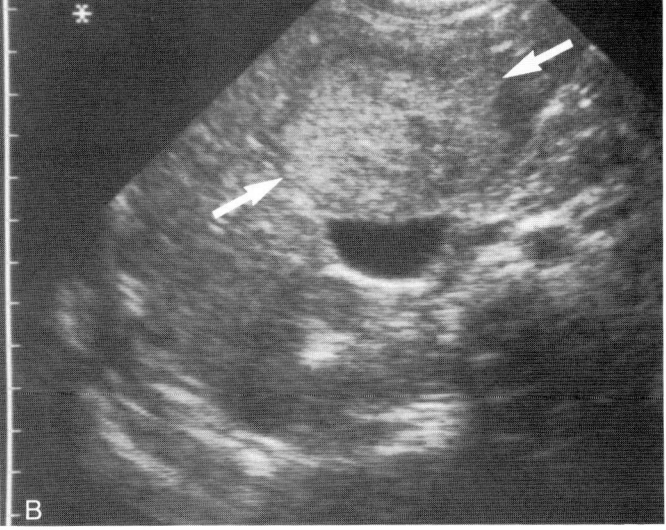

steroids to promote erythroplasia. We screen these children semiannually as well (Fig. 8–71).

Depending on the facilities and expertise available, there are other studies from which to choose when ultrasonography is incompletely diagnostic of an intrahepatic mass. CT scanning demonstrates the number of parenchymal lesions and provides more information regarding vascularity. As mentioned earlier, radionuclide scanning may show uptake of ^{99m}Tc sulfur colloid by focal nodular hyperplasia. The angiographers recommend angiography for differentiation of benign tumors from malignant tumors (Tonkin et al., 1988) and, when needed, for therapeutic delivery of chemotherapy or embolization. Advocates of MRI recommend replacing all these methods with one trip through their scanner. The diagnosis, however, usually rests with histopathologic examination by an experienced pathologist. It is our view that surgeons should go to the operating room with as much information as they feel is necessary to perform the surgery well. In spite of advances in chemotherapy, primary hepatic malignancies are best cured by complete surgical excision.

Mesenchymal Derivatives

Tumors derived from mesenchyma tend to be cystic, multicystic, or mixed solid/cystic on ultrasonic evaluation. The mesenchymal hamartoma is not a true neoplasm but is discussed in this section because it presents clinically as a mass. Derived from the mesenchyma around portal tracts, it includes hepatocytes, abnormal bile ducts, and immature mesenchyma (Ros et al., 1986a). Most hamartomas present during the first 2 years of life as asymptomatic right-sided masses. Most involve the right lobe of the liver (Stanley et al., 1986). Calcification is *not* a feature of these growths. Their characteristic appearance on ultrasonography is of a multiseptate cystic mass. The cysts, which are thought to represent accumulation of fluid in bile ducts and degeneration of mesenchyma, may be quite large, and one cyst may predominate. Most cases of mesenchymal hamartoma that have been reported in the literature have been avascular. Smith and colleagues (1978) reported a patient who had a vascular mesenchymoma, and we have seen two similar patients. In one of these babies, the large cystic spaces of the growth were filled with echogenic fluid representing blood rather than the clear fluid that is typically present in mesenchymal hamartoma (Figs. 8–72, 8–73). Ros and coauthors (1986a) dismissed the diagnosis of hamartoma in cases in which hypervascularity had been reported. Others adopt a more unifying theme to explain both avascular and vascular mesenchymal hamartomas. Hemangioma and hemangioendothelioma are derived from mesenchymal elements and may overlap in histopathologic

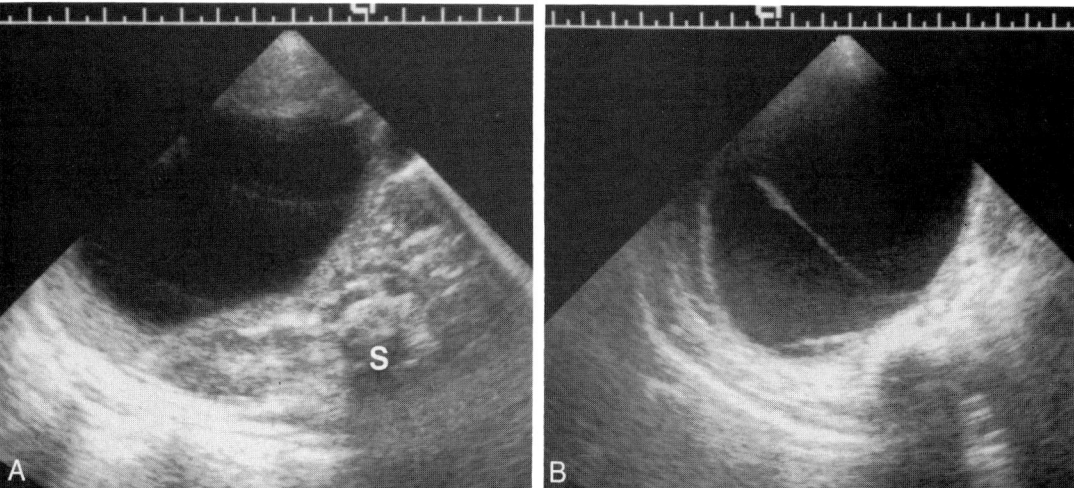

Figure 8–72. Abdominal distention and constipation were the presenting problems in this 10-month-old girl. She was brought to ultrasonography after plain films revealed a huge mass in the right upper quadrant. Transverse **(A)** and longitudinal **(B)** scans show an intrahepatic fluid-filled mass with septations. This was removed and proved to be a mesenchymal hamartoma. In **A**, S = spine.

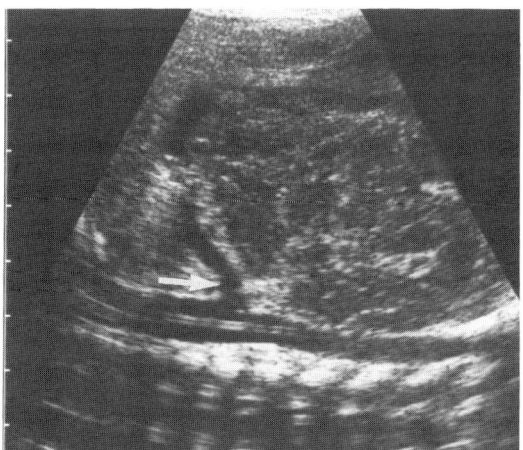

Figure 8–73. A huge mass in the right lobe of the liver in this neonate is shown on this longitudinal scan. An umbilical arterial catheter was in the aorta, which decreased significantly in diameter after giving off a very large hepatic artery (arrow). The mass itself was septated, but the locules did not contain clear fluid. The baby died of massive intracranial hemorrhage, and pathologic examination revealed that the lesion was a septated mass filled with locules of blood. Pathologic diagnosis was of a vascular mesenchymal hamartoma. (From Teele RL, Share JC: The abdominal mass in the neonate. Semin Roentgenol 1988; 23:175–184.)

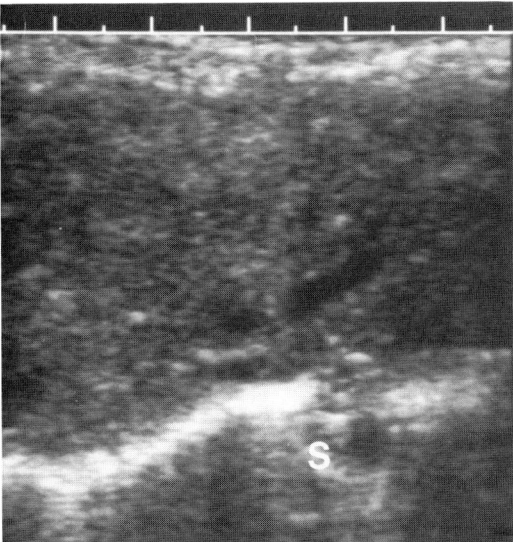

Figure 8–74. This newborn had hemangiomas of the skin and mild respiratory distress. The heart appeared mildly enlarged on initial radiographs. The scans of the liver showed a subtle, blotchy parenchymal pattern, which was associated with mild dilatation of the hepatic veins. The child was not treated with medication or with surgery. We consider the lesions in the liver to be associated with cutaneous hemangiomas and believe that they will regress over time. S = spine.

characteristics with mesenchymal hamartoma. Most vascular lesions in the child's liver appear to be hemangioendotheliomas (Fig. 8–74; Dachman et al., 1983). Cavernous hemangiomas are unusual and in most cases are found only as small incidental lesions during autopsy. Because, in children, *hemangiomas* of the skin are associated with *hemangioendotheliomas* of the liver, confusion regarding terminology has infiltrated the literature. In addition, writers have rarely discriminated between patients on the basis of age; therefore, hemangioma is assumed by many readers to be as common in children as in adults. This is not true. Hepatic hemangioma seems to accompany aging, like simple renal cysts and wrinkles. We prefer to avoid the pathologic labels and use the terms "vascular" and "avascular mesenchymal growth." The vascularity is key, first, in establishing benignancy and, second, in formulating further investigation and management.

It has been our experience that characteristic features of benign vascular masses are (1) enlargement of the celiac axis and common hepatic artery (or the superior mesenteric artery and replaced right hepatic artery), (2) diminution in the caliber of the aorta after the take-off of the hepatic artery, (3) large hepatic veins draining a mass, and (4) usually concomitant clinical evidence of cardiomegaly to indicate arteriovenous shunting (Fig. 8–75). Malignancies derived from the epithelium, although appearing hypervascular on angiography, do not cause such dramatic changes in the caliber of nutritive and draining vessels as do the vascular mesenchymal tumors. On rare occasions, we see a patient who has a true arteriovascular malformation within the liver (Plate X). The liver is filled with echolucent channels that all show a vascular signal on Doppler imaging. There is very little if any stromal component to the vascular malformation, and arterial blood supply may be recruited from multiple vessels, including intercostal branches and renal, adrenal, left gastric, and superior mesenteric arteries, in addition to the hepatic artery from the celiac axis.

We have followed several babies who had received an incidental diagnosis of vascular hepatic mass from scans done in utero, who were asymptomatic after birth, and who had no cutaneous hemangiomas. Each infant had a lesion typical of hemangioendothelioma, and because the normal history of this lesion

270 / EVALUATING AN ABDOMINAL MASS

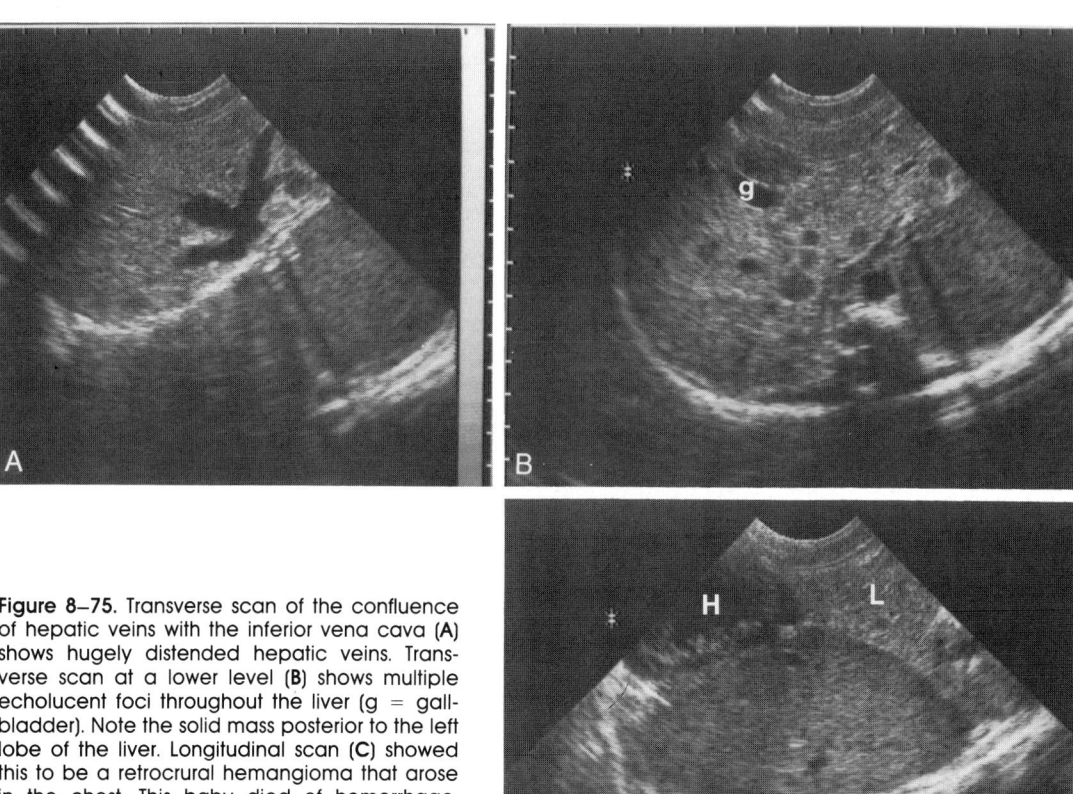

Figure 8–75. Transverse scan of the confluence of hepatic veins with the inferior vena cava (**A**) shows hugely distended hepatic veins. Transverse scan at a lower level (**B**) shows multiple echolucent foci throughout the liver (g = gallbladder). Note the solid mass posterior to the left lobe of the liver. Longitudinal scan (**C**) showed this to be a retrocrural hemangioma that arose in the chest. This baby died of hemorrhage, which possibly resulted from the trapping of platelets. H = heart; L = liver.

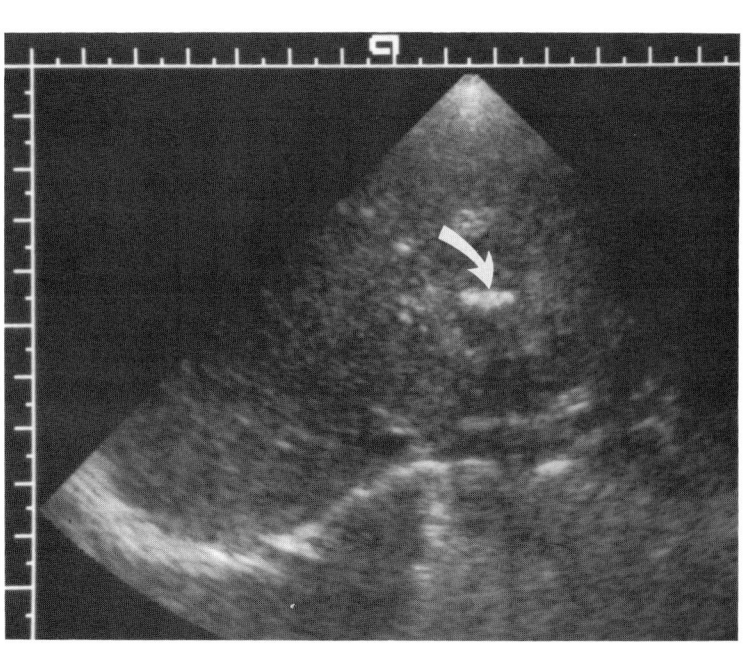

Figure 8–76. Transverse scan of the left lobe of the liver shows a shadowing echogenic focus (arrow). A vascular lesion of the left lobe of the liver had been diagnosed on the basis of prenatal scans, which showed large draining hepatic veins. A biopsy was not performed because the child was relatively asymptomatic. Calcification has gradually developed in the lesion, which indicates that it is involuting.

is regression, no treatment was instituted. Many babies therefore may have silent intrahepatic vascular masses that are unassociated with cutaneous hemangiomas.

Hepatic vascular lesions may be either single and large or multiple and small. The draining hepatic vein appears to arise from the periphery of the lesion, which is usually of mixed echogenicity. Calcification is occasionally present and provides a shadowing focus. Doppler imaging can demonstrate the turbulence and high frequency of blood flow through the lesions. Therapy is based on the number of lesions and the severity of clinical symptoms. An isolated mass in one lobe can be excised surgically; multiple lesions are problematic. Most regress with time, as do cutaneous hemangiomas if associated. However, cardiac failure that is unresponsive to routine medical management requires more drastic measures, as does the trapping of platelets (Kasabach-Merritt syndrome), which is associated with vascular masses in some children. Steroids and radiotherapy have been used with variable response in diminution of the lesions. Angiographic embolization with coils of the feeding hepatic artery does decrease some of the arterial blood flow, but many of these lesions parasitize other vessels. Each case of course has to be managed individually. During therapy, ultrasonography provides information about the size of lesions and the degrees of vascularity.

Some hemangioendotheliomas appear on ultrasonography to have slow blood flow and marginally increased vasculature (Fig. 8–76). Radionuclide scans with labeled red blood cells are very useful in showing the vascular nature of these lesions, as is CT scanning with bolus injection of contrast material. Angiography is reserved for those for whom the diagnosis is still uncertain.

Congenital hepatic cysts are rare lesions in childhood. We scanned one patient who presented after scans in utero had shown a hepatic cyst (Fig. 8–77). It seemed such an unusual diagnosis that we couldn't believe it until a pedunculated cyst was removed from the undersurface of the right lobe of the liver. More common are cystic disorders of the biliary tree (discussed in the section on right upper quadrant pain and jaundice), inflammatory cysts (to be discussed), and cysts in association with autosomal dominant polycystic disease of kidneys.

Malignant mesenchymoma now carries a new label: "undifferentiated (embryonal) sar-

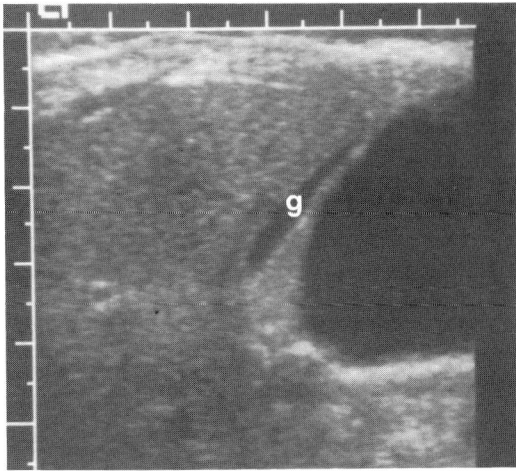

Figure 8–77. A 6-cm cyst was removed from the inferior portion of the left lobe of the liver in this 2-month-old. The preoperative scan shown is a longitudinal view. The cyst is exophytic, extending from the left lobe across the midline to distort the gallbladder (g).

coma" of the liver. Its ultrasonographic appearance is similar to that of mesenchymal hamartoma, although a predominantly echogenic mass, as opposed to multiseptate mass, has been described in two patients (Ros et al., 1986b). The differential diagnosis depends on the age of the patient. The age range of children with undifferentiated sarcoma is much higher (mean age is 11.8 years), in contrast to those with hamartoma, who are usually less than 2 years old at presentation. Levels of alpha-fetoprotein are not elevated, in contrast to those of most patients with malignancies derived from epithelial cells of the liver.

TUMORS OF THE BILIARY TRACT

Only five patients with botryoid rhabdomyosarcoma of the biliary tract were treated at our institution between 1924 and 1990. In spite of its rarity, it is the most common primary tumor of the biliary tract and a major cause of obstructive jaundice in children (Lack et al., 1981). Its pathogenesis is uncertain; the proffered explanation is that the tumor arises from a multipotent splanchnic mesenchyma that is capable of rhabdomyoblastic differentiation. We scanned one patient with such a tumor; it had completely filled the cystic duct and extended in an exophytic manner to occlude the common hepatic and common bile ducts (Patient JL in the study reported by Lack et al., 1981). The gallbladder and intrahepatic ducts were dilated; the tumor extended as a solid cylinder from the porta hepatis to the head of the pancreas.

A study of eight children, diagnosed and treated in France, indicated that no ultrasonographic pattern was pathognomonic of this tumor. On scans, very large tumors could not be traced to an origin in the biliary tract. However, in contrast to hepatoblastoma or hepatocarcinoma, thrombosis of the portal vasculature was not apparent in any patient, levels of alpha-fetoprotein in the blood were not elevated, and calcification was distinctly unusual (Geoffray et al., 1987a).

INFLAMMATORY HEPATIC MASSES

A hepatic abscess is not usually mistaken for a tumor because the affected child presents clinically with fever, with signs of infection, usually with pain, and often with a history that supports the diagnosis. The children with hepatic abscesses can be divided into three groups: those with bacterial or fungal infection, those with amebic abscess, and those with hydatid disease. Each group is discussed separately below.

True prevalence of pyogenic hepatic abscess is unknown. Many individual cases are not reported, and few institutions have large series. Children with immunodeficiency, immunosuppression (see Chapter 18, Hepatic Transplantation), and chronic granulomatous disease (Garel et al., 1984) are particularly susceptible to pyogenic hepatic abscess. Other predisposing situations include appendicitis or other inflammation of the bowel with pylephlebitis, omphalitis or presence of an umbilical venous catheter in neonates (or both), previous trauma, and sepsis.

Early hepatic abscess is usually hypoechogenic and poorly marginated from liver. Much later in the evolution, the liquid pus becomes more defined by an encircling wall of inflammation. Gas in the abscess causes hyperechogenicity. When such a lesion is identified, the portal venous system should be carefully evaluated for possible septic thrombus. Hepatic abscess is treated by percutaneous drainage (Vachon et al., 1986). A No. 9 French or larger pigtail catheter is left in the cavity after fine-needle aspiration of pus has confirmed the diagnosis (Fig. 8–78). Calcification of earlier granuloma or abscess is common.

Children who have candidal sepsis may suffer gradual development of candidal abscesses in the liver and spleen. It seems to take days to a couple of weeks for the microscopic foci to develop into lesions large enough to be identified on ultrasonography. A normal scan does not rule out the possibility of hepatic candidiasis. The foci are multiple and, in our experience, have had a target appearance with a central echogenicity

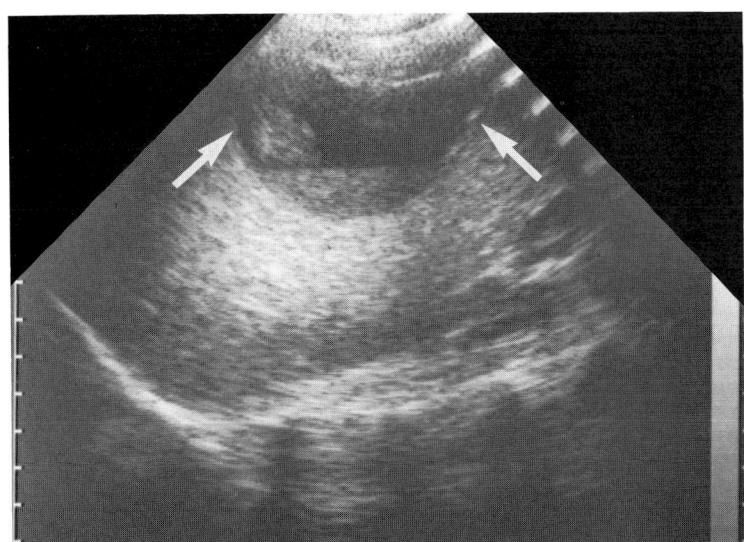

Figure 8–78. This patient presented several months after abdominal trauma. The hepatic abscess with fluid-debris level (arrows) demonstrated on this scan was likely a secondary infection of hepatic hematoma. It was percutaneously drained. Cultures revealed *Staphylococcus aureus*.

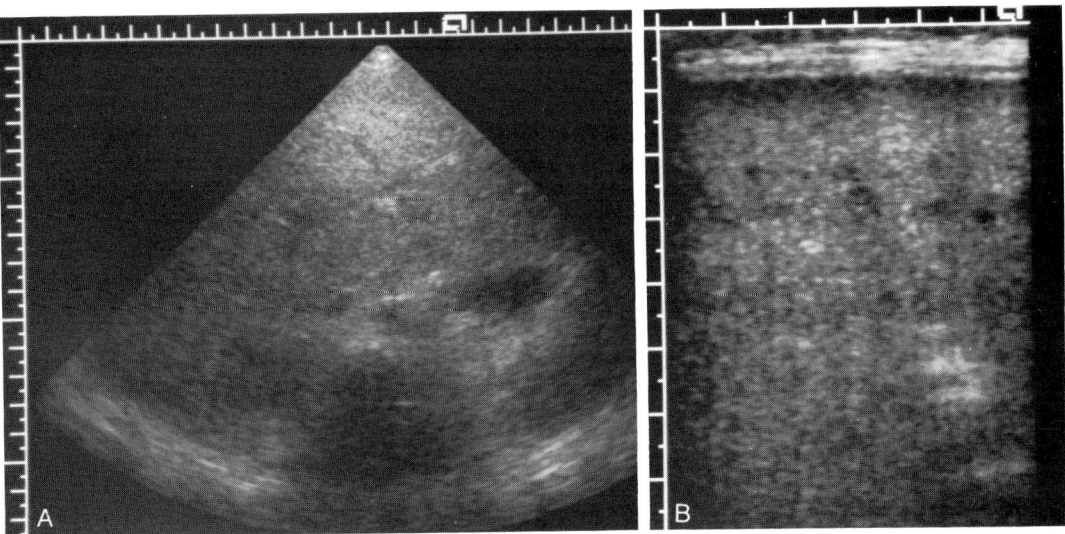

Figure 8-79. The hepatic parenchyma becomes quite echogenic from fat in children who are treated with chemotherapy for acute lymphoblastic leukemia. Routine sector scanning of the liver as shown in **A** may completely miss small focal hypoechoic areas, which are typical for candidal abscess (**B**). For any child at risk for candidal infection, it is important to use transducers with good resolution and perform a careful search of both hepatic and splenic parenchyma.

surrounded by lucent halo. This pattern has also been termed "wheels within wheels" (Pastakia et al., 1988). In our practice, the children who have been affected were severely immunocompromised and had been treated with prolonged antimicrobial therapy for bacterial infections (Fig. 8–79).

Amebic disease is rife in subtropical and tropical underdeveloped countries. Amebic hepatic abscess is the most common manifestation of extraintestinal disease. The trophozoite of *Entamoeba histolytica* invades the wall of an ulcerated bowel and makes its way via the portal system to the liver. Here the protozoan causes focal necrosis by producing proteolytic enzyme and begins establishing an abscess. Multiple abscesses are common in children. Rupture of an abscess into adjacent organs or spaces may result in shock and death (Merten and Kirks, 1984).

Serologic testing is occasionally unreliable in children but should be performed for any child in whom amebic disease is suspected. Ralls and colleagues (1982) compiled a list of features termed "suggestive sonographic pattern" for amebic abscess: (1) lack of significant wall echoes; (2) round or oval configuration; (3) echogenicity that is less than that in normal hepatic parenchyma; (4) peripheral location, contiguous to capsule; and (5) distal acoustic enhancement. Obviously, as these ultrasonographic features are similar to those seen with pyogenic abscess, the most important factor in making the diagnosis of amebic abscess is to think of it in the first place. A child whom we studied was diagnosed only after aspiration of a presumed pyogenic abscess yielded thick green material that grew nothing on standard culture media. Although considered the classic feature of amebic abscess, the "anchovy paste" characterization of the contents is actually uncommon. Further questioning of the family revealed that this child of the suburbs had been on a trip to the Caribbean. Serologic examination yielded positive findings of *Entamoeba histolytica*; serologic test is positive in 94 percent of affected children who are tested. Drainage of the amebic abscess is unnecessary for therapy (Ralls et al., 1987); patients respond well to standard treatment with metronidazole or chloroquine, or both. Aspiration does carry a theoretical risk of peritoneal contamination or superimposed infection. The major indication for drainage is a juxtacardiac abscess that threatens to rupture into the pericardium. This is a rare but life-threatening complication of amebic abscess (Ralls et al., 1987).

HYDATID DISEASE

The adult tapeworm *Echinococcus* resides in the jejunum of a carnivorous mammal such as a dog, and lays eggs that are excreted with the animal's feces. If these eggs are ingested by humans or some other intermediate host, such as sheep, they develop into embryos that pass via the duodenal mucosa to the portal vein. They usually are trapped in the liver or lung but occasionally slip through these sieves and arrive in the brain, kidney, or other organs. Embryos that survive the host's defenses form a laminated cyst. Scoleces develop from brood capsules or outpouchings of the germinal membrane. As scoleces and capsules break away from the membrane, they form hydatid sand. Daughter cysts, which develop within the original cyst, may contain hydatid sand and granddaughter cysts. The stimulus for their development is unknown. If the organs that contain cysts are ingested (for instance, by a dog eating the remains of a sheep), the life cycle of the tapeworm is completed: the scoleces attach to the small intestine of the dog and grow to adulthood.

Ultrasonography of humans (or sheep) who have hydatid cysts may show (1) a simple cyst, (2) a cyst with fine echogenicity from hydatid sand ("falling snowflake" sign), (3) undulating membranes, caused by the separation of a lamellated membrane of the cyst wall, (4) a multiseptate cyst representing daughter cysts, and (5) dense, irregular calcification from collapsed cysts, which have no living scoleces left (Lewall and McCorkell, 1985). The clinician can best demonstrate hydatid sand by shaking the patient during ultrasonography, much as one shakes a glass ball that is filled with fluid and artificial snow.

Most infected humans are probably infected in childhood, when they have eating habits similar to those of sheep! Thus most infected children have simple cysts or cysts with undulating membranes resulting from detachment of some of the endocystic wall.

Percutaneous drainage of echinococcal cyst has been avoided in the past because of the potential, albeit poorly quantified, risk of peritoneal contamination or anaphylactic shock. Hydatid cysts have, however, been drained percutaneously without complication (Mueller et al., 1985). In children, surgical evacuation is the procedure of choice. Biliary obstruction and superinfection are recognized complications.

ANTERIOR ABDOMINAL MASS

A freely movable, anterior abdominal mass usually is related to the gastrointestinal tract. Any large retroperitoneal mass can present in the anterior abdomen, but the examiner is usually able to detect the retroperitoneal anchoring. Ovarian cysts, particularly in babies who have poorly defined pelvic cavities, have a marked propensity to drift into the mid- and upper abdomen. They are discussed later in the section on pelvic masses, but the differential diagnosis of an intra-abdominal mass in a baby girl should include ovarian lesions.

Plain films are very helpful in evaluating anterior abdominal masses because effects on distribution and on the pattern of intestinal gas are common. Very few noninflammatory intraperitoneal masses are calcified. The rarest intraperitoneal lesions are the solid tumors of the mesentery (Fig. 8–80). Fibroma, lipoma, neurofibroma, other benign mesenchymal tumors, and their malignant counterparts can arise from any part of the mesenteric connective tissues (Haller et al., 1978). They are frequently invisible or poorly defined on ultrasonography because of the interposed bowel. CT scanning, after good opacification of the bowel with contrast material, is the appropriate study and should be done if a palpable mass is not visible on ultrasonography.

Peritoneal implants of tumor may be evident on ultrasonography, particularly if malignant ascites is present. Irregularity of the lining surface of the abdominal cavity or irregularly clumped loops of bowel may be apparent. Ovarian teratocarcinoma, Wilms tumor, and medulloblastoma seeded through a ventriculoperitoneal shunt have been responsible for peritoneal implants in affected patients whom we have scanned.

We made the point earlier that teratomas can occur anywhere. We were stumped by a noncalcified anterior abdominal mass that, during surgery, was found to be a teratoma that arose from the anterior abdominal wall

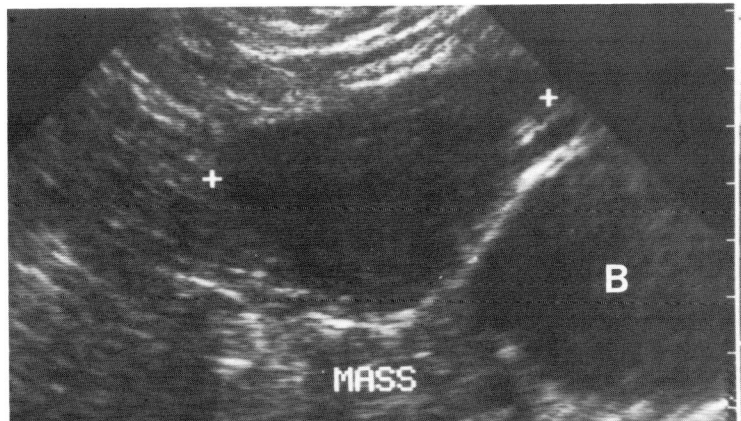

Figure 8–80. This anterior abdominal mass, marked by crosses in this longitudinal scan, was a mesenteric desmoid tumor. It was relatively hypoechoic. The patient had a predisposition to tumors of connective tissues because of underlying Gardner syndrome. B = bladder.

(Teele and Share, 1988). Other masses of the abdominal wall include rhabdomyomas (think of tuberous sclerosis in association), lipomas, fibromas, and rhabdomyosarcomas. None has specific diagnostic characteristics on ultrasonography, although lipomas may be quite echogenic. As with masses related to the thoracic wall, CT often better enables the radiologist to characterize the contents and extent of a lesion. Teratomas can involve the gut and, in boys, have a peculiar affinity for the stomach. Virtually all reported cases of gastric teratomas are in baby boys (Earnshaw, 1985). Other unusual tumors of the stomach include leiomyoma and carcinoma. If a mass in the anterior left upper quadrant is identified on ultrasonography, the patient's stomach should be filled with water and the patient positioned so as to avoid superimposed air during scanning. On the basis of the findings, fluoroscopy with contrast material or CT with contrast material can follow. Gastric trichobezoar may present the confusing ultrasonographic picture of a densely shadowing gastric mass (Newman and Girdany, 1990). Plain radiographs and studies with barium are usually diagnostic.

In general, one can classify the rest of the

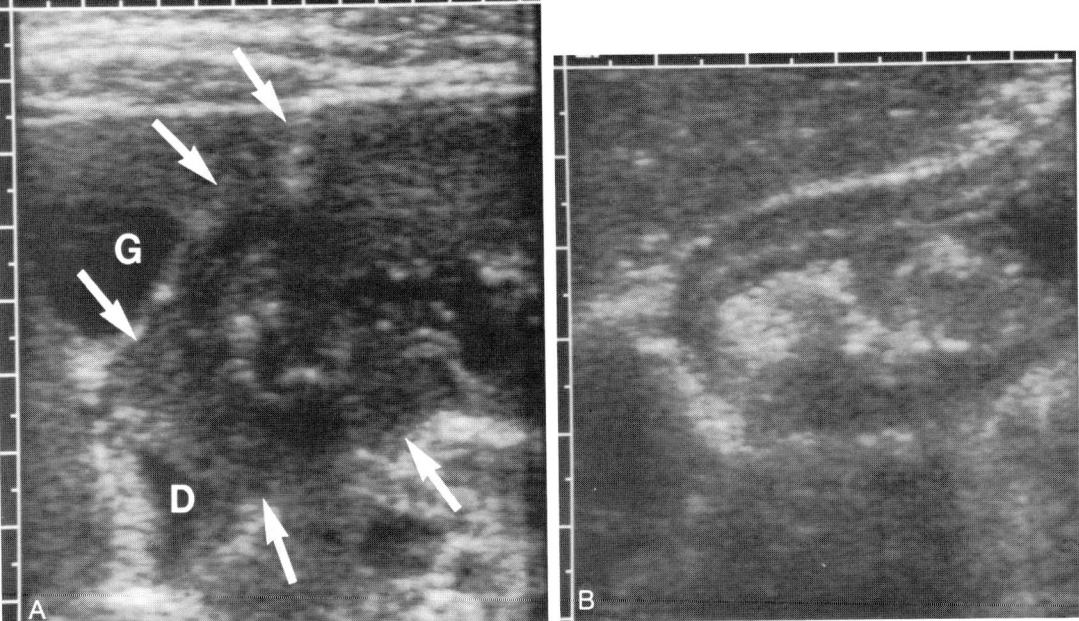

Figure 8–81. Transverse scan at the level of the gastric outlet (A) shows marked circumferential thickening of the gastric wall (arrows). G = gallbladder; D = duodenal cap. This patient had Burkitt lymphoma involving the stomach. Two weeks later, after aggressive chemotherapy (B), the anterior gastric wall was returning to normal thickness. The posterior wall is shadowed by gastric contents.

intraperitoneal masses as cysts or doughnut lesions. Any mass or process (inflammatory, allergic, vascular, neoplastic, infiltrative) that involves the wall of the gut tends to thicken the wall in a circumferential manner and compress the lumen. The wall is relatively echolucent; the lumen is echogenic because of reflection from mucosal surfaces, mucus, and air. In New England, ultrasonographic cross-sections of involved gut look like doughnuts. (Walter Berdon of Babies Hospital has told us that in New York, the cross-sectional scans resemble bagels instead!) The term "pseudokidney" has also been used in this regard, but we believe it to be confusing and, in any case, would prefer that food rather than water be associated with the gastrointestinal tract.

Primary carcinoma of the colon is common in adults but rare in children. Colonic carcinoma may arise in the bowel mucosa adjacent to a ureterosigmoidostomy and in the colon of patients who have familial adenomatous polyps or Gardner syndrome. Ultrasonography is not an appropriate screening method for these patients; colonoscopy and double contrast enema are.

In children, lymphoma is the most common tumor to affect the bowel. Primary lymphoma typically is situated in the distal ileum and the right colon, although it can arise from any part of the gut (Fig. 8–81). American Burkitt lymphoma is characterized by a mass that increases rapidly in size: its doubling time is 24 hours. Large lucent nodes in the mesentery may be matted together, extra-

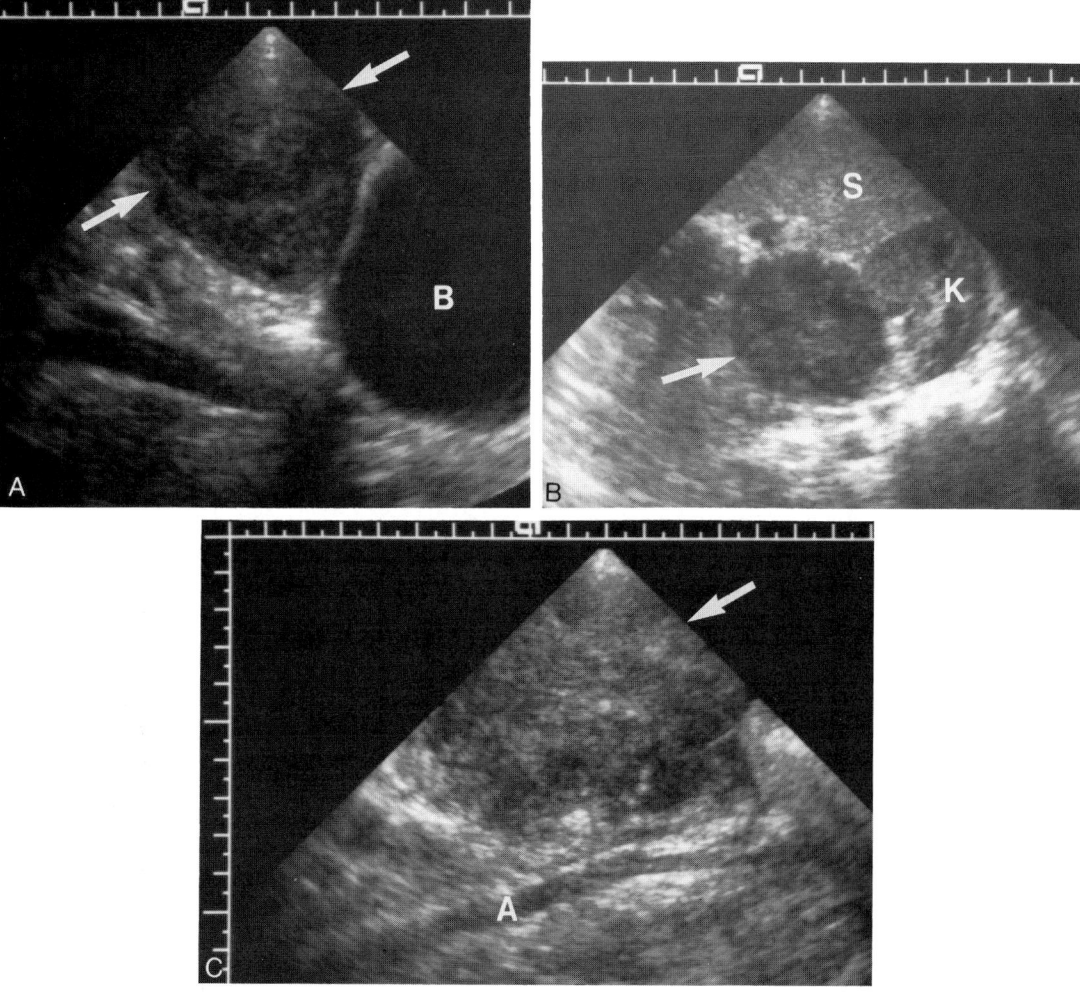

Figure 8–82. Huge, lucent masses of Burkitt lymphoma were present throughout the abdomen in this child who presented after only 3 weeks of symptoms. Longitudinal scan of the pelvis **(A)** shows a large mass (arrows) superior to the bladder **(B)**. **B** is a transverse view of the spleen **(S)**, the kidney **(K)**, and a large hilar mass of lymphoma (arrow). Coronal view **(C)** of the aorta **(A)** shows another large mass (arrow). Burkitt lymphoma is characterized by large masses that increase rapidly in size.

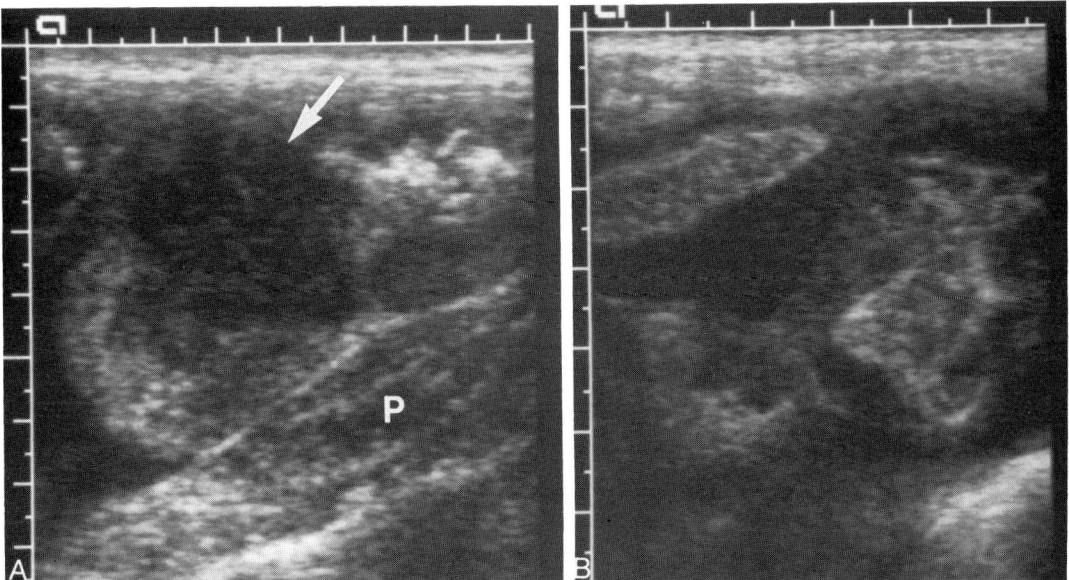

Figure 8–83. This 12-year-old patient presented with right lower quadrant pain and a mass. Appendicitis was a consideration in the differential diagnosis, but it was apparent both from clinical examination and from ultrasonography that the right lower quadrant mass was much larger and less tender than the typical appendiceal abscess. Longitudinal scan **(A)** along the right psoas (P) shows an ill-defined lucent mass (arrow) that, as shown on a more medial scan **(B)**, envelops loops of the small bowel and colon. This was Burkitt lymphoma arising in the right lower quadrant.

nodal mass may engulf loops of intestine, and lucent deposits may be present in the liver, spleen, kidneys, and gonads. Because its stroma is deficient and sheets of malignant cells grow rapidly, lucent masses are characteristic of Burkitt lymphoma (Figs. 8–82, 8–83).

Lymphoma that infiltrates the gastric or intestinal wall tends to be bulky (Fig. 8–84). Tuberculosis of the bowel may be associated with adjacent, extensive adenopathy but is rare in developed countries. Crohn disease may affect any area of the intestinal tract but is typically not associated with as much mass

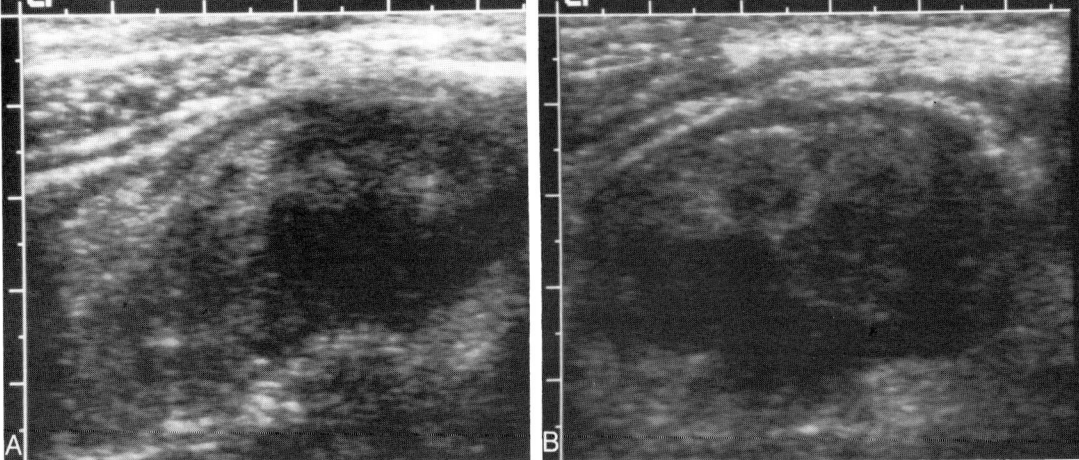

Figure 8–84. A poorly defined, bulky, echolucent mass surrounds the bowel in the right lower quadrant in this 9-year-old boy, who presented with chronic diarrhea. Longitudinal **(A)** and transverse **(B)** views are of the cecum, which is pushed anteriorly by non-Hodgkin lymphoma. It would be atypical for Crohn disease to be associated with such an extensive extraluminal mass.

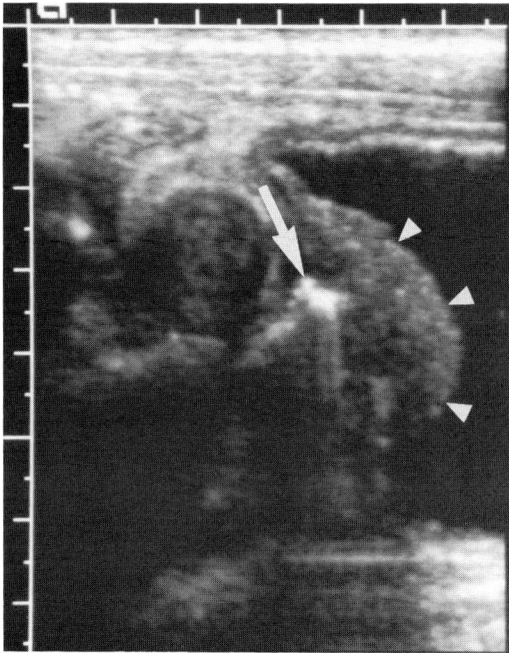

Figure 8–85. Longitudinal scan of the pelvis shows extraluminal gas (arrow) associated with marked thickening of the mucosa of the bladder (arrowheads). This patient, known to have Crohn disease, presented with pneumaturia from enterovesical fistula.

as is lymphoma. Crohn disease is not usually diagnosed on ultrasonography. Rather, patients are scanned as part of an evaluation to rule out abscess or other complications of known disease (Fig. 8–85). Thickening of the intestinal wall in the right lower quadrant is common, inasmuch as most pediatric patients who have Crohn disease have ileocolic disease (Fig. 8–86). The wall of the normal small bowel should not exceed 5 mm in thickness and, in most cases, its thickness is 3 mm or less. The colonic wall is difficult to measure, and its width changes, depending on colonic distention. In one study, children who had colonic involvement with Crohn disease had colonic walls measuring 0.8 to 1.7 cm in thickness (Fig. 8–87; Dinkel et al., 1986). Acute ulcerative colitis, in spite of being a mucosal rather than transmural inflammatory disease, also results in colonic thickening from edema and, occasionally, from pseudopolyps (Fig. 8–88). We have found that the best method of evaluating the bowel is with linear array transducers of high frequency. Gradual, gentle pressure over an area of interest will displace other intestinal loops with their gas. If there is a marked

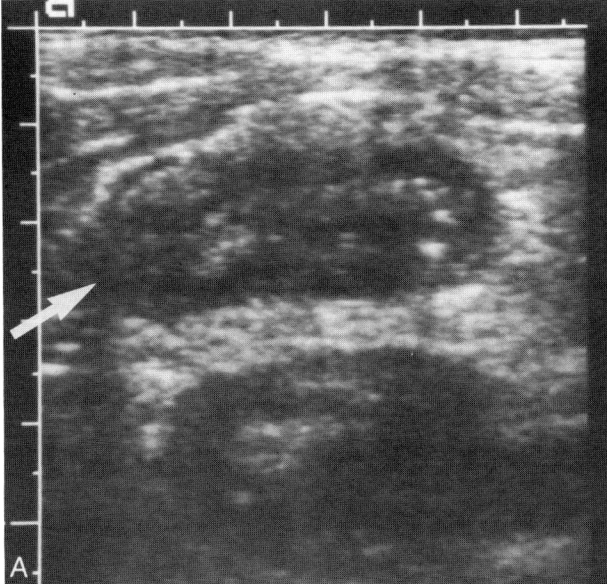
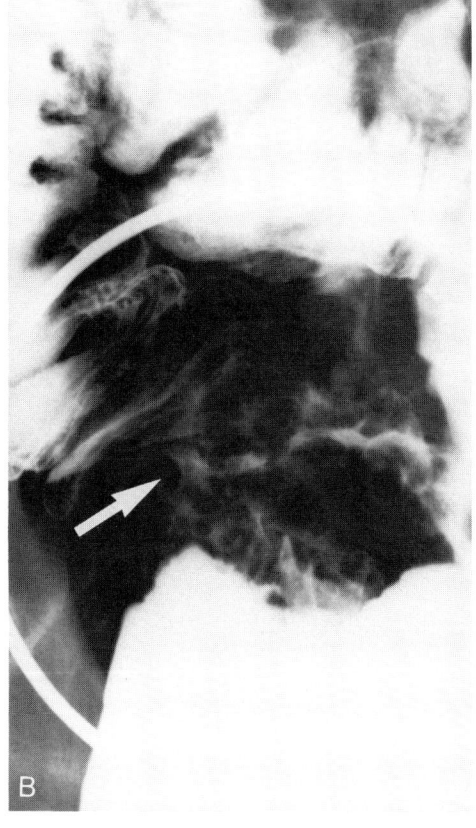

Figure 8–86. Transverse scan (**A**) of the terminal ileum is from a patient with Crohn disease. The wall is irregularly thickened and lucent. In some areas, it is more than 5 mm thick. Corresponding spot film from the patient's gastrointestinal series is shown for comparison (**B**). Arrow points to area of ileocecal junction on both **A** and **B**.

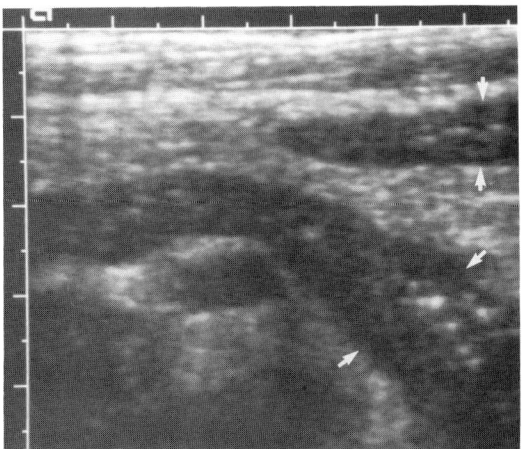

Figure 8–87. The colonic lumen is barely discernible in this adolescent girl, who has diffuse Crohn disease of the colon. This longitudinal scan of the left lower quadrant cuts across two loops of colon and shows circumferential thickening of the colonic wall (arrows).

ileus, coronal scans through the flank below the air-fluid level in the bowel can be used. Valvulae conniventes extend circumferentially around the small intestine and differentiate it from the large bowel, which has haustra only (Fig. 8–89).

Other inflammatory diseases cause mural thickening of the bowel. Chronic granulomatous disease of childhood is notorious for its associated antral involvement. This area is easy to study with ultrasonography because one can fill the antrum with fluid by placing the patient in an oblique position. The scanning is performed in the same manner as in evaluating a baby with pyloric stenosis (Fig. 8–90). Because antral thickening can decrease when the child is treated with antimicrobial therapy (and even resolves, in some cases, without therapy), we have followed the resolution of mural thickening with serial ultrasonograms. This avoids repeated fluoroscopic examinations of the stomach.

Peptic disease in childhood is uncommon, but inflammation and ulceration of the gastric mucosa may cause the gastric lining to thicken (Fig. 8–91; Hayden et al., 1987). We studied one child who had a walled-off perforated ulcer. An inflammatory mass surrounded the antrum in the area of perforation and was the cause of the ultrasonic "doughnut" (Teele, 1984).

Ménétrier disease in children may be an inflammatory disorder. It certainly produces thickening of the gastric wall from edema (Bar-Ziv et al., 1988). There is an association of Ménétrier disease with cytomegalovirus, but cause and effect has not been proved (Coud and Shah, 1986). Follow-up with ultrasonography can be used to document recovery. Other diseases that produce edematous or hemorrhagic intestinal wall include Henoch-Schönlein purpura (HSP), hemolytic uremic syndrome, hereditary angioneurotic

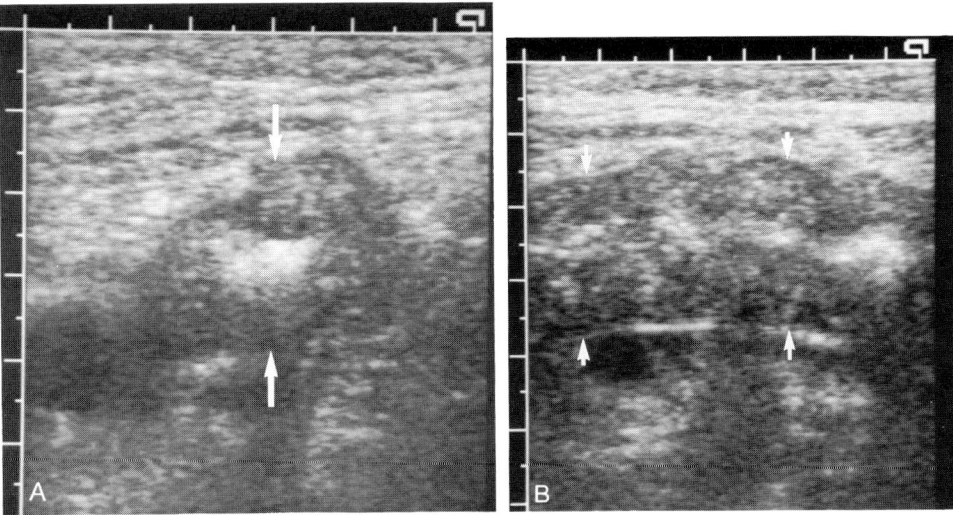

Figure 8–88. Transverse (A) and longitudinal (B) scans are of the descending colon in a child with ulcerative colitis. The lumen is defined by the echogenic mucosa and contents. Circumferential thickening of the wall (arrows) is secondary to edema.

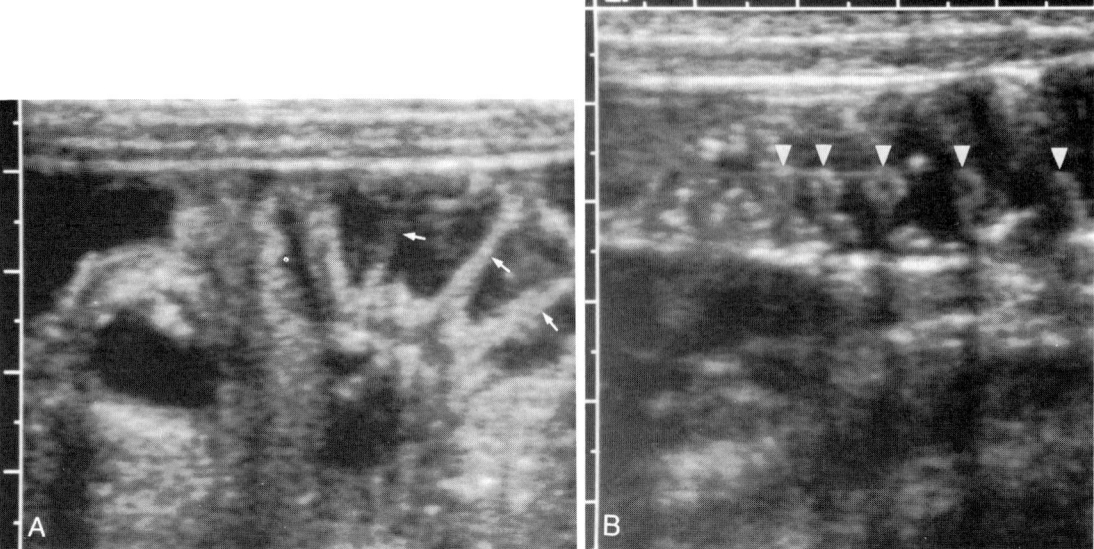

Figure 8–89. A shows fluid-filled, dilated small bowel in which the valvulae conniventes (arrows) extend across the lumen. B shows fluid in the normal colon of a baby boy. Note the haustra (arrowheads), which do not extend across the entire width of bowel.

edema (C1 cholinesterase deficiency), ischemia from vascular compromise, coagulopathies, severe infectious enteritis, and typhlitis. None of these conditions is likely to be diagnosed primarily by ultrasonography. Usually, scans are done for other reasons or to confirm a diagnosis. We missed a chance at diagnosing HSP in a child who was undergoing ultrasonography for severe upper abdominal pain. He had no rash and had a periduodenal mass. By the time anyone thought of the diagnosis, the characteristic rash had appeared! An immunosuppressed child who presents with clinical signs of typhlitis, a necrotizing inflammatory condition of the cecum, has rather characteristic scans that allow one to support the clinical impression and rule out the major differential

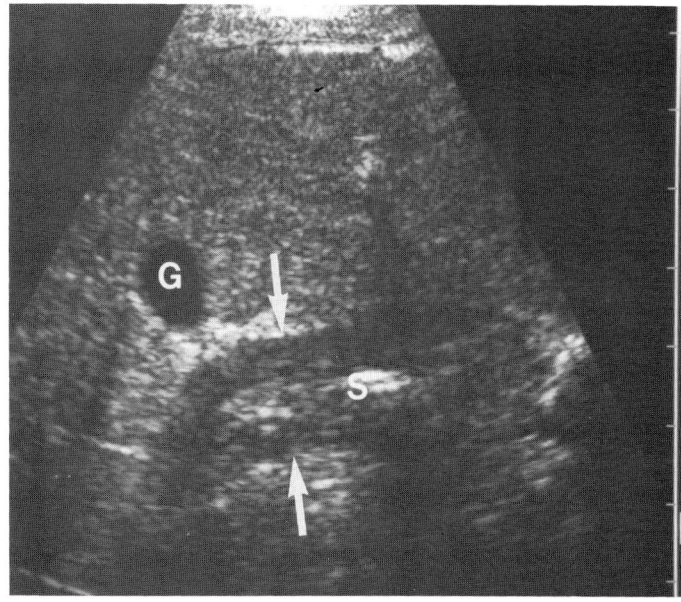

Figure 8–90. This 2-year-old boy, known to have chronic granulomatous disease, presented with vomiting. The transverse scan of the gastric antral area shows circumferential thickening of the gastric wall (arrows). G = gallbladder; S = lumen of stomach.

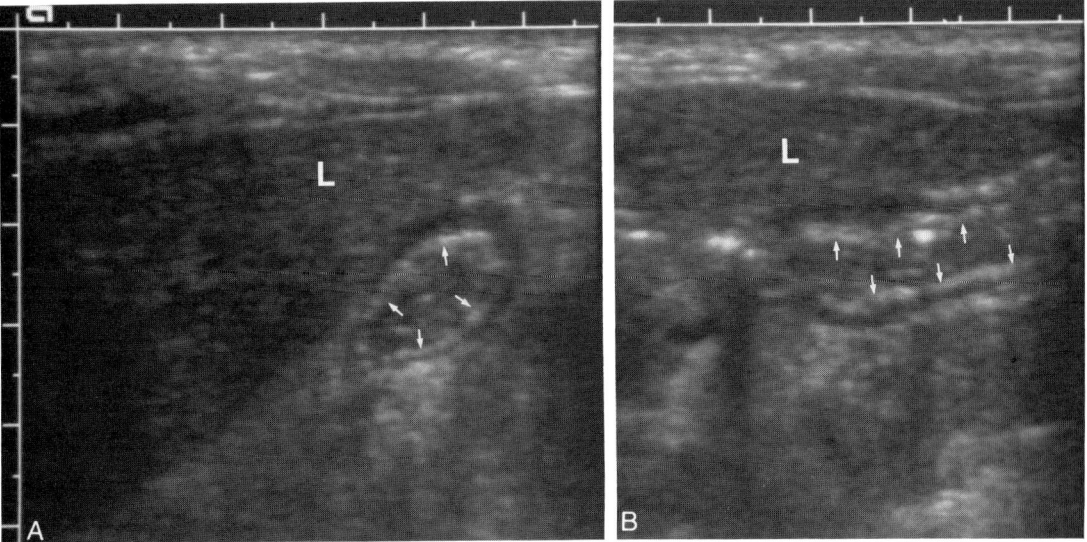

Figure 8–91. This little boy had biopsy-proven gastritis of the antrum of the stomach. Longitudinal (A) and transverse (B) abdominal scans show marked prominence of the gastric mucosa (arrows). This patient was being treated with steroids for astrocytoma of the brain. He presented with vomiting. L = left lobe of liver.

diagnosis of appendicitis. In typhlitis, much of the thickened cecal wall is echogenic mucosa (Alexander et al., 1988).

The gasless abdomen in the severely ill neonate is ideally suited to ultrasonic investigation as Seibert and associates (1986) pointed out. The wall of the bowel, edged by intraluminal fluid, is easily measured and evaluated. Vascular compromise, either from volvulus or from preceding shock, causes edematous mural thickening.

Hematoma of the bowel is usually caused by trauma, but in patients who have hemophilia or other types of coagulopathy, hematoma may be spontaneous. Duodenal hematoma is commonly associated with a fall onto the handlebars of a bicycle or with direct trauma during sports. Unexplained duodenal or other enteric hematoma in young children should prompt consideration of nonaccidental injury (i.e., child abuse; Kleinman et al., 1986). The child may present with vomiting or a mass several days after the injury. Ultrasonography cannot document integrity of the intestinal wall; for this reason, radiographic studies are commonly needed. Scans are very useful in establishing the diagnosis of duodenal hematoma, if it has not been made clinically. Questioning the patient while he or she is on the table during ultrasonography often uncovers a history of recent trauma. In addition, scans can be used to evaluate the pancreas and biliary tree. Pancreatitis is a common sequel to midabdominal trauma, and follow-up is keyed to the complications of pancreatitis as well as to documenting a decrease in duodenal hematoma (see Chapter 15).

INTUSSUSCEPTION

Idiopathic intussusception is a purely pediatric disease, and most cases occur in children who are 6 months to 3 years of age. Intussusception is usually ileocolic, and according to textbook descriptions, children present with colicky pain, bloody stool, and an abdominal mass. In actuality, however, many do not, and the diagnostic dilemma is compounded if radiographs are nonspecific. What happens next varies among institutions. Swischuk and colleagues (1985) strongly recommend that every child who is clinically suspected of having intussusception should undergo ultrasonography as a first study. Most institutions still rely on plain films, even if they are not completely sensitive. There are practical matters to be considered.

Intussusception is not always the cause of abdominal pain; plain films may show another abnormality or, if normal, encourage the physician to reassess the clinical situation. Plain radiographs, and the expertise to read them properly, are more often available than is expertly performed ultrasonography. A normal ultrasonogram cannot prevent an enema with air or contrast media if there is enough clinical suspicion of the diagnosis.

If the baby has an ultrasonographic study—and our policy is to reserve scanning for unusual situations and not screen every child—one should look for the characteristic appearance of concentric rings or a large doughnut, beginning scanning in the right lower quadrant and moving clockwise around the abdomen. Concentric rims mark the mucosal and serosal interfaces in early intussusception. When the telescoping has stayed fixed for some time, the wall of the intussusceptum becomes edematous, its lumen is compressed, and the intussuscipiens becomes stretched around this mass (Swischuk et al., 1985). An axial cross-section of the bowel at this stage shows a round, thick-walled doughnut; a longitudinal cross-section shows an oval, thick-walled doughnut (Fig. 8–92).

We have often commented that ultrasonography may confirm the diagnosis of intussusception but that radiology is still needed in order to perform hydrostatic reduction. Now that statement has been challenged. Saline enema under ultrasonic guidance was used in 377 cases of intussusception with successful reduction in 95.5 percent (Wang and Liu, 1988), and ultrasonographic monitoring of reduction with air has been reported by another group (Todani et al., 1990). We still believe that the child is best served by studies that the doctor performs best. If there is the opportunity to see and perform many studies for intussusception in an institution, then radiologists can gain experience with different techniques and train others in their use. However, one cannot gain experience and feel comfortable in doing studies in a manner completely different from previous practice if patients with intussusception are few and far between.

On occasion, intussusception is found during ultrasonographic examination before the diagnosis is made clinically. One baby was referred to us because of a mass that was thought to be an enlarged gallbladder; intussusception was otherwise silent. Another little girl was being evaluated for abdominal pain when her ultrasonograms revealed an intussuscepted bowel. The telescoping may be quite dynamic in early stages and the mass may disappear, only to reappear as the intussusception recurs. In children with Henoch-Schönlein purpura, the bowel may become intussuscepted. This typically occurs in the small bowel and is associated with intramural hematoma, which may be obscured by the edema of the intussusceptum. Lymphosarcoma of the bowel may be a lead point for intussusception, and this complication typically affects boys. Inspissated stool acts as a lead point in children with cystic fibrosis. In these latter situations, the children are usually all past the age when idiopathic intussusception occurs. Any child 5 years or older who presents with intussusception should be suspected of having a lead point other than a hypertrophied Peyer patch.

An intra-abdominal mass that is purely cystic is virtually always benign. The differ-

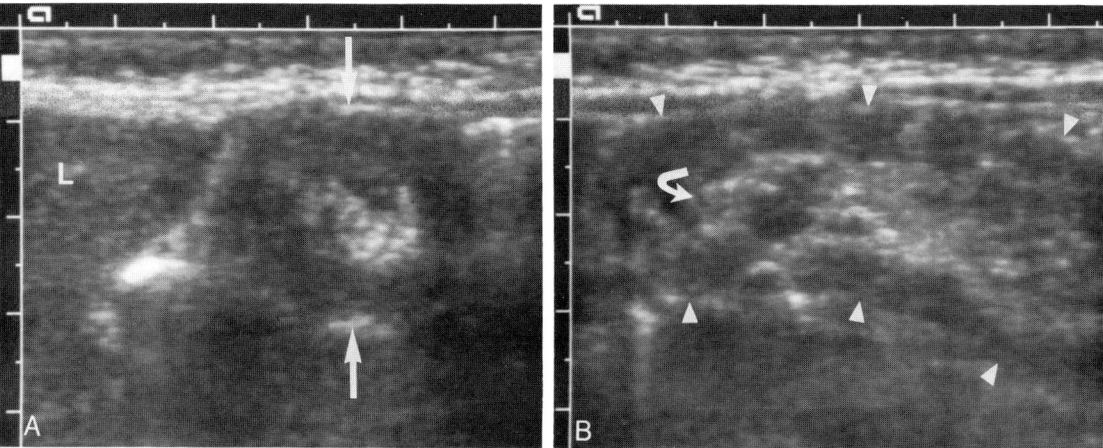

Figure 8–92. Ultrasonography was the first study of this 4-month-old, who presented after 24 hours of vomiting and irritability and with a mass in the left upper quadrant. The longitudinal scan **(A)** actually shows the intussuscepted bowel in cross-section. The appearance is that of a thick-walled doughnut (arrows). L = left lobe of liver. The transverse view **(B)** shows the intussusceptum (curved arrow) within the intussuscipiens (arrowheads). This was an idiopathic ileocolic intussusception. It was reduced with contrast enema.

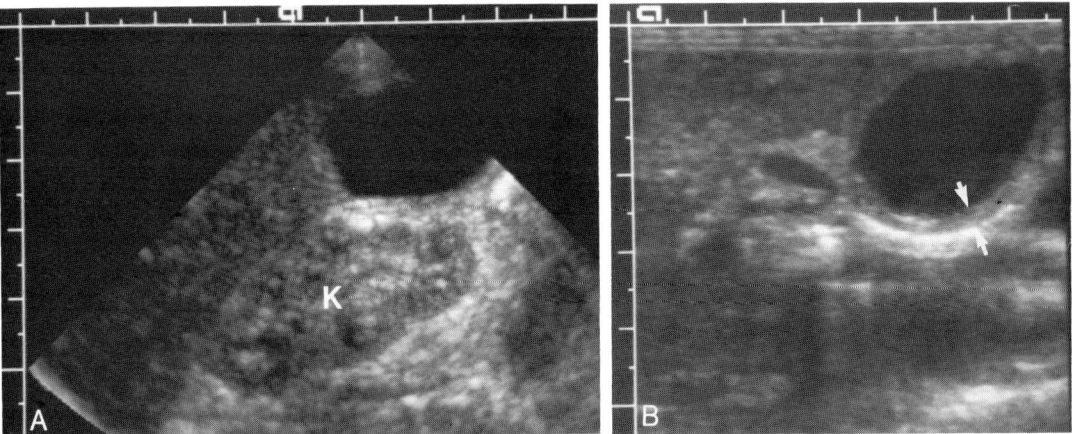

Figure 8-93. A cystic abdominal mass had been prenatally diagnosed in this baby boy. These postnatal scans are longitudinal views (**A** and **B**). Note the thick wall (arrows) of the cyst, which is apparent with use of linear array transducer (**B**). This proved to be an ileal duplication. In **A**, K = kidney.

ential diagnosis of an intraperitoneal cyst includes duplication cyst of the gastrointestinal tract, mesenteric or omental cyst, ovarian cyst, urachal cyst, and loculated cerebrospinal fluid.

A duplication cyst at the gastroesophageal junction is likely to be part of the spectrum of bronchopulmonary foregut malformations. Duplication cysts of the distal stomach, small bowel, and colon may be enteric or neurenteric in origin (Fig. 8-93). Enteric cysts probably form from an extra channel as the solid cord of the gut canalizes. If associated with anomalies of spinal cord or vertebrae, a duplication cyst is blamed on persistence of the neurenteric canal, which normally disappears in early intrauterine life. All duplication cysts have some alimentary epithelial lining, and the most proximal cysts often have elements of respiratory epithelium as well. Ectopic mucosa, usually gastric, is present in 20 percent of cysts (Egelhoff et al., 1986). Duplication cysts larger than 6 cm in diameter are uncommon; the most common duplication is at the level of the ileocecal valve or the terminal ileum (Fig. 8-94; Teele et al., 1980). The duplications that are extensive and represent virtually doubling of an organ, such as the colon, tend to communicate with the primary lumen. Babies and children who have a duplication cyst may present with obstruction of the small bowel, bleeding, or an asymptomatic mass. The cause of the bleeding is poorly explained. These masses may act as lead points for intussusception if they are located in the distal small bowel or at the ileocecal valve. The cyst is anechoic on ultrasonography, unless there has been ulceration and bleeding caused by presence of acid-producing gastric mucosa. The wall of the cyst is usually 2 to 3 mm thick because it is composed of mucosa and smooth muscle. The mucosa produces a rather characteristic echogenic lining to the cyst. The major differential diagnosis in a girl is of ovarian cyst. The exact location of the cyst, unless obviously in the stomach or duodenum, can be determined only with radiographic studies. The ileocecal duplication cyst appears to favor a subhepatic location. The presence of an ileocecal cyst possibly prevents normal fixation of the cecum in the right lower quadrant during intrauterine life.

Mesenteric and omental cysts generally are larger than duplication cysts, have thinner walls, are septated, and displace rather than obstruct the bowel. Despite these generalizations, one of our patients, who was a diagnostic puzzle, was an adolescent girl who had a cyst deep in the pelvis and coincident small bowel obstruction. Her mesenteric cyst hung across the ileum like saddlebags, thereby compressing the lumen and producing symptoms of obstruction. Most children who present with mesenteric cyst are boys who present with an asymptomatic mass or increasing abdominal girth. The cyst may be mistakenly diagnosed in clinical examination as ascites. As with duplications, hemorrhage into the cyst may produce the appearance of a complex mass on ultrasonic

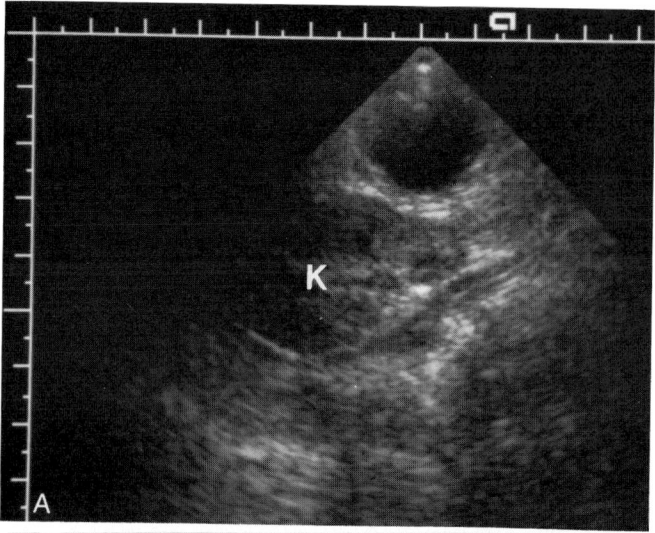

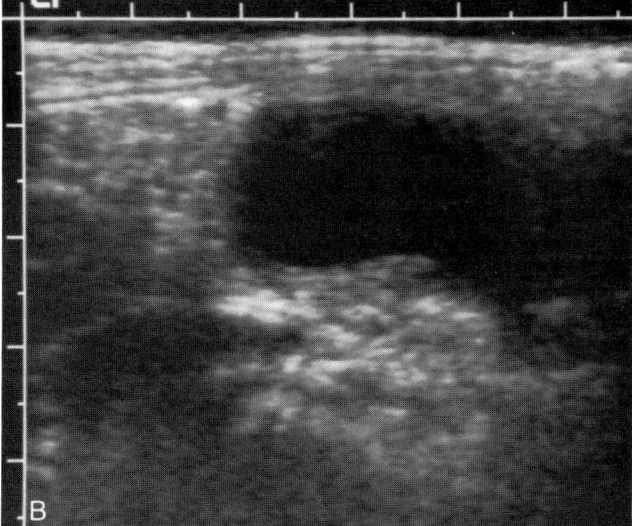

Figure 8–94. The pediatrician palpated a mass in the right upper quadrant when he saw this 4½-month-old girl at her well-baby check-up. Transverse scan (**A**) shows a cystic mass anterior to the kidney (K). The longitudinal scan, performed with the linear array transducer, is shown in **B**. This was a cecal duplication, presenting in the right upper quadrant. Ileocecal duplication cysts appear to prevent normal fixation of the cecum in the right lower quadrant.

Figure 8–95. A multilocular cystic mass filled the entire abdomen of this 2½-year-old girl. It was discovered accidentally when the child presented for treatment of fever and sore throat. During surgery, this proved to be a large lymphangioma, part of the spectrum of mesenteric cysts.

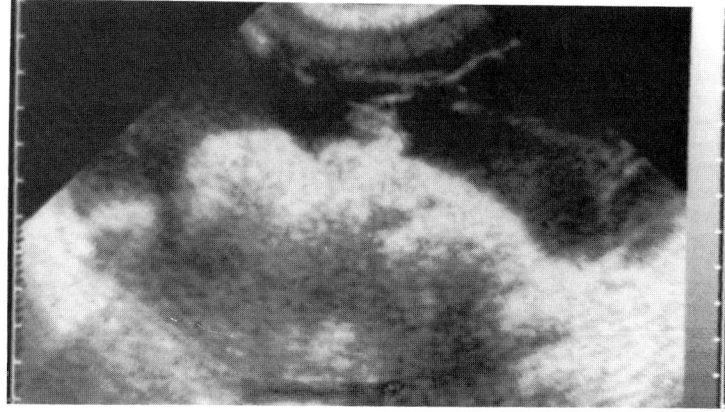

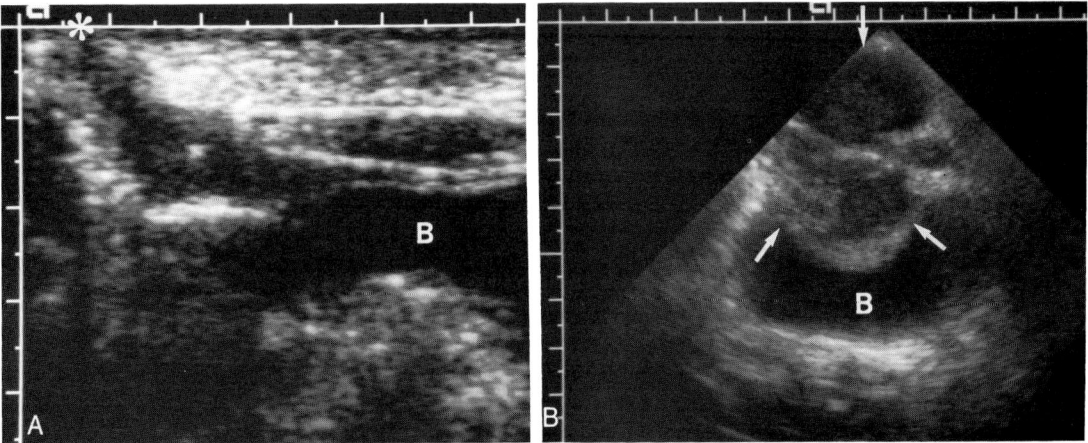

Figure 8-96. Longitudinal scan in the midline of the lower abdomen of this 3-month-old was requested when he presented with intermittent umbilical drainage. Scan (**A**) shows irregular lucency related to urachal sinus. B = bladder. Asterisk marks umbilicus. Because no cystic mass was identified at the time, the tract was treated with cauterization only. **B** is a transverse scan of another 3-year-old child. Pus was drained from the large complex mass (arrows) that indented the upper margin of the bladder. Pus had been oozing from the umbilicus. After the abscess was treated, the child was readmitted for elective removal of what proved to be a urachal remnant extending from the umbilicus to the dome of the bladder. B = bladder.

examination and may be quite confusing. Although trauma has been invoked as an etiologic factor in the development of cysts, most are likely lymphatic malformations: hamartomatous growths of the lymphatic system (Fig. 8-95). A mesenteric cyst may coexist with lymphangiectasia.

Although the urachal cyst belongs to the genitourinary tract, it is palpated as an anterior abdominal mass in the midline, below the umbilicus. Careful transverse and sagittal scanning may show its extension to the umbilicus through a fibrous cord and its relationship to the dome of the bladder. Infection in urachal cysts has been reported (Boyle et al., 1988), and we have also seen a similar patient (Fig. 8-96).

Development of loculated cerebrospinal fluid around the peritoneal tip of ventriculoperitoneal shunts is recognized as a complication of the shunting procedure. Scans are usually performed after radiographic "shunt series" show soft tissue density adjacent to the tip of the catheter. Adjacent loculated fluid also prevents the tip from moving freely in the peritoneal cavity, and so sequential radiographs that show no change in position of the catheter also prompt ultrasonographic follow-up. Local peritoneal irritation and loculation may be chemically or mechanically induced; when infection is associated, the loculated collections acquire debris and septations. Shunt catheters may crack or pull apart anywhere along their course and leak cerebrospinal fluid at the site of disruption. Ultrasonography can be used to evaluate subcutaneous collections, but clinically the problem is usually obvious and confirmed with radiographs. Children with normally functioning ventriculoperitoneal shunts commonly have a moderate amount of fluid in the cul-de-sac. Many of these children are being followed up with abdominal ultrasonography for other problems (e.g., follow-up studies of the urinary tract in patients with meningomyelocele). It is important to know that a shunt is present and not to misinterpret the intraperitoneal fluid as a sign of some other intra-abdominal process (see Chapter 14).

EVALUATING A PELVIC MASS

The ideal examination of the pelvis is modified by what can happen with a baby or toddler who is not toilet-trained. We ask that the child be well hydrated, and we try to catch appropriate views when the bladder is full enough to give us a window. Older

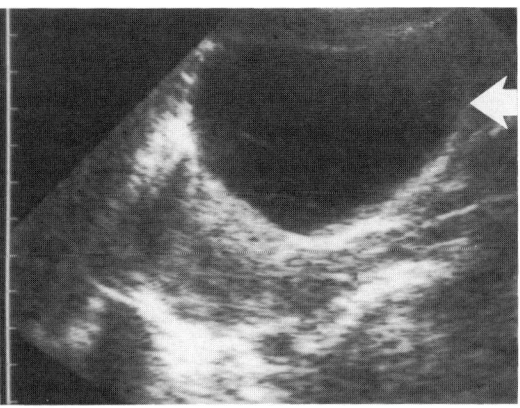

Figure 8–97. This longitudinal scan of the pelvis of a 16-year-old girl shows a corpus luteum cyst (arrow) simulating the bladder. The wall of an ovarian cyst is usually thinner than that of the bladder. In addition, the uterus usually indents the posterior aspect of the bladder.

children and adolescents are usually cooperative and are able to drink enough fluids before the study to fill the bladder to capacity. We do not favor catheterizing the bladder in order to fill it quickly unless a situation is urgent: we encourage the view that ultrasonography is noninvasive, and catheterization is considered invasive. The literature of the late 1980s advocated the use of transvaginal ultrasonography in cases of suspected ectopic pregnancy (Dashefsky et al., 1988); we therefore believe that adolescents who are at risk should have this procedure rather than transvesical scanning. This is a problem for many hospitals that are free-standing pediatric units and do not have appropriate equipment. Some relationship with an obstetric service is necessary to provide the appropriate care for these girls, and in a general facility, the expertise in transvaginal ultrasonography is usually available.

There are some particular pitfalls in evaluating pelvic structures with ultrasonography. An ovarian cyst may mimic the bladder when the bladder is empty (Fig. 8–97). It may also displace the bladder and can present superior, posterior, or anterior to the bladder. One can artifactually create two images of the same structure (Kremkau, 1989) and, for example, mistakenly diagnose didelphia, when only a single uterine cavity is actually present. Tissue planes are altered by inflammation, previous surgery, radiation, and bleeding, and the delineation of organs may be quite difficult in those situations. A large mass may distort normal anatomy to the point of nonrecognition. Furthermore, with a retrovesical mass, one is often hard put to localize it further (i.e., retrorectal vs. prerectal). Therefore, particularly for young children, we also rely on radiographic techniques to limit the list of differential diagnoses.

NORMAL ANATOMY

The uterus should be identifiable in girls of all ages. In neonates, the uterus is quite prominent, measuring up to 5 cm in length (Nussbaum et al., 1986). As the maternal hormonal influence wanes, the uterus decreases in size and loses its endometrial differentiation. The prepubertal uterus measures 2 to 3.3 cm long and 0.5 to 1 cm wide (Orsini et al., 1984). With the onset of puberty, not only does the uterus enlarge, but it changes shape. The fundus becomes bulbous in comparison with the cervix, and central echogenicity representing endometrial proliferation becomes apparent (Fig. 8–98).

Each ovary in prepubertal girls generally has a volume of less than 1 cm^3 (Fig. 8–99). Follicular cysts may be present in neonates, tend to disappear in childhood, and tend to reappear just before puberty. It is always a problem when an ovarian cyst of 1 or 2 cm in diameter is found in an otherwise normal infant. On the basis of several cases that we have studied, we believe that these cysts are transient and benign (Fig. 8–100). The ovary is a cystic organ. The normal adolescent has mean ovarian volumes of 4 cm^3, and cysts may reach 3 or 4 cm in diameter and be completely asymptomatic (Fig. 8–101). We generally tend to downplay the importance

---

Figure 8–98. All of these scans are of normal children. Arrows delineate the uterus on longitudinal scans. **A** and **B** are longitudinal and transverse views of the uterus in a girl less than 24 hours old. The uterus is 5 cm long and has a very prominent endometrial reaction. The neonatal uterus often is mistaken for a mass. **C** and **D** are longitudinal and transverse views of a normal 2-month-old whose uterus measures 3 cm. The endometrial interface is no longer apparent. **E** and **F** are scans of an adolescent girl who is in early puberty. Note that the uterus has lengthened, but endometrial reaction is not evident. **G** and **H** are longitudinal and transverse views of the typical pubertal uterus. Notice that the fundus is bulbous in relation to the lower segment and cervix. An endometrial echo is present. The vaginal stripe is apparent inferior to the uterus, paralleling the posterior wall of the bladder.

EVALUATING AN ABDOMINAL MASS / 287

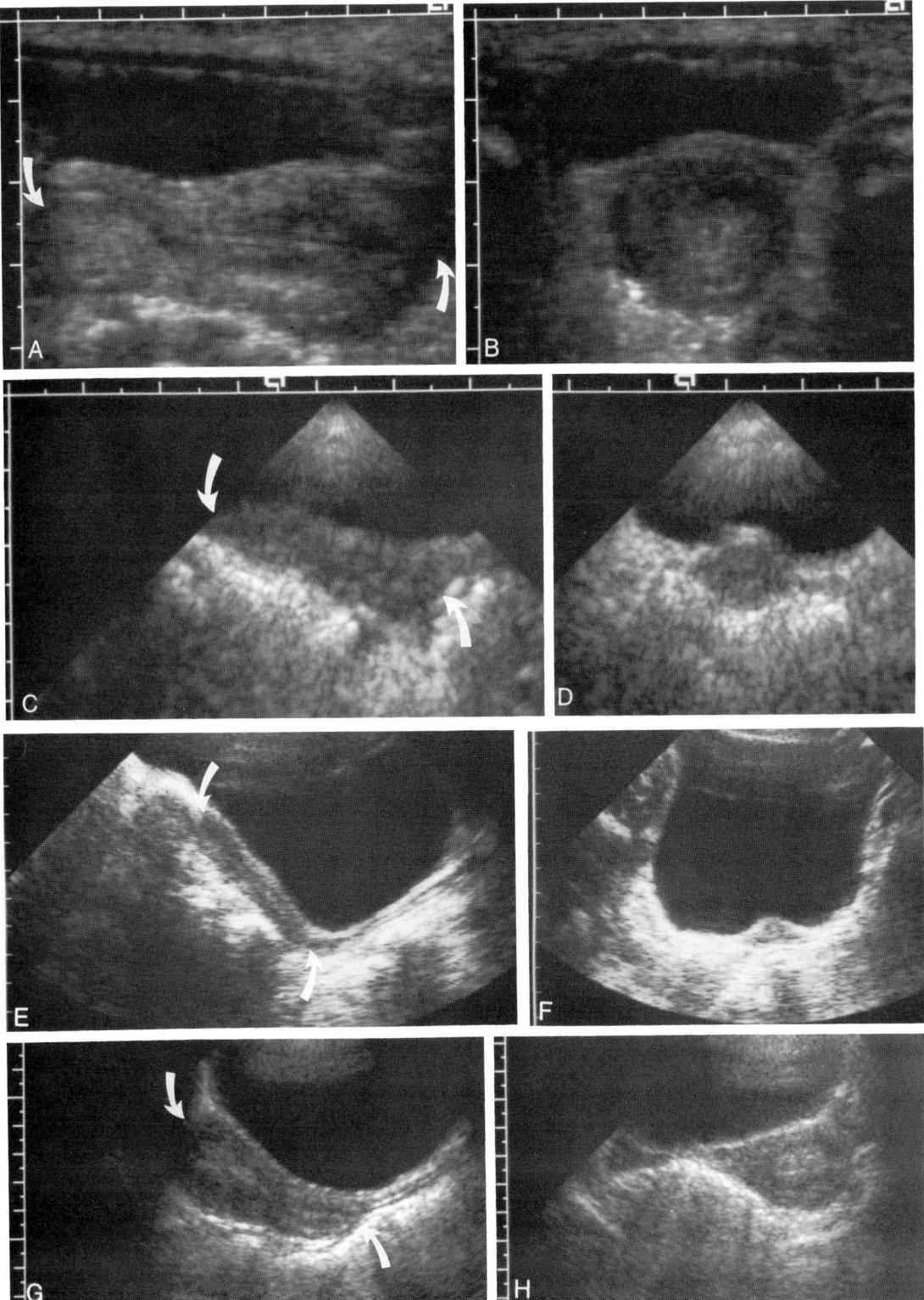

Figure 8–98 *See legend on opposite page*

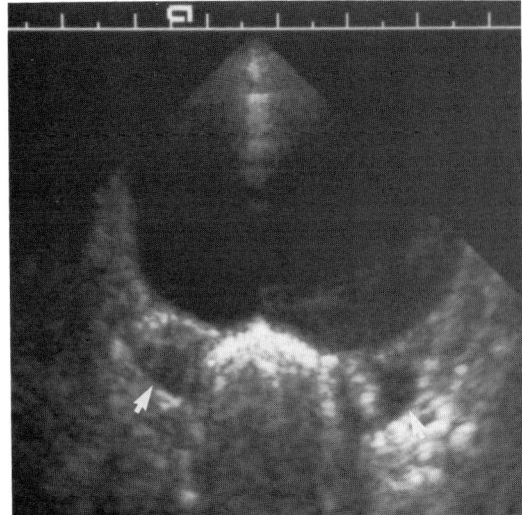

Figure 8–99. The ovaries of prepubertal girls are often very difficult to find. In this 8-year-old girl, each normal ovary (arrows) is less than 1 cm^3 in volume.

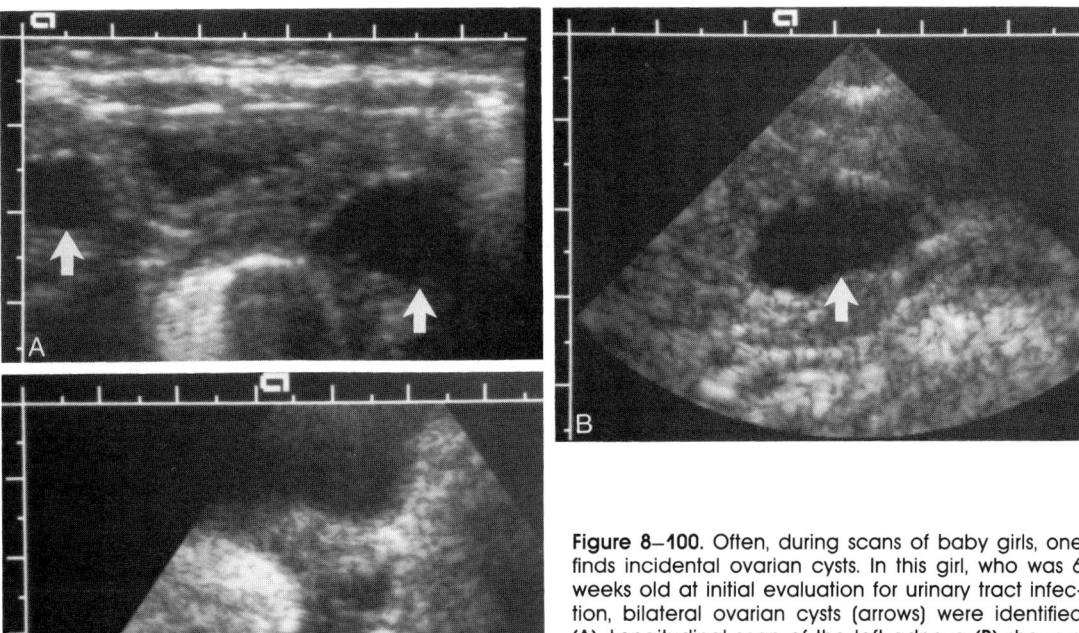

Figure 8–100. Often, during scans of baby girls, one finds incidental ovarian cysts. In this girl, who was 6 weeks old at initial evaluation for urinary tract infection, bilateral ovarian cysts (arrows) were identified (**A**). Longitudinal scan of the left adnexa (**B**) shows a cyst measuring 2 × 1 cm (arrow). The follow-up scan of this child 2 months later (**C**) shows a much smaller left ovary and only a tiny residual cyst (arrow).

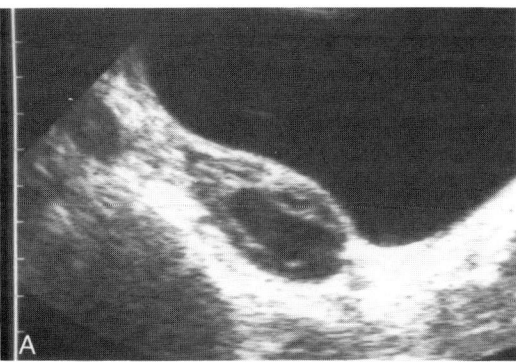

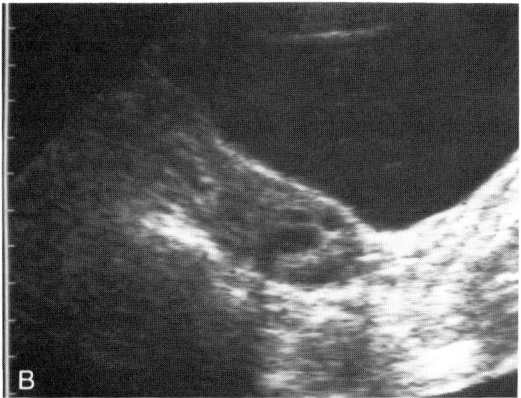

Figure 8–101. Longitudinal scans of right (A) and left (B) ovaries in this normal adolescent girl show typical, small, bilateral follicular cysts.

of an asymptomatic cyst unless the diameter reaches 5 cm or more or if the contents are other than completely echofree.

In boys the normal prostate is evident as an area of hypolucency at the base of the bladder only if angled transverse scans are directed under the symphysis pubis (Fig. 8–102). The normal seminal vesicles are too small to identify.

With any pelvic scan, we also survey the child's kidneys. If a pelvic mass is present, we want to document its effect on the ureters and show hydronephrosis if present. For girls who have a complex pelvic mass, absence of a kidney secures a diagnosis of obstructed anomalous genital tract. Renal agenesis in boys coexists with anomalies of seminal vesicles and other wolffian derivatives. And, of course, a pelvic kidney presenting as a pelvic mass has an empty ipsilateral renal fossa.

As a general rule, when we are evaluating a pelvic mass in a baby or young child, we immediately consider congenital anomalies and neoplasms as diagnostic possibilities. When an adolescent girl presents with a pelvic mass, we think first of gynecologic disorders with ovarian cysts and inflammatory disease heading the list. Therefore, this section is really in three parts: discussing the baby first and then the older child and adolescent girl. A pelvic mass in an adolescent boy is unusual indeed and, if not an abscess from appendicitis, also tends to fall under the categories of congenital anomaly and neoplasm.

PELVIC MASSES IN BABIES

Sacrococcygeal teratoma is the most blatant of pelvic masses in neonates, typically affect-

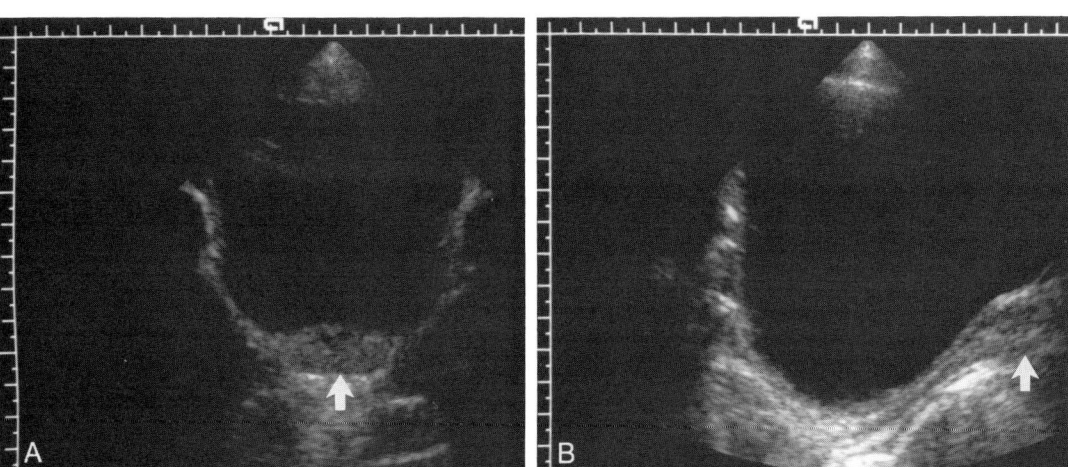

Figure 8–102. In young boys, the normal prostate is not usually imaged. In the adolescent male, the prostate is quite evident, as in this patient. Angled transverse (A) and longitudinal (B) scans show prostatic tissue at the base of the bladder (arrow).

290 / EVALUATING AN ABDOMINAL MASS

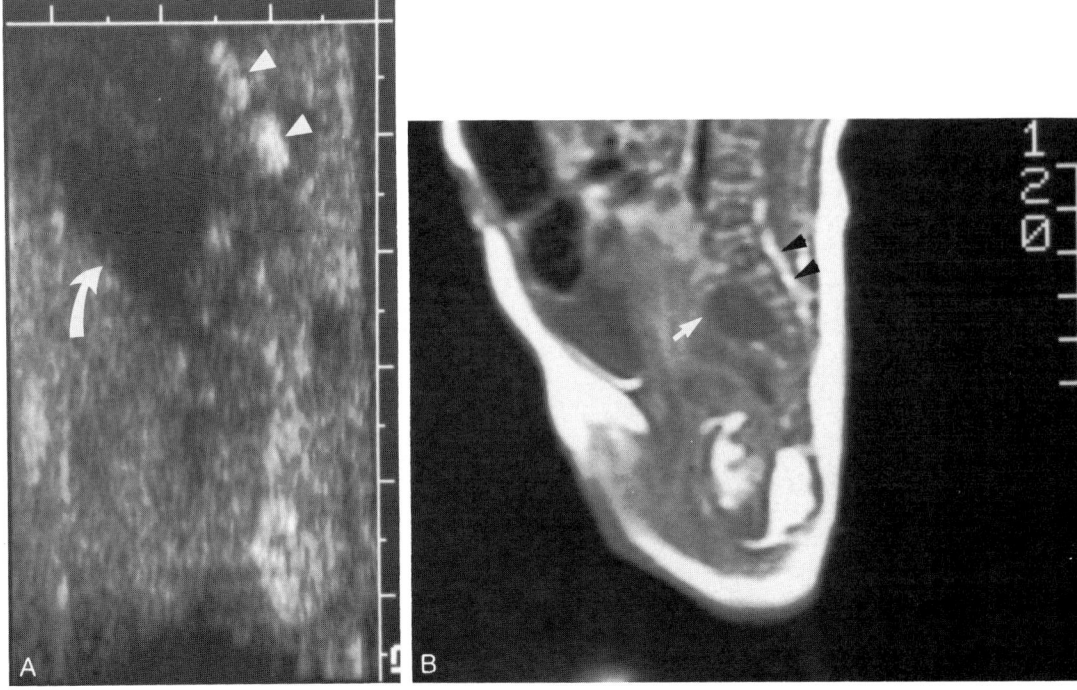

Figure 8–103. When this girl was born, it was obvious that there was a mass extending between the buttocks from the lower sacrum. The longitudinal scan of the back (A) has an orientation similar to that of the subsequent magnetic resonance imaging (MRI) scan (B). The mass, predominantly solid, extended inferiorly from the sacrum. A cystic component of the mass (arrow) was intrapelvic. None of the mass extended above S–1. It was removed in toto and proved to be a benign teratoma. Arrowheads mark lower sacrum.

ing girls more than boys in a 4:1 ratio (Sty and Wells, 1988). The tumor arises from pluripotential cells anterior to the coccyx and generally emerges behind the anus as an exophytic mass. It may, however, have a significant intrapelvic extent and rarely may extend into the spinal canal. Calcifications and predominantly cystic composition tend to indicate benignancy; 90 percent of sacrococcygeal teratomas are benign if they are removed immediately after birth. The longer the tumor remains in place, the greater the

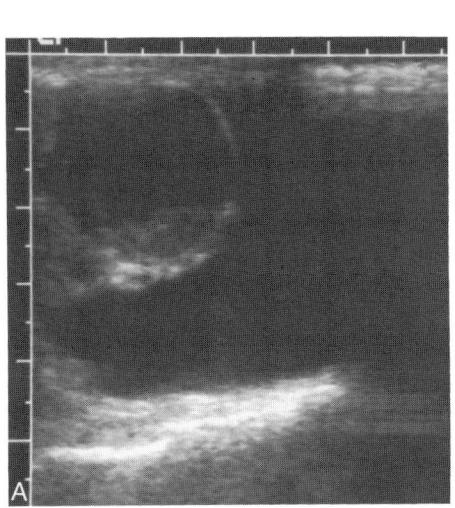
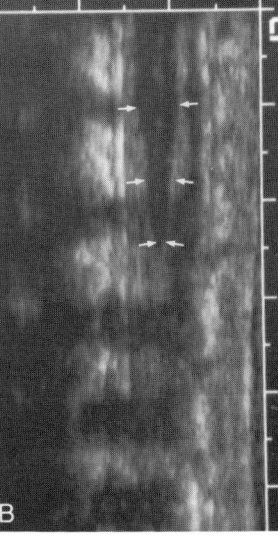

Figure 8–104. Examination revealed a huge sacrococcygeal mass in this newborn girl. Longitudinal scan directly over the mass showed it to be predominately cystic, typical of sacrococcygeal teratoma (A). There was no evidence of intrapelvic extension. Scans of the spinal canal were normal (B). Arrows outline the conus medullaris. No other imaging was done before surgery, at which time the ultrasonographic diagnosis was confirmed.

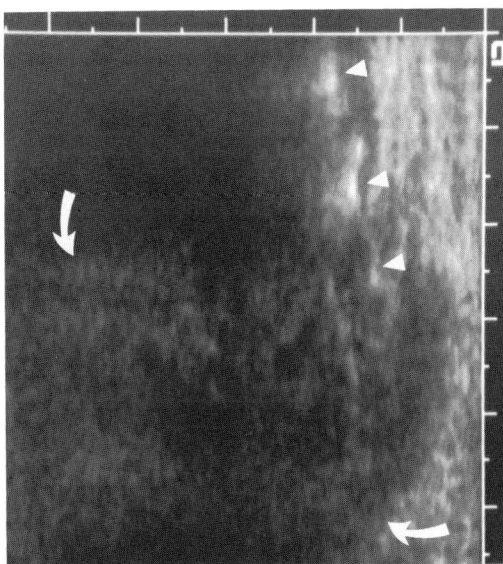

Figure 8–105. The ultrasonographic study of this 17-month-old with an intragluteal mass did not reveal the expected cystic component of a sacrococcygeal teratoma. Rather, the mass (arrows) appeared unusually irregular and solid. Pulmonary metastases were present. A biopsy of this mass proved it to be an endodermal sinus tumor. Arrowheads outline the sacrum. The scan is oriented so that craniad is at the top.

incidence of malignancy. The surgical approach to this tumor is through an incision over the lower back, removal of the coccyx, and the establishment of a plane of dissection between the mass and spine until the top of the mass is reached. Therefore, ultrasonography is directed primarily toward evaluating the intrapelvic tumoral extent and, secondarily, to characterizing the mass as predominately cystic or solid (Figs. 8–103, 8–104). In cases in which the tumor extends above the sacrum, both anterior and perineal surgical approaches may be necessary. If infiltration of ureters or the bladder is suggested by ultrasonograms, or if the anatomy is not fully displayed, CT or MRI scanning should follow (Fig. 8–105).

Other retrorectal masses in young children and babies tend to be purely intrapelvic. Anterior meningocele is not always associated with obvious bony defect. A cystic mass in the posterior pelvis mandates examination of the spinal canal: by ultrasonography if there is a window for scanning or, if not, by CT or MRI. In the absence of MRI, sagittal CT is ideal if the child is small enough to be

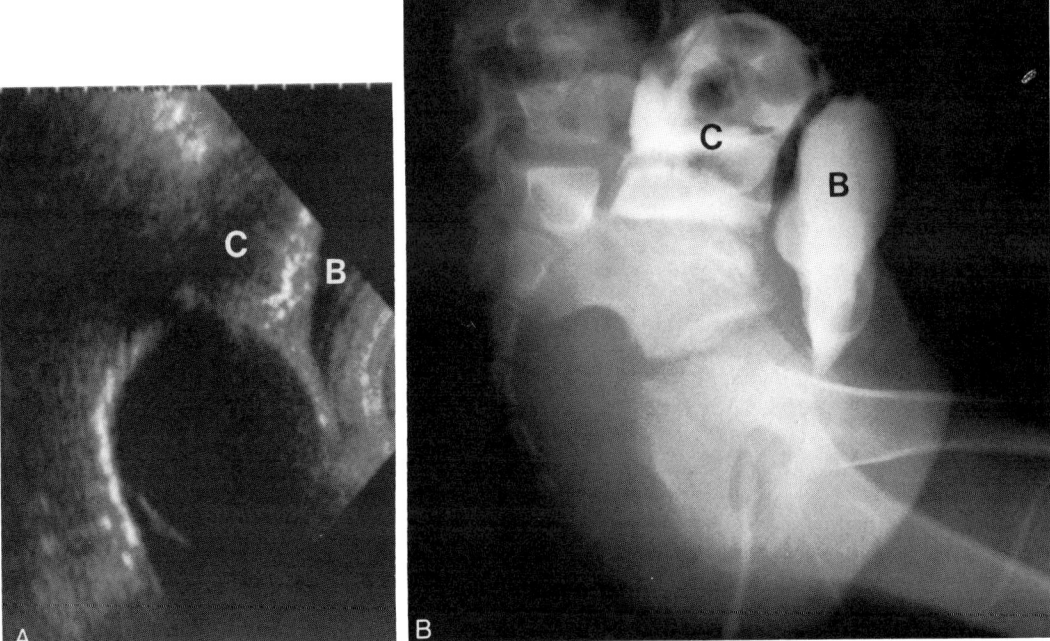

Figure 8–106. This longitudinal scan of the pelvis (A) is oriented to match the accompanying contrast study (B). It shows a cystic mass posterior to the bladder. This 6-year-old girl presented with urinary retention. She also had a history of constipation. Combined contrast enema and cystogram (B) showed this cystic mass to be retrorectal, and, during surgery, rectal duplication was excised. B = bladder; C = colon.

placed crosswise in the gantry. Rectal duplication also presents as a cystic or complex mass in the posterior pelvis (Fig. 8–106). Other retrorectal masses include cysts of residual tailgut, dermoids, abscesses, neuroblastomas, and, rarely, ependymomas, chordomas, hemangiomas, rhabdomyosarcomas, and bone tumors. A remnant of tailgut may persist as a cystic mass and be indistinguishable from a rectal duplication cyst or a dermoid cyst. Dermoid cysts are more typically dorsal to the spine, rather than ventral. Abscesses are a complication of Crohn disease, previous rectal surgery, and, occasionally, penetrating injury (thermometer, stick, child abuse).

Masses that are rectal in origin might be apparent with ultrasonography but are usually appropriately diagnosed with plain radiographs or contrast enemas before ultrasonography is performed. For example, ileocolic intussusception may extend down to the rectum, and a large juvenile polyp, if surrounded by liquid, might be apparent as an intrarectal mass. We have seen one child whose dilated sigmoid colon, palpable as a pelvic mass, was secondary to previously unrecognized Hirschsprung disease, but these types of cases are few and far between. As a rule, plain radiographs should precede ultrasonography when young children present with a pelvic mass.

Prerectal masses in girls almost always arise from the genital tract. Congenital anomalies associated with obstruction are typically evident in the first few days of life. Hydrometrocolpos is most commonly due to an imperforate hymen, and the bulging hymen is usually obvious on physical examination. Vaginal and cervical stenosis and atresia are less apparent on physical examination because the introitus appears normal. When the uterus or vagina is distended, the base of the bladder is pushed anteriorly, and there is frequently coexistent outlet obstruction. The full bladder provides a good scanning window. We always begin with transverse views. The uterus may deviate toward the right or the left; thus sagittal scans of the organs are often oblique scans of the pelvis. Coronal views also allow recognition of duplex systems. Duplication of the uterus or vagina, or both, commonly coexists with cloacal anomalies (Fig. 8–107). When the uterus is distended, its wall becomes quite thin. If the obstruction is distal to the cervix, the cervix becomes dilated, and uterine and vaginal cavities coalesce. In the presence of obstruction, the fallopian tubes may dilate as well but are difficult to differentiate as such on ultrasonography. The contents of the obstructed uterus and vagina may be clear if there is reflux of urine into the system (through the cloaca) or echogenic if meconium or cellular debris is mixed in. The role of ultrasonography in these situations is to prove that a mass is gynecologic in origin, to identify a single or duplex genital tract, to show the extent of dilatation in order to locate the level of obstruction (cervix, midvagina, distal vagina), to characterize fluid behind the obstruction, and to document the effect of the mass on the bladder. Then a vaginogram or genitogram with water-soluble contrast can be used to further define the relationship of the urethra, vagina, and rectum. The kidneys should always be scanned in order to assess degree of hydronephrosis from extrinsic compression of ureters and to document anomalies.

Although many girls who have an anomalous gynecologic tract present as neonates, some are not identified until puberty. It appears that levels of maternal estrogen, known to vary widely among pregnant women, are the deciding factor for the early detection of anomalies. If maternal estrogen levels during pregnancy are high, the fetal endocervical glands secrete a large volume of fluid that becomes trapped behind an obstruction. Babies whose mothers have had low levels of estrogen would be expected to show no obstructive signs until their own menarche (Burbige and Hensle, 1984).

An ovarian cyst may present as a pelvic mass in a neonatal girl. To be accurate, most ovarian cysts in neonates present as an abdominal, rather than pelvic, mass. This type of mass, which was once considered rare, has become more commonly detected with the use of prenatal ultrasonography, and controversy concerning the appropriate ther-

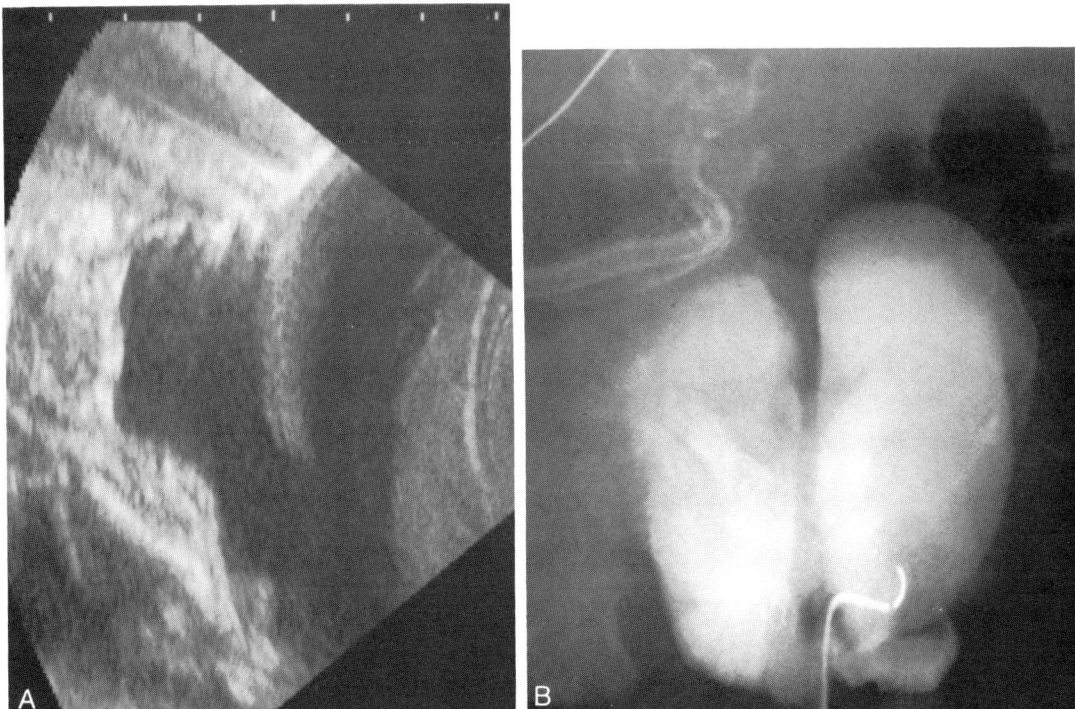

Figure 8–107. Abdominal distention, esophageal atresia, tracheoesophageal fistula, and imperforate anus had already been diagnosed in this newborn girl. The ultrasonograms that were requested to evaluate the abdomen showed a septated cystic mass. The coronal scan (**A**) is of a fluid-filled duplicated vagina. This baby had a cloacal anomaly, which commonly is associated with duplication of the genital tract. The scan is oriented to match the subsequent contrast vaginogram (**B**). An obstructed vagina associated with a cloacal anomaly can extend to the level of the xiphoid process. The septation may be missed if the scans are not performed in a plane perpendicular to the septum. Coronal scans are ideal for demonstrating the anatomy. In this baby, a single kidney was present. Renal anomalies are common associated problems in children who have cloacal anomalies.

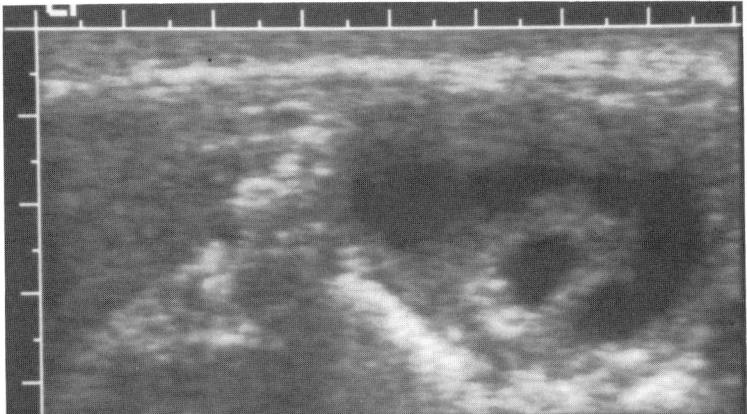

Figure 8–108. A prenatal diagnosis of a cystic abdominal mass in this baby had been made. This longitudinal ultrasonogram of the upper abdomen was done when the girl was 2 months old. It shows a complex mass in the middle of the upper abdomen. During surgery, no left ovary could be identified in the pelvis. The mass had a pedicle based on the omentum. We assume that the hemorrhagic cyst represents the left ovary, which had undergone torsion in utero and then parasitized the omental blood supply. (From Teele RL, Share JC: The abdominal mass in the neonate. Semin Roentgenol 1988; 23:175–184.)

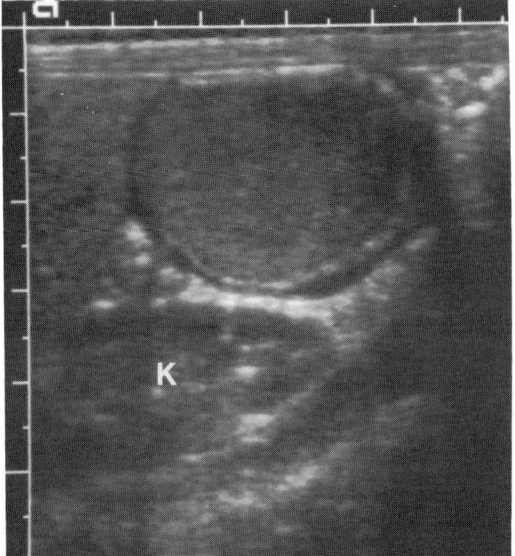

Figure 8–109. A cystic abdominal mass had been prenatally diagnosed in this girl. By the time this postnatal scan was obtained, when she was 3 weeks old, the mass had become solid. A postnatal hemorrhagic cyst seems to be typical of prenatal torsion of the ovary. K = kidney.

apy has arisen (Suita et al., 1990). There are likely two etiologies for neonatal ovarian cyst: hormonal stimulation from the mother and perinatal torsion of the ovary. Spontaneous resolution of large ovarian cysts has been reported (Amodio et al., 1987), but other authors advocate removal of large cysts to avoid the potential complication of secondary torsion (Ikeda et al., 1988). In our experience, as in others' (Nussbaum et al., 1988), primary torsion has been marked by a cyst containing fluid-debris level, a retracting clot, or complex/solid contents (Figs. 8–108, 8–109). To date, all neonatal ovarian cysts greater than 4 cm in diameter have been surgically treated in our institution. However, we think that a conservative approach is warranted for baby girls who have an asymptomatic, purely cystic mass. If follow-up ultrasonography reveals that the cyst has not disappeared within 6 months, surgical treatment is warranted. For patients with complex cysts, surgical treatment is appropriate to rule out the very small possibility of tumor and to check the other ovary.

PELVIC MASSES IN CHILDREN

In young girls and in boys, the most common malignant pelvic tumor is embryonal rhabdomyosarcoma. It usually arises from the prostate or the trigone of the bladder in boys and from the vagina or the uterus in girls. When the tumor extends into a lumen, it usually assumes a botryoid appearance. Typical clinical presentation in boys is of difficulty with urination or pain resulting from obstruction at the bladder neck, fever from superimposed urinary infection, or hematuria. A large mass in girls, low in the

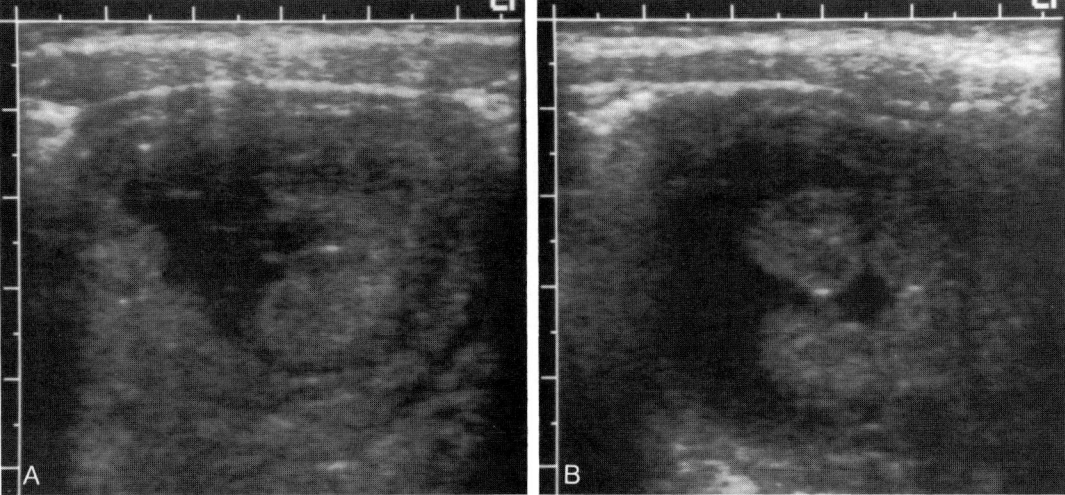

Figure 8–110. Transverse (A) and longitudinal scans (B) of the bladder were done in this 2½-year-old boy after he presented with a 2-week history of dysuria and frequency. Scans show a lobulated mass within the bladder. It arose from the trigone, and a biopsy showed it to be an embryonal rhabdomyosarcoma.

vagina, also causes urinary obstruction. Vaginal discharge and evidence of the mass at the introitus are other presentations in girls. Ultrasonograms may not enable the clinician to classify the disease adequately because regional and retroperitoneal nodes may be involved before the child presents with symptoms. The literature suggests that 20 percent of patients with genitourinary tumors present with local involvement of lymph nodes (Geoffray et al., 1987b). The ultrasonograms are, however, usually diagnostic of embryonal rhabdomyosarcoma because it has such a characteristic multilobular appearance when it grows into the lumen of the bladder. The mass is usually quite solid in pattern but transmits sound well because the cells are quite monotonous. In boys, it almost always involves the trigone and prostatic area (Fig. 8–110). Apparent attachment to the anterior wall of the bladder results if the tumor is on a stalk or if the bladder is not fully distended. A tumor in the vagina or uterus appears simply as a solid mass invading and distorting one or both organs (Figs. 8–111, 8–112). Its botryoid nature is apparent when fluid surrounds it. Because chemotherapy is instituted early after microscopic diagnosis is made from tissue, ultrasonography is ideal for following up regression of the tumor with time. Because this

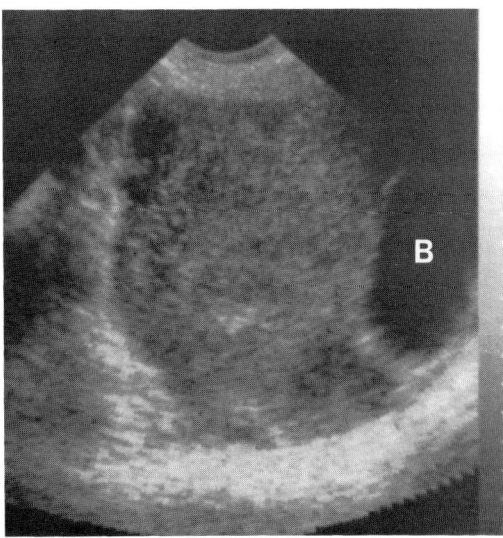

Figure 8–112. Rhabdomyosarcoma of the uterus often completely distorts the anatomy of the pelvis. This 3-year-old child presented with a lower abdominal mass of 10 days' duration. The longitudinal scan shows a large, solid mass in the midline that extends above the partially filled bladder. This is rhabdomyosarcoma of the uterus. A solid mass in the pelvis of a young girl is more likely to be uterine than ovarian in origin. B = bladder.

type of rhabdomyosarcoma is truly pelvic in origin, it may obstruct the ureters, either from its intraluminal component in the bladder or from extrinsic compression when the tumor is primary in the vagina or uterus. The ultrasonograms are directed toward identifying the mass and its origin (if possible), establishing the presence of local spread when the nodes are obviously enlarged, documenting degree of ureteral obstruction if any, and surveying the liver for metastatic disease. We also perform prevoiding and postvoiding scans of the bladder in order to judge how severely the outlet of the bladder is obstructed by the mass. CT is necessary to classify regional spread to pelvic and retroperitoneal nodes, but a good baseline study with ultrasonography allows better follow-up during chemotherapy.

Ovarian tumors in infancy and childhood are rare, but approximately half of the total number are malignant (Fig. 8–113). Tumors are classified according to their cellular origin: germ cells, mesenchymal stromal cells, or epithelial cells. Most originate from germ cells, and many of these are benign teratomas. According to a large retrospective review from our institution, 16 of 94 ovarian teratomas were malignant (Tapper and Lack,

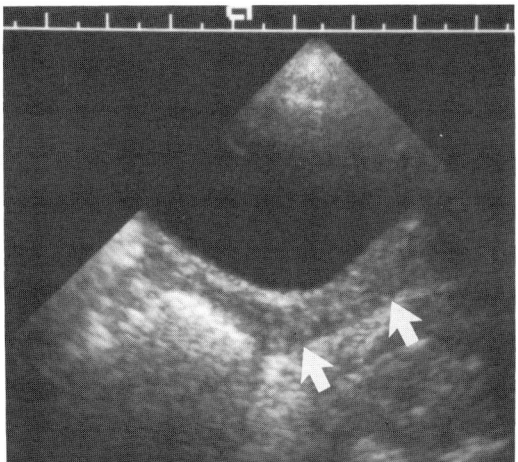

Figure 8–111. The primary site of pelvic rhabdomyosarcoma in girls is typically the vagina or the uterus. This 3-year-old girl had rhabdomyosarcoma of the vagina, shown here on a longitudinal scan as widening of the vaginal vault (arrows). The botryoid nature of rhabdomyosarcoma can be appreciated only when it is surrounded by fluid. This girl presented with vaginal bleeding, a typical presentation of this tumor in girls.

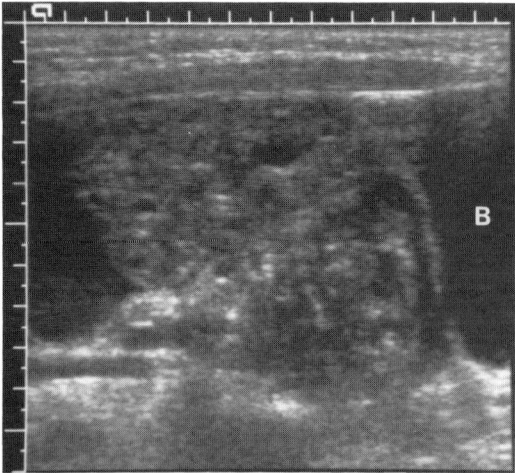

Figure 8–113. For 1 week before her admission to the hospital, abdominal fullness had been noticed by this 12-year-old girl. The scans of the lower abdomen showed a poorly defined mass associated with ascites. The mass seemed to arise from the pelvis. This ultrasonic appearance is very suggestive of immature teratoma. Histologic examination proved this to be a grade II immature teratoma. B = bladder.

lignant tumors from stromal cells include granulosa-theca cell tumor (84 percent of the total), androblastoma, and gynandroblastoma. Precocious puberty is associated with 70 to 75 percent of granulosa-theca cell tumors; virilization may be due to androblastoma. Gonadoblastoma, which is a mixture of both germ cells and stromal cells, develops in the abnormal gonads of patients with mixed gonadal dysgenesis. This tumor may be benign or malignant. Tumors of epithelial origin are rarely encountered before adolescence.

On ultrasonography, with the exception of "classic" teratoma, none of these ovarian tumors can be differentiated from one another with any certainty. The combination of densely shadowing focus and cystic components in a well-defined ovarian mass is typical of a teratoma containing a bone or a tooth (Fig. 8–114). Shadowing echogenicity, more diffuse in appearance, also results from hair or fat, or both, in the teratoma. If the cystic component is missing, the mass is difficult to find among adjacent loops of bowel (Fig. 8–115).

Ovarian torsion can simulate a neoplasm because it presents on ultrasonography as a solid ovarian mass. However, the typical clinical presentation is of acute or recurrent abdominal pain and fever of low grade to the extent that right-sided torsion simulates appendicitis. The clue on ultrasonography is the presence of prominent follicles around the margin of the ovary, which occurs in more than 50 percent of patients (Graif and Itzchak, 1988) (Figs. 8–116, 8–117). Although

1983). The biologic behaviors of tumors of germ cell origin vary with age and site of the tumor. Young girls with ovarian teratoma are more likely to have malignant than benign tumors. The presence of yolk sac (endodermal sinus) components is associated with aggressive tumoral behavior (Harms and Jänig, 1986). Other tumors of germ cell origin include dysgerminoma, embryonal carcinoma, choriocarcinoma, and pure endodermal sinus (yolk sac) tumor. Benign and ma-

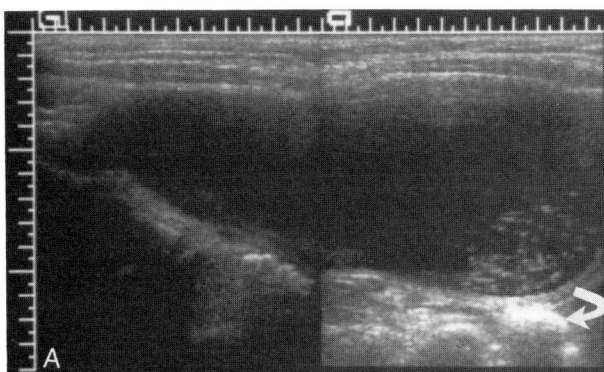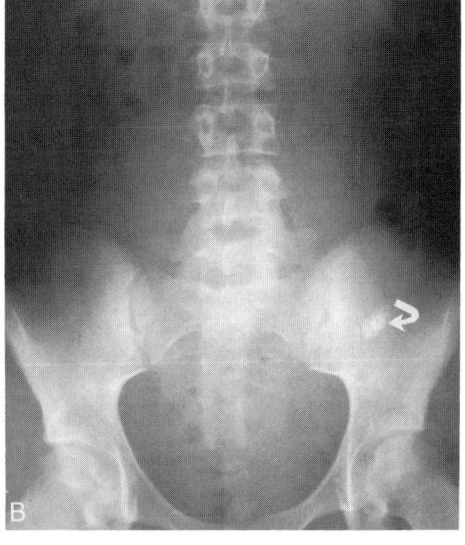

Figure 8–114. Benign teratoma or benign dermoid is the most common ovarian mass occurring in adolescents. The longitudinal scan (A) of this 14-year-old, who had noticed left lower quadrant fullness, shows a huge, predominantly cystic mass. The densely reflective area (arrow) at the inferior edge of the mass proved to be calcification (arrow) on the subsequent abdominal radiograph (B).

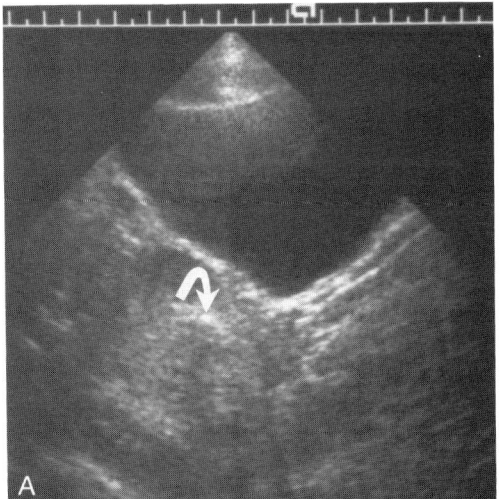
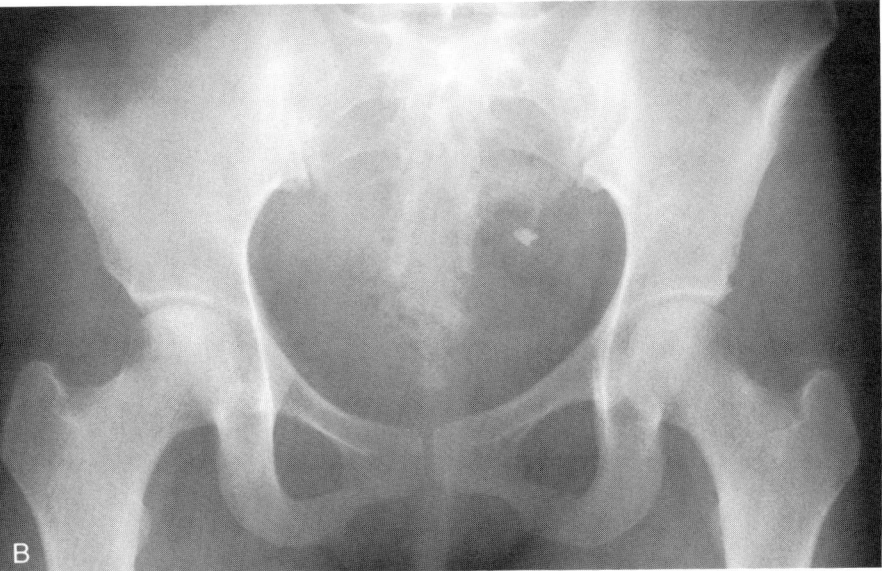

Figure 8–115. If a dermoid has very few cystic components, it may be very difficult to distinguish it as a discrete mass. This patient presented with a left adnexal mass. The longitudinal scan (A) shows diffuse, poorly defined echogenicity associated with one area of shadowing density (arrow). An abdominal radiograph was then obtained (B). The calcification associated with a rather fatty dermoid is evident on the plain film. Hair within a dermoid can also cast an acoustic shadow on ultrasonograms.

torsion is reportedly more common in early adolescence, we have scanned children as young as 2 years of age who have presented with acute abdominal pain, and it is apparent that perinatal torsion is more common than once thought (Nussbaum et al., 1988).

Ovarian masses that are associated with ascites are more likely to be malignant. Our ultrasonographic evaluation is aimed at (1) identifying the mass as ovarian in source, (2) characterizing its appearance, (3) looking for the other ovary in order to document its normalcy (bilateral tumors can occur with granulosa-theca cell tumor, teratoma, dysgerminoma, and gonadoblastoma), (4) evaluating the peritoneal space for the presence of ascites, and (5) if ascites is present, scanning peritoneal surfaces to look for peritoneal implants and scanning the liver for metastases.

Disease that is metastatic to the ovaries affects only children who have lymphoproliferative disease. Usually both ovaries are involved, but asymmetric enlargement can oc-

298 / EVALUATING AN ABDOMINAL MASS

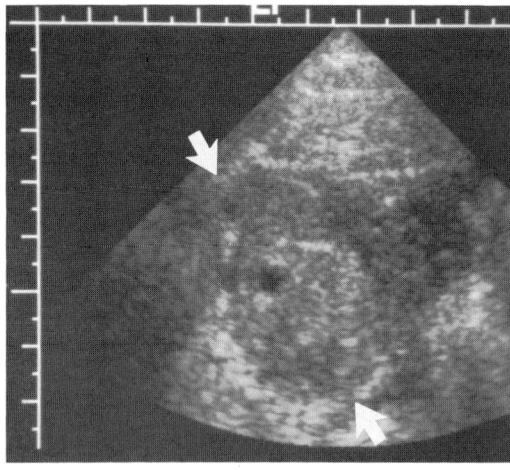

Figure 8–116. Scans of the pelvis in infants and toddlers are difficult because young children cannot hold much urine in the bladder. This is a transverse view of the pelvis in a little girl who had a 2-day history of severe lower abdominal pain and pain in the rectum. The white blood cell count was elevated at 25,000. This right adnexal mass (arrows) proved to be hemorrhagic infarction of the ovary and fallopian tube secondary to torsion.

Figure 8–117 This 6-year-old presented to the emergency room with a 4-day history of nausea and vomiting and a temperature of 40°C. An experienced examiner thought her presentation atypical for appendicitis and requested ultrasonography. It showed an unusual, complex mass in the right adnexa. During surgery, this proved to be torsion of the right ovary and fallopian tube. It is common in girls aged 6–12 years for the clinical presentation of ovarian torsion to simulate that of appendicitis.

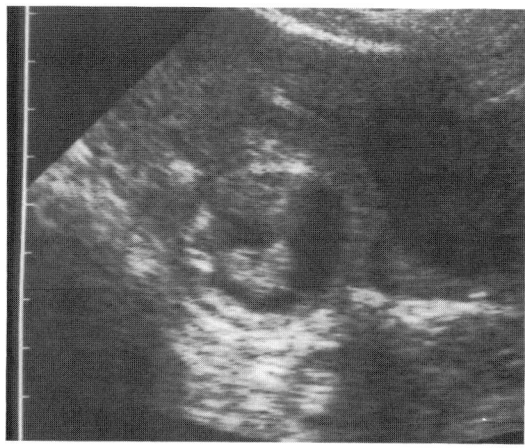

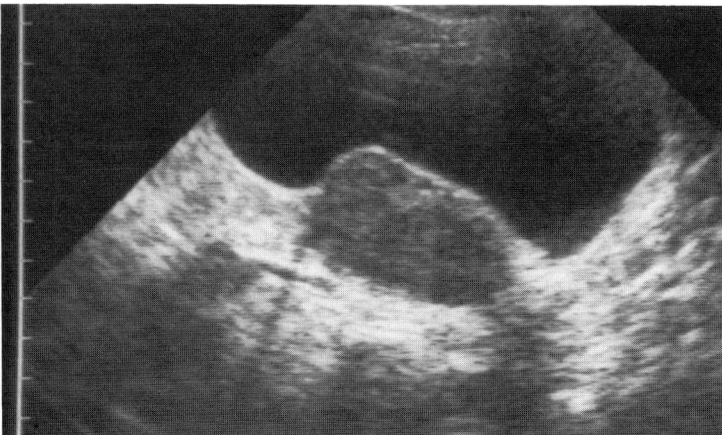

Figure 8–118. Suprapubic pain that followed mild trauma was associated with a mass in the cul-de-sac in this 9-year-old girl. A uniformly homogeneous mass representing the right ovary was found on ultrasonography. This longitudinal scan shows the size of the right ovary and its indentation of the bladder. During surgery, this proved to be a large-cell lymphoma of the right ovary.

cur, as with testicular involvement in boys who have acute lymphoblastic leukemia (Fig. 8–118; Lane and Birdwell, 1986).

PELVIC MASSES IN ADOLESCENTS

The older girl and adolescent who present with an uncomplicated pelvic mass generally come straight to ultrasonography, bypassing radiography. Plain films are usually nondiagnostic for this age group, and there is always the chance that we might be radiographing an early pregnancy. Having said that, we discourage ultrasonography for the diagnosis of early pregnancy. The urinary tests that are now available are cheaper and faster than scheduling scans. Children and adolescents do come to ultrasonography for assessment of gestational age of a pregnancy when dates are uncertain or when ectopic pregnancy is considered possible. The criteria for a complete fetal survey should be followed because fetal anomalies are more frequent in the pregnancies of adolescents. As mentioned in the introduction, we believe that transvaginal scanning, where available, is superior to transvesical scanning in the diagnosis of ectopic pregnancy. The reader is referred to the standard obstetric textbooks and literature for more information regarding this adult disease. We add a footnote: diagnosis of pregnancy in a girl or young adolescent is not usually a happy occasion. We have experienced some difficult times in an examining room either with the patients themselves or with the patients' parents. When an unsuspected pregnancy is discovered, or when a therapeutic abortion is being considered, we try to be as efficient as possible in obtaining the study and getting the patient back to her doctor for consultation. In these situations, we try to deflect the viewing screen away from the patient so that the psychologic impact is lessened. We do not discuss the findings unless directly asked to by the patient or her parents; we prefer that the referring physician who has met or who knows the family relay all the necessary information.

Girls who have imperforate hymen may present at birth, but some do not come to medical attention until the time of menarche. Then the obstructing hymen causes retention of blood and gradual enlargement of the vagina and uterus. The girl typically has monthly pelvic pain and, of course, is amenorrheic. Clinical examination is diagnostic, and incision of the membrane is curative. The few such patients who have made their way to ultrasonography in our hospital have had an incomplete physical examination. Scans show a mass low in the pelvis, which represents the blood-filled vagina. The uterus is variably dilated and the cervix in-

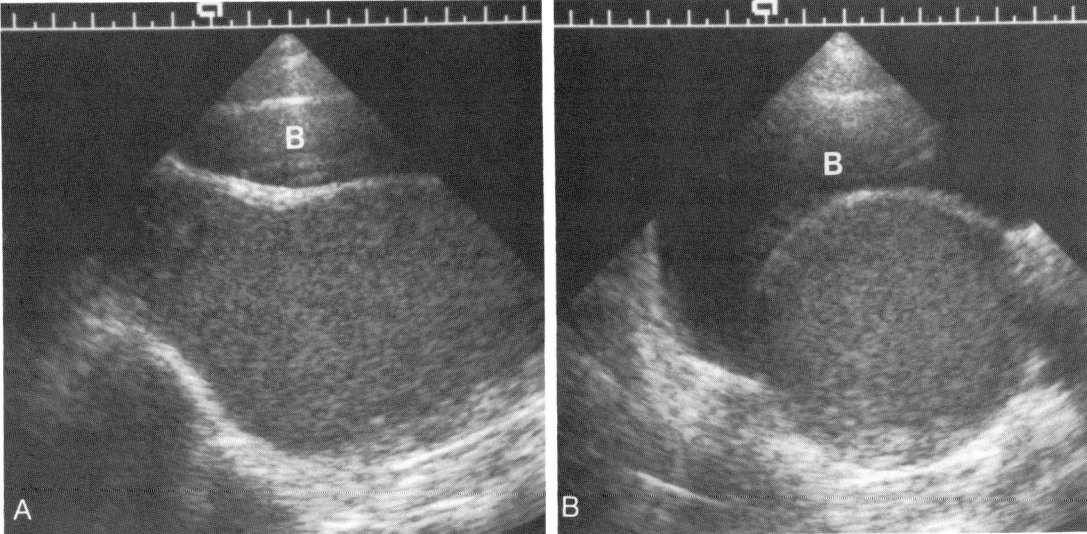

Figure 8–119. Longitudinal (**A**) and transverse (**B**) scans of the lower pelvis show the typical appearance of distended vagina, secondary to imperforate hymen. This 12-year-old girl had had monthly pain for 1 year. Five hundred milliliters of blood were drained after hymenectomy. B = bladder.

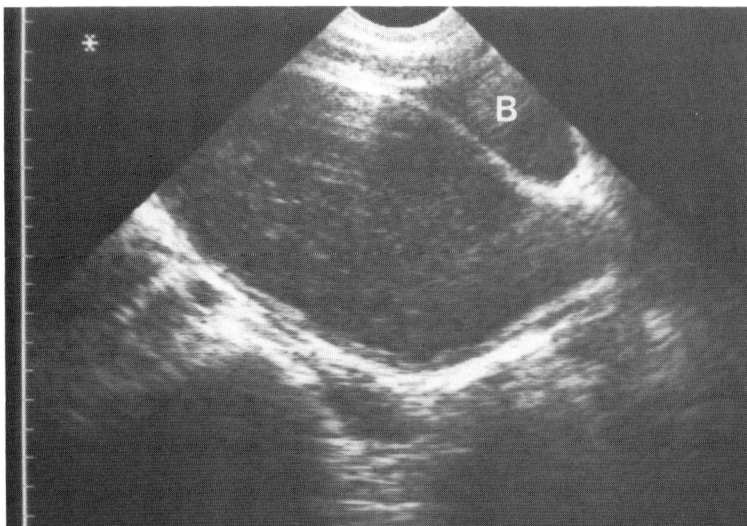

Figure 8–120. Hematometrocolpos may result from duplication of the genital tract and obstruction of one half of the tract at the level of the vagina. This child had a septated vagina and left-sided hematometrocolpos resulting from distal obstruction. Urinary anomalies—specifically, renal agenesis on the side of the obstruction—are frequently associated as was the case in this child. Scans of the kidneys should always accompany scans of the pelvis. B = bladder.

competent, depending on the duration of the obstruction after menarche (Fig. 8–119). Occlusion of the vagina at any level by a membrane and atresia of the cervix or upper vagina are rare embryologic faults in müllerian development. The introitus may be normal, but the patient presents with increasing pelvic mass, pain, and amenorrhea. Complete vaginal atresia results in the same symptoms. The ultrasonograms may be diagnostic of the level of obstruction. Vaginal atresia commonly coexists with an abnormal uterus or occurs in the absence of a uterus, and this spectrum of embryologic failure is termed Mayer-Rokitansky-Küster syndrome. When no uterus or a hypoplastic uterus is apparent, the girl presents with amenorrhea unassociated with pelvic mass (see Chapter 9). The kidneys and skeleton are frequently anomalous in girls who have gynecologic anomalies. Renal anomalies include unilateral agenesis, horseshoe kidney, and cross-fused ectopia.

Duplication of the genital tract is often complicated by obstruction of one unit. Typically, the obstruction is at the level of the distal vagina. The obstructed system causes periodic pain, but the unobstructed system allows monthly menses to occur. Only when the pain becomes severe, or the mass obvious, does the girl come to medical attention. Unilateral renal agenesis on the side of

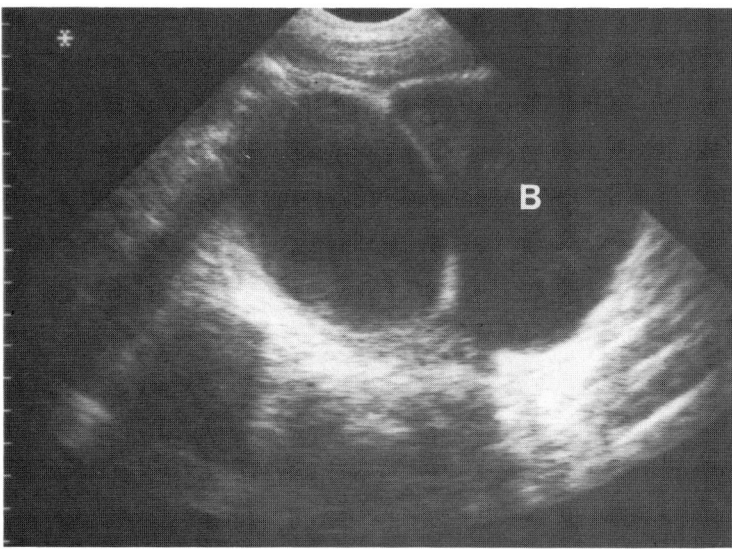

Figure 8–121. Follicular cysts may reach gigantic proportions. This longitudinal scan shows an 8-cm cyst, which during surgery proved to be a follicular cyst. Simple or follicular cysts of the ovary occasionally may extend to the umbilicus or even to the xiphoid process. B = bladder.

the hematometrocolpos is a common association (Fig. 8–120; Gilsanz and Cleveland, 1982).

By far the most common pelvic masses in adolescent girls are ovarian in origin. Of these, follicular and simple ovarian cysts are most frequent (Wu and Siegel, 1987). Both are unilocular and thin-walled and have no internal echoes. Most are 3 to 6 cm in diameter, but some simple cysts can fill the abdomen from the xiphoid process to the pubis. In most cases, unilocular cysts are managed with hormonal therapy and follow-up ultrasonography. Surgery is reserved for patients in whom there is persistence of a large cyst for more than 2 months and for patients who have pain and presumed torsion of the cyst (Figs. 8–121, 8–122, 8–123).

There are two groups of patients in whom cysts tend not to change with time (because they are not under hormonal control). Some girls have a paraovarian cyst originating from the wolffian remnants. Although these cysts are located in the broad ligaments, they may be adjacent to an ovary and may simulate an ovarian cyst (Fig. 8–124). The other group includes girls who have undergone pelvic surgery or trauma. Ovarian fluid produced by ruptured follicles may be trapped by peritoneal adhesions and simulate ovarian cysts. These inclusion cysts should be managed with conservative therapy rather than with salpingo-oophorectomy (Hoffer et al., 1988).

A septated cystic ovarian mass is more of a diagnostic problem than is a simple cyst. Septations have been noted in cystadenoma, teratoma, simple cyst, and corpus luteum cyst with previous hemorrhage (Figs. 8–125, 8–126). The failure to be able to make a specific diagnosis in many cases extends to the group of girls who have a solid or mixed cystic/solid adnexal mass. The differential list

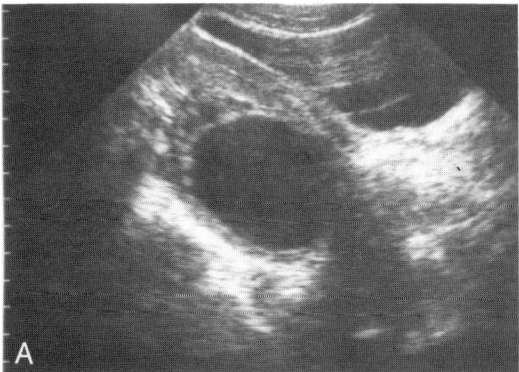

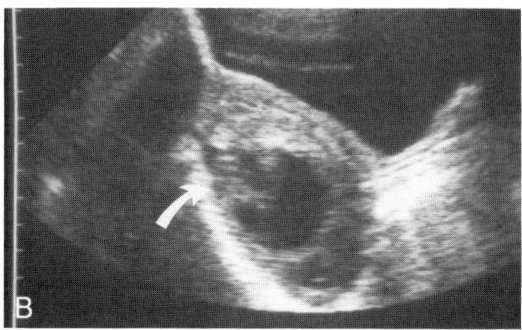

Figure 8–123. Although physicians are often cavalier about the diagnosis of ovarian cyst, one should always remember that a cyst may be a focus for torsion. This 12-year-old child had right lower quadrant pain, and in ultrasonographic evaluation, a right-sided adnexal cyst was identified (A). She was treated with birth control pills, but the episodes of acute right lower quadrant pain persisted. She was taken to the operating room after a second study (B) suggested that there was bleeding into the cyst (arrow). Surgical examination revealed torsion of the right fallopian tube, presumably resulting from the presence of the ovarian cyst.

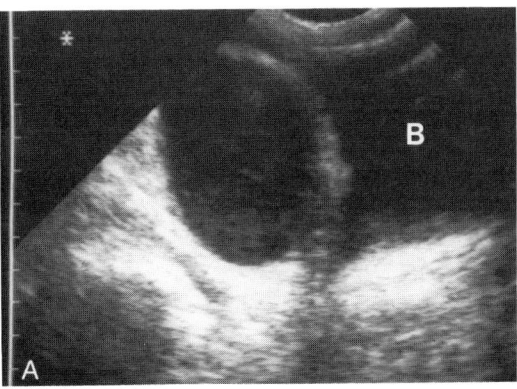

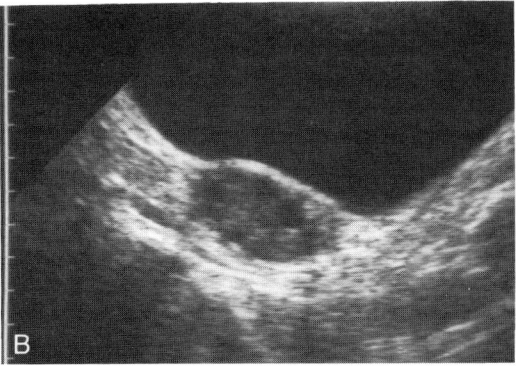

Figure 8–122. Usually, ovarian cysts that measure 5 cm or less in diameter are managed conservatively. This child, whose longitudinal scan initially showed a right ovarian cyst (A), had a normal follow-up study of the right adnexa 2 months later (B). In A, B = bladder.

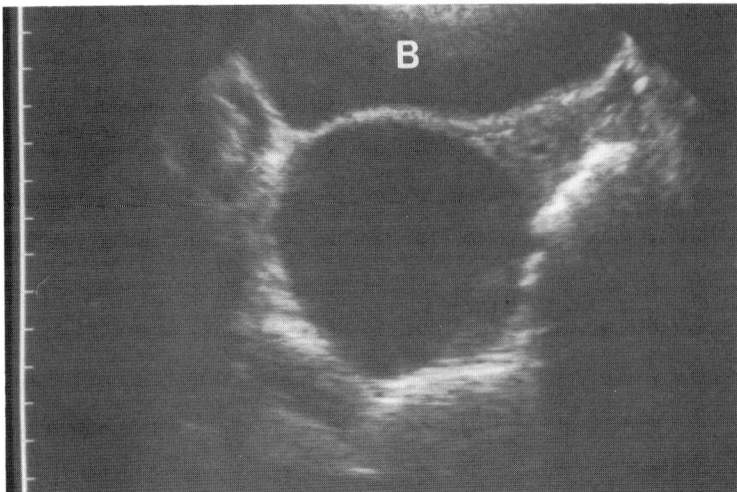

Figure 8–124. Usually, a cystic adnexal mass is thought to be ovarian in origin. Paraovarian cyst, a remnant of the wolffian ductal system, may be present in girls as an adnexal mass. This 13-year-old, who had pelvic pain, had a persistent right-sided adnexal mass. It did not change throughout the menstrual cycle. A paraovarian cyst, 7 cm in diameter, was surgically removed. B = bladder.

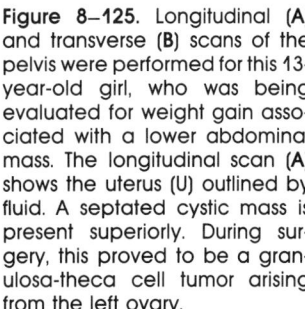

Figure 8–125. Longitudinal (A) and transverse (B) scans of the pelvis were performed for this 13-year-old girl, who was being evaluated for weight gain associated with a lower abdominal mass. The longitudinal scan (A) shows the uterus (U) outlined by fluid. A septated cystic mass is present superiorly. During surgery, this proved to be a granulosa-theca cell tumor arising from the left ovary.

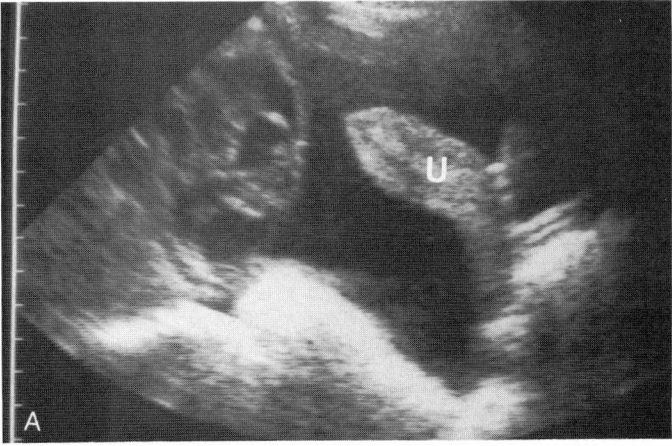

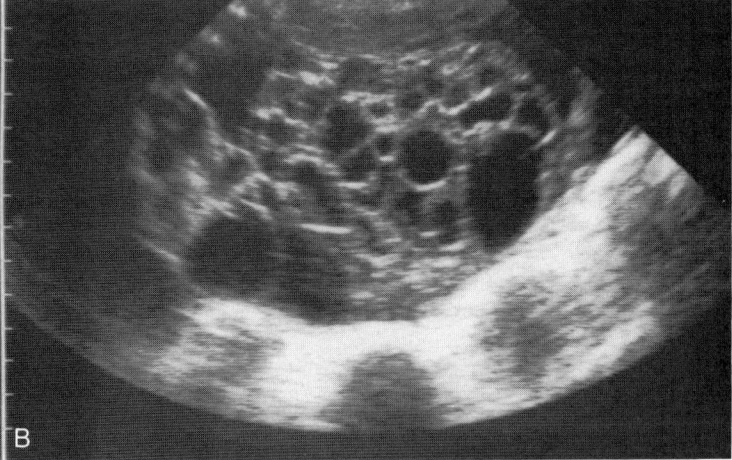

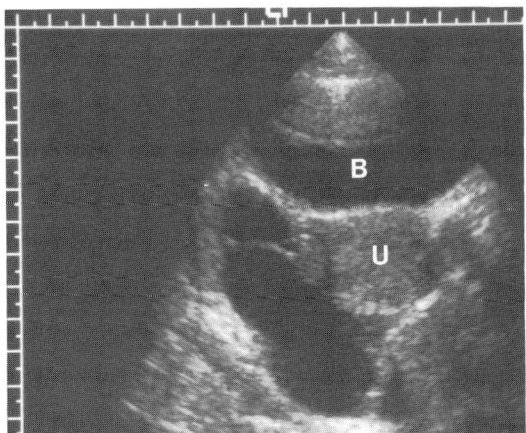

Figure 8–126. This transverse scan shows a septated adnexal mass, which was removed at surgery and shown to be a simple ovarian cyst. B = bladder; U = uterus.

is extensive and includes ectopic pregnancy, hemorrhage into an ovarian cyst, ovarian torsion, ovarian neoplasm, endometrioma, tubo-ovarian abscess, and periappendiceal abscess. Without some information from the patient's history, a clinical examination, and laboratory data, reaching a diagnosis is achieved with chance alone (Figs. 8–127, 8–128, 8–129, 8–130).

Bleeding into an ovarian cyst (typically a luteal cyst) can result in a mass that appears truly solid. As the clot forms and then retracts, the ultrasonograms follow this progression by showing a mixed mass and then a return to a cystic mass. Other features of hemorrhagic ovarian cyst include thick-rimmed masses, septations, and fluid in the cul-de-sac. If the patient is stable, is not pregnant, and can be followed closely, ultrasonography will show the progression of changes that establish the diagnosis (Fig. 8–131; Bass et al., 1984).

Ovarian torsion of a normal adnexa can occur around the time of puberty as well as at younger ages, and its cause is unknown. The pattern of a swollen echogenic ovary with peripheral follicles that are quite prominent is diagnostic. Fluid in the cul-de-sac is present in small amounts (Graif and Itzchak, 1988).

Although most often it is a teratoma, as in the younger age group, an ovarian neoplasm in an adolescent may be a tumor of epithelial origin. These tumors, usually benign and only rarely malignant, include serous, mucinous, and endometrioid cystadenoma. There is no reasonable way to differentiate them from each other or from other ovarian tumors.

The degree of involvement and complications of pelvic inflammatory disease (PID) are so variable that attempts at diagnosis with ultrasonography can be quite frustrating. Edema and inflammation blur tissue planes, and adnexal enlargement is common (Golden

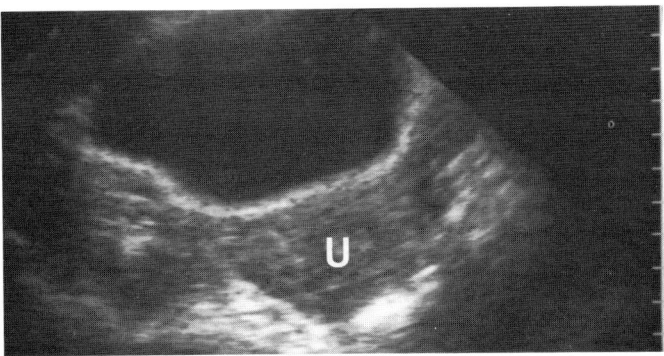

Figure 8–127. Ectopic pregnancy should always be considered in the differential diagnosis of a complex or solid adnexal mass. This 16-year-old patient had a positive pregnancy test and vaginal bleeding associated with right lower quadrant pain. The transverse scan shows the uterus (U) slightly to the left of midline and an inhomogeneous mass in the right adnexa. The tubal pregnancy was removed during laparotomy. Note that there is no free fluid in the cul-de-sac in this particular patient, although free fluid often accompanies ectopic pregnancy. Transvaginal scanning is the method of choice in evaluating patients who may have an ectopic pregnancy. (Reprinted by permission of Elsevier Science Publishing Co. from Share JC, Teele, RL: Ultrasound of the pediatric and adolescent patient. Clin Pract Gynecol 1989; 1[3]:72–92. Copyright 1989 by Elsevier Science Publishing Co., Inc.)

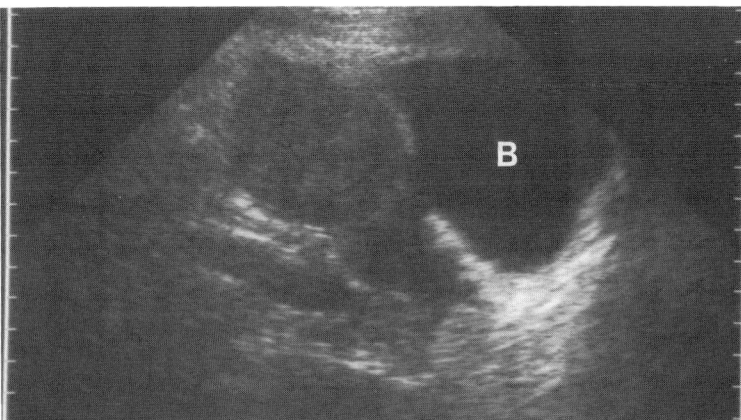

Figure 8–128. Patients who are taking anticoagulants seem to be particularly prone to bleeding into a corpus luteum cyst. This 19-year-old was taking sodium warfarin (Coumadin) because of earlier cardiac surgery. Her presentation this time was with right lower quadrant pain and vomiting. The echogenic mass indenting the bladder was assumed to be bleeding into a corpus luteum cyst. She was treated conservatively without surgery, and the mass disappeared. B = bladder.

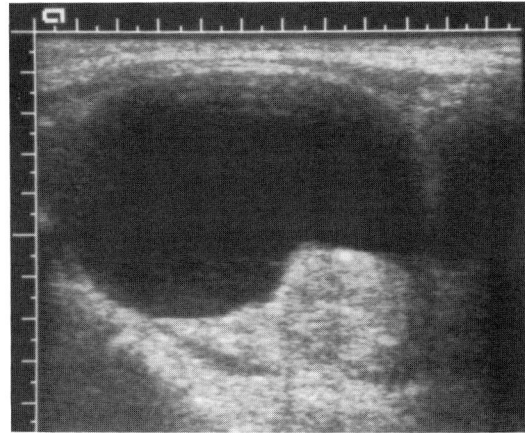

Figure 8–129. Simple ovarian cyst is more common in adolescents, but in this 8-year-old girl, it was the cause of abdominal pain, nausea, and vomiting. The large cyst shown here on a transverse scan of the left hemiabdomen was found, during surgery, to be associated with torsion of the left adnexa.

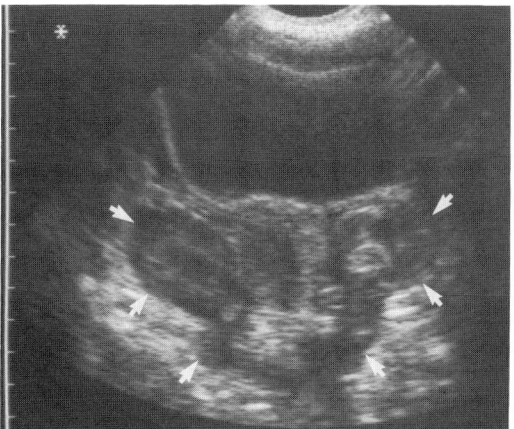

Figure 8–130. Thrombocytopenia, pallor, and fatigue brought this child to medical attention. A platelet count of 26,000 and a hematocrit of 25 resulted in a bone marrow aspiration, which contained small, round tumor cells. Abdominal evaluation included this ultrasonogram, which on the transverse view shows unusual appearance of both adnexa. There is lucent material encasing the ovaries and extending posterior to the uterus (arrows). During surgery, malignant carcinomatosis of the peritoneum engulfing the ovaries was identified, and a diagnosis of alveolar rhabdomyosarcoma was ultimately made on the basis of electromicroscopy of biopsy specimens.

EVALUATING AN ABDOMINAL MASS / 305

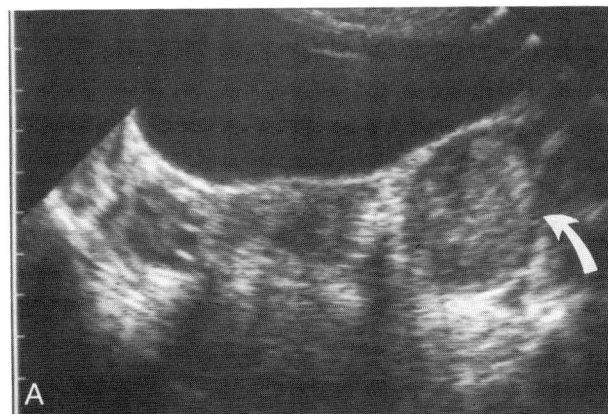

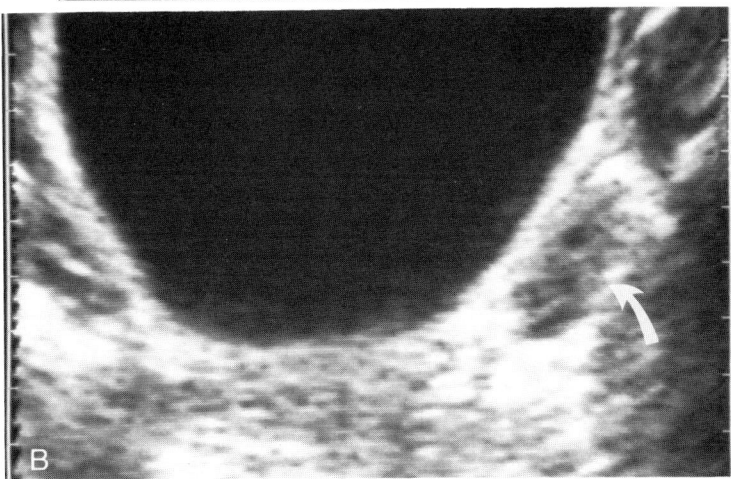

Figure 8–131. The echogenic left adnexal mass (arrow) seen in **A** resolved completely 26 days later (arrow, **B**). This is the typical appearance of hemorrhage into a corpus luteum cyst.

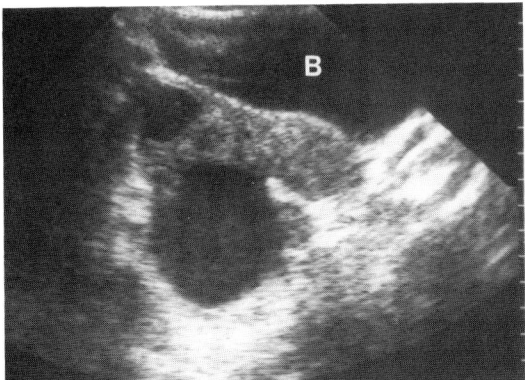

Figure 8–132. This longitudinal scan followed clinical examination, which revealed a right-sided adnexal mass in a girl who had a high sedimentation rate, elevation of the white blood cell count, and cervical cultures for positive gonococcus. Diagnosis of tubo-ovarian abscess was made on the basis of these scans. It resolved with antibiotic therapy only. In general, when the diagnosis of pelvic inflammatory disease of venereal origin is made, we prefer to reserve ultrasonography for those patients who do not respond immediately to antibiotic therapy. B = bladder.

et al., 1989). We rarely define, with certainty, a tubo-ovarian abscess unless it is chronic and well defined. Because aggressive medical therapy, rather than surgical intervention, is the rule in most cases, we prefer to reserve ultrasonography for patients who have a persistent mass after a course of antimicrobial therapy (Figs. 8–132, 8–133). The diagnosis in the acute situation should be made with cultures, not with transducers. There is one situation in which the ultrasonographer can make the diagnosis before clinical suspicions have been raised: the adolescent with severe pain in the right upper quadrant may have perihepatitis from infection traveling along the paracolic gutter. In the days of compound scanners, one could actually show the thickening of peritoneal and juxtaperitoneal soft tissues from the inflammatory response. This is less evident with real-time units, but an otherwise normal scan of a girl who has tenderness over the right upper abdomen should provoke an ultrasonic look at the

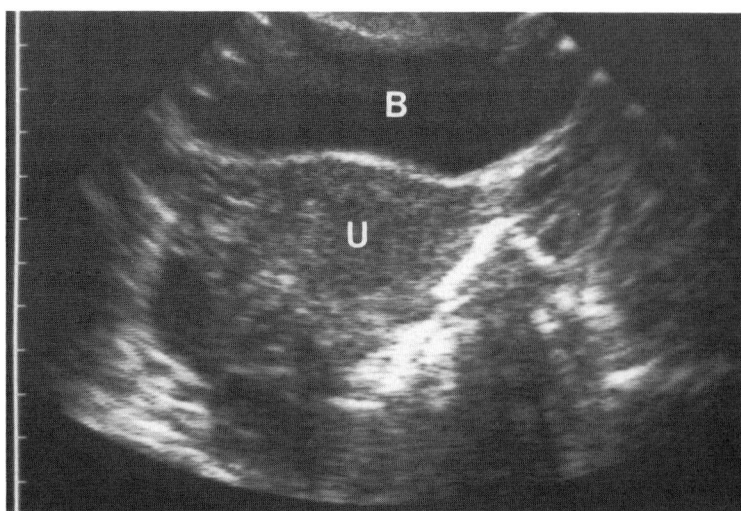

Figure 8–133. Pelvic inflammatory disease is associated with adnexal enlargement and poor delineation of tissue planes. This 17-year-old patient responded to antibiotics. Transverse scan of the pelvis shows poorly defined but enlarged right adnexa. B = bladder; U = uterus.

pelvis as well as stimulate clinical interest in the possibility of pelvic inflammatory disease.

We usually think of PID in terms of venereal disease, but complications of appendiceal inflammation are a common cause of pelvic infection in the pediatric age group. Adnexal mass may represent a walled-off appendiceal abscess and, without a helpful clinical history, may be indistinguishable from primary ovarian pathology. If the patient is young, is not sexually active, and has signs or symptoms indicating infection, pelvic abscess from appendicitis should be the first diagnosis considered (Figs. 8–134, 8–135).

A primary uterine mass is a rare problem in adolescence. Pregnancy is the most com-

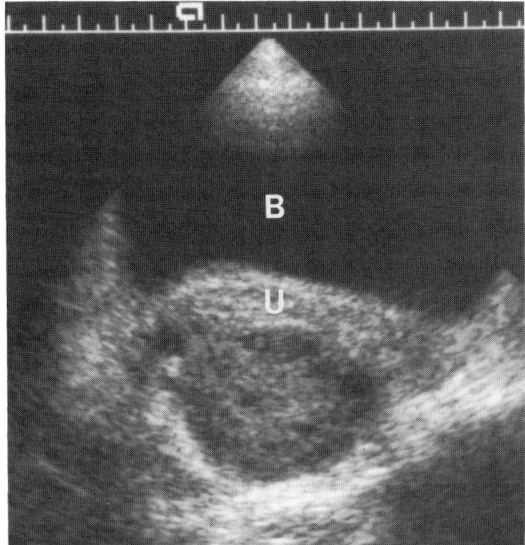

Figure 8–134. Appendicitis and its complications are always in the differential diagnosis with gynecologic disease and vice versa. This 16-year-old, who had had right lower quadrant pain and a temperature up to 40°C for several days, had this longitudinal ultrasonogram, which shows a right-sided complex mass posterior to the bladder and uterus. During surgery, this proved to be a periappendiceal abscess around a perforated appendix. Differentiating appendiceal disease from inflammatory disease of the ovary and fallopian tube is often extremely difficult. B = bladder; U = uterus.

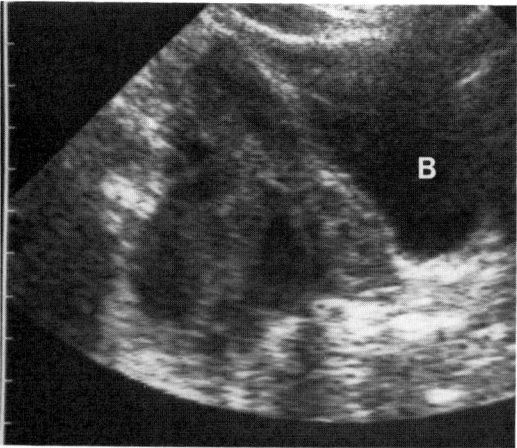

Figure 8–135. This longitudinal scan of a 14-year-old child with right-sided abdominal pain beginning 1 week before admission, temperature up to 39°C, and decreased appetite strongly supported the possibility of perforated appendicitis. However, during surgery, bicornuate uterus and an enlarged right fallopian tube filled with endometriosis were found to be the cause of the patient's right-sided adnexal mass. The entire right tube was removed. B = bladder.

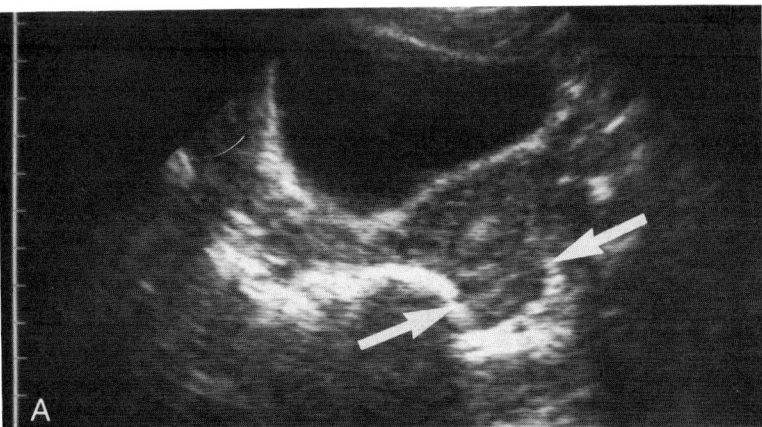

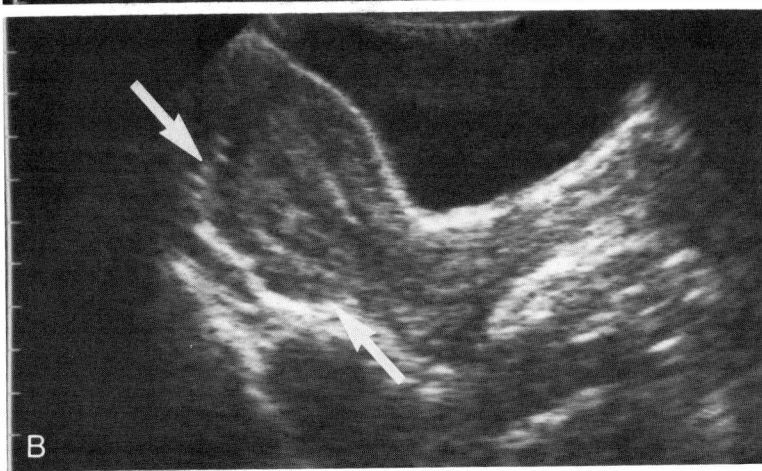

Figure 8–136. Fibroid of the uterus is uncommon in the pediatric population. Patients in whom we have identified a fibroid uterus have been black. These transverse (**A**) and longitudinal (**B**) studies of the pelvis show a leiomyoma, or fibroid of the uterus (arrows), which on rectal examination was palpated as a midline mass.

mon cause of uterine enlargement. Leiomyomas may occur in a few adolescent patients, most of whom are black. Ultrasonographic features of leiomyoma include uterine enlargement, textural alteration, and distortion of the uterine contour (Figs. 8–136, 8–137). Bicornuate uterus may present as a bulky uterus on physical examination: transverse

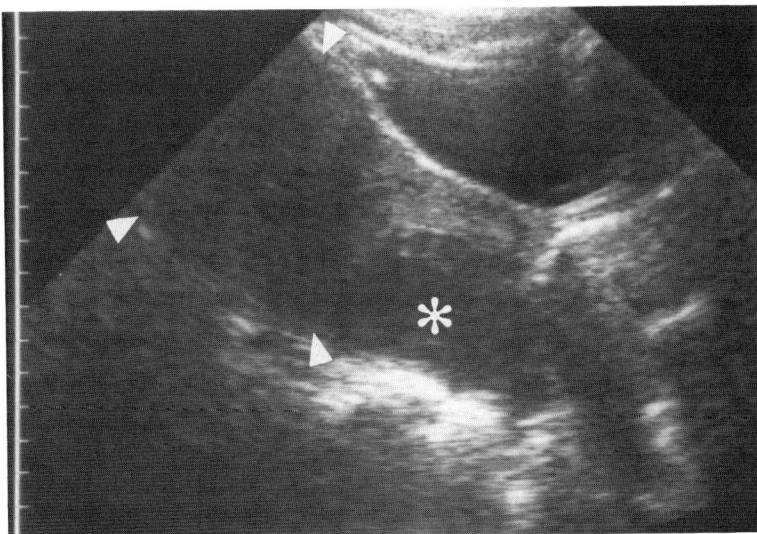

Figure 8–137. Longitudinal scan showed a very large hypoechoic mass (arrowheads) arising from the uterine fundus. There is free fluid in the cul-de-sac (asterisk), which is mildly echogenic. We were concerned about the possibility of malignancy, but surgery revealed that this patient had a large fibroid of the uterus. The fluid in the pelvis was 250 cc of blood from a ruptured right ovarian cyst.

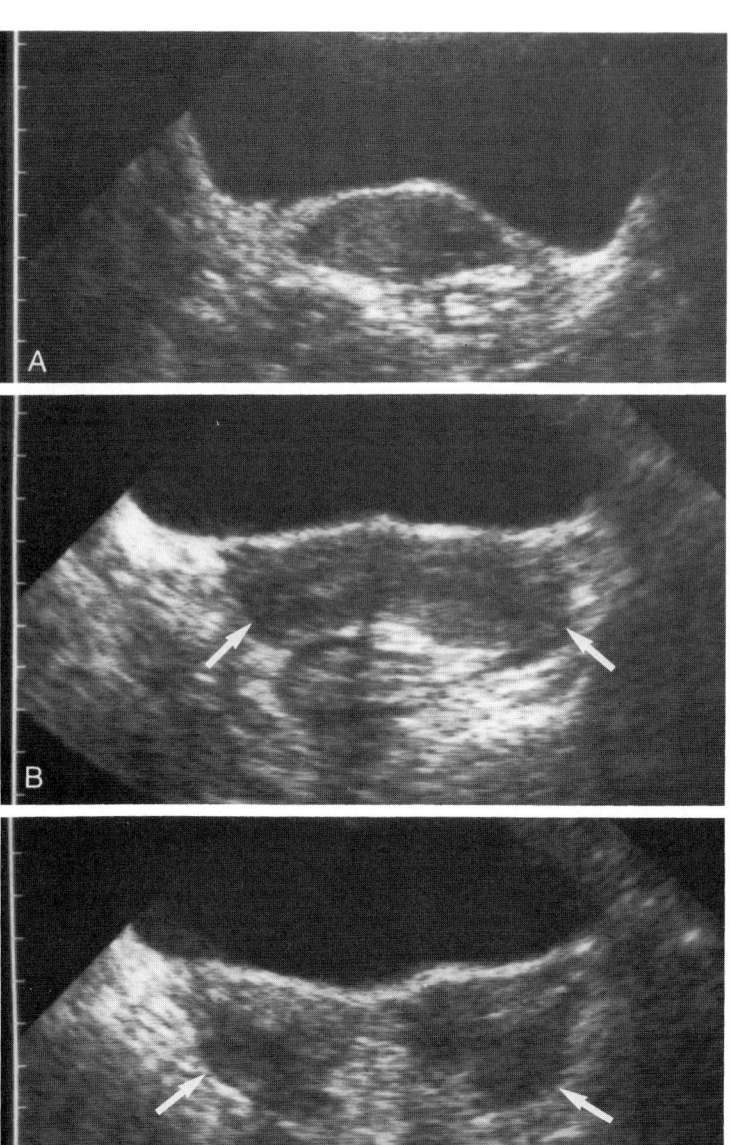

Figure 8-138. This series of transverse scans of the pelvis from inferior (**A**) to superior (**C**) shows a bicornuate uterus (arrows, **B** and **C**). This patient had coincidental horseshoe kidney. Renal anomalies commonly coexist with anomalies of the genital tract.

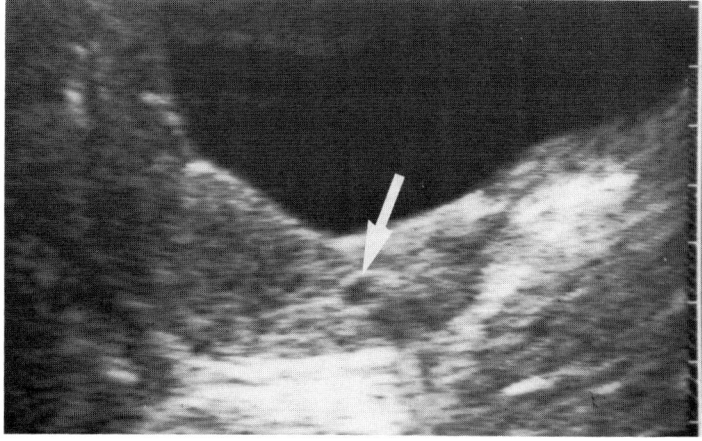

Figure 8-139. Cyst of the cervical canal or nabothian cyst is an incidental finding on ultrasonography. This longitudinal scan shows a small cyst (arrow) in the cervical canal of this adolescent girl. Transvaginal scanning commonly shows these cysts and small cystic remnants of the wolffian ductal system (Gartner cysts), which are paracervical.

scans are best for identifying two endometrial cavities (Fig. 8–138). Vaginal duplication has to be diagnosed clinically. Incidental cysts can be identified in the cervix or vaginal wall in many adolescents and young adults (Fig. 8–139). The advent of transvaginal scanning has shown that these cysts are more frequent in normal persons than originally thought. Gartner cysts, remnants of the inferior portions of wolffian ducts, can grow to be quite large and present as anechoic masses low in the pelvis.

We are now seeing some patients who have undergone genitourinary reconstructive surgery for the repair of cloacal deformities and presented as adolescents with a pelvic mass, often accompanied by pain. In all, obstruction of some part of the genital tract, usually the uterus, was the cause of their symptoms.

In boys, cysts of the seminal vesicle coexist with an ipsilateral renal anomaly, typically renal agenesis or a dysplastic pelvic kidney that enters the seminal vesicle. A retrovesical cyst in a boy should provoke scans of the testis as well as of the ipsilateral renal fossa. Chronic obstruction of the vas deferens, associated with abnormal wolffian ductal development, may be present and may cause textural changes or diminution in size of the testis.

Other cystic masses in the male pelvis are distinctly unusual. Masses that originate in the urinary tract, intestine or mesentery, or abdominal wall should be considered sites of origin (Fig. 8–140).

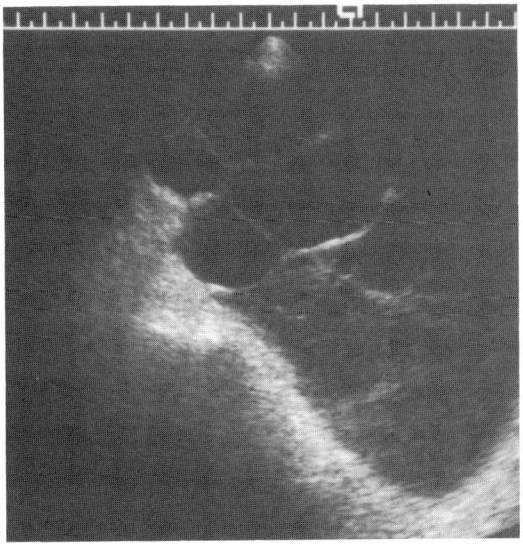

Figure 8–140. A pelvic mass is an unusual occurrence in an adolescent boy. This 19-year-old, who presented with lower abdominal pain, tenesmus, and diarrhea, had a large, multilocular cystic mass extending low in the pelvis and around the rectum. The mass was removed and proved to be a cystic hygroma. On this longitudinal scan, it has the typical ultrasonographic appearance of a multiseptate cystic mass. Its initial presentation in this age group, however, is distinctly unusual.

REFERENCES

General

Bove KE: Pathology of selected abdominal masses in children. Semin Roentgenol 1988; 23:147–160.

Didier D, Racle A, Etievent JP, et al: Tumor thrombus of the inferior vena cava secondary to malignant abdominal neoplasms: US and CT evaluation. Radiology 1987; 162:83–89.

Merten DF, Kirks DR: Diagnostic imaging of pediatric abdominal masses. Pediatr Clin North Am 1985; 32:1397–1425.

Rosenberg HK, Boyle GK: Abdominal masses. Clin Diagn Ultrasound 1989; 24:43–76.

Seidel FG: Imaging of a pediatric abdominal mass. Semin Surg Oncol 1986; 2:125–138.

Teele RL, Henschke C: Ultrasonography in the evaluation of 482 children with abdominal masses. Clin Diagn Ultrasound 1984; 14:141–165.

Teele RL, Share JC: The abdominal mass in the neonate. Semin Roentgenol 1988; 23:175–184.

Retroperitoneal Masses

Hydronephrosis and Related Conditions

Ahmed S, LeQuesne GW: Urological anomalies detected on antenatal ultrasound: A 9 year review. Aust Paediatr J 1988; 24:178–183.

Arnold AJ, Rickwood AM: Natural history of pelviureteric obstruction detected by prenatal sonography. Br J Urol 1990; 65:91–96.

Avni EF, Thoua Y, Lalmand B, et al: Multicystic dysplastic kidney: Natural history from in utero diagnosis and postnatal followup. J Urol 1987; 138:1420–1424.

Babut JM, Frémond B, Sameh A, et al: Primary megaureter in the neonate with prenatal or postnatal diagnosis. Z Kinderchir 1988; 43:150–153.

Bernstein GT, Mandell J, Lebowitz RL, et al: Ureteropelvic junction obstruction in the neonate. J Urol 1988; 140:1216–1221.

Blane CE, DiPietro MA, Bloom DA, et al: Percutaneous nephrostogram in the newborn with bilateral renal cystic disease. Am J Dis Child 1988; 142:1349–1351.

Brown T, Mandell J, Lebowitz RL: Neonatal hydronephrosis in the era of sonography. AJR 1987; 148:959–963.

Burbige KA, Amodio J, Berdon WE, et al: Prune belly syndrome: 35 years of experience. J Urol 1987; 137:86–90.

Carey PO, Howards SS: Multicystic dysplastic kidneys and diagnostic confusion on renal scan. J Urol 1988; 139:83–84.

Cerniglia FR Jr, Gonzales ET Jr, Roth DR: Posterior urethral valves: Twelve years of experience [abstract]. J Urol 1988; 139 (4, Pt 2):165A.

Chopra A, Teele RL: Hydronephrosis in children: Narrowing the diagnosis with ultrasound. JCU 1980; 8:473–478.

Connor JP, Hensle TW, Berdon W, et al: Contained neonatal urinoma: management and functional results. J Urol 1988; 140:1319–1322.

Cremin BJ: A review of the ultrasonic appearances of posterior urethral valve and ureteroceles. Pediatr Radiol 1986; 16:357–364.

Ebel KD, Bliesener JA, Gharib M: Imaging of ureteropelvic junction obstruction with stimulated diuresis: With consideration of the reliability of ultrasonography. Pediatr Radiol 1988; 18:54–56.

Eklöf O, Parkkulainen K, Thönell S, et al: Ectopic ureterocele in the male. Ann Radiol 1987; 30:486–490.

Elder JS, Duckett JW: Management of the fetus and neonate with hydronephrosis detected by prenatal ultrasonography. Pediatr Ann 1988; 17:19–28.

Felson B, Cussen LJ: The hydronephrotic type of unilateral congenital multicystic disease of the kidney. Semin Roentgenol 1975; 10:113–123.

Geary DF, MacLusky IB, Churchill BM, McLorie G: A broader spectrum of abnormalities in the prune belly syndrome. J Urol 1986; 135:324–326.

Ghidini A, Sirtori M, Vergani P, et al: Ureteropelvic junction obstruction in utero and ex utero. Obstet Gynecol 1990; 75:805–808.

Gordon AC, Thomas DFM, Arthur RJ, et al: Multicystic dysplastic kidney: Is nephrectomy still appropriate? J Urol 1988; 140 (Pt 2):1231–1234.

Gordon AC, Thomas DFM, Arthur RJ, et al: Prenatally diagnosed reflux: A follow-up study. Br J Urol 1990; 65:407–412.

Gottlieb RH, Luhmann K 4th, Oates RP: Duplex ultrasound evaluation of normal native kidneys and native kidneys with urinary tract obstruction. J Ultrasound Med 1989; 8:609–611.

Greskovich FJ III, Nyberg LM Jr: The prune belly syndrome: A review of its etiology, defects, treatment and prognosis. J Urol 1988; 140:707–712.

Griscom NT, Vawter GF, Fellers FX: Pelvoinfundibular atresia: The usual form of multicystic kidney: 44 unilateral and two bilateral cases. Semin Roentgenol 1975; 10:125–131.

Guys JM, Borella F, Monfort G: Ureteropelvic junction obstruction: Prenatal diagnosis and neonatal surgery in 47 cases. J Pediatr Surg 1988; 23:156–158.

Hodson CJ, Heptinstall RH, Winberg J: *Reflux Nephropathy Update: 1983*. New York: Karger Basel, 1984.

Homsy YL, Mehta PH, Huot D, et al: Intermittent hydronephrosis: A diagnostic challenge. J Urol 1988; 140 (Pt 2):1222–1226.

Homsy YL, Saad F, Laberge I, et al: Transitional hydronephrosis of the newborn and infant. J Urol 1990; 144:579–583.

Jones BE, Hoffer FA, Teele RL, et al: Pitfalls in pediatric urinary sonography. Urology 1990; 35:38–44.

Kessler RM, Altman DH: Real-time sonographic detection of vesicoureteral reflux in children. AJR 1982; 138:1033–1036.

Kleiner B, Filly RA, Mack L, et al: Multicystic dysplastic kidney: Observations of contralateral disease in the fetal population. Radiology 1986; 161:27–29.

Kullendorf CM: Surgery in unilateral multicystic kidney. Z Kinderchir 1990; 45:235–237.

Laing FC, Burke VD, Wing VW, et al: Postpartum evaluation of fetal hydronephrosis: Optimal timing for follow-up sonography. Radiology 1984; 152:423–424.

Lebowitz RL: Pediatric uroradiology. Pediatr Clin North Am 1985; 32:1353–1362.

Lebowitz RL, Teele RL: Fetal and neonatal hydronephrosis. Urol Radiol 1983; 5:185–188.

Macpherson RI, Leithiser RE, Gordon L, et al: Posterior urethral valves: An update and review. Radiographics 1986; 6:753–791.

Mandell GA, Snyder HM III, Heyman S, et al: Association of congenital megacalycosis and ipsilateral segmental megaureter. Pediatr Radiol 1986; 17:28–33.

Mandell J, Colodny AH, Lebowitz R, et al: Ureteroceles in infants and children. J Urol 1980; 123:921–926.

Mandell J, Docimo SG, Lebowitz RL, et al: Congenital midureteral obstruction in children [abstract]. J Urol 1988; 139(4, Pt 2): 218A.

McGrath MA, Estroff J, Lebowitz RL: Coexistence of obstruction at the ureteropelvic and ureterovesical junctions. AJR 1987; 149:403–406.

Mellins HZ: Cystic dilatations of the upper urinary tract: A radiologist's developmental model. Radiology 1984; 153:291–301.

Najmaldin A, Burge DM, Atwell JD: Fetal vesicoureteric reflux. Br J Urol 1990; 65:403–406.

Nussbaum AR, Dorst JP, Jeffs RD, et al: Ectopic ureter and ureterocele: Their varied sonographic manifestations. Radiology 1986; 159:227–235.

Paltiel HJ, Lebowitz RL: Neonatal hydronephrosis due to primary vesicoureteral reflux: Trends in diagnosis and treatment. Radiology 1989; 170:787–789.

Peters CA, Mandell J, Lebowitz RL, et al: Congenital obstructive megaureter in early infancy: Diagnosis and treatment [abstract]. J Urol 1988; 139(4, Pt 2): 444A.

Peters PC, Johnson DE, Jackson JH Jr: The incidence of vesicoureteral reflux in the premature child. J Urol 1967; 97:259–260.

Platt JF, Rubin JM, Ellis JH: Distinction between obstructive and nonobstructive pyelocaliectasis with duplex Doppler sonography. AJR 1989; 153:997–1000.

Preston A, Lebowitz RL: What's new in pediatric uroradiology. Urol Radiol 1989; 11:217–220.

Ransley PG, Dhillon HK, Gordon I, et al: The postnatal management of hydronephrosis diagnosed by prenatal ultrasound. J Urol 1990; 144:584–587.

Reinberg Y, Aliabadi H, Johnson P, et al: Congenital ureteral valves in children: Case report and review of the literature. J Ped Surg 1987; 22:379–381.

Reznik VM, Kaplan GW, Murphy JL, et al: Follow-up of infants with bilateral renal disease detected in utero: Growth and renal function. Am J Dis Child 1988; 142:453–456.

Rittenberg MH, Hurlbert WC, Snyder HM III, et al: Protective factors in posterior urethral valves. J Urol 1988; 140:993–996.

Schifter T, Heller RM: Bilateral multicystic dysplastic kidneys. Pediatr Radiol 1988; 18:242–244.

Schneider K, Jablonski C, Weissner M, et al: Screening for vesicoureteral reflux in children using real-time sonography. Pediatr Radiol 1984; 14:400–403.

Schneider K, Martin W, Helmig FJ, et al: Infundibulopelvic stenosis—Evaluation of diagnostic imaging. Eur J Radiol 1988; 8:172–174.

Share JC, Lebowitz RL: Ectopic ureterocele without ureteral calyceal dilatation (ureterocele disproportion): Findings on urography and sonography. AJR 1989; 152:567–571.

Share JC, Lebowitz RL: The unsuspected double collecting system on imaging studies and at cystoscopy. AJR 1990; 155:561–564.

Sheih CP, Liu MB, Hung CS, et al: Renal abnormalities in school children. Pediatrics 1989; 84:1086–1090.

Sholder AJ, Maizels M, Depp R, et al: Caution in antenatal intervention. J Urol 1988; 139:1026–1029.

Silverstein JI, Pena A, Aguire J, et al: Genitourinary manifestations of persistent cloaca [abstract]. J Urol 1988; 139(4, Pt 2):236A.

Stanley P, Bear JW, Reid BS: Percutaneous nephrostomy in infants and children. AJR 1983; 141:473–477.

Steinhart JM, Kuhn JP, Eisenberg B, et al: Ultrasound screening of healthy infants for urinary tract abnormalities. Pediatrics 1988; 82:609–614.

Trulock TS, Finnerty DP, Woodard JR: Neonatal bladder rupture: Case report and review of literature. J Urol 1985; 133:271–273.

Vinocur L, Slovis TL, Perlmutter AD, et al: Follow-up studies of multicystic dysplastic kidneys. Radiology 1988; 167:311–313.

Watson AR, Readett D, Nelson CS, et al: Dilemmas associated with antenatally detected urinary tract abnormalities. Arch Dis Child 1988; 63:719–722.

Willi U, Lebowitz RL: The so-called megaureter-megacystis syndrome. AJR 1979; 133:409–416.

Winfield AC, Kirchner SG, Brun ME, et al: Percutaneous nephrostomy in neonates, infants, and children. Radiology 1984; 151:617–619.

Winters WD, Lebowitz RL: Importance of prenatal detection of hydronephrosis of the upper pole. AJR 1990; 155:125–129.

Wood BP, Ben-Ami T, Teele RL, et al: Ureterovesical obstruction and megaloureter: Diagnosis by real-time ultrasound. Radiology 1985; 156:79–81.

Adrenal Glands

Atkinson GO Jr, Kodroff MB, Gay BB Jr, et al: Adrenal abscess in the neonate. Radiology 1985; 155:101–104.

Bryan PJ, Caldamone AA, Morrison SC, et al: Ultrasound findings in the adreno-genital syndrome (congenital adrenal hyperplasia). J Ultrasound Med 1988; 7:675–679.

Cohen EK, Daneman A, Stringer D, et al: Focal adrenal hemorrhage: A new US appearance. Radiology 1986; 161:631–633.

Daneman A: Adrenal neoplasms in children. Semin Roentgenol 1988; 23:205–215.

Daneman A, Chan HSL, Martin DJ: Adrenal carcinoma and adenoma in children: A review of 17 patients. Pediatr Radiol 1983; 13:11–18.

Dutton RV: Wolman's disease: Ultrasound and CT diagnosis. Pediatr Radiol 1985; 15:144–146.

Farrelly CA, Daneman A, Martin DJ, et al: Pheochromocytoma in childhood: The important role of computed tomography in tumour localization. Pediatr Radiol 1984; 14:210–214.

Ghiacy S, Dubbins PA, Baumer H: Ultrasound demonstration of congenital adrenal hyperplasia. JCU 1985; 13:419–420.

Gotoh T, Adachi Y, Nounaka O, et al: Adrenal hemorrhage in the newborn with evidence of bleeding in utero. J Urol 1989; 141:1145–1147.

Hamper VM, Fishman EK, Hartman DS, et al: Primary adrenocortical carcinoma: Sonographic evaluation with clinical and pathologic correlation in 26 patients. AJR 1987; 148:915–919.

Hata K, Nagata H, Nishigaki A, et al: Ultrasonographic evaluation of adrenal involution during antenatal and neonatal periods. Gynecol Obstet Invest 1988; 26:29–32.

Hauffa BP, Menzel D, Stolecke H: Age-related changes in adrenal size during the first year of life in normal newborns, infants and patients with congenital adrenal hyperplasia due to 21-hydroxylase deficiency: Comparison of ultrasound and hormonal parameters. Eur J Pediatr 1988; 148:43–49.

Heij HA, Taets van Amerongen AH, Ekkelkamp S, et al: Diagnosis and management of neonatal adrenal hemorrhage. Pediatr Radiol 1989; 19:391–394.

Kangarloo H, Diament MJ, Gold RH, et al: Sonography of adrenal glands in neonates and children: Changes in appearance with age. JCU 1986; 14:43–47.

Kenny PJ, Stanley RJ: Calcified adrenal masses. Urol Radiol 1987; 9:9–15.

Lawson EE, Teele RL: Diagnosis of adrenal hemorrhage by ultrasound. J Pediatr 1978; 92:423–426.

Menzel D, Hauffa BP: Changes in size and sonographic characteristics of the adrenal glands during the first year of life and the sonographic diagnosis of adrenal hyperplasia in infants with 21-hydroxylase deficiency. JCU 1990; 18:619–625.

Nissenbaum M, Jequier S: Enlargement of adrenal glands preceding adrenal hemorrhage. JCU 1988; 16:349–352.

Prando A, Wallace S, Marins JLC, et al: Sonographic findings of adrenal cortical carcinomas in children. Pediatr Radiol 1990; 20:163–165.

Sarnaik AP, Sanfilippo DJ, Slovis TL: Ultrasound diagnosis of adrenal hemorrhage in meningococcemia. Pediatr Radiol 1988; 18:427–428.

Scott EM, Thomas A, McGarrigle HHG, et al: Serial adrenal ultrasonography in normal neonates. J Ultrasound Med 1990; 9:279–283.

Volberg FM, Dillard R, Sumner T: Ultrasonography of discoid adrenals in Potter's syndrome: Report of three cases. Am J Perinatol 1989; 6:326–328.

Wright JE, Bear JW: Adrenal hemorrhage presenting as an abdominal mass in the newborn. Aust Paediatr J 1987; 23:305–307.

Wu CC: Sonographic spectrum of neonatal adrenal hemorrhage: Report of a case simulating solid tumor. JCU 1989; 17:45–49.

Neuroblastoma

Armstrong EA, Harwood-Nash DCF, Fitz CR: CT of neuroblastomas and ganglioneuromas in children. AJR 1981; 139:571–576.

Atkinson GO, Zaatari GS, Lorenzo RL, et al: Cystic neuroblastoma in infants: Radiographic and pathologic features. AJR 1986; 146:113–117.

Baker ME, Kirks DR, Korobkin M, et al: The association of neuroblastoma and myoclonic encephalopathy: An imaging approach. Pediatr Radiol 1985; 15:185–189.

Beckwith JB, Perrin EV: In situ neuroblastomas: A contribution to the natural history of neural crest tumors. Am J Pathol 1963; 43:1089–1104.

Bousvaros A, Kirks DR, Grossman H: Imaging of neuroblastoma: An overview. Pediatr Radiol 1986; 16:89–106.

Dershaw DD, Helson L: Sonographic diagnosis and follow-up of abdominal neuroblastoma. Urol Radiol 1988; 10:80–84.

Evans AE, D'Angio GJ, Randolph J: A proposed staging for children with neuroblastoma. Cancer 1971; 27:374–378.

Evans AE: Staging and treatment of neuroblastoma. Cancer 1980; 45:1799–1802.

Farrelly C, Daneman A, Chan HSL, et al: Occult neuroblastoma presenting with opsomyoclonus: Utility of computed tomography. AJR 1984; 142:807–810.

Forman HP, Leonidas JC, Berdon WE, et al: Congenital neuroblastoma: Evaluation with multimodality imaging. Radiology 1990; 175:365–368.

Franken EA Jr, Smith WL, Cohen MD, et al: Hepatic imaging in stage IV-S neuroblastoma. Pediatr Radiol 1986; 16:107–109.

Fujioka M, Saiki N, Aihara T, et al: Imaging evaluation of infants with neuroblastoma detected by VMA screening spot test. Pediatr Radiol 1988; 18:479–483.

Guin GH, Gilbert EF, Jones B: Incidental neuroblastoma in infants. Am J Clin Path 1969; 51:126–136.

Ikeda Y, Lister J, Bouton JM, Buyukpamukcu M: Congenital neuroblastoma, neuroblastoma in situ, and the normal fetal development of the adrenal. J Pediatr Surg 1981; 16(Suppl 1):636–644.

Neuenschwander S, Ollivier L, Toubeau M, et al: Local evaluation of abdominal neuroblastoma stage III and IV: Use of US, CT, and 123 I-meta-iodobenzylguanidine (MIBG) scintigraphy. Ann Radiol 1987; 30:491–496.

Rosenfield NS, Leonidas JC, Barwick KW: Aggressive neuroblastoma simulating Wilms' tumor. Radiology 1988; 166:165–167.

Shimada H, Chatten J, Newton WA Jr, et al: Histopathologic prognostic factors in neuroblastic tumors: Definition of subtypes of ganglioneuroblastoma and an age-linked classification of neuroblastomas. JNCI 1984; 73:405–416.

Turkel SB, Itabashi HH: The natural history of neuroblastic cells in the fetal adrenal gland. Am J Pathol 1974; 76:225–244.

Wilms Tumor and Other Renal Malignancies

Beckwith JB, Palmer NF: Histopathology and prognosis of Wilms tumor: Results from the first national Wilms' tumor study. Cancer 1978; 41:1937–1948.

Billiet I, Van Poppel H, Baert L: Actual approach to cystic nephroma. Eur Urol 1988; 14:280–286.

Bonnin J, Rubenstein LJ, Palmer N, et al: The association of embryonal tumors originating in the kidney and in the brain: A report of seven cases. Cancer 1984; 54:2137–2146.

Bove KE: Pathology of selected abdominal masses in children. Semin Roentgenol 1988; 23:147–160.

Cassady JR, Filler R, Jaffe N, et al: Carcinoma of the kidney in children. Radiology 1974; 112:691–693.

Chan HSL, Daneman A, Gribbin M, et al: Renal cell carcinoma in the first two decades of life. Pediatr Radiol 1983; 13:324–328.

Chan HSL, Cheng M-Y, Mancer K, et al: Congenital mesoblastic nephroma: A clinicoradiologic study of 17 cases representing the pathologic spectrum of the disease. J Pediatr 1987; 111:64–70.

D'Angio GJ, Evans AE, Breslow N, et al: Results of the third national Wilms' tumor study (NWTS-3): A preliminary report. Abst 723 Proc Amer Assoc Cancer Res 1984; 25:183.

Davis CJ Jr: Pathology of renal neoplasms. Semin Roentgenol 1987; 22:233–240.

Donaldson JS, Shkolnik A: Pediatric renal masses. Semin Roentgenol 1988; 23:194–204.

Farrell TP, Boal DK, Wood BP, et al: Unilateral abdominal mass: An unusual presentation of autosomal dominant polycystic kidney disease in children. Pediatr Radiol 1984; 14:349–352.

Fernbach SK, Feinstein KA, Donaldson JS, et al: Nephroblastomatosis: Comparison of CT with US and urography. Radiology 1988; 166:153–156.

Ferraro EM, Klein SA, Fakhry J, et al: Hypercalcemia in association with mesoblastic nephroma: Report of a case and review of the literature. Pediatr Radiol 1986; 16:516–517.

Kirks DR, Kaufman RA, Babcock DS: Renal neoplasms in infants and children. Semin Roentgenol 1987; 22:292–302.

Kirks DR, Kaufman RA: Function within mesoblastic nephroma: Imaging-pathologic correlation. Pediatr Radiol 1989; 19:136–139.

Mesrobian H-GJ: Wilms' tumor: Past, present, future. J Urol 1988; 140:231–238.

Nakayama DK, Ortega W, D'Angio GJ, et al: The nonopacified kidney with Wilms' tumor. J Pediatr Surg 1988; 23:152–155.

Pickering SP, Fletcher BD, Bryan PJ, et al: Renal lymphangioma: A cause of neonatal nephromegaly. Pediatr Radiol 1988; 14:445–448.

Ramos IM, Taylor KJ, Kier R, et al: Tumor vascular signals in renal masses: Detection with Doppler US. Radiology 1988; 168:633–637.

Ritchey ML, Kelalis PP, Breslow N, et al: Intracaval and atrial involvement with nephroblastoma: Review of national Wilms' tumor study-3. J Urol 1988; 140:1113–1118.

Sandler MA, Beute GH, Madrazo BL, et al: Ultrasound case of the day. Multilocular cystic nephroma. Radiographics 1988; 8:188–190.

Sisler CL, Siegal MJ: Malignant rhabdoid tumor of the kidney: Radiologic features. Radiology 1989; 172:211–212.

Weinberger E, Rosenbaum DM, Pendergrass TW: Renal involvement in children with lymphoma: Comparison of CT with sonography. AJR 1990; 155:347–349.

Other Retroperitoneal Masses

Blumhagen JD, Wood BJ, Rosenbaum DM: Sonographic evaluation of abdominal lymphangiomas in children. J Ultrasound Med 1987; 6:487–495.

Bowen A, Gaisie G, Bron K: Retroperitoneal lipoma in children: Choosing among diagnostic imaging modalities. Pediatr Radiol 1982; 12:221–225.

Bradford BF, Abdenour GE Jr, Frank JL, et al: Usual and unusual radiologic manifestations of acquired immunodeficiency syndrome (AIDS) and human immunodeficiency virus (HIV) infection in children. Radiol Clin North Am 1988; 26:341–353.

Buck BE, Scott GB, Valdeo-Dapena M, et al: Kaposi sarcoma in two infants with acquired immune deficiency syndrome. J Pediatr 1983; 103:911–913.

Cohen MD, Siddiqui A, Weetman R, et al: Hodgkin disease and non-Hodgkin lymphomas in children: Utilization of radiological modalities. Radiology 1986; 158:499–505.

Davidson AJ, Hartman DS: Lymphangioma of the retroperitoneum: CT and sonographic characteristics. Radiology 1990; 175:507–510.

Goldman SM, Davidson AJ, Neal J: Retroperitoneal and pelvic hemangiopericytomas: Clinical, radiologic, and pathological correlation. Radiology 1988; 168:13–17.

Gore RM, Shkolnik A: Abdominal manifestations of pediatric leukemias: Sonographic assessment. Radiology 1982; 143:207–210.

Graif M, Martinovitz U, Strauss S, et al: Sonographic localization of hematomas in hemophilic patients with positive iliopsoas sign. AJR 1987; 148:121–123.

Grünebaum M, Ziv N, Kornreich L: The sonographic evaluation of the great vessels' interspace in the pediatric retroperitoneum. Pediatr Radiol 1986; 16:384–387.

Heifetz SA, Alrabeeah A, Brown BS, et al: Fetus in fetu: A fetiform teratoma. Pediatr Pathol 1988; 8:215–226.

Hoffer FA, Shamberger RC, Teele RL: Ilio-psoas abscess: Diagnosis and management. Pediatr Radiol 1987; 17:23–27.

Knowles MC, Magid D, Fishman EK, et al: Case report 612: Rhabdomyosarcoma of the right psoas muscle. Skeletal Radiol 1990; 19:299–301.

Leventhal BG, Donaldson SS: Hodgkin's disease. In Pizzo PA, Poplack DG (eds): Principles and Practice of Pediatric Oncology. Philadelphia: JB Lippincott, 1989, 457–476.

Magrath IT: Malignant non-Hodgkin's lymphomas. In Pizzo PA, Poplack DG (eds): Principles and Practice of Pediatric Oncology. Philadelphia: JB Lippincott, 1989, 415–455.

Ransom JL, Pratt CB, Hustu HO, et al: Retroperitoneal rhabdomyosarcoma in children: Results of multimodality therapy. Cancer 1980; 45:845–850.

Schey WL, Vesely JJ, Radkowski MA: Shard-like calcifications in retroperitoneal teratomas. Pediatr Radiol 1986; 16:82–84.

Hepatic Masses*

Epithelial Tumors

Atkinson GO Jr, Kodroff M, Sones JP, et al: Focal nodular hyperplasia of the liver in children: A report of three new cases. Radiology 1980; 137:171–174.

Bedi DG, Kumar R, Morettin LB, et al: Fibrolamellar carcinoma of the liver: CT, ultrasound and angiography. Case report. Eur J Radiol 1988; 8:109–112.

Boechat MI, Kangarloo H, Gilsanz V: Hepatic masses in children. Semin Roentgenol 1988; 23:185–193.

Brunelle F, Chaumont P: Hepatic tumors in children: Ultrasonic differentiation of malignant from benign lesions. Radiology 1984; 150:695–699.

Brunelle F, Tammam S, Odievre M, et al: Liver adenomas in glycogen storage disease in children: Ultrasound and angiographic study. Pediatr Radiol 1984; 14:94–101.

Cosgrove DO, Arger PH, Coleman BG: Ultrasonic anatomy of hepatic veins. JCU 1987; 15:231–235.

Craig JR, Peters RL, Edmondson HA, et al: Fibrolamellar carcinoma of the liver: A tumor of adolescents and young adults with distinctive clinico-pathologic features. Cancer 1980; 46:372–379.

De Campo M, De Campo JF: Ultrasound of primary hepatic tumours in childhood. Pediatr Radiol 1988; 19:19–24.

D'Souza VJ, Sumner TE, Watson NE, et al: Focal nodular hyperplasia of the liver imaging by differing modalities. Pediatr Radiol 1983; 13:77–81.

Exelby PR, Filler RM, Grosfield JL: Liver tumors in children in the particular reference to hepatoblastoma and hepatocellular carcinoma: American Academy of Pediatrics Surgical Section Survey— 1974. J Pediatr Surg 1975; 10:329–337.

Friedman AC, Lichtenstein JE, Goodman Z, et al: Fibrolamellar hepatocellular carcinoma. Radiology 1985; 157:583–587.

Koufos A, Hansen MF, Copeland NG, et al: Loss of heterozygosity in three embryonal tumours suggests a common pathogenetic mechanism. Nature 1985; 316:330–334.

Li FP, Thurber WA, Seddon J, et al: Hepatoblastoma in families with polyposis coli. JAMA 1987; 257:2475–2477.

Miller JH, Greenspan BS: Integrated imaging of hepatic tumors in childhood. Part I: Malignant lesions (primary and metastatic). Radiology 1985a; 154:83–90.

Miller JH, Greenspan BS: Integrated imaging of hepatic tumors in childhood. Part II: Benign lesions (congenital, reparative and inflammatory). Radiology 1985; 154:91–100.

Miller ST, Wollner N, Meyers PA, et al: Primary hepatic or hepatosplenic non-Hodgkin's lymphoma in children. Cancer 1983; 52:2285–2288.

Rak K, Hopper KD, Parker SH: The "starry sky" liver with Burkitt's lymphoma. J Ultrasound Med 1988; 7:279–281.

Smith WL, Franken EA, Mitros FA: Liver tumors in children. Semin Roentgenol 1983; 18:136–148.

Thomas BL, Krummel TM, Parker GA, et al: Use of intraoperative ultrasound during hepatic resection in pediatric patients. J Pediatr Surg 1989; 24:690–692.

Titelbaum DS, Burke DR, Meranze SG, et al: Fibromellar hepatocellular carcinoma: Pitfalls in nonoperative diagnosis. Radiology 1988; 167:25–30.

Tonkin IL, Wrenn EL Jr, Hollabaugh RS: The continued value of angiography in planning surgical resection of benign and malignant hepatic tumors in children. Pediatr Radiol 1988; 18:35–44.

Mesenchymal Tumors

Abramson SJ, Lack EE, Teele RL: Benign vascular tumors of the liver in infants: Sonographic appearances. AJR 1982; 138:629–632.

Dachman AH, Lichtenstein JE, Friedman AC, et al: Infantile hemangioendothelioma of the liver: A radiologic-pathologic clinical correlation. AJR 1983; 140:1091–1096.

Dehner LP, Ishak KG: Vascular tumors of the liver in infants and children. Arch Pathol 1971; 92:101–111.

Leary DL, Weiskittel DA, Blane CE, et al: Follow-up imaging of benign pediatric liver tumors. Pediatr Radiol 1989; 19:234–236.

Ros PR, Goodman ZD, Ishak KG, et al: Mesenchymal hamartoma of the liver: Radiologic-pathologic correlation. Radiology 1986a; 159:619–624.

Ros PR, Olmsted WW, Dachman AH, et al: Undifferentiated (embryonal) sarcoma of the liver: Radiologic-pathologic correlation. Radiology 1986b; 161:141–145.

Smith WL, Ballantine TVN, Gonzalez-Crussi F: Hepatic mesenchymal hamartoma causing heart failure in the neonate. J Ped Surg 1978; 13:183–185.

Smith WL, Franken EA, Mitros FA: Liver tumors in children. Semin Roentgenol 1983; 18:136–148.

Stanley P, Hall TR, Wooley MM: Mesenchymal hamartomas of the liver in childhood: Sonographic and CT findings. AJR 1986; 147:1035–1039.

Stanley RJ, Dehner LP, Hesker AE: Primary malignant mesenchymal tumors (mesenchymoma) of the liver in childhood: An angiographic–pathologic study of three cases. Cancer 1973; 32:973–984.

Weber TR, Connors RH, Tracy TF Jr, et al: Complex hemangiomas of infants and children. Individualized management in 22 cases. Arch Surg 1990; 125:1017–1020.

Tumors of the Biliary Tract

Geoffray A, Couanet D, Montagne JP, et al: Ultrasonography and computed tomography for diagnosis and follow-up of biliary duct rhabdomyosarcomas in children. Pediatr Radiol 1987a; 17:127–131.

Lack EE, Perez-Atayde AR, Schuster SR: Botryoid rhabdomyosarcoma of the biliary tract: Report of five cases with ultrastructural observations and literature review. Am J Surg Pathol 1981; 5:643–652.

---

*See Chapter 13 for hepatic hematoma associated with trauma.

Williams AG Jr, Sheward SE: Ultrasound appearance of biliary rhabdomyosarcoma. JCU 1986; 14:63–65.

Hepatic Abscess

Ahmed L, Salama ZA, el Rooby A, et al: Ultrasonographic resolution time for amebic liver abscess. Am J Trop Med Hyg 1989; 41:406–410.

Arya LS, Ghani R, Abdali S, et al: Pyogenic liver abscesses in children. Clin Pediatr 1982; 21:89–93.

Berry M, Bazaz R, Bhargava S: Amebic liver abscess: Sonographic diagnosis and management. JCU 1986; 14:239–242.

Chung W-M: Antenatal detection of hepatic cyst. JCU 1986; 14:217–219.

Chusid MJ: Pyogenic hepatic abscess in infancy and childhood. Pediatrics 1978; 62:554–559.

Esfahani F, Rooholamini SA, Vessal K: Ultrasonography of hepatic hydatid cysts: New diagnostic signs. J Ultrasound Med 1988; 7:443–450.

Frider B, Losada CA, Larrieu E, et al: Asymptomatic abdominal hydatidosis detected by ultrasonography. Acta Radiol 1988; 29:431–434.

Garel LA, Pariente DM, Nezelof C, et al: Liver involvement in chronic granulomatous disease: The role of ultrasound in diagnosis and treatment. Radiology 1984; 153:117–121.

Laurin S, Kaude JV: Diagnosis of liver-spleen abscesses in children—with emphasis on ultrasound for the initial and follow-up examinations. Pediatr Radiol 1984; 14:198–204.

Lewall DB, McCorkell SJ: Hepatic echinococcal cysts: Sonographic appearance and classification. Radiology 1985; 155:773–775.

Liu KW, Fitzgerald RJ, Blake NS: An alternative approach to pyogenic hepatic abscesses in childhood. J Paediatr Child Health 1990; 26:92–94.

Marti-Bonmati L, Menor Serrano F: Complications of hepatic hydatid cysts: Ultrasound, computed tomography, and magnetic resonance diagnosis. Gastrointest Radiol 1990; 15:119–125.

Maxwell AJ, Mamtora H: Fungal liver abscesses in acute leukaemia—a report of two cases. Clin Radiol 1988; 39:197–201.

Merten DF, Kirks DR: Amebic liver abscess in children: The role of diagnostic imaging. AJR 1984; 143:1325–1329.

Miller JH, Greenfield LD, Wald BR: Candidiasis of the liver and spleen in childhood. Radiology 1982; 142:375–384.

Moss TJ, Pysher TJ: Hepatic abscess in neonates. Am J Dis Child 1981; 135:726–728.

Mueller PR, Dawson SL, Ferrucci JT Jr, et al: Hepatic echinococcal cyst: Successful percutaneous drainage. Radiology 1985; 155:627–628.

Oleszczuk-Raszke K, Cremin BJ, Fisher RM, et al: Ultrasonic features of pyogenic and amoebic hepatic abscesses. Pediatr Radiol 1989; 19:230–233.

Palmer PES: Diagnostic imaging in parastic infections. Pediatr Clin North Am 1985; 32:1019–1040.

Pastakia B, Shawker TH, Thaler M, et al: Hepatosplenic candidiasis: Wheels within wheels. Radiology 1988; 166:417–421.

Pineiro-Carrero VM, Andres JM: Morbidity and mortality in children with pyogenic liver abscess. Am J Dis Child 1989; 143:1424–1427.

Ralls PW, Barnes PF, Johnson MB, et al: Medical treatment of hepatic amebic abscess: Rare need for percutaneous drainage. Radiology 1987; 165:805–807.

Ralls PW, Mikity VG, Colletti P, et al: Sonography in the diagnosis and management of hepatic amebic abscess in children. Pediatr Radiol 1982; 12:239–243.

Taguchi T, Ikeda K, Yakabe S, et al: Percutaneous drainage for post-traumatic hepatic abscess in children under ultrasound imaging. Pediatr Radiol 1988; 18:85–87.

Vachon L, Diament MJ, Stanley P: Percutaneous drainage of hepatic abscesses in children. J Pediatr Surg 1986; 21:366–368.

Van Sonnenberg E, Mueller PR, Schiffman HR: Intrahepatic amebic abscess: Indications for and results of percutaneous catheter drainage. Radiology 1985; 156:631–635.

Anterior Abdominal Masses

Gastrointestinal Masses

Alexander JE, Williamson SL, Seibert JJ, et al: The ultrasonographic diagnosis of typhlitis (neutropenic colitis). Pediatr Radiol 1988; 18:200–204.

Barr LL, Hayden CK Jr, Stansberry SD, et al: Enteric duplication cysts in children: Are their ultrasonographic wall characteristics diagnostic? Pediatr Radiol 1990; 20:326–328.

Bar-Ziv J, Barki Y, Weizman Z, et al: Transient protein-losing gastropathy (Menetrier's disease) in childhood. Pediatr Radiol 1988; 18:82–84.

Bisset GS 3d, Kirks DR: Intussusception in infants and children: Diagnosis and therapy. Radiology 1988; 168:141–145.

Bowen A, Mazer J, Zarabi M: Cystic meconium peritonitis: Ultrasonographic features. Pediatr Radiol 1984; 14:18–22.

Bowen B, Ros PR, McCarthy PJ: Gastrointestinal teratomas: CT and US appearance with pathologic correlation. Radiology 1987; 62:431–433.

Cajozzo A, Perricone R, Abbadessa V, et al: Primary gastrointestinal involvement in non-Hodgkin's lymphomas. Acta Haematol (Basel) 1987; 78(Suppl 1):151–156.

Coud NA, Shah KJ: Menetrier's disease in childhood associated with cytomegalovirus infection: A case report and review of the literature. Br J Radiol 1986; 59:615–620.

Dinkel E, Dittrich M, Peters H, et al: Real-time ultrasound in Crohn's disease: Characteristic features and clinical implications. Pediatr Radiol 1986; 16:8–12.

Earnshaw JJ: Gastric teratoma in infancy. J R Coll Surg Edin 1985; 30:199–200.

Egelhoff JC, Bisset GS 3rd, Strife JL: Multiple enteric duplications in an infant. Pediatr Radiol 1986; 16:160–161.

Hayden CK Jr, Swischuk LE, Rytting JE: Gastric ulcer disease in infants: US findings. Radiology 1987; 164:131–134.

Hernanz-Schulman M, Genieser NB, Ambrosino M: Sonographic diagnosis of intramural duodenal hematoma. J Ultrasound Med 1989; 8:273–276.

Kleinman PK, Brill PW, Winchester P: Resolving duodenal-jejunal hematoma in abused children. Radiology 1986; 160:747–750.

Kopen PA, McAlister WH: Upper gastrointestinal and ultrasound examinations of gastric antral involvement in chronic granulomatous disease. Pediatr Radiol 1984; 14:91–93.

Lee HC, Yeh HJ, Leu YJ: Intussusception: The sonographic diagnosis and its clinical value. J Pediatr Gastroenterol Nutr 1989; 8:343–347.

Malpani A, Ramani SK, Wolverson MK: Role of sonography in trichobezoars. J Ultrasound Med 1988; 7:661–663.

Martinez-Frontanilla LA, Silverman L, Meagher DP Jr: Intussusception in Henoch-Schönlein purpura: Diag-

nosis with ultrasound. J Pediatr Surg 1988; 23:375–376.
McAlister WH, Siegal MJ: Pediatric radiology case of the day. Duodenal duplication. AJR 1989; 152:1328–1329.
McCracken S, Jongeward R, Silver TM, et al: Gastric trichobezoar: Sonographic findings. Radiology 1986; 161:123–124.
Miyamoto Y, Fukuda Y, Urushibara K, et al: Ultrasonographic findings in duodenum caused by Schönlein-Henoch purpura. JCU 1989; 17:299–303.
Morimoto K, Hashimoto T, Choi S, et al: Ultrasonographic evaluation of intramural gastric and duodenal hematoma in hemophiliacs. JCU 1988; 16:108–113.
Newman B, Girdany BR: Gastric trichobezoars—Sonographic and computed tomographic appearance. Pediatr Radiol 1990; 20:526–527.
Orel SG, Nussbrum AR, Sheth S, et al: Duodenal hematoma in child abuse: Sonographic detection. AJR 1988; 161:147–149.
Pracros JP, Tran-Minh VA, Morin de Finfe CH, et al: Acute intestinal intussusception in children: Contribution of ultrasonography (145 cases). Ann Radiol 1987; 30:525–530.
Seibert JJ, Williamson SL, Golladay ES: The distended gasless abdomen: A fertile field for ultrasound. J Ultrasound Med 1986; 5:301–308.
Swischuk LE, Hayden CK, Boulden T: Intussusception: Indications for ultrasonography and an explanation of the doughnut and pseudokidney signs. Pediatr Radiol 1985; 15:388–391.
Teele RL, Henschke CI, Tapper D: The radiographic and ultrasonographic evaluation of enteric duplication cysts. Pediatr Radiol 1980; 10:9–14.
Teele RL: A dozen ultrasonographic donuts. Mt Sinai J Med 1984; 51:528–534.
Todani T, Sato Y, Watanabe Y, et al: Air reduction for intussusception in infancy and childhood: Ultrasonographic diagnosis and management without X-ray exposure. Z Kinderchir 1990; 45:222–226.
Vade A, Blanc CE: Imaging of Burkitt Lymphoma in pediatric patients. Pediatr Radiol 1985; 15:123–126.
Wang GD, Liu SJ: Enema reduction of intussusception by hydrostatic pressure under ultrasound guidance: A report of 377 cases. J Pediatr Surg 1988; 23:814–818.
Worlicek H, Lutz H, Heyder N, et al: Ultrasound findings in Crohn's disease and ulcerative colitis: A prospective study. JCU 1987; 15:153–163.

Intraperitoneal Masses*

Avni EF, Matos C, Diard F, et al: Midline omphalovesical anomalies in children: Contribution of ultrasound imaging. Urol Radiol 1988; 10:189–194.
Borgia G, Ciampi R, Nappa S, et al: Tuberculous mesenteric lymphadenitis clinically presenting as abdominal mass: CT and sonographic findings. JCU 1985; 13:491–493.
Boyle G, Rosenberg HK, O'Neill J: An unusual presentation of an infected urachal cyst: Review of urachal anomalies. Clin Pediatr 1988; 27:130–134.
Bryant MS, Bremer AM, Tepas JJ 3d, et al: Abdominal complications of ventriculoperitoneal shunts: Case reports and review of the literature. Am Surg 1988; 54:50–55.
Cacciarelli AA, Kass EJ, Yang SS: Urachal remnants: Sonographic demonstration in children. Radiology 1990; 174:473–475.
Geer LL, Mittelstaedt CA, Staab EV, et al: Mesenteric

---

*For splenic masses, see Chapter 16.

cyst: Sonographic appearance with CT correlation. Pediatr Radiol 1984; 14:102–104.
Grünebaum M, Ziv N, Kornreich L, et al: The sonographic signs of the peritoneal pseudocyst obstructing the ventriculo-peritoneal shunt in children. Neuroradiology 1988; 30:433–448.
Haller JO, Schneider M, Kassner EG, et al: Sonographic evaluation of mesenteric and omental masses in children. AJR 1978; 130:269–274.
Hornback NB, Shidnia H: Rhabdomyosarcoma in the pediatric age group. AJR 1976; 126:542–560.
Mantello MT, Haller JO, Marquis JR: Sonography of abdominal desmoid tumors in adolescents. J Ultrasound Med 1989; 8:467–470.
Ros PR, Olmsted WW, Moser RP Jr: Mesenteric and omental cysts: Histologic classification with imaging correlation. Radiology 1987; 164: 327–332.
Sty JR, Wells RG: Other abdominal and pelvic masses in children. Semin Roentgenol 1988; 23:216–231.
Teele RL, Share JC: The abdominal mass in the neonate. Semin Roentgenol 1988; 23:175–184.

Evaluating a Pelvic Mass

Normal Pelvic Anatomy in Girls

Cohen HL, Tice HM, Mandel FS: Ovarian volumes measured by US: Bigger than we think. Radiology 1990; 177:189–192.
Curtis EM: Normal ovarian histology in infancy and childhood. Obstet Gynecol (NY) 1962; 19:444–454.
Dashefsky SM, Lyons EA, Levi CS, et al: Suspected ectopic pregnancy: Endovaginal and transvesical US. Radiology 1988; 169:181–184.
De Sa DJ: Follicular ovarian cysts in stillbirths and neonates. Arch Dis Child 1975; 50:45–50.
Ivarsson S-A, Nilsson KO, Persson P-H: Ultrasonography of the pelvic organs in prepubertal and postpubertal girls. Arch Dis Child 1983; 58:352–354.
Kremkau FW: Diagnostic Ultrasound. Principles, Instruments, and Exercises (3rd ed). Philadelphia: WB Saunders, 1989, 155.
Nussbaum AR, Sanders RC, Jones MD: Neonatal uterine morphology as seen on real-time US. Radiology 1986; 160:641–643.
Orsini LF, Salardi S, Pilu G, et al: Pelvic organs in premenarcheal girls: Real-time ultrasonography. Radiology 1984; 153:113–116.
Renaud RL, Macler J, Dervain I, et al: Echographic study of follicular maturation and ovulation during the normal menstrual cycle. Fertil Steril 1980; 33:272–276.
Share JC, Teele RL: Ultrasound of the pediatric and adolescent patient. Clin Pract Gynecol 1989; 3:72–92.

Pelvic Masses in Children

Alrabeesh A, Galliani CA, Giacomantonio M, et al: Neonatal ovarian torsion: Report of three cases and review of the literature. Pediatr Pathol 1988; 8:143–149.
Ammerman S, Shafer MA, Snyder D: Ectopic pregnancy in adolescents: A clinical review for pediatricians. J Pediatr 1990; 117:677–686.
Amodio J, Abramson S, Berdon W, et al: Postnatal resolution of large ovarian cysts detected in utero. Report of two cases. Pediatr Radiol 1987; 17:467–469.
Bahnson RR, Zaontz MR, Maizels M, et al: Ultrasonography and diagnosis of pediatric genitourinary rhabdomyosarcoma. Urology 1989; 33:64–68.
Bale PM: Sacrococcygeal developmental abnormalities

and tumors in children. Perspect Pediatr Pathol 1984; 1:9–56.

Burbige KA, Hensle TW: Uterus didelphys and vaginal duplication with unilateral obstruction presenting as a newborn abdominal mass. J Urol 1984; 132:1195–1198.

Cohen HL, Haller JO: Pediatric and adolescent genital abnormalities. Clin Diagn Ultrasound 1989; 24:187–215.

Davis AJ, Feins NR: Subsequent asynchronous torsion of normal adnexa in children. J Pediatr Surg 1990; 25:687–689.

Dehner LP: Gonadal and extragonadal germ cell neoplasia of childhood. Hum Pathol 1983; 14:493–511.

Denes FT, Montellato NID, Lopes RN, et al: Seminal vesicle cyst and ipsilateral renal agenesis. Urology 1986; 28:313–315.

Farrell TP, Boal DK, Teele RL, et al: Acute torsion of normal uterine adnexa in children: Sonographic demonstration. AJR 1982; 139:1223–1225.

Geoffray A, Couanet D, Montagne JP, et al: Ultrasonography and computed tomography for diagnosis and follow-up of pelvic rhabdomyosarcomas in children. Pediatr Radiol 1987b; 17:132–136.

Gilsanz V, Cleveland RH: Duplication of the Müllerian ducts and genitourinary malformations. Radiology 1982; 144:793–801.

Graif M, Shalev S, Strauss S, et al: Torsion of the ovary: Sonographic features. AJR 1984; 143:1331–1334.

Graif M, Itzchak Y: Sonographic evaluation of ovarian torsion in childhood and adolescence. AJR 1988; 150:647–649.

Grapin C, Montagne JP, Sirinelli D, et al: Diagnosis of ovarian cysts in the perinatal period and therapeutic implications (20 cases). Ann Radiol 1987; 30:497–502.

Gray SW, Skandalakis JE: Embryology for Surgeons. The Embryological Basis for the Treatment of Congenital Defects. Philadelphia: WB Saunders, 1972, 195–196.

Haller JO, Bass IS, Friedman AP: Pelvic masses in girls: An 8-year retrospective analysis stressing ultrasound as the prime imaging modality. Pediatr Radiol 1984; 14:363–368.

Harms D, Jänig U: Germ cell tumours of childhood. Report of 170 cases including 59 pure and partial yolk-sac tumours. Virchows Arch [A] 1986; 409:223–239.

Ikeda K, Suita S, Nakano H: Management of ovarian cyst detected antenatally. J Pediatr Surg 1988; 23:432–435.

King DR: Ovarian cysts and tumors. In Welch KJ, Randolph JG, Ravitch MM, et al (eds): Pediatric Surgery (4th ed). Chicago: Year Book Medical Publishers, 1986, 1341–1352.

Lane DM, Birdwell RL: Ovarian leukemia detected by pelvic sonography. A case report. Cancer 1986; 58:2338–2342.

Lindeque BG, du Toit JP, Muller LM, et al: Ultrasonographic criteria for the conservative management of antenatally diagnosed fetal ovarian cysts. J Reprod Med 1988; 33:196–198.

Mandell J, Stevens PS, Lucey DJ: Diagnosis and management of hydrometrocolpos in infancy. J Urol 1978; 120:262–265.

McKeever PA, Andrews H: Fetal ovarian cysts: A report of five cases. J Pediatr Surg 1988; 23:354–355.

Nussbaum AR, Sanders RC, Hartman DS, et al: Neonatal ovarian cysts: Sonographic-pathologic correlation. Radiology 1988; 168:817–821.

O'Sullivan P, Daneman A, Chan HSL, et al: Extragonadal endodermal sinus tumors in children: A review of 24 cases. Pediatr Radiol 1983; 13:249–257.

Pringle KC, Weiner CP, Soper RT, et al: Sacrococcygeal teratoma. Fetal Ther 1987; 2:80–87.

Shawis RN, El Gohary A, Cook RCM: Ovarian cysts and tumours in infancy and childhood. Ann R Coll Surg Engl 1985; 67:17–19.

Sheth S, Nussbaum AR, Sanders RC, et al: Prenatal diagnosis of sacrococcygeal teratoma: Sonographic-pathologic correlation. Radiology 1988; 169:131–136.

Sty JR, Wells RG: Other abdominal and pelvic masses in children. Semin Roentgenol 1988; 23:216–231.

Suita S, Sakaguchi T, Ikeda K, Nakano H: Therapeutic dilemmas associated with antenatally detected ovarian cysts. Surg Gynecol Obstet 1990; 171:502–508.

Tannous WN, Azouz EM, Homsy YL, et al: CT and ultrasound imaging of pelvic rhabdomyosarcoma in children. A review of 56 patients. Pediatr Radiol 1989; 19:530–534.

Tapper D, Lack EE: Teratomas in infancy and childhood. A 54-year experience at the Children's Hospital Medical Center. Ann Surg 1983; 198:398–410.

Widdowson DJ, Pilling DW, Cook RC: Neonatal ovarian cysts: Therapeutic dilemma. Arch Dis Child 1988; 63:737–742.

Wu A, Siegel MJ: Sonography of pelvic masses in children: Diagnostic predictability. AJR 1987; 148:1199–1202.

Zachariou Z, Roth H, Boos R, et al: Three years' experience with large ovarian cysts diagnosed in utero. J Pediatr Surg 1989; 24:478–482.

Gynecologic Masses in Adolescents

Bass IS, Haller JO, Friedman AP, et al: The sonographic appearance of the hemorrhagic ovarian cyst in adolescents. J Ultrasound Med 1984; 3:509–513.

Burgos FJ, Matorras R, Rivera M, et al: Double uterus associated with unilateral vaginal obstruction and ipsilateral renal agenesis: Ultrasonographic diagnosis. JCU 1989; 17:296–298.

Golden N, Neuhoff S, Cohen H: Pelvic inflammatory disease in adolescents. J Pediatr 1989; 114:138–143.

Han BK, Towbin RB, Ball WS Jr: Pediatric case of the day. Infected ovarian cyst. Radiographics 1988; 8:813–817.

Hoffer FA, Kozakewich H, Colodny A, et al: Peritoneal inclusion cysts: Ovarian fluid in peritoneal adhesions. Radiology 1988; 169:189–191.

Rimsza HE: An illustrated guide to adolescent gynecology. Pediatr Clin North Am 1989; 36:639–663.

Risser WL, Pokorny SF, Maklad NF: Ultrasound examination of adolescent females with lower abdominal pain. J Adolesc Health Care 1988; 9:407–410.

Rosenberg HK, Sherman NH, Tarry WF: Mayer-Rokitansky-Kuster-Hauser syndrome: US aid to diagnosis. Radiology 1986; 161:815–819.

Sisler CL, Siegel MJ: Ovarian teratomas: A comparison of the sonographic appearance in prepubertal and postpubertal girls. AJR 1990; 154:139–141.

Swayne LC, Love MB, Karasick SR: Pelvic inflammatory disease: Sonographic-pathologic correlation. Radiology 1984; 151:751–755.

Sty JR, Wells RG: Other abdominal and pelvic masses in children. Semin Roentgenol 1988; 23:216–231.

Thind CR, Carty HM, Pilling DW: The role of ultrasound in the management of ovarian masses in children. Clin Radiol 1989; 40:180–182.

Tolete-Velcek F, Hansbrough F, Kugaczewski J, et al: Utero vaginal malformations: A trap for the unsuspecting surgeon. J Pediatr Surg 1989; 24:736–740.

CHAPTER 9

ENDOCRINOLOGIC ULTRASONOGRAPHY

EVALUATION OF THE BABY WHO HAS AMBIGUOUS GENITALIA

It is a pediatric emergency if an obstetrician or family practitioner is unable to determine the sex of a baby upon its delivery. Clinicians consider the following genital phenotypes ambiguous: (1) hypospadias with no palpable gonad, (2) hypospadias with one palpable gonad, and (3) micropenis with no palpable gonad (Pagon, 1987). If at all possible, the affected infant should be referred to an institution where pediatric endocrinology, surgery, and radiology are available. If the genital abnormalities are an isolated problem and not associated with obvious other malformations (trisomy 13, triploidy, 13q− syndromes, camptomelic dysplasia, Smith-Lemli-Opitz syndrome, and cryptophthalmos are all associated with genital ambiguity), the clinician should prepare to answer three questions: (1) What is the chromosomal sex? (2) What is the gonadal sex? (3) What is the phenotypic sex? Ultrasonography is used primarily to answer the third question.

Purely phenotypic abnormalities are those in which there is either masculinization of a genetic female or undermasculinization of a genetic male, both of whom have normal chromosomes and normal (albeit hidden) gonads. Masculinization of a girl may result either from exposure in utero to exogenous androgens or from ongoing exposure to endogenous androgens, such as occurs with inherited defects in corticosteroid metabolism. In the adrenal glands, the fault may be in deficiency of 21-hydroxylase or 11β-hydroxylase. Salt wasting occurs in two thirds of those with the more common 21-hydroxylase deficiency. Undermasculinization of a boy occurs if production of testosterone is inadequate, if synthesis of testosterone is defective, if conversion of testosterone to dihydrotestosterone is faulty, or if binding of androgen to genital tissues is absent or faulty. This last syndrome is termed "testicular feminization," but only 10 percent of affected babies present with genital ambiguity. The other 90 percent appear phenotypically female and come to attention later in life when it becomes apparent that they do not have müllerian derivatives such as a vagina or a uterus and are not developing secondary sexual characteristics.

For babies who have genital ambiguity, pelvic ultrasonography is performed to de-

317

termine whether a normal-appearing uterus is present. If a normal uterus is seen, then müllerian development has occurred, and *functioning* testicular tissue with Sertoli cells (which produce müllerian-inhibiting factor) is not present. The gonads may be some combination of ovary, streak gonad, ovotestis, or dysgenetic testis. A unicornuate uterus may be associated with ipsilateral ovary or ovotestis and with contralateral testis. Differentiation between a normal uterus and a unicornuate uterus may be very difficult in the newborn, and this potential pitfall should be kept in mind by the clinician. In the newborn, gonads may not be identifiable on ultrasonography, although, if seen, a cyst associated with a gonad indicates that ovarian tissue is present. Gonads that are palpable in the scrotum or lower inguinal canal are either ovotestes or normal testes. Circulating androgens do not cause descent of normal ovaries. Streak gonads cannot be reliably identified with ultrasonography.

Adrenal glands should be evaluated in all babies who present with ambiguous genitalia. Hypertrophy of adrenal cortex can be detected on scans of many infants with defects in corticosteroid synthesis (Hauffa, 1988). (See the section on adrenal glands in Chapter 8.) Scanning the adrenal glands also reminds one to look at the kidneys. There is a rare sporadic condition of female pseudohermaphroditism with imperforate anus, müllerian anomalies, and renal malformation (Wenstrup and Pagon, 1985). We also examined one baby boy who had severe penile-scrotal hypoplasia, rectal stenosis, a right pelvic kidney, and a tethered spinal cord. Therefore, it is important to consider all the neighboring organs when evaluating children who have ambiguous genitalia.

In our practice, we often combine ultrasonography with voiding urethrography (Fig. 9–1). The urethrogram is another means of showing wolffian derivatives, such as the prostate, or müllerian derivatives, such as the utricle. Scans are performed after the bladder has been filled with contrast material. We simply wheel the ultrasonic unit to the fluoroscopy room. The full bladder provides a good ultrasonographic window only if care has been taken to introduce no air at the time of catheterization. Air bubbles can be relocated superiorly by adjustment of the fluoroscopy table to place the child in reverse Trendelenburg position until scanning is finished.

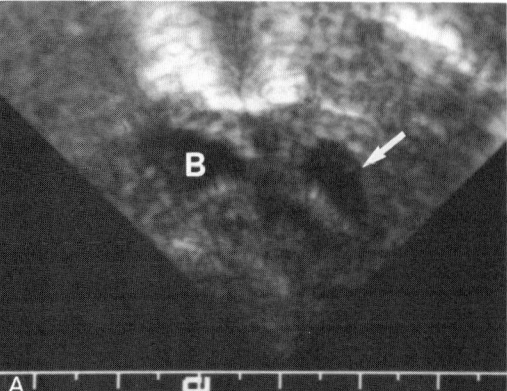

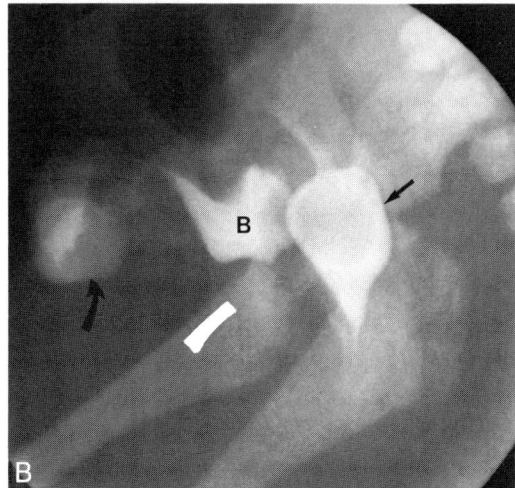

Figure 9–1. Pelvic ultrasonography was combined with genitography to evaluate ambiguous genitalia in this 5-day-old. Sagittal scan through the perineum (**A**) is oriented to match the genitogram (**B**). It shows fluid in the bladder (B) and a fluid-filled structure behind it that likely represents a müllerian derivative (arrow). No uterus was identified. Genitogram (**B**) showed filling of the bladder (B) and enlarged prostatic utricle (straight arrow). In addition, an anterior saccular structure was filled (curved arrow) and at surgery was found to contain an ovary. Chromosomal analysis revealed mosaicism; the baby is being reared as a boy.

SEXUAL DEVELOPMENTAL PRECOCITY

Precocious Puberty in Girls

The group of girls with sexual developmental precocity includes those with true precocious puberty and those with premature thelarche or premature adrenarche. True precocious puberty is complete sexual development before the age of 8 years, and the primary etiology is premature maturation of the hypothalamic-pituitary axis. Other etiologies include tumors and other disorders of the central nervous system. Premature thelarche is premature development of breasts. Although this is usually a benign, self-limited occurrence in young children, autonomous ovarian cysts or an ovarian neoplasm may be the source of estrogen that results in premature thelarche. Premature appearance of pubic hair or axillary hair or both—adrenarche—is usually a benign situation associated with slightly advanced bone and height age and normal age of onset of menses. However, if clitoral enlargement is also evident, adrenal tumor or virilizing ovarian tumor may well be the cause.

Pediatric endocrinologists use ultrasonography early in the evaluation of girls referred because of precocious puberty. Ultrasonography is used as a screening procedure in part because serologic tests of hormonal function take a long time to process. If a final diagnosis of hypothalamic-induced precocious puberty is made, the girl is followed with pelvic ultrasonography as part of a protocol for the use of gonadotropin-releasing hormone (Gn-RH) analog in treating the hypothalamic disorder (Hall et al., 1986).

All scans are performed when the child's bladder is full enough to permit easy viewing of the pelvic organs. This is not so easy in 2-year-olds who are not toilet trained. We supply liberal fluids by mouth and often spend a morning performing intermittent scanning in order to catch the right moment. Although it is stated that girls with precocious puberty act appropriately for their age, we have found that they often are difficult to manage.

For all girls who present with any form of sexual precocity, our ultrasonographic checklist is as follows: (1) Are the uterus and cervix enlarged or "mature" in comparison with normal, and is the endometrial interface prominent? In the normal prepubertal child, the uterus and cervix are similar in size and, together, are less than 4 cm long (Fig. 9–2). Fundal swelling and development of endometrial tissue indicate an effect of estrogen. (2) Are ovaries visible, what is their size, and

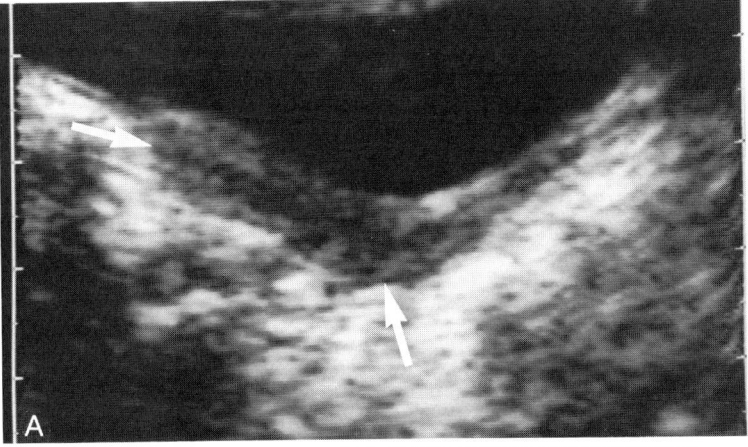
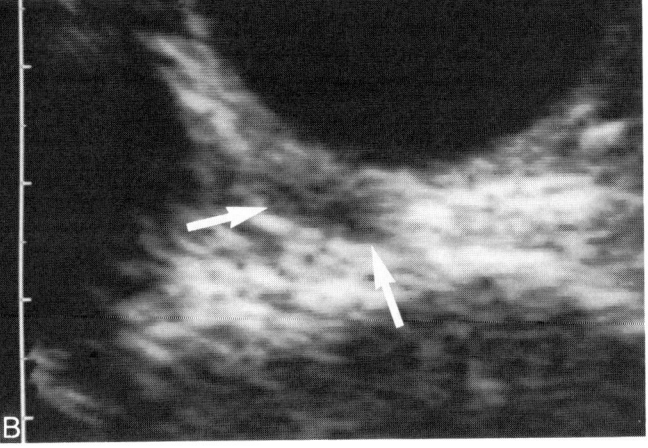

Figure 9–2. An 18-month-old girl presented with premature thelarche. A longitudinal scan (A) shows a uterus (arrows) that is 3.5 cm long. There was no well-defined endometrial echo, and the cervical portion was similar in configuration to the fundus. A longitudinal scan of the right adnexal area (B) shows a small ovary (arrows) that measures less than 1 cm in all dimensions. The left ovary was identical in appearance. No cyst or mass was present. These are normal prepubertal scans.

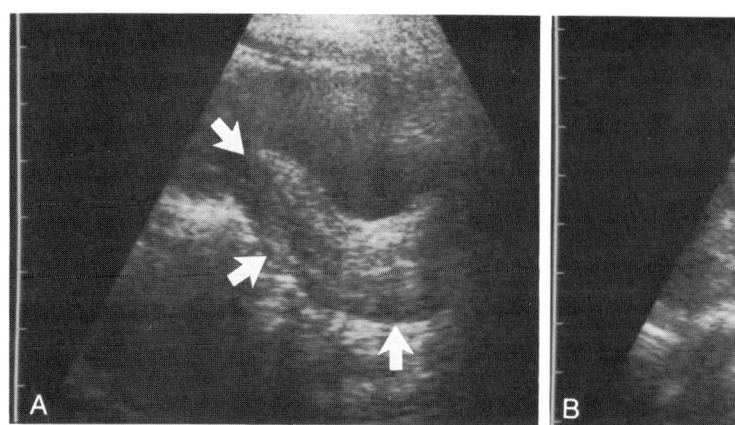

Figure 9–3. Hematuria in this 6-month-old girl actually was vaginal bleeding heralding the onset of precocious puberty. Longitudinal scan of the pelvis (A) shows a bulky uterus (arrows) that was 5.5 cm long. Normal ovarian tissue was not identified, but a cyst, 6 cm in diameter, lay just anterior to the left kidney (K), as shown on the upper abdominal scan (B). A functional ovarian cyst was removed, and follow-up studies showed that the uterus had returned to its normal prepubertal size.

are any cysts or masses present (Fig. 9–3)? We have learned that the normal ovary is difficult to find, even in cooperative patients, if they are less than 6 or 7 years old. Small cysts may be present in normal girls. In our practice, those that have proved to be autonomously functioning have been larger than 2 cm in diameter. Of importance is that they have not disappeared on follow-up studies 6 to 8 weeks later. Ovarian tumors that can secrete estrogen include granulosa or theca cell tumors, gonadoblastomas, cystadenomas, and ovarian carcinomas. Ovarian sources of androgen include arrhenoblastoma, lipoid tumor, cystadenoma, carcinoma, and gonadoblastoma. (3) Are adrenal glands normal? It is imperative to include adrenals in the scanning if the patient has virilization. Even when ultrasonography is completely normal, computed tomography (CT) scanning should be done if the results of hormonal studies point to the adrenal gland as the source of trouble. (See the section on the adrenal gland in Chapter 8.)

In those girls who have true precocious puberty, the pelvic scans show pelvic organs of the same size as that in normally pubertal adolescents (Figs. 9–4, 9–5). After treatment with Gn-RH analog, the size of the organs decreases, although ovarian size tends to be greater than that in the normal age-peer group (Hall et al., 1986). The scans of most girls who present with premature thelarche or premature adrenarche appear normal for the girls' age, and, if the hormonal studies add no additional information, they are considered to have idiopathic "benign" incomplete precocious puberty and receive no therapy. Persistent ovarian cyst, ovarian tumor, and adrenal tumor are surgically removed from the very few patients in whom they are discovered.

Precocious Puberty in Boys

Precocious adrenarche in boys is the isolated development of pubic hair at an early age (usually before 8 years). The condition is harmless and no treatment is needed, as long as the testes and penis are normal for age and the results of hormonal studies are normal. Diagnosis of precocious puberty is based on premature testicular and penile enlargement, as well as development of pubic hair. The disorder may be idiopathic and related to premature development of the hypothalamic-pituitary axis. It is more often secondary to a serious disorder of the central nervous system, to a gonadotropin-secreting tumor, or to an adrenal or testicular tumor (typically Leydig cell tumor). Initial ultrasonographic evaluation therefore includes scans of the adrenal glands, the liver and retroperitoneum (as hepatoblastoma and retroperitoneal tumors have been reported as secreting gonadotropins), and the testes. Boys who have precocious puberty have testicular scans for two reasons. First, we have to rule in or out a Leydig tumor that may be stimulating development of secondary sexual characteristics by its production of testoster-

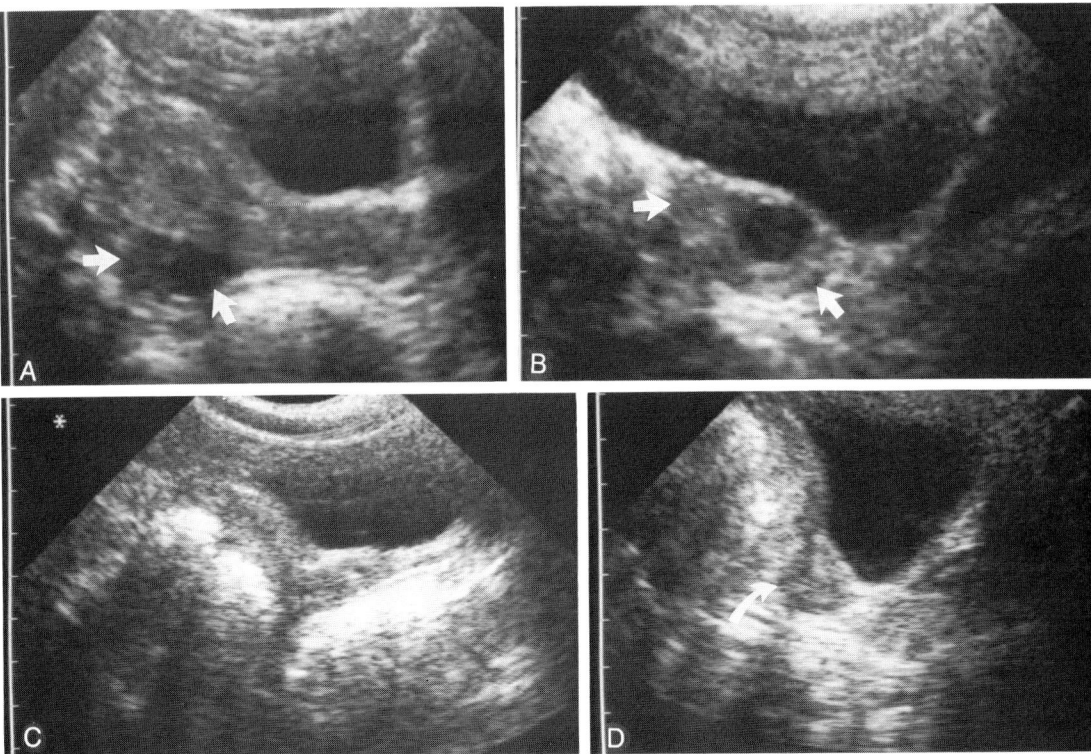

Figure 9–4. Longitudinal scan (A) of the uterus of a 2-year-old girl who presented with precocious puberty of hypothalamic origin shows fundal swelling and endometrial reaction. There was a small amount of free fluid in the cul-de-sac (arrows). The left ovary (arrows, B) had a central cyst. Three months later, after treatment with gonadotropin-releasing hormone analog, the uterus (C) had returned to normal prepubertal size. In D the left adnexa (arrow) no longer shows a central ovarian cyst.

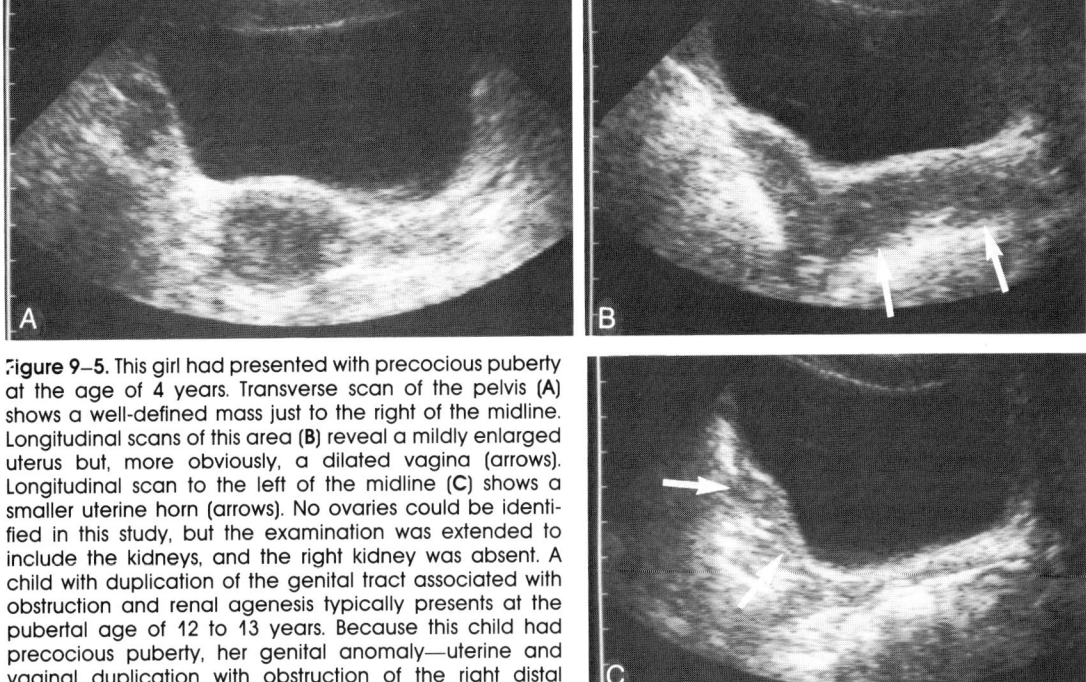

Figure 9–5. This girl had presented with precocious puberty at the age of 4 years. Transverse scan of the pelvis (A) shows a well-defined mass just to the right of the midline. Longitudinal scans of this area (B) reveal a mildly enlarged uterus but, more obviously, a dilated vagina (arrows). Longitudinal scan to the left of the midline (C) shows a smaller uterine horn (arrows). No ovaries could be identified in this study, but the examination was extended to include the kidneys, and the right kidney was absent. A child with duplication of the genital tract associated with obstruction and renal agenesis typically presents at the pubertal age of 12 to 13 years. Because this child had precocious puberty, her genital anomaly—uterine and vaginal duplication with obstruction of the right distal vagina—was discovered early.

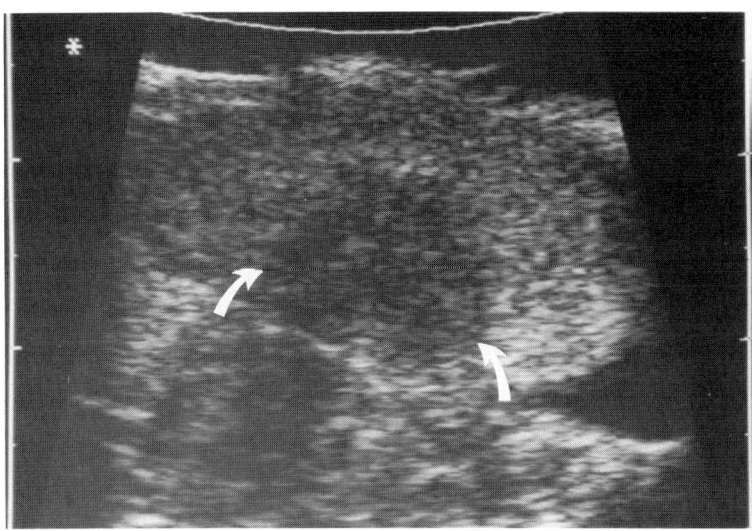

Figure 9-6. At age 9 years, this boy already had pubic hair, and his penis was large for his age. A few months later, a right testicular nodule was detected, and ultrasonography and serologic studies were obtained. This longitudinal scan of the right testis shows an echo-poor mass (arrows). Biopsy revealed a Leydig cell tumor. At the time, the patient had pubertal levels of serum testosterone.

one (Fig. 9-6). Second, we also obtain careful measurements of testicular size to provide quantitative data to endocrinologists who are treating and following this group of patients.

SCROTAL ULTRASONOGRAPHY

Scrotal ultrasonography in babies and young boys is technically difficult, simply because of the small size of the testes and surrounding structures. As a boy becomes pubertal, scans are easier to perform and interpret. It is most important that the patient be comfortable during the examination. This is an embarrassing procedure for any boy of school age, and having an audience should be discouraged. We use towels to support and stabilize the undersurface of the boy's scrotum as he lies supine on the examining table. We keep the lower abdomen covered by a sheet—for reasons of both warmth and modesty—and encourage the child to look at the ultrasonic monitor in order to keep him distracted. Warm gel for acoustic coupling is a must, as is gentle pressure from the transducer. We favor the use of linear array transducers. Particularly for transverse scans, they allow comparison between right and left scrotum more easily than do sector scans. Time gain compensation curves and gain should be based on the normal testis at the beginning of the procedure and not changed. Otherwise, comparisons between normal and abnormal parenchymal texture are lost. The normal side, if there is one, should be scanned first. The thickness of scrotal skin and muscle, testicular texture and size, and epididymal texture and size are noted for comparison with the abnormal side. If the patient has painful unilateral swelling, he is more likely to comply with a request for a complete study if the painful area is examined last.

Normal scrotal contents consist of the testis and epididymis, a thin layer of fluid in the cavity of tunica vaginalis, pampiniform venous plexus, spermatic artery, and vas deferens. The remnants of the müllerian ducts in the groove at the superior margin of the epididymis and testis cannot ordinarily be identified (Fig. 9-7).

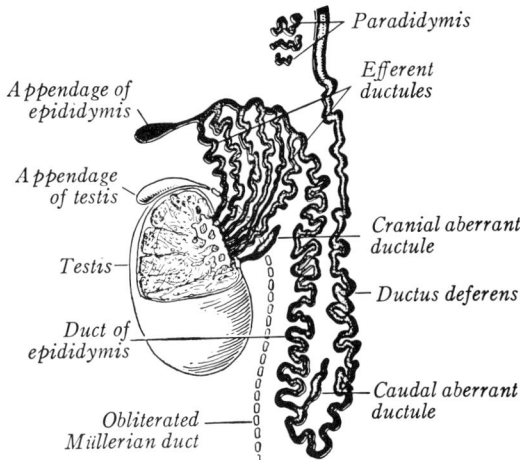

Figure 9-7. Anatomic diagram of the normal testicle. (From Arey LB: Developmental Anatomy, 7th ed. Philadelphia: WB Saunders, 1974.)

On ultrasonography, the normal testis is an oval organ of uniform echogenicity. The mediastinum testis occasionally presents as an echogenic line in the center of the testis. The epididymis is situated posterior to the testis if the testis is lying in anatomic position. Often, the scrotal contents are distorted by the towels used for support and also by contralateral pathology. The epididymis may appear to be more superior or, occasionally, more inferior in such situations. It is less well defined than the testis and appears as a thick plaque of tissue, slightly more echogenic than adjacent testis. Testicular size varies, of course, depending on the age and sexual development of the boy. Generally accepted normal values are as follows: 2 cm³ until age 11 years; 2 to 5 cm³ at 12 years; 5 to 10 cm³ at 13 years; and 12 to 14 cm³ at 15 years (Fig. 9–8; Fonkalsrud, 1987).

Requests for scrotal ultrasonography are made when a boy presents with the following clinical problems: (1) cryptorchidism, (2) painless unilateral mass, (3) painful unilateral swelling, (4) swelling that follows trauma, (5) diffuse bilateral scrotal swelling, (6) varicocele, and (7) precocious puberty. In some of these situations, we are able to answer all the questions posed; in others, ultrasonography has grave limitations and either should not be used or should be used only in concert with other studies, such as scintigraphy.

Cryptorchidism

Normal testicular development and descent depend on a complex series of endocrinologic and mechanical interactions both in utero and ex utero. Descent normally oc-

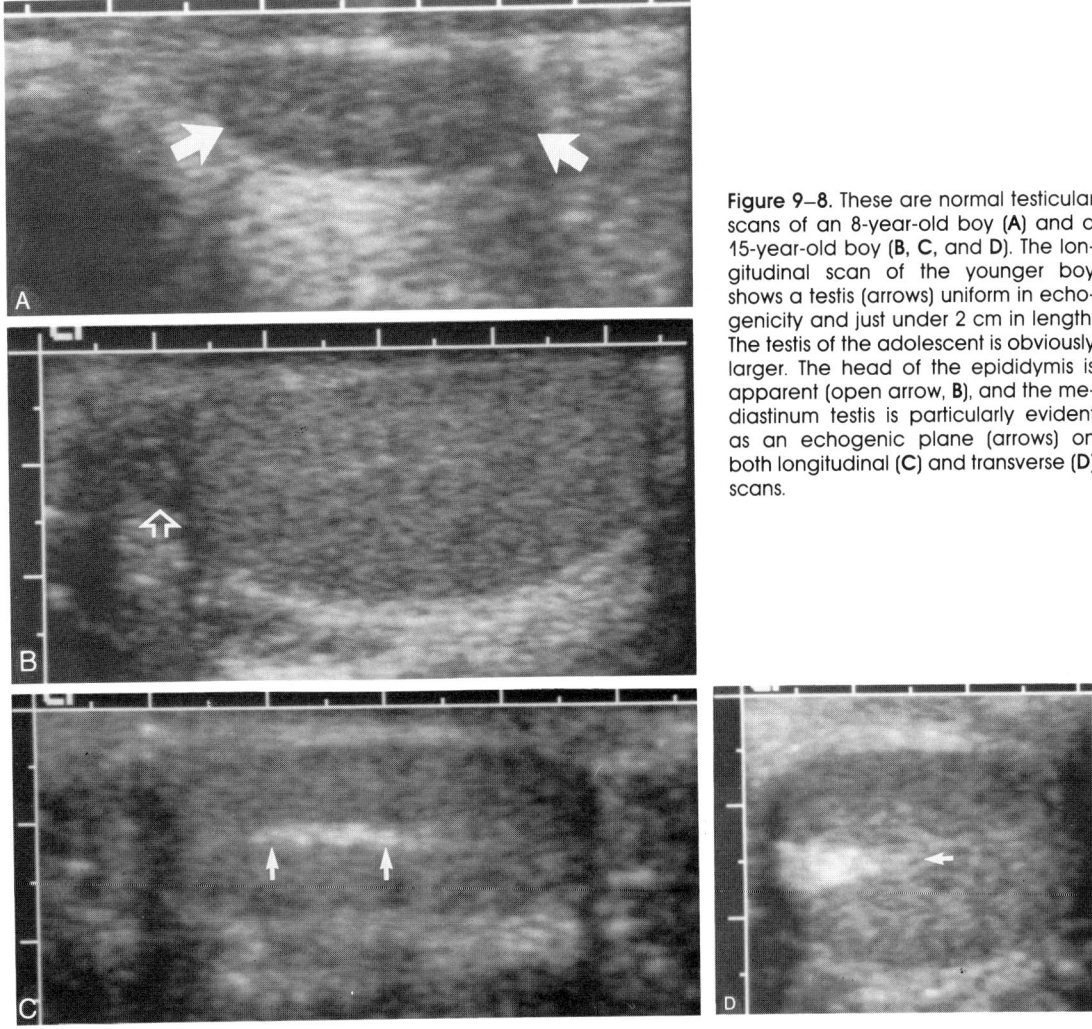

Figure 9–8. These are normal testicular scans of an 8-year-old boy (**A**) and a 15-year-old boy (**B, C,** and **D**). The longitudinal scan of the younger boy shows a testis (arrows) uniform in echogenicity and just under 2 cm in length. The testis of the adolescent is obviously larger. The head of the epididymis is apparent (open arrow, **B**), and the mediastinum testis is particularly evident as an echogenic plane (arrows) on both longitudinal (**C**) and transverse (**D**) scans.

curs in the last trimester of gestation. Four percent of newborn boys have an undescended testis, but this number decreases to 1.8 percent at 1 month and 0.8 percent at 9 months of age. Presumably, withdrawal of maternal estrogen allows a surge of luteinizing hormone and follicle-stimulating hormone after birth and a corresponding rise in testosterone, which stimulates descent. No one would have to worry about cryptorchidism if we were creatures of the sea; only ground-based mammals have developed testicular descent (Elder, 1987).

Because undescended testes show histologic changes, referable to spermatogenesis, after 18 months of extrascrotal location, orchiopexy usually is performed between 1 and 2 years of age. Other reasons for orchiopexy include increased risk of malignancy in the cryptorchid testis (35 to 48 times the risk in a normal testis); degenerative changes of the normal testis, which apparently are caused by the undescended testis; preservation of fertility; correction of associated hernia; and cosmetic appearance. Although orchiopexy does not completely prevent malignancy, it seems to lessen the risk (Blandy, 1982).

The location of the cryptorchid testis is classified as (1) intra-abdominal (inside internal inguinal ring), (2) canalicular (between internal and external inguinal rings), (3) ectopic (outside normal pathway of descent), or (4) retractile (moving between scrotum and external ring).

It is estimated that 20 percent of children with cryptorchidism have an impalpable testis. However, an experienced pediatric urologist or surgeon may be able to palpate an undescended testis when other clinicians have failed to do so. Of impalpable testes, 50 percent are canalicular, 20 to 25 percent are intra-abdominal, 15 percent are at the external inguinal ring, and 10 percent are absent as a result of either in utero torsion or agenesis.

When is ultrasonography appropriate in evaluating the child with cryptorchidism? Ultrasonography of a palpable testis adds no information but unnecessary expense. Proving the absence of a testis is impossible; therefore, its nonvisualization on ultrasonography does not prevent exploration. False-positive results of scans occur when a residual gubernaculum is mistaken for a testis (Weiss et al., 1986). The gubernaculum (from the Latin, meaning "helm" or "rudder") is a cylindrical structure, adherent to the fetal testis and epididymis, that appears to lead or steer them into their final position. Having performed this function, the gubernaculum atrophies and becomes unrecognizable on ultrasonographic scans. In young babies, it may be evident as a small nubbin adjacent to the inferior margin of the testis and epididymis. It is possible that androgenic receptors, on the genitofemoral nerve that accompanies the leading edge of the gubernaculum, are stimulated by testosterone and, in turn, encourage gubernacular motility (Beasley and Hutson, 1988).

Boys who have an impalpable testis and who are obese can be scanned if physical examination results are difficult to interpret. In addition, ultrasonography can discriminate between a testis and a lymph node, if this is a clinical problem. However, we are not enthusiastic about using routine ultrasonography for those with an impalpable testis, as our results do not appear to change the surgical approach taken by our urologic colleagues. Because of the current pressure on surgeons to operate on very young boys with

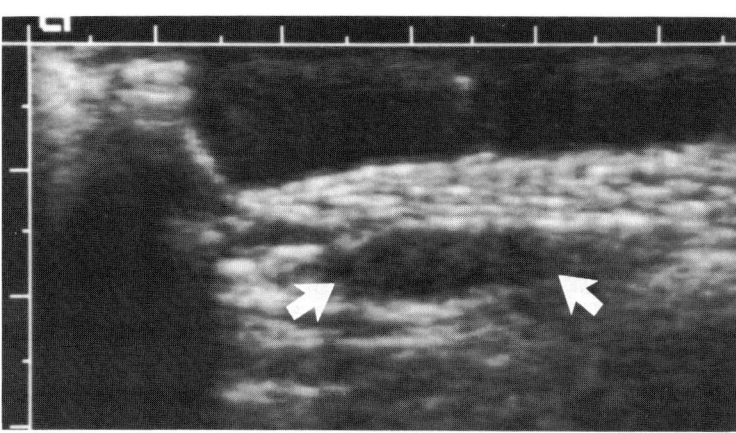

Figure 9–9. One begins the hunt for the undescended testis by establishing the size and parenchymal pattern of the normal testis. This undescended testis (arrows) was in the inguinal canal and was palpable on repeat clinical evaluation. Note the use of tissue standoff material, which can help in defining the anterior soft planes to better advantage.

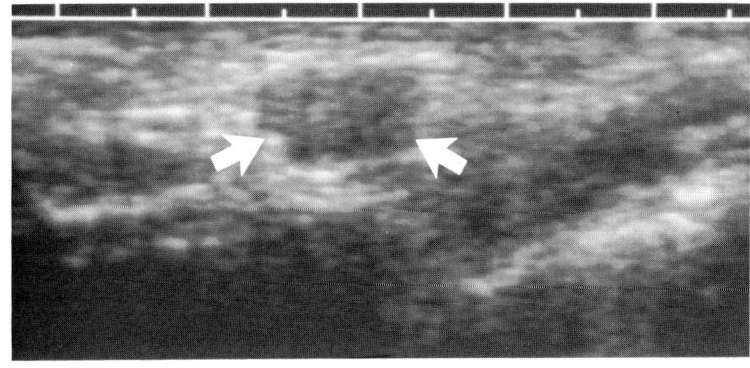

Figure 9–10. If there is no testis in either scrotal sac, it is twice as difficult to find them! This child had no apparent testis on the right side. We found a small, possibly dysplastic testis (arrows) in the left inguinal canal. Orchiopexy was performed.

cryptorchidism, an undescended and usually smaller than normal testis is very hard to find with ultrasonography even when it is canalicular.

It should be realized that many of the published reports of successful ultrasonography for patients with undescended testes included those who had palpable testes or patients who were quite old at presentation.

There is now evidence from the literature that magnetic resonance imaging (MRI) is far more sensitive than ultrasonography in localizing an abdominal testis. Boys must be sedated if very young but diagnostic accuracy in one series of 23 patients was 90 percent when MRI was used after unsuccessful ultrasonography (Beomonte et al., 1990).

When we do perform ultrasonography, we begin with scanning the normal testis, and establish its size and parenchymal pattern (Fig. 9–9). Slow, careful search of the other scrotum, the inguinal canal, and the iliac vessels follows (Fig. 9–10). If the ectopic testis is located in the canal, the transducer can be used to push the testis into the scrotum. If this is possible, the testis is retractile rather than canalicular. The very rare ectopic testis, which may be found in the perineum, in the abdominal wall, at the base of the penis, in the thigh, or in the opposite scrotal sac, has probably followed a wayward gubernaculum and gone astray from the main path of normal descent.

In a review of cryptorchid boys, Pappis and colleagues (1988) reported a high incidence of associated renal anomalies, but earlier surveys have shown no such correlation (Elder, 1987). We have made it a policy to consider the genitourinary tract as a single unit, and when genital anomalies or abnormalities arise (in girls as well as boys), we take the small amount of extra time needed to screen their kidneys and bladder.

One interesting association was noted by Elder (1987). Twelve percent of boys with a posterior urethral valve have an undescended testis. We saw one baby boy, operated on for hernia and an undescended testis, present during the postoperative period with acute urinary obstruction from a previously undiagnosed posterior urethral valve. Usually, the converse occurs and an undescended testis is noted during the evaluation of urinary obstructive symptoms.

Painless Unilateral Scrotal Mass

The list of causes for painless unilateral scrotal mass includes benign and malignant lesions (Table 9–1). The clinical examination with transillumination is quite accurate in separating boys who have a simple hydrocele from those with other pathologic conditions. Occasionally, however, a hydrocele does not transmit light well, tumors may transilluminate (Kaplan et al., 1988), and sometimes the scrotum is too distended to allow good examination of its contents. Ultrasonography

Table 9–1. PAINLESS UNILATERAL SCROTAL MASS

Hydrocele: primary and secondary
Hematocele (old trauma)
Varicocele
Epididymal cyst
Cyst (hydrocele) of spermatic cord
Hernia
Bilobed testis or polyorchidism
Simple testicular cyst
Epidermoid cyst of testis
Testicular carcinoma
Paratesticular tumor
Perinatal testicular torsion
Adrenal rest
Splenogonadal fusion

can enable one to determine the intra- or extratesticular location of the palpable mass and further define the nature of the mass.

Benign Scrotal Mass

There is no question that hydroceles are very common in newborn boys, and their waxing and waning size along with brilliant transillumination makes ultrasonographic evaluation superfluous. A congenital hydrocele is a reminder of the embryologic history of the descending testis. The peritoneal diverticulum, the processus vaginalis (which accompanies the testis), normally seals itself off from the peritoneal cavity to become the tunica vaginalis, a potential space only, anterior to the testis. A completely open processus vaginalis not only allows fluid to collect around the testis but provides the route for a hernia to occur (Fig. 9–11). Only if the hydrocele persists into the 2nd year of life or is associated with a hernia is surgical intervention needed. In most babies, the patent processus vaginalis gradually, spontaneously closes. Incomplete closure of the processus may result in a hydrocele of the spermatic cord (Fig. 9–12).

Late onset of a hydrocele—that is, a hydrocele developing after the 2nd year of life—can be associated with previous trauma and represent a resolved hematocele or be secondary to congestive heart failure or hypoalbuminemia, obstructed lymphatics from fibrosis, infection, or tumor. Primary or idiopathic hydrocele is more common in men than in boys, but, not infrequently, we see a pubertal boy with a hydrocele unassociated with any other problem. Aspiration by the urologist is usually done for both diagnostic and therapeutic purposes. Recurrence of a hydrocele is common, and if this is bothersome to the patient, the capacious sac is removed surgically.

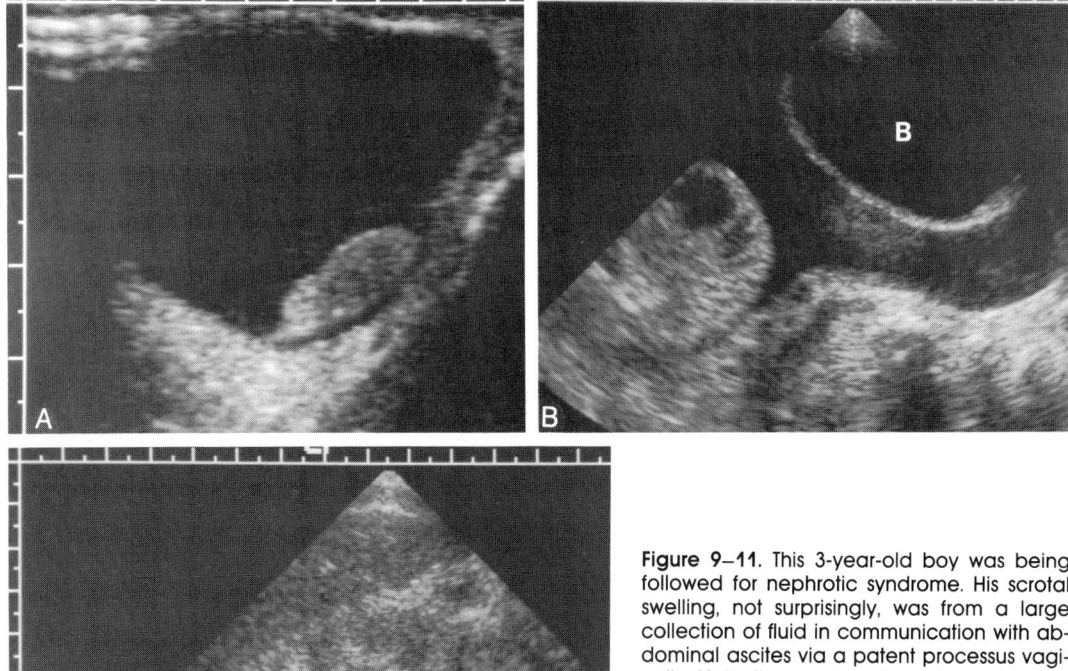

Figure 9–11. This 3-year-old boy was being followed for nephrotic syndrome. His scrotal swelling, not surprisingly, was from a large collection of fluid in communication with abdominal ascites via a patent processus vaginalis. Note the small testis and more echogenic head of epididymis in the base of the scrotal sac (A). Longitudinal scan of the pelvis (B) shows the bladder (B) surrounded by fluid. The echogenic parenchyma of the abnormal kidney is shown in C.

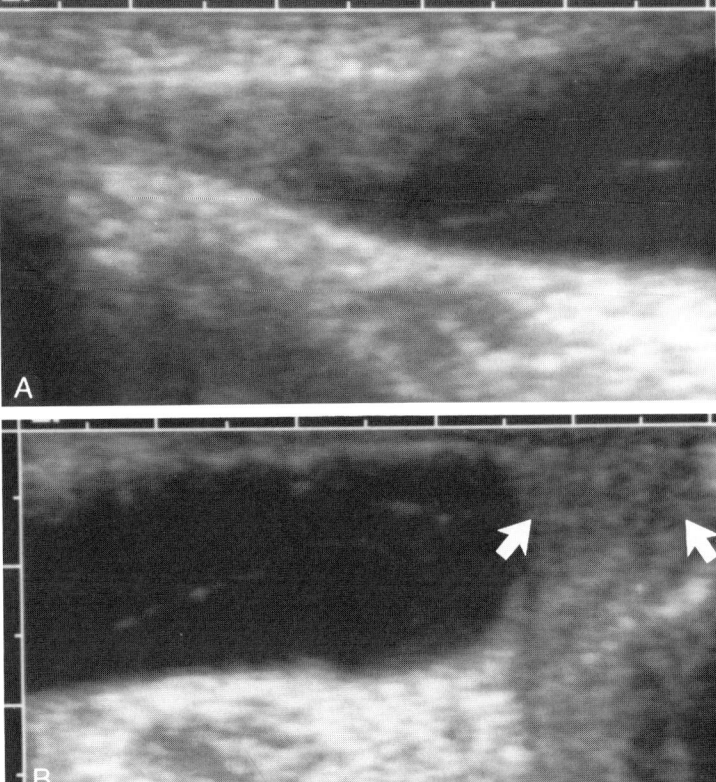

Figure 9–12. A well-defined sac of fluid containing a few echogenic strands extended superiorly along the inguinal canal (A), pushing the testis (arrows) low into the scrotum (B). This was a hydrocele of the spermatic cord.

A hernia, presenting as a scrotal mass, is usually diagnosed as such during clinical examination. Occasionally, we notice while scanning a patient that the extratesticular mass in question has peristaltic activity. The bladder and omentum are much less commonly present in the hernial contents than the bowel (Fig. 9–13).

Presence of a varicocele, dilatation of the pampiniform plexus of veins in the scrotum, is due to increased pressure in the left spermatic vein or its tributaries and reversal of

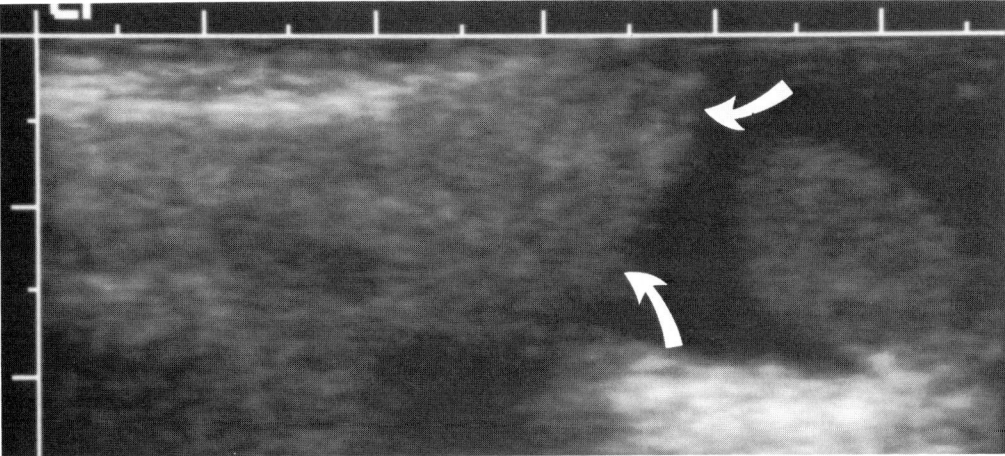

Figure 9–13. When this 4-year-old was being scanned for acute swelling of the scrotum, it was apparent that the soft tissue in the upper portion of the scrotal sac (arrows) was changing throughout the examination. During surgery, this was found to be an omental hernia. The testis is low in the scrotal sac surrounded by hydrocele.

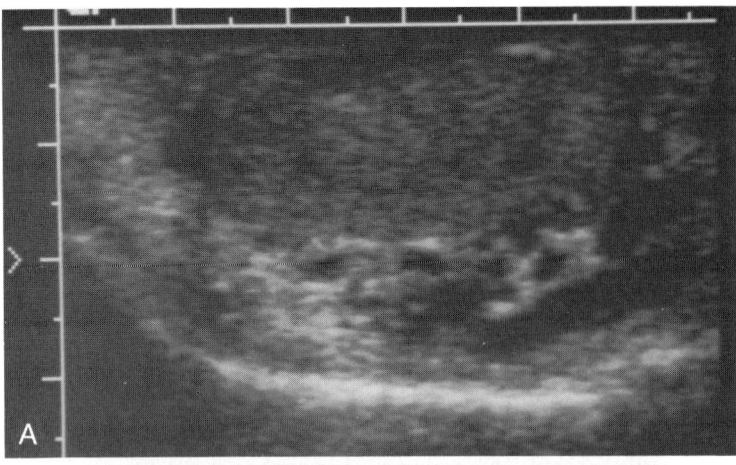

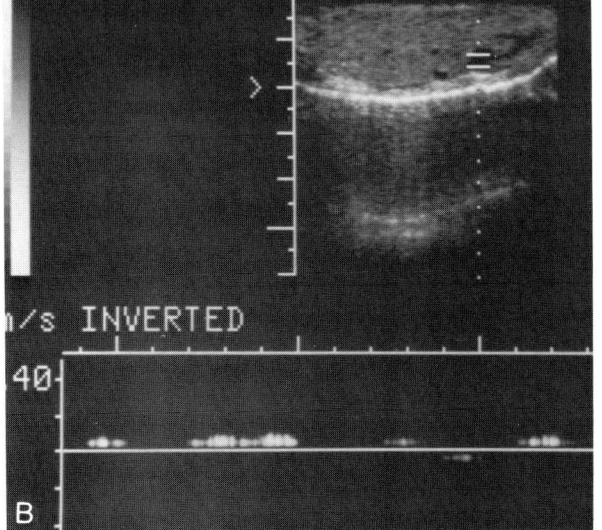

Figure 9–14. This 19-year-old male, who had congenital heart disease, presented with unilateral left scrotal swelling. Longitudinal scan of the left hemiscrotum shows tubular serpiginous structures surrounding the left testis (A). Doppler ultrasonography of these structures showed them to be venous and therefore to constitute a varicocele (B).

venous blood flow. This vascular mass, found almost always on the left, is evident as a mass of tubular anechoic areas that are shown on Doppler examination to have venous blood flow (Fig. 9–14). On clinical evaluation, a Valsalva maneuver increases the size of the mass, as does the erect position. Therefore, ultrasonographic evaluation is not needed for diagnosis. There are two reasons for scanning. First, there is the rare child who presents early (i.e., before puberty) with a varicocele and who has a lesion at the left renal hilum obstructing gonadal venous drainage. We diagnosed a splenic cyst in one young boy who presented with varicocele. The cyst was so situated that it partly obstructed left renal venous blood flow at the hilum of the kidney. Second, there is also increasing concern that the presence of a varicocele, especially prepubertal, is associated with ipsilateral smaller testicular volume. This may have implications regarding later fertility (Sayfan et al., 1988). If testicular volumes are different in a patient with a varicocele, surgical ligation of the veins is recommended (Finkelstein et al., 1986). Radiologists have become interested in producing nonoperative obliteration of the veins by embolization or obstruction of the veins with coils by means of retrograde catheterization of the gonadal vein. Quantitative, "significant" difference in testicular volumes in prepubertal patients has not been established, but postpubertal volumes should not differ by more than 1 cm^3 (Sayfan et al., 1988).

Small cysts of the epididymis may occur at any age, although they seem to be more common as the patient gets older (Fig. 9–15). The epididymis, derived from the mesonephros, consists of vasa efferentia that coalesce

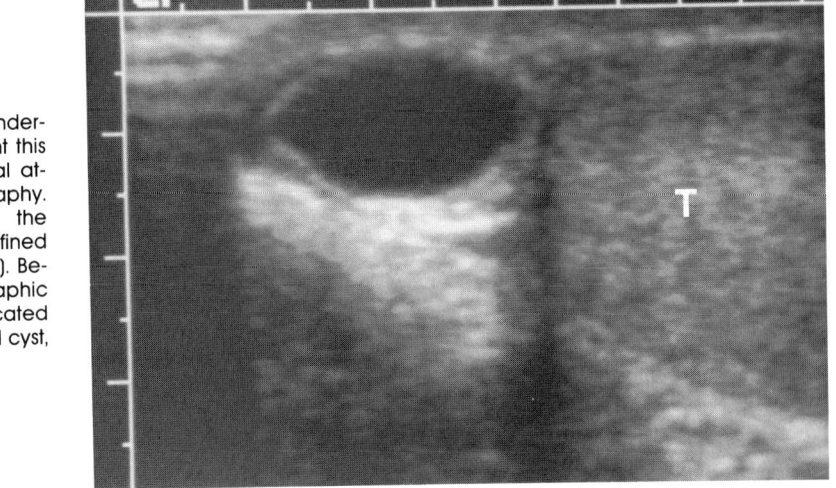

Figure 9–15. Occasional tenderness in the scrotum brought this adolescent boy to medical attention and ultrasonography. The longitudinal scan of the scrotum shows a well-defined cyst superior to the testis (T). Because both the ultrasonographic and clinical diagnosis indicated that this was an epididymal cyst, no surgery was performed.

into a single coiled duct. This duct loops superiorly in relation to the posterior testis and then inferiorly to become the vas deferens, which accompanies spermatic vessels through the inguinal canal.

Simple intratesticular cysts have been described (Altadonna et al., 1988), as have cysts of the tunica albuginea (Hamm et al., 1988). A sharply defined, completely cystic mass can be shelled out of the testis and the remaining parenchyma preserved. Epidermoid cyst is a well-defined, usually spherical mass within the testis, but it has both cystic and solid components. It is difficult to definitely rule out teratoma or malignancy because of the solid matter that is present. The wall appears quite thick because of its fibrotic nature, squamous epithelium, and keratinized debris. Although 86 percent of patients present between the second and fourth decades of life (Fig. 9–16; Nichols et al., 1985), we have seen two infant boys with this lesion. Teratoma consists of all three germ layers, which may be quite differentiated, with, for example, bone, cartilage, skin, and gastrointestinal tract evident on histologic examination. Almost all reported teratomas occurred before 5 years of age; there is a single case report of a 12-year-old boy (Mosli et al., 1985).

Polyorchidism or bilobed testis is a rare cause for a scrotal mass. If the mass has the same homogeneous parenchymal pattern as the ipsilateral and contralateral testes, this rare anomaly is probably present. The accessory testis is usually inferior and smaller. Other rare benign masses include adrenal rest and splenogonadal fusion. Adrenal rest may hypertrophy in boys who have congenital adrenal hyperplasia.

Malignant Scrotal Mass

Although malignancy is foremost in mind when a child presents with a painless scrotal mass, testicular or paratesticular carcinoma

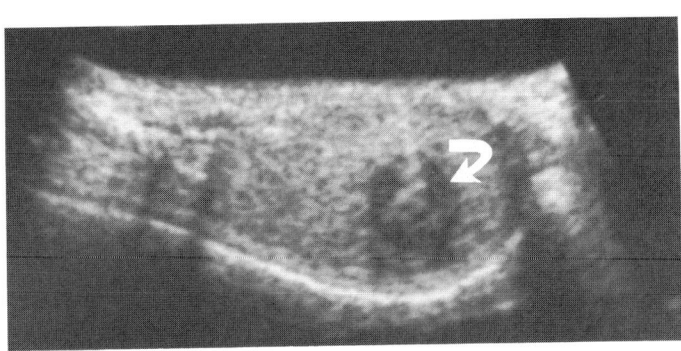

Figure 9–16. This is a longitudinal scan of the testis in an adolescent boy who had noticed a painless testicular mass for several weeks before evaluation. The scan shows a well-defined lesion of mixed echogenicity (arrow). Although the lesion proved to be a benign epidermoid cyst, the possibility of malignancy could not be ruled out preoperatively.

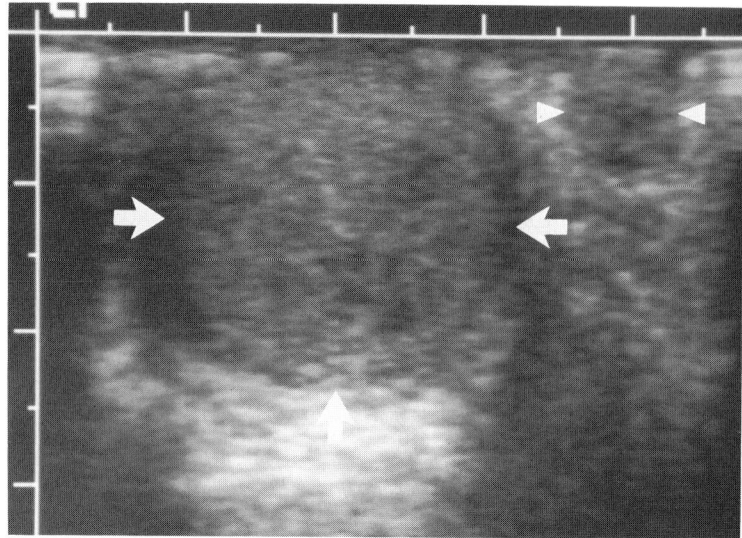

Figure 9–17. Note the marked difference in size between the right testis (arrows) and the left testis (arrowheads) on this transverse scan. This 5-month-old presented with scrotal swelling, and after removal of the right testis, an endodermal sinus tumor was diagnosed.

is a rarity. In black and Asian children, the incidence is particularly low. In boys less than 3 years of age, endodermal sinus tumor (also known as yolk sac tumor and embryonal adenocarcinoma) can occur (Fig. 9–17). It produces high levels in serum of alpha-fetoprotein. These levels fail to return to normal after orchiectomy if metastatic disease is present.

From age 3 years until puberty, the likelihood of testicular carcinoma is very small. Germinal tumors of the testis, when they arise in early puberty, tend to be embryonal carcinoma and teratocarcinoma (Fig. 9–18; Exelby, 1980). Leydig cell tumors may be present in the pediatric age group but are invariably benign. They may present as a testicular mass associated with virilization and are a rare cause of precocious puberty in boys (Fig. 9–6). Sertoli cell tumor, usually benign and another rarity, is associated with gynecomastia. We know of no specific ultrasonographic pattern that allows differentiation between these tumors. Neoplasms of mesenchymal tissue around the testis are all rare. Embryonal rhabdomyosarcoma may arise from the epididymis or spermatic cord. A solid mass, encompassing adnexal structures but separate from testis, was present in one affected child whom we examined (Barth et al., 1984).

It is common to find a benign etiology for painless scrotal mass. However, hydrocele coexists with 25 percent of testicular neoplasms (Exelby, 1980). Any boy who has diagnosed hydrocele and abnormal testis on clinical examination should undergo ultrasonography. If a solid intratesticular mass is diagnosed with ultrasonography, the examination should be expanded to include regions

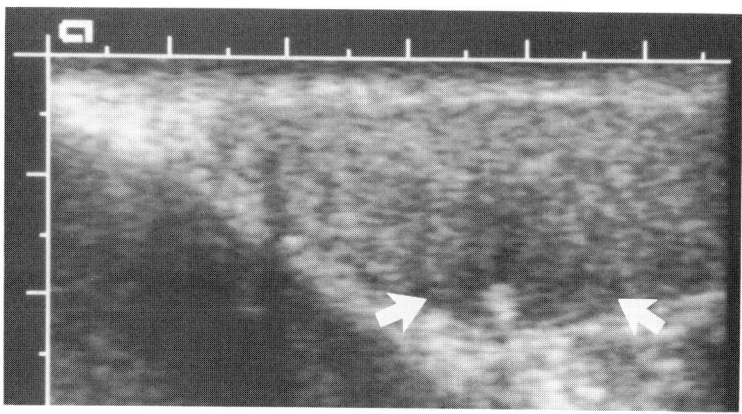

Figure 9–18. A 15-year-old boy presented after 2 months of hemoptysis and weight loss of 30 pounds. Radiographs of the chest, performed to evaluate the pulmonary symptoms, showed multiple metastatic nodules. Sonography of the scrotum was requested as part of a search for a primary tumor. Longitudinal scan of the right testis shows inhomogeneity (arrows) of the inferior portion of the testis. This proved to be embryonal cell carcinoma.

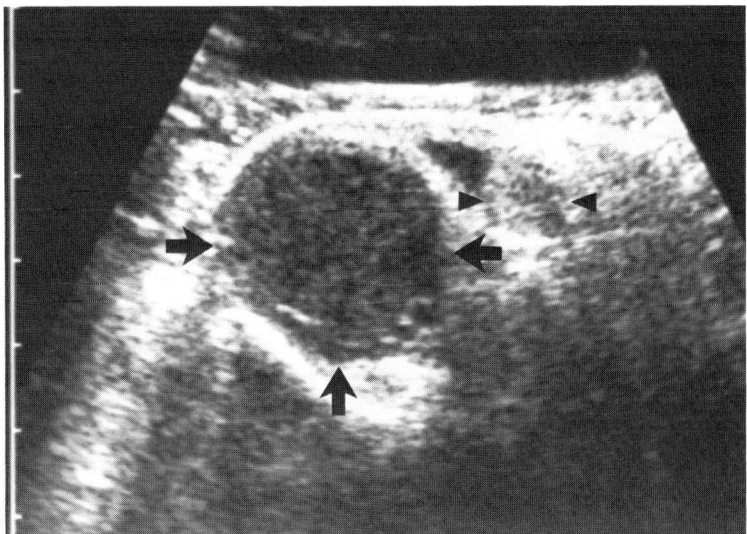

Figure 9-19. An increase in size and abnormal pattern throughout the right testis (arrows), as seen on this transverse ultrasonogram, heralded relapse of acute myelogenous leukemia in this little boy. Arrowheads mark left testis for comparison.

of lymphatic drainage of the testis. In particular, the left renal hilum should be evaluated if a left testicular mass is found. The lymphatics accompany the spermatic cord to the internal ring and then continue cephalad along the spermatic vessels. After crossing the ipsilateral ureter, the channels fan out to periaortic and pericaval nodes up to the level of the renal vessels. Ultrasonography may be able to identify large nodes, but it cannot rule out lymphadenopathy. CT is mandatory for complete evaluation when testicular malignancy is considered likely.

Metastatic disease in the testes occurs with leukemia/lymphoma and, in rare instances, Ewing sarcoma and neuroblastoma (Fig. 9-19). There appears to be an association between leukemic testicular infiltration and renal involvement. Of males with testicular disease, 80 percent have renal infiltration (Sullivan, 1973). Leukemic relapse may present as unilateral or bilateral testicular enlargement. Microscopic involvement is present in both testes, but one testis may be clinically larger. On scans of the larger testis, the leukemic infiltration causes a diffuse decrease in normal parenchymal echogenicity, in comparison with the less involved organ, which may look completely normal (Klein et al., 1986). Neuroblastoma causes a blotchy parenchymal pattern associated with testicular enlargement (Fig. 9-20; Casola et al., 1984).

Painful Unilateral Scrotal Mass

Common causes of painful scrotal mass are listed in Table 9-2. If there has been a history

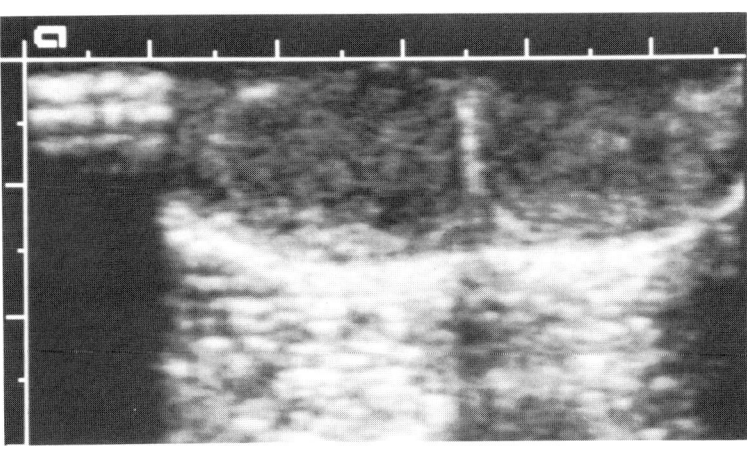

Figure 9-20. Neuroblastoma had already been diagnosed in this child, who had originally presented with a retroperitoneal mass. This transverse scrotal scan shows patchy testicular tissue representing metastatic involvement.

Table 9–2. PAINFUL UNILATERAL SCROTAL MASS

Torsion of testis
Torsion of appendix testis
Epididymitis
Orchitis
Hernia: incarcerated
Trauma

of obvious trauma, the diagnosis and evaluation is directed toward confirming or ruling out testicular rupture. The usual clinical problem is in differentiating those boys with testicular torsion from all others. We have not been enthusiastic, in the past, about using ultrasonography to examine the acutely painful scrotum. A coordinated approach between nuclear medicine and ultrasonography has been recommended (Mueller et al., 1988), and more recently we have been examining more patients who present urgently to the urologist.

Clinicians do get some clues from physical examination of the patient, but their considerations in the differential diagnosis always seem to be the same: torsion versus epididymo-orchitis versus torsion of appendix testis. It has been noted that the cremasteric reflex disappears with torsion (Rabinowitz, 1984). However, it also variably disappears with other conditions that do not necessarily require surgery (Melekos et al., 1988). A history of urinary tract anomalies, infections, or surgery supports a diagnosis of epididymo-orchitis, but in most cases, epididymitis is idiopathic (Gislason et al., 1980; Jarvi et al., 1988). A blue dot, seen through scrotal skin or with transillumination, appears to be specific for torsion of the appendix testis, but it is present in only approximately 20 percent of patients with this condition (Melekos et al., 1988). If the question of testicular torsion is raised, it has to be answered promptly to allow surgical salvage of the affected testicle. Nuclear scintigraphy generally provides reliable physiologic information regarding the presence or absence of blood circulation to the affected side (Majd, 1985). Doppler ultrasonography has been variably successful in the diagnosis of torsion (Bickerstaff et al., 1988). It is important to note that different equipment has been used in different studies. Continuous-wave Doppler ultrasonography records all vascular flow in the path of the beam. Gated, pulsed Doppler ultrasonography records only vascular flow in the area of sampling. A transducer sending out continuous waves may pick up flow from superficial scrotal vessels or from vessels proximal to occlusion if it is not properly angled. Conversely, a gated system will miss flow that is present if the sampled area is just to the side of the vessel. We have found it difficult, with pulsed Doppler scanning only, to establish the presence of testicular vascular flow even in cooperative normal boys. Thus, proving absence of flow is quite a challenge. Color Doppler scanning should make this much less of a problem (Jensen et al., 1990). We have noticed that inflammatory disease increases the color signal because of the stimulation of vascular flow, and this may prove to be very helpful in differential diagnosis.

Early parenchymal changes after torsion are variable and, in our experience, have not been helpful in differentiating inflammatory from vascular insult. In missed torsion and in the neonatal group in which torsion occurred in utero, the testis is firm with a bull's-eye appearance on transverse scans (Fig. 9–21; Zerin et al., 1990). In neonates, torsion tends to be extravaginal. The spermatic cord is less firmly anchored in the inguinal canal, and the cord can twist more easily than in

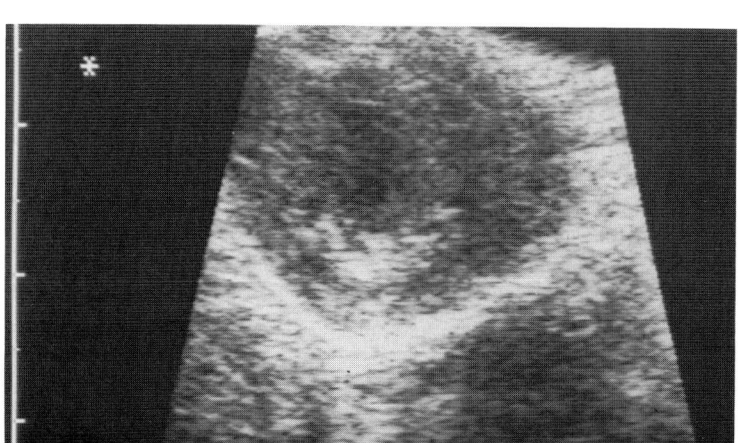

Figure 9–21. The mother noticed asymmetry of the testes in this newborn boy. The left testis was large and, on ultrasonography, displayed the "bull's eye" or "target" appearance typical of intrauterine torsion of the testis.

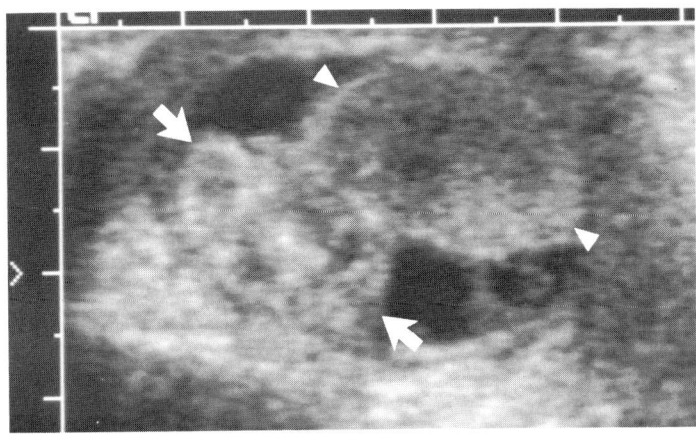

Figure 9–22. Transverse ultrasonogram of the left scrotal sac shows a markedly enlarged epididymis (arrows), inhomogeneous pattern of the testis (arrowheads), and associated hydrocele. This 11-year-old patient had presented with left-sided scrotal pain, nausea, and vomiting. Doppler study was not diagnostic of torsion, but the radionuclide study was. In the operating room, torsion of the entire testicle was apparent. Because it was not necrotic, it was not removed. Orchiopexy was performed on the right side.

the older child or adolescent. In a study of 100 boys who presented with acute scrotal pain, the 42 who had testicular torsion presented either as neonates or around puberty, with a peak incidence at 13 years (Figs. 9–22, 9–23; Melekos et al., 1988). In the older boys, redundant tunica vaginalis ("bell-clapper" deformity) or loose attachment of the epididymis to the testis is thought to predispose the testis to intravaginal torsion. It is of note that in a a report of 7 patients with unilateral anorchism, 5 of 6 operated upon had the bell-clapper deformity of abnormal testicular fixation (Bellinger, 1985). The absence of one testis may be a sign of generalized maldevelopment that predisposes the other testis to torsion.

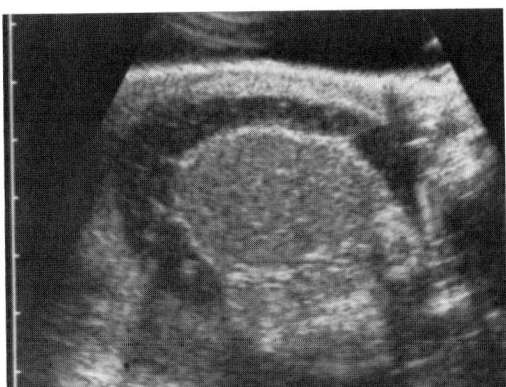

Figure 9–23. Right scrotal edema and pain were the presenting symptoms in this 16-year-old boy. Radionuclide scan showed flow to the right testis at the time, and a diagnosis of epididymitis was made. Increasing pain brought him back to the hospital, at which time he was treated with intravenous antibiotics without resolution of symptoms. Ultrasonography shows the scrotal sac to be filled with echogenic fluid representing hematocele. Hemorrhagic infarction of the testis from torsion resulted in removal of the testis.

Epididymitis and orchitis, although historically linked with previous urinary tract anomalies, infections, and surgery, are in our practice much more common than the old textbooks suggest and typically not secondary to known causes. In one study of 41 patients with suspected torsion, 15 had epididymitis, and only 4 of these patients were older than 18 years (Bickerstaff et al., 1988). In another study, 12 percent of pediatric patients who presented with an acutely painful scrotum had epididymitis or orchitis or both (Melekos et al., 1988). In yet another study of 25 boys who had acute epididymitis, only 3 were identified as having predisposing urologic problems (Gislason et al., 1980). Since the vaccine against mumps has come into use in the United States, orchitis from mumps is a rarity. Other viruses (e.g., coxsackie) can cause either unilateral or bilateral testicular swelling. Pure epididymitis usually results in a swollen, relatively echolucent mass replacing the normal epididymis. A reactive hydrocele may be present. The adjacent testis may be blotchy in pattern, either from edema or from primary involvement (Fig. 9–24). Nuclear scintigraphy typically shows a hotly perfused area corresponding to the epididymis and testis and reflecting the hyperemia from inflammation.

Ultrasonography is most useful (1) in diagnosing suspected testicular abscess in patients who do not respond to antibiotics or (2) in suggesting the diagnosis of inflammation when a patient has relatively few symptoms but presents with scrotal swelling. Abscess is often very painful. It is similar to renal abscess in its appearance and progression; an obvious wall develops only late in the course.

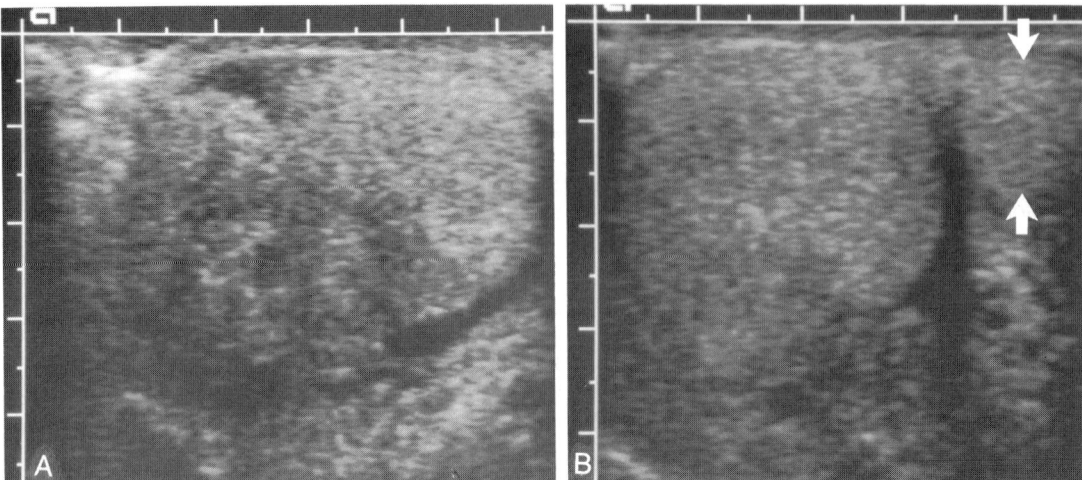

Figure 9–24. Longitudinal (**A**) and transverse (**B**) scans of the right hemiscrotum show marked enlargement and inhomogeneity of the right testis and epididymis with a small reactive hydrocele. The left testis (arrows, **B**) is normal. Radionuclide study showed perfusion of both testes. The condition improved with antibiotics. No underlying etiology for the patient's epididymo-orchitis was found. Note how similar these scans are to those in Figures 9–22 and 9–23.

The appendix testis, also called the hydatid (Latin for "drop of water") of Morgagni, is the vestige of the embryonic müllerian duct. It occupies the superior groove between the testis and epididymis. Its torsion results in scrotal pain and a clinical picture often indistinguishable from that of testicular torsion. In addition, on ultrasonography, it is often difficult to distinguish appendicular torsion from epididymitis with a reactive hydrocele (Fig. 9–25). The radionuclide scans usually rule out testicular torsion in such cases, and treatment is supportive rather than surgical for both epididymitis and appendicular torsion.

Acute trauma, usually from a direct blow, is a surgical problem if the testis has ruptured. Ultrasonographic scans in multiple

Figure 9–25. Confusing history and findings on physical examination seem to be the rule when boys present with painful scrotal swelling. This 11½-year-old boy had suffered mild blunt trauma to the right hemiscrotum 2 days previously. Examination revealed enlargement of the hemiscrotum. The skin was red and indurated. Radionuclide scans had shown bilateral perfusion of testicular tissue. The longitudinal scan shows an echogenic mass (arrow) adjacent to the testis (arrowheads). There is a small reactive hydrocele present. Note the thickening of the skin. During surgery, inflammatory epididymitis secondary to torsion of the appendix testis was discovered. The testis itself was normal.

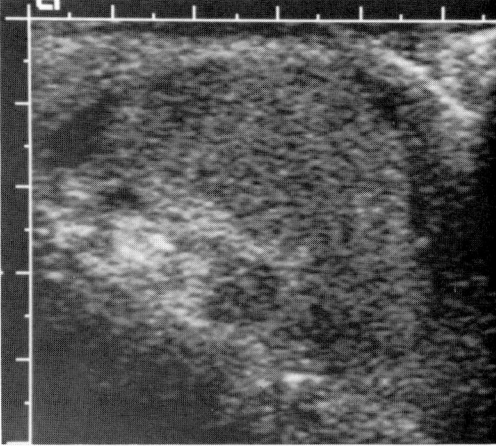

Figure 9–26. This 19-year-old had been kicked in the groin 2 hours before admission to the hospital. Ultrasonography was performed immediately. The testicular margins are indistinct, which indicates that the tunica albuginea was no longer intact. In the operating room, necrotic seminiferous tubules were found to be extruding from the testis. These were excised, and the tunica was sutured.

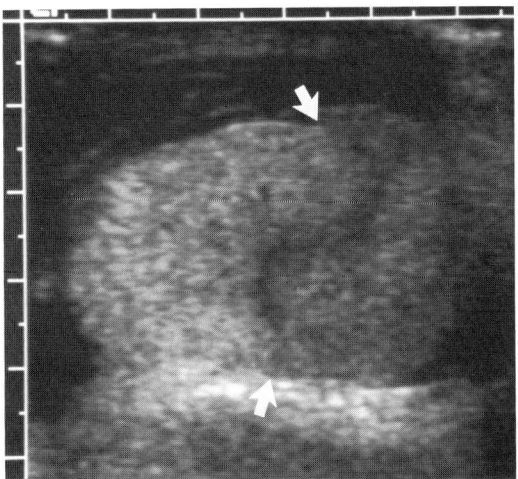

Figure 9–27. There is a fracture line (arrows) through the testis. This injury to a 16-year-old resulted from a line drive in a baseball game. Often, after trauma, there is so much hemorrhage in the scrotal sac that it is difficult to differentiate the testis from associated and adjacent hematocele.

planes are directed toward confirming or ruling out integrity of the tunica albuginea, determining whether normal, undisturbed parenchymal homogeneity is present, and, if possible, documenting arterial flow to the testis (Figs. 9–26, 9–27). Hematoma typically envelops the testis, and the epididymis usually cannot be differentiated as a discrete structure. Minor trauma that results in a hematocele should always raise the question of underlying tumor, and subsequent scans should be viewed with a high degree of suspicion.

In summary, for those boys with an acutely painful scrotal mass, nuclear scintigraphy, with ^{99m}Tc-pertechnetate, is the first study of choice. The examination takes about 20 minutes and generally distinguishes testicular torsion from inflammatory disease. Ultrasonography may be helpful for boys who have indeterminate scintiscans or whose scintigraphic results are at odds with the clinical impression. In boys with recent acute trauma, careful ultrasonography can confirm or rule out testicular rupture. Examinations with Doppler ultrasonography should be compared with those of the normal side, and one should take into consideration the type of equipment used for this technique.

Miscellaneous

Bilateral scrotal swelling that is uncomfortable rather than painful is the clinical picture of idiopathic scrotal edema. This unusual condition, which may be a localized presentation of angioneurotic edema, causes edema of scrotal skin and contents, may be associated with eosinophilia, and tends to affect young boys. Tissue planes are indistinct, and the ultrasonographic picture is of fuzzy borders and poorly defined structures. This is not a technical problem but rather the result of diffuse edema (Fig. 9–28). Surgery is not indicated; the condition is self-limited and has no apparent sequelae. Erysipelas causes edema but is associated with obvious inflammation of the soft tissues. Postoperative scrotal edema may follow otherwise uncomplicated repair of inguinal hernias (Archer et al., 1988). Testicular microlithiasis is an uncommon entity that results in echogenic flecks within the parenchyma of the testes (Fig. 9–29). It may be associated with chromosomal abnormalities in some patients (Jaramillo et al., 1989).

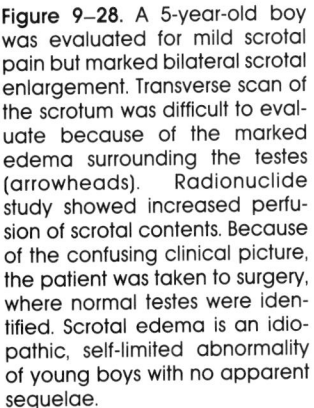

Figure 9–28. A 5-year-old boy was evaluated for mild scrotal pain but marked bilateral scrotal enlargement. Transverse scan of the scrotum was difficult to evaluate because of the marked edema surrounding the testes (arrowheads). Radionuclide study showed increased perfusion of scrotal contents. Because of the confusing clinical picture, the patient was taken to surgery, where normal testes were identified. Scrotal edema is an idiopathic, self-limited abnormality of young boys with no apparent sequelae.

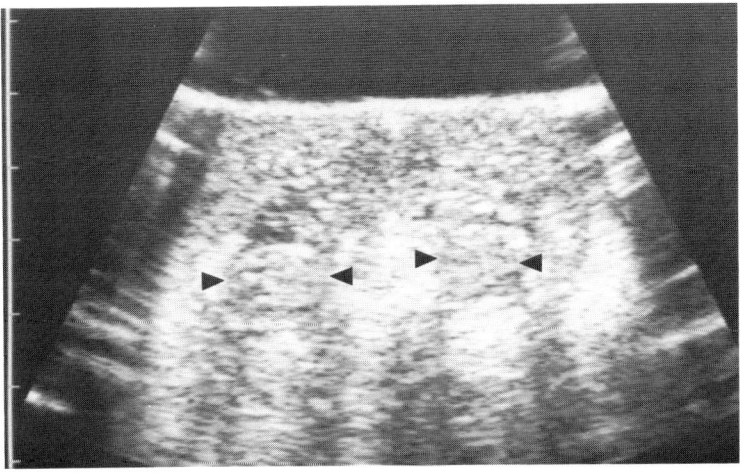

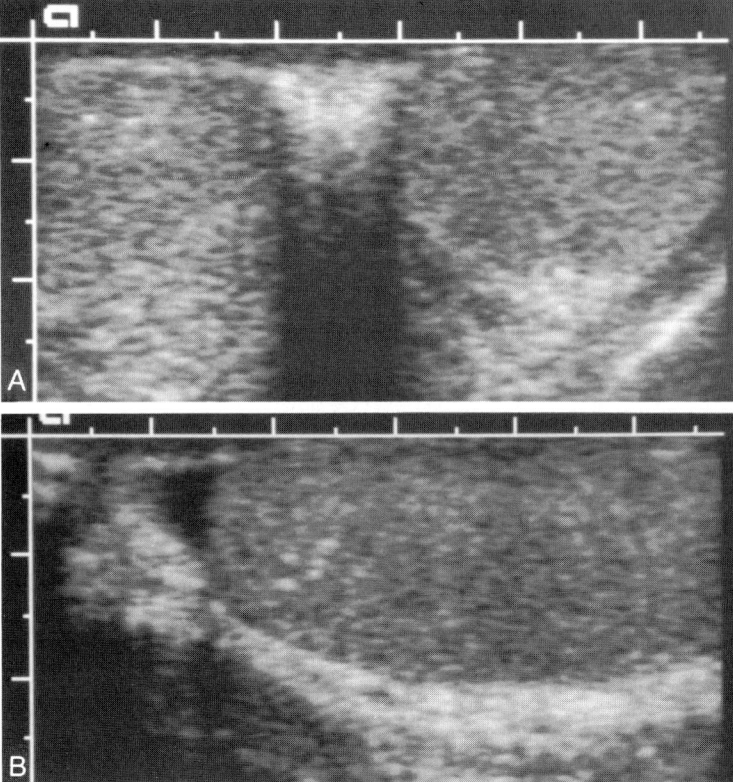

Figure 9–29. Transverse (A) and longitudinal (B) scans of the left testis in a 14-year-old boy, who presented with intermittent mild pain in the groin, show speckles of increased echogenicity indicative of testicular microlithiasis. Often, this is of unknown etiology. It may, however, be associated with chromosomal anomalies.

PRIMARY AND SECONDARY AMENORRHEA

For the adolescent girl who has primary amenorrhea, the major role for ultrasonography is to document anatomy. Are both ovaries, the uterus, and the cervix present? Presentation with amenorrhea and pelvic mass is discussed in Chapter 8.

Primary amenorrhea exists when an adolescent girl fails to achieve menarche by the age of 16 years (Soules, 1987). Thelarche and adrenarche should occur before the age of 14 years. The etiologies of primary amenorrhea could fill an entire page, and in fine print, but the six main divisions are (1) general disorders of the central nervous system; (2) general medical conditions (including adrenal abnormalities); (3) hypothalamic disorders; (4) pituitary masses or other abnormalities; (5) gonadal dysgenesis, agenesis, tumor, or insensitivity; and (6) uterine-vaginal anomalies.

Failure of stimulation of normal ovarian tissue because of faults in the hormonal loop that connects hypothalamus, pituitary, and gonad results in ultrasonographic findings of a small uterus (i.e., prepubertal) and ovaries that are each less than 1 cm^3 in volume. For example, Kallmann syndrome is characterized by sexual infantilism and anosmia. It is a very unusual cause of primary amenorrhea, but it is associated with a small uterus and prepubertal ovaries. The fault lies in the brain with partial or complete agenesis of the olfactory bulb and hypothalamic abnormalities. It belongs in the grouping of hypothalamic disorders. Because follicle-stimulating hormone is the first gonadotropin to increase in puberty, its absence prevents development of obvious follicles, and the ovaries appear acystic and are of relatively uniform echogenicity. Proving that ovaries are absent or dysgenetic is difficult because the normal prepubertal ovaries may be poorly discriminated from the adjacent fallopian tube, bowel, or even lymph nodes.

Gonadal dysgenesis accounts for approximately one third of all cases of primary amenorrhea (Soules, 1987). Most patients who have dysgenetic gonads have a diagnostic chromosomal abnormality: about one half of this group have classic Turner syndrome (45,X0); the rest have a variety of other ab-

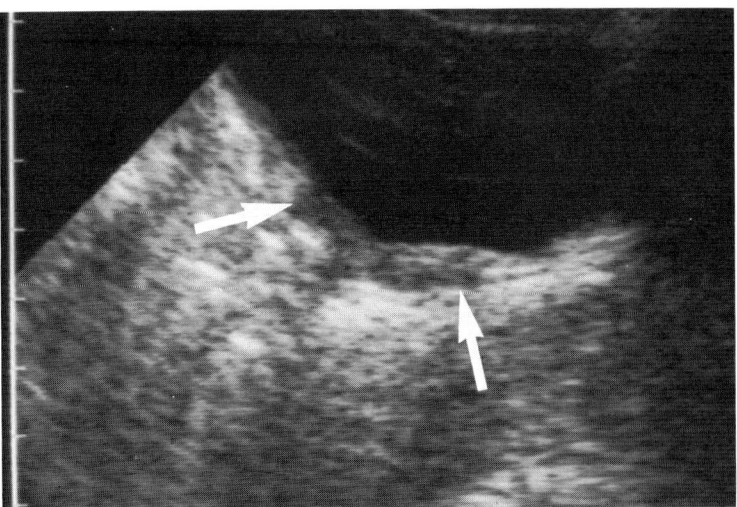

Figure 9–30. This 14-year-old girl with classic Turner syndrome had ultrasonograms of the pelvis that showed no discernible ovarian tissue. The longitudinal scan through the bladder shows a tiny uterus (arrows).

normalities of the X chromosome. Ultrasonography in those with classic Turner syndrome usually reveals a uterus of prepubertal size and "absence" of ovaries, as streak ovaries cannot be visualized as such. Ultrasonograms of patients who have chromosomal mosaicism or other alterations of the X chromosome are variably abnormal. Ovaries may be absent or small or may appear normal. The uterus ranges in size from prepubertal to adult (Fig. 9–30). Mixed gonadal dysgenesis associated with the presence of a Y chromosome predisposes the carrier to gonadoblastoma. Affected children usually have presented in the neonatal period with ambiguous genitalia. Because of the frequent association of renal anomalies with gonadal dysgenesis, kidneys should always be scanned.

Absence of the uterus as a cause of primary amenorrhea is uncommon. Mayer-Rokitansky-Küster-Hauser syndrome and testicular feminization are the two conditions to be considered in this situation. Although rare, Mayer-Rokitansky-Küster-Hauser syndrome is the second most common structural cause of primary amenorrhea. The ovaries are normal; therefore, the girl has developed secondary sex characteristics. Congenital absence of the vagina and absence or hypoplasia of the uterus are secondary to failure of development of normal müllerian derivatives (Fig. 9–31). Because of time-related embryologic faults, the kidneys and the skeleton are affected in 50 and 12 percent of patients, respectively. Renal anomalies include unilateral agenesis, horseshoe kidney, and cross-fused ectopia. The skel-

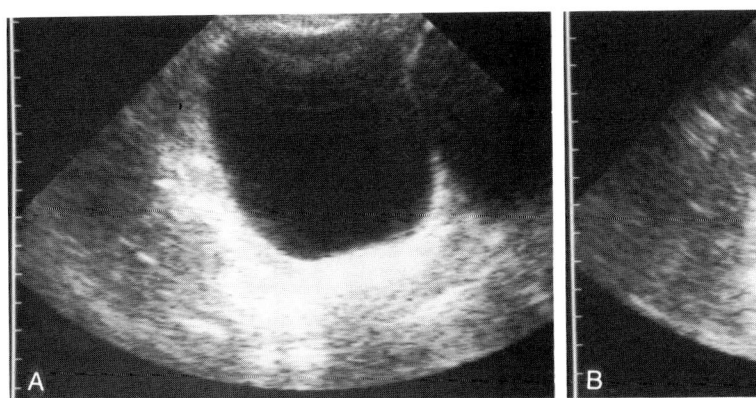
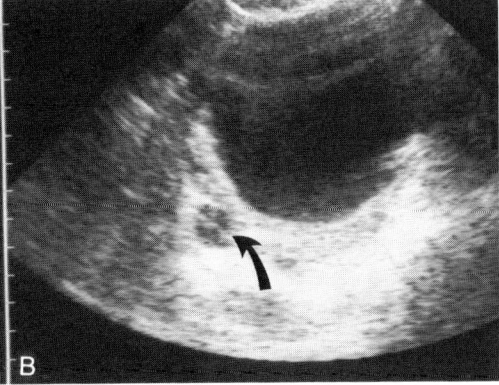

Figure 9–31. These scans are of a 15-year-old girl who had secondary sex characteristics but primary amenorrhea. Physical examination had suggested vaginal and uterine agenesis. This was confirmed on the longitudinal line scan of the pelvis (A), which shows no uterine tissue. Longitudinal scan of the right adnexa (B) shows an ovary (arrow). Scans of the left adnexa were similar.

etal anomalies are usually spinal and include segmentation defects and wedge and rudimentary vertebrae (Rosenberg et al., 1986). This syndrome, therefore, merges with the MURCS complex (*m*üllerian, *r*enal, and *c*ervical *s*omite anomalies).

Patients who have testicular feminization are genotypically male (XY) but phenotypically female because they have end-organ insensitivity to testosterone. They have neither a uterus nor ovaries and therefore do not develop breasts unless given exogenous estrogen. Intra-abdominal testes are present and may be found in the pelvis as small masses of soft tissue (Kangarloo, 1980).

Primary amenorrhea is also caused by radiotherapy or chemotherapy. An increasing number of girls who have survived malignancy in childhood are presenting to gynecologists and endocrinologists because of pubertal failure. Ovarian failure occurs in most patients who have had either a single dose of radiation (650 to 750 rad) or a fractionated dose of between 1500 and 2500 rad (Perez, 1984). We suspect that arrest of uterine growth may be a direct result of radiotherapy. Uterine hypoplasia caused by lack of hormonal stimulation is an indirect result of pelvic irradiation (Fig. 9–32). We are interested in following previously irradiated girls who are receiving therapy with hormonal replacement, to determine whether the uterus can respond in size to exogenous estrogen and progesterone. We also are following one adolescent who underwent transplantation of one ovary into the armpit before extensive pelvic and abdominal irradiation. At puberty, the transplanted ovary began to enlarge, and apparent follicular cysts developed. The girl has secondary sexual characteristics but is amenorrheic, probably because of the uterine hypoplasia (Fig. 9–33).

Pregnancy is the most common reason for secondary amenorrhea. Ultrasonography is not advocated as a means of diagnosis; currently available urinary and serologic testing is the appropriate method.

Approximately 50 percent of patients with

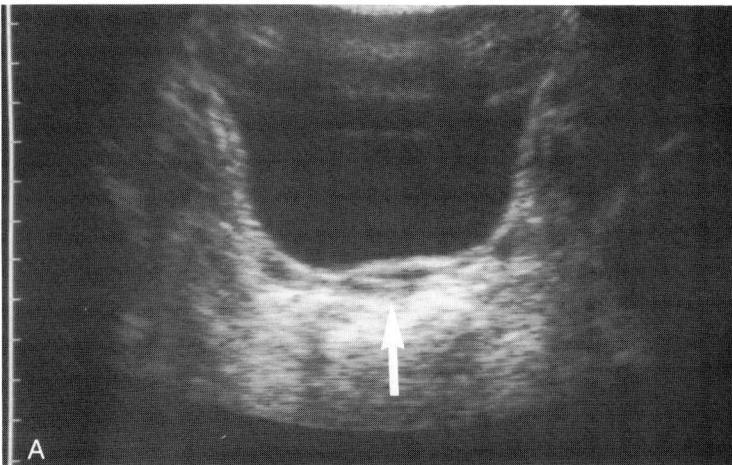
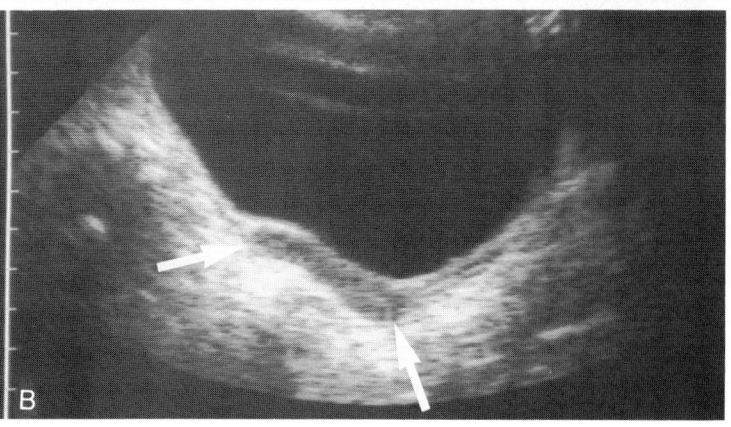

Figure 9–32. Total body irradiation and chemotherapy had been given for acute lymphoblastic leukemia when this 16-year-old girl was a child. She presented with delayed puberty. Her transverse (**A**) and longitudinal (**B**) scans of the pelvis show a very small uterus (arrows) and tiny adnexa with no evidence of follicular cysts. Uterine hypoplasia is likely secondary to both the irradiation and the lack of hormonal stimulation.

Figure 9–33. At the time of surgery for Wilms tumor in this girl, the surgeons (S. Schuster and J. Upton) removed one ovary and transplanted it to the armpit; vascular anastomosis was also performed. She then received total abdominal irradiation. Painful swelling of the transplanted ovary occurred when the patient was 12 years old. On the scan of her arm (A), the ovary (arrows) appears large and cystic with one large cyst predominating. The scans of the pelvis (B), however, show a small uterus (arrows) with no evidence of endometrial reaction.

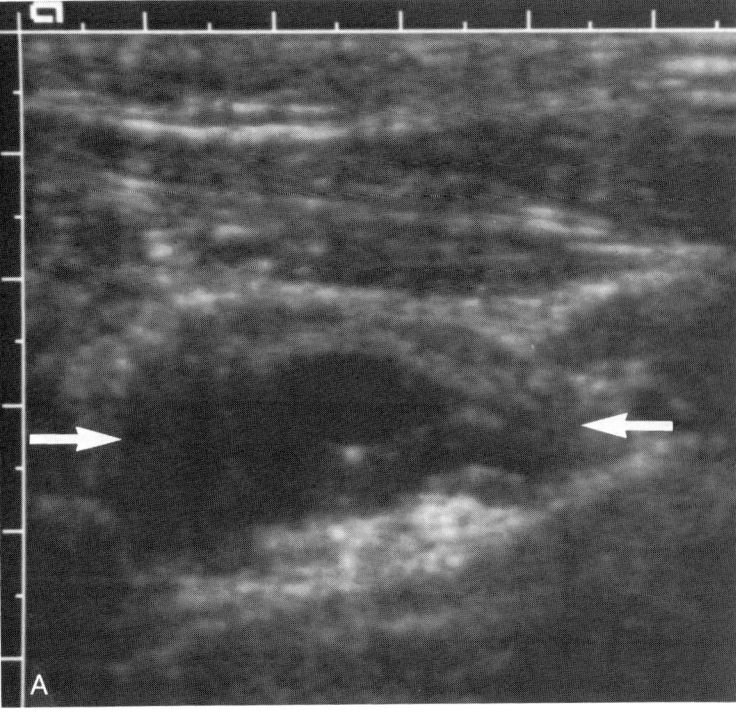

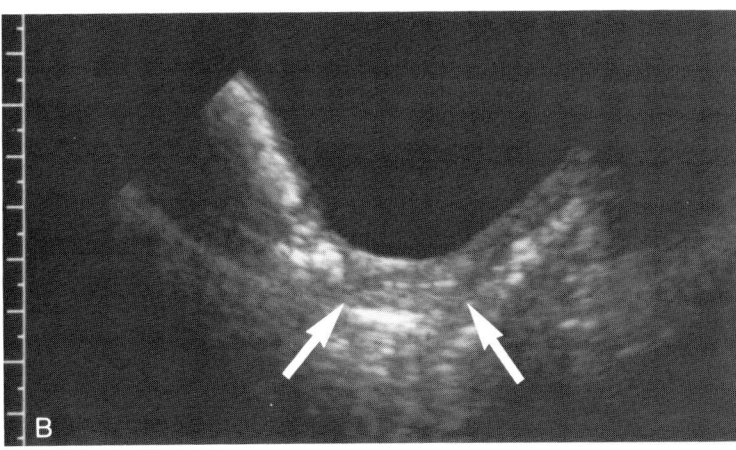

polycystic disease of the ovaries experience amenorrhea, usually secondary (Goldzieher, 1981). The syndrome is no longer defined only by the triad of oligomenorrhea, obesity, and hirsutism associated with very large ovaries, which has been labeled Stein-Leventhal syndrome. An elevated level of luteinizing hormone and an elevated ratio of luteinizing hormone to follicle-stimulating hormone reflects the abnormal feedback loop between pituitary, hypothalamus, and ovaries, which now defines the syndrome. In most large series, the ovaries are normal in size in about one third of patients. In affected adolescent patients whose ovarian changes secondary to the abnormal hormonal influences have not yet fully developed, it is common to find normal-appearing ovaries on ultrasonography. Our role is not to make the diagnosis of polycystic disease, although we do become interested when we see multiple cysts in large ovaries (Fig. 9–34). Rather, we are attempting to rule out primary virilizing tumors and, in those with an established diagnosis, to rule out secondary neoplasm. Ovarian tumors of all types occur with increased frequency in patients with polycystic disease of the ovaries. This frequency has been estimated in the literature to range from 4.6 to 20 percent of affected persons (Babak-

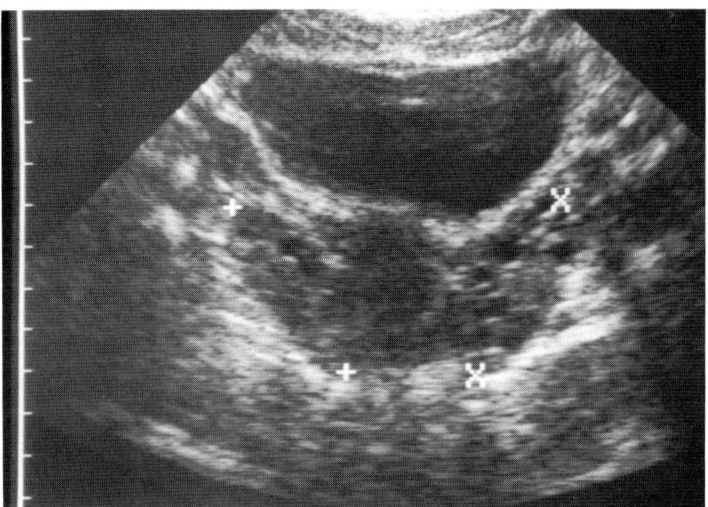

Figure 9-34. A 17-year-old girl with menstrual irregularity had this transverse pelvic scan, which shows very large ovaries containing multiple small cysts. The ratio of luteinizing hormone to follicle-stimulating hormone was more than 3:1, which is also typical of polycystic ovaries (normal is approximately 1:1). The major role of ultrasonography for patients who present with abnormal hormonal studies in the presence of irregular or absent menses is to rule out primary tumors of the ovary. The left ovary is between the plus signs, and the right ovary is between the X signs. (Reprinted by permission of Elsevier Science Publishing Co. from Share JC, Teele RL: Ultrasound of the pediatric and adolescent patient. Clin Pract Gynecol 1989; 1(2):72–92. Copyright 1989 by Elsevier Science Publishing Co., Inc.)

nia, 1978). However, the true incidence, now that the ultrasonographic spectrum of disease has been widened but the hormonal criteria have been more strictly defined, is unknown.

Secondary amenorrhea is associated with weight loss in athletes who are physically active and in anorectic young women who are getting inadequate nutrition. Enlarged ovaries with multiple follicles have been described in women with hypothalamic-ovarian dysfunction secondary to weight loss. Thus on ultrasonography their ovaries look similar to those of many patients who have polycystic disease (Futterweit, 1988).

Secondary amenorrhea can be caused by both virilizing and feminizing ovarian tumors. These include androblastoma (also called "arrhenoblastoma") and granulosa-theca cell tumors, respectively. Cystadenoma, cystadenofibroma, and dysgerminoma are occasionally hormonally active as well.

In summary, the complete ultrasonographic examination for a girl who presents with primary amenorrhea should include good views of uterus and ovaries if present, characterization of ovarian tissue (i.e., obvious follicles present or inapparent), and scans of each kidney and each adrenal area. Small tumors of the adrenal gland and adrenal hyperplasia cannot be ruled out from a normal result of an ultrasonographic study. If there is concern regarding an androgen-secreting tumor, CT scanning is recommended.

The ultrasonograms *must* be related to the endocrinologic findings. In addition, it is important that rectal examination be done before the ultrasonography. If the clinician is doubtful that a uterus is present, the ultrasonographic study that proves its absence should be done and discussed with the family immediately. This is a very emotion-laden problem for both patient and parents, and ultrasonographers should be circumspect in their comments during the examination.

REFERENCES

Ambiguous Genitalia

Donahoe PK, Crawford JD: Ambiguous genitalia in the newborn. *In* Welch KJ, Randolph JG, Ravitch MM et al (eds): Pediatric Surgery (4th ed). Chicago, Year Book Medical Publishers 1986, 1363–1376.

Hauffa BP, Menzel D, Stolecke H: Age-related changes in adrenal size during the first year of life in normal newborns, infants and patients with congenital adrenal hyperplasia due to 21-hydroxylase deficiency: Comparison of ultrasound and hormonal parameters. Eur J Pediatr 1988; 148:43–49.

Pagon RA: Diagnostic approach to the newborn with ambiguous genitalia. Ped Clin North Am 1987; 34:1019–1031.

Wenstrup RJ, Pagon RA: Female pseudo-hermaphroditism with anorectal, müllerian duct, and urinary tract malformations: Report of four cases. J Pediatr 1985; 107:751–754.

Sexual Precocity

Fakhry J, Khoury A, Kotval PS, et al: Sonography of autonomous follicular ovarian cysts in precocious pseudopuberty. J Ultrasound Med 1988; 7:597–603.

Hall DA, Crowley WF, Wierman ME, et al: Sonographic monitoring of LHRH analogue therapy in idiopathic precocious puberty in young girls. JCU 1986; 14:331–338.

Share JC, Teele RL: Ultrasound of the pediatric and adolescent patient. Clin Pract Gynecol 1989; 3:72–92.
Styne DM, Kaplan SL: Normal and abnormal puberty in the female. Pediatr Clin North Am 1979; 26:123–148.

Scrotal Ultrasonography

Cryptorchidism

Arey LB: Developmental Anatomy (7th ed). Philadelphia: WB Saunders 1974, 335.
Beasley SW, Hutson JM: The role of the gubernaculum in testicular descent. J Urol 1988: 140:1191–1193.
Beomonte ZB, Vicentini C, Masciocchi C, et al: Magnetic resonance imaging in the localization of undescended abdominal testes. Eur Urol 1990; 17:145–148.
Blandy J: Lecture Notes on Urology (3rd ed). London: Blackwell Scientific Publications 1982.
Elder JS: Cryptorchidism: Isolated and associated with other genitourinary defects. Pediatr Clin North Am 1987; 34:1033–1053.
Fallon B, Welton M, Hawtrey C: Congenital anomalies associated with cryptorchidism. J Urol 1982; 127:91–93.
Fonkalsrud EW: Testicular undescent and torsion. Pediatr Clin North Am 1987; 34:1305–1317.
Friedland GW, Chang P: The role of imaging in the management of the impalpable undescended testis. AJR 1988; 151:1107–1111.
Johansen TE, Larmo A: Ultrasonography in undescended testes. Acta Radiol 1988; 29:159–163.
Kier R, McCarthy S, Rosenfield AT, et al: Nonpalpable testes in young boys: Evaluation with MR imaging. Radiology 1988; 169:429–433.
Pappis CH, Argianas SA, Bousgas D, et al: Unsuspected urological anomalies in asymptomatic cryptorchid boys. Pediatr Radiol 1988; 18:51–53.
Penny R: The testis. Pediatr Clin North Am 1979; 26:107–121.
Rosenfield AT, Blair DN, McCarthy S, et al: Society of Uroradiology Award paper. The pars infravaginalis gubernaculi: Importance in the identification of the undescended testis. AJR 1989; 153:775–778.
Weiss RM, Carter AR, Rosenfield AT: High resolution real-time ultrasonography in the localization of the undescended testis. J Urol 1986; 135:936–938.

Painless Unilateral Scrotal Mass

Altadonna V, Snyder HM 3d, Rosenberg HK, et al: Simple cysts of the testis in children: Preoperative diagnosis by ultrasound and excision with testicular preservation. J Urol 1988; 140:1505–1507.
Bahnson RR, Slasky BS, Ernstoff MS, et al: Sonographic characteristics of epidermoid cyst of testicle. Urology 1990; 35:508–510.
Baker WC, Bishai MB, Devere White RW: Misleading testicular masses. Urology 1988; 31:111–113.
Barth RA, Teele RL, Colodny A, et al: Asymptomatic scrotal masses in children. Radiology 1984; 152:65–68.
Casola G, Scheible W, Leopold GR: Neuroblastoma metastatic to the testis: Ultrasonographic screening as an aid to clinical staging. Radiology 1984; 151:475–476.
Exelby PR: Testicular cancer in children. Cancer 1980; 45:1803–1809.
Finkelstein MS, Rosenberg HK, Snyder HM 3d, et al: Ultrasound evaluation of scrotum in pediatrics. Urology 1986; 27:1–9.
Hamm B, Fobbe F, Loy V: Testicular cysts: Differentiation with US and clinical findings. Radiology 1988; 168:19–23.
Howe D, Foster ME, Gateley C, et al: Clinical value of scrotal ultrasound in the investigation of scrotal pathology. Br J Urol 1988; 62:263–266.
Kaplan GW, Cromie WC, Kelalis PP, et al: Prepubertal yolk sac testicular tumors—Report of the testicular tumor registry. J Urol 1988; 140:1109–1112.
Klein EA, Kay R, Norris DG, et al: Noninvasive testicular screening in childhood leukemia. J Urol 1986; 136:864–866.
Kromann-Anderson B, Hansen LB, Larsen PN, et al: Clinical versus ultrasonographic evaluation of scrotal disorders. Br J Urol 1988; 61:350–353.
Krone KD, Carroll BA: Scrotal ultrasound. Radiol Clin North Am 1985; 23:121–139.
McAlister WH, Manley CB: Bilobed testicle. Pediatr Radiol 1987; 17:82.
Mosli HA, Carpenter B, Schillinger JF: Teratoma of the testis in a pubertal child. J Urol 1985; 133:105–106.
Nichols J, Kandzari S, Elyaderani MK, et al: Epidermoid cyst of testis: A report of 3 cases. J Urol 1985; 133:286–287.
Rifkin MD, Kurtz AB, Goldberg BB: Epididymis examined by ultrasound. Correlation with pathology. Radiology 1984; 151:187–190.
Ring KS, Axelrod SL, Burbige KA, et al: Meconium hydrocele: An unusual etiology of a scrotal mass in the newborn. J Urol 1989; 141:1172–1173.
Sayfan J, Soffer Y, Manor H, et al: Varicocele in youth. A therapeutic dilemma. Ann Surg 1988; 207:223–227.
Simone JV, Rivera G: Management of acute leukemia. In Sutow WW, Fernback DJ, Vietti TJ (eds): Clinical Pediatric Oncology (3rd ed). St Louis: CV Mosby 1984, 394.
Tammala TL, Mattila SI, Hellström PA, et al: Polyorchidism with normal spermatogenesis, diagnosed preoperatively by ultrasound. A case report. Scand J Urol Nephrol 1989; 23:71–73.
Upton JD, Das S: Benign intrascrotal neoplasms. J Urol 1986; 135:504–506.
Wyllie GG: Varicocele and puberty—the critical factor? Br J Urol 1985; 57:194–196.
Zerin JM, DiPietro MA, Grignon A, et al: Testicular infarction in the newborn: Ultrasound findings. Pediatr Radiol 1990; 20:329–330.

Painful Scrotal Mass

Bellinger MF: The blind-ending vas: The fate of the contralateral testis. J Urol 1985; 133:644–645.
Bickerstaff KI, Sethia K, Murie JA: Doppler ultrasonography in the diagnosis of acute scrotal pain. Br J Surg 1988; 75:238–239.
Cooper SG, Sherman SB, Gross RI, et al: Ultrasound diagnosis of acute scrotal hemorrhage in Henoch-Schonlein purpura. J Clin Ultrasound 1988; 16:353–357.
Das S, Singer A: Controversies of perinatal torsion of the spermatic cord: A review, survey and recommendations. J Urol 1990; 143:231–233.
Gislason T, Noronha RFX, Gregory JG: Acute epididymitis in boys: A 5-year retrospective study. J Urol 1980; 124:533–534.
Jarvi K, Churchill BM, McLorie G: Diagnostic yield in childhood epididymitis (Abstract). J Urol 1988; 139(4, part 2):163A.
Jensen MC, Lee KP, Halls JM, et al: Color Doppler sonography in testicular torsion. JCU 1990; 18:446–448.
MacDermott JP, Gray BK, Stewart PA: Traumatic rupture of the testis. Br J Urol 1988; 62:179–181.

Majd M: Radionuclide imaging in pediatrics. Pediatr Clin North Am 1985; 32:1559–1579.

Melekos MD, Asbach HW, Markou SA: Etiology of acute scrotum in 100 boys with regard to age distribution. J Urol 1988; 139:1023–1025.

Mueller DL, Amundson GM, Rubin SZ, et al: Acute scrotal abnormalities in children: Diagnosis by combined sonography and scintigraphy. AJR 1988; 150:643–646.

Rabinowitz R: The importance of the cremasteric reflex in acute scrotal swelling in children. J Urol 1984; 132:89–90.

Miscellaneous

Archer A, Choyke PL, O'Brien W, et al: Scrotal enlargement following inguinal herniorrhaphy: Ultrasound evaluation. Urol Radiol 1988; 9:249–252.

Jaramillo D, Perez-Atayde A, Teele RL: Sonography of testicular microlithiasis. Urol Radiol 1989; 11:55–57.

Melekos MD, Asbach HW, Markou SA: Etiology of acute scrotum in 100 boys with regard to age distribution. J Urol 1988; 139:1023–1025.

Primary and Secondary Amenorrhea

Babaknia A, Calfopoulos P, Jones HW Jr: The Stein-Leventhal syndrome and coincidental ovarian tumors. Obstet Gynecol 1976; 47:223–224.

Futterweit W, Yeh HC, Mechanick JI: Ultrasonographic study of ovaries of 19 women with weight loss-related hypothalamic oligo-amenorrhea. Biomed Pharmacother 1988; 42:279–283.

Futterweit W, Yeh H-C, Thornton JC: Lack of correlation of ultrasonographically determined ovarian size with age, ponderal index, and hormonal factors in 45 patients with polycystic ovarian disease. Int J Fertil 1987; 32:456–459.

Goldzieher JW: Polycystic ovarian disease. Fertil Steril 1981; 35:371–394.

Hann LE, Hall DH, McArdle CR, et al: Polycystic ovarian disease: Sonographic spectrum. Radiology 1984; 150:531–534.

Kangarloo H, Sarti DA, Sample WF: Ultrasound of the pediatric pelvis. Semin Ultrasound 1980; 1:51–60.

Massarano AA, Adams JA, Preece MA, et al: Ovarian ultrasound appearances in Turner syndrome. J Pediatr 1989; 114:568–573.

Perez CA, Thomas PRM: Radiation therapy: basic concepts and clinical applications. In Sutow WW, Fernbach DJ, Vietti TJ (eds): Clinical Pediatric Oncology. St. Louis: CV Mosby 1984, pp. 198–199.

Polson DW, Adams J, Wadsworth J, et al: Polycystic ovaries—a common finding in normal women. Lancet 1988; 1(8590):870–872.

Rosenberg HK, Sherman NH, Tarry WF: Mayer-Rokitansky-Kuster-Hauser syndrome: US aid to diagnosis. Radiology 1986; 161:815–819.

Shawker TH, Garra BS, Loriaux DL et al: Ultrasonography of Turner's syndrome. J Ultrasound Med 1986; 5:125–129.

Soules MR: Adolescent amenorrhea. Ped Clin North Am 1987; 34:1083–1103.

Treasure JL, Wheeler M, King EA, et al: Weight gain and reproductive function: Ultrasonographic and endocrine features in anorexia nervosa. Clin Endocrinol 1988; 29:607–616.

Yeh H-C, Futterweit W, Thornton JC: Polycystic ovarian disease: US features in 104 patients. Radiology 1987; 163:111–116.

CHAPTER

RECURRENT ABDOMINAL PAIN

Recurrent abdominal pain affects 10 to 15 percent of school children in Great Britain and the United States. Discussions of etiology and treatment are usually published in the pediatric literature (Levine and Rappaport, 1984; Schecter, 1984). Faced with a child who has recurrent abdominal pain, the clinician is usually concerned that there is some serious abdominal disorder that may be overlooked if a complete diagnostic evaluation is not undertaken. In the past, this complete evaluation included such radiologic imaging as barium enema, an upper gastrointestinal series, and intravenous urography. Normal results were the rule unless abnormalities were present on clinical examination or laboratory tests: weight loss or loss of appetite; change in function or progression of symptoms in a specific system; abnormalities of complete blood count, bleeding, or abnormal urinalysis or culture results; compelling family history of predisposition (e.g., ulcer, pancreatitis); or constitutional signs or symptoms (e.g., recurrent fever, growth failure, swollen joints). These features have been termed "red flags," signalling a need for further medical evaluation (Levine and Rappaport, 1984).

Because ultrasonography is noninvasive, it has been adopted by many clinicians as a replacement for studies in which ionizing radiation is used. Reports in the literature that have perhaps overstated the role of ultrasonography in the diagnosis of pancreatitis, as well as others that demonstrate only the positive results from ultrasonography, have encouraged its use in the evaluation of children who have abdominal pain. Having now seen hundreds of children who have had recurrent abdominal pain and completely normal ultrasonograms, we cannot support the use of ultrasonography in any positive sense. However, there is certainly value in a "negative" study. Many families are worried that chronic abdominal pain may mean cancer. Reassurance from ultrasonography that the solid organs appear anatomically normal is often very useful. Documentation of the *absence* of gallstones, hydronephrosis, and mass is the role of ultrasonography. In the rare situation in which an anomaly or abnormality has been discovered on ultrasonography, it is apparent that a red flag had been overlooked, clinical examination had been cursory, or the pain had been localized and specific. John Apley (1982), who as a general pediatrician took a special interest in children with recurrent pains, is particularly remembered for two comments: (1) "the nearer the pain is to the umbilicus, the less likely is a pathologic explanation," and (2) "little bellyachers grow up to be big bellyachers"!

When a child who has recurrent pain is referred for abdominal ultrasonography, we ask the child to describe the pain and to point out its location. After an evaluation that includes standard views of the liver in transverse and longitudinal planes and of the

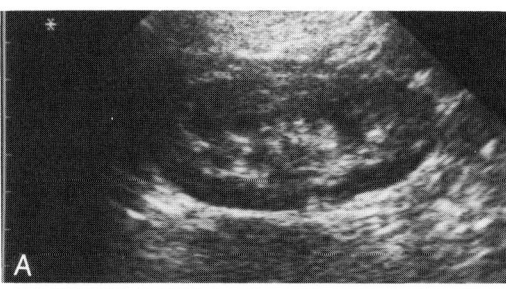

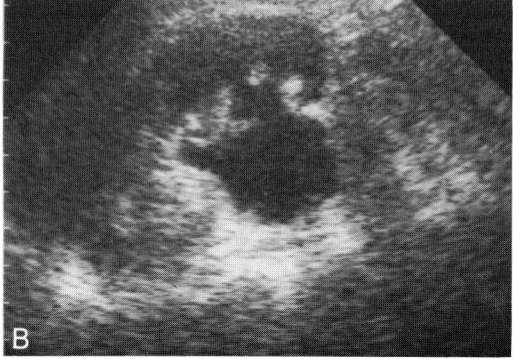

Figure 10–1. Between episodes of abdominal pain, this patient had a normal-appearing kidney on the longitudinal scan (**A**). During an episode of abdominal pain, there was dilatation of the calices and renal pelvis from obstruction by a crossing vessel at the ureteropelvic junction (**B**).

gallbladder, pancreas, both kidneys, and spleen, we specifically scan over the area of pain and document this view on hard copy. Usually the image is of gas-filled bowel, but every so often, when the pain is localized away from the umbilicus, we find an organic cause for the pain. We well remember a boy with recurrent left lower quadrant pain who had symptoms from intermittent obstruction of the left pelvic kidney. Intermittent obstruction of the ureteropelvic junction in a kidney that is normal in position is likely caused by a crossing vessel or an extrinsic band (Fig. 10–1; Homsy et al., 1988). This is a difficult diagnosis to make unless the child is acutely symptomatic at the time of scanning (Byrne et al., 1985). Between episodes of obstruction, the kidney looks quite normal except that the redundant collecting system contributes more echoes to the central sinus. Renal pain tends to be localized along the flank, in the costovertebral angle, or at least to one side of the abdomen. If intermittent obstruction is suspected, diuresis induced by furosemide may produce the hydronephrosis and replicate the pain. Diagnosis can be made with ultrasonography or with radionuclide imaging.

Although we know that an atypical relationship of the superior mesenteric artery to the superior mesenteric vein is not present in all cases of malrotation, we use transverse views to document the position of these vessels at the root of the mesentery. The normal relationship is of the superior mesenteric vein paralleling the artery and lying to the right of the artery until it is joined by the splenic vein and becomes the portal vein (Fig. 10–2). A vein anterior or to the left of the artery should raise the strong possibility of malrotation of the bowel (Fig. 10–3; Gaines et al., 1987). Although most children who develop volvulus of the midgut secondary to malrotation present in the first 3 months of life, there are some who have chronic symptomatology throughout childhood from partial intermittent obstruction (Brandt et al., 1985).

The adolescent with recurrent abdominal pains is much less common a visitor to ultrasonography than the prepubertal child. When the patient is a girl, we include a study of the pelvis and gynecologic tract, but rarely is any abnormality found when pain alone is present. Ovaries are cystic organs, and small or moderately sized cysts are normal findings in pubertal girls. For prepubertal girls and boys, we include one or two views of the

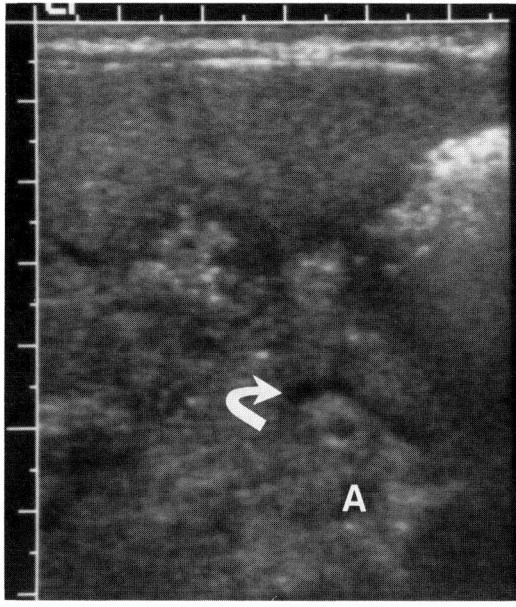

Figure 10–2. On this transverse scan one can see the normal relationship of the superior mesenteric artery (SMA) to the superior mesenteric vein (SMV). The splenic vein crosses anterior to the SMA to join the SMV (arrow) on the right. A = aorta.

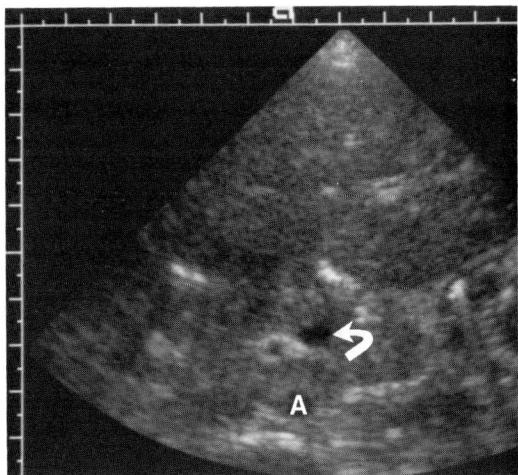

Figure 10–3. The SMV (arrow) is to the left of the SMA in this patient with proven malrotation. A = aorta.

bladder to document its thickness and to evaluate the retrovesical space for fluid. Although we do not advocate ultrasonography as a technique for diagnosing constipation, some children who retain stool also retain urine. They typically have a markedly enlarged bladder with anterior displacement of the base by a stool-filled, distended rectum.

When we begin a study of a child who has chronic abdominal pain, we explain to parents and patient what we shall scan, what we cannot evaluate (i.e., the gastrointestinal tract), and that we are defining anatomy, not assessing physiology.

Expectations of some parents as to the ability of ultrasonography to result in microscopic pathologic diagnoses would make salespersons of ultrasonographic equipment very happy indeed. At the conclusion of a study, we explain what we have or have not found and answer the parents' or child's questions about the scans. Occasionally, we obtain information to relay to the clinician: one little girl had been worried that she had the same gallstones as her ill grandmother, of whom she was very fond. Although we discourage routine ultrasonography for children with recurrent, nonspecific abdominal pain, we understand that clinicians in many parts of the world are under pressure to rule out, as opposed to confirming, diagnoses. A good, thorough ultrasonographic study with normal results is reassuring to the child, family, and physician, and for these reasons we like to think that it is therapeutic as well as diagnostic.

REFERENCES

Apley J: One child. *In* Apley J, Ounsted C (eds.): One Child (Clinics in Developmental Medicine Ser., Vol. 80). Philadelphia, JB Lippincott, 1982; 23–47.

Brandt ML, Pokorny WJ, McGill CW, et al: Late presentations of midgut malrotation in children. Am J Surg 1985; 150:767–771.

Byrne WJ, Arnold WC, Stannard MW, et al: Ureteropelvic junction obstruction presenting with recurrent abdominal pain: Diagnosis by ultrasound. Pediatrics 1985; 76:934–937.

Crossley RB: Hospital admissions for abdominal pain in childhood. J R Soc Med 1982; 75:772–776.

Gaines PA, Saunders AJS, Drake D: Midgut malrotation diagnosed by ultrasound. Clinical Radiology 1987; 38:51–53.

Homsy YL, Mehta PH, Huot D, et al: Intermittent hydronephrosis: A diagnostic challenge. J Urol 1988; 140 (Part 2):1222–1226.

Levine MD, Rappaport LA: Recurrent abdominal pain in school children: The loneliness of the long distance physician. Pediatr Clin North Am 1984; 31:969–991.

Schechter NL: Recurrent pains in children: An overview and an approach. Pediatr Clin North Am 1984; 31:949–968.

Shanon A, Martin DJ, Feldman W: Ultrasonographic studies in the management of recurrent abdominal pain. Pediatrics 1990; 86:35–38.

CHAPTER 11

APPENDICITIS AND OTHER CAUSES OF INTRA-ABDOMINAL INFLAMMATION

APPENDICITIS

The diagnosis of appendicitis, early in its clinical course, has perplexed clinicians for years. In the 1880s Reginald Fitz, pathologist at Harvard Medical School, presented his classic paper on the perforating ulcer of the vermiform appendix, in which he emphasized its diagnosis and treatment, and Charles McBurney described the sign that bears his name (Fitz, 1886; McBurney, 1889). Since then, there has been ongoing debate as to which children should be operated on and which ones can be spared a "negative" exploration. The rate of negative exploration is usually about 20 percent but ranges between 14 and 45 percent, depending on the series (Alvarado, 1986). The rate tends to be higher in female patients because some gynecologic conditions simulate appendicitis.

In an attempt to quantify the clinical examination, Alvarado (1986) developed a practical score with which to evaluate a patient with possible appendicitis (Table 11–1). This has been helpful to us in ultrasonography because the mnemonic reminds us of the specific clinical features of the disease. A score of 5 or 6 is compatible with a diagnosis of appendicitis, 7 or 8 indicates probable appendicitis, and 9 or 10 indicates *very* probable appendicitis. Rectal examination is neither a sensitive nor a specific test for appendicitis. It is noteworthy that patients who have a gangrenous appendix tend to have a slightly lower mean score than patients whose appendix is in the suppurative phase of inflammation.

In spite of enthusiastic medical press that has suggested that ultrasonography is the answer to this clinical dilemma, we still find that the diagnosis of pain in the right lower quadrant may be difficult no matter what technique is used. The differential diagnosis

Table 11–1. ALVARADO SCORE FOR APPENDICITIS

M	Migration of pain	1
A	Anorexia or acetone	1
N	Nausea or vomiting	1
T	Tenderness in right lower quadrant	2
R	Rebound pain	1
E	Elevated temperature	1
L	Leucocytosis >10,000	2
S	Shift to left >75%	1
		10

Score of 5 or 6 = compatible
       7 or 8 = probable
       9 or 10 = very probable

From Alvarado A: A practical score for the early diagnosis of acute appendicitis. Ann Emerg Med 1986; 15:557–564.

includes uncomplicated appendicitis, ruptured appendicitis, yersinial or other inflammatory ileitis, mesenteric adenitis, omental infarct, Crohn disease, lymphoma, and renal obstruction. When the patient is a girl, the diagnosis is expanded to include ovarian torsion, ovarian cyst, pelvic inflammatory disease, and ectopic pregnancy. For many children, no diagnosis is made during the acute episode of pain, and the child recovers spontaneously. In a large series that included adults, 53 percent had no final diagnosis for their abdominal pain (Gaensler et al., 1989). We prefer to scan only those children who do not have the classic clinical presentation of appendicitis, ultrasonography thereby being used as an ancillary diagnostic tool (Pearson, 1988; Larson et al., 1989). Scans of an inflamed appendix in a child who has presented in typical clinical fashion only delay the surgery. Rupture of the appendix occurs within 24 to 48 hours of acute inflammation and results in significant morbidity and occasionally even death.

We admit that the demonstration of shadowing fecalith, intraluminal fluid, and thickened appendiceal wall makes for beautiful ultrasonograms (Fig. 11–1; Puylaert, 1986; Puylaert et al., 1987; Jeffrey et al., 1988; Kao et al., 1989). A negative ultrasonographic

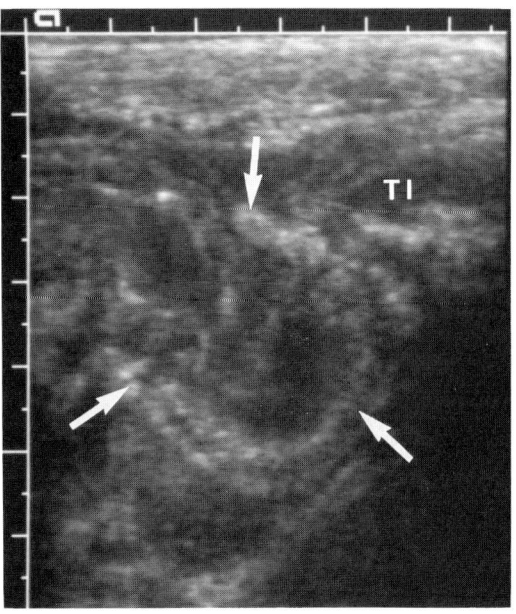

Figure 11–2. When we scanned the right lower quadrant in this 6-year-old girl, the pain there was not as severe as it had been earlier in the day. We saw a thick-walled cecum (arrows) outlined by echogenic fluid. We could not find the appendix in spite of careful searching. During surgery, this girl was found to have a perforated appendix and early periappendiceal abscess. TI = terminal ileum.

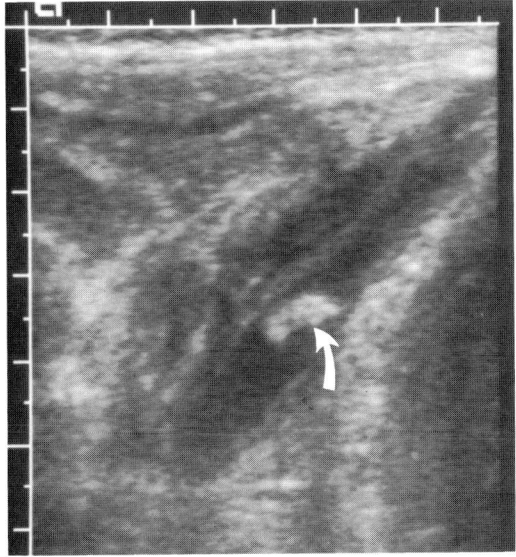

Figure 11–1. This is a longitudinal view of the inflamed appendix of a 3-year-old girl. She had had a 2½-day history of abdominal pain, nausea, and vomiting. The white blood cell count was 18,000. Note the irregular thickening of the appendiceal wall. There is a localized bulge anteriorly. Immediately below the bulge is the faintly shadowing appendicolith (arrow).

finding does not always mean that appendicitis is *not* present (Adams et al., 1988; Fa and Cronan, 1989). Good communication between radiologist and surgeon is of paramount importance to avoid misinterpretation of scans within the specific clinical situation. We are certain that much of the diagnostic success of the series reporting ultrasonographic and surgical findings in patients with appendicitis has been generated by the close communication between the two clinical services.

When the appendix ruptures, the ultrasonographic signs of appendicitis disappear for a variable time. The fluid-filled obstructed lumen is the reason why an inflamed appendix becomes visible on ultrasonograms. As the tip blows out, the appendix becomes difficult to identify, and only when enough fluid accumulates can an appendiceal abscess be identified (Fig. 11–2). If there is heavy reliance on "negative" ultrasonograms, the recently ruptured appendix is missed. Conversely, other diseases may produce free fluid and localized pain. We have been impressed with the symptoms and signs of omental infarction and how they simulate

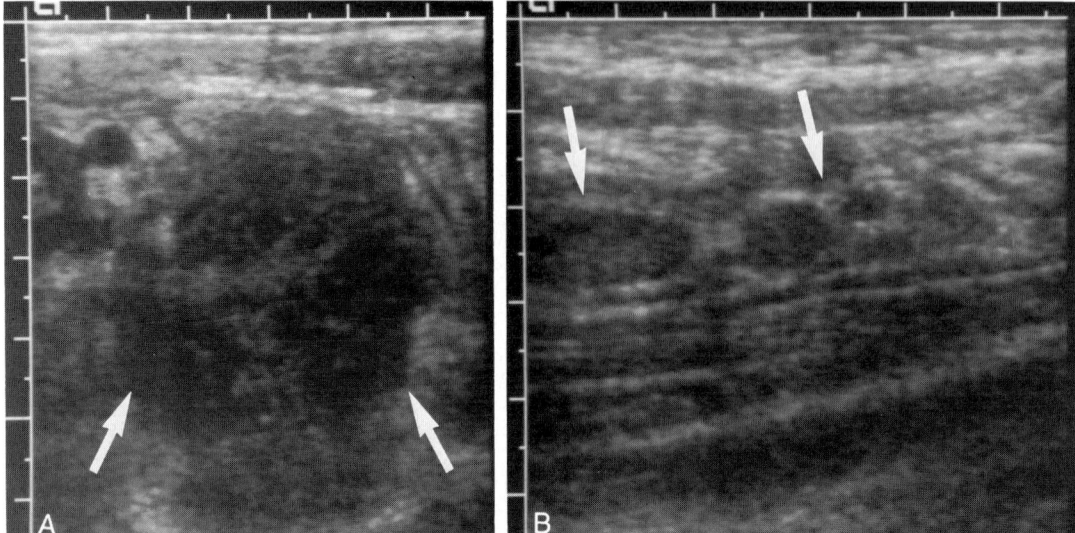

Figure 11–3. This 11-year-old girl presented with fever, diarrhea, and vomiting. Ten days before admission to the hospital, she had been seen by a physician because of abdominal pain. She had been partially treated with antibiotics for a presumed strep throat in the interim. When she presented to the hospital, she again had pain in the right lower quadrant, especially when we pressed the transducer over the area. **A** shows the right lower quadrant abscess (arrows), which was quickly identified. The appendix could not be visualized at all. In scans along the psoas **(B)**, multiple lymph nodes (arrows) were apparent. The child's appendix had ruptured 1 week before admission, but her symptoms had been masked by the antibiotics that she had been given.

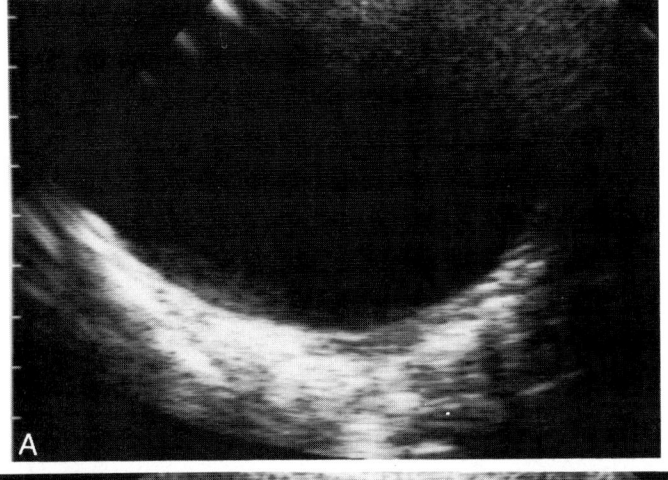

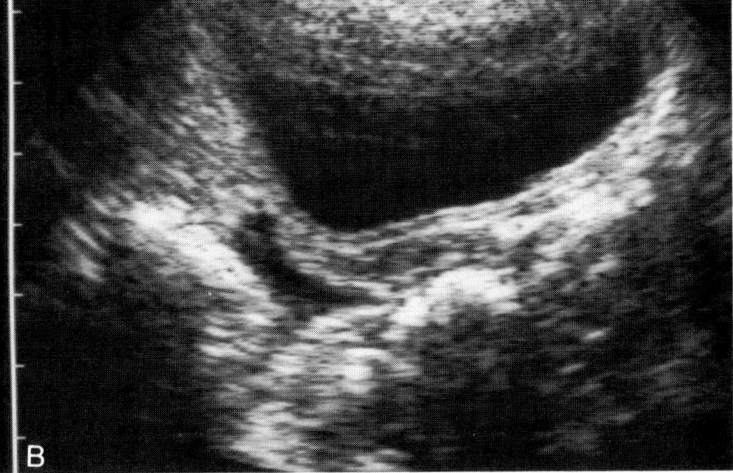

Figure 11–4. Longitudinal views of the pelvis before **(A)** and after **(B)** partial voiding show how an extremely full bladder can "iron out" a small amount of intraperitoneal fluid.

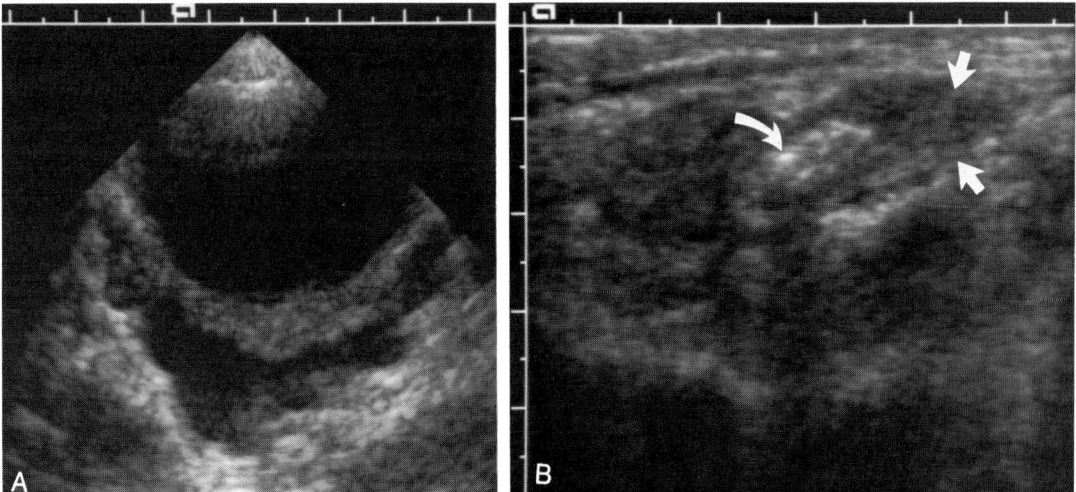

Figure 11–5. Transverse scan of the pelvis in this little girl shows free fluid pooling behind the bladder **(A)**. The longitudinal scan of the right lower quadrant **(B)** shows a shadowing appendicolith (curved arrow) in a thick-walled appendix, which is typical of appendicitis. Straight arrows outline the appendiceal tip, which looks ready to perforate. Free fluid in the pelvis always increases the suspicion of appendicitis.

those of appendicitis. There is one group of patients whom we really have helped: children who have entered the hospital with vague or specific pain in the right lower quadrant but who are not acutely ill. Proving the presence of an appendiceal abscess and then piecing together the clinical history to support a diagnosis of earlier appendiceal rupture is a very satisfying diagnostic exercise (Fig. 11–3). Typically, the patient has had a 7- to 10-day history beginning with periumbilical pain, anorexia, and then right-sided pain. This is followed by relief of symptoms, then gradual recurrence of lower abdominal pain, change in appetite and bowel movements, and intermittent fevers. The child may have had therapy with antibiotics, which serve to obscure the diagnosis while simultaneously helping to wall off the infection. Common diseases present in an uncommon fashion, and in no condition is this more true than in appendicitis.

When evaluating a child who has pain in the right lower quadrant, we begin by scanning the pelvis. The child must have a full bladder, and so a bolus of intravenous fluid is given before the child is sent to ultrasonography. Free abdominal fluid tends to pool in the cul-de-sac, but severe distention of the bladder irons out the cul-de-sac and pushes fluid superiorly (Fig. 11–4). In girls we pay special attention to the uterus and ovaries. Appendicitis is more common in boys, and inflammatory disease of the gynecologic tract commonly simulates appendicitis in girls

(see Chapter 8). The presence of free fluid, whether clear or echogenic, increases our level of suspicion for intraperitoneal inflammation (Figs. 11–5, 11–6). We also scan the

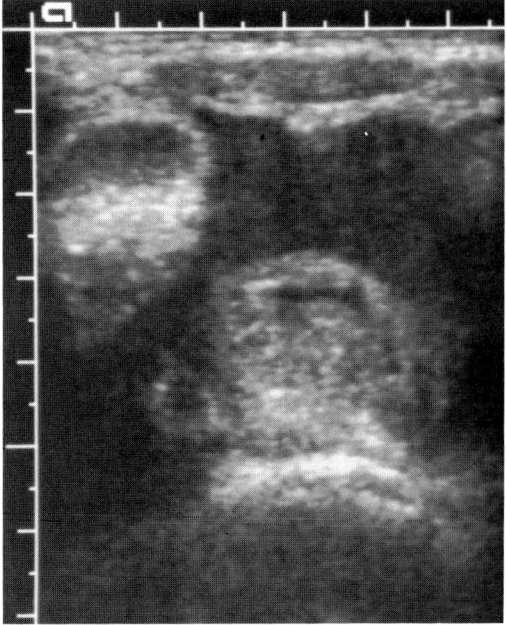

Figure 11–6. This 3-year-old boy had severe abdominal pain. The scans of the right lower abdomen showed dilated loops of bowel filled with debris. Echogenic fluid surrounded the bowel loops. Although the appendix could not be identified, appendicitis was considered the likely etiology for the peritoneal fluid, and a ruptured appendix with peritonitis was found during surgery.

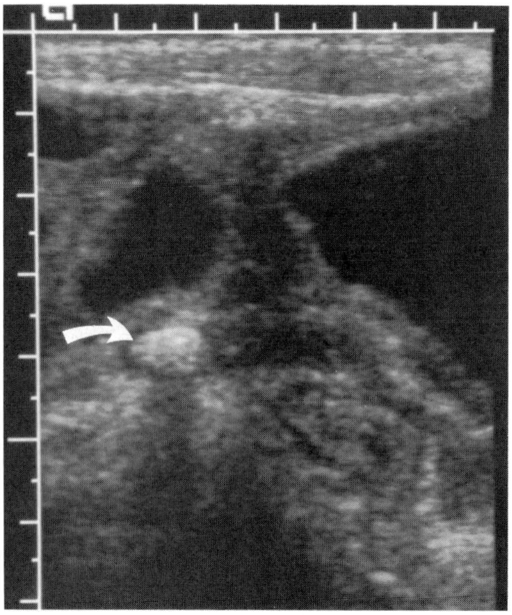

Figure 11-7. Scan of the right lower quadrant in this little boy shows a shadowing appendicolith (arrow). The bladder is to the right in the illustration. A bowel loop filled with clear fluid is just anterior to the appendix. A radiograph of this patient had appeared normal with no evidence of calcification.

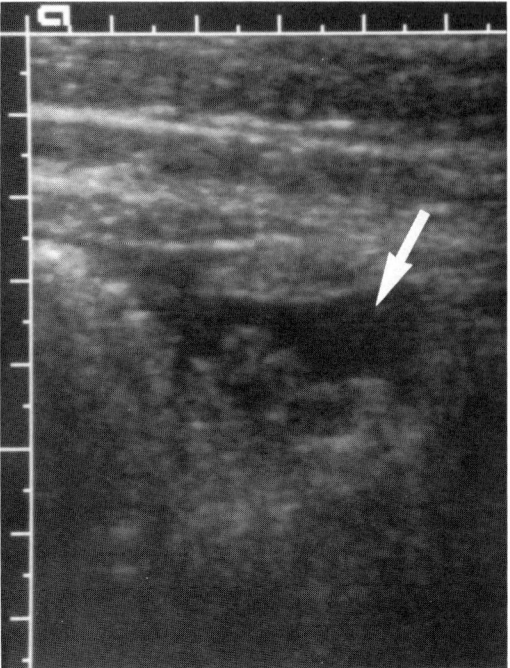

Figure 11-8. When we saw this 6-year-old boy, he had severe right-sided pain and a small amount of free fluid in the right lower quadrant (arrow). In spite of careful searching, we could not find a thick-walled appendix or an appendicolith. Interestingly, his pain seemed a little higher in location than is usual in appendicitis, but he was definitely ill. During surgery, an omental infarct was diagnosed. We have been impressed with how symptoms of omental infarcts are similar to those of appendicitis. Also, it seems that those children who have had omental infarcts are heavier than average.

right upper quadrant to check the gallbladder and kidney, and then we switch from using a sector transducer to using a high-frequency, linear array probe. If the child is able to tolerate continuing the examination with a full bladder, we prefer doing it in this way. The full bladder pushes the bowel out of the pelvis and makes it more accessible to compression. The transducer is gradually passed from superior to inferior as the abdominal wall is compressed. The cecum tends to lie lateral to the psoas muscle. The appendix extends from the cecum as a variably long, blind-ending tube. We generally cannot visualize the normal appendix. The diagnosis of

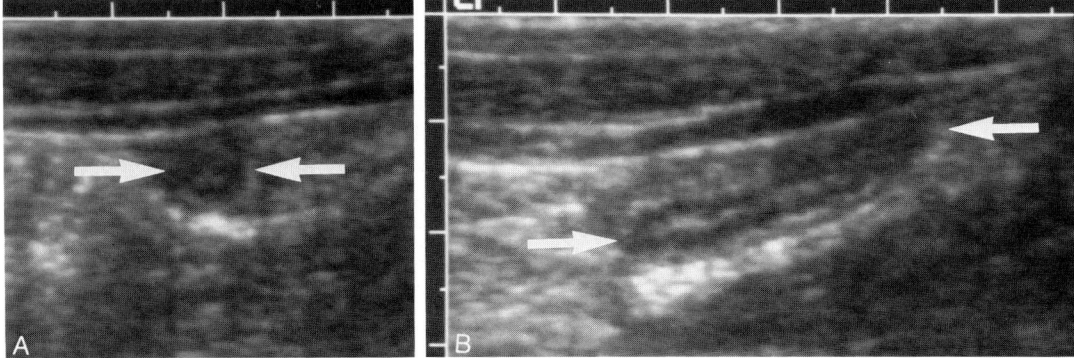

Figure 11-9. Transverse (A) and longitudinal (B) scans of the right lower quadrant did demonstrate the appendix (arrows) in this patient, but the lumen was not distended, and the appendix was barely 6 mm in diameter. Although the patient was not febrile, her white blood cell count was elevated to 19,080. She had had 4 days of abdominal pain, anorexia, and vomiting. Because of her symptoms, she was taken to the operating room. Acute appendicitis without perforation was present, and the appendix was removed.

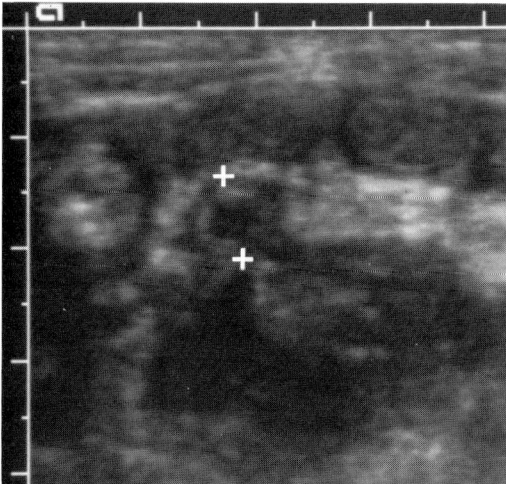

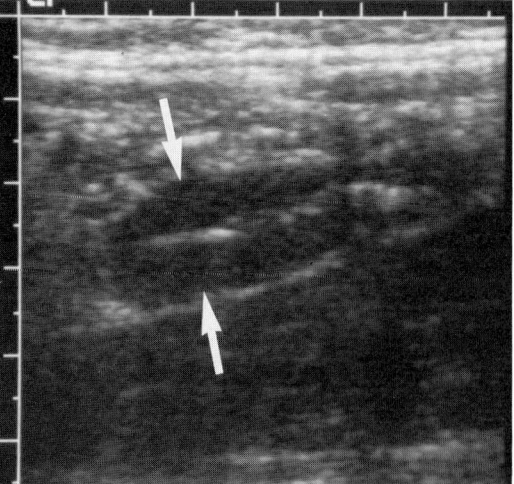

Figure 11–10. We had trouble compressing the appendix in this patient, as it was retrocecal in location. It is marked by the crosses on this transverse view. Its diameter was 8 mm, and the lumen was obviously distended. No shadowing appendicolith could be identified. This patient has cystic fibrosis and he presented with right lower quadrant pain. He was already receiving therapy with antibiotics for pulmonary disease, and we were in the difficult situation of determining whether he had acute appendicitis. Persistent right lower quadrant pain resulted in his being taken to surgery. A normal appendix filled with thick stool, typical in patients with cystic fibrosis, was removed. The diagnosis, therefore, was a false-positive one.

Figure 11–11. In this patient, the appendiceal wall was thickened, and the overall diameter of the appendix measured nearly 2 cm (arrows). The lumen is represented by an echogenic line on this longitudinal scan. The patient had neutropenic colitis associated with therapy for acute lymphoblastic leukemia. Conservative, supportive therapy was instituted, and the right lower quadrant pain as well as the ultrasonographic findings resolved in 2 weeks. He did not go to surgery.

appendicitis relies on visualizing a noncompressible appendix that is more than 6 mm in diameter (Jeffrey et al., 1988). The wall of the inflamed appendix is usually thicker than 2 mm. Asymmetric thickening is indicative of inflammation. The contents of the lumen are usually hypoechoic; one or more appendicoliths within the lumen are echogenic and cast a shadow, whether they are calcified or not (Fig. 11–7). In rare instances, gas is present within the wall of the appendix (Kao et al., 1989). Fluid around the tip indicates imminent rupture. Compression directly over the inflamed appendix usually results in expressions of pain by all but the most stoic of children. However, we have had our share of false-negative, false-positive, and borderline cases (Figs. 11–8 to 11–13).

If a child continues to be febrile after appendectomy, abdominal scans are useful to

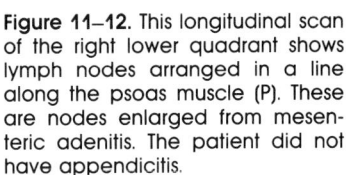

Figure 11–12. This longitudinal scan of the right lower quadrant shows lymph nodes arranged in a line along the psoas muscle (P). These are nodes enlarged from mesenteric adenitis. The patient did not have appendicitis.

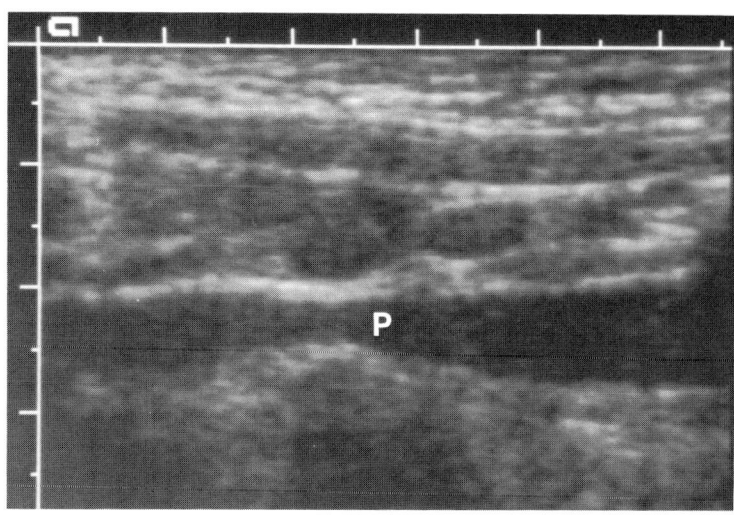

352 / APPENDICITIS AND OTHER CAUSES OF INTRA-ABDOMINAL INFLAMMATION

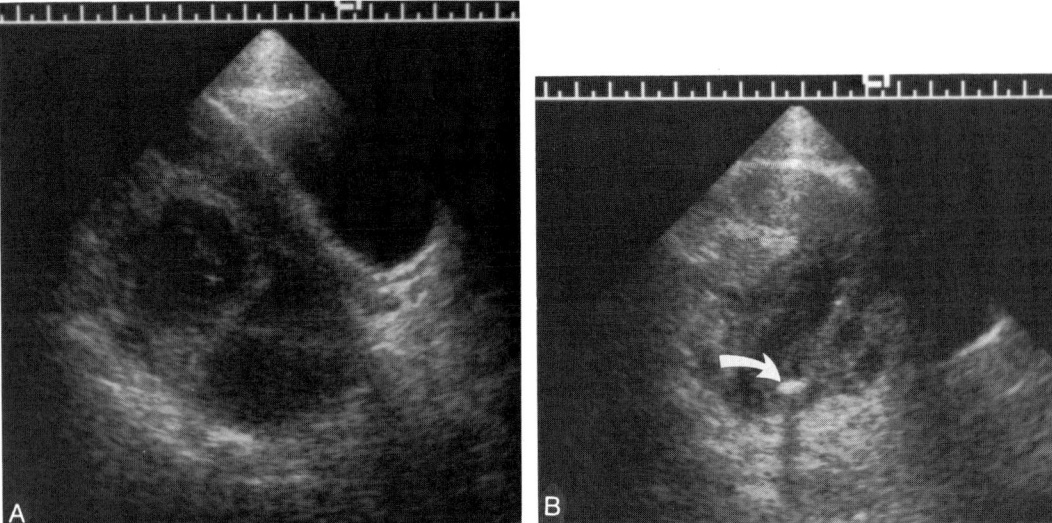

Figure 11-13. Thirty-six hours of crampy abdominal pain brought this 15-year-old girl to the emergency room. Her white blood cell count was 17,000. She denied having had sexual activity, but a right-sided adnexal mass was apparent (A). Further scanning revealed an echogenic sulcus at the periphery of the mass (B) with a shadowing echogenic focus (arrow). Because an appendicolith can escape from the appendix when the appendix ruptures, we thought that an abscess associated with previous appendicitis was the likely cause of her symptoms. However, during surgery, she was found to haave hydrosalpinx and periovarian abscess. Of importance is the clinical history that this girl was a competitive diver. It is possible that her pelvic inflammatory disease was secondary to influx of bacteria during diving practice. We have no explanation for the shadowing density that we saw on ultrasonography and no calcification could be identified at surgery.

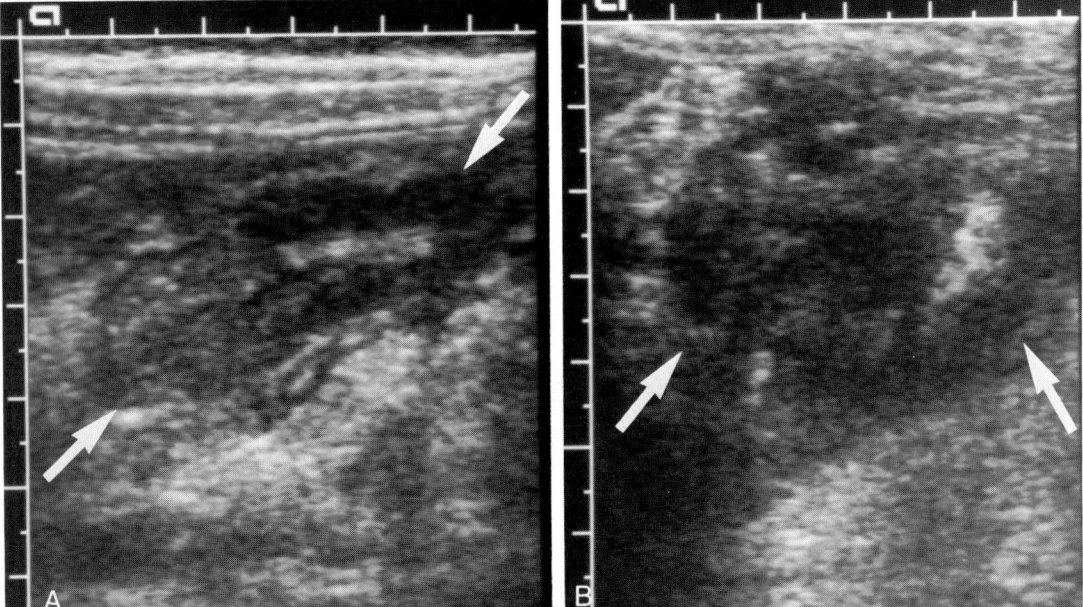

Figure 11-14. One week after surgery for acute appendicitis, this patient re-presented with pain in the right lower quadrant and with fever. The initial scan (A) before surgery had shown an irregularly thickened appendiceal wall (arrows). Lack of luminal distention suggested that the appendix had probably already perforated, although a discrete abscess could not be identified. B shows the right lower quadrant abscess (arrows) that was apparent 1 week later. This was drained percutaneously and resolved.

evaluate first the site of the operation and the area around the incision and then the peritoneal cavity for loculated collections of fluid. The pelvis, subhepatic area, Morison pouch, and perisplenic region are usual sites for development of an abscess after perforation of an appendix (Fig. 11–14). In fact, James Morison, a British surgeon of the 19th century, described the peritoneal recess that bears his name in reference to an abscess from a perforated appendix. Intraloop abscesses are difficult to find, and computed tomography (CT) is better able to locate them. Small collections of fluid are not unusual after surgery for appendicitis (Baker et al., 1986). However, collections that are spherical, associated with local pain or obstruction of bowel, or increasing in size are defined as abscesses and are treated with antibiotics (Fig. 11–15). An abscess can be drained percutaneously if there is no response to antibiotics (Fig. 11–16). The catheter (9 French or larger) is left in place until drainage ceases, generally in 3 to 7 days.

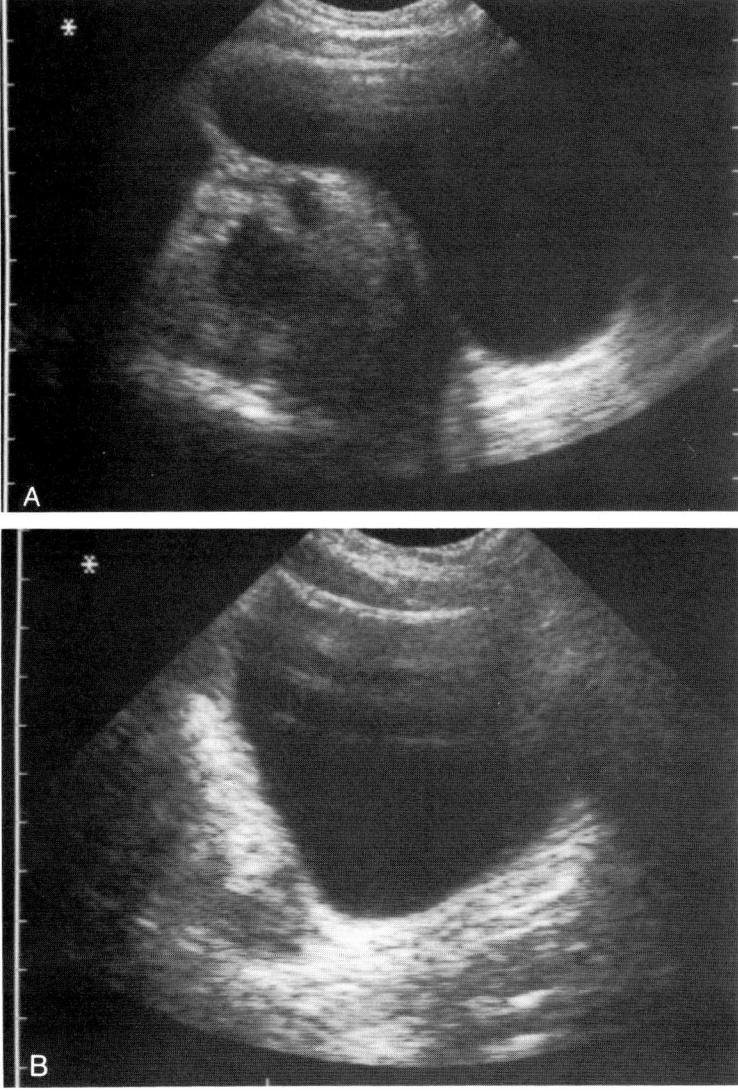

Figure 11–15. A gangrenous appendix was removed from this 10-year-old girl, who had presented with abdominal pain and a 7-day history of nausea, vomiting, and temperatures up to 39°C. After surgery, she was treated with intravenous antibiotics for 4 days and then oral antibiotics for 5 days. Persisting low-grade fevers and continued pain in the right lower quadrant caused her readmission 3 weeks after surgery. An ill-defined right adnexal mass was identified on ultrasonography (A). Ten days of treatment with intravenous antibiotics resulted in resolution of the right adnexal inflammatory mass (B).

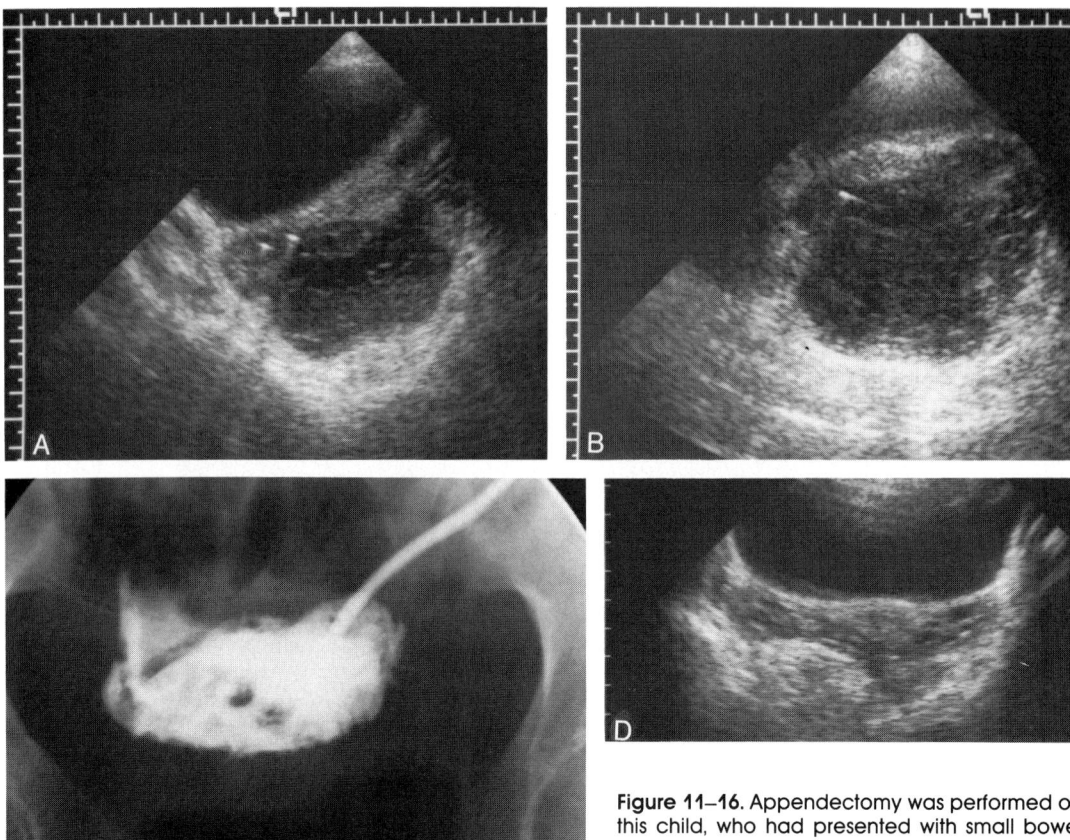

Figure 11–16. Appendectomy was performed on this child, who had presented with small bowel obstruction and temperatures up to 39.5°C. Her white blood cell count was 29,000, and her admission to the hospital had been preceded by 3 days of diffuse abdominal pain, nausea, and vomiting. The appendix had perforated, and in spite of intravenous antibiotics given postoperatively, the white blood cell count remained elevated. Follow-up ultrasonography of the pelvis showed fluid collection that continued to increase in size (**A and B**). This was drained percutaneously (**C**). Follow-up studies showed complete resolution of the pelvic abscess (**D**).

OTHER INTRAPERITONEAL INFLAMMATORY DISEASES

Crohn disease is particularly crippling in children whose growth and development are affected by this so-called benign disease. We generally see such children in ultrasonography only after the diagnosis has been made on radiologic examination. In series of adults, the diagnosis has been made with ultrasonography when affected patients presented with signs and symptoms simulating appendicitis (Puylaert et al., 1988b; Gaensler et al., 1989). Thickening of the wall of the small bowel in the right lower quadrant (≥4 mm), occasionally with involvement of cecum, is typical of Crohn disease (Worlicek et al., 1987). It is not specific; bacterial ileitis also presents with thickening of the wall of the small bowel. Yersinial enteritis is the major differential diagnosis (Puylaert et al., 1989). A psoas abscess may be the presenting abnormality in a very small percentage of patients who have Crohn disease (see Chapter 8).

Fever of Unknown Origin

Children who have fever with no source documented after extensive clinical and laboratory evaluation and who have no localizing abdominal signs rarely have abnormal abdominal ultrasonograms. We can think of only a handful of patients for whom ultrasonography was a useful diagnostic adjunct. If and when we are persuaded to do the scans, we do a complete abdominal survey and pay special attention to hepatic and splenic parenchyma. Small focal parenchymal lucencies or inhomogeneities may be

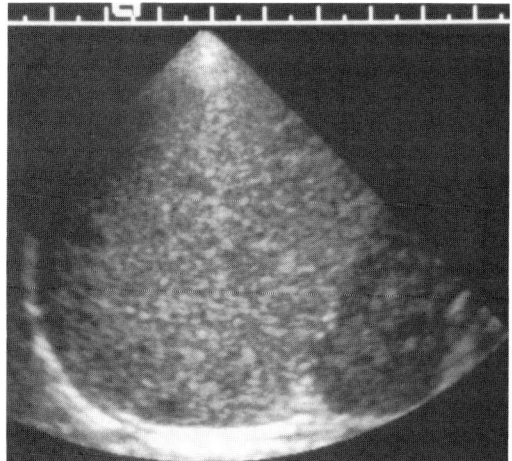

Figure 11–17. Osteomyelitis of a lower lumbar vertebral body had been diagnosed on computed tomography (CT) scans and from histologic examination of a bone biopsy. However, no organism ever grew from cultures. The patient's spiking fevers continued despite intensive antibiotic therapy. Abdominal scans revealed small, focal parenchymal lucencies throughout the spleen. The CT scan that followed confirmed these abnormalities and suggested that a similar abnormality affected the liver. The liver was biopsied, and microabscesses were identified. Further changes in antibiotic therapy followed, although no organism ever grew from cultures. The fevers finally disappeared. We speculated about the possibility of cat-scratch disease, but we could not confirm this with serologic studies.

caused by microabscesses or granulomas (Fig. 11–17). Splenomegaly is a nonspecific but occasional sign of viral illness or connective tissue disorder such as systemic rheumatoid arthritis. We look for free or loculated collections of fluid but are surprised when we find any. Usually such children have had earlier abdominal surgery or a known predisposing disease. CT scanning is better able to evaluate all the abdominal contents when

occult abscess is being sought. Furthermore, it is the appropriate technique with which to evaluate bone and soft tissue.

Abdominal Involvement with Acquired Immunodeficiency Syndrome (AIDS)

Most of the radiologic imaging for patients who have infection with human immunodeficiency virus (HIV) is done with plain films. CT or magnetic resonance imaging (MRI) scanning of the brain is added if necessary. We do not perform routine abdominal screening of children with AIDS; we use ultrasonography when a child has abdominal symptoms or signs that cannot be explained. Hepatosplenomegaly may result from infection with cytomegalovirus, or, possibly, from primary infection with HIV or modification of other hepatitic agents by the presence of HIV. Increased echogenicity of the liver from fatty infiltration results when the patient is severely malnourished. Lymphadenopathy is not unusual and may represent reactive lymphoid hyperplasia or infection with *Mycobacterium avium-intracellulare* (Fig. 11–18). Lymphoma and Kaposi sarcoma are not common in the pediatric population but have been reported (Bradford et al., 1988; Genieser et al., 1988). It is worth using the transducer to look at the pericardial space if one is evaluating the abdomen of an infected child. One quarter of a prospectively screened group of children had pericardial effusion without tamponade (Lipshultz et al., 1989).

Of course, a child who has AIDS is also at risk for all the routine problems of childhood.

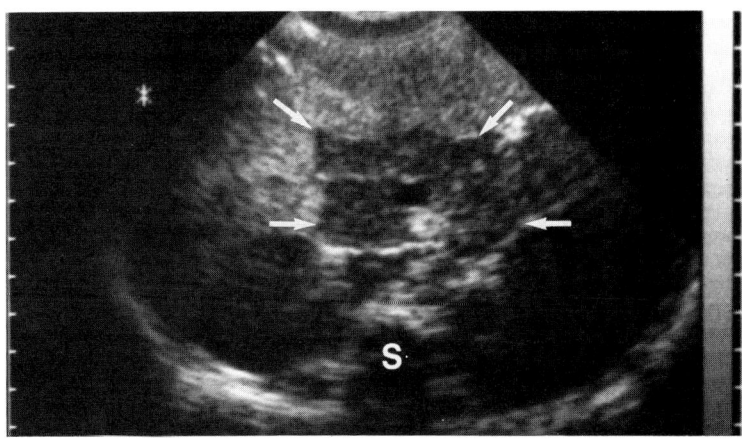

Figure 11–18. Intermittent fevers were documented in this little girl who was known to have acquired immunodeficiency syndrome (AIDS). Peripancreatic adenopathy is evident (arrows); there was no other abnormality present. Adenopathy related to human immunodeficiency virus or infection with *Mycobacterium avium intracellulare* are the most common causes of nodal enlargement with AIDS. Lymphoma and Kaposi sarcoma are rare in pediatric patients. S = spine.

Clinicians should approach ultrasonographic examinations of such a child as they would for any other child who presents with similar symptoms. Then they should evaluate the findings in light of the child's immunodeficiency. We use gloves and gowns when examining children with AIDS if they have open wounds or secretions (e.g., gastrostomy tubes), and we take appropriate protective measures to guard against "splash" contamination (Johnson, 1988). We wear masks to protect the child from infection if we have upper respiratory symptoms. We wash transducers thoroughly, both before and after the procedure, with germicidal fluid. And we fervently hope, when future books are written, that the chapter on AIDS will be relegated to a historical description of this modern human plague.

REFERENCES

Appendicitis

Adams DH, Fine C, Brooks DC: High-resolution real-time ultrasonography. A new tool in the diagnosis of acute appendicitis. Am J Surg 1988; 155:93–97.

Alvarado A: A practical score for the early diagnosis of acute appendicitis. Ann Emerg Med 1986; 15: 557–564.

Amland PF, Skaane P, Ronnigen H, et al: Ultrasonography and parameters of inflammation in acute appendicitis. A comparison with clinical findings. Acta Chirug Scand 1989; 155:185–189.

Baker DE, Silver TM, Coran AG, et al: Postappendectomy fluid collections in children: Incidence, nature, and evolution evaluated using US. Radiology 1986; 161:341–344.

Borushok KF, Jeffrey RB Jr, Laing FC et al: Sonographic diagnosis of perforation in patients with acute appendicitis. AJR 1990; 154:275–278.

Fa EM, Cronan JJ: Compression ultrasonography as an aid in the differential diagnosis of appendicitis. Surg Gynecol Obstet 1989; 169:290–298.

Fitz RH. Perforating inflammation of the vermiform appendix with special reference to its early diagnosis and treatment. Am J Med Sci 1886; 92:321–346.

Gaensler EH, Jeffrey RB Jr, Laing FC, Townsend RR: Sonography in patients with suspected acute appendicitis: Value in establishing alternative diagnoses. AJR 1989; 152:49–51.

Jeffrey RB Jr, Laing FC, Townsend RR: Acute appendicitis: Sonographic criteria based on 250 cases. Radiology 1988; 167:327–329.

Kang WM, Lee CH, Chou YH, et al: A clinical evaluation of ultrasonography in the diagnosis of acute appendicitis. Surgery 1989; 105:154–159.

Kao SCS, Smith WL, Abu-Yousef MM, et al: Acute appendicitis in children: Sonographic findings. AJR 1989; 153:375–379.

Larson JM, Peirce JC, Ellinger DM, et al: The validity and utility of sonography in the diagnosis of appendicitis in the community setting. AJR 1989; 153:687–691.

McBurney C: Disease of the vermiform appendix. NY Med J 1889; 50:676–684.

Pearson RH: Ultrasonography for diagnosing appendicitis. Br Med J 1988; 297:309–310.

Puylaert JBCM: Acute appendicitis: US evaluation using graded compression. Radiology 1986; 158:355–360.

Puylaert JBCM, Lalisang RI, van der Werf SDJ, et al: Campylobacter ileocolitis mimicking acute appendicitis: Differentiation with graded-compression US. Radiology 1988a; 166:737–740.

Puylaert JBCM, Rutgers P, Lalisang RI, et al: A prospective study of ultrasonography in the diagnosis of appendicitis. N Engl J Med 1987; 317:666–669.

Slovis TL, Haller JO, Cohen HL, et al: Complicated appendiceal inflammatory disease in children: Pylephlebitis and liver abscess. Radiology 1989; 171:823–825.

Worrell JA, Drolshagen LF, Kelly TC, et al: Graded compression ultrasound in the diagnosis of appendicitis. A comparison of diagnostic criteria. J Ultrasound Med 1990; 9:145–150.

Intra-Abdominal Inflammation

Belli AM, Joseph AE: The renal rind sign: A new ultrasound indication of inflammatory disease in the abdomen. Br J Radiol 1988; 61:806–810.

Gaisie G, Jaques PF, Mauro MA: Radiologic management of fluid collections in children. Pediatr Radiol 1987; 17:143–146.

Hoffer FA, Fellows KE, Wyly JB, et al: Therapeutic catheter procedures in pediatrics. Pediatr Clin North Am 1985; 32:1461–1476.

Liu P, Daneman A, Stringer DA, et al: Percutaneous aspiration, drainage, and biopsy in children. J Pediatr Surg 1989; 24:865–866.

Puylaert JBCM, van der Werf SDJ, Ulrich C, et al: Crohn disease of the ileocecal region: US visualization of the appendix. Radiology 1988b; 166:741–743.

Puylaert JBCM, Vermeijden RJ, van der Werf SDJ, et al: Incidence and sonographic diagnosis of bacterial ileocaecitis masquerading as appendicitis. Lancet 1989; 2:84–86.

Towbin RB, Ball WS: Pediatric interventional radiology. Radiol Clin North Am 1988; 26:419–440.

Worlicek H, Lutz H, Heyder N, et al: Ultrasound findings in Crohn's disease and ulcerative colitis: A prospective study. 1987; 15:153–163.

AIDS

Amodio JB, Abramson S, Berdon WE, et al: Pediatric AIDS. Semin Roentgenol 1987; 22:66–76.

Bradford BF, Abdenour GE Jr, Frank JL, et al: Usual and unusual radiologic manifestations of acquired immunodeficiency syndrome (AIDS) and human immunodeficiency virus (HIV) infection in children. Radiol Clin North Am 1988; 26:341–353.

Genieser NB, Hernanz-Schulman M, Krasinski K, et al: Pediatric AIDS. In Radiology of AIDS. Federle MP, Megibow AJ, Naidich DP (eds): New York: Raven Press, 1988; 131:142.

Graif M, Kessler A, Neumann Y, et al: Pancreatic Burkitt lymphoma in AIDS: Sonographic appearance [letter]. AJR 1987; 149:1290–1291.

Johnson MAG: Handling AIDS patients in the radiology department. In Radiology of AIDS. Federle MP, Megibow AJ, Naidich DP (eds): New York: Raven Press, 1988, 143–146.

Lipshultz SE, Chanock S, Sanders SP, et al: Cardiovascular manifestations of human immunodeficiency virus infection in infants and children. Am J Cardiol 1989; 63:1489–1497.

CHAPTER 12

GASTRODUODENAL ULTRASONOGRAPHY

There are those who advocate ultrasonography for all babies who come to medical attention because of persistent vomiting. This does not appear to be a particularly cost-effective method, because many patients need radiographic study with barium (Foley et al., 1989). We like to consider a patient's entire clinical situation before embarking on the diagnostic evaluation. We still own a fluoroscopist's apron as well as wearing an ultrasonographic hat! There is no question, however, that the instruction to rule out pyloric stenosis is on many requisitions that come our way and the focus of this discussion is directed first to the subject of pyloric stenosis and then to the diagnosis of other causes of vomiting.

PYLORIC STENOSIS

In reviewing the literature on hypertrophic pyloric stenosis, one quickly realizes that ultrasonic criteria for the diagnosis have been fine-tuned but that the etiology of this common pediatric disorder is still obscure. Why should an otherwise healthy baby begin vomiting because of hypertrophy of smooth muscle in a localized portion of the gastrointestinal tract? The answer has evaded the medical community to date. Furthermore, the surgical approach for relief of the obstruction has not changed much since 1912, when Wilhelm Ramstedt described the procedure that bears his name. What *has* changed is the method of diagnosis. There is increasing reliance on imaging, particularly ultrasonography, in the diagnosis of pyloric stenosis. We, like others ("Is Ultrasound Really Necessary," 1988), are of the opinion that imaging is replacing careful clinical examination in the evaluation of vomiting infants at risk for pyloric stenosis. With new generations of house officers less rigorously trained in the art of clinical examination, we see no likelihood of reversing this trend. Having concluded this pessimistic preamble, we ask: which children are at risk and which should be evaluated?

Nonbilious vomiting by a 5- to 6-week-old boy is the classic presentation of pyloric stenosis and, unlike some other "classic" situations in medicine, is actually typical. Projectile vomiting, because of its dramatic nature, always gains mention in the clinical textbooks, but this sign is variably present in our

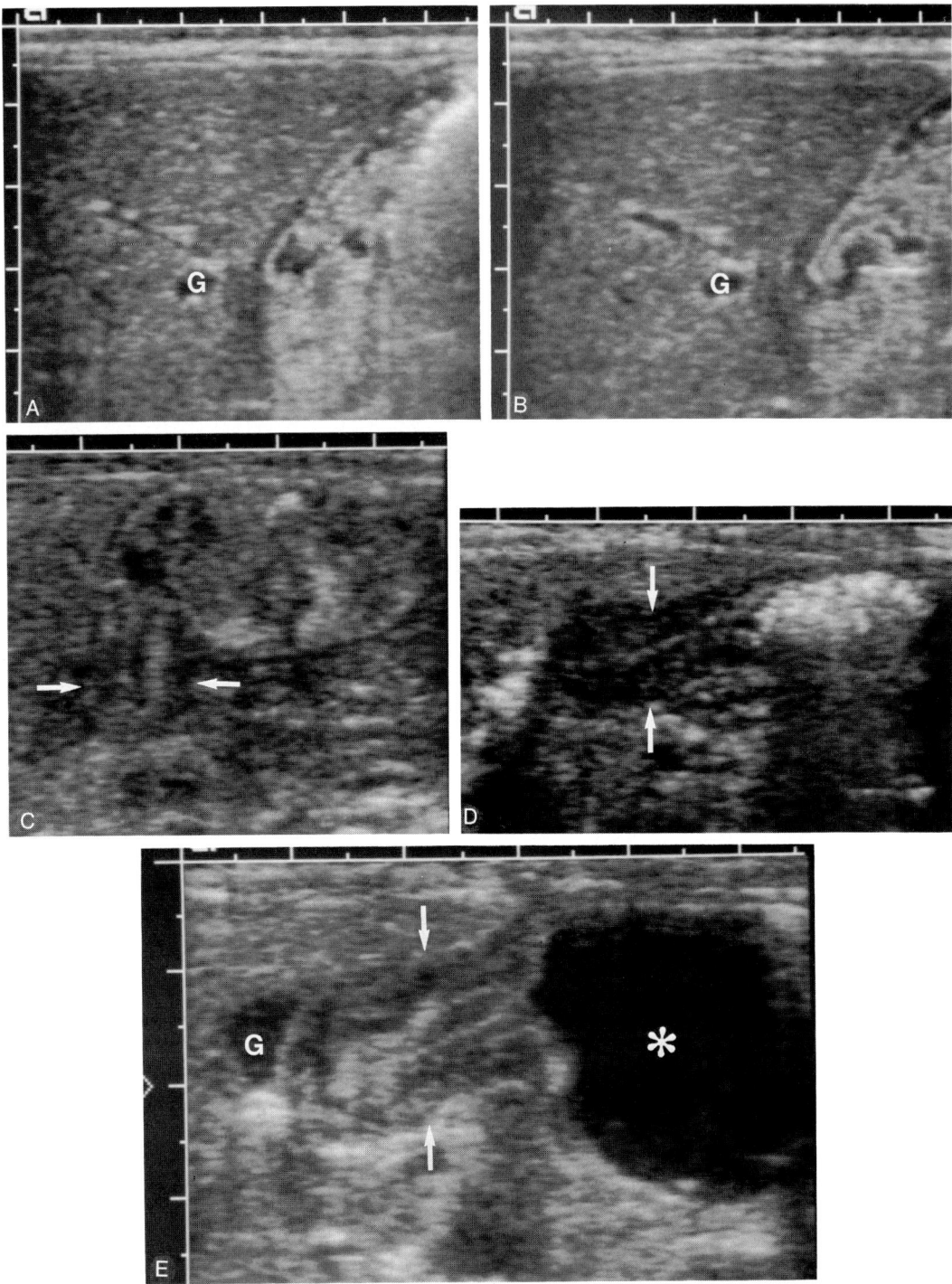

Figure 12–1. The normal pylorus has no thickening of its muscular wall, and gastric contents move into duodenum with each peristaltic push. Note the change in appearance between **A** and **B**. The gallbladder (G) is a good landmark of the gastroduodenal junction. When the pyloric muscle thickens, the canal becomes elongated and peristalsis ends abruptly at the hypertrophied muscle. If the pylorus is directed posteriorly, it may be difficult to image (arrows, **C**) unless one moves the transducer further lateral on the baby's abdominal wall (**D**). This allows identification of the thickened pylorus (arrows) because it lies perpendicular to the ultrasonic beam and permits more accurate measurements. In another baby, note that the presence of clear fluid in the stomach (asterisk, **E**) allows much better delineation of the thickened pylorus. He was given glucose water to drink during the study. The mucosal surface is represented by white or echogenic lines through the gray of the hypertrophied muscle. Arrows mark the diameter of the pylorus. G = gallbladder.

experience. Random occurrence of pyloric stenosis in the general population is considered to be 0.3 percent. The male-to-female ratio of occurrence is 4 or 5 to 1, depending on the series cited. Genetic predisposition to pyloric stenosis is well recognized, but the mode of inheritance is uncertain. Carter and Evans (1969) traced a huge series of families in which one parent had pyloric stenosis. They found that 20 percent of sons and 7 percent of daughters of an affected woman had pyloric stenosis, and 5 percent of sons and 2.5 percent of daughters of an affected man had pyloric stenosis. We have scanned twins and triplets who each had pyloric stenosis, but of a pair of monozygotic twins, both do not invariably have the disease when one twin is diagnosed (Hicks et al., 1981). This raises questions about postnatal influences that may trigger the hypertrophy.

Ideally, imaging is reserved for those babies in whom an experienced examiner cannot feel the "olive" that represents the hypertrophied pyloric muscle. Diagnosis can be made with ultrasonography or contrast examination of the stomach. A little more practice is required for ultrasonic examination of the pylorus than the literature suggests. If the presentation is atypical and the ultrasonograms are difficult to interpret, there is no shame in repeating the study (after clinical examination) in 24 hours or in performing an upper gastrointestinal series instead. Any baby who is vomiting should be managed medically to prevent dehydration; surgery for pyloric stenosis is not an emergency procedure.

For the ultrasonographic study, we position the baby supinely on the examining table and put a rolled towel under the left side of the abdomen, thereby placing the baby in a right posterior oblique position. This encourages distention of the antrum with fluid and allows easier localization of the gastric outlet. The gallbladder is a good landmark, as it tends to sit on the duodenal cap. We slowly move a transducer of high frequency (5 MHz or higher), preferably linear array or wide sector, and hold it in transverse orientation, along the right upper abdominal wall. When the pyloric channel is found, we rotate and angle the transducer so that it is aligned with the long axis of the channel (Fig. 12–1). If there is no fluid in the antrum, we feed the baby 20 to 30 ml of glucose water, through a nipple. We prefer feeding the infant, rather than instilling water through a nasogastric tube, because the normal physiology of swallowing and subsequent gastric peristalsis aids in evaluating antral emptying. Overdistention of the stomach pushes the pylorus posteriorly and makes its identification more difficult. However, a hugely distended stomach, 3 or more hours after the baby has been fed, is corroborative evidence of obstruction at the gastric outlet.

In infants with pyloric stenosis, gastric peristalsis squeezes down on the antrum but stops at the hypertrophied pyloric muscle, which indents the fluid-filled antrum. The gastric mucosa is echogenic, probably from its glycoprotein layer of mucus, and it continues as echogenic streaks through the hypertrophied muscle, which is more lucent. If one is looking with the transducer down the "barrel" of the pyloric channel, the outer borders of the muscle are less distinct because of refraction. It is preferable to have the transducer perpendicular to the pyloric muscle and aligned with the center of the channel. Incomplete obstruction of the gastric outlet in some babies who have pyloric stenosis means that some fluid occasionally dribbles into the duodenum and fills the duodenal cap. More often, the coadapted mucosal surfaces of the empty cap produce an echogenic triangle that marks the end of the pylorus. Active peristalsis against the obstructing muscle is often associated with the baby's grimacing, frowning, and becoming restless. An examiner's warm hands, warm gel, light pressure, and constancy of position of the transducer are necessary to document failure of antral emptying and lack of change in the pyloric muscle.

The ultrasonographic criteria for diagnosis of pyloric stenosis vary slightly between institutions; some advocate primary reliance on measurements of muscle thickness, and others on length of channel.

When we began using ultrasonography in the diagnosis of pyloric stenosis, we used static B-scanners and could measure only the diameter of the muscle with any precision (Teele and Smith, 1977). Anecdotally, if the son of our colleague Ed Smith had not been vomiting at the time, we probably would not have considered using ultrasonography for the diagnosis of pyloric stenosis. The "old" measurements (before 1983) should be ignored, as there are many more recent studies in which measurements were taken from real-time scanning. We tend to use measurements to support the subjective impression

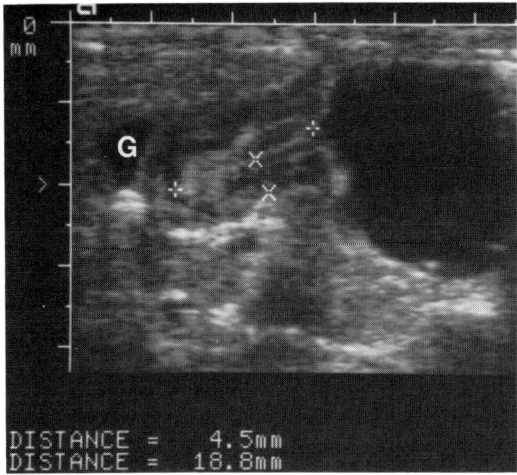

Figure 12-2. Measurements are included on this scan, which is identical to that shown in Figure 12-1E. The distance between plus signs marks the length of the channel, and the distance between X signs marks the thickness of one wall—actually, the radius of the pylorus, as opposed to the diameter. G = gallbladder.

that pyloric hypertrophy is present. Our composite score includes muscle thickness ≥3.5 mm, channel length ≥17 mm, little if any passage of gastric contents, and gastric peristalsis that stops abruptly at the pyloric muscle (Fig. 12-2). Table 12-1 lists the measurements that have been published in recent literature. Note that some authors measured length of muscle and others measured length of channel. There are references in the literature suggesting increased likelihood of renal anomalies in those with pyloric stenosis (Atwell and Levick, 1981). It is very easy to scan both kidneys at the time of the study for pyloric stenosis to rule in or out major anomalies.

Surgery for pyloric stenosis entails using a transverse abdominal incision, delivering the pylorus into the wound, splitting and then spreading the hypertrophied muscle, and checking for mucosal integrity before replacing the pylorus into the peritoneal cavity and closing the incision. A notched appearance of the muscle may be evident on a postoperative transverse scan of the pylorus. Ultrasonic and radiographic signs of pyloric stenosis, except for delayed gastric emptying, may persist up to 6 weeks postoperatively (Sauerbrei and Paloschi, 1983; Jamroz et al., 1986).

If we find no evidence of pyloric stenosis in a baby suspected of having it, we survey the abdomen in the hope of diagnosing another cause for vomiting.

OTHER CAUSES OF VOMITING IN NEONATES

Hayden and colleagues (1987) stated that gastritis can be diagnosed with ultrasonography when the mucosal thickness increases to 4 mm and is associated with no or minimal muscular hypertrophy (Fig. 12-3).

Antral web is a variably occluding membrane that bridges the antrum in the prepyloric area. If the gastric antrum is filled with clear fluid, the web, if present, should be evident as a linear echogenic band. A duodenal web has been diagnosed with ultrasonography because it was outlined on both sides by fluid (Cremin and Solomon, 1987). Strands of mucus should not be mistaken for a web. They are more irregular, quite mobile, and usually multiple.

We have examined two babies who had cystic duplication, one of the distal stomach, the other of the duodenum. Both presented with vomiting in the neonatal period, and ultrasonography for both infants revealed a cystic mass at the gastric outlet (Fig. 12-4).

Annular pancreas (which usually coexists with duodenal stenosis or atresia) may be diagnosed on ultrasonography if, on transverse scans, fluid in the duodenum is noted to pass through the middle of a prominent

Table 12-1. MEASUREMENTS FOR DIAGNOSIS OF PYLORIC STENOSIS

Reference	Muscle Thickness	Muscle Diameter	Muscle Length	Channel Length
Blumhagen and Noble (1983)	≥4	—	—	—
Blumhagen et al. (1988)	≥3.2	—	—	—
Bowen (1988)	≥5	≥15	—	≥17
Haller and Cohen (1986)	≥4	≥15	—	≥18
Lund Kofoed et al. (1988)	≥4	≥10	≥19	—
Stunden et al. (1986)	>3	≥14	—	≥17
Tunell and Wilson (1984)	>4	≥14	≥19	—

Note: All measurements are in millimeters.

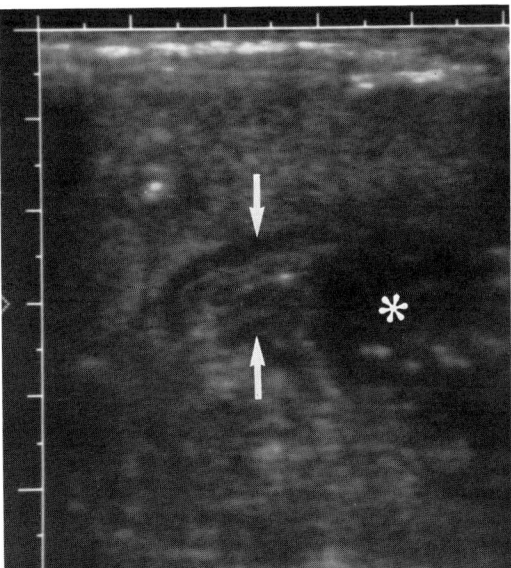

Figure 12–3. In this baby, who had gastritis as proved by biopsy, the echogenic mucosal surface is thickened, but the more lucent muscle is not. Arrows mark the diameter of the antropyloric region. Asterisk marks gastric lumen filled with fluid and debris.

pancreatic bulge (U. Willi, personal communication, April 1987). Pancreatitis as a cause for vomiting is rare in babies unless associated with an anomaly of the foregut, but the pancreas is in the neighborhood and easy to scan.

There are multiple other causes for vomiting by babies, conditions that are unassociated with structural abnormalities of stomach or duodenum. In fact, vomiting is a very nonspecific sign, and in many cases no obvious etiology is found. In rare instances, gallstones in neonates may be associated with vomiting and may be diagnosed with ultrasonography. On one occasion we examined a baby who was thought to have pyloric stenosis because of his projectile vomitus. Ultrasonography showed no abnormality of the gastric antrum but allowed diagnosis of urosepsis secondary to bilateral obstruction at the ureterovesical junction.

Proving the presence of gastroesophageal reflux on ultrasonography by showing fluid entering the lower esophagus (Wright et al., 1988) simply reinforces the parents' history of their baby's vomiting or regurgitating and does nothing to prove its cause.

Arguments revolve around the subject that we have saved for last: the use of ultrasonography to diagnose malrotation. Malrotation is incomplete rotation of the fetal intestine, which results in (1) shortening of the mesenteric base, which normally lies obliquely across the retroperitoneum; (2) formation of abnormal mesenteric attachments (Ladd bands); and (3) absence of the ligament of Treitz (a suspensory ligament of connective tissue and smooth muscle that extends from the root of the superior mesenteric artery (SMA) to the third and fourth portions of the

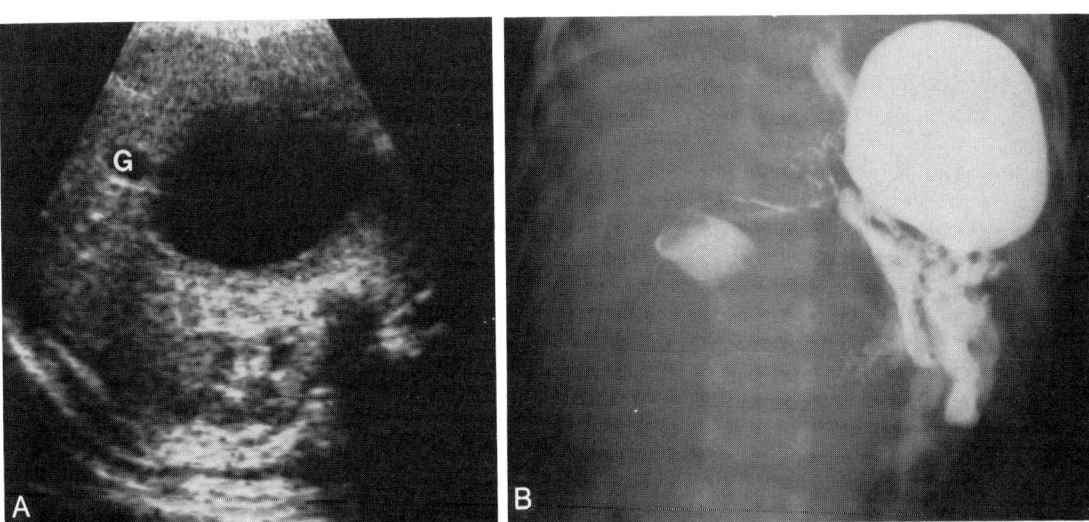

Figure 12–4. Gastric duplication cyst is an unusual cause of obstruction. Transverse scan of the upper abdomen **(A)** shows the cyst adjacent to the gallbladder (G). Confirmatory study with barium **(B)** shows partial obstruction from distortion of the gastric antrum by the large cyst. (From Teele RL and Share JC: The abdominal mass in the neonate. Semin Roentgenol 1988; 23:175–184.)

duodenum). Obstruction of the duodenum may be caused by Ladd bands or by a volvulus of the midgut around the narrow pedicle that carries the superior mesenteric vessels. A dilated, fluid-filled duodenum that narrows to a beak is the ultrasonographic picture of a midgut volvulus (Hayden et al., 1984; Haller and Cohen, 1986; Cohen et al., 1987). However, a volvulus can be an intermittent event, and there is an unknown number of children with malrotation who may or may not be symptomatic at the time of medical examination. Ruling out malrotation on the basis of a normal ultrasonogram, which cannot identify mesenteric attachments, places a great deal of faith in ultrasonography. However, to add more confusion to the issue are reports in which children with proven malrotation were shown to have a relationship of superior mesenteric vessels that was different from normal (Gaines et al., 1987; Loyer and Eggli, 1989). In each, on transverse scans, the superior mesenteric vein (SMV) was anterior to, or to the left of, the SMA rather than lying to the right (Fig. 12–5). There is, at present, no large study to show how reliable a sign of malrotation this might be. We have anecdotal experience with false-positive and false-negative scans. One child with malrotation proven at surgery had a completely normal relationship of superior mesenteric vessels (Fig. 12–6). In three others with proven malrotation, there was an abnormal relationship with the SMV anterior to, or to the left of, the SMA. In another child who had an abnormally related SMV/SMA, two gastrointestinal studies with barium yielded normal results, and the child was not taken to the operating room. However, we do consider it worth scanning the pancreas and vascular relationships in babies or children who are vomiting. If the clinical situation or ultrasonographic findings are at all suspicious, we recommend following ultrasonography with contrast radiography.

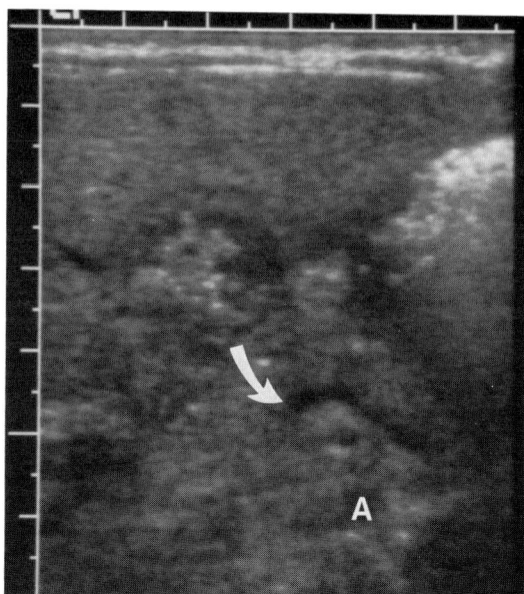

Figure 12–6. The normal relationship of the SMA to the confluence of the SMV with the splenic vein is shown on this transverse scan. Arrow points to venous confluence. A = aorta.

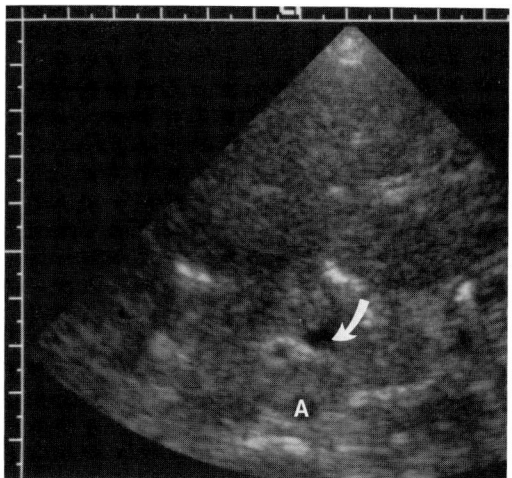

Figure 12–5. This baby had malrotation associated with reversal of normal relationships between the superior mesenteric artery (SMA) and the superior mesenteric vein (SMV). On this transverse scan, the SMV (arrow) is to the left of the SMA. A = aorta.

REFERENCES

Pyloric Stenosis

Atwell JD, Levick P: Congenital hypertrophic pyloric stenosis and associated anomalies in the genitourinary tract. J Pediatr Surg 1981; 16:1029–1035.

Ball TI, Atkinson GO Jr, Gay BB Jr: Ultrasound diagnosis of hypertrophic pyloric stenosis: Real-time application and the demonstration of a new sonographic sign. Radiology 1983; 147:499–502.

Blumhagen JD, Noble HGS: Muscle thickness in hypertrophic pyloric stenosis: Sonographic determination. AJR 1983; 140:221–223.

Blumhagen JD: Invited commentary: The role of ultrasonography in the evaluation of vomiting in infants [with introduction by WE Berdon]. Pediatr Radiol 16:267–70, 1986

Blumhagen JD, Maclin L, Krauter D, et al: Sonographic diagnosis of hypertrophic pyloric stenosis. AJR 1988; 150:1367–1370.

Bowen A: The vomiting infant: Recent advances and unsettled issues in imaging. Radiol Clin North Am 1988; 26:377–392.

Breaux CW Jr, Georgeson KE, Royal SA, et al: Changing patterns in the diagnosis of hypertrophic pyloric stenosis. Pediatrics 1988; 81:213–217.

Carroll BA: US of the gastrointestinal tract. Radiology 1989; 172:605–608.

Carter CO, Evans KA: Inheritance of congenital pyloric stenosis. J Med Genet 1969; 6:233–254.

Carver RA, Okorie M, Steiner GM, et al: Infantile hypertrophic pyloric stenosis—diagnosis from the pyloric muscle index. Clin Radiol 1987; 38:625–627.

Dawson KP: The use of ultrasound in the diagnosis of congenital pyloric stenosis. NZ Med J 1988; 101:1–2.

Foley LC, Slovis TL, Campbell JB, et al: Evaluation of the vomiting infant. Am J Dis Child 1989; 143:660–661.

Forman GP, Leonidas JC, Kronfeld GD: A rational approach to the diagnosis of hypertrophic pyloric stenosis: Do the results match the claims? J Pediatr Surg 1990; 25:262–266.

Haller JO, Cohen HL: Hypertrophic pyloric stenosis: Diagnosis using ultrasound. Radiology 1986; 161:335–339.

Hicks LM, Morgan A, Anderson MR: Pyloric stenosis—A report of triplet females and notes on its inheritance. J Pediatr Surg 1981; 16:739–743.

Is ultrasound really necessary for the diagnosis of hypertrophic pyloric stenosis? [editorial]. Lancet 1988; 1:1146.

Jamroz GA, Blocker SH, McAlister WH: Radiographic findings after incomplete pyloromyotomy. Gastrointest Radiol 1986; 11:139–141.

Keller H, Waldmann D, Greiner P: Comparison of preoperative sonography with intraoperative findings in congenital hypertrophic pyloric stenosis. J Pediatr Surg 1987; 22:950–952.

Lund Kofoed PE, Høst A, Elle B, Larsen C: Hypertrophic pyloric stenosis: Determination of muscle dimensions by ultrasound. Br J Radiol 1988; 61:19–20.

McKeown T, MacMahon B: Infantile hypertrophic pyloric stenosis in parent and child. Arch Dis Child 1955; 30:497–500.

Okorie NM, Dickson JA, Carver RA, et al: What happens to the pylorus after pyloromyotomy? Arch Dis Child 1988; 63:1339–1341.

Sauerbrei EE, Paloschi GGB: The ultrasonic features of hypertrophic pyloric stenosis, with emphasis on the postoperative appearance. Radiology 1983; 147:499–502.

Stunden RJ, LeQuesne GW, Little KET: The improved ultrasound diagnosis of hypertrophic pyloric stenosis. Pediatr Radiol 1986; 16:200–205.

Swischuk LE, Hayden CK Jr, Stansberry SD: Sonographic pitfalls in imaging of the antropyloric region in infants. Radiographics 1989; 9:437–447.

Teele RL, Smith EH: Ultrasound in the diagnosis of idiopathic hypertrophic pyloric stenosis. N Engl J Med 1977; 296:1149–1150.

Tunell WP, Wilson DA: Pyloric stenosis: Diagnosis by real time sonography, the pyloric muscle length method. J Pediatr Surg 1984; 19:795–799.

Weiskittel DA, Leary DL, Blane CE: Ultrasound diagnosis of evolving pyloric stenosis. Gastrointest Radiol 1989; 14:22–24.

Yip WC, Tay JS, Wong HB: Sonographic diagnosis of infantile hypertrophic pyloric stenosis: Critical appraisal of reliability and diagnostic criteria. JCU 1985; 13:329–332.

Other Causes for Vomiting in the Neonate

Bisset RA, Gupta SC, Zammit-Maempel I: Radiographic and ultrasound appearances of an intra-mural haematoma of the pylorus. Clin Radiol 1988; 39:316–318.

Cohen HL, Haller JO, Mestel AL, et al: Neonatal duodenum: Fluid-aided US examination. Radiology 1987; 164:805–809.

Cremin BJ, Solomon DJ: Ultrasonic diagnosis of duodenal diaphragm. Pediatr Radiol 1987; 17:489–490.

Gaines PA, Saunders AJS, Drake D: Midgut malrotation diagnosed by ultrasound. Clin Radiol 1987; 38:51–53.

Hayden CK Jr, Boulden TF, Swischuk LE, et al: Sonographic demonstration of duodenal obstruction with midgut volvulus. AJR 1984; 143:9–10.

Hayden CK Jr, Swischuk LE, Rytting JE: Gastric ulcer disease in infants: US findings. Radiology 1987; 164:131–134.

Lambrecht L, Robberecht E, Deschynkel K, et al: Ultrasonic evaluation of gastric clearing in young infants. Pediatr Radiol 1988; 18:314–318.

Loyer E, Eggli KD: Sonographic evaluation of superior mesenteric vascular relationship in malrotation. Pediatr Radiol 1989; 19:173–175.

McAlister WH, Katz ME, Perlman JM, et al: Sonography of focal foveolar hyperplasia causing obstruction in an infant. Pediatr Radiol 1988; 18:79–81.

Shaw D: Value of ultrasound in differentiating causes of persistent vomiting in infants. [letter] Arch Dis Child 1989; 64:889.

Swischuk LE, Fawcett HD, Hayden CK Jr, et al: Gastroesophageal reflux: How much imaging is required? Radiographics 1988; 8:1137–1145.

Wright LL, Baker KR, Meny RG: Ultrasound demonstration of gastroesophageal reflux. J Ultrasound Med 1988; 7:471–475.

CHAPTER 13

BLUNT ABDOMINAL TRAUMA

The diagnostic approach to the child who has suffered blunt abdominal trauma depends on the facilities that are available, the expertise and experience of the clinicians who are evaluating the patient, and the specific skills of the radiologist who is involved. One must consider the size of the child and the type and severity of trauma to which that child has been exposed. In a community that legislates and enforces mandatory usage of seat belts in automobiles, fewer children are at risk in car accidents; in a farming community, children may be at risk from falls and from using farm equipment. A referral center with an established reputation for handling victims of trauma will attract more such referrals and develop protocols for treating severely injured children. The reader must look critically at his or her own situation within a hospital or practice and then choose the best approach for that situation. Large studies of traumatized patients have been reported in the literature, and, not surprisingly, there is no consensus on a single best way to evaluate the injured child (Filiatrault et al., 1987; Kaufman et al., 1984; Kuhn, 1985; Grüessner et al., 1989).

The recommendations of the experts notwithstanding, it is best to do what one does best. To provide some guidelines for evaluation, we begin in the emergency room, where clinical examination takes place and samples of the patient's blood and urine are acquired. The type and severity of trauma are key information to be obtained from the child or a witness to the injury. Acute deceleration during an automobile accident, while the child is immobilized solely by a lap belt, puts spinal cord and renal pedicles at risk. A hard fall onto the handlebars of a bicycle can result in duodenal hematoma and pancreatitis. Crush injuries of the upper abdomen typically cause lacerations or contusions of the liver. Blunt trauma to the left side injures the spleen. Evidence of bruising or other dermal injury is often minimal. A child who is unconscious as a result of head injury is unable to localize pain. Others with multiple injuries, but who are conscious, may extinguish all but one painful stimulus. Ileus is a typical sequela of trauma; therefore, the abdomen is tympanitic and distended. Because of the difficulty in interpreting the physical examination of a patient who has sustained trauma, many physicians in emergency rooms have relied on peritoneal lavage to assess the need for immediate surgical intervention. In neither our hospital nor most other pediatric hospitals is peritoneal lavage a routine procedure (Filiatrault et al., 1987). Complete blood count, and amylase, serum glutamate oxaloacetic transaminase (SGOT), blood urea nitrogen, creatinine, and electrolyte levels are the basic studies on blood. Urinalysis (microscopic evaluation, not simply dipstick) is done on a sample from a catheterized bladder if the patient cannot void. Plain films of chest and abdomen, although typically non-diagnostic, can be most helpful when results are positive. Free intraperitoneal air, in the absence of pneumomediastinum, implies perforation of the gastrointestinal tract. Rib fractures suggest hepatic injury if right-sided and splenic injury if left-sided. Fractures of transverse processes direct attention to the urinary tract. Pleural and pulmonary parenchymal opacities are associated with infradiaphragmatic injury 50 to 66 percent of the time, especially when left-sided (Kaufman et al., 1984).

When the historical information and results from clinical, laboratory, and radiographic examinations have been assembled, the decision regarding further imaging is made. If the child's condition is unstable and hemostasis cannot be achieved, emergent laparotomy follows. If injury has apparently involved more than one organ, computed tomography (CT) scanning is the most efficient next procedure if it is available immediately. This is particularly true when intracranial injury is also suspected. The head and abdomen can be scanned sequentially. Any child who has suspected injury to the spinal cord coexistent with abdominal trauma should have CT scanning. It is worth noting that axial sections, provided by CT, may not show a vertebral compression fracture. A lateral view of the spine is recommended for those children who have had injury involving the back (Taylor and Eggli, 1988).

Judging that more than one organ has been injured is not easy. In one study of 170 children, 50 percent of those with abnormalities had more than one lesion (Filiatrault et al., 1987). In another study, only 18 percent of 62 patients had multiple injuries (Kaufman et al., 1984).

If the clinicians are reasonably sure that only one organ has been injured, the imaging can be tailored. There are some centers that are skilled and experienced in scintigraphy and use radionuclide scanning for suspected splenic injury. However, probably 7 to 10 percent of scans are falsely positive, and an indeterminate number of scans are falsely negative; these studies, in comparison with CT, tend to miss small lesions (Kaufman et al., 1984). Injured splenic tissue is not removed unless the patient cannot maintain hemostasis with conservative measures.

Ultrasonic scanning of the traumatized spleen is not as reliable as CT scanning, although, in experienced hands, the accuracy of diagnosis can approach 90 percent. The most useful sign of splenic injury is free intraperitoneal fluid. Small lacerations and subcapsular collections are easily missed. Because the patient tends to splint the injured side, the ribs are close together, narrowing the ultrasonic windows.

Elevation of hepatic enzymes in serum flags the liver as a site of injury (Fig. 13–1). The liver can be evaluated with scintigraphy, although not as completely nor as accurately as with CT. Ultrasonography and scintigraphy can be falsely negative or underestimate the extent of hepatic trauma, in comparison with CT. Free intraperitoneal fluid, although more frequently a sign of splenic trauma, also may result from hepatic injury.

There is one situation in which ultrasonography has been very useful: for the neonate who has hepatic hematoma that follows sepsis, asphyxia, or resuscitative efforts (Share et al., 1990). Such babies are generally in too unstable a condition to travel to a CT scanner. Ultrasonography can confirm the diagnosis in an affected neonate, who typically presents with increasing abdominal girth and dropping hematocrit (Fig. 13–2).

One report suggested that in patients with suspected renal injury only, intravenous urography should be the study of choice but be reserved for those children whose urinalysis shows more than 20 red blood cells per high-power field. Of 78 children who had had renal trauma and were seen in an emergency room, 26 (33 percent) had an abnormal intravenous urogram (Lieu et al., 1988). Half of those 26 children had an underlying congenital anomaly that was uncovered by the traumatic episode. Similar results were reported by Stalker and colleagues (1990), who relied primarily on analysis of CT scans. Urography provides both physiologic and anatomic information. Ultrasonography, with the addition of Doppler imaging, has not been used for enough traumatized patients for clinicians to know its possibilities or limitations. There is no question that a kidney may look close to normal on routine ultrasonic scanning and yet be acutely ischemic. We saw one little girl who had hematuria, a dubious history of trauma, and a kidney that appeared normal on standard ultrasonography but was found to be completely nonfunctional as a result of arterial injury and thrombosis, on urography (Jones et al., 1990). We have used ultrasonography to follow patients whose renal injury has been diagnosed with CT scanning or urog-

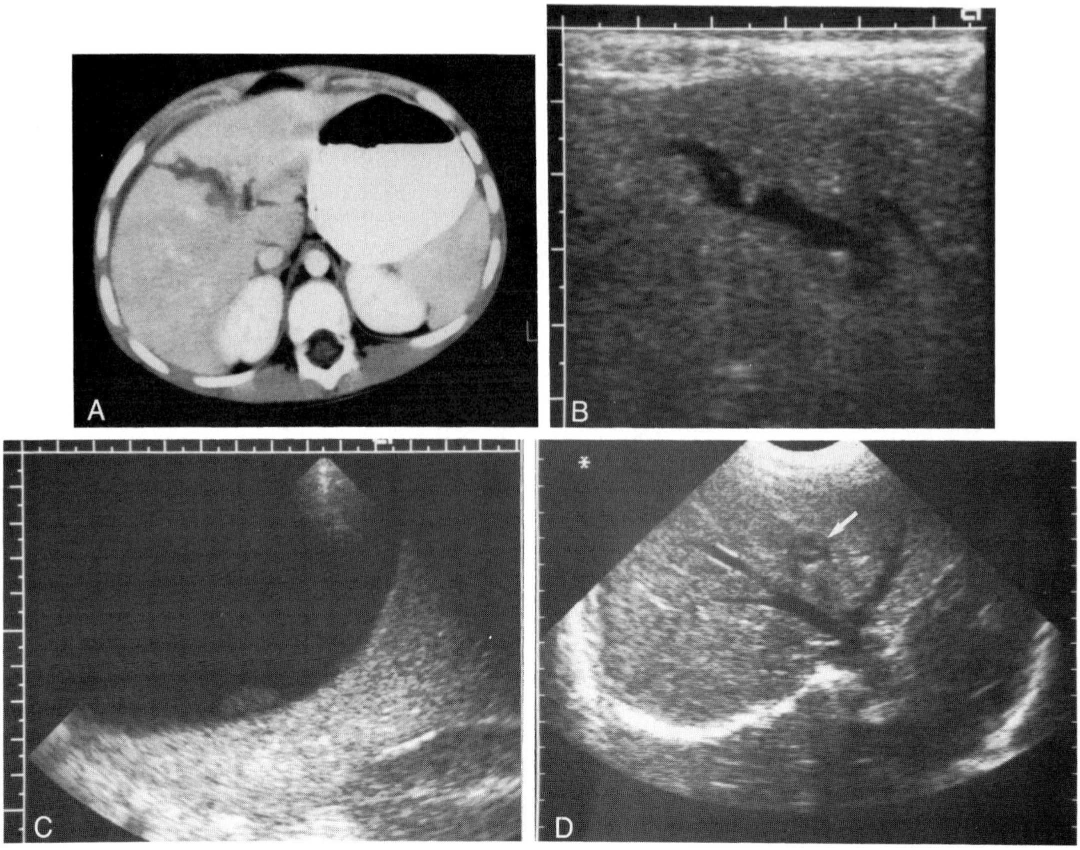

Figure 13–1. This 5-year-old boy fell onto the handlebars of his bicycle. He was admitted to the hospital, and the computed tomography (CT) scan was done emergently after clinical examination revealed severe right upper quadrant tenderness and elevation of liver enzymes. The laceration in the right lobe of the liver is obvious on the contrast-enhanced CT scan **(A)**. He was managed conservatively while in the hospital. Twelve days later, the ultrasonogram **(B)** showed continued abnormality in the right lobe of the liver. Compare the irregular lucency representing the liver laceration with the preceding CT scan. In addition, a large collection of fluid was also identified in the superolateral subcapsular region **(C)**. When percutaneously drained, this fluid proved to be bile. A catheter was left in place for 10 days, after which drainage ceased. A follow-up scan 3 weeks later showed persisting lucency in the liver (arrow) from the laceration but resolution of the biloma **(D)**.

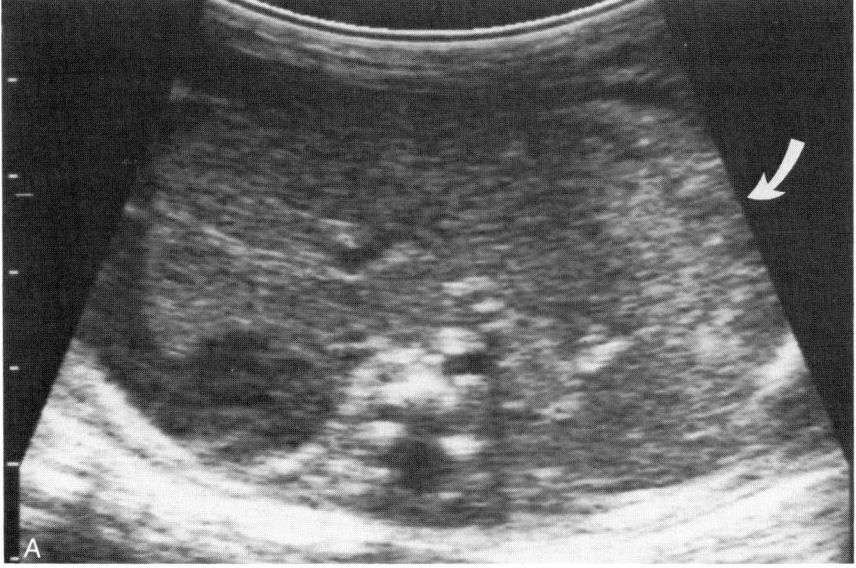

Figure 13–2 *See legend on opposite page*

366

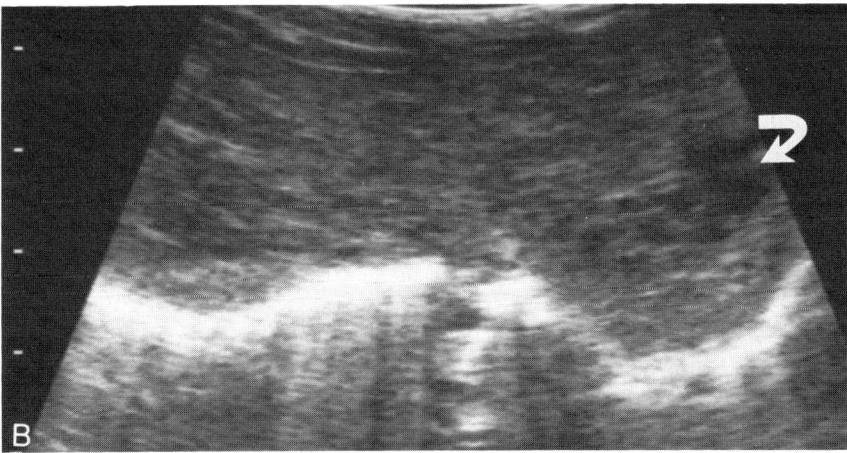

Figure 13–2 *Continued* Portable scans were performed for this 1-day-old girl. She had had a difficult delivery and gradually developed abdominal distention associated with decreasing hematocrit. On the initial transverse scan of upper abdomen **(A)**, there was an echogenic focus (arrow) in the left lobe of the liver associated with free intraperitoneal fluid. After conservative management, a follow-up scan 13 days later **(B)**, showed irregular lucency (arrow) in the left lobe of the liver resulting from the preceding liver laceration. (From Share JC, Pursley D, Teele RL: Unsuspected hepatic injury in the neonate—Diagnosis by ultrasonography. Pediatr Radiol 1990;20:320–322.)

raphy and who have been managed nonoperatively (Fig. 13–3).

For those with suspected pancreatoduodenal injury, the typical story is of previous blunt anterior abdominal trauma. When there is increased amylase in serum and the child is vomiting, coexisting duodenal perforation has to be diagnosed or ruled out. Examination with contrast will show the intramural mass of a duodenal hematoma, if present, but may not demonstrate perforation if hematoma is tamponading the rent. CT has not been foolproof in the diagnosis of duodenal rupture (Cook et al., 1986), and

Figure 13–3. This 10-year-old boy fell 4 feet out of a tree, had a momentary loss of consciousness, and began complaining of increasing right-sided abdominal pain when he arrived at the emergency room. His initial hematocrit was 36. He had visible hematuria. The CT scan that followed **(A)** shows an irregular right renal contour associated with a perinephric hematoma. The lower pole was nonfunctional. While he was in the hospital, the hematocrit continued to fall to 26. Ultrasonography was requested to determine whether the perinephric hematoma was increasing in size. The orientation of the transverse scan **(B)** is equivalent to that of the cross-sectional view shown on the preceding CT scan. The size of the perinephric hematoma was similar to that in the preceding radiographic study. Coronal scan of the right kidney **(C)** shows the irregular echogenicity (arrows) that represents the renal contusion in the lower pole.

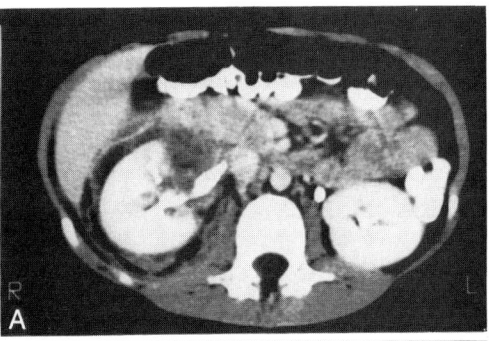
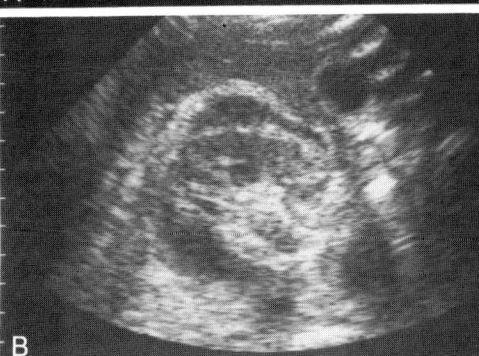
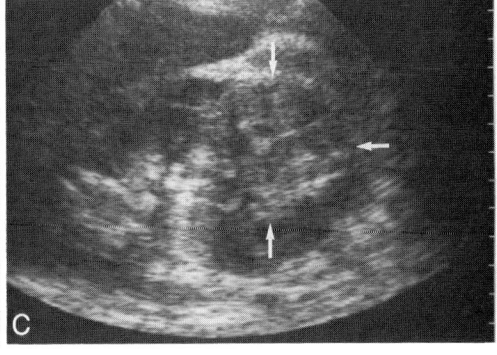

ultrasonography is even less reliable. Each child with duodenal hematoma must be watched carefully during the 7 to 10 days after the trauma, even though perforation is a rare complication. Ultrasonography is a good method with which to follow resolution of duodenal and pancreatic abnormalities and to diagnose pseudocyst which results in 50 percent of patients, generally 7 to 10 days after the trauma (see Chapter 15).

Having written this rather negative overview of ultrasonography vis-à-vis the evaluation of an acutely injured child, we will pretend that the reader has no other option but to use ultrasonography in evaluating a child and highlight important points of the examination. Human nature being as it is, an ultrasonographic examination will be much more revealing if one knows that there is no recourse to CT, scintigraphy, or other imaging.

First is the search for free intraperitoneal fluid. Free fluid may pool in the pelvis behind the bladder, track into Morison pouch, or flow around the spleen. Large amounts of clear fluid signal possible pancreatic ductal laceration or a ruptured bladder. Echogenic fluid may be blood or intestinal contents. However, it is unusual to have traumatic perforation of the intraperitoneal gut without free intraperitoneal air. Clotting blood may be echogenic and difficult to appreciate, especially if pooled in the pelvis around a catheterized and, therefore, empty bladder (Fig. 13–4). Examination of the liver must be systematic and include both lobes. The areas usually missed by ultrasonography are the lateral segment of the left lobe and the dome of the liver. Hematoma associated with lacerations can be hypoechogenic or hyperechogenic (Fig. 13–5). The border of the liver on all sides should be evaluated for subcapsular

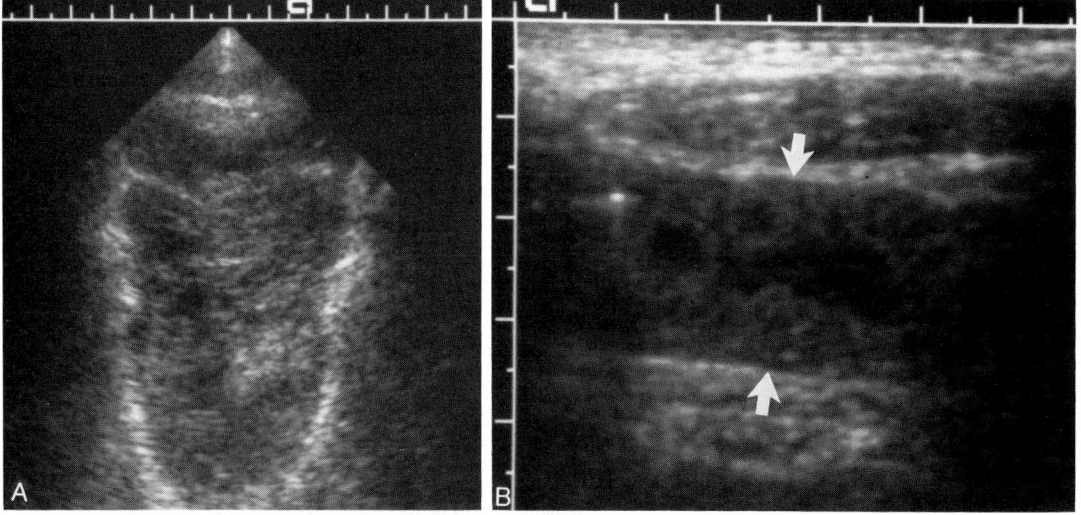

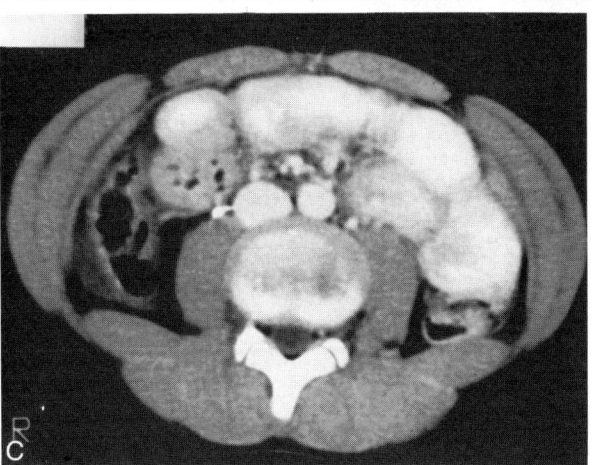

Figure 13–4. The important history of this 12-year-old boy, who was in a motor vehicle accident, was the fact that he had been secured by a loose lap belt. The rapid-deceleration injury resulted in trauma to the bowel, tearing of mesenteric vessels, and free blood flow into the peritoneal cavity. Blood pooled in the pelvis around bowel loops may be a poorly defined echogenic mass, as seen on the transverse scan of the pelvis (A). The bladder was virtually empty at the time, and thus there was no scanning "window." Transverse scan of the upper abdomen (B) shows the thickened jejunal wall (arrows) associated with jejunal hematoma. A CT scan (C) had preceded ultrasonography, and in retrospect, one can detect the same mural thickening of small bowel in the upper abdomen just posterior to the rectus muscles.

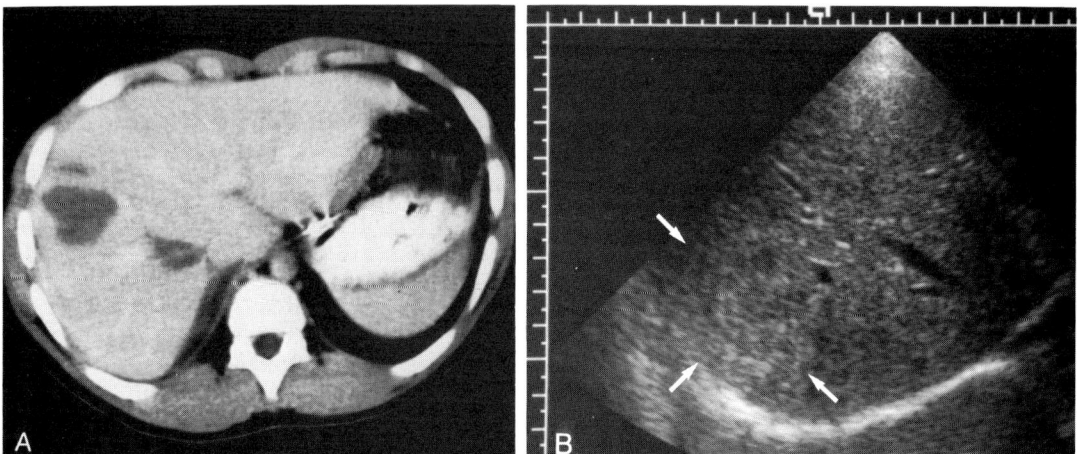

Figure 13-5. Injury to the liver is readily visible on this transverse section from a contrast-enhanced CT scan **(A)**. This injury to a 9-year-old boy occurred when he was struck by a car. Because he had persisting abdominal pain, ultrasonography was requested five days later **(B)**. The area of injury is represented by only a subtle inhomogeneity in the periphery of the liver (arrows). This might be very difficult to detect without the preceding CT scan. This patient was treated conservatively and had no complication from his hepatic trauma.

collections of blood. The diaphragm may have ruptured and appear discontinuous on scans. Pleural fluid should be evident, if present, as should the solid mass of pulmonary parenchymal contusion, if it is adjacent to diaphragm.

The best way to examine the spleen is in transverse and coronal planes through the interspaces of the 10th and 11th ribs. If the child can move his or her arm with the hand above the head, the interspaces will open up a little more. Transducers of high frequency, preferably linear array, should be used. Any irregularity in the splenic parenchyma is suspect, and it may be apparent in only one plane. Sections have to include all splenic tissue, posterior to anterior, and superior to inferior. A double linear interface of the splenic outline suggests a subcapsular collection of blood. Depending on the stage of bleeding and clotting, intraparenchymal or perisplenic collections may be echogenic, lucent or mixed (Fig. 13-6).

The kidneys normally move with deep

Figure 13-6. Two weeks before this coronal scan of the left upper quadrant, this 15-year-old boy had been struck by a car while he was riding his bicycle. CT scan that immediately followed the trauma had shown splenic fracture associated with a large amount of intraperitoneal fluid. Follow-up ultrasonography was performed because the boy had persisting pain. The large perisplenic collection is mixed in its echogenicity. Depending on the stage of bleeding and clotting, there is a wide variation in appearance of intraperitoneal and perisplenic hematomas. No intervention occurred, and the hematoma gradually resorbed.

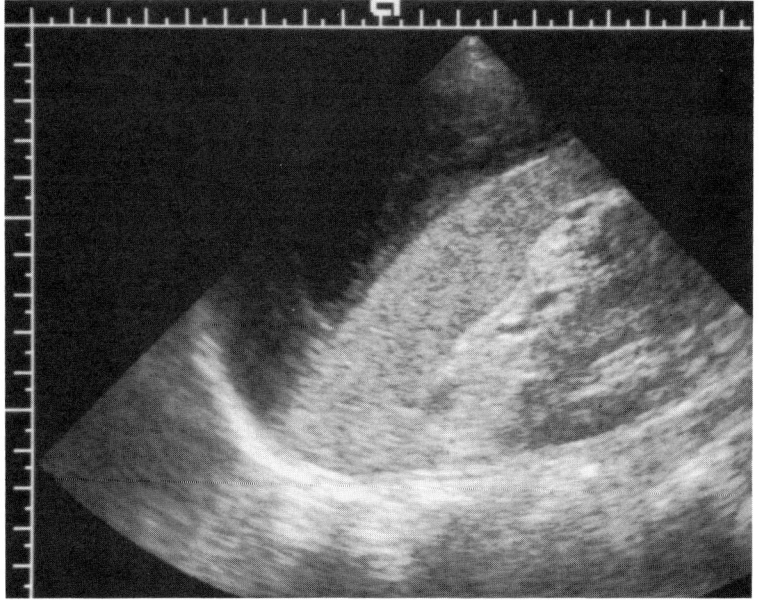

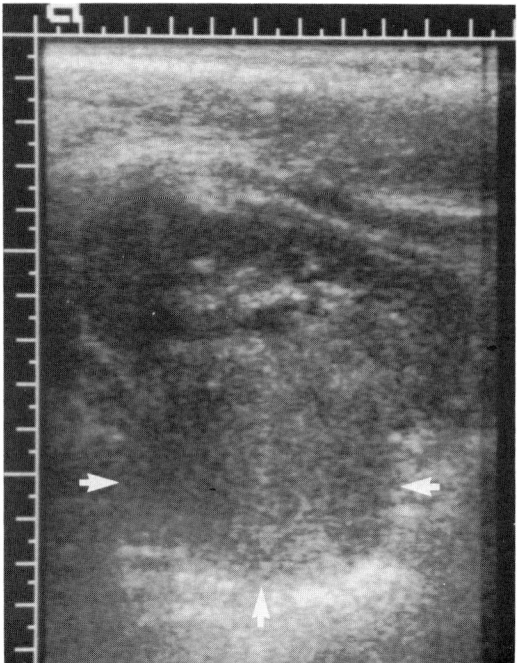

Figure 13–7. Minor trauma resulted in this child's presenting to the emergency room with gross hematuria. The patient was 7 years old and had been kicked by his brother. Longitudinal scan of the left kidney shows a 5 × 8 cm echogenic mass (arrows) extending anteriorly from the kidney. Further evaluation revealed this to be an avascular exophytic mass, which during surgery was found to be a Wilms tumor. Minor trauma may result in gross hematuria if there is an underlying renal mass or anomaly.

inspiratory and expiratory efforts. Immobility of a kidney after trauma indicates perinephric hematoma. Perinephric blood tends to accumulate around the area of renal laceration and then track inferiorly within the fascia of Gerota. A subcapsular hematoma produces a double linear interface if the beam of sound is directly perpendicular to the renal border. If not, the appearance of the subcapsular collection is of a fuzzy rind blending with the renal cortex. Renal laceration tends to produce a linear echogenicity when the ultrasonic beam is perpendicular to the crack. Renal contusion causes a blotchy echogenicity of affected parenchyma. Collections of clear fluid in retroperitoneum are usually urine that has extravasated from a ruptured calix or the pelvis. Hydronephrosis may be caused by an obstructing hematoma but is more often related to an underlying anomaly or abnormality of kidney that predisposed the kidney to trauma. In reported study, 4 to 23 percent of intravenous urograms, performed because of preceding trauma, showed an underlying abnormality (Lieu et al., 1988). Any kidney that has been traumatized should be inspected for a possible anomaly or tumor (Fig. 13–7). The contralateral renal fossa should also be scanned. A big lumpy kidney may actually be cross-fused ectopia, and the other fossa may be empty.

We know of two or three children who

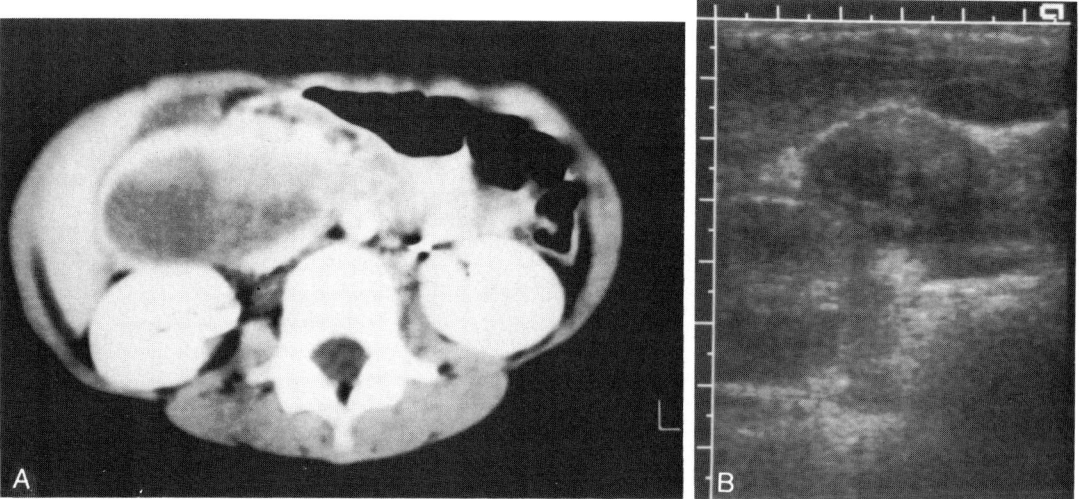

Figure 13–8. Two days before admission to the hospital, this patient fell from his bicycle. At presentation he was vomiting and had an amylase level of 1160. The CT scan performed on admission **(A)** shows a large duodenal hematoma immediately anterior to the kidney. Follow-up ultrasonograms were performed in order to monitor the resolution of the hematoma and to evaluate the pancreas for development of a pseudocyst. The hematoma gradually decreased in size, as shown on the transverse ultrasonogram **(B)**. No pancreatic pseudocyst developed.

had adrenal hematoma after trauma to the flank. None had surgery, and therefore we cannot rule out the possibility of a pre-existing lesion in their adrenal glands. Evaluating the adrenal area in addition to the kidney is worthwhile when a child presents with a history of retroperitoneal trauma.

In evaluations of the duodenum and pancreas, the patient should be rolled, if possible, into a partial right decubitus position, so as to move gastric fluid into the antrum. The gallbladder is a good signpost for the pyloriduodenal junction, and the intraluminal fluid can be followed down to the descending duodenum. Mural hematoma of the duodenum is usually large, echolucent, and laterally eccentric in relation to the compressed lumen of the descending duodenum, which presents as a thick echogenic line on sagittal scans and a circular blotch on transverse views (Fig. 13–8). Hematoma can also occur in the transverse duodenum and the ascending limb of duodenum but is decidedly less common in those areas. The common bile duct tends to be dilated and the gallbladder quite large. The head of the pancreas is usually swollen, as is the body and, variably, the tail in such cases. If the pancreatic duct can be traced in its entirety, there is only proximal obstruction without ductal laceration. A collection of fluid in the lesser sac or free fluid in the peritoneum immediately after trauma indicates ductal injury.

It is not unusual for duodenal hematoma and pancreatic injury to be identified as the source for a patient's pain and vomiting some days after the injury occurred. The actual traumatic episode may not have been reported by the child to parents. Bruising of the skin is often minimal or absent. We examined one child who told us of being stepped on by a horse several days before admission, and we were the first to hear this particularly pertinent history! Jejunal injury may follow automobile trauma when the lap belt crosses the child's waist rather than the pelvis (Fig. 13–4). Hematoma of the bowel may be followed by perforation.

Other situations that predispose a patient to duodenal or jejunal hematoma are earlier endoscopic biopsy and disorders of coagulation. The possibility that a small child has been battered should be considered if the child has no, or a suspicious, history of abdominal trauma but presents with hematoma in the wall of the bowel.

REFERENCES

Adler DD, Blane CE, Coran AG, et al: Splenic trauma in the pediatric patient: The integrated roles of ultrasound and computed tomography. Pediatrics 1986; 78:576–580.

Chambers JA, Pilbrow WJ: Ultrasound in abdominal trauma: An alternative to peritoneal lavage. Arch Emerg Med 1988; 5:26–33.

Cook DE, Walsh JW, Vick CW, et al: Upper abdominal trauma: Pitfalls in CT diagnosis. Radiology 1986; 159:65–69.

Filiatrault D, Longpre D, Patriquin H, et al: Investigation of childhood blunt abdominal trauma: A practical approach using ultrasound as the initial diagnostic modality. Pediatr Radiol 1987; 17:373–379.

Foley C, Teele RL: Duodenal and pancreatic injuries following blunt trauma: Evaluation by ultrasound. AJR 1979; 132:593–598.

Furtschegger A, Egender G, Jakse G: The value of sonography in the diagnosis and follow-up of patients with blunt renal trauma. Br J Urol 1988; 62:110–116.

Grüessner R, Mentges B, Düber C, et al: Sonography versus peritoneal lavage in blunt abdominal trauma. J Trauma 1989; 29:242–244.

Jones BE, Hoffer FA, Teele RL, et al: Pitfalls in pediatric urinary sonography. Urology 1990; 35:38–44.

Kaufman RA, Towbin R, Babcock D, et al: Upper abdominal trauma in children: Imaging evaluation. AJR 1984; 142:449–460.

Kuhn JP: Diagnostic imaging for the evaluation of abdominal trauma in children. Pediatr Clin North Am 1985; 32:1427–1447.

Leppäniemi A, Haapiainen R, Standertskjöld-Nordenstam CG, et al: Delayed presentation of blunt splenic injury. Am J Surg 1988; 155:745–749.

Lieu TA, Fleisher GR, Mahboubi S, et al: Hematuria and clinical findings as indications for intravenous pyelography in pediatric blunt renal trauma. Pediatrics 1988; 82:216–222.

Share JC, Pursley D, Teele RL: Unsuspected hepatic injury in the neonate—diagnosis by ultrasonography. Pediatr Radiol 1990; 20:320–322.

Stalker HP, Kaufman RA, Stedje K: The significance of hematuria in children after blunt abdominal trauma. AJR 1990; 154:569–571.

Taylor GA, Eggli KD: Lap-belt injuries of the lumbar spine in children: A pitfall in CT diagnosis. AJR 1988; 150:1355–1358.

CHAPTER 14

ASCITES AND OTHER ABDOMINAL PROBLEMS

Some topics do not fit comfortably into the problem-oriented chapters that we have created. This chapter, therefore, is a collection of ultrasonographic miscellany. It includes discussions of problems associated with ascites, abdominal vasculature, and imperforate anus.

EVALUATING THE CHILD WHO HAS ASCITES

Usually, the baby or child in whom ascites is diagnosed on clinical examination has a known underlying disease. Occasionally, ascites is the presenting sign of a problem, and even more rarely, ascites is found incidentally on abdominal ultrasonography. In this chapter we outline the causes of ascites in children. We begin with a discussion of the quantitation and characterization of ascitic fluid.

Under experimental conditions, with the pig as an animal model, ultrasonography can detect as little as 10 ml of fluid in the peritoneal cavity. In a series of experiments, this amount could be demonstrated behind the pig's bladder if the animal were held upright for scanning. With the pig in supine position, it took 20 ml of fluid to result in a positive scan. When 30 ml was injected, fluid could be identified in the perihepatic region. With 60 ml, loops of bowel were free floating (Dinkel et al., 1984).

Fluid ascends the pericolic gutters from the pelvis regardless of whether the patient is erect or supine, possibly because hydrostatic pressure is less in the upper abdomen (Proto et al., 1976). The distribution of intraperitoneal fluid is primarily defined by mesenteric attachments and peritoneal reflections (Meyers, 1970). Other factors include the site of origin of the fluid, the amount of fluid, the patient's position, the presence of adhesions, and anomalies of mesenteric attachment.

Ascitic fluid can be divided into two categories: simple (echofree) and complex (mildly to grossly echogenic). Simple ascitic fluid results from transudate, urine, cerebrospinal fluid (CSF), and, rarely, bile. Transudate results from an imbalance among capillary hydrostatic pressure, colloid oncotic pressure, and capillary permeability. The occurrence of increased capillary hydrostatic pressure is secondary to congestive heart failure, constrictive pericarditis, portal hypertension, Budd-Chiari syndrome, or any other situation that impedes abdominal venous return of blood to the heart. Decreased oncotic pressure results from a fall in levels of albumin in serum. Fluid escapes into extracellular spaces, and the intravascular volume decreases. This contraction of the vascular bed triggers retention of sodium and water, which leads to further accumulation of extravascular fluid. Severe malnutrition, hepatic disease, nephrosis, and protein-losing enteropathy are typical situations associated with hypoalbuminemia. Increase in permeability of capillaries may occur with allergic, inflammatory, and malignant diseases. Hormonally mediated inappropriate retention of sodium and water occurs in some patients with chronic severe anemia, renal failure, hepatic cirrhosis, and congestive heart failure (Newman and Teele, 1984). Urinary ascites typically results from obstruction of the urinary tract, perforation of a renal fornix, and decompression of the resultant retroperitoneal urinoma into the peritoneal space. On rare occasions, urinary ascites occurs from rupture of the bladder secondary to posterior urethral valves or from pelvic trauma. Instrumentation of the bladder, particularly of the augmented bladder, can also cause its perforation.

Cerebrospinal fluid (CSF) may develop into a loculated collection around the tip of a peritoneal shunt catheter or, in some cases, may fill the abdomen. Overproduction of CSF (from papilloma of the choroid plexus) or failure of the peritoneal surface to absorb fluid are the two major causes of overt ascites associated with peritoneal shunts.

Bile ascites in neonates is the result of perforation of the common bile duct (Balsam and Wasserstein, 1990; Haller et al., 1989). Biliary leakage that may follow hepatic trauma, surgery on the biliary tree, or percutaneous biopsy of the liver generally affects older children and tends to loculate in the right upper quadrant.

Complex ascitic fluid is usually an exudate with protein or blood causing the echogenic component. Chylous, hemorrhagic, inflammatory, and neoplastic ascites are the major causes of complex ascitic fluid. Perforation of the bowel is rarely diagnosed by the ultrasonographer because such a situation is usually quickly recognized as an acute surgical emergency on the basis of clinical and radiographic findings. Complex ascites is more likely to loculate than is simple ascites. Differentiating locules of echogenic ascites from fluid-filled loops of bowel is an ultrasonographic challenge. Computed tomography (CT) scanning, after thorough filling of the gastrointestinal tract with contrast, is superior in this diagnostic situation.

The major causes of ascites in the fetus and neonate are listed in Table 14–1 (Figs. 14–1 to 14–5). The causes of ascites in childhood overlap those of the neonate but are more often related to acquired disease rather than to congenital anomalies or infections. In Table 14–2 we list the problems and mechanisms of production associated with ascites in children who are outside the neonatal age group (Figs. 14–6 to 14–15). It is apparent, after a review of these lengthy tables, that a baby or child who has ascites needs a complete abdominal scan at presentation. One can go further and suggest that the heart and head should also be scanned if the abdominal scans are unrevealing. Structural cardiac disease or arrhythmias may be responsible for abdominal signs and symptoms. A baby who has an intracranial arteriovenous malformation can present with congestive heart failure and ascites.

Clinical information and results of laboratory tests can help to focus an ultrasonic examination. Following are a few tips that we have learned from experience.

1. A child with a huge mesenteric or ovarian cyst may be clinically diagnosed as having ascites. Displacement of the bowel and indentation of the bladder are characteristic effects of enclosed collections of intraabdominal fluid.

2. When extensive ascites is present, loops of air-filled bowel float to the anterior midabdomen. The fluid-filled bowel sinks to the posterior abdomen, as does the spleen. Coronal scans from the flanks are often most useful in avoiding the air-filled bowel.

3. Inability to obtain good images of liver from an anterior approach suggests that subcutaneous or free intraperitoneal air is present.

4. Dense shadowing from calcifications, which result from meconium peritonitis, tend to be right-sided and perihepatic and, in boys, also may be scrotal. Plain radiographs may underestimate the amount and location of calcification present.

5. Chylous ascites may be subtly echogenic when the patient has been following a normal diet that includes fat.

6. Hemorrhagic ascites, depending on the hematocrit of the ascitic fluid and the frequency of the transducer, is variably echogenic. Acute bleeding, such as occurs when the spleen ruptures, may be quite lucent.

7. The presence of fibrinous strands in an ascitic collection represents clotting blood or

Text continued on page 384

Table 14-1. MAJOR CAUSES OF ASCITES IN THE FETUS AND NEONATE

Etiology	Mechanism	Special Ultrasonographic Features
Genitourinary (Fig. 14-1)		
Obstruction of urinary tract, most commonly posterior urethral valve	Rupture of caliceal fornix with formation of retroperitoneal urinoma, which ruptures into peritoneum	Hydronephrosis, hydroureters, distended thickened bladder, and sometimes dilated posterior urethra may be apparent
Rupture of bladder secondary to birth trauma or occasionally bladder outlet obstruction	Urine enters peritoneal cavity directly	Bladder is irregular, small, or both
Congenital nephrosis	Proteinuria leads to hypoalbuminemia and decreased oncotic pressure	Kidneys may be unusually echogenic
Gastrointestinal (Figs. 14-2, 14-3)		
Meconium peritonitis due to perforation of bowel secondary to atresia, stenosis, intussusception, volvulus, hernia, meconium ileus, or duplication	Direct	Localized or widespread peritoneal calcifications
Fetal appendicitis with rupture	Increased capillary fluid loss due to inflammation	Free or loculated fluid collections
Perforation of Meckel diverticulum		Obstructed loops of bowel
		Obstructed fluid-filled loops
Portohepatic (Fig. 14-4)		
Biliary atresia	(i) Increased portal and intrahepatic hydrostatic pressure	Liver may be enlarged and unusual in its parenchymal pattern
Congenital infection		
Glycogen storage disease	(ii) Hypoproteinemia and decreased oncotic pressure	Spleen enlarges with increased portal pressure
Metabolic diseases		
Transplacental hepatitis	(iii) Sodium retention and impaired water excretion	
Fibrocystic disease		
Common duct perforation	Bile peritonitis	
Cardiac		
Rh disease	Ascites usually precedes hydrops fetalis	Enlarged, dilated, or malformed heart
Severe anemia secondary to thalassemia, hemorrhage	(i) Major mechanism is probably congestive heart failure	Pleural effusions
Major congenital heart disease	(ii) Hypoproteinemia	When hydrops is present, scalp and body wall edema, hepatosplenomegaly, polyhydramnios, and placentomegaly may be apparent in utero
Arrhythmia (e.g., supraventricular tachycardia)	(iii) Hepatic congestion and intrahepatic erythropoiesis may cause liver dysfunction	
		Abnormal rhythm can be detected on real-time or Doppler study in utero
Arteriovenous malformation	High output failure	Arteriovenous malformation in liver, head, or placenta
Chylous Ascites		
Lymphatic obstruction due to congenital malformation (e.g., cystic lymphangioma, lymphangiectasia, malrotation, neoplasm, inflammation)	Lymphatic leak	Ascites may contain echogenic particles
Traumatic disruption of thoracic duct		Underlying mass or malformation may be apparent
Infections		
Congenital syphilis, cytomegalovirus, and toxoplasmosis	(i) Peritonitis and increased capillary permeability	Hepatosplenomegaly
	(ii) Associated hepatic and cardiac pathology	
	(iii) Hemorrhagic disorder	
Tumors		
E.g., hepatoblastoma	Bleeding	Image underlying neoplasm
	Portal hypertension	
Intraperitoneal Bleeding (Fig. 14-5)	Ischemic bowel, coagulopathy, trauma	Echogenic ascites

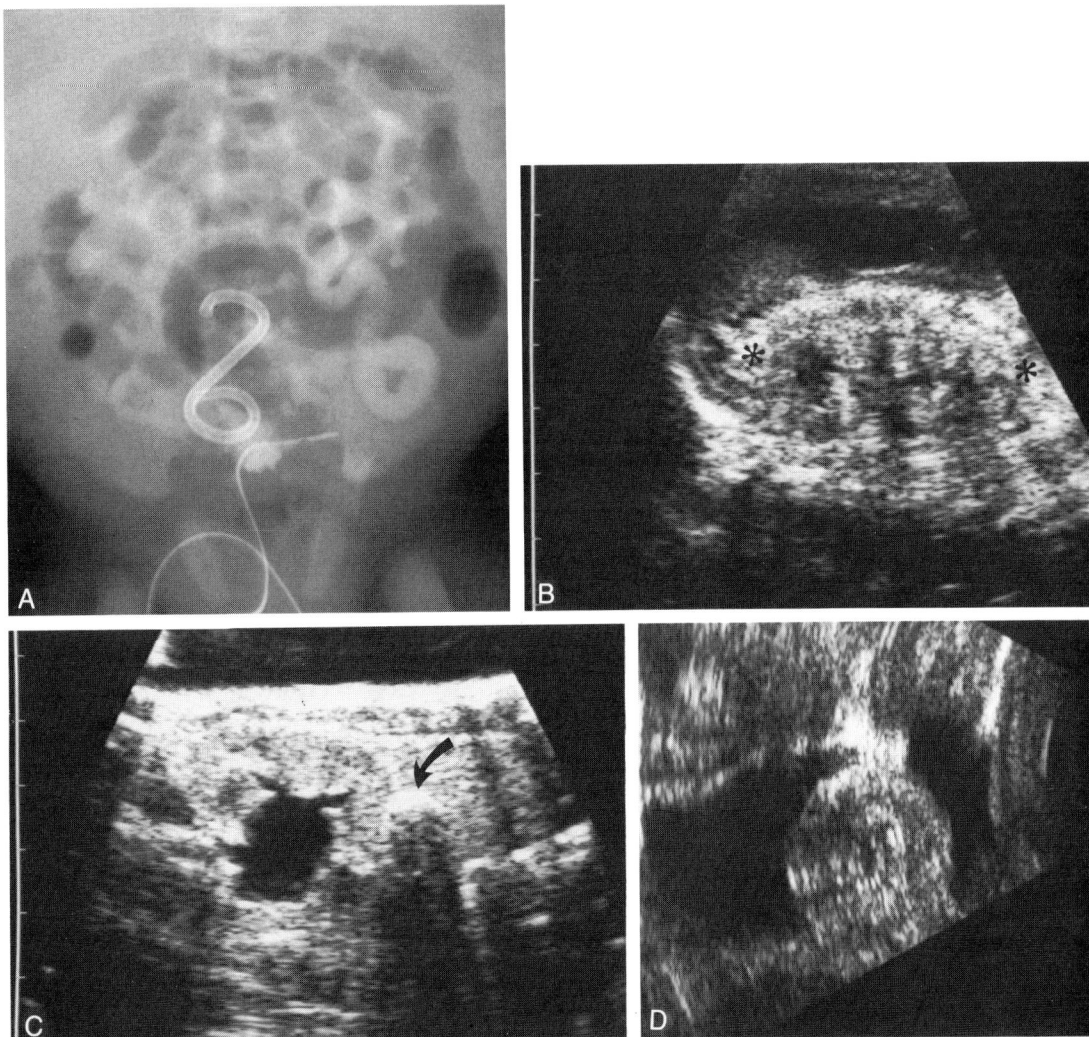

Figure 14-1. At 26 weeks' gestation, this baby had a prenatal diagnosis of hydronephrosis, secondary to posterior urethral valve. Because the mother developed oligohydramnios, intervention to decompress the fetal urinary tract was initiated. A catheter was placed percutaneously to drain the fetal bladder into the amniotic sac. The catheter worked for some time but then retracted and resulted in the fetal bladder's draining into the fetal peritoneal cavity **(A)**. Thus this baby had urinary ascites that was iatrogenically induced. The left kidney is poorly outlined and echogenic **(B)**. It was removed later because it had no function. (Here, as in other figures in this chapter, asterisks outline the kidney.) The right kidney is shown on a prone transverse view **(C)**. Arrow points to the upper end of the catheter. A coronal scan, not in the plane of the catheter, shows the thick-walled bladder outlined by ascites **(D)**. The picture is oriented like the anteroposterior (AP) radiograph of the abdomen.

376 / ASCITES AND OTHER ABDOMINAL PROBLEMS

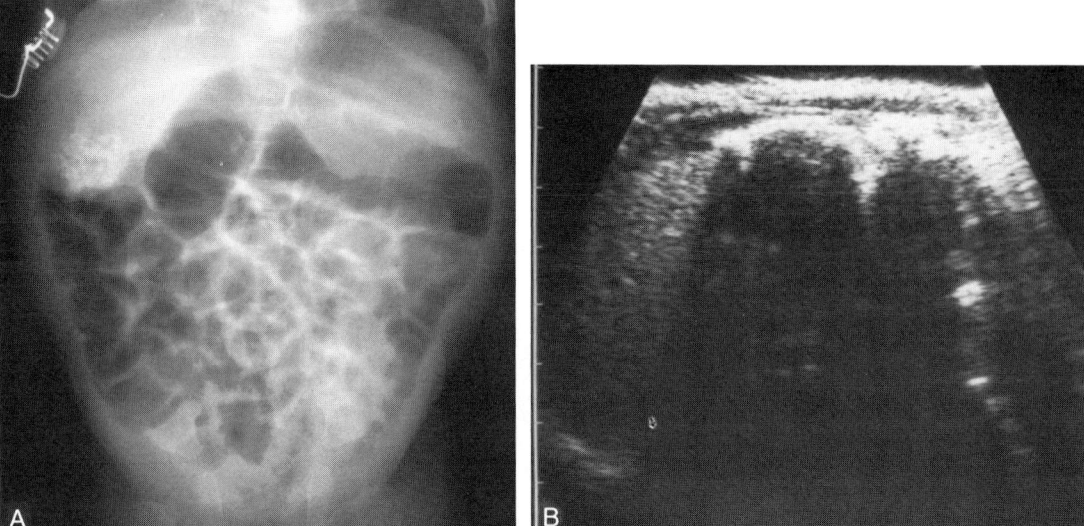

Figure 14–2. AP radiograph of the abdomen (**A**) of this 3-month-old preceded scans that were requested after a mass was felt in the right upper quadrant. Dense calcification is easily detected in the right upper abdomen. This study was followed by ultrasonogram (**B**), which shows the calcification to be in the peritoneal space around the liver. Although meconium peritonitis usually is associated with perforation and obstruction of the bowel, it is occasionally an incidental finding, as in this baby. (From Teele RL, Share JC: The abdominal mass in the neonate. Semin Roentgenol 1988; 23:175–184.)

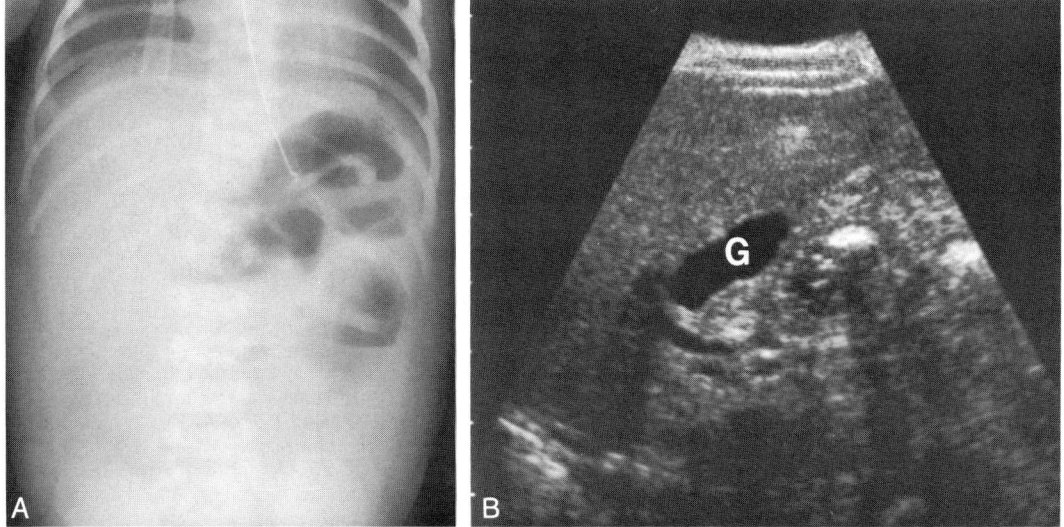

Figure 14–3. Ultrasonography was requested after a palpable mass was detected. The plain radiograph showed air-fluid levels in bowel dilated from obstruction (**A**). The ultrasonogram (**B**) revealed calcification, shown here as echogenic foci around loops of bowel and inferior to the gallbladder (G). The dilation of bowel associated with the peritoneal calcification was responsible for the mass. Notice how the plain films do not reveal the presence of calcification in this child, who had ileal atresia with meconium peritonitis.

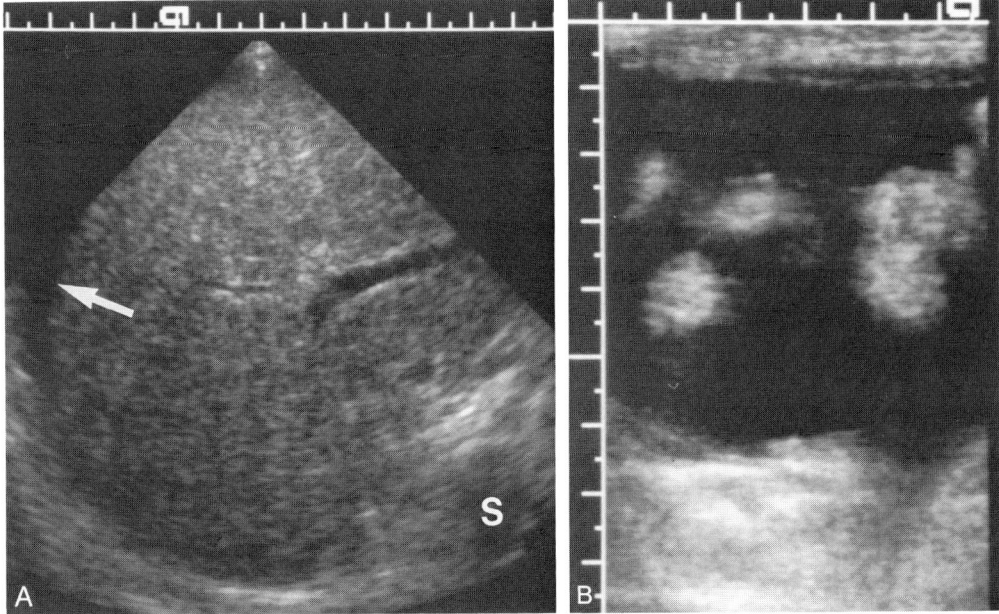

Figure 14–4. When this baby originally presented, she was being evaluated for hepatomegaly. The transverse view of the liver (**A**) shows a rim of fluid around it (arrow). Most of the ascitic fluid, however, was pooled in the pelvis (**B**). Note that the hepatic parenchyma is diffusely echogenic; this is typical of fatty infiltration of the liver. This baby proved to have tyrosinemia. In the ensuing months, adenomatous change within the liver occurred. The baby underwent liver transplantation at 2 years of age. S = spine.

Figure 14–5. Intraperitoneal bleeding may result from ischemia of the bowel or diffuse coagulopathy or trauma. This scan is of the left upper quadrant in a baby who had received extracorporeal membrane oxygenation (ECMO). Hemorrhage into the peritoneum is the mixed echogenicity anterior to the kidney. The baby was heparinized and had severe intestinal ischemia resulting from underlying persistent pulmonary hypertension of the neonate. Hemorrhage within the abdomen can be difficult to diagnose once it starts to clot.

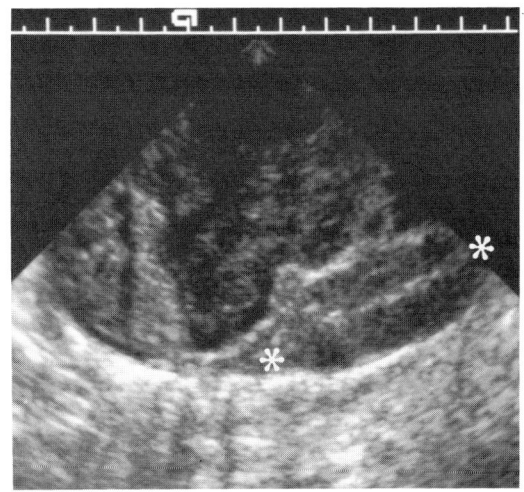

Table 14-2. MAJOR CAUSES OF ASCITES IN CHILDHOOD

Etiology	Mechanism	Special Ultrasonographic Features

Cardiac (Fig. 14-6)
Congestive heart failure of varying etiologies, including
    Congenital heart disease
    Rheumatic heart disease
    Cardiomyopathy
    Constrictive pericarditis
    Severe anemia
	(i) Increased hydrostatic pressure due to pump failure
	(ii) Abnormal sodium and water retention
	(iii) Congestive hepatic dysfunction
		Dilated, enlarged, or malformed heart may be apparent
		Pleural effusions or anasarca

Hepatic (Fig. 14-7)
Cirrhosis:
    Alpha$_1$-antitrypsin deficiency
    Biliary atresia
    Cardiac cirrhosis
    Chronic active hepatitis
    Biliary cirrhosis
Extrahepatic portal hypertension
Budd-Chiari syndrome
	(i) Increased portal and hepatic hydrostatic pressures
	(ii) Hypoproteinemia and decreased oncotic pressures
	(iii) Sodium retention and impaired water excretion
	(iv) Impaired clotting with hemorrhage
		Liver may be enlarged and its parenchymal pattern unusual
		Spleen enlarges with portal hypertension
		Ascites can be clear or echogenic, if bloody

Genitourinary (Fig. 14-8)
Acute and chronic renal failure; e.g.,
    Glomerulonephritis
    Reflux nephropathy
    Metabolic diseases
    Nephrotic syndrome
	(i) Proteinuria and hypoalbuminemia cause decreased oncotic pressure
	(ii) Impaired handling of sodium and water
		Kidneys may be small or large, depending on etiology, and also unusually echogenic

Perforation of bladder	Instrumentation	Evidence of previous urinary tract surgery
Gastrointestinal (Figs. 14-9, 14-10) Perforated hollow viscus Ischemic or infarcted bowel Inflammatory bowel disease Protein-losing enteropathy/lymphangiectasia	Multiple, including hypoproteinemia, increased capillary permeability, and direct spill of bowel contents	Ascites may be free or loculated and can evolve into an abscess (e.g., perforated appendix) Thickened dilated bowel loops Inability to image abdomen should suggest free air; confirm by radiograph

Peritoneal (Figs. 14-11, 14-12)
Intraperitoneal bleeding
Chylous ascites
    Obstruction
    Lymphangiectasia
    Traumatic
Inflammatory peritonitis:
    Primary
    Secondary to, e.g., ruptured viscus, surgery, pelvic inflammation
    Tuberculous
	Coagulopathy, varices, trauma
	Lymphatic leak
	
	Multiple, including direct spill and capillary leak
		Echogenic fluid
		Clear, echogenic, or loculated ascites
		
		Clear, echogenic, free, or loculated ascites or abscess

Pancreatitis	Extravasation of fluid from inflamed pancreas or from ruptured duct	Free fluid tends to loculate into pseudocyst or abscess; site may be remote from pancreas Large hypoechoic pancreas in acute pancreatitis Dilated pancreatic duct

Neoplastic (Figs. 14-13, 14-14, 14-15)
    Ovarian cyst or fibroma (Meig syndrome)
    Ovarian tumor
    Lymphoma
    Medulloblastoma with shunt and peritoneal implants
		Cystic or solid mass
		Metastases; e.g., peritoneal implants and nodal and hepatic masses

Miscellaneous (Fig. 14-15)
CSF shunt with pseudocyst
 	
Malnutrition (kwashiorkor)
Collagen vascular disease, such as
    Juvenile rheumatoid arthritis
    Lupus erythematosus
	
	Hypoalbuminemia
	Polyserositis
		Collection can be free or loculated around tip of shunt tube
		Fatty (echogenic) liver
		Splenomegaly may be present

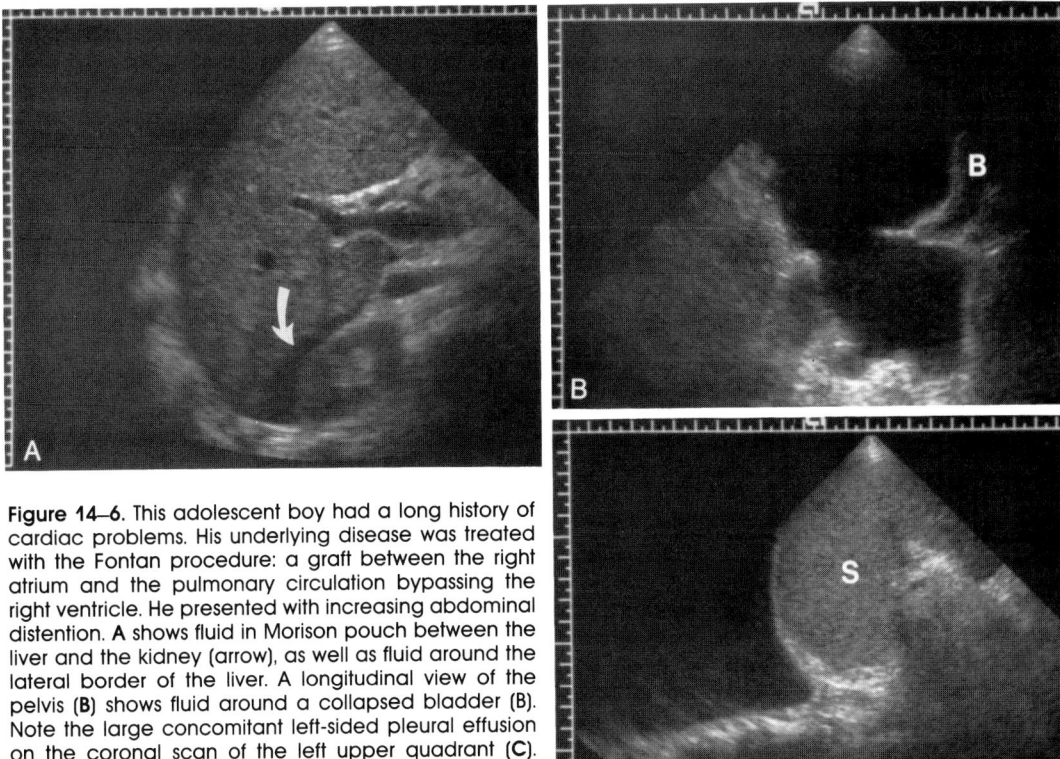

Figure 14–6. This adolescent boy had a long history of cardiac problems. His underlying disease was treated with the Fontan procedure: a graft between the right atrium and the pulmonary circulation bypassing the right ventricle. He presented with increasing abdominal distention. A shows fluid in Morison pouch between the liver and the kidney (arrow), as well as fluid around the lateral border of the liver. A longitudinal view of the pelvis (B) shows fluid around a collapsed bladder (B). Note the large concomitant left-sided pleural effusion on the coronal scan of the left upper quadrant (C). S = spleen.

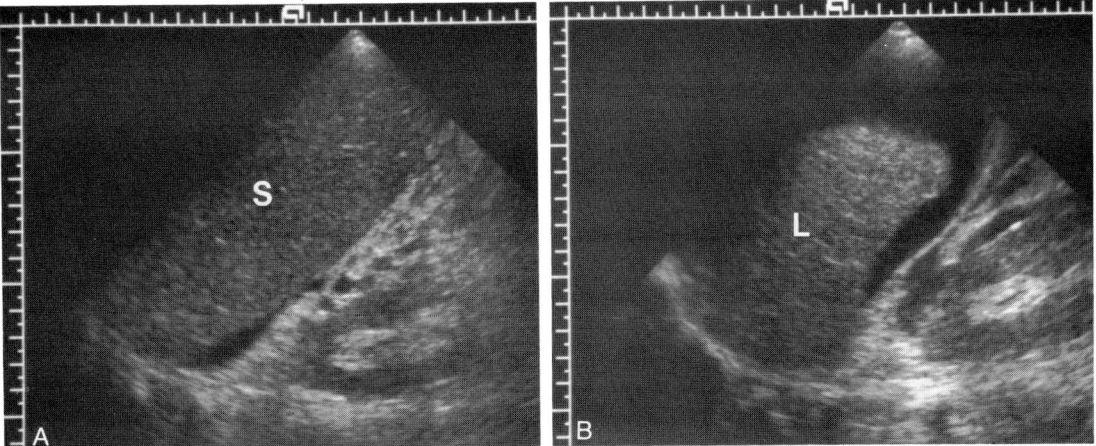

Figure 14–7. Longitudinal scans of the left upper quadrant (A) and the right upper quadrant (B) show, in addition to ascites, the significant splenomegaly and small, shrunken liver of this patient, who had portal hypertension. He died before his cryptogenic cirrhosis could be evaluated. In A, S = spleen. In B, L = liver.

380 / ASCITES AND OTHER ABDOMINAL PROBLEMS

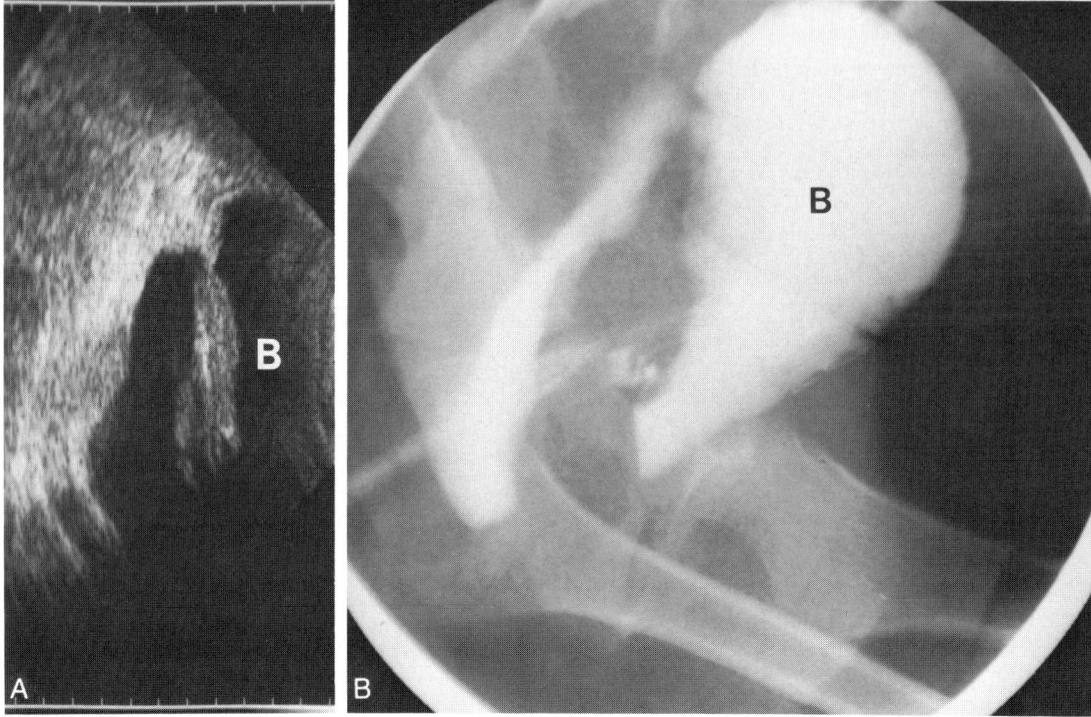

Figure 14–8. Multiple operative procedures on the genitourinary tract of this child, who had underlying myelodysplasia, resulted in augmentation of the bladder with the stomach to provide the child with an adequate capacity for storing urine. She reentered the hospital shortly after surgery, complaining of fever and abdominal pain. The ultrasonogram (**A**), oriented to match the cystogram (**B**), shows a loculated collection of fluid immediately posterior to the bladder. This proved to be perforation of the bladder at the suture line between the stomach and the normal bladder mucosa. It is common in such children, when perforation does occur, for urine to loculate in the pelvis because they have multiple adhesions from previous operations. Free ascites in this child was also present, but she had the confounding situation of a ventriculoperitoneal shunt, the tip of which was in the upper abdomen. B = bladder.

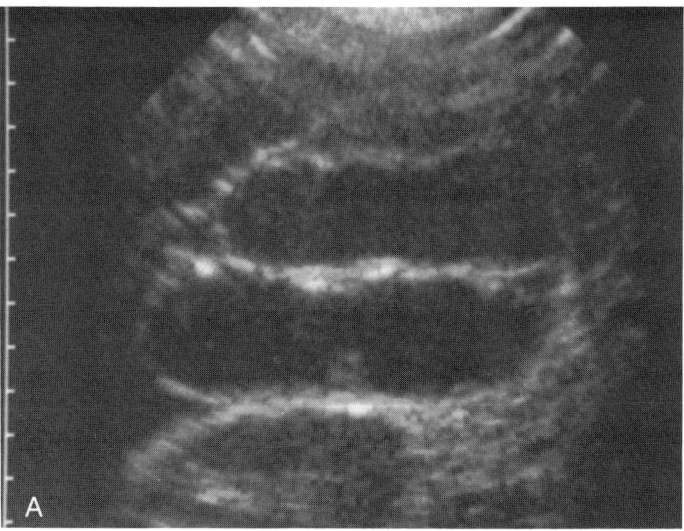

Figure 14–9. Portable ultrasonographic study was requested for this child, who was known to have Crohn disease and who had acute symptoms with abdominal pain. It was apparent that the walls of dilated fluid-filled loops of small bowel in the right hemiabdomen (**A**) were thinner than the walls of a loop of bowel in the left hemiabdomen (**B**), which was the site of the patient's pain. Echogenic fluid (asterisk) surrounded the thickened bowel loop. The patient was taken to surgery shortly thereafter. A volvulus of the left-sided small bowel around adhesions from previous surgical resection was the cause of his acute symptoms. The thick-walled bowel was ischemic and had to be removed. The echogenic ascites proved to be bloody fluid.

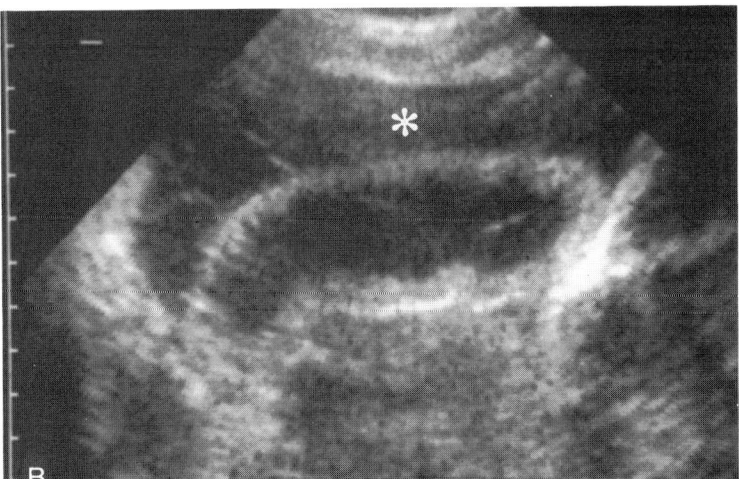

Figure 14-9 Continued.

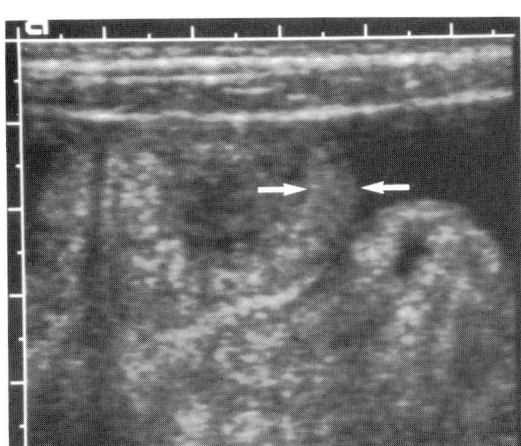

Figure 14-10. We have had only the rare chance to evaluate a patient with lymphangiectasia. Abdominal scans of this child, who had chylous ascites, revealed obvious thickening of the wall of the small bowel (arrows).

Figure 14-11. In spite of our extensive list of causes for ascites, it is difficult to pigeonhole this particular patient. Note the echogenic fluid surrounding the bowel loops (asterisks) in the right upper abdomen of this patient. His scan was taken after bone marrow transplant for Gaucher disease. He had severe hepatic dysfunction. Just before this study, he had undergone sclerosis of esophageal varices. An acute increase in his abdominal girth ensued. Whether the bloody ascites was related to coagulopathy, the recent sclerosis, or another cause was unknown. He was managed conservatively with replacement of blood and without surgical intervention.

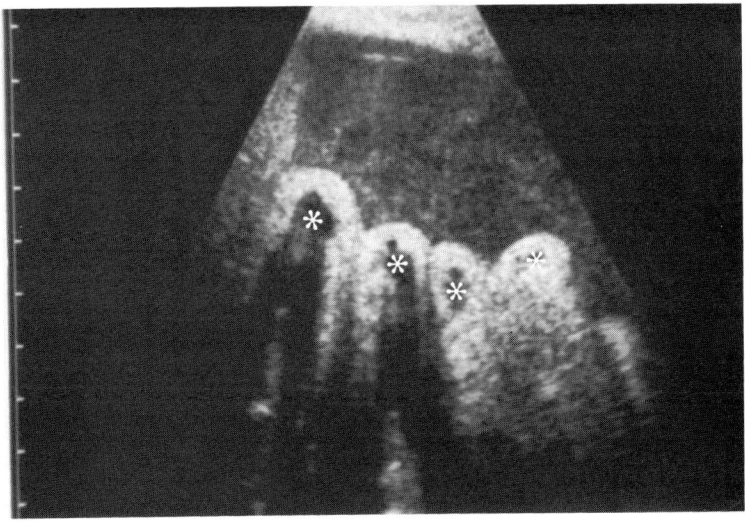

382 / ASCITES AND OTHER ABDOMINAL PROBLEMS

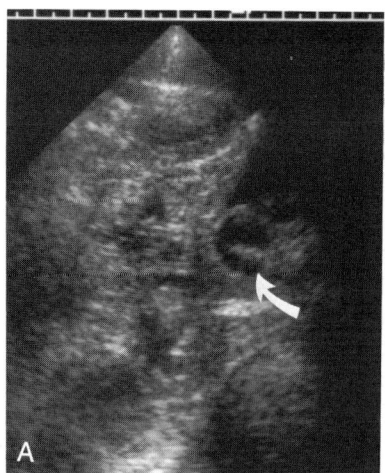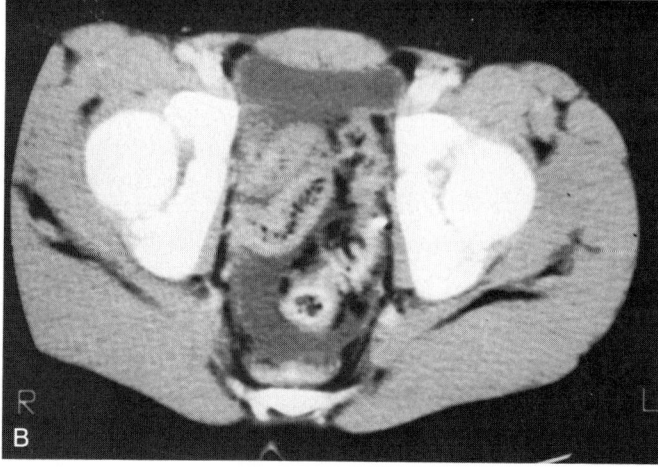

Figure 14–12. After injury to the jejunum from a lap seat belt, this boy had bleeding that pooled in the pelvis and then clotted. This longitudinal scan (A) shows how difficult it can be to discriminate between the bowel and clotted blood. Arrow points to the Foley catheter, which is in the bladder. The presence of blood was confirmed on the computed tomography (CT) scan (B).

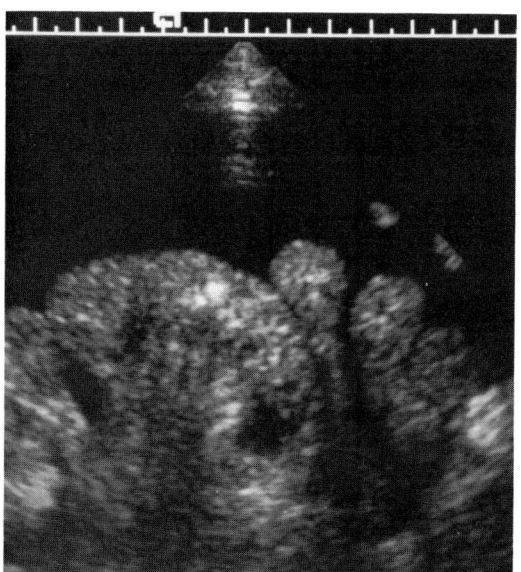

Figure 14–13. Ascites associated with malignancy may be echo free or echogenic on ultrasonographic evaluation. This abdominal scan is from a man who proved to have metastatic peritoneal carcinomatosis, the primary site of which was unknown. He had been followed since childhood at our hospital because of agammaglobulinemia and because of previous lymphoma that had been treated with radiotherapy and chemotherapy 15 years before this study.

Figure 14–15. These three scans belong to different patients, each of whom has a ventriculoperitoneal shunt in place. The first shows the stacked-coin appearance of the coiled ventriculoperitoneal shunt tubing (A). There is no loculation of fluid around the shunt tubing. A plain radiograph was necessary to prove that there was a twist or a knot in the tubing. When loculated cerebrospinal fluid (CSF) accumulates around the tip of the shunt, signs and symptoms of increased intracranial pressure develop. B shows the tip of the shunt tubing with a loculated collection of fluid. This fluid was drained percutaneously in order to determine whether infection was also present. Culture results were negative. When a CSF pseudocyst becomes very large, it may present as an abdominal mass (C). Externalization of this child's shunt followed the diagnosis of a CSF pseudocyst on ultrasonography.

ASCITES AND OTHER ABDOMINAL PROBLEMS / 383

Figure 14–14. Echogenic fluid anterior and posterior to the uterus in this little girl preceded the diagnosis of diffuse peritoneal spread of alveolar rhabdomyosarcoma. Although we attempt to find peritoneal implants with ultrasonography, their diagnosis is difficult unless they are large lesions. In neither of the scans shown here or in Figure 14–13 were we able to detect metastatic deposits on the peritoneal surface.

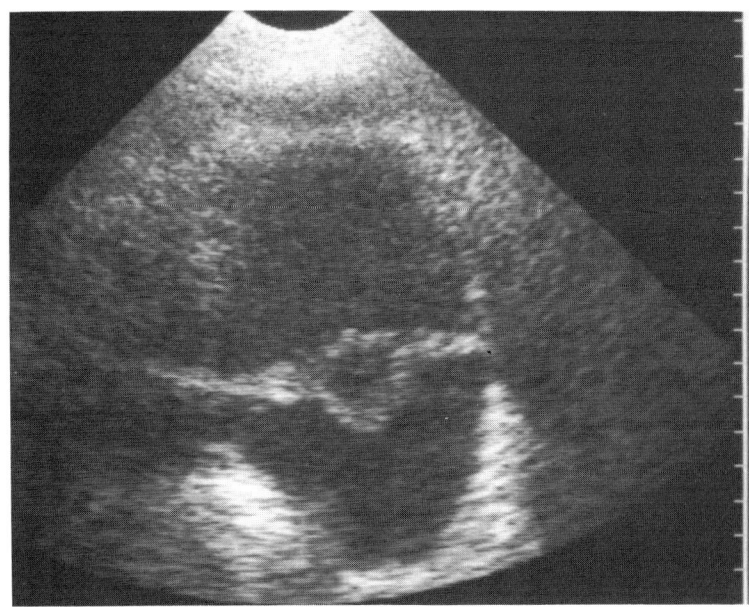

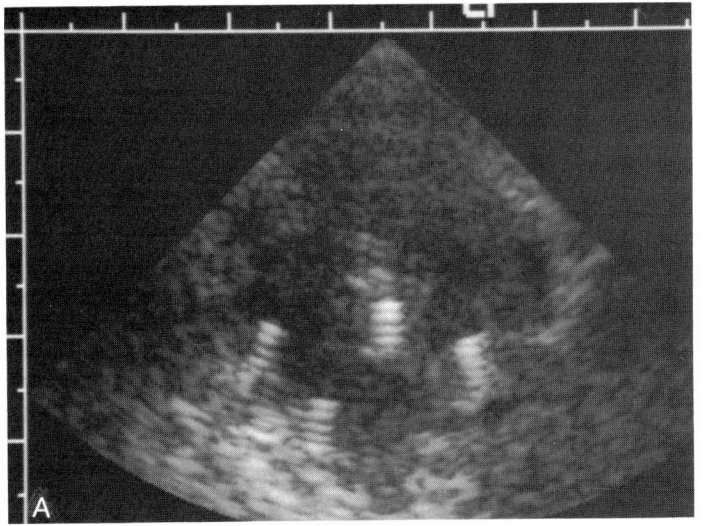

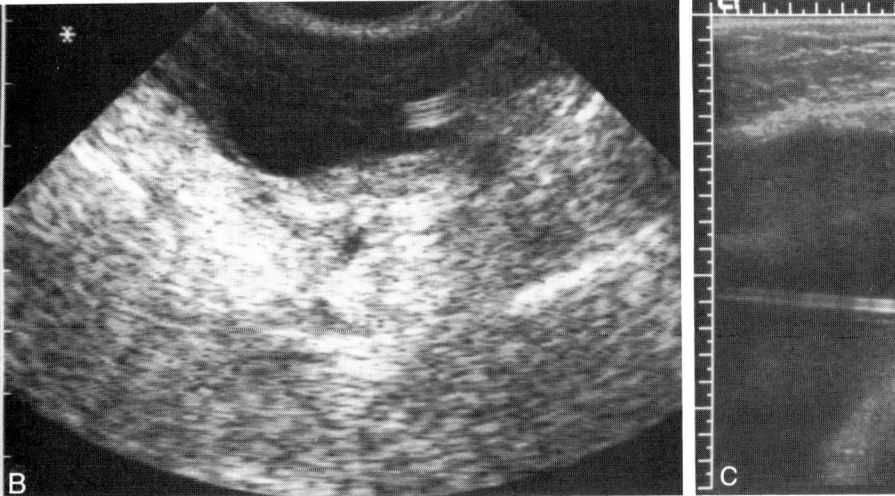

Figure 14–15 See legend on opposite page

infected ascites. When we see this webbing in association with a ventriculoperitoneal shunt, we assume that the fluid is infected.

8. Free fluid in the abdomen is common in children who have a normally functioning ventriculoperitoneal shunt (Fig. 14–16).

9. A small amount of clear fluid in the cul-de-sac (about 5 ml) is common in pubertal girls and is likely related to follicular rupture (Fig. 14–17). Unfortunately, a small or moderate amount of fluid in the cul-de-sac may also result from adjacent appendicitis, pelvic inflammatory disease, or pancreatitis.

10. The presence of moderate ascites should stimulate examination of pleural spaces so as to document pleural effusions if present.

At the conclusion of the ultrasonographic study, the examining physician should be able to quantify, in general terms, the amount of ascitic fluid, give a qualitative judgment as to whether it is simple or complex, and localize an appropriate area for paracentesis if the etiology of the ascitic fluid is in doubt. Aspiration can be done in the examining room after informed consent is obtained from the patient or the parent, or both. Sedation is usually needed for children who are younger than 5 years of age. Local anesthesia of the skin and soft tissues is followed by peritoneal puncture with a 20-gauge needle or with a needle/catheter system that is attached to a 10- or 20-ml syringe. Fluid should be sent for Gram stain, culture and sensitivities, and cell count with differential cytologic examination when risk of tumor is present; and evaluation of levels of amylase, glucose, lactate dehydrogenase, total protein, and albumin.

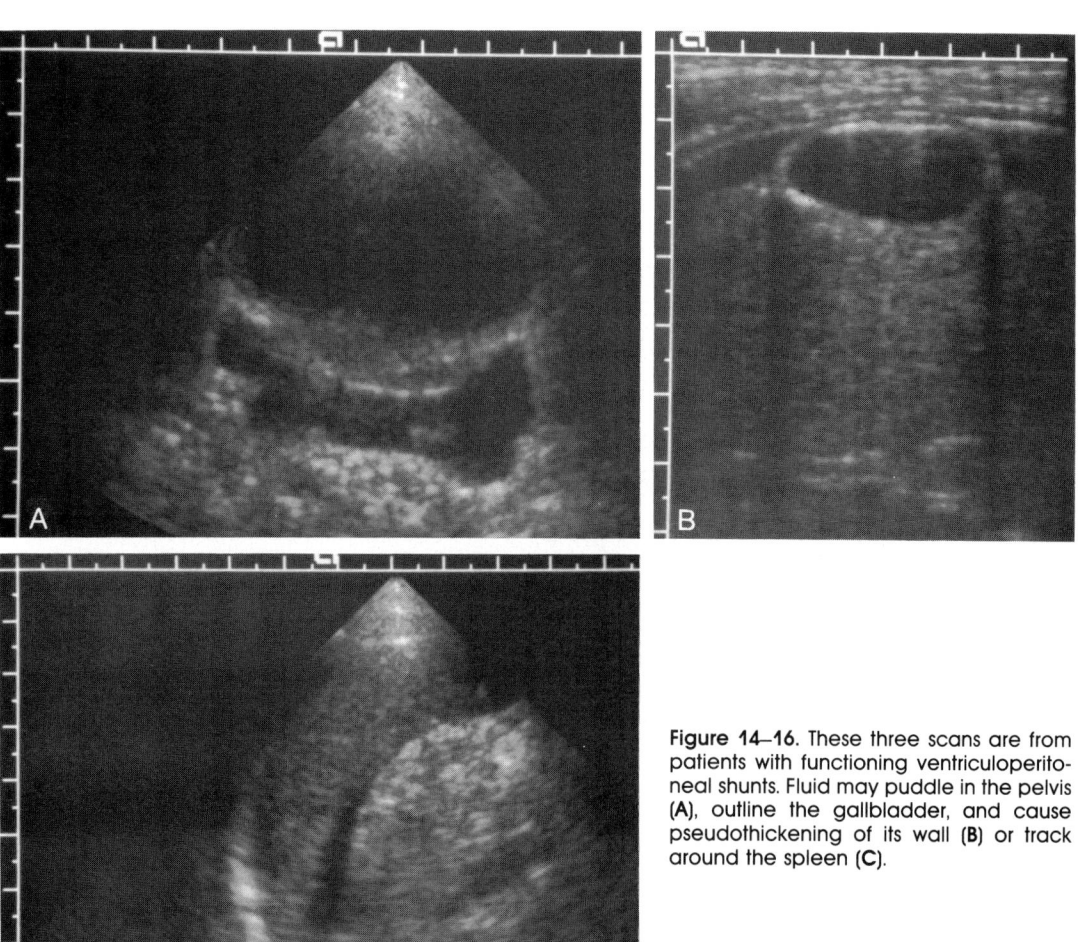

Figure 14–16. These three scans are from patients with functioning ventriculoperitoneal shunts. Fluid may puddle in the pelvis (A), outline the gallbladder, and cause pseudothickening of its wall (B) or track around the spleen (C).

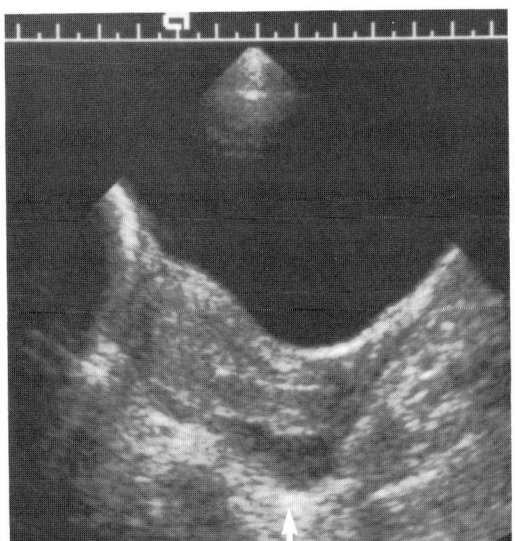

Figure 14–17. A small amount of fluid in the pelvis of pubertal girls is common and likely related to follicular rupture. This longitudinal scan of the pelvis shows a small amount of fluid (arrow) in the cul-de-sac. We accept this amount of fluid as normal.

ABDOMINAL VASCULATURE

A bullet-shaped calcification to the right of midline, high in the abdomen, is the well-known radiographic sign of inferior vena caval thrombosis. It is assumed that intrauterine events are responsible for the development of this thrombosis. However, there seem to be no clinical sequelae. The calcified clot is both a radiographic and an ultrasonographic curiosity. A shadowing echogenicity within the lumen of the cava can be demonstrated on scans of the right upper abdomen (Sandler et al., 1986). We have also seen a patient whose calcification was in thrombus in the renal vein (Fig. 14–18).

Calcification of an arterial aneurysm is distinctly unusual in the pediatric population. A mesenchymal abnormality (e.g., Ehlers-Danlos syndrome, homocystinuria) associated with the aneurysm may be the predisposing situation. Preceding trauma to a renal pedicle—specifically, hyperextension injury—may result in arterial injury and an aneurysm in the renal hilum. A mycotic aneurysm, which will rupture before it has time to calcify, is often the result of arterial injury (from catheterization) in the presence of sepsis (Fig. 14–19; Tran-Minh et al., 1989; Kirpekar et al., 1989). Idiopathic congenital abdominal aortic aneurysm has also been reported (Latter et al., 1989). Coarctation of the abdominal vasculature is a sign of neurofibromatosis until proved otherwise. In affected children, the aorta may narrow to a thin string; hypertension is the typical presentation.

Portal venous gas can be detected quite easily with ultrasonography because the microbubbles create an obvious interface in the otherwise echofree portal vein (Merritt et al., 1984; Robberecht et al., 1988). Necrotizing

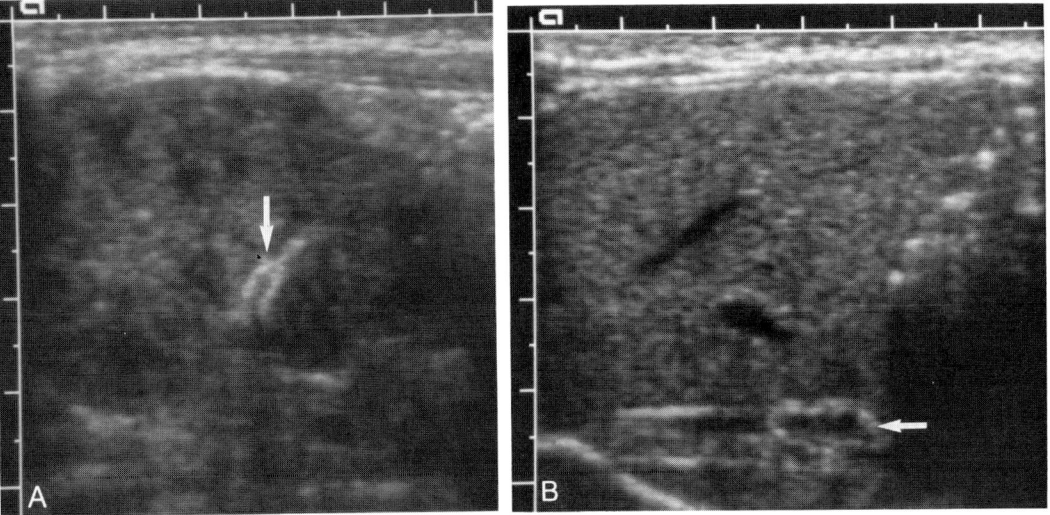

Figure 14–18. Renal venous thrombosis may calcify (arrow, **A**), as in this baby, whose scans were taken 3 days after he presented with gross hematuria. The caval extension of the clot (arrow, **B**) has not calcified.

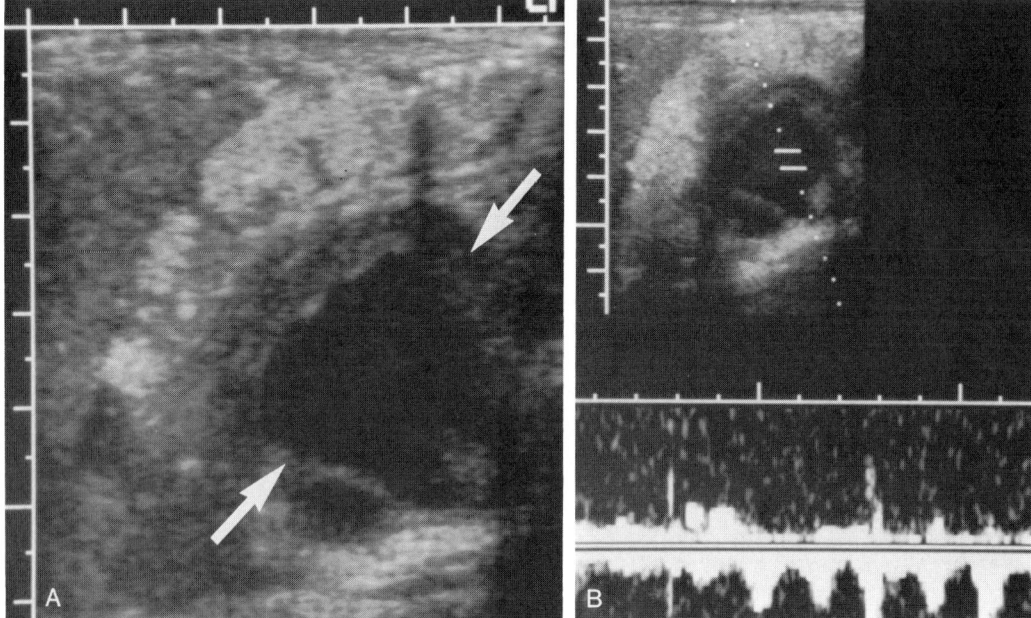

Figure 14–19. Previous umbilical arterial catheterization and an episode of sepsis preceded, by 5 days, the development of this mycotic aneurysm of the right iliac artery just below the aortic bifurcation. The mass (arrows, **A**) is displacing the bowel anteriorly. The Doppler tracing (**B**) shows the arterial signal within the aneurysm. The surgeons were able to resect the aneurysm and perform a primary repair of the artery.

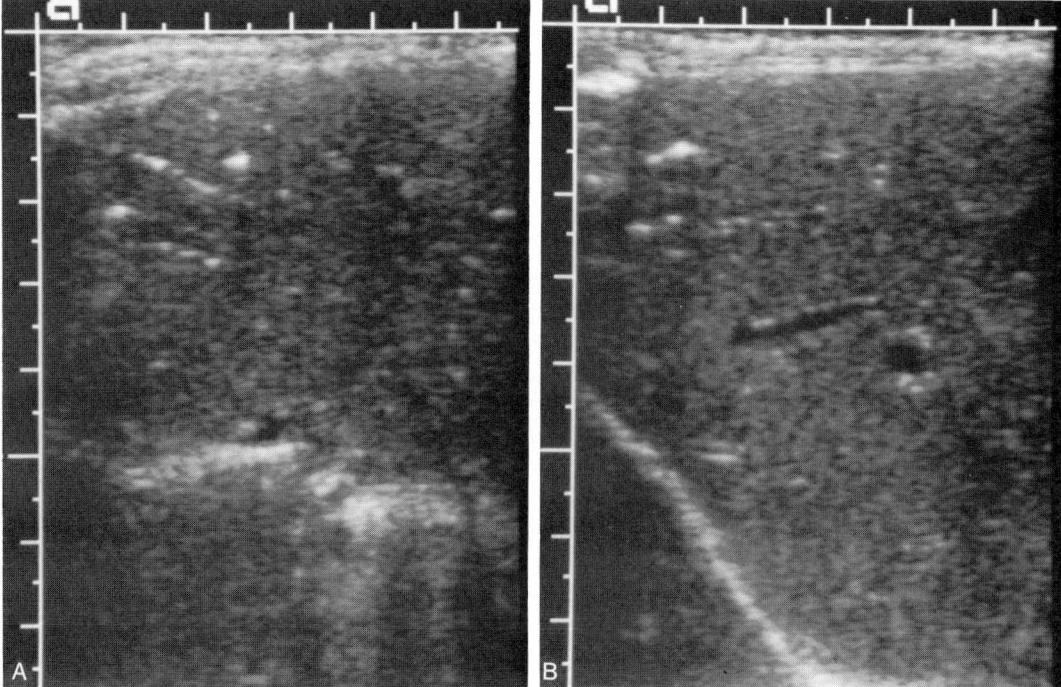

Figure 14–20. Portal venous gas, associated with necrotizing enterocolitis in this 2-week-old prematurely born baby, creates echogenic flecks in the periphery of the liver. **A** is a transverse scan, and **B** is a longitudinal scan.

enterocolitis probably allows gas from the lumen of the bowel to pass into the mesenteric venous drainage as the mucosal surface of the gut becomes eroded. The discovery of portal venous gas on ultrasonography does not necessarily indicate a fulminating course, and the decision to perform surgical intervention is not based on this finding alone (Fig. 14–20). Therefore, we are not enthusiastic about evaluating every baby who has abdominal distention; we rely heavily on radiographic and clinical information instead. Necrotizing enterocolitis is a disease of sick premature infants, who also are at risk for developing patent ductus arteriosus. Doppler scanning of the splanchnic arterial supply has been performed for small groups of both healthy and sick neonates, and, as might be expected, there are differences in velocities of blood flow between groups (Van Bel et al., 1990). The differences may be due to changes in the vasculature supplying the bowel but may equally be reflecting the presence of coincident cardiac complications such as patent ductus arteriosus or myocardial ischemia. A single baby is its own best control subject, and studies with Doppler scanning of normal neonates before and after feeding show a definite increase in velocity of blood flow and a drop in the resistive index 45 minutes after the feeding (Leidig, 1989).

IMPERFORATE ANUS

In babies who have an imperforate anus, the level of the distal rectal pouch is not as important as the location of the pouch in relation to the pubolevator sling. A low imperforate anus requires treatment with a simple anoplasty; a high imperforate anus requires a diverting colostomy and a later "pull-through" operation to position the rectum centrally within the sphincteric musculature. Ultrasonographic evaluation is subject to the same problems as the radiographic studies; the distance from pouch to perineum is not always indicative of whether the imperforate anus is high or low. There are guidelines, however. Our experience as well as others' suggests that the distance from pouch to perineum is less than 10 mm in a baby who has a low imperforate anus. Distances of 10 to 15 mm are in a gray zone; distances greater than 15 mm indicate a high imperforate anus (Fig. 14–21; Schuster and

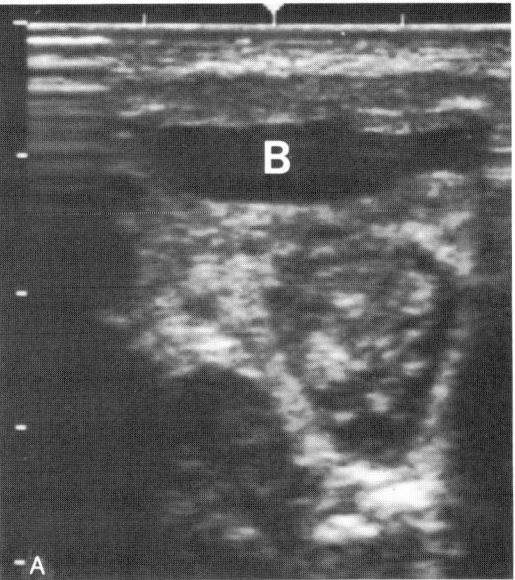

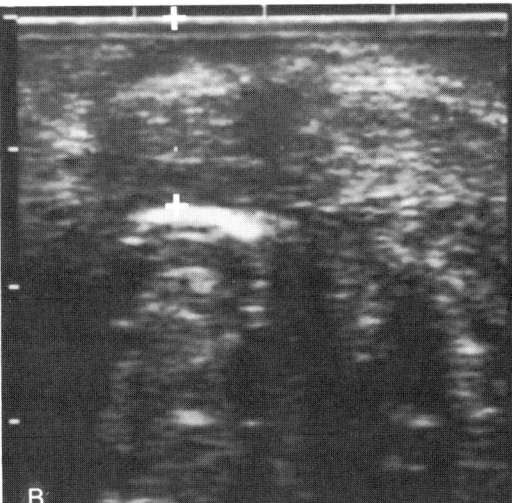

Figure 14–21. Imperforate anus was obvious on clinical examination of this baby, who also had Down syndrome. The transverse scan of the pelvis (A) shows the rectum behind the bladder (B). Scan through the perineum (B) shows a distance of 14 mm between skin and the rectal pouch, which is identified by a reflective interface. Crosses mark the skin surface and the distal extent of rectal pouch. For such a scan, the baby is placed in lithotomy position and kept as calm as possible to avoid descent of the pouch, which is caused by crying. A measurement of less than 1 cm indicates a low lesion. The measurement of 14 mm is in the gray zone; this patient had a high imperforate anus.

Teele, 1979; Donaldson et al., 1989). However, other information is available on ultrasonography. The kidneys can be scanned for associated renal anomalies. In addition, the spinal canal should be scanned for the presence of a tethered cord or some other malformation (Karrer et al., 1988).

REFERENCES

Ascites

Balsam D, Wasserstein GJ: Spontaneous perforation of the common bile duct [letter]. Radiology 1990; 174:578.

Dinkel E, Lehnart R, Tröger J, et al: Sonographic evidence of intraperitoneal fluid: An experimental study and its clinical implications. Pediatr Radiol 1984; 14:299–303.

Haller JO, Condon VR, Berdon WE, et al: Spontaneous perforation of the common bile duct in children. Radiology 1989; 172:621–624.

Meyers MA: The spread and localization of acute intraperitoneal effusions. Radiology 1970; 95:547–554.

Newman B, Teele RL: Ascites in the fetus, neonate, and young child: Emphasis on ultrasonographic evaluation. Semin Ultrasound CT & MR 1984; 5:85–101.

Proto AV, Lane EJ, Marangola JP: A new concept of ascitic fluid distribution. AJR 1976; 126:974–980.

Wu CC: Sonographic findings of generalized meconium peritonitis presenting as neonatal ascites. JCU 1988; 16:48–51.

Shunt-Related Intraperitoneal Loculation of Cerebrospinal Fluid (CSF Pseudocyst)

Bryant MS, Bremer AM, Tepas JJ 3d, et al: Abdominal complications of ventriculoperitoneal shunts: Case reports and review of the literature. Am Surg 1988; 54:50–55.

Egelhoff J, Babcock DS, McLaurin R: Cerebrospinal fluid pseudocysts: Sonographic appearance and clinical management. Pediatr Neurosci 1985–1986; 12:80–86.

Grünebaum M, Ziv N, Kornreich L, et al: The sonographic signs of the peritoneal pseudocyst obstructing the ventriculo-peritoneal shunt in children. Neuroradiology 1988; 30:433–438.

Abdominal Vasculature

Kirpekar M, Augenstein H, Abiri M: Sequential development of multiple aortic aneurysms in a neonate post umbilical arterial catheter insertion. Pediatr Radiol 1989; 19:452–453.

Latter D, Béland MJ, Batten A, et al: Congenital abdominal aortic aneurysm. Can J Surg 1989; 32:135–138.

Leidig E: Pulsed Doppler ultrasound blood flow measurements in the superior mesenteric artery of the newborn. Pediatr Radiol 1989; 19:169–172.

Merritt CRB, Goldsmith JP, Sharp MJ: Sonographic detection of portal venous gas in infants with necrotizing enterocolitis. AJR 1984; 143:1059–1062.

Robberecht EA, Afschrift M, De Bel CE: Sonographic demonstration of portal venous gas in necrotizing enterocolitis. Eur J Pediatr 1988; 147:192–194.

Sandler MA, Beute GH, Madrazo BL, et al: Ultrasound case of the day. Inferior vena cava calcification (calcified thrombus). Radiographics 1986; 6:512–514.

Starinsky R, Graif M, Lotan D, et al: Thrombus calcification of renal vein in neonate: Ultrasound and CT diagnosis. J Comput Assist Tomogr 1989; 13:545–546.

Tran-Minh VA, Le Gall C, Pasquier JM, et al: Mycotic aneurysm of the abdominal aorta in the neonate. JCU 1989; 17:37–39.

Van Bel F, Van Zwieten PH, Guit GL, et al: Superior mesenteric artery blood flow velocity and estimated volume flow: Duplex Doppler US study of preterm and term neonates. Radiology 1990; 174:165–169.

Imperforate Anus

Donaldson JS, Black CT, Reynolds M, et al: Ultrasonography of the distal pouch in infants with imperforate anus. J Pediatr Surg 1989; 24:465–468.

Karrer FM, Flannery AM, Nelson MD, et al: Anorectal malformations: Evaluation of associated spinal dysraphic syndromes. J Ped Surg 1988; 23:45–48.

Schuster S, Teele RL: An analysis of ultrasound scanning as a guide in determination of "high" or "low" imperforate anus. J Pediatr Surg 1979; 14:798–800.

CHAPTER 15

THE PANCREAS

PANCREATITIS

Pancreatic ultrasonography is requested by clinicians when a child is found to have hyperamylasemia, upper abdominal pain, or an upper abdominal mass. We always scan the pancreas when a child presents with pain or jaundice. The pancreas sits at a busy intersection of blood vessels, lymphatics, the common bile duct, and the duodenum. It is retroperitoneal, but it is pushed into the anterior abdomen by the spine. It is amazing how, on ultrasonography of thin children, one can demonstrate the pancreas just under the surface of the skin. The left lobe of the liver is prominent in young children and often provides a good window to the tail of the pancreas. A fast of 4 hours before scanning usually prevents the stomach from obscuring the view of head and body. Occasionally, we have to sit a child upright, or give him or her a glass of water, to allow visualization of the pancreas without there being gastrointestinal gas superimposed. Because ileus is common with pancreatitis, we prefer scanning a child after decompression of the gut has been achieved with a nasogastric tube. The diagnosis of pancreatitis is a clinical one. The situation is rarely so urgent that scanning cannot be delayed 6 to 8 hours while the gastrointestinal tract is decompressed.

In comparison with that of most adults, the pancreas of a child tends to be more transverse in orientation. Shallow oblique scans of the upper abdomen usually allow evaluation of the entire gland along its axis. The pancreatic tail is often prominent in width and is often a bit thicker than the body of the pancreas, which in some people may be only a thin sliver of tissue (Fig. 15–1). Standard dimensions of the pancreas have been published (Siegel et al., 1987) and are reprinted in Table 15–1. As a rule, the pancreas is usually considered enlarged when, at any age, the body of the pancreas is greater than 1.5 cm in its anteroposterior dimension.

It is distinctly unusual for the pancreatic duct to be identified as anything but a fine single or double linear interface in the central portion of the gland (Fig. 15–2). A measurable ductal diameter of 1.5 mm or more should be considered abnormal until proved otherwise (Fig. 15–3). The normal pancreatic texture is of moderate echogenicity with, on occasion, a pattern slightly coarser than that of the adjacent normal liver. However, there is wide variation in normal children. Furthermore, increased lucency, representing edematous pancreatic tissue, does not always occur with inflammation of the pancreas (Siegel et al., 1987). Increased echogenicity, to the extent that the pancreatic outline becomes virtually obliterated, occurs when fat,

390 / THE PANCREAS

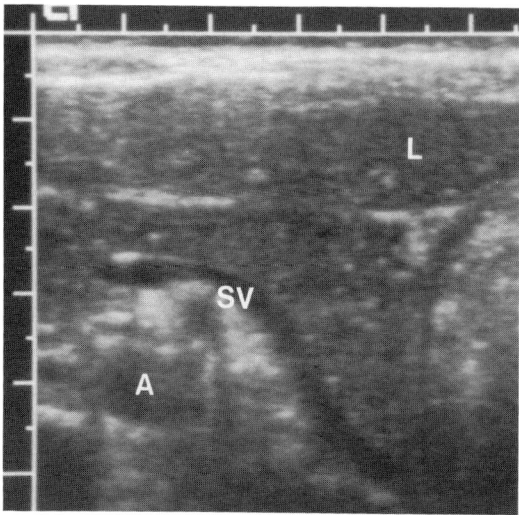

Figure 15–1. Shallow oblique view of the pancreas in a normal child shows the prominence of the pancreatic tail in comparison with the body. The left lobe of liver (L) provides the scanning window to the pancreas in children. The pancreas courses anterior to the splenic vein (SV). A = aorta.

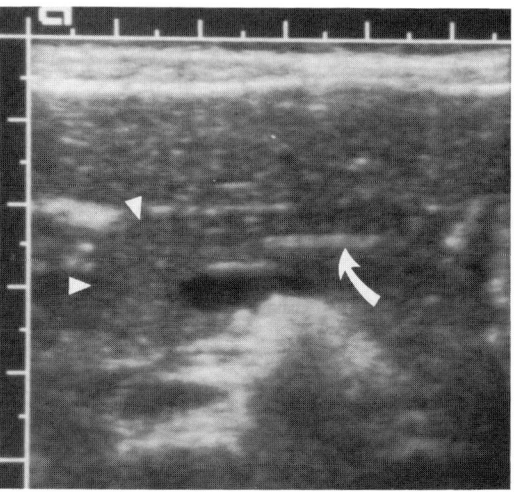

Figure 15–2. Transverse view of the head and body of the pancreas in a normal 8-year-old. Note the double linear interface of the normal pancreatic duct (arrow) just anterior to the confluence of the splenic and superior mesenteric veins. The head of the pancreas is outlined by arrowheads.

Table 15–1. NORMAL DIMENSIONS OF THE PANCREAS AS A FUNCTION OF AGE

Patient Age	No. of Patients	Maximum Anteroposterior Dimensions of Pancreas*		
		Head	Body	Tail
<1 month	15	1.0 ± 0.4	0.6 ± 0.2	1.0 ± 0.4
1 month to 1 year	23	1.5 ± 0.5	0.8 ± 0.3	1.2 ± 0.4
1–5 years	49	1.7 ± 0.3	1.0 ± 0.2	1.8 ± 0.4
5–10 years	69	1.6 ± 0.4	1.0 ± 0.3	1.8 ± 0.4
10–19 years	117	2.0 ± 0.5	1.1 ± 0.3	2.0 ± 0.4

From Siegel MJ, Martin KW, Worthington JL: Normal and abnormal pancreas in children: US studies. Radiology 1987; 165:15–18.
*In centimeters ± one standard deviation.

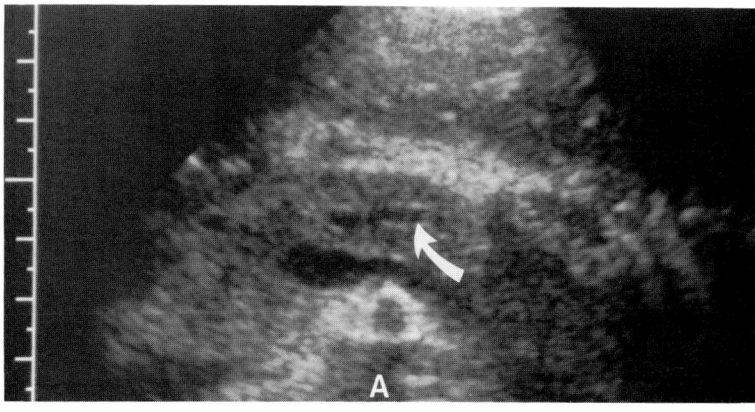

Figure 15–3. The ductal diameter was 3 mm in this 19-year-old adolescent boy, who presented with epigastric pain, vomiting, and an amylase level of over 2400. He had a long history of alcoholism and no other reason for acute pancreatitis. The duct is indicated by arrow. A = aorta.

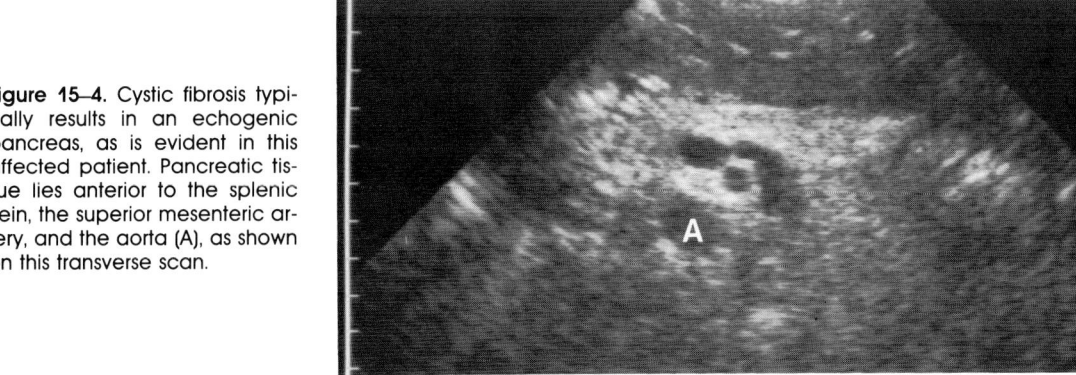

Figure 15–4. Cystic fibrosis typically results in an echogenic pancreas, as is evident in this affected patient. Pancreatic tissue lies anterior to the splenic vein, the superior mesenteric artery, and the aorta (A), as shown on this transverse scan.

fibrosis, or hemosiderin is infiltrating the gland (Schneider et al., 1987). These situations occur with cystic fibrosis, chronic pancreatitis, administration of steroids, hemosiderosis, and Shwachman syndrome (idiopathic pancreatic insufficiency and neutropenia; Figs. 15–4, 15–5). We have also noted that the waterlogged pancreas, in the presence of severe, diffuse edema of the abdominal wall and abdominal contents, can be quite echogenic. In scans of babies who are paralyzed while on respirators, this echogenicity appears because much of their bodily fluid leaks into extravascular spaces (Fig. 15–6).

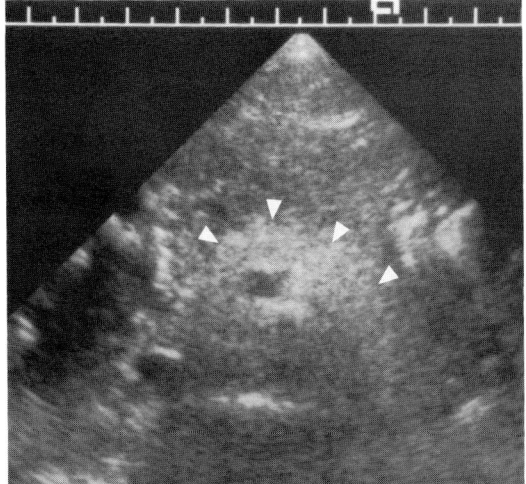

Figure 15–5. Shwachman-Diamond syndrome is an association of pancreatic insufficiency and neutropenia. This little girl had presented with failure to thrive, breast abscess, and otitis media. This transverse scan shows poorly defined echogenicity replacing the normal pancreas. Fat or fibrosis, or both, is likely responsible for this appearance. The head and body of the pancreas are outlined by arrowheads.

For most clinical situations related to the pancreas, ultrasonography is the first examination of choice. The major pancreatic disorders of childhood are inflammatory in nature. Serum or urine, or both, should be sampled for levels of amylase and lipase because they are the most reliable tests with which to establish the presence of pancreatitis. Pancreatitis should not be diagnosed primarily by ultrasonography. However, the diagnosis can be supported by demonstration of a dilated pancreatic duct, diffuse swelling of the pancreas, and obviously abnormal texture of tissue. Of all these ultrasonic findings, ductal dilatation is the most reliable sign of pancreatitis. It is important that the ultrasonographer search for a reason for the pancreatitis or show complications of the inflammatory episode (Fig. 15–7).

Pancreatitis in the pediatric population has multiple etiologies: trauma, infection (particularly viral, e.g., mumps), toxins (specifically agents such as L-asparaginase, valproic acid, and alcohol), peptic disease, obstruction related to anomalies or diseases of the biliary tree and pancreatic ducts, cystic fibrosis, and hereditary pancreatitis. There is also a sizable number of patients for whom no cause of the disease is discovered.

In children, pancreatitis is frequently traumatic in origin and may coexist with duodenal hematoma (see Chapter 13). The pancreas may be irregularly echogenic from bleeding or edema, and vascular landmarks are often distorted or indistinct. The common bile duct and gallbladder are variably dilated from edema in the head of the pancreas. Large collections of fluid in the lesser sac, porta hepatis, or Morison pouch or free fluid in the abdomen occur when the pancreas has

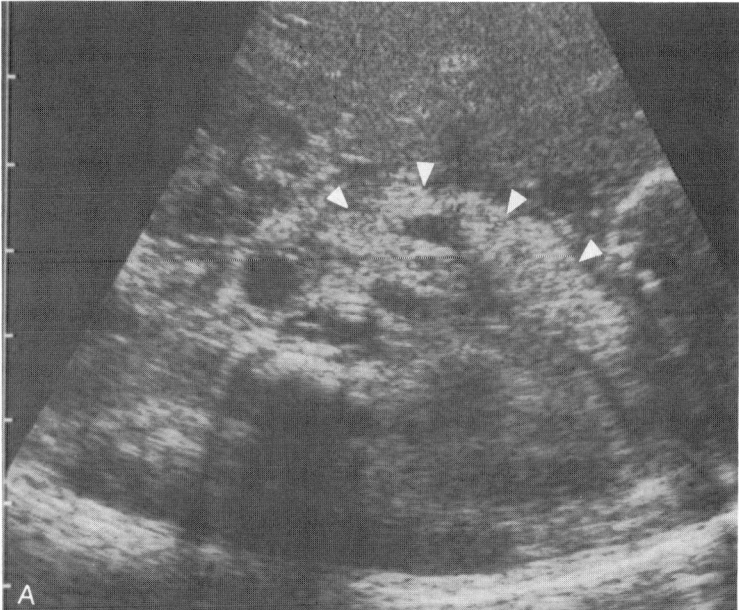

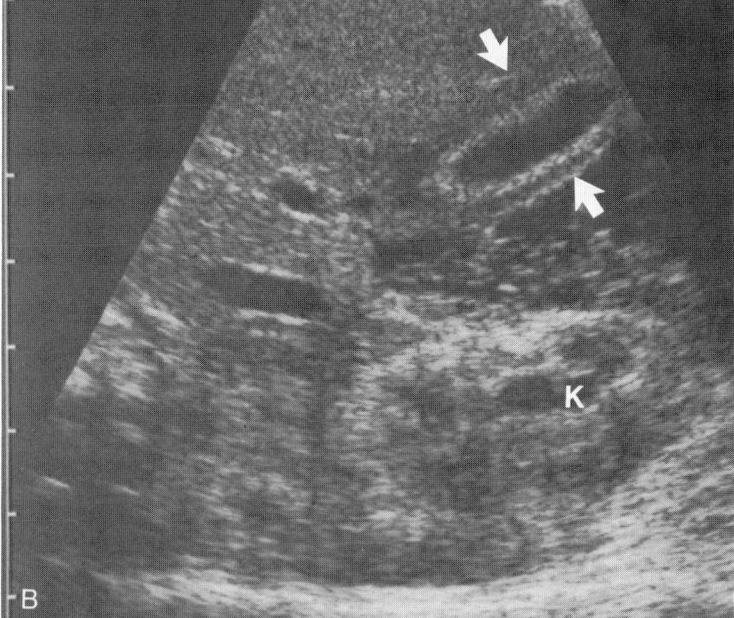

Figure 15–6. Transverse (A) and longitudinal (B) scans are of a 2-week-old who had cardiac anomalies, congestive heart failure, and significant retroperitoneal edema, as well as ascites. Pancreatic echogenicity is related to increased fluid within the retroperitoneum. The pancreas is outlined by arrowheads in A. Longitudinal scan (B) shows thickening of the gallbladder wall (arrows) and increased echogenicity around the right kidney (K) from edematous connective tissue within the fascia of Gerota.

been fractured with disruption of a major duct (Fig. 15–8). Pseudocysts are common sequela to traumatic pancreatitis but do not generally develop until 1 to 3 weeks after the injury.

Severe upper abdominal trauma, particularly from crush injury, is best evaluated with contrast-enhanced computed tomography (CT) scanning. A fractured pancreas is easier to identify on CT scans than with ultrasonography (Jeffrey et al., 1986a). In general, surgery follows to remove the distal portion of the gland and oversew the pancreatic duct. There is one report of percutaneous drainage that resulted in spontaneous healing of a lacerated duct (Garel et al., 1983). Our experience with one similarly injured child was of continued drainage, by catheter, of large amounts of pancreatic secretions that did not decrease with time and therefore required surgical intervention. The pediatric surgical literature recommends surgical intervention

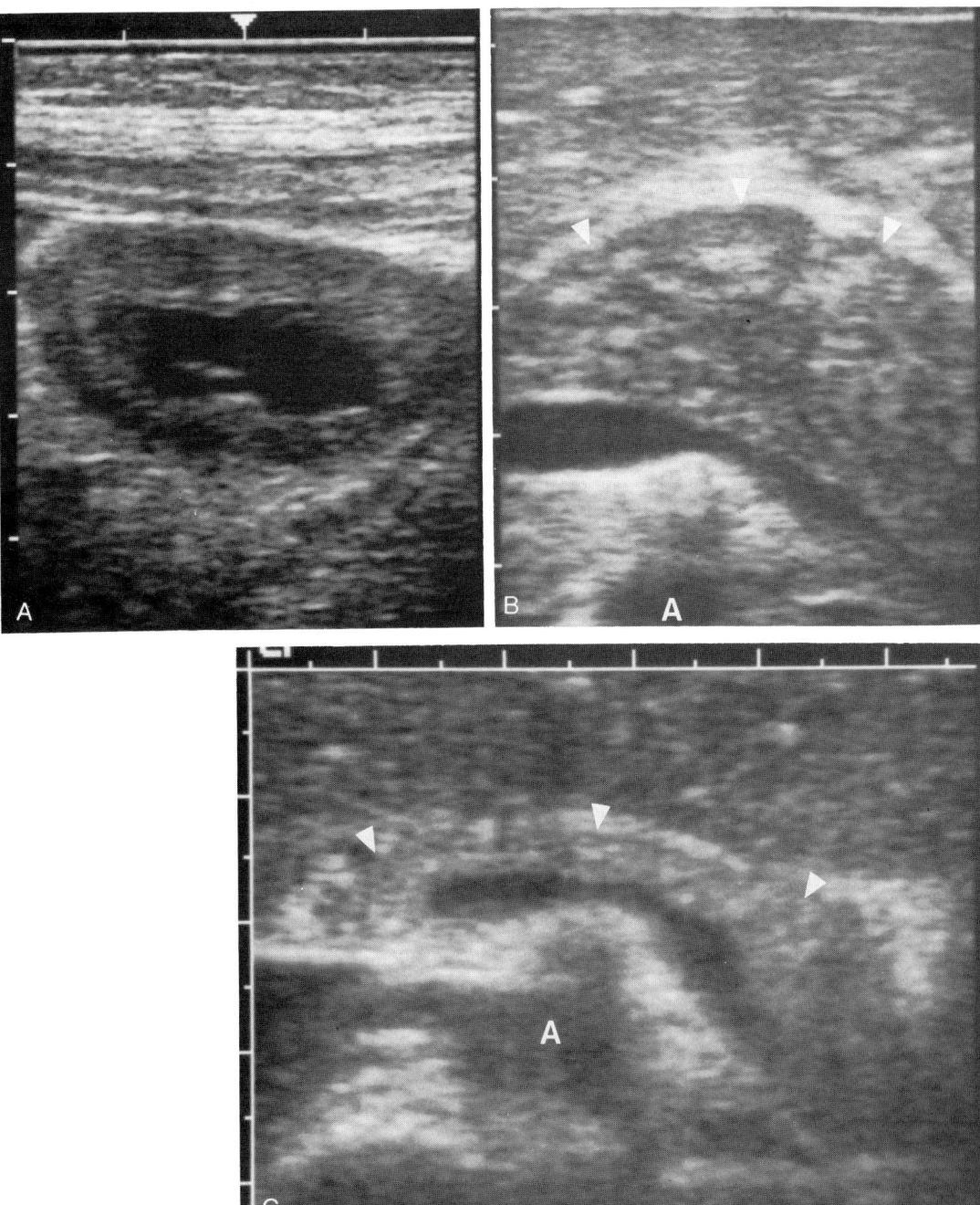

Figure 15–7. A 4-day history of bloody diarrhea, vomiting, and decreasing urinary output preceded this child's admission to the hospital. Her white blood cell count was elevated, as was the level of amylase in her serum. Scans were requested when she became obtunded and anuric. Transverse scan of the left lower quadrant (A) shows marked thickening of the colonic wall secondary to the microangiopathy of hemolytic uremic syndrome. Scans of the pancreas showed marked enlargement associated with a coarsened parenchymal pattern. The transverse view of the pancreatic body (B) shows pancreatic tissue immediately anterior to the splenic vein and the confluence of the splenic vein with the superior mesenteric vein. The anterior margin of the pancreas is outlined by arrowheads. A = aorta. This patient recovered with supportive therapy, and several weeks later, a transverse scan of the pancreas (C) showed marked diminution in the size of the pancreas. The parenchymal pattern is now more echogenic; however, the patient has not developed signs of pancreatic insufficiency. The anterior margin of the pancreas is outlined with arrowheads. A = aorta.

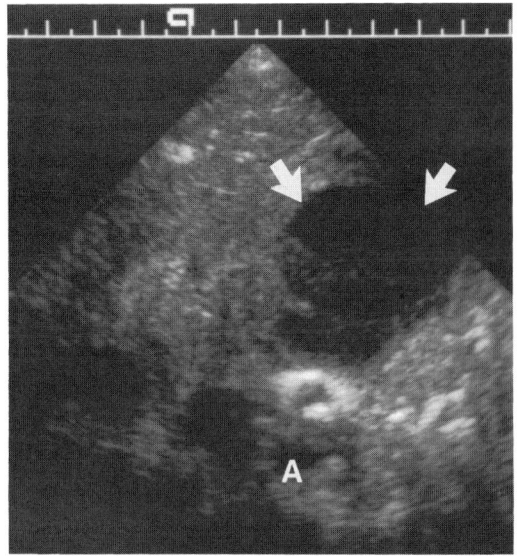

Figure 15-8. Transverse scan of the upper abdomen in this 6-year-old boy was performed 4 days after he fell onto the handlebars of his bicycle. There was a large collection of fluid (arrows) immediately anterior to the superior mesenteric artery. The pancreatic outline was poorly defined. Catheterization of this collection was performed, but drainage persisted in large volumes. A computed tomography (CT) scan performed 4 days after the intervention showed a fracture of the body of the pancreas. The boy went to surgery for removal of the distal pancreas and for oversewing of the lacerated duct.

when a duct is obviously lacerated (Bass et al., 1988).

In children who have uncomplicated traumatic pancreatitis, we recommend a follow-up scan 7 to 10 days after the injury (Fig. 15–9). Pseudocysts occur in approximately 30 percent of injured patients (Bass et al., 1988), and at least half of those resolve spontaneously with conservative treatment. The development of pseudocysts is not re-

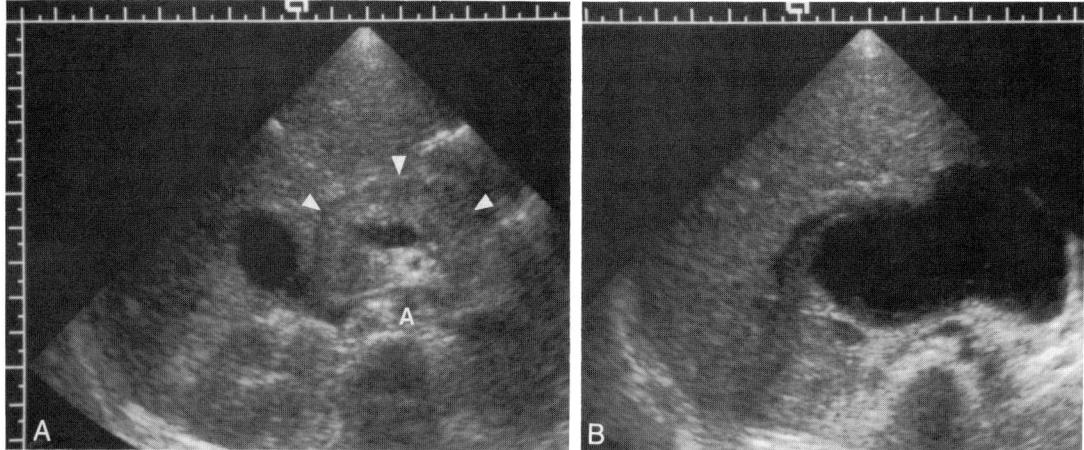

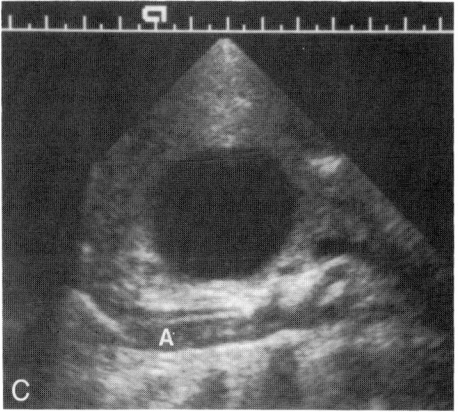

Figure 15-9. This child underwent exploratory laparotomy for a hemoperitoneum associated with a lacerated mesentery after blunt abdominal trauma to the abdomen. The level of serum amylase was elevated, and 10 days later, ultrasonograms of the abdomen revealed a pseudocyst immediately superior to the pancreas. **A** is a transverse view at the level of the head and body of the pancreas. The anterior margin of the gland is outlined by arrowheads. A = aorta. There is mild enlargement of the pancreas but no ductal dilation. The pancreatic pseudocyst is shown on transverse **(B)** and longitudinal **(C)** scans. Conservative therapy to shrink the pseudocyst was unsuccessful; 3 weeks later the patient underwent percutaneous drainage, and the pseudocyst resolved.

stricted to traumatic pancreatitis; it can follow pancreatitis of any etiology (Fig. 15–10). Pseudocysts are collections of pancreatic fluid, necrotic glandular tissue, and blood that escape from the gland when a pancreatic duct is obstructed. The thickness of the fibrous capsule that develops around the collection 4 to 6 weeks after injury is best delineated by CT. We have tended to underestimate its thickness on ultrasonography. The appearance of the surrounding capsule is of importance only if surgical intervention, with the creation of a cyst-gastrostomy, is contemplated. Percutaneous drainage of pseudocysts is now a popular alternative to surgery (Burnweit et al., 1990; Jaffe et al., 1989; Bass et al., 1988). For most children, catheterization is performed only after 3 to 4 weeks of conservative treatment has failed to bring about spontaneous resolution of the pseudocyst or if the child becomes febrile and superinfection of the pseudocyst is considered likely. In a study of seven children, managed with drainage by

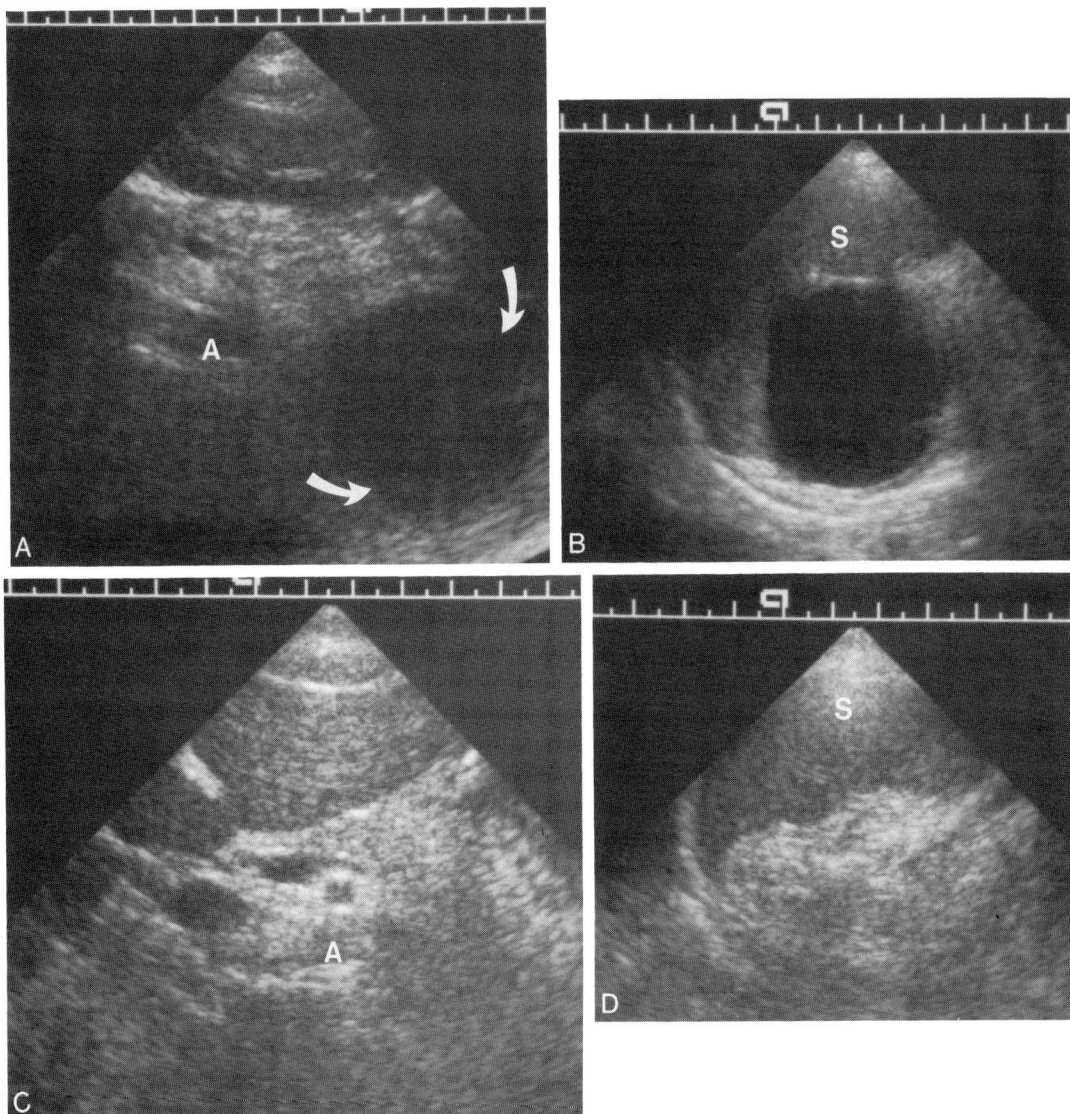

Figure 15–10. The pseudocyst shown in **A** and **B** is secondary to therapy with L-asparaginase in a 7-year-old boy, whose acute lymphocytic leukemia had been treated with this drug. After episodes of pancreatitis, a 6 × 5 cm pseudocyst (arrows) was identified in the tail of the pancreas on the transverse (**A**) and coronal (**B**) scans. In **A**, A = aorta. In **B**, S = spleen. He was asymptomatic at the time; only conservative therapy was instituted. Follow-up transverse (**C**) and longitudinal (**D**) scans 1 month later showed spontaneous resolution of the pseudocyst. In **C**, A = aorta. In **D**, S = spleen.

percutaneous catheter, catheters were left in place until drainage ceased (mean of 25 days), and no complications followed removal of the catheter (Jaffe et al., 1989). Transgastric, transcutaneous, and transhepatic approaches have all been used without sequelae (Figs. 15–11, 15–12).

Infectious, drug-related, and hereditary pancreatitis may result in some swelling of the gland but may be otherwise "silent" on ultrasonography. Ancillary but variably present signs of pancreatitis may be found with careful scanning. These include intra-abdominal fluid, fluid in the lesser sac, and echogenicity around the pancreas and kidneys that represents edema of the transverse mesocolon and the perirenal fascia (Fig. 15–13; Jeffrey et al., 1986b; Swischuk and Hayden, 1985). Perirenal echogenicity is not pathognomonic of pancreatitis. It is evident whenever there is diffuse abdominal edema and when adjacent appendicitis or some other localized inflammatory process causes inflammation of the perirenal fat and connective tissues.

Peptic disease associated with pancreatitis can leave clues to its presence on abdominal scans. Fluid in the gastric antrum retained as a result of obstruction to the gastric outlet is easy to detect. Chronic ulceration may result in thickening of the mucosa of the stomach or duodenum. Endoscopy or radiographic studies should follow the ultrasonograms in such cases.

Causes of pancreatitis that are unusual in the U.S. but more often found in developing

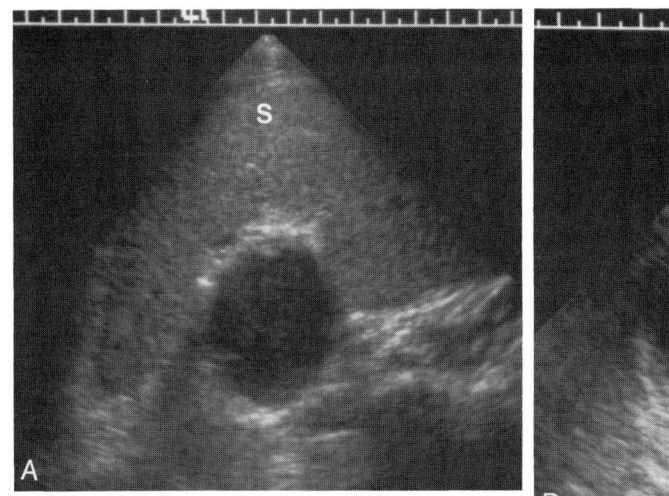
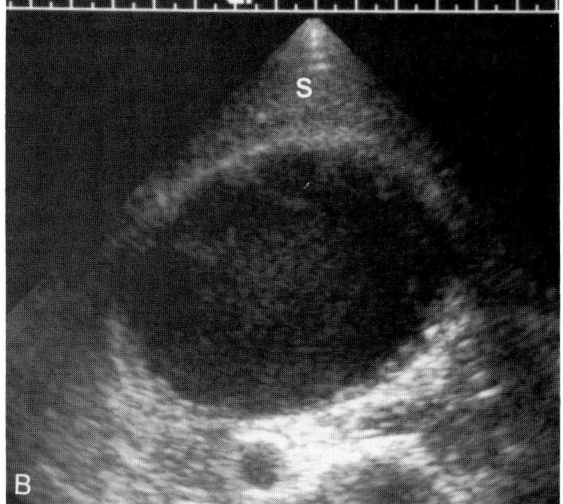
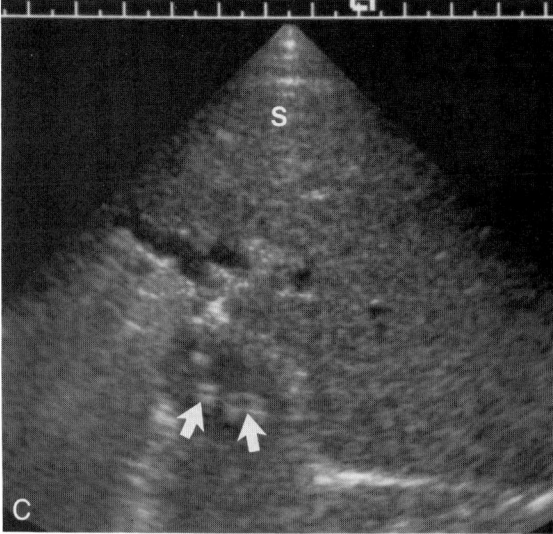

Figure 15–11. A small pseudocyst in the tail of the pancreas near the hilum of the spleen (S) increased in size over 2 months (**A** and **B**). The pseudocyst was drained percutaneously. **C** shows decompression of the cyst with a pigtail catheter (arrows) in place. S = spleen. Pancreatitis in this patient was associated with chronic renal failure. We have seen several children who have been on renal dialysis develop pancreatitis.

Figure 15–12. This longitudinal scan shows the markers from the biopsy transducer superimposed over a pseudocyst that followed pancreatitis associated with battering. In this baby, a transhepatic route for catheter drainage was used. The catheter is outlined by arrows.

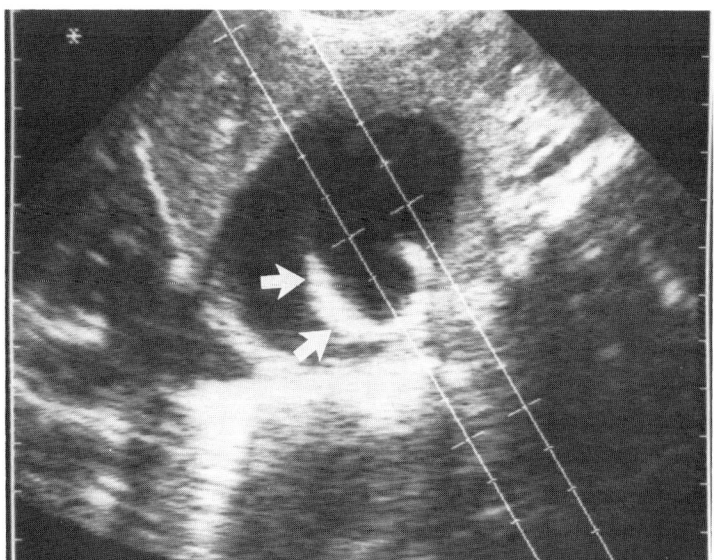

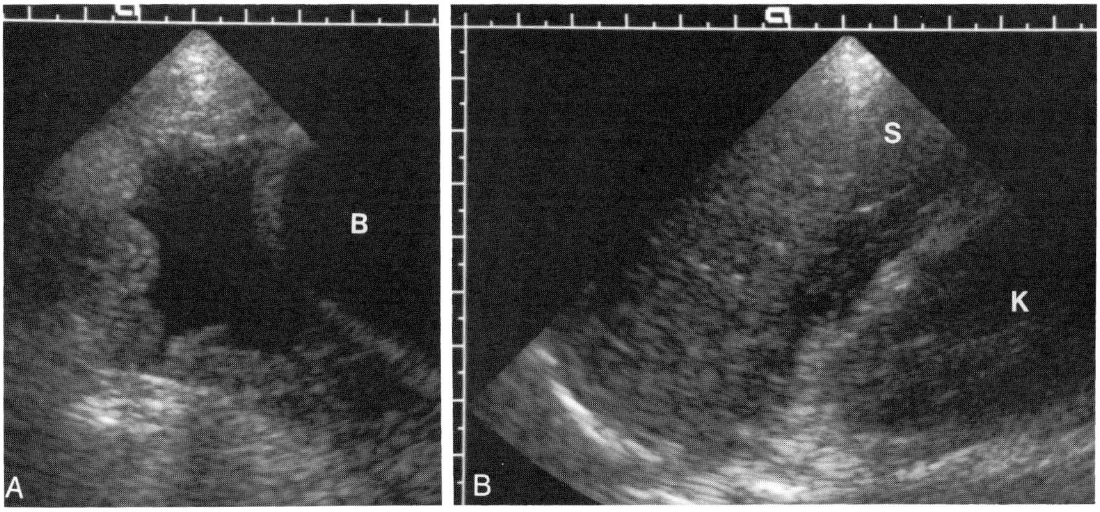

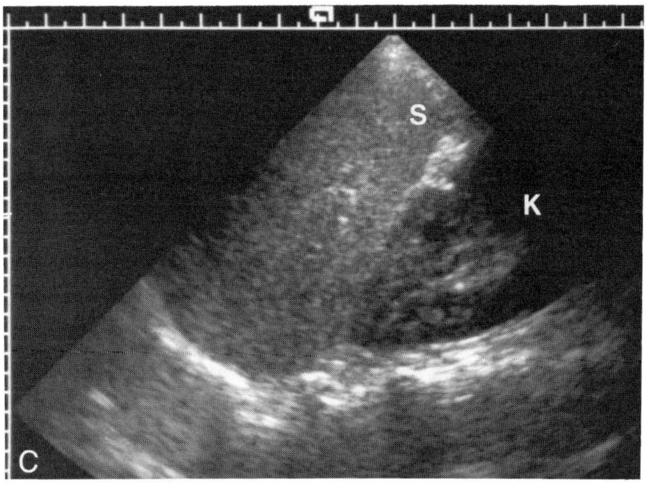

Figure 15–13. Free fluid adjacent to the bladder (B) is apparent on the longitudinal scan (A) of the pelvis in a child treated with L-asparaginase for acute lymphocytic leukemia. Coronal scan of the left upper quadrant (B) shows echogenic ring around the upper pole of the left kidney (K) secondary to retroperitoneal edema. S = spleen. Follow-up scan (C) shows resolution of the perinephric edema several weeks later when the child had recovered from the episode of pancreatitis. S = spleen. K = kidney.

nations include schistosomiasis and ascariasis. In fact, a worm was discovered within the pancreatic duct of one patient, and his ultrasonograms were published (Leung et al., 1987).

For any patient with pancreatitis, the gallbladder and biliary tree must be scanned. Although relatively uncommon in the pediatric population, gallstone-associated pancreatitis has been reported (Albu et al., 1987), and we have seen several such patients. Impacted stone, stones that intermittently obstruct the pancreatic duct as they pass through the ampulla of Vater, or predisposing congenital anomalies of the ductal systems appear to be the etiologic factors. Pancreatitis, rather than jaundice, may be the presentation of a choledochal cyst. An anomalous relationship of pancreatic and biliary ducts without the cystic ectasia of choledochus also predisposes a child to pancreatitis, but these anomalous ductal relationships are unlikely to be diagnosed with ultrasonography (Suarez et al., 1987). Endoscopic retrograde cholangiopancreatography (ERCP) usually follows ultrasonography when a child has pancreatitis with no obvious cause (Allendorph et al., 1987). ERCP is performed when the child is fully recovered from the acute illness. The aims of ERCP are (1) to outline ductal anatomy, both pancreatic and biliary; (2) to identify features of chronic pancreatitis, if present; and (3) to provide guidance for further medical or surgical therapy. The discussion of pancreatic ductal anomalies brings us to the controversy of pancreas divisum and its role in predisposing a child to pancreatitis. Pancreas divisum is found in 4 to 14 percent of autopsy series. It is defined as failure of fusion between the duct of Santorini and the duct of Wirsung. In pancreas divisum, secretions from the body and tail of the pancreas are drained into the duodenum through a variably sized duct (Santorini) that enters the duodenum proximal to the ampulla. The ventral pancreas drains through the ampulla of Vater. The incidence of pancreas divisum is stated as being 6 percent in the general population. In one large series of 5357 patients (apparently adults), there was no increased incidence of pancreatitis diagnosed in patients who on ERCP were found to have pancreas divisum (Delhaye et al., 1985). Other researchers, however, believe that pancreas divisum is one of three anatomic situations that predispose a patient to partial obstruction of pancreatic drainage; the other two are complete absence of the ventral duct and incomplete communication between ventral and dorsal ducts. These three anatomic variants are termed "dominant dorsal ducts" and are present in approximately 10 percent of Western populations (Warshaw et al., 1990). We have seen several children who had ductal anomalies associated with pancreatitis and are inclined to believe that an anomalous ductal system predisposes the child to pancreatitis. We have not been able to make the diagnosis of pancreas divisum with ultrasonography, but it is possible that stimulation of pancreatic juices by exogenous secretin might distend ductal systems differently and allow, in some cases, recognition of two ductal systems (Tulassay et al., 1988). Complete duplication of the ventral pancreatic system has been reported (Agha, 1987), and with increasing use of ERCP for children, other variations on normal anatomy may be recognized earlier in life. In our pediatric practice, a patient with "idiopathic pancreatitis" is always evaluated with ERCP.

An annular pancreas is usually associated with duodenal stenosis or atresia. In patients without overt obstruction in the neonatal period, the anomaly may be discovered later in childhood. On ultrasonograms, the appearance is that of a globular pancreatic head with the duodenum coursing through it rather than around it. This is one situation in which, if the anomaly is suspected, the child should be given fluid to drink during the examination in order that the proximal duodenum be distended.

Aberrant pancreatic tissue, found in approximately 2 percent of autopsies, is usually situated along the greater curvature of the stomach or in the duodenum. It is typically nodular or microscopic and is often recognized only incidentally on air-contrast studies of the stomach. Its presence is rarely associated with clinical pancreatitis, and we know of no cases (to date) in which aberrant pancreatic tissue has been diagnosed primarily by ultrasonography.

When children have a history of recurrent episodes of pancreatitis unassociated with chemotherapy, they usually belong to one of three groups: those who have cystic fibrosis, some who have hereditary pancreatitis, and the majority, whose pancreatitis is idiopathic. Follow-up scans are directed toward establishing size and appearance of the gland for comparison with previous studies, docu-

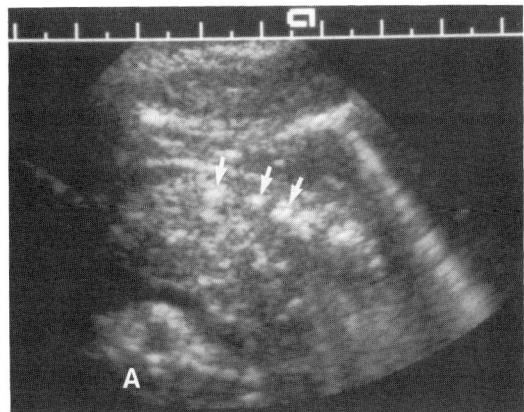

Figure 15–14. Transverse scan of the body and tail of the pancreas shows multiple echogenic foci (arrows) representing stones within the pancreas in a child who has been hospitalized repeatedly for familial pancreatitis. A cousin is also affected. A = aorta.

menting ductal dilatation, if present, and searching for parenchymal or ductal calcifications, pseudocysts, and splenic venous thrombosis (Fig. 15–14). Over time, chronic fibrosis or fatty replacement of the pancreas results in the gland's being echogenic and indistinguishable from surrounding connective tissue. This is particularly true in children with cystic fibrosis. Calcifications may be evident as shadowing foci but can get lost in a fibrotic parenchyma. Although splenic venous thrombosis is a rare complication of chronic pancreatitis in childhood, it has been reported in adults and is not always associated with splenomegaly (Zalcman et al., 1987). If Doppler ultrasonography is available, scanning of splenic, superior mesenteric, and portal veins should be included as part of the examination of the pancreas.

We have been interested in establishing, in children, whether exogenous administration of secretin produces ductal dilatation in patients with presumed chronic pancreatitis. In normal young adults, intravenous injection of secretin produces overt dilation of the duct to the extent that it typically doubles in size within 5 minutes (Glaser et al., 1987). Because secretin is given to children immediately before ERCP in order to allow immediate identification of the ampulla and easier cannulation, ultrasonography may be used to measure ductal diameter immediately after the dose is given. In adults who have chronic pancreatitis, there is typically no, poor, or delayed response to secretin as measured by changes in ductal diameter.

Chronic fibrosing pancreatitis is an unusual, low-grade inflammatory process that is characterized by collagenous bands enclosing normal acini in the absence of necrosis, hemorrhage, or pseudocyst. Both in ultrasonography and at surgery, the resultant mass simulates a tumor (Fig. 15–15). If it involves the head of the pancreas, it may obstruct the biliary tree (Atkinson et al., 1988).

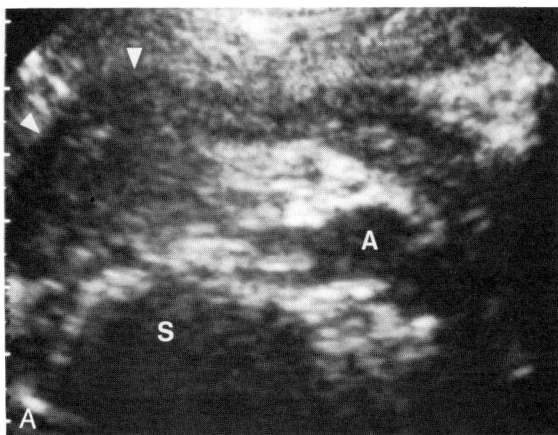
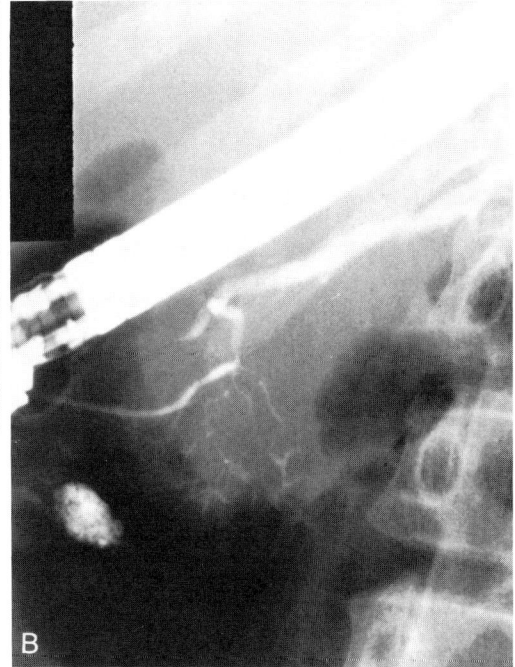

Figure 15–15. Recurrent abdominal pain brought this 10-year-old girl to medical attention. The head of the pancreas was enlarged (A), and the parenchymal pattern was irregular. A = aorta. S = spine. Arrowheads point to head of pancreas. Because of the concern that this was a tumor, the patient went to surgery after endoscopic retrograde cholangiopancreatography (ERCP) showed a narrowed irregular proximal duct (B). Chronic fibrosing pancreatitis was diagnosed from a biopsy of the head of the pancreas.

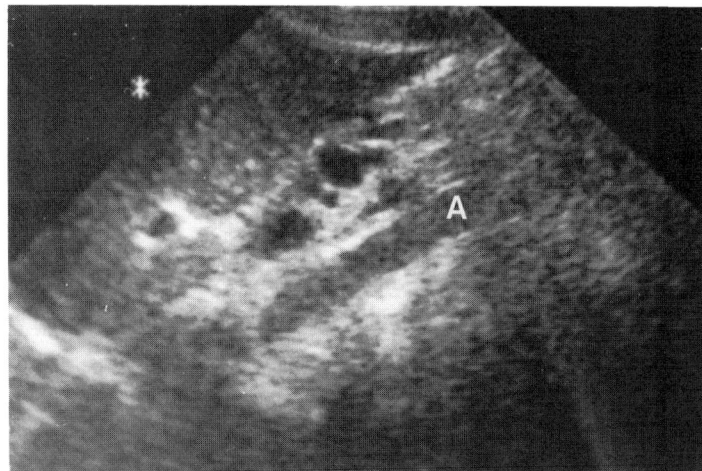

Figure 15–16. Scans were requested for this young woman, who was known to have von Hippel-Lindau disease. She was asymptomatic at the time of the study. Cysts are obvious in the head of the pancreas on this longitudinal scan. A = aorta.

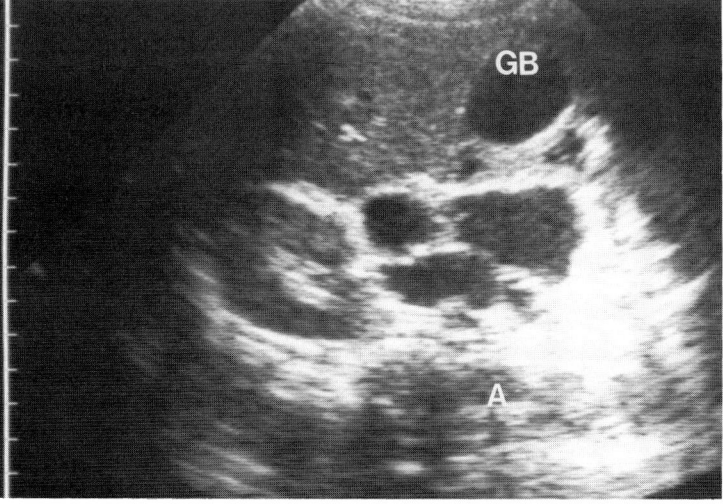

Figure 15–17. Large cysts replaced the head of the pancreas in this 14-year-old girl, who was known to have cystic fibrosis. The transverse scan is an angled view through the right lobe of the liver. A = aorta. GB = gallbladder.

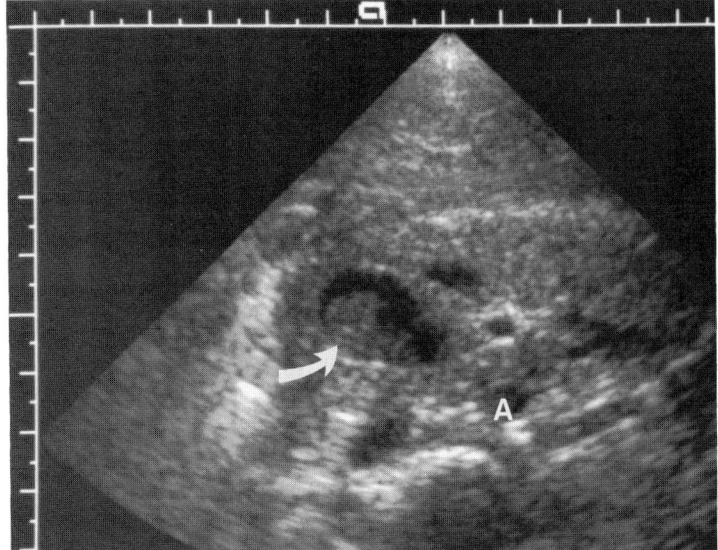

Figure 15–18. Intermittent fever and abdominal pain in this baby boy were unexplained. Exploration for presumed appendicitis resulted in the removal of a normal appendix but the discovery of a retroperitoneal hematoma, which was evacuated. Postoperative evaluation included ultrasonography and ERCP. There was a cyst, filled with echogenic debris, in the head of the pancreas on this transverse scan (arrow). (ERCP revealed that this communicated with the main pancreatic duct.) During surgery, a duplication cyst lined with gastric mucosa was treated by removal of the gastric lining and drainage of the region via Roux-en-Y loop from the jejunum. A = aorta.

PANCREATIC MASSES

Pseudocysts are the most common cystic masses related to the pancreas, and their nature is usually obvious because of a history and clinical evidence of pancreatitis. Other cysts can occur: 5 to 10 percent of patients with autosomal dominant kidney disease have pancreatic cysts; these usually develop after adolescence and do not interfere with pancreatic function. Similarly, patients with von Hippel-Lindau syndrome develop pancreatic cysts (Fig. 15–16). A solitary congenital pancreatic cyst is a rare anomaly (Welch, 1986). It is indistinguishable from a mesenteric or an omental cyst if it is large. It may be recognized as being pancreatic in origin only when its contents, aspirated during surgery, are found to have high levels of amylase. Large cysts that virtually replace the entire pancreas have been found in a few patients who have cystic fibrosis (Hernanz-Shulman et al., 1986), but the occurrence of such cysts in this disease is decidedly uncommon (Fig. 15–17). One type of cystic mass of the pancreas can be a real diagnostic puzzle because it may wax and wane between examinations. A duplication cyst of the foregut can be enveloped in pancreatic tissue and may communicate with the ductal system of the pancreas. It can cause obstruction to normal flow of pancreatic juices or it may ulcerate and bleed, resulting in a solid intrapancreatic mass. This anomaly may be suspected on ultrasonography, in which it presents as an atypical cyst, irregular in contour with a variably thickened wall and, occasionally, intraluminal debris (Fig. 15–18). ERCP, alone or in combination with CT, is diagnostic if the cyst freely communicates with the ductal system (Black et al., 1986).

Neoplasms of the pancreas, benign and malignant, are, fortunately, rare in children (Fig. 15–19; Plate XI). There are isolated reports of children who have received a diagnosis of hamartoma (Burt et al., 1983), adenocarcinoma (Robey et al., 1983), or islet cell (nonfunctioning) carcinoma (Moynan et al., 1964). To classify a malignant pancreatic neoplasm as being derived from ductal, acinar, or islet cells is often difficult and accounts for the overlap in classification between pathologic reviews of the same material. To date, the number of reported cases of carcinoma totals about 50. In our hospital, one patient with pancreatic adenocarcinoma presented with duodenal obstruction years after orthovoltage radiotherapy for Wilms tumor. As mentioned previously, fibrosing pancreatitis can appear as a solid parenchymal mass and be indistinguishable from a primary tumor (Fig. 15–15). If an echogenic intrapancreatic mass is identified with ultrasonography, the portal system should be carefully scanned for thrombus, and the hepatic parenchyma should be surveyed for metastatic deposits (Fig. 15–19).

In contrast to primary neoplasms, it is much more common for neuroblastoma, lymphoma, and the adenopathy or tumor associated with acquired immunodeficiency syndrome (AIDS; Graif et al., 1987) or with other

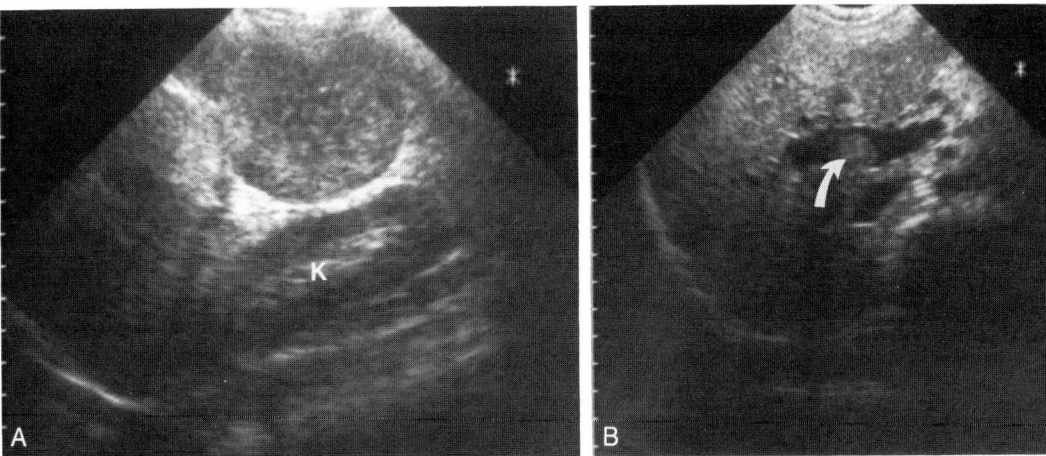

Figure 15–19. Longitudinal (**A**) scan of the right upper quadrant followed discovery of a mass in this 5-year-old boy, who had adenocarcinoma of the pancreas. The mass replaced the head of the pancreas and was immediately anterior to the kidney (K). Transverse scan (**B**) revealed a thrombus of tumor (arrow) within the portal vein.

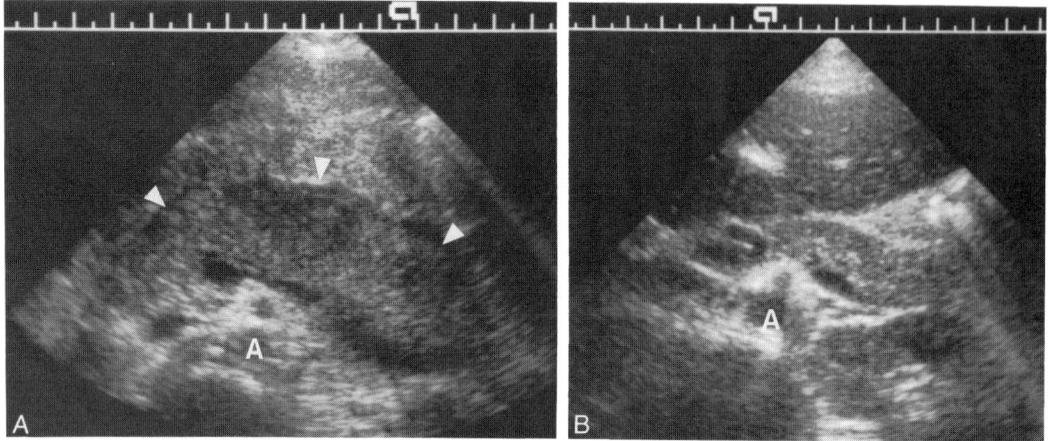

Figure 15–20. Pancreatic enlargement seen on the transverse scan of the pancreas (A) in this 12-year-old boy heralded relapse of his Burkitt lymphoma. Note the bulky and irregular contour of the pancreas as outlined by arrowheads. A = aorta. He was switched to a different protocol for chemotherapy. Follow-up scans 4 months later show resolution of the lymphadenopathy around the pancreas (B). A = aorta.

immunodeficiencies to affect the pancreas. Although they do not arise from the pancreas, these retroperitoneal tumors or nodes distort or silhouette the gland (Figs. 15–20, 15–21). The function of the pancreas is unaffected by the masses around it. Benign lymphangioma of the root of the mesentery may appear to involve the pancreas if it is immediately adjacent to it. Lymphangioma, if it is more stromal than cystic in consistency, may appear quite echogenic on scans. It tends to adapt to the shape of the normal organs and structures around it rather than to displace or invade them. Concomitant lymphangiectasia or other lymphatic abnormalities may be present, inasmuch as lymphangioma is often part of a generalized hamartomatous malformation of the lymphatic system.

Two diseases of the pancreas cause severe hypoglycemia in infancy and childhood. One is nesidioblastosis, which is hyperplasia of insulin-producing beta cells in or around acinar elements, outside the islets of Langerhans. Only when stains specific for insulin were developed were pathologists able to differentiate nesidioblastosis from the normal pancreas (Yakovac et al., 1971). It appears

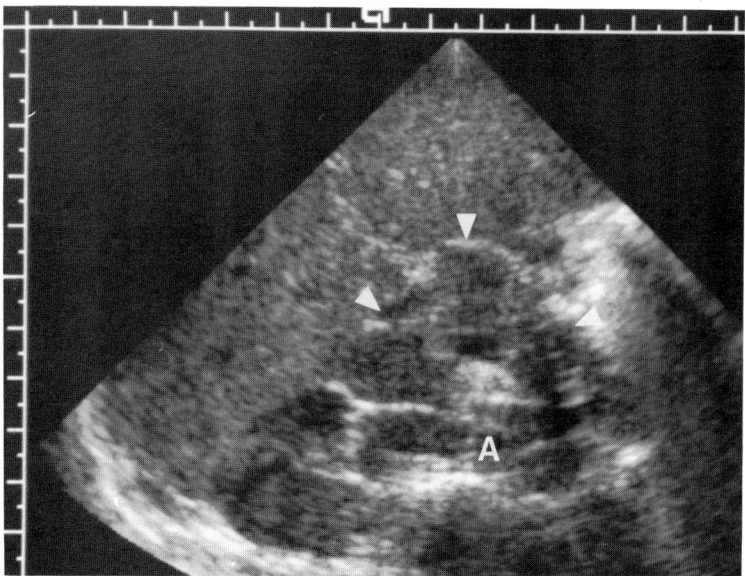

Figure 15–21. This 17-month-old girl was suspected of having acquired immunodeficiency syndrome (AIDS) when she presented with pancytopenia, diffuse adenopathy, and hepatosplenomegaly. All results of serologic testing for the human immunodeficiency virus have been normal. She has an as-yet-undefined immunodeficiency. The transverse scan of the upper abdomen shows an irregular pancreatic contour from adjacent adenopathy (arrowheads). A = aorta.

that nesidioblastosis is a perpetuation of the embryologic state, in which beta cells, which produce insulin, are continuously arising from the exocrine pancreas. With ultrasonography, not surprisingly, we have been unable to differentiate nesidioblastosis from a normal pancreas. The other lesion to cause hyperinsulinemia is pancreatic insulinoma. In the ultrasonographic literature, it is generally described as a small, solitary, hypoechoic mass. Identification of insulinoma in adult patients is facilitated by the fact that aging is associated with increasing echogenicity of pancreatic tissue. In children, whose pancreatic parenchyma is usually of low to moderate echogenicity, finding the tumor is a real challenge. If a patient has multiple endocrine neoplasia, type I, multiple insulinomas may be present (Telander et al., 1986). Intraoperative pancreatic ultrasonography is well worth considering if transducers of high frequency can be placed into a fluid bath (saline) around the pancreas. Ultrasonography in the operating room can occasionally enable the clinician to diagnose a nonpalpable lesion, can demonstrate the location of multiple lesions, and can show the relationship of an insulinoma to the pancreatic duct, common bile duct, and blood vessels (Gorman et al., 1986). It is not foolproof, especially for children whose anatomy is small to start with and in whom lesions tend to be isoechoic with pancreatic parenchyma. Hyperechoic insulinoma has been reported, but only in 2 of a series of 29, primarily adult, patients (Gorman et al., 1986).

In any situation in which the pancreas is poorly visualized by ultrasonography, when severe trauma has occurred, and when an intrapancreatic mass is discovered, further evaluation with CT is appropriate.

REFERENCES

Pancreatitis

Agha FP: Duplex ventral pancreas. Gastrointest Radiol 1987; 12:23–25.
Albu E, Buiumsohn A, Lopez R, et al: Gallstone pancreatitis in adolescents. J Pediatr Surg 1987; 22:960–962.
Allendorph M, Werlin SL, Geenen JE, et al: Endoscopic retrograde cholangiopancreatography in children. J Pediatr 1987; 110:206–211.
Atkinson GO Jr, Wyly JB, Gay BB Jr, et al: Idiopathic fibrosing pancreatitis: A cause of obstructive jaundice in childhood. Pediatr Radiol 1988; 18:28–31.
Bass J, Di Lorenzo M, Desjardins JG, et al: Blunt pancreatic injuries in children: The role of percutaneous external drainage in the treatment of pancreatic pseudocysts. J Pediatr Surg 1988; 23:721–724.
Bolondi L, Li Bassi S, Gaiani S, et al: Impaired response of main pancreatic duct to secretin stimulation in early chronic pancreatitis. Dig Dis Sci 1989; 34:834–840.
Burnweit C, Wesson D, Stringer D, Filler R: Percutaneous drainage of traumatic pancreatic pseudocysts in children. J Trauma 1990; 30:1273–1277.
Coleman BG, Ayer PH, Rosenberg HK: Gray-scale sonographic assessment of pancreatitis in children. Radiology 1983; 146:145–150.
Delhaye M, Engelholm L, Cremer M: Pancreas divisum: Congenital anatomic variant or anomaly? Contribution of endoscopic retrograde dorsal pancreatography. Gastroenterology 1985; 89:951–958.
Fleischer AC, Parker P, Kirchner SG: Sonographic findings of pancreatitis in children. Radiology 1983; 146:151–155.
Garel L, Brunelle F, Lallemand D, et al: Pseudocysts of the pancreas in children: Which cases require surgery? Pediatr Radiol 1983; 13:120–124.
Glaser J, Högemann B, Krummenerl T, et al: Sonographic imaging of the pancreatic duct: New diagnostic possibilities using secretin stimulation. Dig Dis Sci 1987; 32:1075–1081.
Gorenstein A, O'Halpin D, Wesson DE, et al: Blunt injury to the pancreas in children: Selective management based on ultrasound. J Pediatr Surg 1987; 22:1110–1116.
Jaffe RB, Arata JA Jr, Matlak ME: Percutaneous drainage of traumatic pancreatic pseudocysts in children. AJR 1989; 152:591–595.
Jeffrey RB Jr, Laing FC, Wing VW: Ultrasound in acute pancreatic trauma. Gastrointest Radiol 1986a; 11:44–46.
Jeffrey RB Jr, Laing FC, Wing VW: Extrapancreatic spread of acute pancreatitis: New observations with real-time US. Radiology 1986b; 159:707–711.
Lawson TL: Acute pancreatitis and its complications: Computed tomography and sonography. Radiol Clin North Am 1983; 21:495–513.
Leung JWC, Mok SD, Metreweli C: Ascaris-induced pancreatitis. AJR 1987; 149:511–512.
Mallory A, Kern F Jr: Drug-induced pancreatitis: A critical review. Gastroenterology 1980; 78:813–820.
McHugo JM, McKeown C, Brown MT, et al: Ultrasound findings in children with cystic fibrosis. Br J Radiol 1987; 60:137–141.
Rosenberg HK, Ortega W: Hemorrhagic pancreatitis in a young child following valproic acid therapy. Clinical and ultrasonic assessment. Clin Pediatr 1987; 26:98–101.
Schneider K, Harms K, Fendel H: The increased echogenicity of the pancreas in infants and children: The white pancreas. Eur J Pediatr 1987; 146:508–511.
Siegel MJ, Martin KW, Worthington JL: Normal and abnormal pancreas in children: US studies. Radiology 1987; 165:15–18.
Stoler J, Biller JA, Grand RJ: Pancreatitis in Kawasaki disease. Am J Dis Child 1987; 141:306–308.
Suarez F, Bernard O, Gauthier F, et al: Bilio-pancreatic common channel in children: Clinical, biological and radiological findings in 12 children. Pediatr Radiol 1987; 17:206–211.
Swischuk LE, Hayden CK Jr: Pararenal space hyperechogenicity in childhood pancreatitis. AJR 1985; 145:1085–1086.
Tulassay Z, Gupta R, Keleman E, et al: Secretin provocation ultrasonography in the assessment of papillary

obstruction in pancreas divisum [Abstract]. Gastroenterol 94 pt 2:A467, 1988.
Veda D: Sonographic measurement of the pancreas in children. JCU 1989; 17:417–423.
Van Steenbergen W, Samain H, Pouillon M, et al: Transection of the pancreas demonstrated by ultrasound and computed tomography. Gastrointest Radiol 1987; 12:128–130.
Warshaw AL, Simeone JF, Schapiro RH, et al: Evaluation and treatment of the dominant dorsal duct syndrome (pancreas divisum redefined). Am J Surg 1990; 159:59–64.
Willi UV, Reddish JM, Teele RL: Cystic fibrosis: Its characteristic appearance on abdominal sonography. AJR 1980; 134:1005–1010.
Zalcman M, Van Gansbeke D, Matos C, et al: Sonographic demonstration of portal venous system thromboses secondary to inflammatory diseases of the pancreas. Gastrointest Radiol 1987; 12:114–116.

Pancreatic Masses

Baker LL, Hartman GE, Northway WH: Sonographic detection of congenital pancreatic cysts in the newborn: Report of a case and review of the literature. Pediatr Radiol 1990; 20:488–490.
Black PR, Welch KJ, Eraklis AJ: Juxtapancreatic intestinal duplications with pancreatic ductal communication: A cause of pancreatitis and recurrent abdominal pain in childhood. J Pediatr Surg 1986; 21:257–261.
Bowerman RA, McCracken S, Silver TM, et al: Abdominal and miscellaneous applications of intra-operative ultrasound. Radiol Clin North Am 1985; 23:107–119.
Burt TB, Condon VR, Matlak ME: Fetal pancreatic hamartoma. Pediatr Radiol 1983; 13:287–289.
Frable WJ, Still WJS, Kay S: Carcinoma of the pancreas, infantile type. A light and electron microscopic study. Cancer 1971; 27:667–673.
Gauderer M, Stanley CA, Baker L, et al: Pancreatic adenomas in infants and children: Current surgical management. J Pediatr Surg 1978; 13:591–596.
Gorman B, Charboneau JW, James EM, et al: Benign pancreatic insulinoma: Preoperative and intraoperative sonographic localization. AJR 1986; 147:929–934.
Graif M, Kessler A, Neumann Y, et al: Pancreatic Burkitt lymphoma in AIDS: Sonographic appearance [letter]. AJR 1987; 149:1290–1291.
Hernanz-Schulman M, Teele RL, Perez-Atayde A, et al: Pancreatic cystosis in cystic fibrosis. Radiology 1986; 629–631.
Moynan RW, Neerhout RC, Johnson TS: Pancreatic carcinoma in childhood. Case report and review. J Pediatr 1964; 65:711–720.
Robey G, Daneman A, Martin DJ: Pancreatic carcinoma in a neonate. Pediatr Radiol 1983; 13:284–286.
Telander RL, Charboneau JW, Haymond MW: Intraoperative ultrasonography of the pancreas in children. J Pediatr Surg 1986; 21:262–266.
Welch KJ: The pancreas. In Welch KJ, Randolph JG, Ravitch MM, et al (eds): Pediatric Surgery (Vol 2, 4th ed). Chicago: Year Book Medical Publishers, 1986, 1086–1106.
Yakovac WC, Baker L, Hummeler K: Beta cell nesidioblastosis in idiopathic hypoglycemia of infancy. J Pediatr 1971; 79:226–231.

CHAPTER 16

THE SPLEEN

Of the solid intra-abdominal organs, the spleen is the most difficult to image. It is hidden under the ribs (which, in some children, are ticklish to the touch) and shadowed by gastric air. Oblique scans of the upper left flank result in coronal views of the spleen. The splenic hilum is the reference point for the midplane of the organ. In order to achieve scans through the longest coronal plane, the child can be rolled onto the right side. The left arm, held over the head, tends to widen the intercostal scanning windows. Children do not like the pressure of the transducer over their ribs, but use of a firm hand while angling the transducer is the only way for the ultrasonographer to get a reasonable view. In a general abdominal survey, we tend to leave examination of the spleen until near the end, in order to keep the child's cooperation for the entire examination.

Splenic shape is neither oval nor pyramidal; thus its size is difficult to gauge. Although some authors have proposed volumetric measures to assess splenic size (Dittrich et al., 1983), we find that we rely on experience and a few general rules. Rarely is a baby's spleen longer than 6 cm. In children 6 to 12 years old, splenic length is 8 to 10 cm. In adolescents, splenic length should be less than 12 cm. A good rule is the following: maximal splenic length in centimeters is 6 + 1/3 of a person's age in years until the age of 21 years (Fig. 16–1). A spleen that has a rounded lower border and that extends beyond the lower pole of a normal left kidney is always suspect (Fig. 16–2).

We do not rely on transverse views of the spleen to any great degree unless we are searching for parenchymal abnormalities such as inflammatory or ischemic lesions, or tumoral deposits, hematomas, or lacerations. Perisplenic collections of fluid can be visualized more easily in the coronal plane. As discussed in Chapter 13, we prefer other imaging in the emergent evaluation of a child presumed to have suffered splenic trauma. Any ultrasonographic examination of a child who has suffered injury to the left upper quadrant should include coronal and transverse views of the spleen, the left kidney, and the pancreas and a check of Morison pouch and the retrovesical space for the presence of free fluid (Fig. 16–3; Booth et al., 1987).

The spleen is first cousin to the hematopoietic system and second cousin to the liver. It should never be evaluated in isolation. The most common causes of splenomegaly in our practice are chronic hepatic diseases and leukemia/lymphoma (Fig. 16–4). Viral illnesses of all types and especially infection with the Epstein-Barr virus can cause splenic enlargement. Other pediatric diseases that cause splenomegaly are collagen vascular disor-

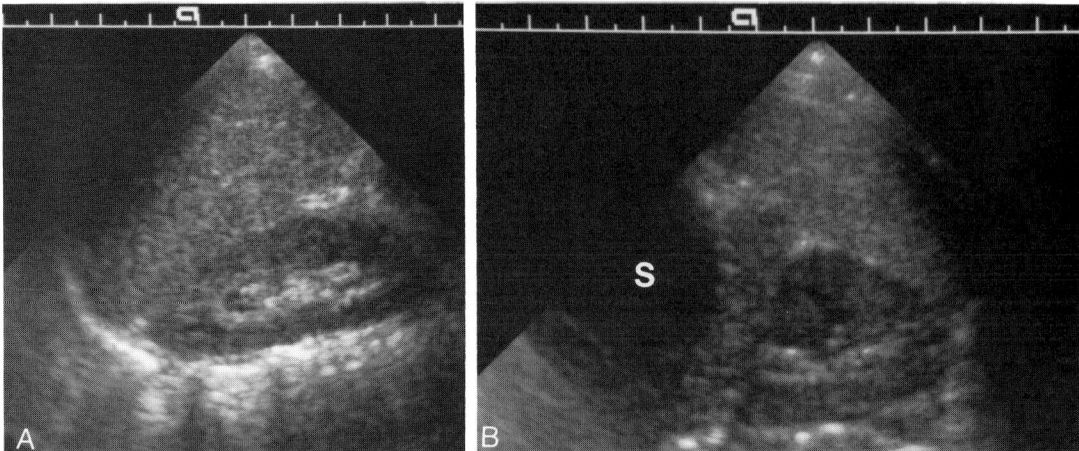

Figure 16–1. Coronal (A) and transverse (B) scans of the spleen in a 2-year-old girl show normal size, configuration, and texture of the organ. S = stomach.

ders, storage diseases such as Gaucher disease, infections (granulomatous and parasitic in developing nations), and the hemolytic anemias.

Evaluation of the spleen in patients with chronic hepatic disease and possible or established portal hypertension should include documentation of size with reasonable other landmarks on scans (e.g., the left kidney, the splenic hilum) in order that follow-up studies can duplicate the views; notation of splenic parenchymal pattern because with increasing hypertension, the spleen becomes more echogenic from fibrosis; and documentation of splenic arterial and venous blood flow. Because the splenic artery is quite tortuous, even in children, it is best to investigate splenic vessels at the hilum, through a coronal approach. The vessels are so closely related that the Doppler signals often register on the same image. In normal children, the arterial blood flow (splenopetal) is on the opposite side of the baseline as the venous (splenofugal) flow (Fig. 16–5).

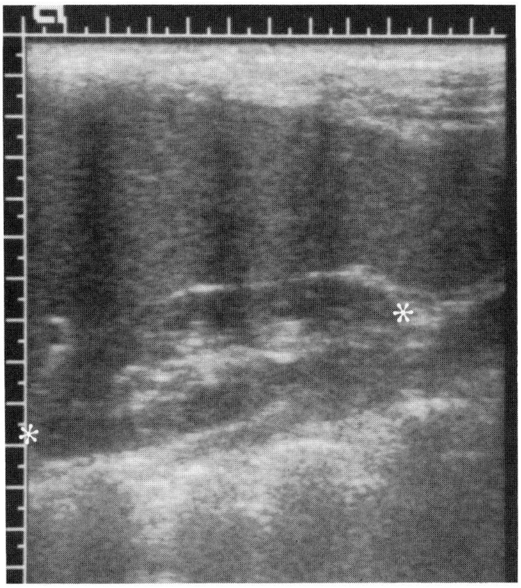

Figure 16–2. Coronal view shows the spleen extending below the inferior edge of the left kidney. This 12-year-old girl had presented with pain in the left upper quadrant. She had previously received a diagnosis of acute lymphocytic leukemia, and her acute splenic enlargement was from leukemic infiltration associated with relapse. (Asterisks delineate upper and lower margins of left kidney.)

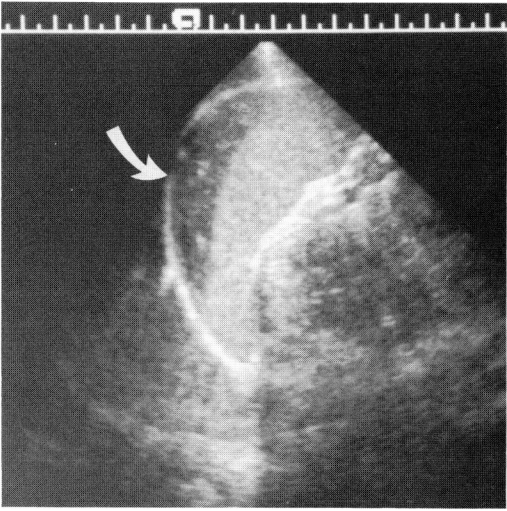

Figure 16–3. The subcapsular hematoma (arrow) in this 15-year-old boy, who had been in an automobile accident, was best seen on coronal scans through the left intercostal spaces.

THE SPLEEN / 407

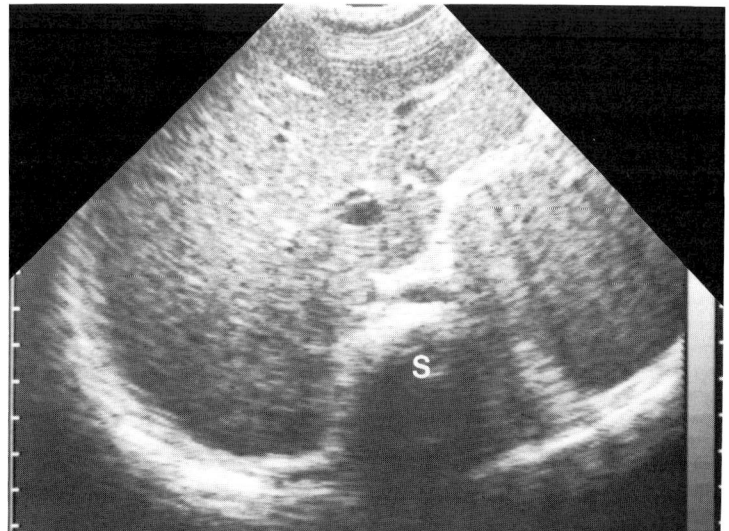

Figure 16–4. Severe hepatosplenomegaly, demonstrated on this transverse scan, was the presenting sign of leukemia in this 2-year-old girl. S = spine.

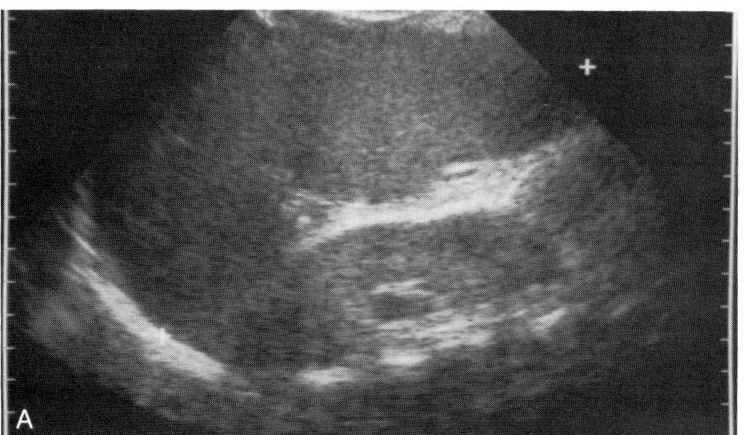

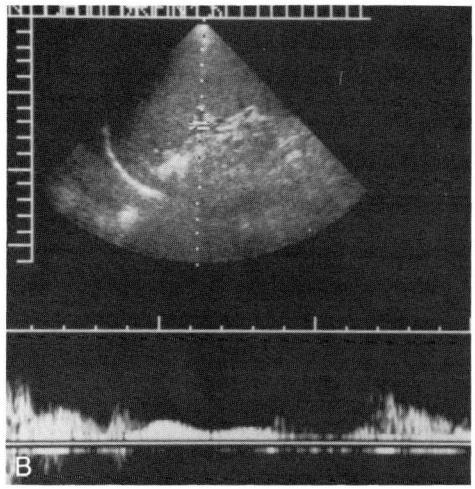

Figure 16–5. At the age of 2 years, this girl had had a right-sided Wilms tumor removed. Hepatic disease developed, probably as a secondary result of radiotherapy of the right upper quadrant and possibly chemotherapy. She presented at age 9 with esophageal varices. These scans were done a year later. The scans show splenomegaly (A) and splenic venous and arterial blood flow on the same side of the baseline (B). Because of hypersplenism, she underwent splenectomy with a splenorenal shunt. The abnormal splenopetal nature of the venous flow was confirmed at surgery.

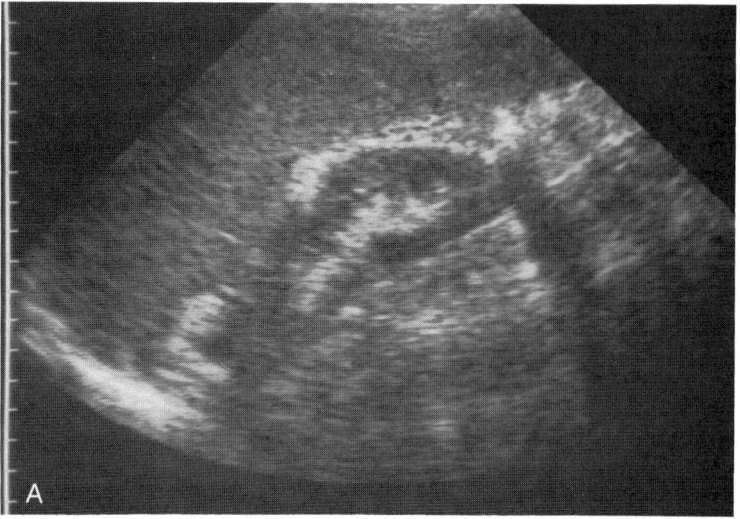
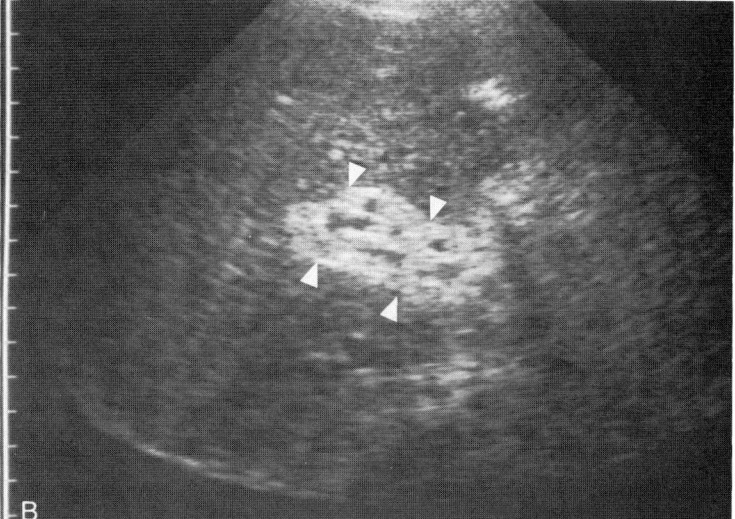
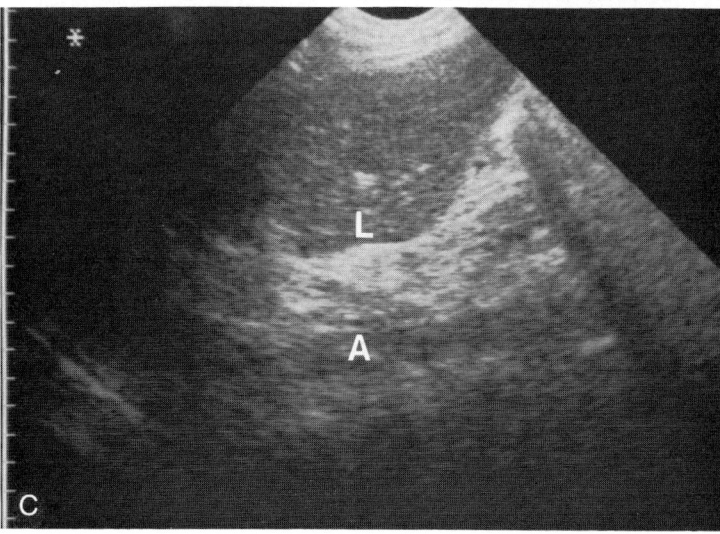

Figure 16–6. Splenomegaly was the only clinical finding in this 12-year-old boy. His initial referral was from oncologists who were concerned that he might have lymphoproliferative disease. Coronal scan of the left upper quadrant shows a very large spleen (**A**). Further evaluation of the liver (**B**) revealed cavernous transformation of the portal vein (arrowheads). Increased distance between aorta (A) and left lobe of liver (L) was due to esophageal varices' occupying this space (**C**). Presumably, he had neonatal thrombosis of the portal vein, which resulted in presinusoidal portal hypertension and resulting splenomegaly. Several years later, hypersplenism and bleeding esophageal varices necessitated placement of a splenorenal shunt. Since then, he has been asymptomatic.

Many of our patients who have had neonatal thrombosis of the portal vein have presented only with splenomegaly (Fig. 16–6). On occasion, splenomegaly has been the first sign of undiagnosed chronic liver disease with portal hypertension. The evaluation of splenomegaly should always include real-time scanning of the liver and the splenic and portal veins. Doppler study should follow, if the equipment is available.

Enlargement from infiltration with leukemic cells or from non-Hodgkin lymphoma can be quite dramatic, but in affected patients the diagnosis has usually been made before splenic scanning is performed. With enlargement, the spleen loses its beveled inferior tip to become more rounded in all dimensions. The parenchyma may be slightly less echoic than normal, but this is difficult to detect when there is no baseline for comparison. Typically, the parenchyma has a uniform pattern although focal, hypoechoic deposits may occur, and echogenic deposits have also been described (Solbiati et al., 1983). Ultrasonography has great difficulty in distinguishing the focal deposits of Hodgkin disease from normal splenic parenchyma and cannot be used as a reliable screening method for patients with this tumor (King et al., 1985).

Mild splenic enlargement may accompany viral illnesses. We also have scanned patients whose diagnosis was juvenile rheumatoid arthritis or Crohn disease and who had mild splenomegaly, presumably associated with their underlying illness. Immunosuppressed patients may develop both hepatomegaly and splenomegaly with diffuse candidal infection. Ultrasonography can distinguish the candidal abscesses only when their size increases beyond the microscopic range (Fig. 16–7). We have seen patients in whom can-

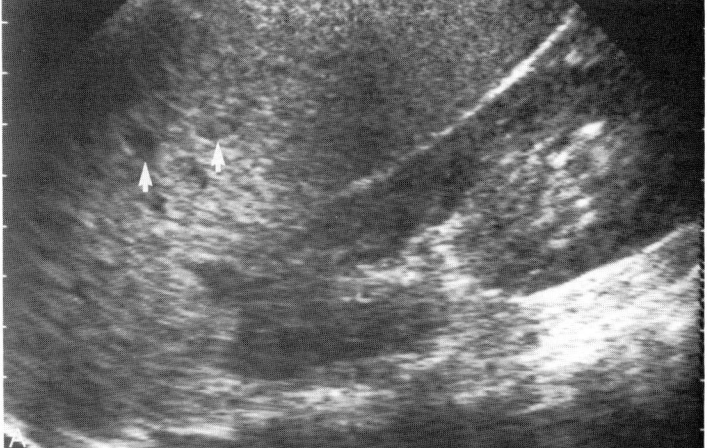

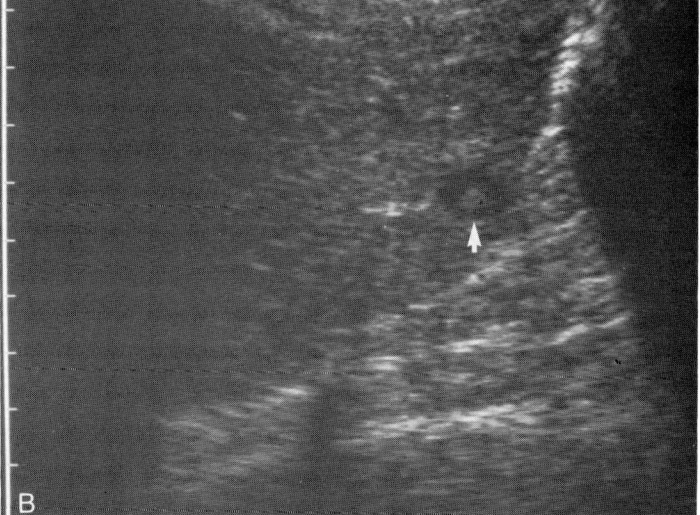

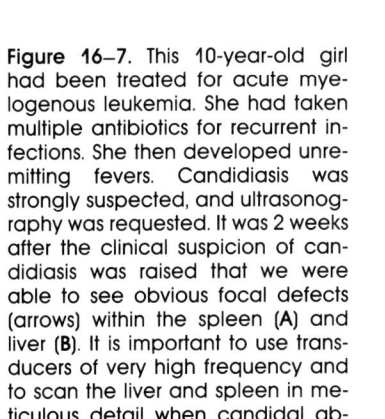

Figure 16–7. This 10-year-old girl had been treated for acute myelogenous leukemia. She had taken multiple antibiotics for recurrent infections. She then developed unremitting fevers. Candidiasis was strongly suspected, and ultrasonography was requested. It was 2 weeks after the clinical suspicion of candidiasis was raised that we were able to see obvious focal defects (arrows) within the spleen (A) and liver (B). It is important to use transducers of very high frequency and to scan the liver and spleen in meticulous detail when candidal abscesses are suspected.

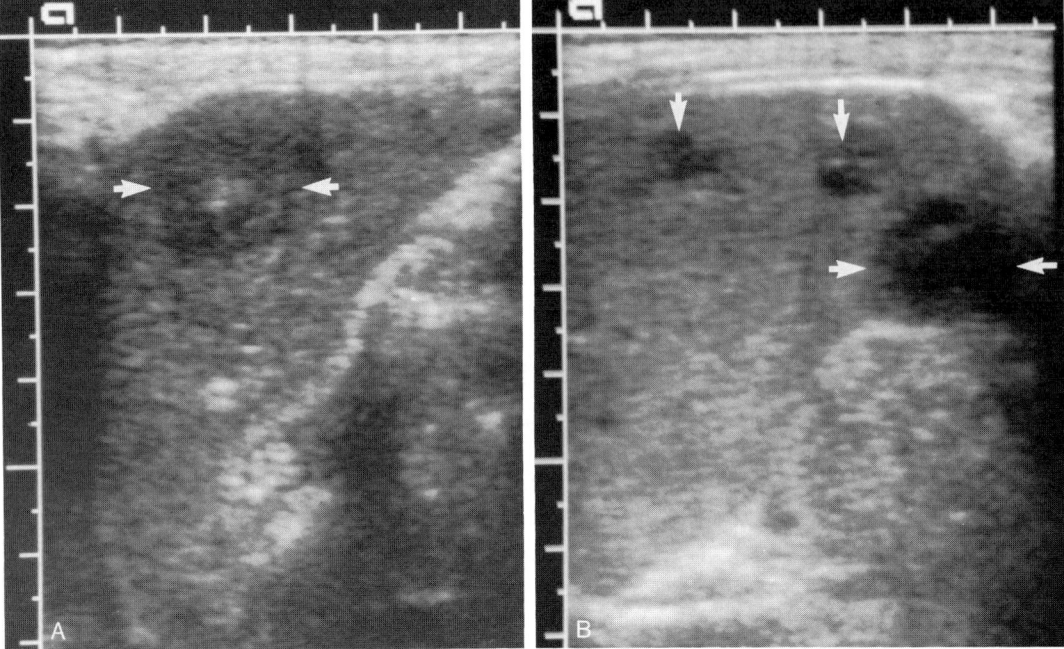

Figure 16–8. This 2½-year-old girl had a fever for 40 days. Intermittently, it would rise to 39.5°C. Her sedimentation rate was elevated at 23. Ultrasonographic evaluation showed multiple, lucent foci (arrows) in the liver (**A**) and spleen (**B**). These were biopsied and proved under the microscope to be noncaseating granulomas. An etiology for the patient's granulomatous disease was never identified, and she eventually became afebrile without therapy.

didal sepsis was suspected 2 weeks before we were able to demonstrate an abnormal appearance of the liver and spleen on ultrasonograms. Cat-scratch disease should be included in the differential diagnosis of multiple splenic abscesses (Cox et al., 1989).

It is not unusual for small focal calcifications within the spleen to be an incidental finding, unassociated with any other abnormality. Some are probably residua of previous granulomatous infection. Occasionally we see a child, acutely ill, in whom granulomatous hepatitis and concomitant splenic granulomas are diagnosed but the infectious agent has not been isolated (Fig. 16–8). Chronic granulomatous disease of childhood, histoplasmosis, and tuberculosis are typically associated with calcified granulomata, but in many patients, a cause for intrasplenic calcifications is never found (Fig. 16–9).

Other focal splenic masses in the pediatric age group may result from epidermoid or congenital cyst; posttraumatic cyst (pseudocyst); or hydatid cyst, abscess, infarct, arteriovenous malformation, and metastatic disease. Multiple cysts associated with autosomal dominant polycystic kidney disease are unusual in childhood.

Epidermoid cyst is a congenital cyst of the spleen. Its epithelial lining differentiates it from a pseudocyst that is secondary to previous trauma or infarction. It is more common in girls than in boys and can be found

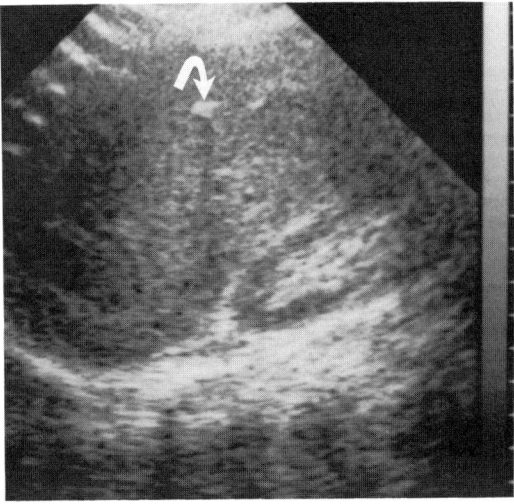

Figure 16–9. Multiple small echogenic foci within the spleen of this patient were secondary to calcified granulomata associated with chronic granulomatous disease of childhood. One is shown (arrow) on this coronal scan. The spleen has always been moderately enlarged in this patient, whom we have now followed for more than 17 years.

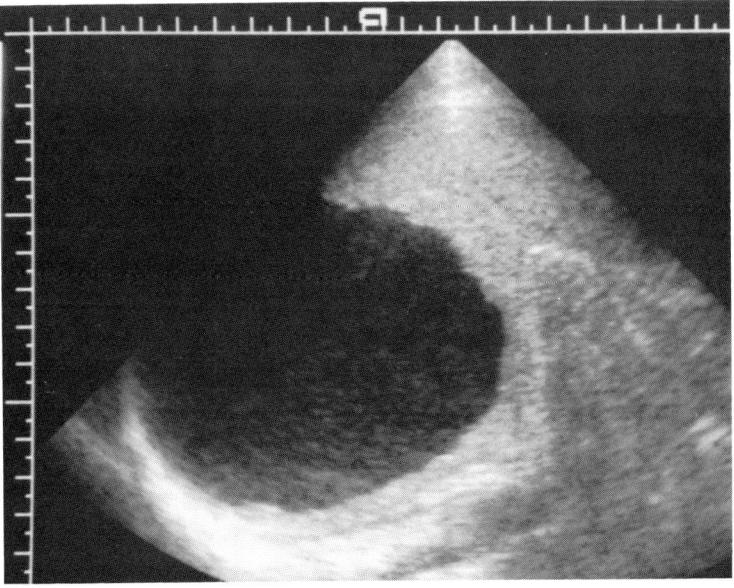

Figure 16–10. This large splenic cyst, which proved to be an epidermoid cyst, was discovered by the patient as a mass in the left upper quadrant. Hemisplenectomy was performed so that splenic tissue could be retained.

at any age, typically as an asymptomatic mass. Ultrasonography shows a smooth-walled unilocular cyst in most cases; the contents may be slightly echogenic if the cyst contains droplets of fat, cholesterol crystals, or desquamated cells or if superimposed hemorrhage or infection is present (Fig. 16–10; Daneman and Martin, 1982). Its large size in some affected patients may lead to secondary effects on the adjacent kidney. One little boy, who was referred to our hospital for evaluation of a varicocele, had a large epidermoid cyst of the spleen, with compressed renal and gonadal veins at the left renal hilum (Fig. 16–11).

Splenic pseudocysts have been rare in our experience. In one child, a partially calcified cyst at the splenic hilum, presumed to be a result of previous trauma, may have been splenic in origin but, equally likely, may have arisen from the pancreatic tail. Another child, who had had normal previous splenic ultrasonograms, developed an intrasplenic cyst after surgery to remove a left renal tumor. Trauma to the spleen during the operation was assumed to be causative.

Parasitic cysts, specifically hydatid cysts, are likely the most common splenic mass in the world. The hydatid cyst in the spleen undergoes the same evolution as does the more common hepatic lesion: unilocular cyst with later development of hydatid sand, membranous proliferation, and daughter cysts (Beggs, 1985).

Differentiating an abscess from an infarct is not easy. The patient prone to infarction is often equally prone to infection. In the pediatric population this is typically an older child with cyanotic cardiac disease who is polycythemic and also susceptible to endocarditis, or it is a child who is immunosuppressed (Fig. 16–12). However, we scanned one patient who had primary staphylococcal splenic abscess and no obvious predisposing reasons for his rather dramatic infection (Fig. 16–13). The generally low incidence of splenic abscess is related to the active phagocytic activity of the reticuloendothelial system and leukocytes within the spleen.

Splenic abscess may have mixed echogenicity or be relatively hypoechoic in comparison with splenic parenchyma. Infarction, although classically described as producing a wedge-shaped (as opposed to spherical) defect in the spleen, can simulate abscess on ultrasonography. Both are more likely to be multifocal than solitary. Fine-needle aspiration under ultrasonic guidance has been recommended for diagnosis in difficult cases, and although we have not yet had the occasion to do this, we would support that suggestion from the literature (Hertzanu et al., 1983; Solbiati et al., 1983).

We studied two patients who proved to have total splenic infarction. One child, severely immunosuppressed and in renal failure, had diffuse intra-abdominal ischemia after a severe hypotensive episode (Fig. 16–

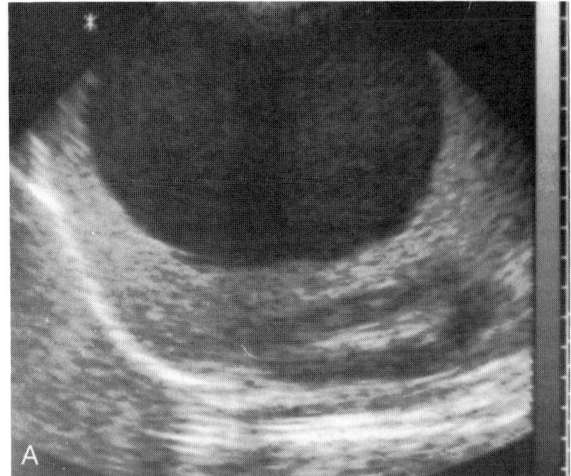
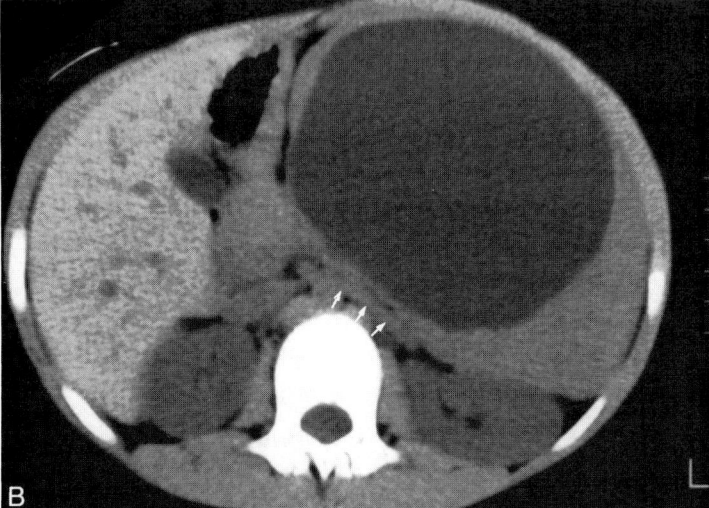

Figure 16–11. The large epidermoid cyst of the spleen in this boy (A) is shown by computed tomography (CT) scan (B) to compress the left renal vein (arrows). The boy presented with varicocele.

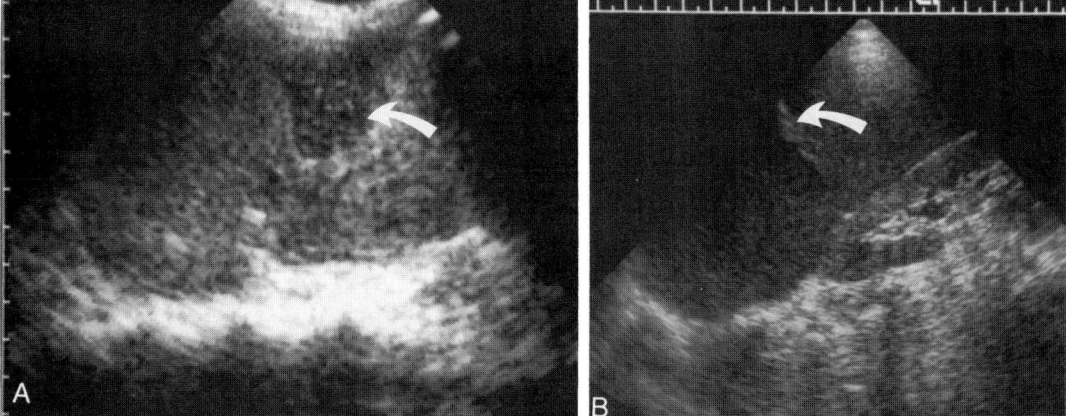

Figure 16–12. This adolescent girl had cyanotic cardiac disease. She presented with fever and increasing splenomegaly. The hypoechoic area in the spleen (arrow), obvious on ultrasonography (A), presented the diagnostic dilemma of whether this was splenic abscess or infarct. She was treated aggressively with antibiotics. Her cardiac disease prevented consideration of abdominal surgery. Months later (B), the only evidence of the previous insult was an echogenic scar in the spleen (arrow).

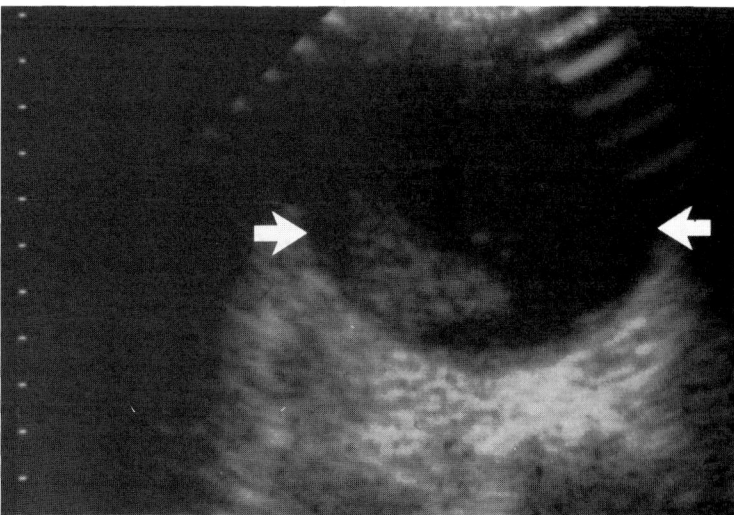

Figure 16–13. This 4-year-old boy presented with epigastric pain and mild fever. The coronal scan shows virtually complete destruction of the spleen by a mass (arrows). Radionuclide study showed only a small amount of residual splenic uptake. Laparotomy examination revealed that a splenic abscess had replaced the spleen. Cultures of the contents grew *Staphylococcus aureus*.

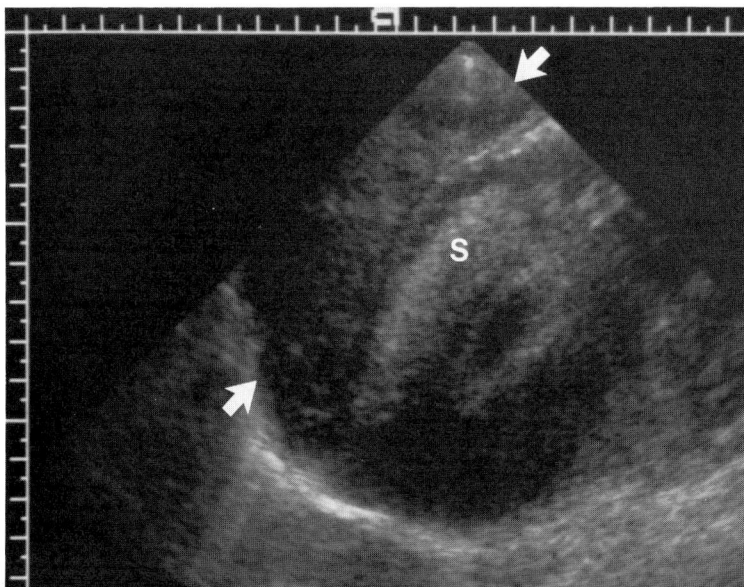

Figure 16–14. This coronal view is of the spleen (arrows) in a severely immunosuppressed child whose sepsis and subsequent shock resulted in thrombosis of splenic vein. The spleen was completely infarcted. S = stomach.

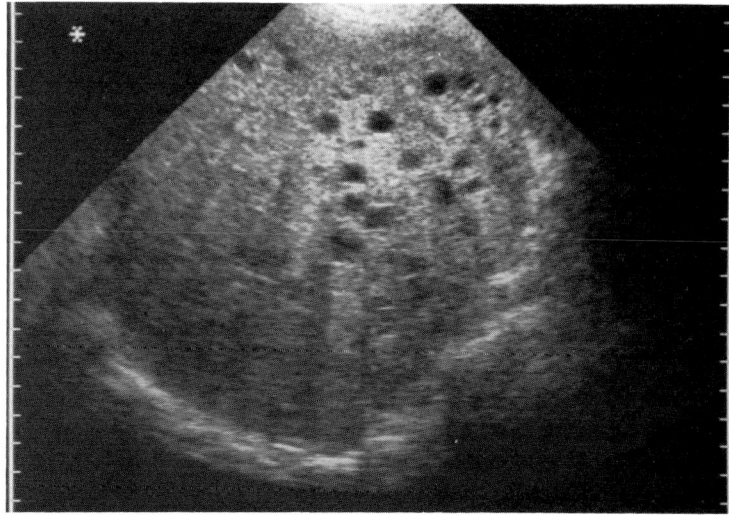

Figure 16–15. Cystic lesions throughout the spleen shown on this scan were not enhanced on CT scanning, which followed intravenous contrast. This patient with Klippel-Trenaunay syndrome has venous and lymphatic malformations that involve multiple organs and soft tissues.

14). The other child had thrombosis of the splenic vein after transplantation of the liver. In both children, the spleen became quite obviously hypoechoic after the vascular insult.

Arteriovenous malformation of the spleen is characterized by large nutritive and draining vessels that can be investigated with Doppler ultrasonography. Lymphangioma (lymphatic malformation) may be primarily unilocular (Cornaglia-Ferraris et al., 1982) or have a Swiss cheese–like appearance (Fig. 16–15). Metastatic involvement of the splenic parenchyma is almost unheard of in pediatrics. We have seen only one patient, an adolescent boy, with splenic metastases, and these were from widespread malignant melanoma.

NO SPLEEN OR TOO MANY SPLEENS

Anomalies of the spleen usually coexist with other congenital anomalies, specifically those affecting the heart. Proving that no splenic tissue is present may be difficult with ultrasonography alone; radionuclide studies are definitive. Microgastria is associated with asplenia. Splenic tissue may be present within the abdomen but in an unusual location. Connections with hepatic, gonadal, or nephric tissue, which are normal in utero but abnormal when they persist postnatally, result in splenohepatic, splenogonadal (Mandell et al., 1983), or splenorenal fusions, respectively.

"Wandering spleen" (also termed "ectopic spleen"), is probably due to deficient or absent gastrosplenic and phrenicosplenic ligaments. Torsion around the splenic pedicle results in acute pain. Partial occlusion of vessels causes intermittent symptoms. Absence of splenic tissue in the left upper quadrant associated with a spleenlike mass discovered elsewhere in the abdomen on ultrasonography is diagnostic of wandering spleen (Setiawan et al., 1982).

It is easier to diagnose polysplenia than asplenia with ultrasonography. It too is strongly associated with cardiac malformations. In 10 percent of cases of biliary atresia, there is coincident polysplenia (Abramson et al., 1987). Multiple spleens accompany the gastric fundus; therefore, polysplenia in the right upper quadrant is associated with a right-sided stomach. The discovery of polysplenia should provoke an extensive evaluation of abdominal vasculature. A preduodenal portal vein, an unusual course of the inferior vena cava, and other anomalies may be present as part of the syndrome of abdominal heterotaxia (Fig. 16–16; Hernanz-Schulman et al., 1990).

Accessory spleen is not an infrequent finding (10 to 30 percent of autopsy studies) and is typically revealed on ultrasonograms as a spherical mass in the splenic hilum or near the lower border of the spleen. Rarely is it lower in position than the left renal pedicle. An accessory spleen should not be mistaken for adenopathy or some other mass (Fig. 16–17). After a traumatically ruptured spleen is removed, spilled splenic pulp may parasitize

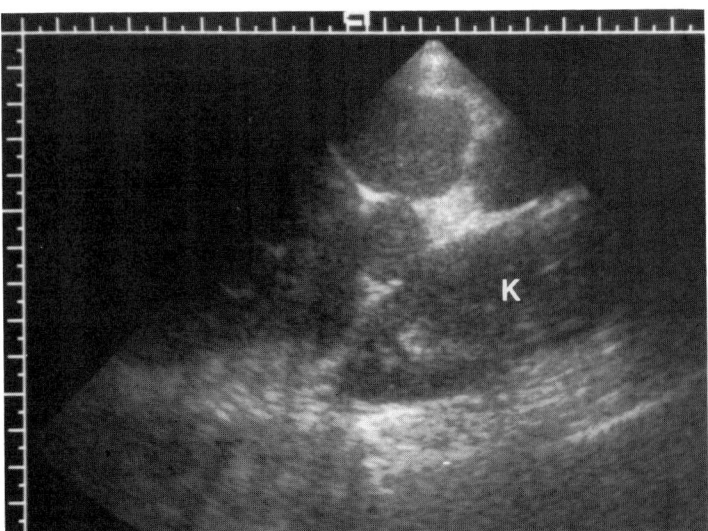

Figure 16–16. Multiple spleens were an incidental but not unexpected finding in this baby, who was undergoing abdominal ultrasonography before cardiac transplantation. He had a single right ventricle associated with heterotaxia. Multiple spleens are always on the same side as the gastric fundus. K = kidney.

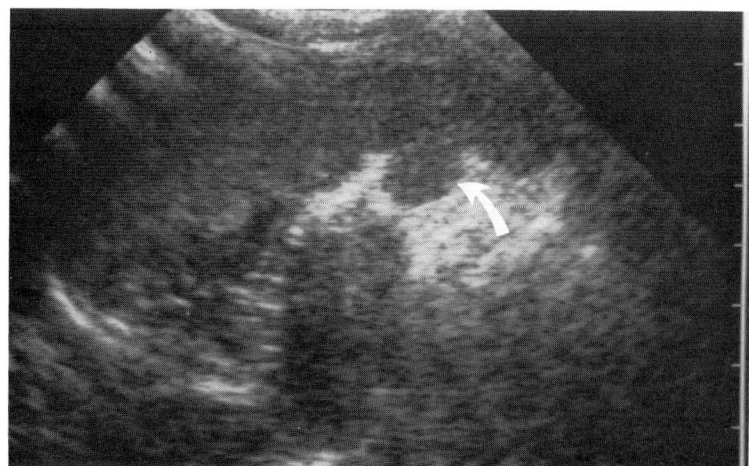

Figure 16–17. This coronal scan shows the typical appearance of an accessory spleen (arrow).

peritoneal vessels, grow into nodules 1 to 4 cm in diameter (splenosis), and also be mistaken for masses.

REFERENCES

Splenomegaly, Splenic Masses

Beggs I: The radiology of hydatid disease. AJR 1985; 145:639–648.

Bollinger B, Lorentzen T: Torsion of a wandering spleen: Ultrasonographic findings. JCU 1990; 18:510–511.

Booth AJ, Bruce DI, Steiner GM: Ultrasound diagnosis of splenic injuries in children—The importance of free peritoneal fluid. Clin Radiol 1987; 38:395–398.

Cornaglia-Ferraris P, Perlino GF, Barabino A, et al: Cystic lymphangioma of the spleen. Report of CT scan findings. Pediatr Radiol 1982; 12:94–95.

Corthouts B, De Schepper A: Ultrasonography of a splenic abscess due to Listeria monocytogenes. J Belge Radiol 1988; 71:375–376.

Cox F, Perlman S, Sathyanarayana: Splenic abscesses in cat scratch disease: Sonographic diagnosis and follow-up. JCU 1989; 17:511–514.

Daneman A, Martin DJ: Congenital epithelial splenic cysts in children: Emphasis on sonographic appearances and some unusual features. Pediatr Radiol 1982; 12:119–125.

Dittrich M, Milde S, Dinkel E, et al: Sonographic biometry of liver and spleen size in childhood. Pediatr Radiol 1983; 13:206–211.

Filiatrault D, Longpre D, Patriquin H, et al: Investigation of childhood blunt trauma: A practical approach using ultrasound as the initial diagnostic modality. Pediatr Radiol 1987; 17:373–379.

Gore RM, Shkolnik A: Abdominal manifestations of pediatric leukemias: Sonographic assessment. Radiology 1982; 143:207–210.

Hertzanu T, Mendelsohn D, Goodie E, et al: Splenic abscess: A review with the value of ultrasound. Clin Radiol 1983; 34:661–667.

Hill SC, Reinig JW, Barranger JA, et al: Gaucher disease: Sonographic appearance of the spleen. Radiology 1986; 160:631–634.

Jequier S, Guttman F, Lafortune M: Non-surgical treatment of a congenital splenic cyst. Pediatr Radiol 1987; 17:248–249.

King DJ, Dawson AA, Bayliss AP: The value of ultrasonic scanning of the spleen in lymphoma. Clin Radiol 1985; 36:473–474.

Lam AH, Parslow B: Ultrasound of splenic epidermoid cyst in children. Australas Radiol 1985; 29:47–49.

Shirkhoda A, Wallace S, Sokhandan M: Computed tomography and ultrasonography in splenic infarction. J Can Assoc Radiol 1985; 36:29–33.

Solbiati L, Bossi MC, Bellotti E, et al: Focal lesions in the spleen: Sonographic patterns and guided biopsy. AJR 1983; 140:59–65.

Wu CC, Chow KS, Lü TN, et al: Tuberculous splenic abscess: Sonographic detection and follow-up. JCU 1990; 18:205–209.

Splenic Anomalies

Abramson SJ, Berdon WE, Altman RP, et al: Biliary atresia and noncardiac polysplenic syndrome: US and surgical considerations. Radiology 1987; 163:377–379.

Hernanz-Schulman M, Ambrosino MM, Genieser NB, et al: Current evaluation of the patient with abnormal visceroatrial situs. AJR 1990; 154:797–802.

Mandell GA, Heyman S, Alavi A, et al: A case of microgastria in association with splenic-gonadal fusion. Pediatr Radiol 1983; 13:95–98.

Setiawan H, Harrell RS, Perret RS: Ectopic spleen: A sonographic diagnosis. Pediatr Radiol 1982; 12:152–153.

CHAPTER 17

THE LIVER

For many pediatric patients who have pain in the upper right quadrant or jaundice, or both, a diagnosis is immediately evident from ultrasonography. If not, the study aids in the planning of the next diagnostic procedure. One must remember that adequate scans of a child who complains of pain in the right upper quadrant include not only a full survey of liver and biliary tree but also a look at the right hemidiaphragm, the right pleural space, the right kidney, and the perirenal space. The ultrasonographic diagnosis of pneumonia is not routine but always enjoyable! If we have eliminated unusual diaphragmatic masses, made sure that diaphragmatic excursion is normal, found no peritoneal fluid or pleural fluid or pulmonary consolidation, and seen no renal abnormality or perinephric edema from adjacent inflammation (Belli and Joseph, 1988), we focus attention on the biliary tract. The gallbladder is almost always visible in normal children, even when they are not fasting. However, to encourage its dilatation with bile, we try to perform scans 4 to 6 hours after the child has been fed.

In a study by Carroll and colleagues (1982), palpable gallbladders were no different in length from normal gallbladders, but they were definitely wider. Sarnaik and coauthors (1980) published data from scans of a group of children with sickle cell disease. Although this group was not a truly normal population, there was no difference in length of gallbladder between patients with stones and patients without. Mean lengths were 4.3 cm at ages 2 to 4 years, 5.3 cm at 5 to 9 years, 6.2 cm at 10 to 14 years, and 7.2 cm at 15 to 19 years. As a rule, the normal gallbladder is rarely longer than the ipsilateral kidney, but, most important, it is teardrop, not spherical, in shape (Fig. 17–1).

The thickness of the wall of the gallbladder should be 3 mm or less (Patriquin et al., 1983). The contents should be clear. A fatty meal normally results in contraction of the gallbladder within 1 to 2 hours.

The usual location of the gallbladder is in the fossa between right and left lobes. Occasionally, the gallbladder is intrahepatic rather than subhepatic. It has been known to herniate through the foramen of Winslow or to dip into the pelvis. It may be congenitally absent, duplicated, or even interposed, receiving drainage directly from right and left hepatic ducts and connecting to the common bile duct (Stringer et al., 1987).

Finding any of these anomalies with ultrasonography is unusual because their occurrence in the general population is very rare: 1 in 3000 to 4000 people. Veterinary ultrasonographers may have more experience: bilobed or truly duplicated gallbladder is present in 12.5 percent of cats (Fig. 17–2; Boyden, 1926)!

JAUNDICE IN THE NEONATE

Landing, in 1974, proposed the concept of infantile obstructive cholangiopathy, hypothesizing that neonatal hepatitis and biliary

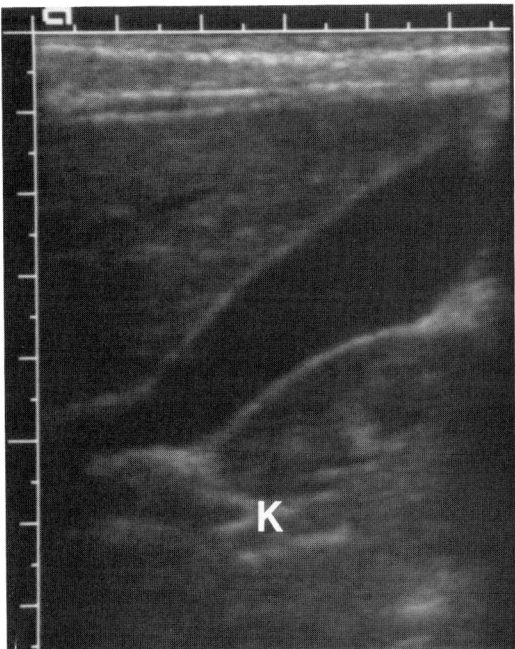

Figure 17–1. This is a longitudinal scan of the gallbladder in a 7-year-old. It is 5.5 cm long and lies anterior to the kidney (K).

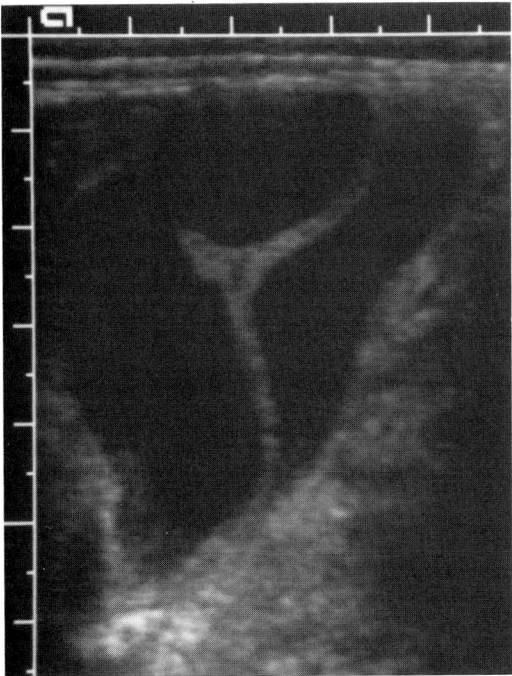

Figure 17–2. Duplication of the gallbladder is a very unusual anomaly. This condition was found incidentally during evaluation of this little girl's abdomen for caval clot. She had recently undergone surgery for complex congenital heart disease. The larger of the two gallbladders is sitting piggyback on the smaller gallbladder. The child had no biliary obstruction and no other intra-abdominal anomalies.

atresia represent the two ends of a spectrum of inflammatory disease. Twenty years later the heterogeneous group of neonatal diseases that cause hepatic dysfunction and, more specifically, that cause cholestasis is still poorly understood. Cholestasis is defined as hyperbilirubinemia greater than 2.0 mg/dl or when the conjugated fraction exceeds 30 percent of the total bilirubin. For ultrasonographers and radiologists, the short question, asked by clinicians, is whether biliary atresia is present. Biliary atresia is the absence of any part of the biliary tree. The disease or diseases that cause some or all of the intrahepatic biliary ducts to disappear are unlikely to be affected by surgery. However, the extrahepatic component of obstruction can be relieved with hepatic portoenterostomy. By allowing better drainage of bile, the toxic effect of bile itself may be removed from the diseased liver. Kasai and associates (1978) reported that 91 percent of patients operated on before 60 days of age had sustained drainage of bile; only 17 percent of patients operated on after the age of 3 months had successful drainage. Thus there has always been a premium on making the diagnosis of biliary atresia early. The clinicians, however, must also consider a page-long list of "medical" causes of cholestasis that encompass infections, metabolic diseases, and toxins (Balistreri, 1985). The initial evaluation of a jaundiced baby includes standard tests of hepatic function; cultures of blood, urine, and spinal fluid; hepatitis B antigen titers; toxoplasmosis, rubella, cytomegalovirus, and herpes simplex titers; Venereal Disease Research Laboratory titers; alpha$_1$-antitrypsin phenotype testing; metabolic screening; a sweat chloride test; examination of stool for color; and, ultimately, ultrasonography and scintigraphy if the diagnosis is still unknown. Our role in ultrasonography is to show anatomy as best we can. Size and parenchymal patterns of liver and spleen should be documented. Any abnormality of the biliary tree should be carefully displayed and ancillary findings, such as a renal anomaly or ascites, shown. In the neonate, normal intrahepatic bile ducts are too small to be visualized. The normal common bile duct is evident not as a channel but rather as an interface or a crack extending into the head of the pancreas from the porta hepatis. The gallbladder must be demonstrated in its longest and widest cross-sections. Although it is unusual for a gallbladder to be of normal size in a baby later shown to have biliary atresia, we are wary of relying solely on ultrasonography to rule out the diagnosis. Ideally, the baby is given a feeding in order that contraction of the gallbladder can be documented. Contraction after feeding implies patency of the ductal system (Ikeda et al., 1989). In most babies with biliary atresia, the gallbladder is hypoplastic (<1.5 cm) or invisible (Abramson et al., 1982). However, in many cases of neonatal hepatitis, the gallbladder is also small, possibly because of underuse. Small size, therefore, is not a reliable discriminatory feature. The presence of multiple spleens or other components of the heterotaxy syndrome are associated with biliary atresia. We have noticed that in neonates who have a choledochal cyst, discovered early in life because of clinical jaundice, concomitant biliary atresia is common (Fig. 17–3; Torrisi et al., 1990).

If ultrasonography of the jaundiced infant fails to reveal any obvious anatomic abnormality, scintigraphic study with one of the iminodiacetic acid analogs follows 3 to 5 days of oral administration of phenobarbital. Percutaneous hepatic biopsy follows if there is failure of radionuclide excretion into the gut. Experienced pathologists can differentiate the features of biliary atresia from neonatal hepatitis in many cases. Most babies at this juncture would go to surgery if the diagnosis were still in doubt or if biliary atresia were considered most likely. There is an alternative route that we consider as potentially very useful if the gallbladder is visible on ultrasonography (Treem et al., 1988). Percutaneous puncture of the gallbladder under ultrasonic control, aspiration of bile for analysis, and then injection of contrast media under fluoroscopy are analogous to the intraoperative cholangiogram that precedes exploration of the porta hepatis. The liver is used as a path of access in order to prevent peritoneal leakage of bile. The bile can be cultured, as well as analyzed, for its components, and it is possible that injection of contrast may be therapeutic in some situations in which plugging of ducts with viscous bile has occurred. There is one potential pitfall: intrahepatic radicles may not be demonstrated if the contrast medium drains rapidly through the cystic duct and common bile duct into the duodenum. In some infants, normal extrahepatic ducts coexist with intrahepatic atresia (Kirks et al., 1984). Failure to demonstrate normal intraheptic radicles re-

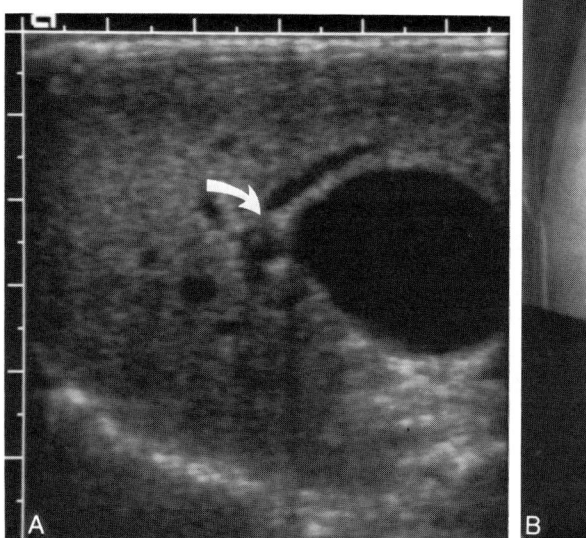
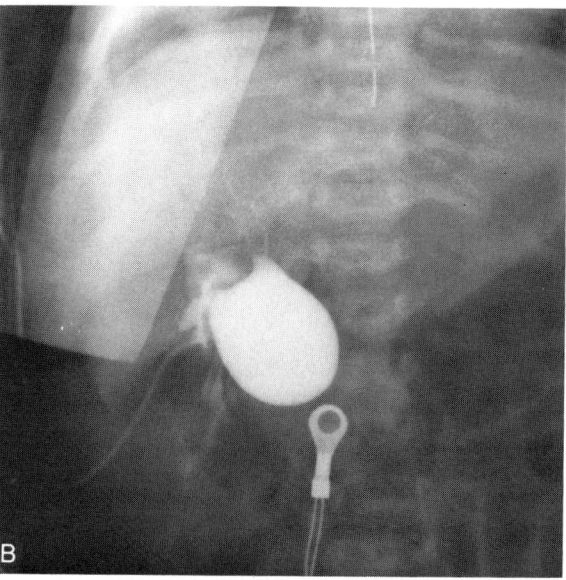

Figure 17–3. Prenatal scans had shown a subhepatic cyst in this baby. After delivery, she seemed perfectly normal. Postnatal follow-up, however, confirmed the presence of a large subhepatic cyst (**A**). The gallbladder seemed to enter the region of the porta hepatis (arrow) just superior to the cyst. There was no ductal dilatation whatsoever. All lucencies within the liver, as shown on this sagittal scan, were venous. Studies done in nuclear medicine showed no excretion of radionuclide from the liver into the gut. Intraoperative cholangiogram (**B**) showed extravasation of contrast around portal triads when the cyst was injected. The baby underwent a formal Kasai procedure for biliary atresia. Although she is now well, she has recurrent episodes of cholangitis and is now developing bile lakes in the liver.

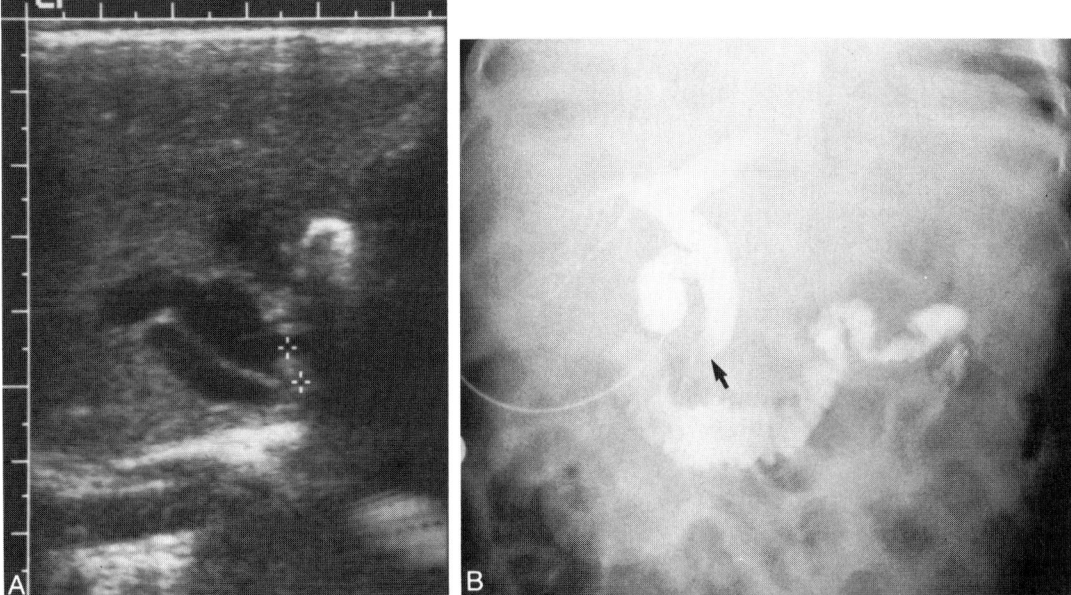

Figure 17–4. A plug of bile (between crosses) in the distal common bile duct obstructed the biliary tree in this 2-month-old (**A**). The scans were done when the baby presented with sepsis and jaundice. Adherent sludge was also present in the gallbladder. Intraoperative cholangiogram (**B**) shows the plug as a filling defect (arrow) in the distal common bile duct. This ball of bile crumbled when removed. The baby was completely asymptomatic afterwards. There was no apparent predisposition to the formation of stones.

quires surgical exploration. Operative cholangiography allows the option of manual compression of distal common bile duct in order that contrast media be forced, retrograde, from the gallbladder and the cystic duct.

If a diagnosis of biliary atresia has been established and portoenterostomy performed, the child is followed clinically. Ultrasonography is performed only when clinical or laboratory data show a change. Specific areas of interest are as follows.

1. Porta hepatis at site of anastomosis: in some patients an antireflux nipple is created in the loop of small bowel that connects liver to bowel. Stasis of bile behind the nipple occurs when it is partially obstructing.

2. Parenchymal pattern of liver: bile lakes and intrahepatic echogenic foci, which may represent biliary sludge, are features of a poorly draining biliary system. Biliary cirrhosis is a common result of biliary atresia, and on ultrasonography the liver tends to become patchily echogenic and lose its homogeneous speckled pattern. Ascending cholangitis is a common complication of portoenterostomy, hence the surgical modification of creating a one-way valve or nipple to prevent reflux of intestinal contents into the liver. It is not possible to make the diagnosis of cholangitis with ultrasonography. And, in spite of obvious bacterial seeding in some children, we have yet to diagnose a liver abscess in any of these patients. If intrahepatic bile lakes are evident, percutaneous puncture and aspiration of bile, which is then sent for microbiologic analysis, allow identification of bacteria, if present, and direct appropriate antimicrobial therapy.

3. Signs of portal hypertension: with biliary cirrhosis come portal hypertension and splenomegaly. Careful evaluation, of both the portal venous system and sites where varices are common, follows.

In babies who have biliary atresia, there is on occasion secondary involvement of kidneys, which appears to be due to hyperfiltration injury. Affected kidneys are large and quite markedly echogenic on ultrasonography (Boechat et al., 1986).

Babies who have a normal biliary tract may present with jaundice if there is obstruction from biliary stone, bile plug, or extrinsic mass. Dilatation of the tract to the level of obstruction is usually obvious (Fig. 17–4). Perforation of the common bile duct, at the level of the cystic duct, may be associated with biliary stones. It is a rare complication, and its presentation is usually dramatic, bile ascites being the result (Fig. 17–5).

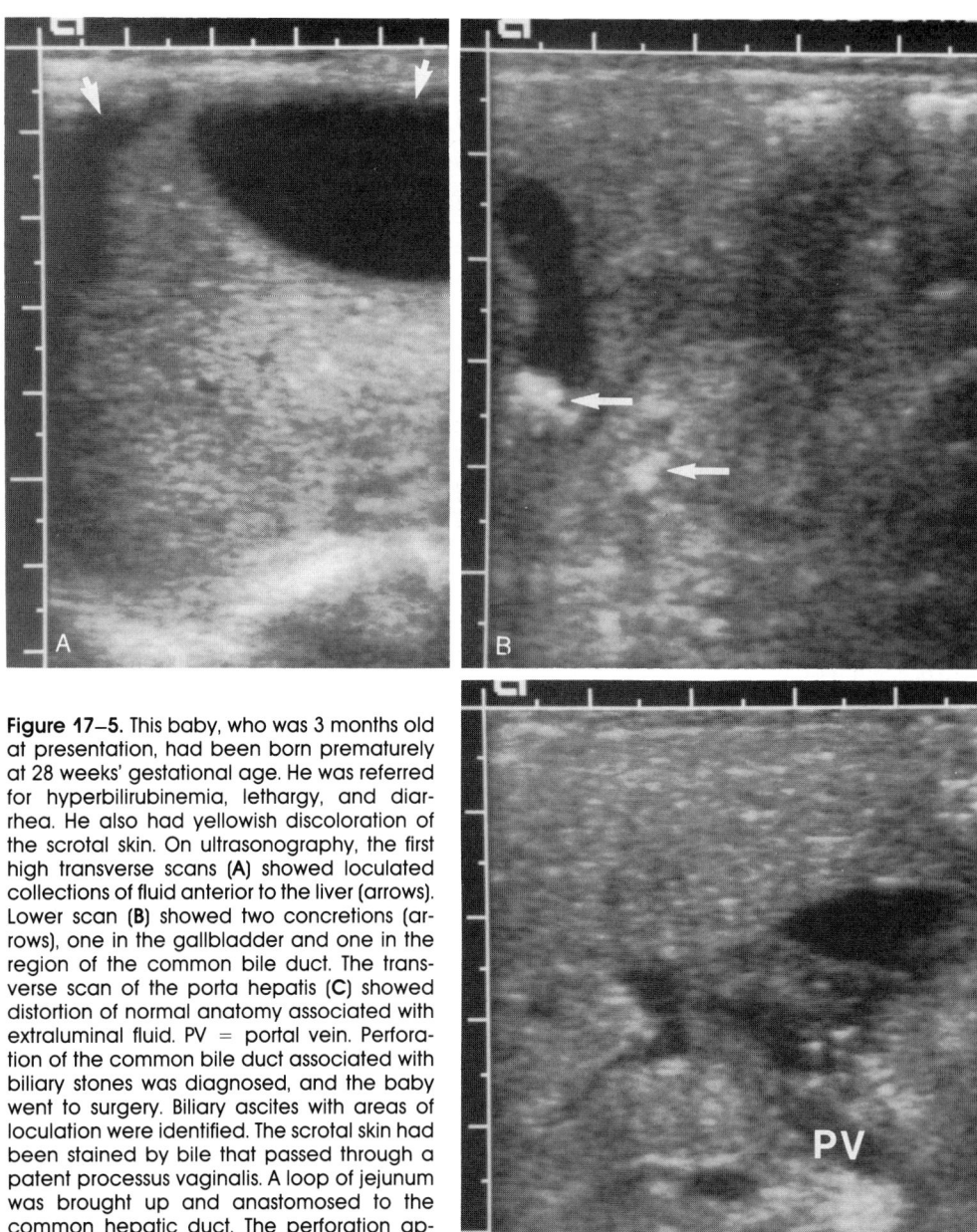

Figure 17–5. This baby, who was 3 months old at presentation, had been born prematurely at 28 weeks' gestational age. He was referred for hyperbilirubinemia, lethargy, and diarrhea. He also had yellowish discoloration of the scrotal skin. On ultrasonography, the first high transverse scans (A) showed loculated collections of fluid anterior to the liver (arrows). Lower scan (B) showed two concretions (arrows), one in the gallbladder and one in the region of the common bile duct. The transverse scan of the porta hepatis (C) showed distortion of normal anatomy associated with extraluminal fluid. PV = portal vein. Perforation of the common bile duct associated with biliary stones was diagnosed, and the baby went to surgery. Biliary ascites with areas of loculation were identified. The scrotal skin had been stained by bile that passed through a patent processus vaginalis. A loop of jejunum was brought up and anastomosed to the common hepatic duct. The perforation appeared to occur at the junction of the common hepatic duct and the cystic duct.

BILIARY ANOMALIES THAT CAUSE PAIN, JAUNDICE, OR BOTH

Infants and children may present with jaundice because they have an underlying anomaly of the biliary tree that prevents normal drainage of bile. The best known of these anomalies is the badly named choledochal cyst. Choledochal cyst is not a true cyst, but ectasia of the choledochus. There has been great interest in explaining this anomaly as a result of proximal insertion of the choledochus on the pancreatic duct. Babbitt proposed this etiology in 1973, and more recent work by Suarez and colleagues (1986) is very persuasive in support of this theory.

Not only did the length of the common channel exceed 1.5 cm in all of their 12 patients, but amylase was present in the bile of all patients so tested. Trypsin was identified in the fluid from a choledochal cyst in each of two neonates (O'Neill et al., 1987). Reflux of pancreatic secretions has been blamed for the obliteration of mucosal lining of the choledochus. Obstruction at the site of insertion of the choledochus is blamed for the proximal dilatation of biliary ducts. However, this explanation does not fit the radiographic picture in every case. Some children with a hugely dilated common bile duct have no intrahepatic dilatation at all, and in almost all patients with choledochal cyst, the gallbladder is normal in size, not distended. It may be that varying degrees of dysplasia involving the entire biliary tree are present in each case and that obstruction is an added factor that is part of, and complicating, the underlying dysplasia. The surgical literature in particular usually recalls the system of classification established in 1959 by Alonso-Lej in which choledochal cysts were divided into three types: type I is ectasia of the entire choledochus, type II is a diverticulum of the common bile duct, and type III (the rarest) is choledochocele. Because modern imaging techniques continually show variations on the theme, it is apparent that this classification is not helpful, inasmuch as most clinicians cannot remember the original definitions anyway! Good description of intrahepatic ducts and extrahepatic tree is much more useful to physician and surgeon alike (Young et al., 1990).

As mentioned earlier, choledochal cyst may be diagnosed in the neonate who presents with cholestatic jaundice. Failure to show contiguity of main right and left hepatic ducts with the dilated choledochus increases the possibility of coexistent biliary atresia (Fig. 17–3). Whether the "cyst" is part of a generalized dysplasia of the biliary tree or causes the intrahepatic changes is unknown (Lilly, 1979). Prenatal diagnosis may help in answering some of the mysteries associated with choledochal cysts, but as the incidence of choledochal cyst in Western populations appears to be 1 in 2 million, it may take some time.

For any patient with a diagnosis of choledochal cyst, the checklist for the ultrasonographer is as follows: (1) Is the cyst truly a dilated choledochus and not a dilated gallbladder or separate hepatic cyst? The gallbladder enters the choledochal cyst via a cystic duct and should be seen as a separate but related structure in all cases of choledochal cyst. (2) Are intrahepatic ducts dilated, and to what extent? Is the dilatation cylindric or saccular? (3) Are there stones in the biliary tree? (4) Is the pancreatic duct dilated, or is there other evidence for pancreatitis? What appears to be a choledochal "cyst" may simply be choledochal obstruction from a distal stone, a stricture, a mass, or pancreatitis. (5) Is the spleen enlarged, and are there signs of portal hypertension? Long-standing biliary cirrhosis will cause these problems; fortunately, a choledochal cyst usually makes its presence known before irreversible hepatic changes occur. Diagnosis is rarely made on the basis of the "classic" triad of pain, jaundice, and a mass. Usually, only one or, at most, two of the triad are present in any one patient (Figs. 17–6 to 17–8).

After the diagnosis of choledochal cyst is made with ultrasonography, it is confirmed and amplified by radionuclide scintigraphy with iminodiacetic acid derivatives (Papanicolau et al., 1985). The radionuclide study provides physiologic information by showing how well hepatocytes extract the radionuclide. It also demonstrates the degree of obstruction at the distal choledochus. Neither preoperative transhepatic cholangiography nor endoscopic retrograde cholangiopancreatography has been performed routinely in our institution, but in published studies these techniques have been valuable in showing the relationship of the pancreatic duct with the choledochus and in showing the dysplasia involving the more proximal pancreatic duct (Wiedmeyer et al., 1989). We do not advocate direct puncture of the choledochus, as this may cause leakage of bile into the peritoneum. The usual surgical treatment of this anomaly is resection of the cyst and creation of a jejunal Roux-en-Y loop to drain bile from the right and left hepatic ducts into the small bowel. Cholangiocarcinoma may develop if the choledochus is bypassed but left in place (O'Neill et al., 1987). Postoperative ultrasonographic evaluation is needed only if the child becomes jaundiced again or develops pain. Anastomotic stricture, obstructing gravel or stones in the ducts, or ascending cholangitis are rare but possible complications after surgery.

"Caroli disease" simply refers to saccular or beadlike dilatation of the intrahepatic bil-

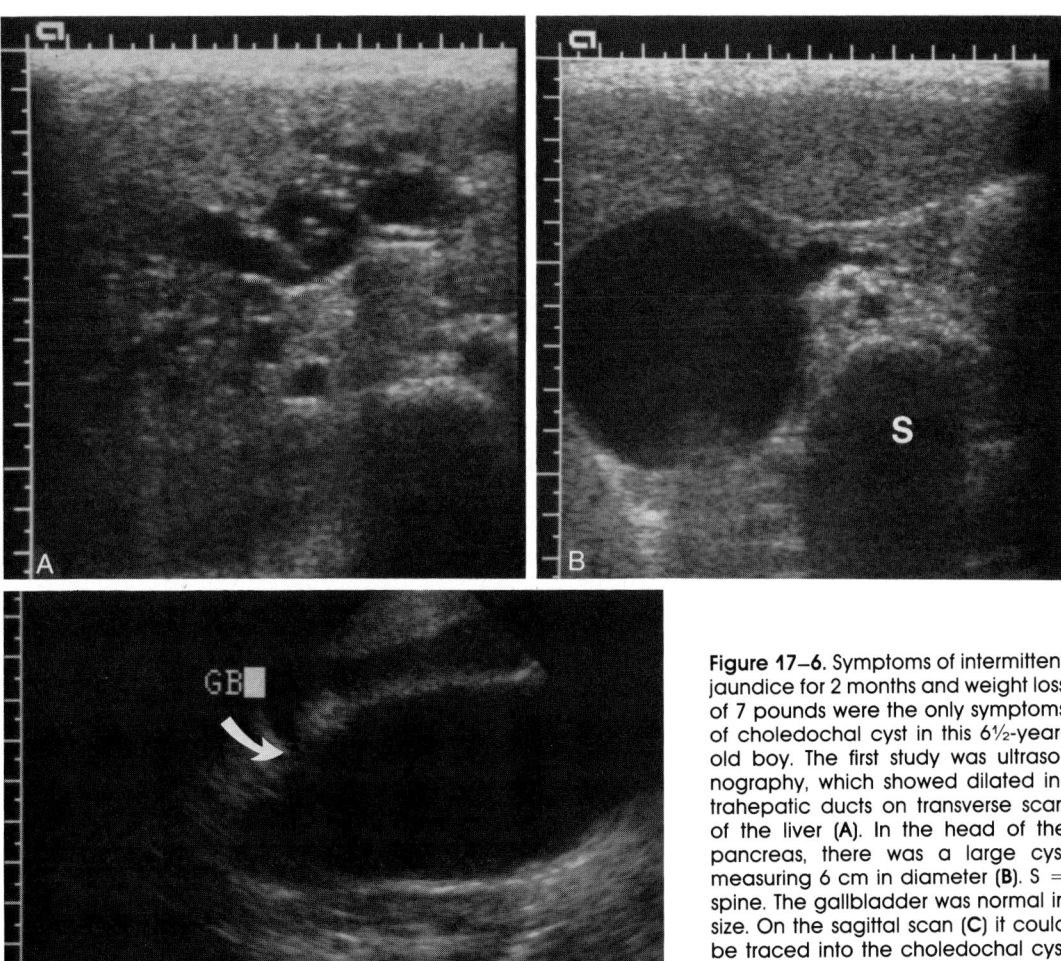

Figure 17–6. Symptoms of intermittent jaundice for 2 months and weight loss of 7 pounds were the only symptoms of choledochal cyst in this 6½-year-old boy. The first study was ultrasonography, which showed dilated intrahepatic ducts on transverse scan of the liver (A). In the head of the pancreas, there was a large cyst measuring 6 cm in diameter (B). S = spine. The gallbladder was normal in size. On the sagittal scan (C) it could be traced into the choledochal cyst (arrow). GB = gallbladder.

iary tree (Caroli et al., 1958; Caroli, 1972); it is a descriptive and nonetiologic term. Intrahepatic dilatation of ducts may or (more typically) may not be associated with ectasia of the choledochus (Fig. 17–9). It is apparent that saccular dilation is associated with congenital hepatic fibrosis, with or without renal cystic disease. Marchal and colleagues (1986) described three infants with Caroli disease. Two babies had autosomal recessive polycystic renal disease, and the other had nephronophthisis. The authors discussed the theoretic pathogenesis of the disease as a malformation in resorption of the embryonic ductal plate, which is the precursor of intrahepatic biliary ducts. Case reports supporting the impression that Caroli disease is part of a spectrum of anomalies affecting biliary tree and kidneys have been published (Davies et al., 1986; McAlister et al., 1989). Diagnosis of Caroli disease with ultrasonography can be tricky because the ectatic ducts may appear to be cysts and may not be recognized as part of a continuous ductal system. Stones or sludge may complicate intrahepatic ductal dysplasia.

Intrahepatic cysts are distinctly uncommon in children; thus any periportal cyst must be considered part of the biliary tract until proved otherwise (Fig. 17–10). Congenital hepatic fibrosis is manifest by densely echogenic bands of collagen paralleling the portal tracts. The thickness of the bands is greater than that seen in children with acquired chronic hepatic disease and cirrhosis. The kidneys should be scanned with care in any

THE LIVER / 423

Figure 17–7. The transverse (**A**) and longitudinal (**B**) scans are of a 6-month-old boy who presented with fever and hepatomegaly. Bilirubin levels were mildly elevated. The transverse scan shows irregular dilation of intrahepatic ducts. Longitudinal scan shows an eccentric choledochal cyst. Arrowheads point to the common hepatic duct. Arrow points to the gallbladder.

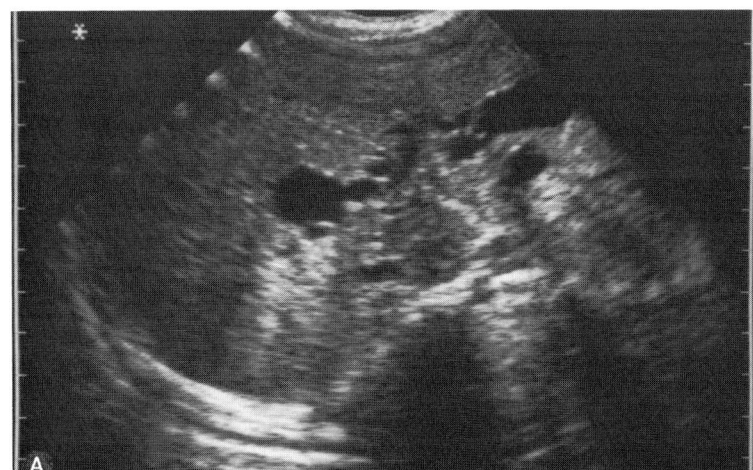
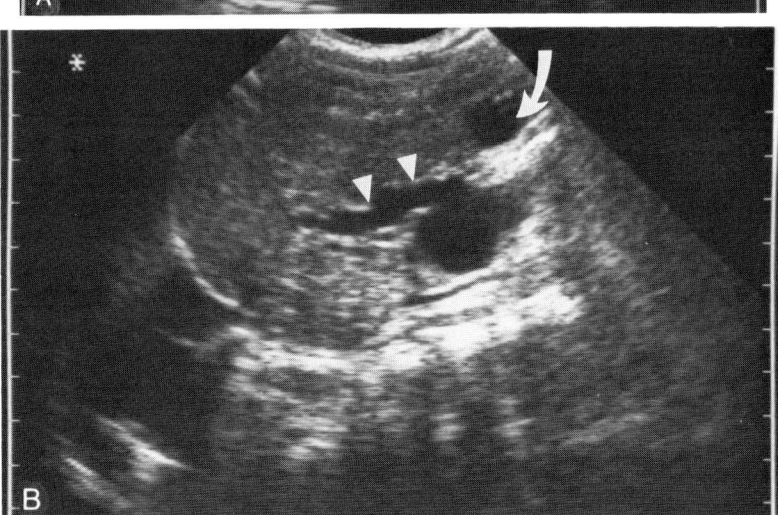

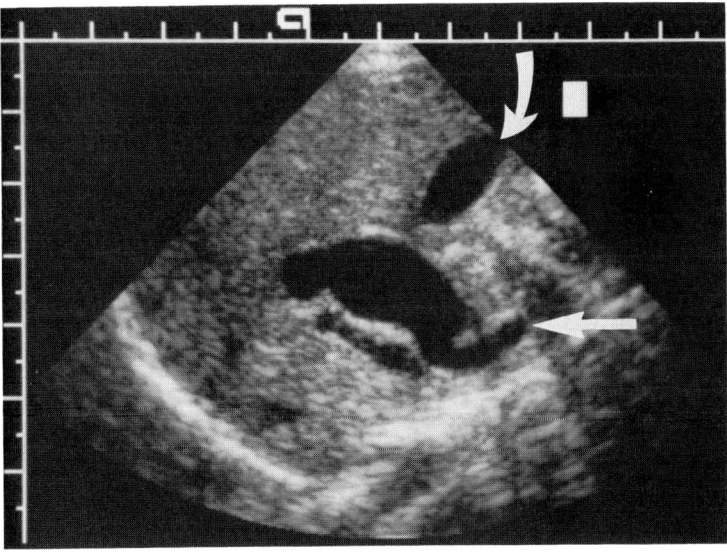

Figure 17–8. Saccular dilation of the common hepatic and common bile ducts is evident on the longitudinal scan of this 4-month-old girl, who presented with vomiting, dehydration, and hyperbilirubinemia. Radionuclide scan showed no excretion of contrast from the dilated duct into the duodenum. During surgery, the choledochal cyst was resected, and a loop of jejunum was anastomosed to the common hepatic duct at the porta hepatis. Straight arrow points to the termination of the choledochus in the head of the pancreas. Note that the distal portion of the choledochus in this particular patient is not as dilated as the proximal portion. The intrahepatic ducts were not dilated. Curved arrow points to the gallbladder.

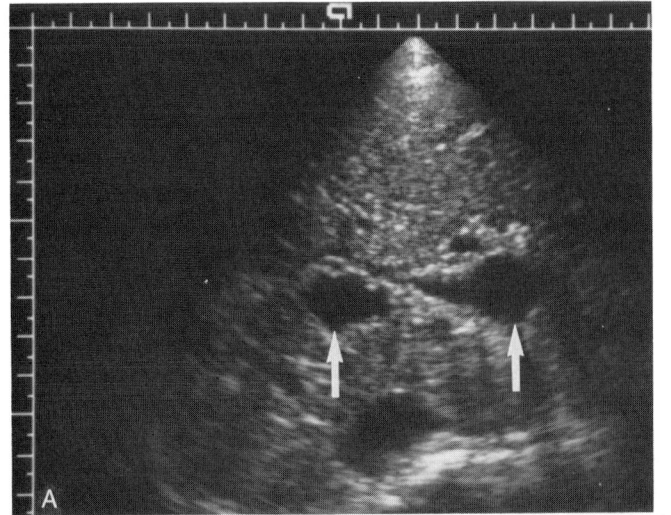
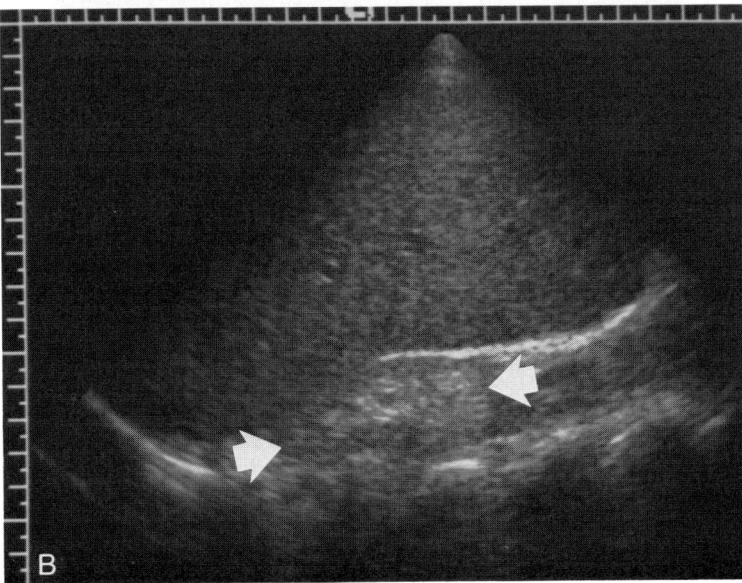

Figure 17-9. Saccular dilatation of the biliary ducts (Caroli disease) was associated with congenital hepatic fibrosis in this little girl. She originally presented because of splenomegaly. The transverse scan (A) shows the beadlike dilated ducts (arrows). The choledochus was not dilated. Coronal scan of the left upper quadrant (B) shows splenomegaly. The kidney (between arrows) is small and echogenic. Her renal disease is uncharacterized but is likely nephronophthisis. The girl is now 14 years old and undergoing renal dialysis.

Figure 17-10. Prenatal ultrasonography identified this intrahepatic cyst (arrow). Radionuclide study showed a normal biliary tract. The baby was completely asymptomatic and has been followed for 2 years with no change in the size of this cyst.

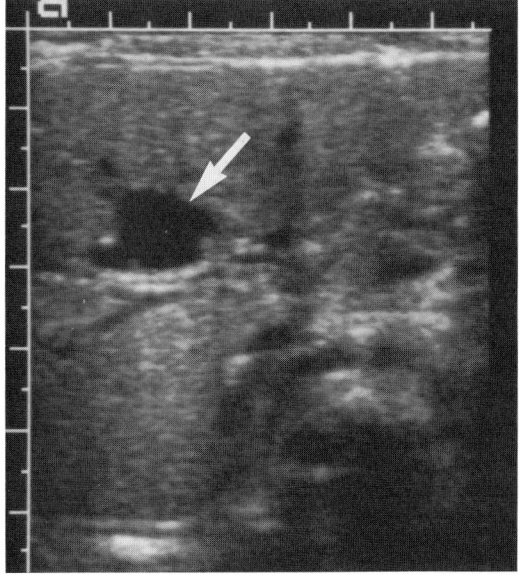

child who receives a diagnosis, by ultrasonography or other means, of hepatic fibrosis or Caroli disease (see Chapter 6). Children with congenital hepatic fibrosis develop portal hypertension. Occasionally, their sole presenting sign is splenomegaly.

GALLSTONES

Ultrasonographers who study adults have trouble understanding our interest in gallstones because cholelithiasis is such a common occurrence in adults. Gallstones are not common in children, but neither are they as rare as once thought. The major predisposing situations or illnesses associated with cholelithiasis in infancy and childhood are listed in Table 17–1. When we reviewed records of 52 patients in whom gallstones were diagnosed by ultrasonography, we found that only 17 percent of children had idiopathic gallstones (Henschke and Teele, 1983). Many stones are calcium bilirubinate or mixed stones; the cholesterol stones of adulthood are unusual in children except in patients who have cystic fibrosis.

The development of gallstones is multifactorial, likely quite complicated, and obviously incompletely understood. However, a variable combination of biliary stasis, immaturity of hepatic function (specifically in neonates), a superimposed added load of bilirubin from the breakdown of red blood cells, immobilization of the patient, disturbed enterohepatic circulation, and abnormal bile is an etiologic explanation for most pediatric patients who have cholelithiasis.

We have followed the development of gallstones in some children. Cholelithiasis begins with sludge in the gallbladder that changes into "bile balls" and then apparently hardens around a nidus into focal, shadowing stones. The development of stones takes weeks to months. A bile ball generally does not have enough protein matrix and mineral content to cause shadowing on ultrasonograms. Ando and Ito (1986) explained the variable appearance of bile balls, with their ability to change into a sludge layer after being shaken, by the principle of thixotropy from the science of colloids. Thus one may see a variable appearance on ultrasonography if one literally shakes the patient!

Gallstones have been diagnosed in utero in a few patients and incidentally in the neonatal period in others. Our policy is conservative: we follow the babies with ultrasonography and hope that the gallstones will disappear on their own (Keller et al., 1985). There is no question, however, that complications from stones or sludge can arise. Perforation of the bile duct is an unusual occurrence, but it occurs at the level or junction of cystic and hepatic ducts in association with obstruction by stones (Hammoudi and Alauddin, 1988). Stones can obstruct the pancreatic and common bile duct by impaction proximal to the sphincter of Oddi. Stones may also be a sign of bacterial infection of the biliary tract (Treem et al., 1989). If stones are within the gallbladder and are not associated with obvious complication, and if the baby is asymptomatic, a decision regarding surgical intervention has to be made by the pediatrician, the parents, and the surgeon. We do not know the consequences of the presence of cholelithiasis in the neonate's gallbladder vis-à-vis later development of cholecystitis or a tumor. One option is simple cholecystotomy, with removal of stones and sampling of bile. Some reports in the literature suggest that the incidence of colonic carcinoma is higher in patients who have had previous cholecystectomy (Vernick and Kuller, 1981). The controversy of "what to do" for neonatal cholelithiasis awaits further elaboration of causes of lithiasis in this age group (Fig. 17–11).

A few babies with transient dysfunction/obstruction of the biliary tree seem to have blockage of the ducts by viscous bile or plugs of bile. We see very little on ultrasonography of these children except for sludge in the gallbladder. Dilatation of ducts may be undetectable because the echogenic bile is in-

Table 17–1. GALLSTONES IN CHILDREN: ASSOCIATED DISEASES

Sickle cell disease
Spherocytosis
Rh and ABO blood incompatibility
Other hemolytic anemias
Previous transfusions of blood
Ongoing hemolysis from artificial cardiac valve
Postoperative orthopedic procedures
Postoperative cardiac surgery
Postoperative intestinal resection
Ileal dysfunction (e.g., Crohn disease)
Sepsis/dehydration/furosemide (in infants)
Total parenteral nutrition
Metabolic liver disease (especially Wilson disease)
Cystic fibrosis
Anomalies of biliary tract
Earlier pregnancy

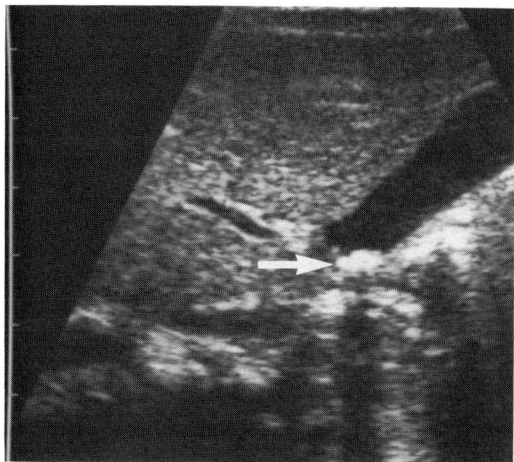

Figure 17-11. Prenatal diagnosis of shadowing echogenicities in the gallbladder prompted ultrasonographic follow-up of this baby. The longitudinal scan was performed when the baby was 6 months old. There is shadowing echogenicity (arrow) in the dependent portion of the gallbladder. The baby is completely asymptomatic, and no intervention has been undertaken.

distinguishable from the adjacent hepatic parenchyma. Babies who have this condition are typically under investigation for possible biliary atresia. It is likely that percutaneous puncture of the gallbladder, aspiration of bile for culture, and injection of ionic water-soluble contrast material would be both diagnostic and therapeutic for these patients.

Older children may present with jaundice, right upper quadrant pain, or pancreatitis as signs of their underlying lithiasis. Many are scanned as part of a screening program for patients known to have hemolytic anemia (Fig. 17-12). The percentage of children whose gallstones are secondary to chronic hemolysis increases with age. In a study of 226 patients who had sickle cell anemia, 12 percent of those 2 to 4 years old and 42 percent of those 15 to 18 years old had cholelithiasis (Sarnaik et al., 1980). The percentage of patients who have cystic fibrosis and hepatic dysfunction increases with age. Ultrasonographic findings include the development of biliary cirrhosis, gallstones, and intrahepatic stones (Fig. 17-13; Willi et al., 1980). Intrahepatic bile ducts may be nondilated but studded with concretions in affected patients (Fig. 17-14). The echogenic foci from these intrahepatic stones may be difficult to recognize as being separate from the echogenic periportal fibrosis, which is commonly present in the same population.

Intrahepatic stones cannot be removed surgically and are associated with a poor prognosis; severe cholestatic jaundice and infection are common complications.

Children who received prolonged parenteral nutrition, which probably causes pigmented gallstones by altering hepatic metabolism and promoting biliary stasis, had a 43 percent prevalence of cholelithiasis, according to a study published by Roslyn and colleagues (1983). Among patients who had undergone previous intestinal resection, the prevalence was 64 percent (Fig. 17-15). In other studies, ileal resection or dysfunction has been blamed for causing lithogenesis (Kirks, 1979) because enterohepatic circulation of bile has been altered.

The period after orthopedic surgery is commonly one of prolonged immobilization. When immobilization is combined with perioperative bleeding and transfusions, which result in delivery of a large load of bilirubin to the liver, cholelithiasis may result (Teele et al., 1987). Cholelithiasis also develops in children who have suffered significant hemolysis during cardiac surgery or who experience ongoing breakdown of red blood cells from an artificial cardiac valve (Fig. 17-16).

Metabolic liver disease is associated with cholelithiasis, probably because excretion and composition of bile is abnormal. Wilson disease has the additional feature of hemolytic anemia, which further promotes formation of stones.

Finally, children with choledochal cyst and related anomalies may present with acute obstruction from gravel or stones, which have developed because of stasis.

Ultrasonographic diagnosis of cholelithiasis relies on demonstration of constant, echogenic focus or foci within the gallbladder. The stones change, in relation to the wall of the gallbladder, as the patient changes position ("rolling stone" sign). Shadowing may not be present if stones are small or have an insufficient protein/mineral matrix. Solid bile balls are usually stones in the making. Follow-up scans (after 4 to 6 weeks) will show whether they are developing into true stones or whether they have broken up and have been excreted in the biliary drainage. The gallbladder must be distended with bile in order to visualize stones optimally. A densely shadowing focus in the fossa between right and left lobes is typical of a gallbladder that is packed with stones but little liquid bile (Fig. 17-13). It is helpful to

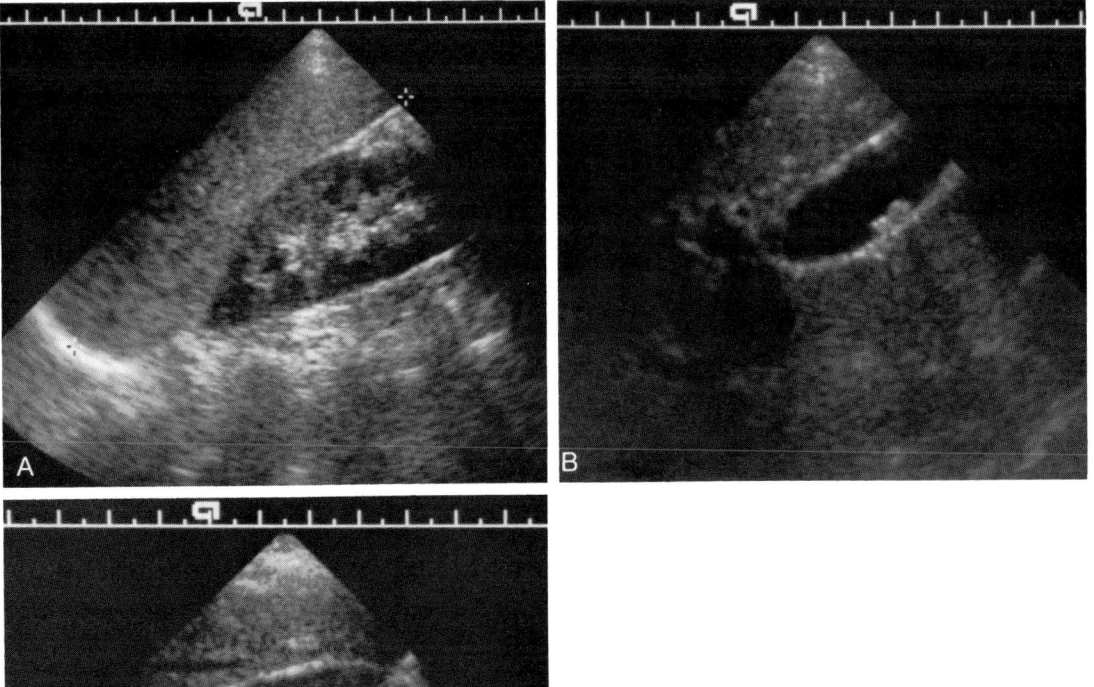

Figure 17–12. This 9-year-old's anemia is secondary to hereditary spherocytosis. Note the splenomegaly on the coronal view of the left upper quadrant (**A**). Changes in the patient's position resulted in the two gallstones' moving within the gallbladder (**B** and **C**).

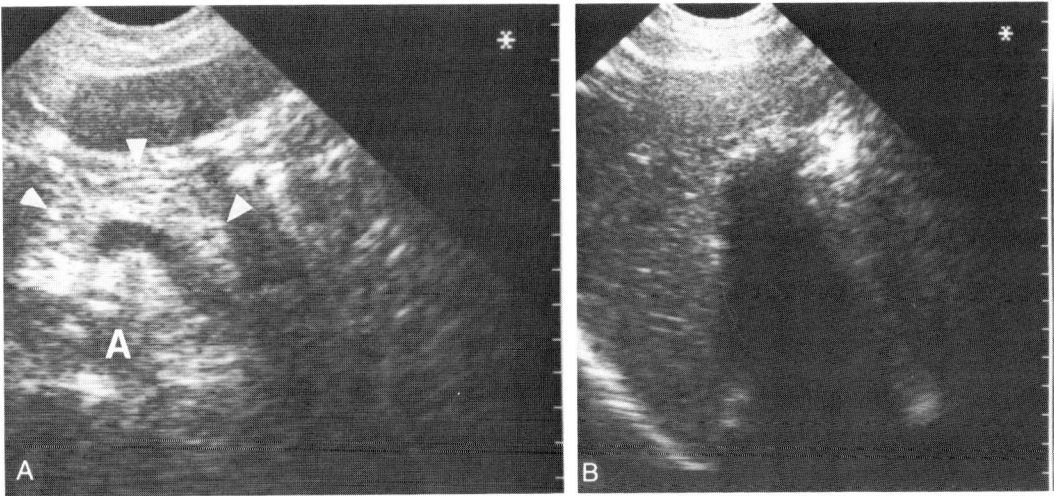

Figure 17–13. Transverse scan through the left lobe of the liver (**A**) shows the echogenic pancreatic head and body (arrowheads) in a patient who has cystic fibrosis. A = aorta. **B** is a longitudinal scan through the right upper quadrant. Stones packing a small gallbladder are creating a distinct shadow.

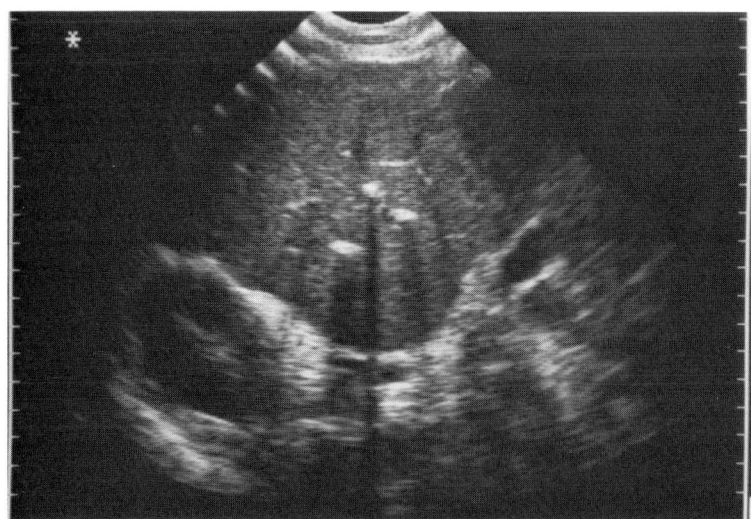

Figure 17–14. Transverse scan of the right lobe of the liver through intercostal spaces shows densely shadowing foci that represent intrahepatic biliary stones. This patient has cystic fibrosis. He is now 22 years old and has had recurrent episodes of jaundice associated with fever that is presumably related to intermittent obstruction from these stones.

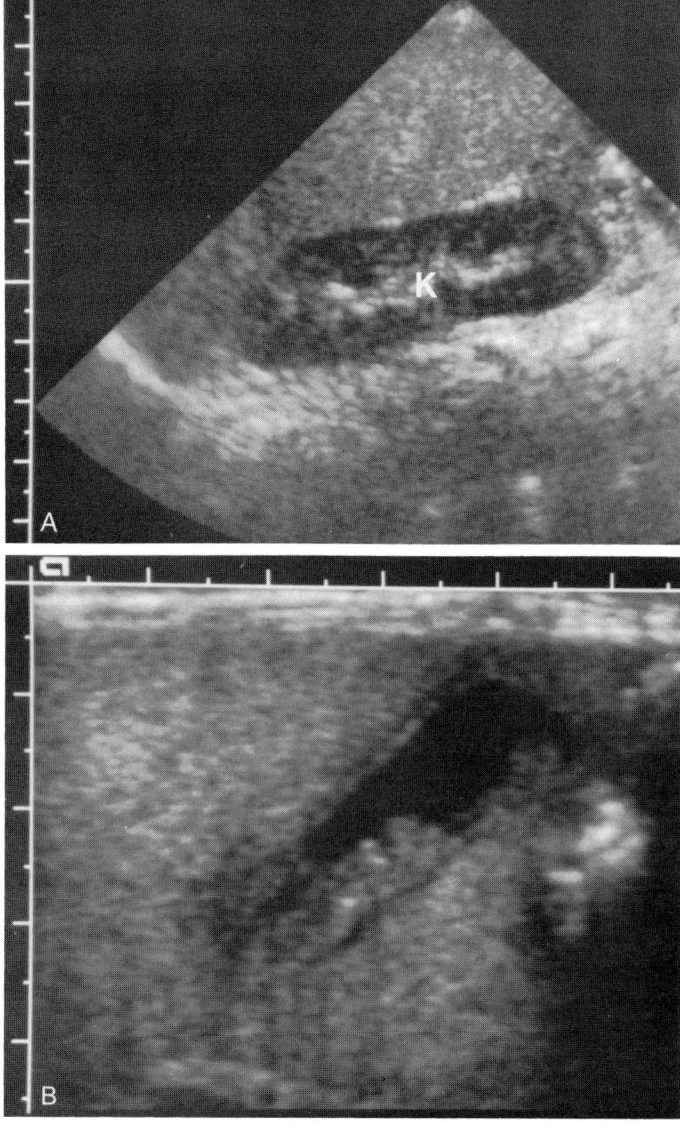

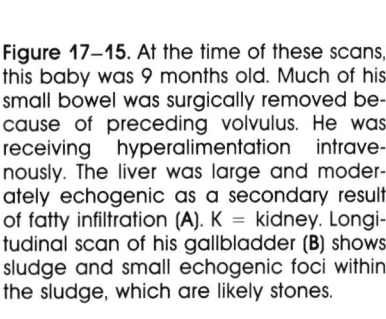

Figure 17–15. At the time of these scans, this baby was 9 months old. Much of his small bowel was surgically removed because of preceding volvulus. He was receiving hyperalimentation intravenously. The liver was large and moderately echogenic as a secondary result of fatty infiltration (**A**). K = kidney. Longitudinal scan of his gallbladder (**B**) shows sludge and small echogenic foci within the sludge, which are likely stones.

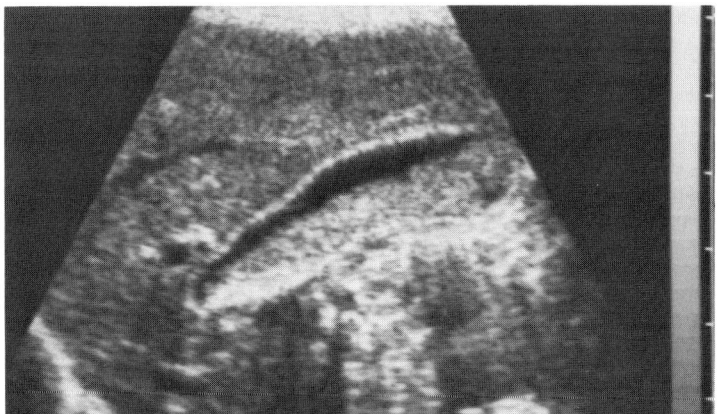

Figure 17–16. This longitudinal view shows debris in several layers within the gallbladder. This baby has Down syndrome and has undergone gastrostomy, repair of duodenal atresia, and cardiac surgery.

rescan such a patient in order not to mistake gas-filled bowel for a stone-filled gallbladder. Some gallstones may "float" or at least be suspended in bile if their specific density is less than that of bile (Fig. 17–17). Most stones, however, are dependent, in relation to the patient's position. When gallstones are identified, hepatic ducts should be evaluated for evidence of distention and stones, the wall of the gallbladder measured, and the pancreas surveyed for any evidence of pancreatitis related to passage of stones.

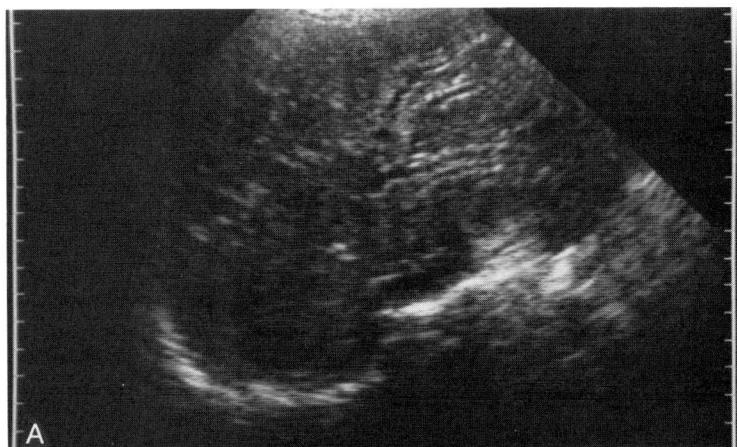
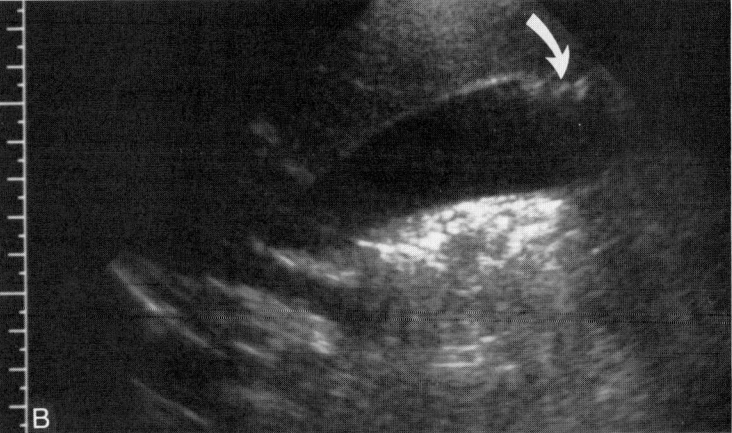

Figure 17–17. This 14-year-old girl presented with severe pain in the right upper quadrant. Transverse scan of her liver (A) shows double tracks within the liver, indicating the presence of dilated ducts. Longitudinal scan of the gallbladder (B) shows no obvious stones in the dependent portion of the gallbladder, but it does show echogenic foci that are floating in the fundus of the gallbladder (arrow). Her gallbladder was removed. It was found on histologic examination to be acutely inflamed; it contained multiple stones. No obstructing stone was present in the common bile duct at the time of surgery.

CHOLECYSTITIS: CALCULOUS AND ACALCULOUS

Children who have cholelithiasis may have episodes of upper abdominal pain, nausea, and intolerance of fatty food. The best ultrasonographic sign of inflammation is the patient's perception of pain when the transducer is pushed into the soft tissues over the gallbladder (the ultrasonic Murphy sign). Cholecystitis is an uncommon cause of mural thickening of gallbladder in the pediatric population. An occasional patient has acute cholecystitis and has the textbook picture of fluid/sludge in the gallbladder, a stone impacted in the cystic duct, mural thickening, and pericolic fluid, but this is the exception rather than the rule in pediatric practice (Fig. 17–18). Thickening of the wall of the gallbladder, greater than the 3 mm that we accept as normal, is more commonly associated with hypoalbuminemia, ascites, obstruction to hepatic venous return, and acute hepatitis (Figs. 17–19, 17–20; Patriquin et al., 1983; Levine et al., 1986).

Acute biliary colic results when a child passes one or more gallstones into the common bile duct. The common bile duct rarely measures more than 6 mm in diameter in the normal adolescent. In younger children, it is a barely visible channel. Ductal dilatation can usually be detected and the duct traced distally to the level of the obstructing stone (Fig. 17–21).

Before we consider the topic of acalculous cholecystitis, we have to discuss the hydropic gallbladder. The terminology of many references in the literature is very confusing because "hydrops" and "acalculous cholecystitis" are used as interchangeable terms. Furthermore, "hydrops of the gallbladder" is an unfortunate label anyway because "hydrops" can refer to edema of tissues or serous distention of a viscus. Neither definition is appropriate to describe a gallbladder distended with bile. We prefer to use the term "cholecystomegaly" when we show, with ultrasonography, a thin-walled gallbladder that is longer than usual for the patient's age and has a spherical, as opposed to teardrop, shape.

In most patients with cholecystomegaly, there is a primary reason for the enlargement. Huge gallbladders have been described in neonates who are not being fed, are septic, or have multiple other medical and surgical problems (El-Shafie and Mah, 1986). Sepsis in older babies, especially with streptococcal infections, is associated with enlargement of the gallbladder (Fig. 17–22). Cholecystomegaly is a cardinal feature of Kawasaki syndrome, but it resolves after the acute illness (Fig. 17–23; Suddleson et al.,

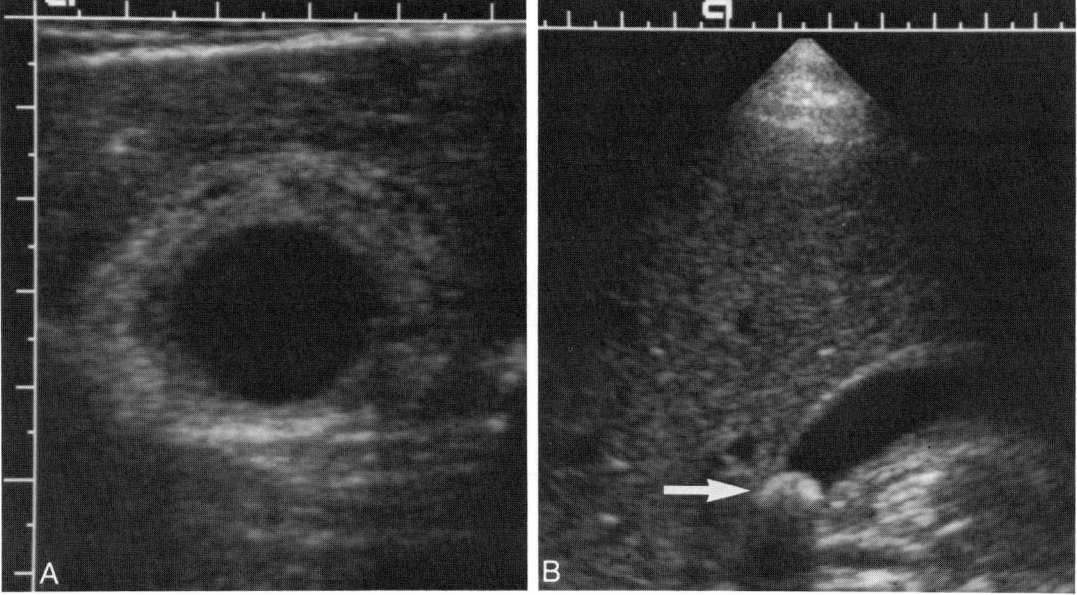

Figure 17–18. Transverse scan with linear array transducer shows pericholic edema in this teenage boy, who presented with severe pain in the right upper quadrant from acute cholecystitis (A). Longitudinal scan of the right upper quadrant (B) shows a stone (arrow) that was thought to be impacted in the neck of the gallbladder because it did not change at all with position. The patient had severe pain with palpation over the gallbladder.

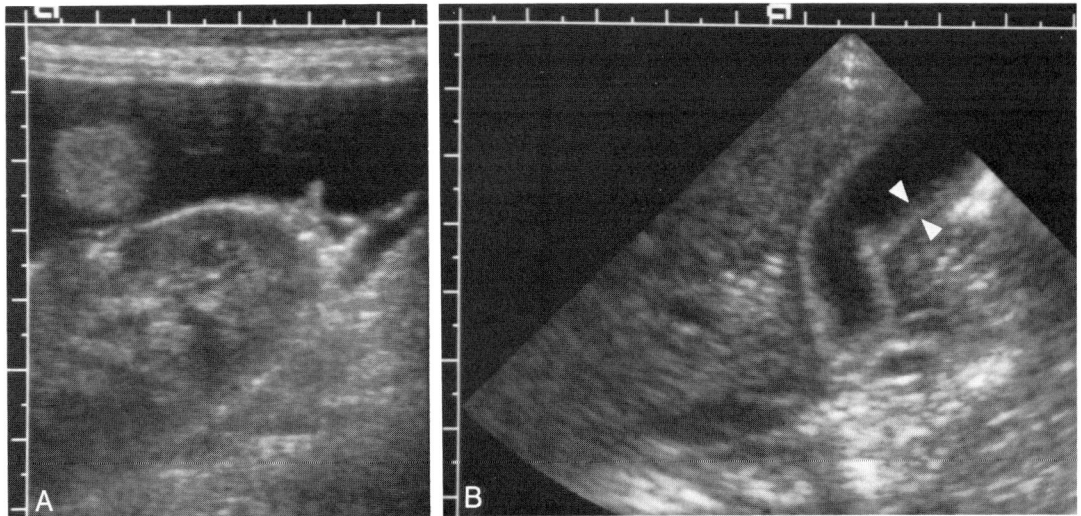

Figure 17–19. Abdominal ascites shown on longitudinal view of the right upper abdomen (**A**) was responsible for thickening of the wall of the gallbladder in this patient. The baby did not have hypoalbuminemia; he did have meningococcemia and capillary leakage of fluid. Longitudinal view of the gallbladder is shown in **B**. The wall (arrowheads) measured 4 mm; 3 mm is the norm.

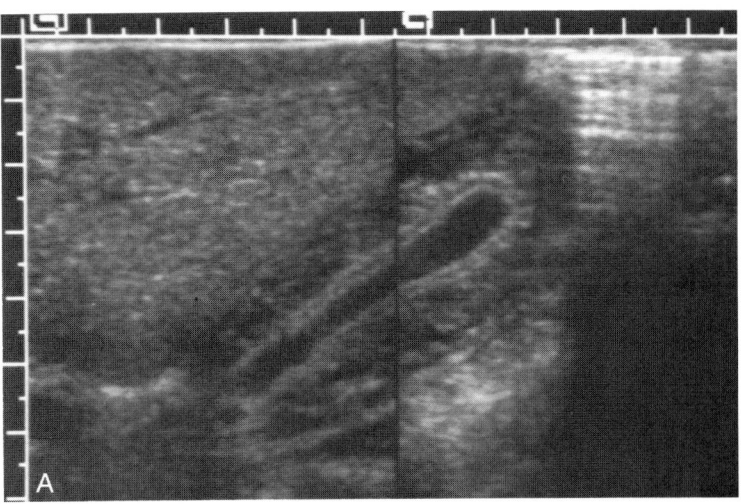
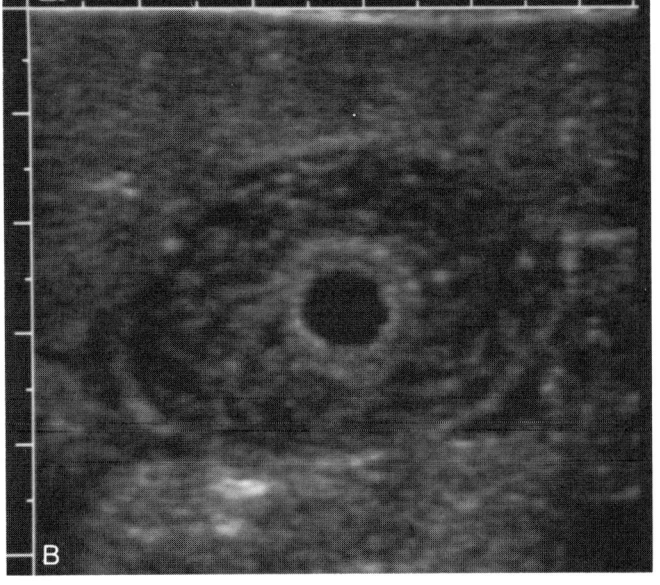

Figure 17–20. Longitudinal (**A**) and transverse (**B**) views of the gallbladder show dramatic thickening of the wall. This patient had acute hepatitis, probably associated with reaction to sulfa-containing drugs.

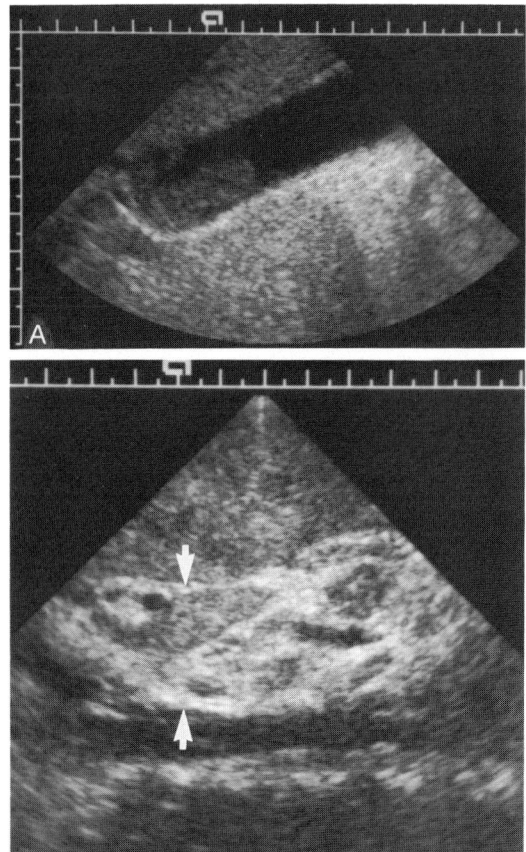
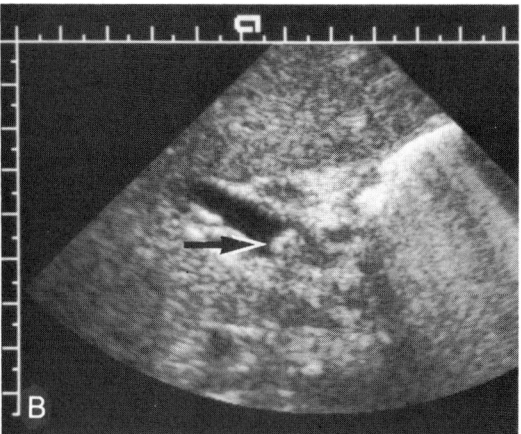

Figure 17–21. This 4½-year-old boy was admitted for pain in the right upper quadrant, fever, and jaundice. Longitudinal scan (**A**) shows sludge within the gallbladder that measures 8 cm. This is large for the patient's age. Intrahepatic ducts were prominent, and the common hepatic duct could be traced to a dilated common bile duct (**B**). A nonshadowing mass (arrow) was present within the distal duct. During surgery, cholecystectomy was performed. A black crumbling stone was present in the common bile duct, obstructing the biliary tree. This patient's history is important: he had had neonatal obstruction of the portal vein. Note that no normal portal venous structure is seen around the porta hepatis in **B**. Longitudinal scan of the aorta (**C**) demonstrates increased space (arrows) between the left lobe of the liver and the aorta. This thickening is associated with esophageal varices. Previous transfusions for gastrointestinal bleeding possibly resulted in biliary calculi.

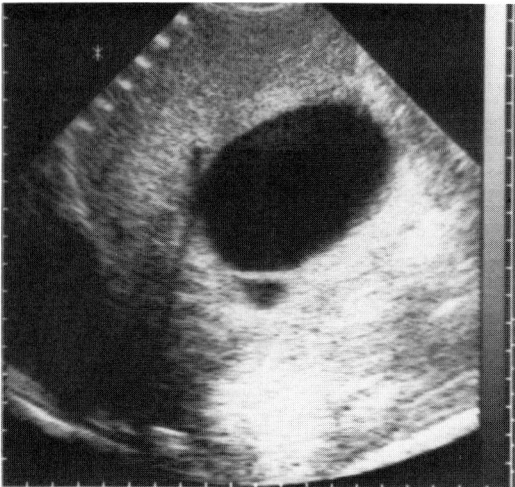

Figure 17–22. Longitudinal scan of the right upper quadrant shows a spherical gallbladder measuring 8.5 cm in this 4½-year-old boy, who was febrile. Infection with group A streptococcus was proved with titers. It took 10 days for the gallbladder to return to normal size.

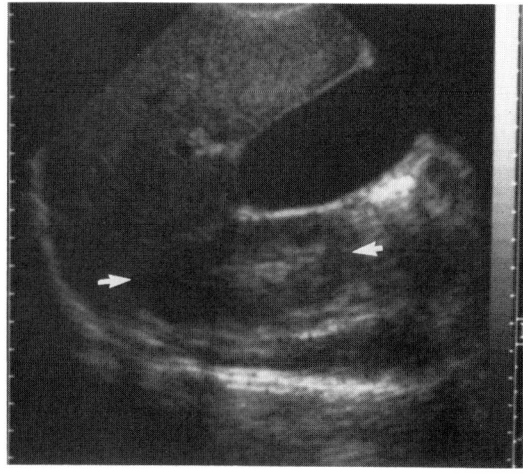

Figure 17–23. Cholecystomegaly is commonly associated with Kawasaki syndrome. This 6-year-old presented with fever and a palpable mass in the right upper quadrant. Note the size of the gallbladder in comparison with the length of adjacent kidney (arrows).

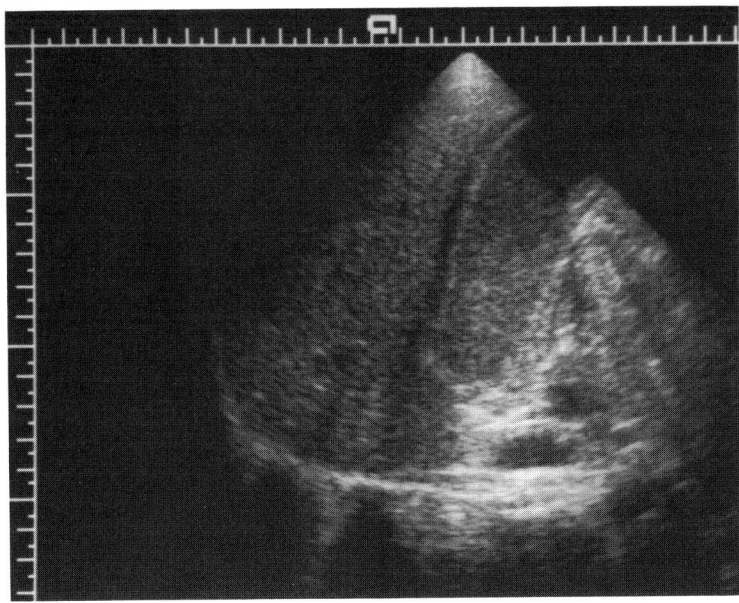

Figure 17-24. Acute acalculous cholecystitis was diagnosed during surgery after an ultrasonogram showed a fluid debris level within a dilated gallbladder in this 17-year-old patient. The patient had pain on palpation over the gallbladder. No stones, only tarry sludge, were identified at surgery. Sixteen days before this episode, the patient had undergone spinal fusion for progressive scoliosis secondary to myelodysplasia.

1987). We also have seen children in whom prolonged vomiting, severe disturbances of electrolytes, or acute hepatitis presented with cholecystomegaly. The dilated gallbladder is painful when touched. It is part of the foregut and, like the bowel, hurts when distended. In fact, we often think of the condition in terms of "gallbladder ileus." If the underlying problems are treated and normal nutrition can be gradually instituted, the gallbladder usually decreases in size and returns to normal. If, however, dilatation is prolonged, ischemia of the wall or sepsis, or both, may supervene, and the patient develops true acalculous cholecystitis.

Acalculous cholecystitis is, therefore, a diagnosis of exclusion, and each patient who presents with cholecystomegaly has to be considered individually (Fig. 17-24). A primary cause for the dilatation should be investigated before surgical intervention is considered. We remember, from many years ago, one child with undiagnosed Wilson disease who presented with cholecystomegaly. Surgical removal of the gallbladder under anesthesia exacerbated the hepatitis, and the child died in the postoperative period.

Any child who has a dilated gallbladder should have a complete examination of the liver and biliary tract in order to rule out an obstructing stone, a stricture, or a mass (Fig. 17-25). Radionuclide scans with iminodiacetic acid derivatives may not differentiate between obstructive and physiologic cholecystomegaly. Abnormal hepatic metabolism and a stagnant biliary system often result in a "positive" radionuclide scan.

Conversely, some children present with pain in the right upper quadrant and have normal ultrasonograms but radionuclide scans that suggest dysfunctional emptying of the gallbladder. We do not understand the underlying physiologic problem in these patients; it is apparent that ultrasonography is able to rule out anatomic abnormalities but provides little physiologic information.

Primary sclerosing cholangitis in children is associated with inflammatory bowel disease in approximately half of reported cases. Histiocytosis and immunodeficiency states are associated in 15 and 10 percent of cases, respectively (Sisto et al., 1987). The ectasia or irregularity of ducts is less than that seen with Caroli disease, and a definitive diagnosis of this entity is made only with cholangiography. Ultrasonography can be suggestive and guide transhepatic cholangiography. Although fibrosis is present, it is much less than the broad bands associated with congenital hepatic fibrosis. Clinical presentation in most affected children is of pain, jaundice, or both.

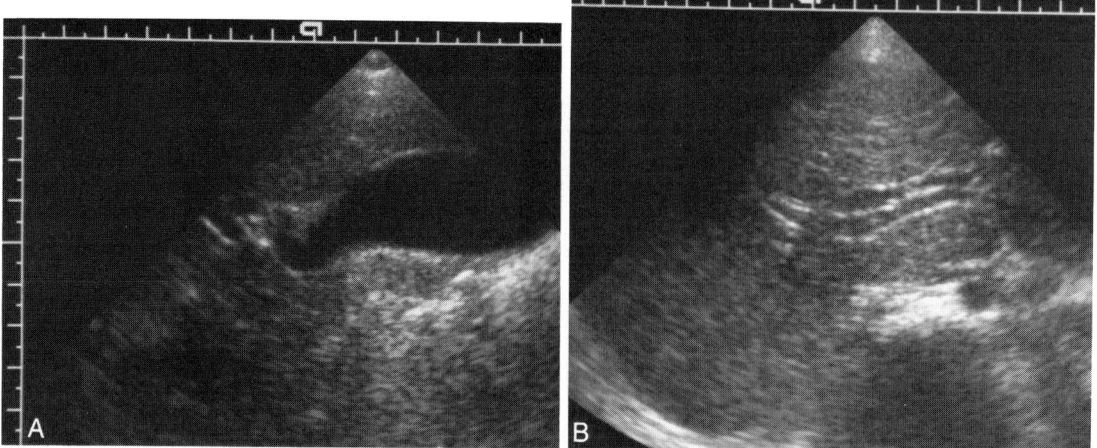

Figure 17–25. Cholecystomegaly (A) was associated with dilated bile ducts (B) in this 9-year-old girl. She had started taking morphine for severe abdominal pain related to graft-versus-host disease after transplantation of bone marrow. No anatomic obstruction was identified, and the biliary tract returned to normal when the patient was weaned from morphine.

HEPATIC PARENCHYMAL DISEASES

Hepatomegaly is a worrisome clinical finding, particularly in babies. However, infiltration with a tumor, as discussed in Chapter 8, is less common than hepatic enlargement caused by inflammation or some other diffuse parenchymal abnormality. The pediatrician is always interested in whether the clinical impression of hepatic enlargement is supported by the scans. Volumetric studies of liver have been done (Dittrich et al., 1983), but these are quite cumbersome to perform, and with a few rules of thumb and some experience, one can judge hepatic size without the aid of computers or equations.

We do use tables that are based on evaluations of normal hepatic scintigrams from our hospital (Markisz et al., 1987). As part of this study, vertical dimension was calculated as a function of both age and weight (Fig. 17–26). Ultrasonographic scans in the sagittal plane can be used to measure vertical dimension. Clinicians palpate the edge of the right lobe of the liver; rarely do they percuss or palpate the left lobe. In babies and young children, the left lobe is relatively large and truly left sided (Fig. 17–27). Transverse scans just below the xiphoid process usually display a plane through the left portal vein. If scans show a confluence of hepatic veins instead, it may be that lungs are hyperinflated and are pushing both the diaphragm

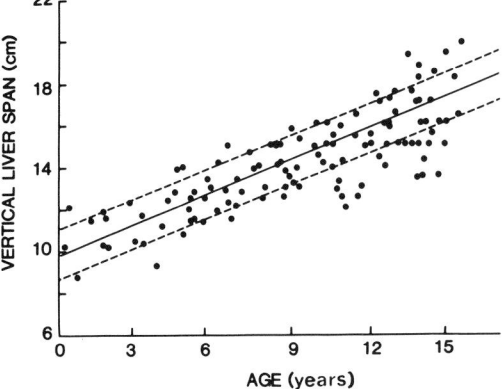
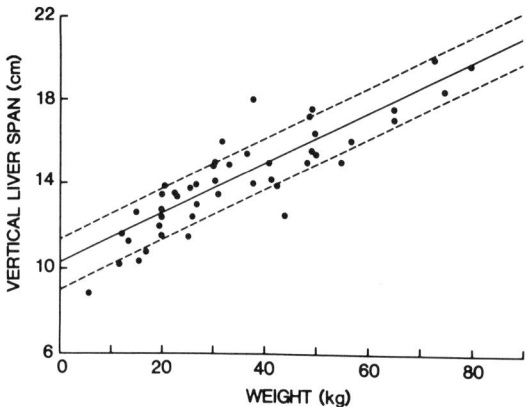

Figure 17–26. Length of the liver is plotted against age and weight on these charts. (From Markisz JA, et al: Normal hepatic and splenic size in children: Scintigraphic determination. Pediatr Radiol 1987;17:273–276.)

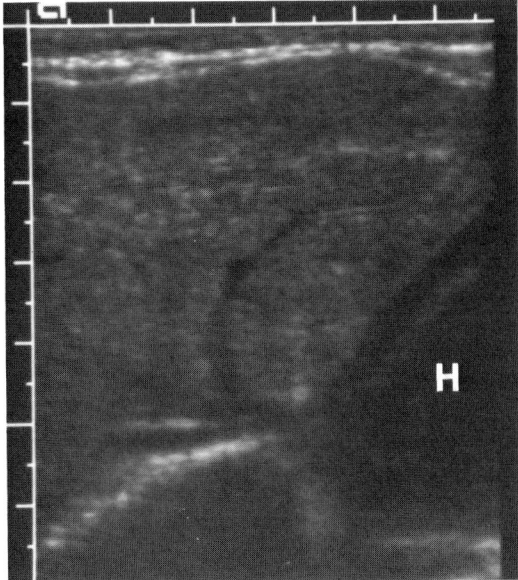

Figure 17–27. Transverse scan high in the abdomen in a 3-month-old shows the left lobe of the liver adjacent to the heart (H).

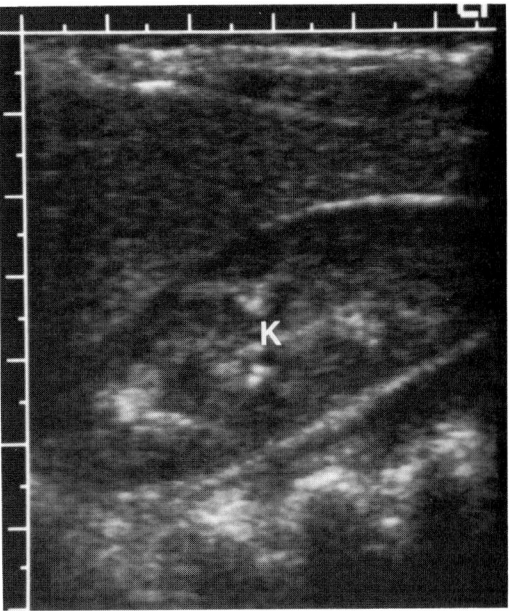

Figure 17–28. Longitudinal scan shows the normal relationship of the right lobe of the liver with the kidney (K) in this child. Echogenicity in central areas in the kidney is from nephrocalcinosis.

and the liver inferiorly. Longitudinal scans of the normal liver show a sharp, V-shaped edge. When the liver is enlarged, the contour becomes rounded. A long, thin tongue from the right lobe (Riedel lobe) is an unusual finding, but its pattern should betray its hepatic origin, and its edge should be sharp. The right lobe of the liver does not normally extend below the inferior margin of the right kidney on sagittal scans (Fig. 17–28). The left lobe does not normally extend below the costal edge on the left. Equally important as size is the parenchymal pattern of the liver. Scans of normal children show a liver with homogeneous gray texture and speckles provided by portal triads (Fig. 17–29).

We have noted obvious lucency of the liver

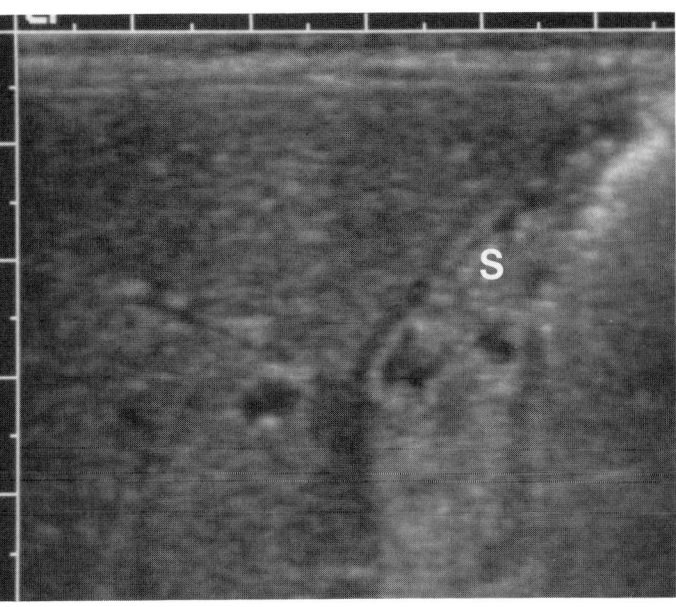

Figure 17–29. Transverse scan of the left lobe of the liver in this baby, who was undergoing evaluation for possible pyloric stenosis, shows the speckled pattern associated with normal hepatic parenchyma. S = stomach.

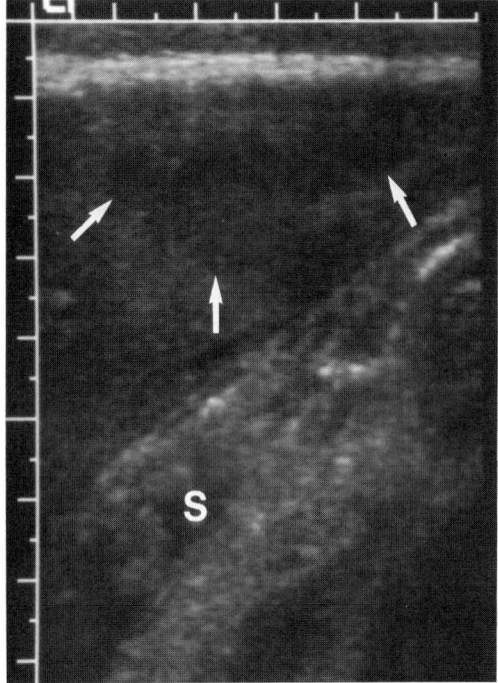

Figure 17–30. Peripheral ischemia of the liver and spleen occurred in this 7-year-old girl, who was immunosuppressed after renal transplantation and then went into shock with sepsis. The left lobe of the liver shows patchy lucency (arrows). On computed tomography (CT) scans, these areas did not enhance with contrast. The gastric mucosa was markedly thickened from gastritis. S = stomach.

Table 17–2. COMMON CAUSES OF ACUTE HEPATITIS

Hepatitis A and B
Delta hepatitis
Hepatitis C
Epstein-Barr virus
Cytomegalovirus
Toxins, drugs
Reye syndrome

in children who suffered severe asphyxia (Fig. 17–30). Presumably, we see edema causing the change in hepatic texture. Why the liver does not become echogenic, thereby similar in appearance to cerebral edema, is unknown. It is interesting that Garra and coauthors (1988) also reported hypoechoic hepatic parenchyma with injury induced by radiation. Viral or other hepatitis provides no clues to its presence (Giorgio et al., 1986). A child with clinically evident infectious hepatitis does not need ultrasonography unless some unusual clinical feature is present. Common causes of acute hepatitis are listed in Table 17–2.

The children who have hepatomegaly, increased reflectivity of hepatic parenchyma, and poor ultrasonic penetration of liver form an interesting group. Our experience, which has been supported by basic research in adults (Taylor et al., 1986), is that fat within hepatocytes, and not fibrosis, causes the ultrasonographic appearance of the diffusely echogenic liver (Henschke et al., 1982). Fat may be microvesicular or macrovesicular. It may be overlooked on routine histologic examination of the liver and detected only if appropriate stains are performed on freshly frozen specimens of tissue. Fat within hepatocytes is a nonspecific marker of injury, but

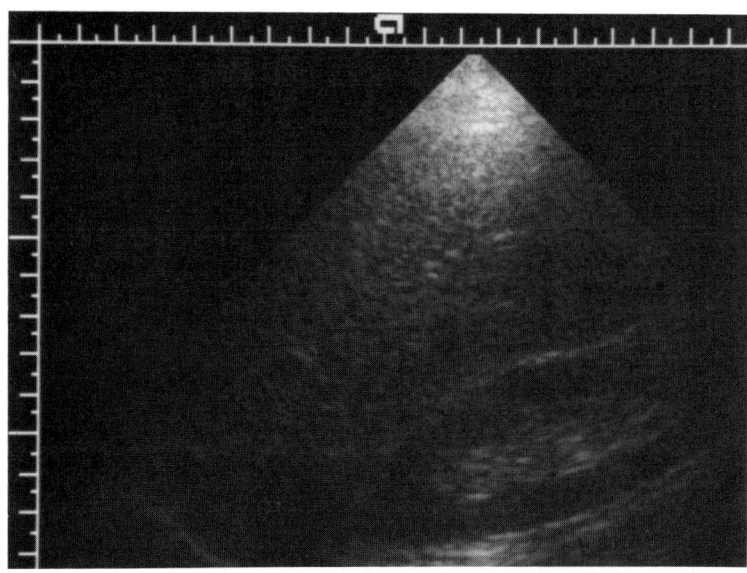

Figure 17–31. A 3.5-MHz transducer was unable to penetrate the liver in this 12-year-old child, who was morbidly obese. Fatty infiltration throughout the liver is a very effective reflector of the ultrasonic beam.

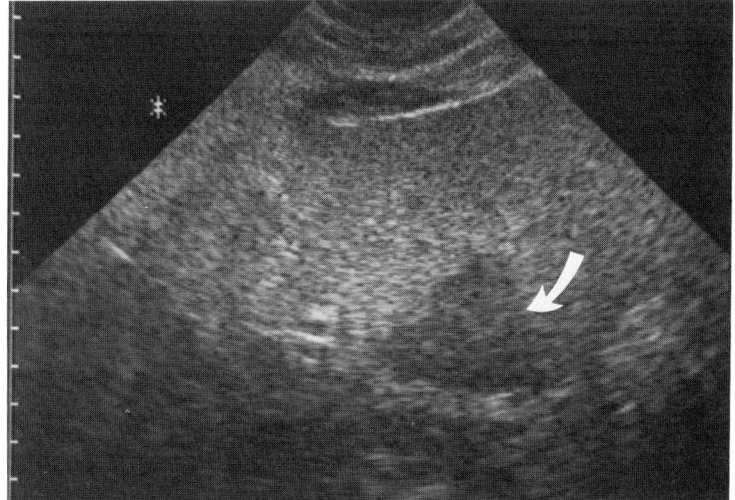

Figure 17–32. The triangular area (arrow) within the liver was an area spared from fatty infiltration associated with marked obesity. Fatty infiltration decreased when the patient adhered to a diet restricted in calories.

the list of differential diagnoses can help guide further evaluation. Obese patients and patients who are receiving hyperalimentation have fatty deposits in the liver (Figs. 17–31, 17–32). Although it seems contradictory, patients who are starving, either because of inadequate intake of calories or from malabsorption (e.g., untreated cystic fibrosis or diabetes mellitus) also develop fatty livers. Chemotherapeutic agents and steroids both

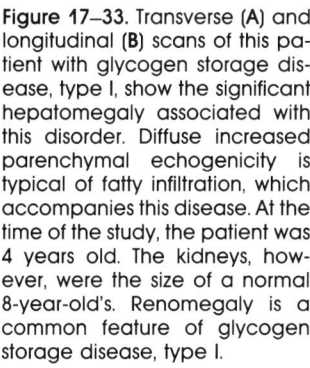

Figure 17–33. Transverse (**A**) and longitudinal (**B**) scans of this patient with glycogen storage disease, type I, show the significant hepatomegaly associated with this disorder. Diffuse increased parenchymal echogenicity is typical of fatty infiltration, which accompanies this disease. At the time of the study, the patient was 4 years old. The kidneys, however, were the size of a normal 8-year-old's. Renomegaly is a common feature of glycogen storage disease, type I.

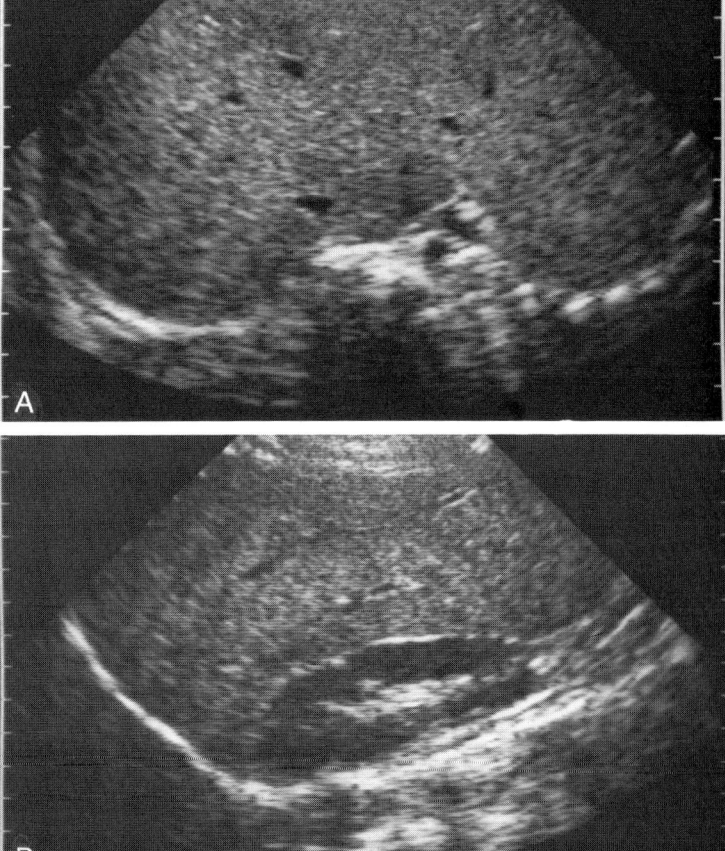

cause fatty liver. Reye syndrome causes acute fatty infiltration that can be evident on scans (Henschke et al., 1982). For adolescents, one should also consider the possibility of alcoholic liver disease. The smallest group of patients with fatty liver is children with metabolic liver disease. Tyrosinemia, fructose intolerance, Wilson disease, and glycogen storage disease, particularly type I (von Gierke disease), produce metabolic disturbances or byproducts that cause hepatocytes to increase their store of fat (Figs. 17–33, 17–34). For all patients who have apparent hepatic infiltration of fat, the ultrasonographic study should be extended to include the kidneys and the spleen and a careful evaluation of the biliary tree. Glycogen storage diseases and tyrosinemia are frequently associated with renomegaly. The spleen is usually normal in size and in pattern unless portal hypertension supervenes. The incidence of biliary calculi is higher than normal in children who have metabolic hepatic disease.

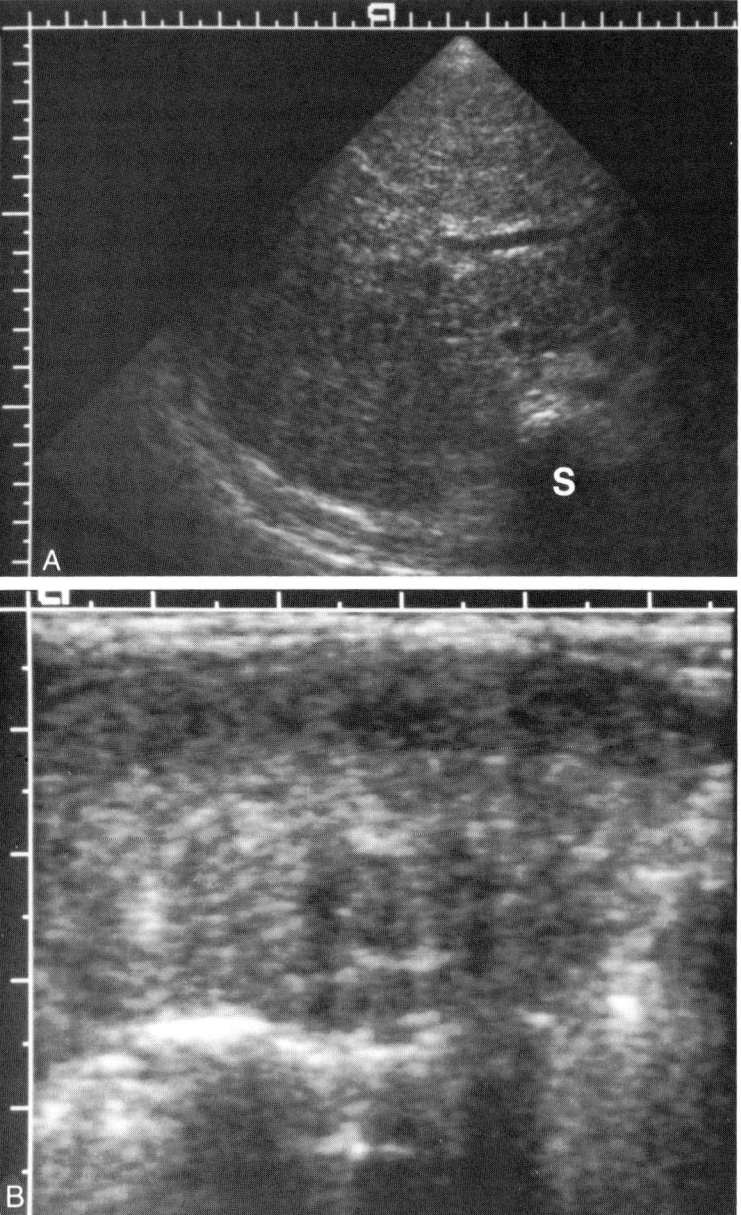

Figure 17–34. Both scans shown are transverse views of the liver. A, a sector scan of the right upper quadrant, shows diffuse increase in echogenicity typical of fatty infiltration. S = spine. B was obtained with a linear array transducer and shows inhomogeneity of the hepatic parenchymal pattern. This patient had tyrosinemia, which was diagnosed in metabolic studies. The inhomogeneity was the harbinger of adenomatous change in the liver.

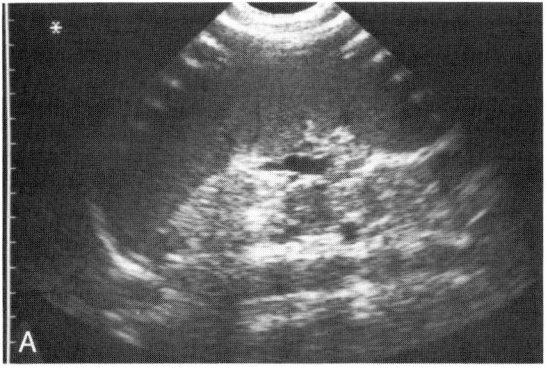
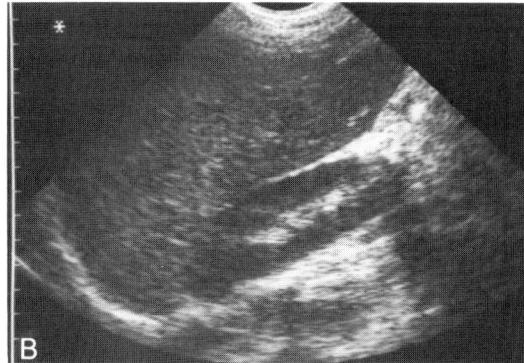
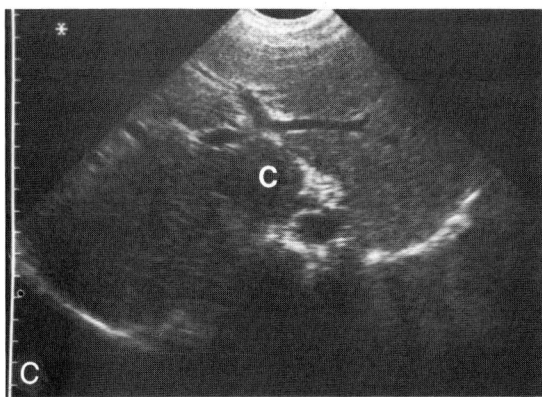

Figure 17–35. These scans are of an 11-year-old girl with chronic active hepatitis and cirrhosis documented by hepatic biopsy. Coronal view through the left upper quadrant (A) shows splenomegaly. Longitudinal view of the right abdomen (B) shows large right hepatic lobe. Its rounded inferior contour extends below the right kidney. Transverse scan of the portal venous system (C) shows a mild increase in periportal echogenicity, in comparison with normal. The caudate lobe (C) is prominent.

CHRONIC HEPATIC DISEASE

The appearance of hepatic parenchyma changes, as do the size and contour of the liver, in children with chronic hepatic disease. Increasing fibrosis around portal triads produces increasing periportal echogenicity (Fig. 17–35). With time, the surface of the liver becomes lobular instead of smooth, and after a variable period of hepatomegaly, the liver contracts in size. One cannot, however, make a diagnosis of cirrhosis from ultrasonic scans alone. As in adults, the caudate lobe may be spared the disruption of normal lobular anatomy that accompanies increasing fibrosis. The caudate lobe may appear relatively lucent and may be prominent in size. Hypertrophy of the caudate may compromise caval blood flow to the degree that a portocaval shunt or a mesocaval shunt may not be successful because intracaval pressure below the liver is high (Fellows et al., 1975). Loss of normal triphasic pattern in the inferior vena cava on examination with Doppler ultrasonography may be a clue to this problem.

The scans can certainly suggest cirrhosis, but confirmatory biopsy is always needed because implications regarding therapy for the child are significant. Chronic hepatic disease may result from many different inflammatory, metabolic, or mechanical insults to the liver. The most common are listed in Table 17–3. Although we have listed it last on our list, schistosomiasis is the most common cause of chronic hepatic fibrosis (Symmers periportal fibrosis) in some countries (Homeida et al., 1988; Abdel-Wahab et al., 1990).

It is rare for chronic hepatic disease to be diagnosed primarily with ultrasonography.

Table 17–3. CONDITIONS THAT MAY PROGRESS TO CHRONIC HEPATIC DISEASE

Hepatitis B
Delta hepatitis
Hepatitis C
Autoimmune chronic active hepatitis (lupoid)
$Alpha_1$-antitrypsin deficiency
Wilson disease
Indian childhood cirrhosis
Hemachromatosis
Tyrosinemia
Cystic fibrosis
Radiation
Biliary atresia
Biliary duct hypoplasia
Sclerosing cholangitis
Schistosomiasis

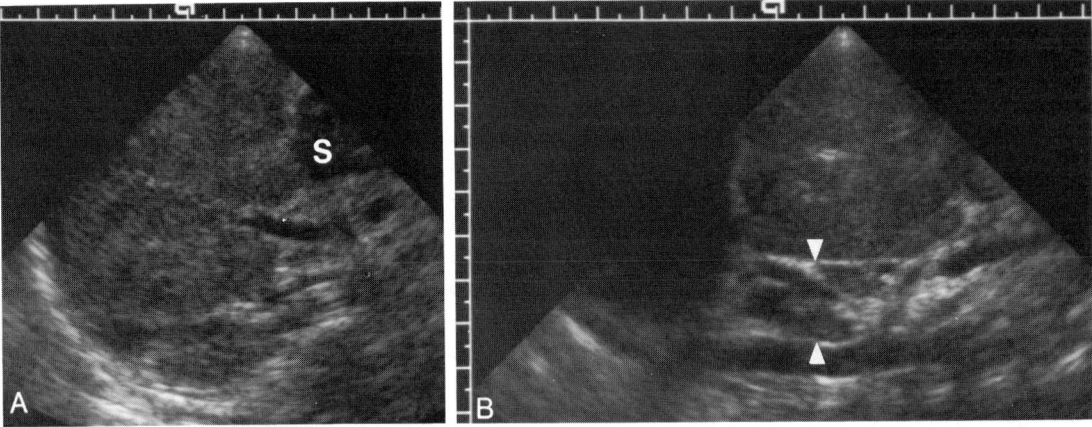

Figure 17-36. This transverse scan (A) shows the portal vein entering the liver. The hepatic parenchymal pattern is irregular. The liver is small. S = stomach. Longitudinal scan (B) shows a significant distance between the undersurface of the left lobe of the liver and the anterior border of the aorta (arrowheads). This patient had rapid deterioration of hepatic function from alpha$_1$-antitrypsin deficiency. The thickening of the preaortic space was secondary to esophageal varices. This patient is currently being considered for hepatic transplantation.

Typically, we are following children who are already known to the clinicians and who are being scanned to document anatomic changes and possible portal hypertension (Fig. 17-36; Plate XII).

After hepatic size and parenchymal pattern are checked, the ultrasonographic study is incomplete unless the hepatic vasculature, biliary tree, and spleen have been completely assessed. Problems related to the biliary tract usually present with pain or jaundice and are discussed in the first section of this chapter. The spleen is first cousin to the liver and should always be scanned when hepatic problems are present and vice versa (see Chapter 16).

HEPATIC VASCULAR ABNORMALITIES

The liver is unique among visceral organs in that it receives both arterial and venous blood flow, mixes it in the sinusoids, and sends the resultant effluent to the right side of the heart. The normal common hepatic artery arises as the right-sided branch of the celiac trunk (Fig. 17-37). In 25 percent of people (Gray, 1985), there is some anomaly of the right hepatic artery. The most common anomaly is that it arises separately, as a "replaced" artery, from the superior mesenteric artery (Fig. 17-38). This normal variation can be shown on ultrasonography even in small babies. The hepatic artery is quite prominent in children and should not be mistaken for a bile duct (Fig. 17-39). Aneurysmal dilatation of the hepatic artery should prompt evaluation of systemic vasculature and suggests abnormality of connective tissues. The portal vein develops from the paired vitelline veins. It receives flow from the splenic, inferior mesenteric, and superior mesenteric veins. The confluence of the splenic and superior mesenteric veins should

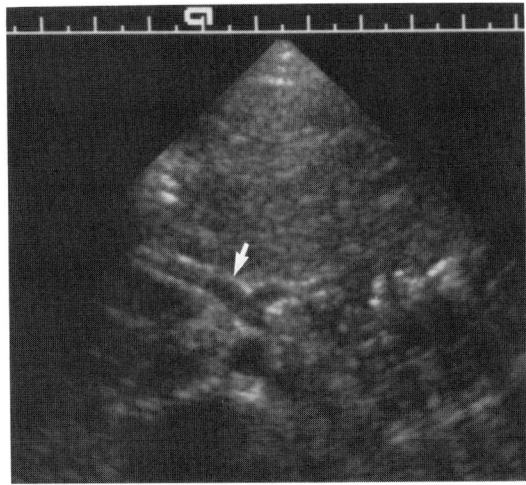

Figure 17-37. Transverse scan of the upper abdomen at the level of T-12 usually shows the very short, stubby celiac axis with its two major arteries, the splenic and the common hepatic (arrow). The left gastric artery is infrequently identified because of its more vertical course and its smaller diameter. The hepatic artery typically runs anterior to the portal vein until it enters the liver.

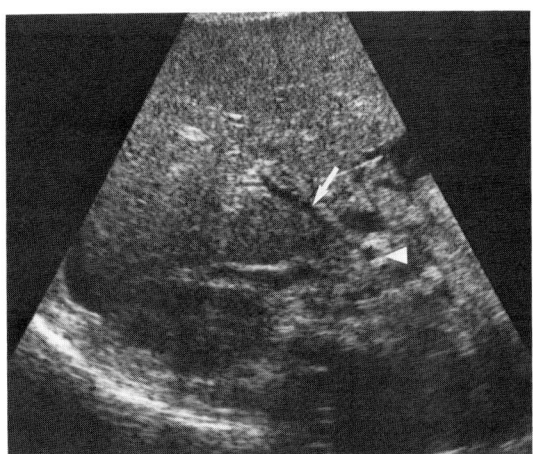

Figure 17-38. Transverse scan at the level of L-1 in this 1-month-old shows a replaced right hepatic artery (arrow) originating from the superior mesenteric artery (arrowhead).

be to the right of the superior mesenteric artery. The normal portal vein passes posterior to the duodenum to enter the liver at the hilum along with the hepatic artery, the common hepatic duct, and the ultrasonographically invisible lymphatic channels. The left portal vein takes an anterior course into the left lobe of the liver, where it branches into lateral and medial vessels (Fig. 17–40). The right portal vein runs a straight lateral course until it divides into posterior and anterior branches (Plate XIII). The hepatic veins, which do not have an echogenic rim from adjacent reticulin and collagen, are equidistant in relation to the branching portal veins. Hepatic veins define the lobar anatomy for the surgeon. The inferior vena cava receives hepatic venous flow as it passes through the diaphragm (Fig. 17–41). Usually, the middle and left hepatic veins join within the liver and enter the cava as a common trunk (Plate XIV). The ligamentum venosum joins the left portal vein with the left hepatic vein. Its path is the border between the caudate lobe and the medial segment of the left hepatic lobe (Fig. 17–42; Auh et al., 1984). In newborns one can occasionally identify the ductus venosus before it closes. The ligamentum teres is the residuum of the umbilical venous connection to the left portal vein. It tends to be a site of deposition of fat and therefore may be a large echogenic focus in children who are obese or receiving steroids (Fig. 17–43). In newborns the umbilical vein may be evident as a patent channel, but it is our experience that the patent umbilical vein in older children is associated with portal hypertension. The falciform ligament, which is the external continuation of the ligamentum teres, divides the left lobe into medial (quadrate lobe) and lateral segments. The boundary between right and left lobes is defined

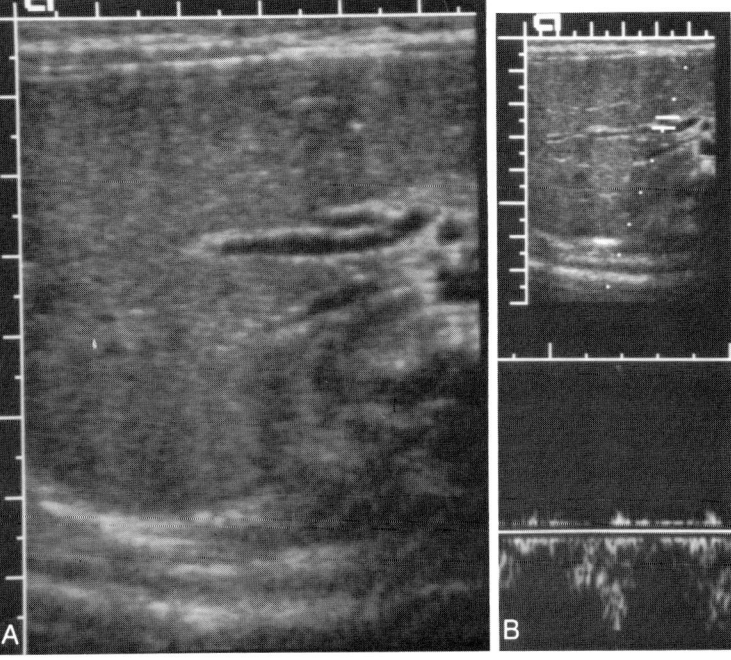

Figure 17-39. Hyperbilirubinemia prompted evaluation of the liver and biliary tree in this 1-month-old. Transverse (A) scan shows a parallel channel sign in the porta hepatis. The more superior of the channels is, however, the hepatic artery, as shown on Doppler tracing (B). Blood flow in the hepatic artery is moving away from the transducer and thus is below the baseline.

442 / THE LIVER

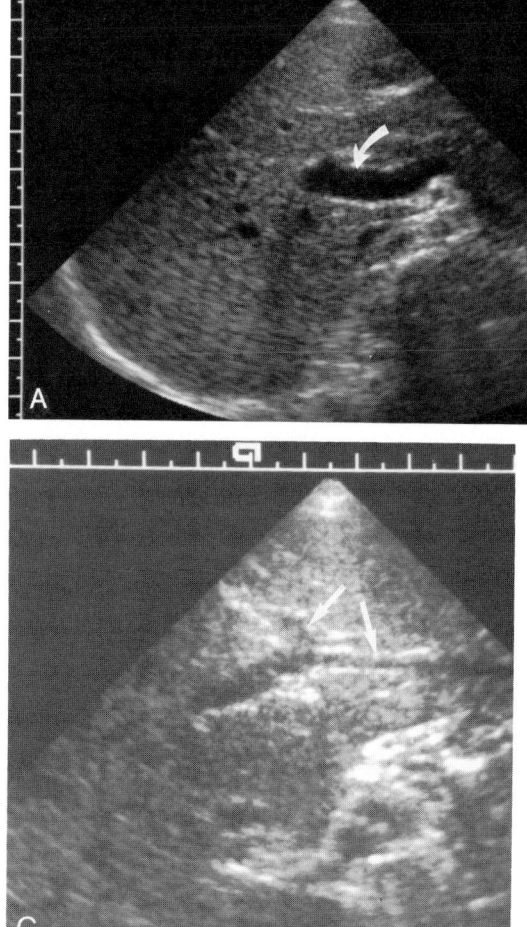

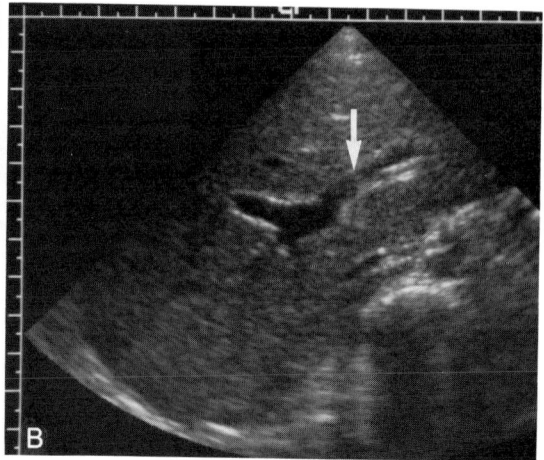

Figure 17–40. Transverse view at the head of the pancreas (**A**) shows the confluence of the superior mesenteric vein and the splenic vein and the resultant portal vein (arrow). The main portal vein is relatively horizontal in children. The right portal vein is a continuation of this horizontal course. The left portal vein (arrow, **B**) takes a more anterior course into left lobe of liver. It branches into medial and lateral segments (arrows, **C**).

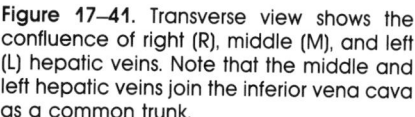

Figure 17–41. Transverse view shows the confluence of right (R), middle (M), and left (L) hepatic veins. Note that the middle and left hepatic veins join the inferior vena cava as a common trunk.

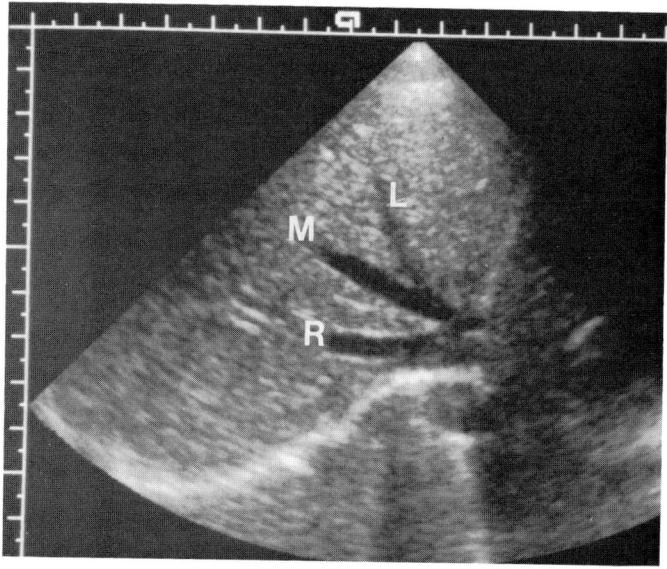

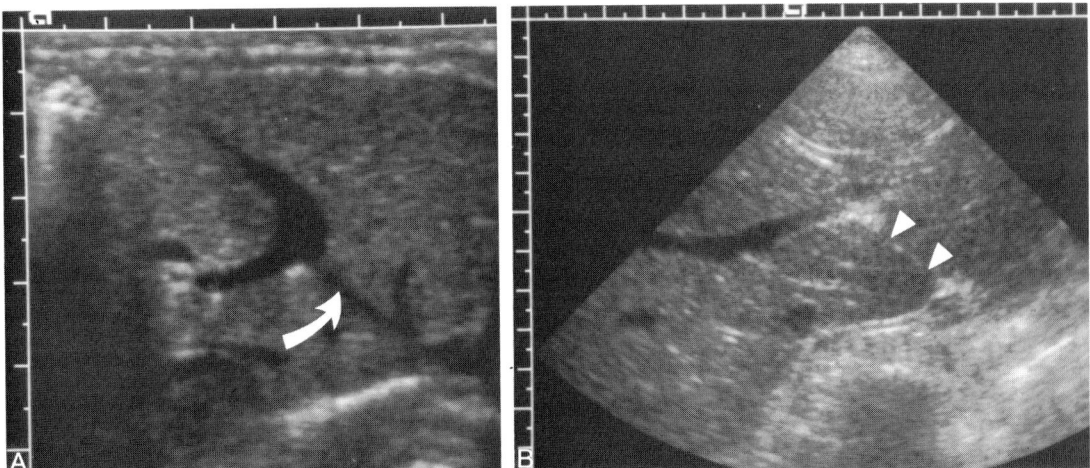

Figure 17-42. The patent ductus venosus (arrow) joins the portal vein with the left hepatic vein in a newborn (**A**). Transverse scan (**B**) at the level of the branching left portal vein shows the posteriorly directed echogenic line (arrowheads), which is the fibrous remnant of the ductus venosus in a 10-year-old.

by a plane that passes through the fossa of the gallbladder to the inferior vena cava (Fig. 17-44).

The portal triad—portal vein, hepatic artery, and bile duct—shows great variation in the relationships of its contents. Only at the porta hepatis is the bile duct usually anterior to the portal vein. As the triad ramifies in the liver, the bile ducts pass posteriorly or wind around the vessels (Bret et al., 1988). Care must be taken not to mistake the hepatic artery for the duct, and in any situation in which this problem arises, Doppler imaging of the channels should be performed.

In spite of the complicated embryology that precedes development of the portal venous system, anomalies of the portal vein are rare. Its absence has been documented in a few infants; splanchnic blood flow makes its way back to the heart through vessels that are remnants of the left vitelline vein, through

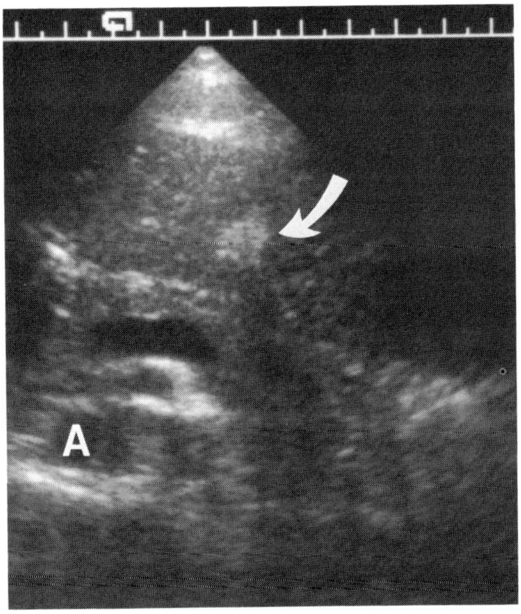

Figure 17-43. Exogenous steroids have resulted in the deposition of fat in the ligamentum teres (arrow). This is a transverse view of the left lobe of liver. The ligamentum teres is the dividing line between the medial and lateral segments of the left lobe. A = aorta.

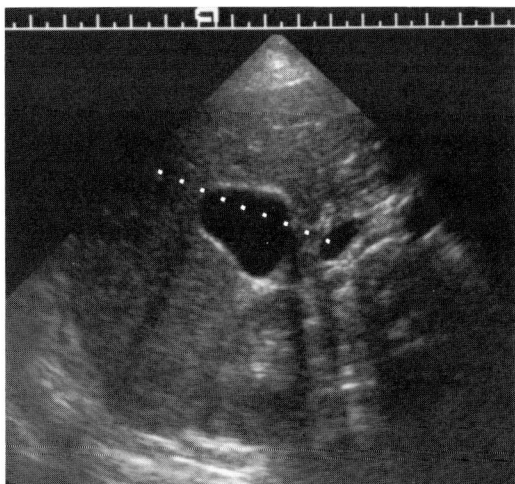

Figure 17-44. The plane between the right and left lobes of the liver is shown on this transverse scan. It passes from the inferior vena cava through the gallbladder.

444 / THE LIVER

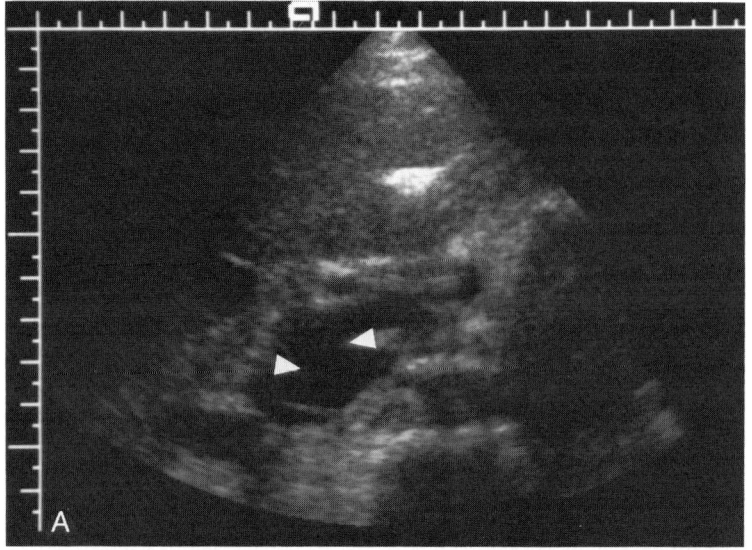

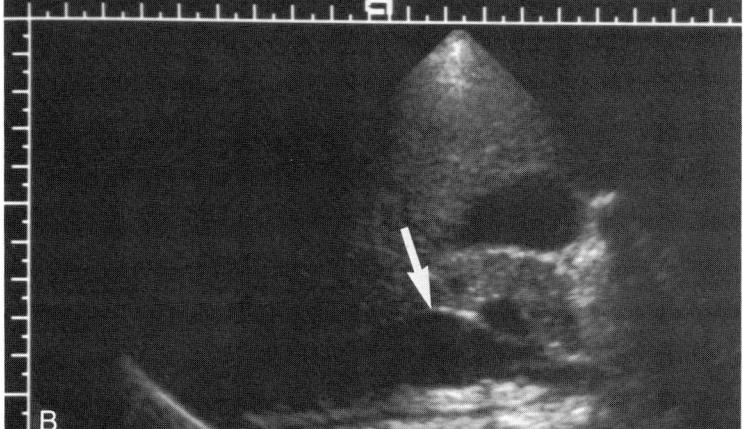

Figure 17–45. Transverse scan of the upper abdomen (**A**) shows the portal vein emptying into the inferior vena cava. The junction is outlined by arrowheads. The longitudinal scan (**B**) shows aneurysmal dilatation (arrow) of the inferior vena cava above the level of portal inflow. This anomaly was an incidental finding in this patient. She was being scanned for renal problems after surgery for aortic stenosis complicated by endocarditis.

Figure 17–46. Transverse scan of the upper abdomen showed no definable portal venous channel in this baby. Rather, the porta hepatis (arrowheads) was slightly more echogenic than normal. Small tubular lucencies probably represent combination of collateral veins and hepatic artery. The baby had previously undergone umbilical venous catheterization, and his portal venous occlusion was thought to be secondary to the intervention.

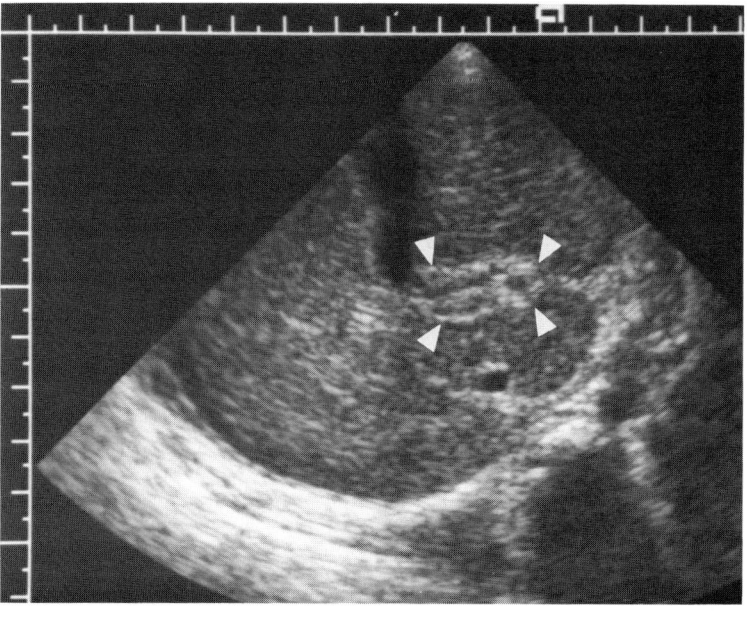

retroperitoneal collaterals, or directly into the inferior vena cava (Morse et al., 1986). Interestingly, cardiomyopathy has been associated with splanchnic bypass of the liver (Fig. 17–45; Bellah et al., 1989).

A preduodenal portal vein is associated with other major anomalies in the area, including duodenal stenosis, annular pancreas, malrotation of the gut, and biliary anomalies, and it is a common component of heterotaxy syndrome. Its position anterior to the duodenum results from persistence of the caudal (ventral) anastomosis between the pair of vitelline veins rather than the middle or dorsal anastomosis (McCarten and Teele, 1978).

"Cavernous transformation of the portal vein" is the misleading name for idiopathic occlusion of the portal vein. The cavernous appearance is from the secondary feature of collaterals that develop in and around the obstructed channel. Thrombosis of the portal vein may be caused by inflammation, associated with neonatal omphalitis, that extends along the course of the umbilical vein. Catheterization of the umbilical vein is known to be a predisposition to thrombosis (Fig. 17–46). Usually, however, there is no obvious cause for portal venous obstruction. Affected children may be completely asymptomatic and come to medical attention because of splenomegaly. They may present at any age with bleeding from gastroesophageal varices. Ultrasonography shows a small portal vein or, more typically, a spongelike pattern in the porta hepatis. This represents the cross-sectional view of multiple collateral channels (Alvarez et al., 1983; Frider et al., 1989). Doppler ultrasonography can show which channels are patent; it can document blood flow and show its direction (Raby and Meire, 1988). There is frequently a very echogenic flare around the vessels, suggesting that previous inflammation with subsequent fibrosis has occurred. The spleen is often large, and splenorenal collaterals may be present, as may retroperitoneal and gastroesophageal collaterals. The cava, if it receives significant collateral blood flow, is widened above the renal veins. The liver is normal in size or slightly small; the hepatic artery tends to be prominent in size because it is carrying the major supply of blood to the liver (Fig. 17–47).

Thrombosis of the portal vein may occur after splenectomy, particularly if the procedure is performed to treat hypersplenism.

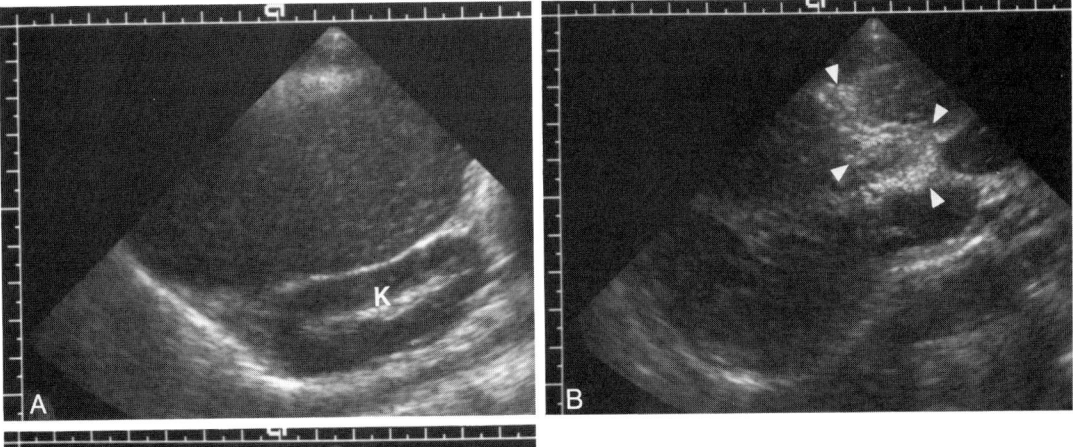
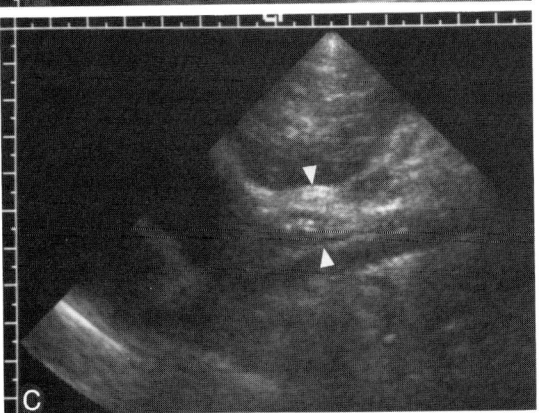

Figure 17–47. This adolescent boy had ultrasonic scans when asymptomatic splenomegaly was discovered during a routine physical examination. The spleen was enlarged, as shown on the coronal view through the left upper quadrant (A). K = kidney. The transverse scan through the porta hepatis (B) shows no identifiable vascular channels and replacement of the porta hepatis by irregular echogenicity (arrowheads). The patient also had widening of the preaortic space (arrowheads, C) associated with esophageal varices, which were documented on endoscopy. The etiology for the patient's portal venous obstruction is unknown.

The rebound in platelet count likely accentuates the normal healing and, in association with the marked changes in portal hemodynamics, causes a clot to propagate along the remaining splenic vein to the portal vein.

Pylephlebitis is now rare, but it used to be a common association with appendicitis in the days before therapy with antibiotics or prompt surgery. Occasionally it may present as a complication of appendicitis or other intra-abdominal inflammatory process, especially when the primary diagnosis has been delayed (Slovis et al., 1989).

Portal venous invasion by a tumor is usually found after the patient presents with a mass, and there should be no confusion with the idiopathic or inflammatory thromboses.

A sievelike portal vein may occur in children who have disorders of vascular growth. For example, we examined a boy with Klippel-Trenaunay syndrome who developed, among other problems, splenomegaly (Fig. 17-48). With ultrasonography, intra-abdominal vasculature can easily be viewed in children who have disorders associated with abnormal vasculature, such as Maffucci and Proteus syndromes.

Portal venous enlargement occurs every day, after every meal, in normal children. We have not tested a series of children, but of 13 normal adult volunteers, the postprandial measurements of the portal vein increased 50 percent over baseline (Bellamy et al., 1984). Portal venous dynamics also change with exercise and position (Ohnishi et al., 1985). Using the diameter of the portal vein to assess the degree of portal hypertension in children is at best simplistic and at worst thoroughly misleading. It is helpful if a series of scans are done under similar conditions in situations in which portal venous diameter is a critical issue. For instance, we examine children with chronic liver disease before hepatic transplantation. Surgery becomes more difficult when the diameter of the vein decreases to less than 5 mm. As part of our routine, we always measure the portal vein immediately distal to the confluence of the superior mesenteric vein and the splenic vein at the porta hepatis. Diagnosis of portal hypertension relies on several factors: direction of blood flow in the portal venous system as ascertained by Doppler imaging, direct or indirect evidence of varices, size of the spleen, and presence of ascites (Plate XV). Most scans are performed while a child is fasting; thus even results from Doppler imaging have to be viewed with care. Stimulation of splanchnic blood flow may change hepatic hemodynamics dramatically. Direct visualization and Doppler imaging of varices is proof of portal hypertension (except in the rare case of downhill varices that develop after obstruction of the superior vena cava). One can obtain indirect evidence of varices by measuring the thickness of the lesser omentum on longitudinal scans of the upper abdomen (Patriquin et al., 1985). The space between the inferior surface of the left lobe of the liver and the anterior wall of the aorta should not exceed 1.7 times the diameter of the aorta (Figs. 17-36, 17-47). Obesity, deposition of fat because of steroid administration, lymphadenopathy, and abnormality of the cardioesophageal junction also cause widening of this space but are usually evident at the time of the study.

The umbilical vein is rarely visualized unless it is patent. Documentation by Doppler imaging of blood flow within the umbilical vein is diagnostic of portal hypertension (Gibson et al., 1989). Thus in a patient for whom ultrasonograms suggest chronic disease of the liver, it is worth searching for the umbilical vein (Plate XII). Hepatopetal blood

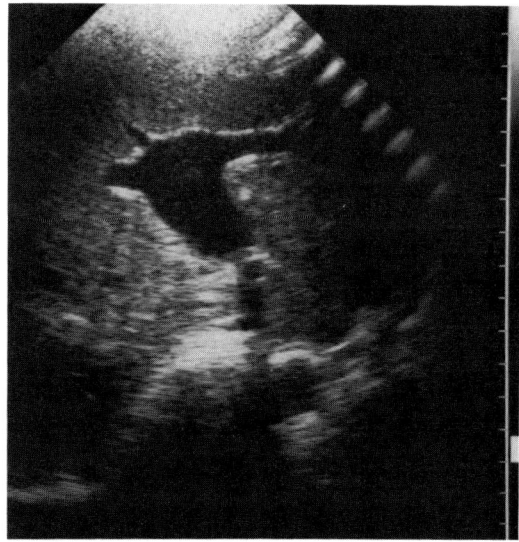

Figure 17-48. This patient, who had an established diagnosis of venous/lymphatic malformation associated with Klippel-Trenaunay syndrome, has irregular portal venous channels in the region of the head of the pancreas that coalesce to form an aneurysmal portal vein, as shown on this transverse scan.

flow through the left portal vein may not be perfusing the liver but may be supplying the venous drainage to a caput medusa around the umbilicus.

In summary, when the portal system in a child with known or suspected chronic hepatic disease is being evaluated, its patency should be assured, the spleen should be measured, and the presence of ascites shown or disproved. Doppler imaging should include investigation of the right, left, and main portal veins; the relationship of the splenic vein and the superior mesenteric vein; and the umbilical vein if it is visible. The lesser omental thickness should be noted, and Doppler sonography of the area attempted in order to document flow in coronal veins. The suprarenal inferior vena cava dilates if enough collateral blood flow reaches it, specifically through the left renal vein. Partial obstruction of the upper inferior vena cava by extrinsic pressure from the hypertrophied caudate lobe obliterates the typical triphasic pattern of its flow (Keller et al., 1989).

A common cause of portal hypertension in developing nations is infection with *Schistosoma*. The ova and, to a lesser extent, worms of *S. japonicum* and *S. mansoni* incite inflammatory and then fibrotic reactions after they reach portal venules from the gastrointestinal tract. Periportal fibrosis, also known as Symmer's or "clay pipestem" fibrosis, occurs in approximately 15.2 percent of older children and adolescents in endemic areas (Homeida et al., 1988).

Ultrasonography has been used as one method of judging the efficacy of chemotherapeutic intervention in endemic areas. Increased echogenicity in portal triads is typical of evolving fibrosis, and late findings on ultrasonography are those of chronic portal hypertension.

Obstruction to hepatic venous outflow has been termed the Budd-Chiari syndrome. The physician George Budd described the medical consequences in 1845, and the pathologist Hans Chiari described the pathology of "endophlebitis obliterans" in 1899 (McDermott et al., 1984). Patients who have an obstruction to hepatic venous outflow may present with insidious onset of hepatomegaly and ascites refractory to treatment or with acute pain in the right upper abdomen. The obstruction may be caused by congenital web in hepatic veins or inferior vena cava, by thrombosis of veins, or by veno-occlusive disease or be secondary to cardiac or pericardial disease. In children, congenital webs are the cause most likely to be diagnosed on ultrasonography (Plate XVI; Gentil-Kocher et al., 1988; Hoffman et al., 1987). In adults, who make up the majority of previously reported series, one is more likely to find tumor, polycythemia vera, paroxysmal nocturnal hemoglobinuria, hypercoagulopathy secondary to oral contraceptives, and so forth, as causes of hepatic venous thrombosis (Tavill et al., 1975; McDermott et al., 1984).

Scans of affected patients can be quite dramatic. The hepatic vein or veins, depending on the level and type of obstruction, can dilate. In chronic obstruction, the caudate lobe hypertrophies. Its venous drainage is directly into the inferior vena cava, and nodular regeneration seems to favor the caudate rather than other lobes (Tavill et al., 1975). Careful scanning of the inferior vena cava and hepatic veins at their juncture with the cava may reveal the web, if present, or the echogenic thrombus, if that is causing the obstruction. Angioplastic dilation of the congenital web may be curative if the vessel can be catheterized. Any child with or without pain but with hepatomegaly and ascites of unknown etiology should therefore be investigated with this syndrome in mind (Fig. 17–49).

Color Doppler ultrasonography has aided the investigation of postoperative shunts in children who have needed surgical intervention to palliate their portal hypertension. Splenorenal shunts are most commonly used in our institution, although we have examined children who have had mesocaval and portocaval anastomoses. Hepatofugal blood flow in the main portal vein is indirect evidence that a shunt is decompressing the portal system. The inferior vena cava usually dilates above the entrance of the shunt whether it is direct, as in portocaval anastomosis, or indirect, as in splenorenal anastomosis. In the latter situation, we are usually able to measure an increased diameter of the left renal vein and show increased blood flow in comparison with the preoperative baseline. Failure of the shunt is associated with clinical signs or symptoms related to variceal distention. Magnetic resonance imaging or angiography can follow ultrasonographic studies if repeat surgery is being considered.

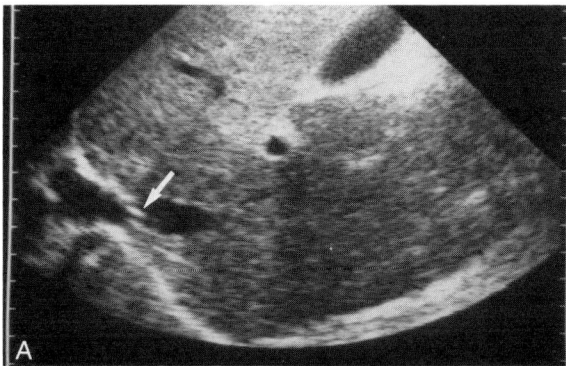
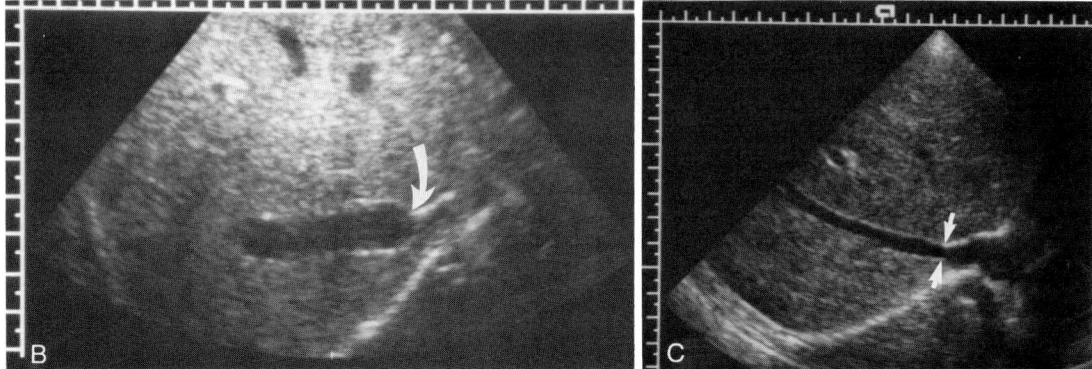

Figure 17–49. The original scans of this patient, who presented with hepatomegaly, failure to thrive, and ascites, showed a linear filling defect within the lumen of the inferior vena cava at its junction with the right hepatic vein. Oblique view (A) shows this filling defect as an echogenic flap (arrow). Transverse scan (B) shows dilation of the right hepatic vein, which narrows at its junction with the inferior vena cava (arrow). The left and middle hepatic veins drained via collaterals into the right hepatic vein. They had no separate insertions into the inferior vena cava. Inferior venacavography confirmed the diagnosis of Budd-Chiari syndrome associated with congenital web. Angioplastic dilation of the orifice of the right hepatic vein was undertaken. This transverse scan taken 1 month later (C) shows normal caliber of the right hepatic vein and the patent junction (arrows) between it and the inferior vena cava.

REFERENCES

Belli AM, Joseph AEA: The renal rind sign: A new ultrasound indication of inflammatory disease in the abdomen. Br J Radiol 1988; 61:806–810.

Boyden EA: The accessory gallbladder—An embryological and comparative study of aberrant biliary vesicles occurring in man and the domestic mammals. Amer J Anat 1926; 38:177–222.

Carroll BA, Oppenheimer DA, Muller HH: High-frequency real-time ultrasound of the neonatal biliary system. Radiology 1982; 145:437–440.

Patriquin HB, DiPietro M, Barber FE, et al: Sonography of thickened gallbladder wall: Causes in children. AJR 1983; 141:57–60.

Sarnaik S, Slovis TL, Corbett DP, et al: Incidence of cholelithiasis in sickle cell anemia using the ultrasonic gray-scale technique. J Pediatr 1980; 96:1005–1008.

Stringer DA, Dobranowski J, Ein SH, et al: Interposition of the gallbladder—or the absent common hepatic duct and cystic duct. Pediatr Radiol 1987; 17:151–153.

Willi U, Teele RL: Hepatic artery and "parallel channel" sign. JCU 1979; 7:125–127.

Jaundice in the Neonate

Abramson SJ, Treves S, Teele RL: The infant with possible biliary atresia: Evaluation by ultrasound and nuclear medicine. Pediatr Radiol 1982; 12:1–5.

Balistreri WF: Neonatal cholestasis. J Pediatr 1985; 106:171–184.

Fitzgerald JF: Cholestatic disorders of infancy. Pediatr Clin North Am 1988; 35:357–373.

Ikeda S, Sera Y, Akagi M: Serial ultrasonic examination to differentiate biliary atresia from neonatal hepatitis—Special reference to changes in size of the gallbladder. Eur J Pediatr 1989; 148:396–400.

Kasai M, Susuki H, Ohashi E, et al: Technique and results of operative management of biliary atresia. World J Surg 1978; 2:571–580.

Kirks DR, Coleman RE, Filston HC, et al: An imaging approach to persistent neonatal jaundice. AJR 1984; 142:461–465.

Landing BH: Considerations on the pathogenesis of neonatal hepatitis, biliary atresia, and choledochal cyst: The concept of infantile obstructive cholangiography. Prog Pediatr Surg 1974; 6:113–139.

McGahan JP, Phillips HE, Cox KL: Sonography of the normal pediatric gallbladder and biliary tract. Radiology 1982; 144:873–875.

Torrisi JM, Haller JO, Velcek FT: Choledochal cyst and biliary atresia in the neonate: Imaging findings in five cases. AJR 1990; 155:1273–1276.

Treem WR, Grant EE, Barth KH, et al: Ultrasound guided percutaneous cholecystocholangiography for early differentiation of cholestatic liver disease in infants. J Pediatr Gastroenterol Nutr 1988; 7:347–352.

Wanek EA, Horgan JG, Karrer FM, et al: Portal venous velocity in biliary atresia. J Pediatr Surg 1990; 25:146–148.

Diseases of the Biliary Tract, Congenital and Acquired

Alonso-Lej F, Rever WB, Pessagno DJ: Congenital choledochal cyst, with a report of 2, and an analysis of 94, cases. International Abstracts of Surgery 1959; 108:1–30.

Ando H, Ito T: Ultrasonic characteristics of tumefactive biliary sludge: A thixotropic phenomenon. JCU 1986; 14:289–292.

Babbit DP: Choledochal cyst: A concept of etiology. AJR 1973; 119:57–62.

Boechat MI, Querfeld U, Dietrich RB, et al: Large echogenic kidneys in biliary atresia. Ann Radiol 1986; 29:660–662.

Bowen AD: Acute gallbladder dilatation in a neonate: Emphasis on ultrasonography. J Pediatr Gastroenterol Nutr 1984; 3:304–306.

Bradford BF, Reid BS, Weinstein BJ, et al: Ultrasonographic evaluation of the gallbladder in mucocutaneous lymph node syndrome. Radiology 1982; 142:381–384.

Callahan J, Haller JO, Cacciarelli AA, et al: Cholelithiasis in infants: Association with total parenteral nutrition and furosemide. Radiology 1982; 143:437–439.

Caroli J: Disease of the intrahepatic biliary tree. Clin Gastroenterol 1972; 2:147–161.

Caroli J, Soupault R, Kossakowski J: La dilatation polykystique congénitale des voies biliares intrahépatiques: Essai de classification. Sem Hop Paris 1958; 34:488–495.

Carroll BA, Oppenheimer DA, Muller HH: High-frequency real-time ultrasound of the neonatal biliary system. Radiology 1982; 145:437–440.

Chang MH, Wang TH, Chen CC, et al: Congenital bile duct dilatation in children. J Pediatr Surg 1986; 21:112–117.

Choi YS, Sharma B: Gallbladder hydrops in mucocutaneous lymph node syndrome. South Med J 1989; 82:397–398.

Cohen EK, Stringer DA, Smith CR, et al: Hydrops of the gallbladder in typhoid fever as demonstrated by sonography. JCU 1986; 14:633–635.

Darweesh RM, Dodds WJ, Hogan WJ, et al: Roscoe Miller award. Fatty-meal sonography for evaluating patients with suspected partial common duct obstruction. AJR 1988; 151:63–68.

Davies CH, Stringer DA, Whyte H, et al: Congenital hepatic fibrosis with saccular dilatation of intrahepatic bile ducts and infantile polycystic kidneys. Pediatr Radiol 1986; 16:302–305.

El-Shafie M, Mah CL: Transient gallbladder distention in sick premature infants: The value of ultrasonography and radionuclide scintigraphy. Pediatr Radiol 1986; 16:468–471.

Ford WD, Sen S, Morris L, LeQuesne G: Spontaneous perforation of the common bile-duct in the neonate: Imaging and treatment. Aust Paediatr J 1988; 24:306–308.

Hammoudi SM, Alauddin A: Idiopathic perforation of the biliary tract in infancy and childhood. J Pediatr Surg 1988; 23:185–187.

Han BK: The biliary tract. Clin Diagn Ultrasound 1989; 24:129–155.

Henschke CI, Teele RL: Cholelithiasis in children: Recent observations. J Ultrasound Med 1983; 2:481–484.

Hyams JS, Baker E, Schwartz AN, et al: Acalculous cholecystitis in Crohn's disease. J Adolesc Health Care 1989; 10:151–154.

Keller MS, Markle BM, Laffey PA, et al: Spontaneous resolution of cholelithiasis in infants. Radiology 1985; 157:345–348.

Kirks DR: John Caffey Award: Lithiasis due to interruption of the enterohepatic circulation of bile salts. AJR 1979; 133:383–388.

Levine J, Seidman E, Teele RL, Walker WA: Gallbladder wall thickening in acute hepatitis. J Pediatr Gastroenterol Nutr 1986; 5:147–149.

Lilly JR: The surgical treatment of choledochal cyst. Surg Gynecol Obstet 1979; 149:36–42.

Marchal GJ, Desmet VJ, Proesmans WC, et al: Caroli disease: High frequency US and pathologic findings. Radiology 1986; 158:507–511.

McAlister WH, Siegel MJ: Pediatric radiology case of the day: Congenital hepatic fibrosis with saccular dilatation of the intrahepatic bile ducts and infantile polycystic kidneys. AJR 1989; 152:1329–1330.

Nzeh DA, Adedoyin MA: Sonographic pattern of gallbladder disease in children with sickle cell anaemia. Pediatr Radiol 1989; 19:290–292.

O'Neill JA, Templeton JM, Schnaufer L, et al: Recent experience with choledochal cyst. Ann Surg 1987; 205:533–540.

Palasciano G, Portincasa P, Vinciguerra V, et al: Gallstone prevalence and gallbladder volume in children and adolescents: An epidemiological ultrasonographic survey and relationship to body mass index. Am J Gastroenterol 1989; 84:1378–1382.

Papanicolau N, Abramson SJ, Teele RL, et al: Specific preoperative diagnosis of choledochal cysts by combined sonography and hepatobiliary scintigraphy. Ann Radiol 1985; 28:276–282.

Pariente D, Bernard O, Gauthier F, et al: Radiological treatment of common bile duct lithiasis in infancy. Pediatr Radiol 1989; 19:104–107.

Patriquin HB, DiPietro M, Barber FE, et al: Sonography of thickened gallbladder wall: Causes in children. AJR 1983; 141:57–60.

Peevy KJ, Wiseman HJ: Neonatal gallbladder distention. Am J Dis Child 1982; 136:1030.

Ramey SL, Williams JL: Nephrolithiasis and cholelithiasis in a premature infant. JCU 1986; 14:203–206.

Robertson JF, Carachi R, Sweet EM, et al: Cholelithiasis in childhood: A follow-up study. J Pediatr Surg 1988; 23:246–249.

Roca M, Sellier N, Mensire A, et al: Acute acalculous cholecystitis in salmonella infection. Pediatr Radiol 1988; 18:421–423.

Roslyn JJ, Berquist WE, Pitt HA, et al: Increased risk of gallstones in children receiving total parenteral nutrition. Pediatrics 1983; 71:784–789.

Rumley TO, Rodgers BM: Hydrops of the gallbladder in children. J Pediatr Surg 1983; 18:138–140.

Sarnaik S, Slovis TL, Corbett DP, et al: Incidence of cholelithiasis in sickle cell anemia using the ultrasonic gray-scale technique. J Pediatr 1980; 96:1005–1008.

Schaad UB, Wedgwood-Krucko J, Tschaeppeler H: Reversible ceftriaxone-associated biliary pseudolithiasis in children. Lancet 1988; 2:1411–1413.

Schroeder D, Smith L, Prain HC: Antenatal diagnosis of choledochal cyst at 15 weeks' gestation: Etiologic implications and management. J Pediatr Surg 1989; 24:936–938.

Sherman P, Kolster E, Davies C, et al: Choledochal cysts: Heterogeneity of clinical presentation. J Pediatr Gastroenterol Nutr 1986; 5:867–872.

Sisto A, Feldman P, Garel L, et al: Primary sclerosing cholangitis in children: Study of five cases and review of the literature. Pediatrics 1987; 80:918–923.

Suarez F, Bernard O, Gauthier F, et al: Bilio-pancreatic

common channel in children: Clinical, biological and radiological findings in 12 children. Pediatr Radiol 1986; 17:206–211.
Suddleson EA, Reid B, Woolley MM, et al: Hydrops of the gallbladder associated with Kawasaki syndrome. J Pediatr Surg 1987; 22:956–959.
Teele RL, Nussbaum AR, Wyly JB, et al: Cholelithiasis after spinal fusion for scoliosis in children. J Pediatr 1987; 111:857–860.
Todani T, Watanabe Y, Fujii T, et al: Anomalous arrangement of the pancreatobiliary ductal system in patients with a choledochal cyst. Am J Surg 1984; 147:672–676.
Treem WR, Malet PF, Gourley GR, et al: Bile and stone analysis in two infants with brown pigment gallstones and infected bile. Gastroenterology 1989; 96:519–523.
Vernick LJ, Kuller LH: Cholecystectomy and right-sided colon cancer: An epidemiological study. Lancet 1981; 1:381–383.
Webb DK, Darby JS, Dunn DT, et al: Gallstones in Jamaican children with homozygous sickle cell disease. Arch Dis Child 1989; 64:693–696.
Wiedmeyer DA, Stewart ET, Dodds WJ, et al: Choledochal cyst: Findings on cholangiopancreatography with emphasis on ectasia of the common channel. AJR 1989; 153:969–972.
Willi U, Reddish J, Teele RL: Cystic fibrosis: Its characteristic appearance on abdominal ultrasound. AJR 1980; 134:1005–1010.

Normal and Abnormal Hepatic Parenchyma

Auh YH, Rubenstein WA, Zirinsky K, et al: Accessory fissures of the liver: CT and sonographic appearance. AJR 1984; 143:565–572.
Cançado ELR, Rocha M de S, Barbosa ER, et al: Abdominal ultrasonography in hepatolenticular degeneration: A study of 33 patients. Arq Neuropsiquiatr 1987; 45:131–136.
Dittrich M, Milde S, Dinkel E, et al: Sonographic biometry of liver and spleen size in childhood. Pediatr Radiol 1983; 13:206–211.
Garra BS, Shawker TH, Chang R, et al: The ultrasound appearance of radiation-induced hepatic injury: Correlation with computed tomography and magnetic resonance imaging. J Ultrasound Med 1988; 7:605–609.
Giorgio A, Amoroso P, Fico P, et al: Ultrasound evaluation of uncomplicated and complicated acute viral hepatitis. JCU 1986; 14:675–679.
Henschke CI, Goldman H, Teele RL: The hyperechogenic liver in children: Cause and sonographic appearance. AJR 1982; 138:841–846.
Madigan SM, Teele RL: Ultrasonography of the liver and biliary tree in children. Semin Ultrasound 1984; 5:68–84.
Markisz JA, Treves ST, Davis RT: Normal hepatic and splenic size in children: Scintigraphic determination. Pediatr Radiol 1987; 17:273–276.
Sexton CC, Zeman RK: Correlation of computed tomography, sonography, and gross anatomy of the liver. AJR 1983; 141:711–718.
Taylor KJ, Riely CA, Hammers L, et al: Quantitative US attenuation in normal liver and in patients with diffuse liver disease: Importance of fat. Radiology 1986; 160:65–71.

Fibrosis/Cirrhosis*

Abdel-Wahab MF, Esmat G, Narooz SI, et al: Sonographic studies of schoolchildren in a village endemic

---

*See also Chapter 18, Hepatic Transplantation.

for *Schistosoma mansoni*. Trans R Soc Trop Med Hyg 1990; 84:69–73.
Fellows KE, Grand RJ, Colodny AH, et al: Combined portal and vena caval hypertension in Gaucher disease: The value of preoperative venography. J Pediatr 1975; 87:739–743.
Homeida MA, Cheever AW, Bennett JC: Diagnosis of pathologically confirmed Symmers' periportal fibrosis by ultrasonography: A prospective blinded study. Am J Trop Med 1988; 38:86–91.
Mitchell SE, Gross BH, Spitz HB: The hypoechoic caudate lobe: An ultrasonic pseudolesion. Radiology 1982; 144:569–572.
Patriquin HB, Roy CC, Weber AM, et al: Liver disease and portal hypertension. Clin Diagn Ultrasound 1989; 24:103–127.

Acquired and Congenital Abnormality of Hepatic Vasculature

Alvarez F, Bernard O, Brunelle F: Portal obstruction in children. J Pediatr 1983; 103:696–702.
Bellah RD, Hayek J, Teele RL: Anomalous portal venous connection to the suprahepatic vena cava: Sonographic demonstration. Pediatr Radiol 1989; 20:115–117.
Bellamy EA, Bossi MC, Cosgrove DO: Ultrasound demonstration of changes in the normal portal venous system following a meal. Br J Radiol 1984; 57:147–149.
Bret PM, de Stempel JV, Atri M, et al: Intrahepatic bile duct and portal vein anatomy revisited. Radiology 1988; 169:405–407.
Frider B, Marin AM, Goldberg A: Ultrasonographic diagnosis of portal vein cavernous transformation in children. J Ultrasound Med 1989; 8:445–449.
Gentil-Kocher S, Bernard O, Brunelle F, et al: Budd-Chiari syndrome in children: Report of 22 cases. J Pediatr 1988; 113:30–38.
Gibson RN, Gibson PR, Donlan JD, et al: Identification of a patent paraumbilical vein by using Doppler sonography: Importance in the diagnosis of portal hypertension. AJR 1989; 153:513–516.
Goyal AK, Pokharna DS, Sharma SK: Effects of a meal on normal and hypertensive portal venous system: A quantitative ultrasonographic assessment. Gastrointest Radiol 1989; 14:164–166.
Goyal AK, Pokharna DS, Sharma SK: Ultrasonic measurements of portal vasculature in diagnosis of portal hypertension: A controversial subject reviewed. J Ultrasound Med 1990; 9:45–48.
Gray H: *Gray's Anatomy* (30th American ed; Clemente C, ed). Philadelphia: Lea & Febiger, 1985, p 735.
Hoffman HD, Stockland B, von der Hayden U: Membranous obstruction of the inferior vena cava with Budd-Chiari syndrome in children: A report of nine cases. J Pediatr Gastroenterol Nutr 1987; 6:878–884.
Keller MS, Taylor KJW, Riely CA: Pseudoportal Doppler signal in the partially obstructed inferior vena cava. Radiology 1989; 170:474–477.
McCarten KM, Teele RL: Preduodenal portal vein: Venography, ultrasonography, and review of the literature. Ann Radiol 1978; 21:155–160.
McDermott WV, Stone MD, Bothe A Jr, et al: Budd-Chiari syndrome. Historical and clinical review with an analysis of surgical corrective procedures. Am J Surg 1984; 147:463–467.
Miller VE, Berland LL: Pulsed Doppler duplex sonography and CT of portal vein thrombosis. AJR 1985; 145:73–76.
Morse SS, Taylor KJW, Strauss EB, et al: Congenital absence of the portal vein in oculoauriculovertebral

dysplasia (Goldenhar syndrome). Pediatr Radiol 1986; 16:437–439.

Nakamura T, Moriyasu F, Ban N, et al: Hemodynamic analysis of postsplenectomy portal thrombosis using ultrasonic Doppler duplex system. Am J Gastroenterol 1987; 82:1212–1216.

Ohnishi K, Saito M, Nakayama T, et al: Portal venous hemodynamics in chronic liver disease: Effects of posture change and exercise. Radiology 1985; 155:757–761.

Pariente D, Gentil S, Brunelle F, et al: Budd-Chiari syndrome in children: Radiologic investigation. Ann Radiol 1987; 30:518–524.

Parvey HR, Eisenberg RL, Giyanani V, et al: Duplex sonography of the portal venous system: Pitfalls and limitations. AJR 1989; 152:765–770.

Patriquin H, Lafortune M, Burns PN, et al: Duplex Doppler examination in portal hypertension: Technique and anatomy. AJR 1987; 149:71–76.

Patriquin H, Tessier G, Grignon A, et al: Lesser omental thickness in normal children: Baseline for detection of portal hypertension. AJR 1985; 145:693–696.

Powell-Jackson PR, Karani J, Ede RJ, et al: Ultrasound scanning and 99mTc sulphur colloid scintigraphy in diagnosis of Budd-Chiari syndrome. Gut 1986; 27:1502–1506.

Raby N, Meire HB: Duplex Doppler ultrasound in the diagnosis of cavernous transformation of the portal vein. Br J Radiol 1988; 61:586–588.

Rizzo AJ, Haller JO, Mulvihill DM, et al: Calcification of the ductus venosus: A cause of right upper quadrant calcification in the newborn. Radiology 1989; 173:89–90.

Salmi A, Paterlini A: Sonographic patent umbilical vein: Lack of specificity for portal hypertension. Am J Gastroenterol 1986; 81:556–558.

Sellier N, Adamsbaum C, Checoury A, et al: Sonographic hepatic arterialisation in newborns receiving parenteral nutrition. Pediatr Radiol 1988; 18:471–473.

Slovis TL, Haller JO, Cohen HL, et al: Complicated appendiceal inflammatory disease in children: Pylephlebitis and liver abscess. Radiology 1989; 171:823–825.

Tavill AS, Wood EJ, Kreel L, et al: The Budd-Chiari syndrome: Correlation between hepatic scintigraphy and the clinical, radiological, and pathological findings in nineteen cases of hepatic venous outflow obstruction. Gastroenterology 1975; 68:509–518.

Tudway D, Sangster G: Ultrasound diagnosis of portal vein thrombosis following splenectomy. Postgrad Med J 1986; 62:1153–1156.

Zalcman M, Van Gansbeke D, Matos C, et al: Sonographic demonstration of portal venous system thromboses secondary to inflammatory diseases of the pancreas. Gastrointest Radiol 1987; 12:114–116.

CHAPTER 18

HEPATIC TRANSPLANTATION

PREOPERATIVE EVALUATION

Of the children who undergo hepatic transplantation at our hospital, many have had hepatic failure from biliary atresia. It is apparent from our data that 60 percent of our patients are included in this category. Many of those who have biliary atresia weigh less than 10 kg when transplantation becomes necessary; thus we are faced with evaluating small babies with their correspondingly small anatomy. The other 40 percent of patients are children who have had unusual diseases such as neonatal hemochromatosis, fulminant hepatitis, metabolic disease, alpha$_1$-antitrypsin deficiency, or cryptogenic cirrhosis. The specific issues to be addressed by the ultrasonographer during the child's evaluation, before transplantation, are listed below.

SIZE, SHAPE, AND PARENCHYMAL PATTERN OF THE LIVER. An overtly small liver, shrunken by cirrhosis, hinders replacement with a normal liver because the abdominal cavity has adapted to the small volume of the diseased liver. The parenchymal pattern of the liver is usually that of increased echogenicity, the intensity of which roughly parallels the degree of hepatic fibrosis.

VOLUME OF ASCITES. This may be either under- or overestimated by the clinician. Gross ascites keeps the abdominal cavity distended and the skin stretched. To some degree this is helpful in placing the graft, which is usually bigger than the recipient's diseased liver. Ascites should be clear—that is, echofree. Bloody or infected ascites is echogenic.

SPLEEN. Splenic size increases as portal hypertension increases. Good baseline scans of the spleen help in tracking postoperative complications such as portosplenic thrombosis with resultant splenic necrosis.

VARICES. Esophageal varices increase the thickness of the lesser omentum (Patriquin et al., 1985). Even when varices are not obvious as discrete channels, Doppler scanning of the area may register a venous signal. Spontaneous splenorenal shunts result in enlargement of the left renal vein and prominence of the inferior vena cava above the renal venous connection (Fig. 18–1). Large varices may also be traced around the pancreas and duodenum to the retroperitoneum, and the umbilical vein may be patent (Plate XII; Gibson et al., 1989). Surgeons appreciate information regarding the presence and extent of varices. Intraoperative bleeding often is related to manipulation of these thin-walled veins. Although there is little that surgeons can do to avoid varices, the patient can undergo plasmapheresis immediately before surgery. This procedure decreases intraoperative bleeding by reversing the coagulopathy. There is one benefit from plentiful collateral shunts: they protect the bowel and spleen from intraoperative ischemia when the patient's portal vein is clamped and cut.

VENOUS AND ARTERIAL SUPPLY TO THE LIVER. Portal hypertension results in gradual diminution of hepatopetal portal venous blood flow. The hepatic artery tends to

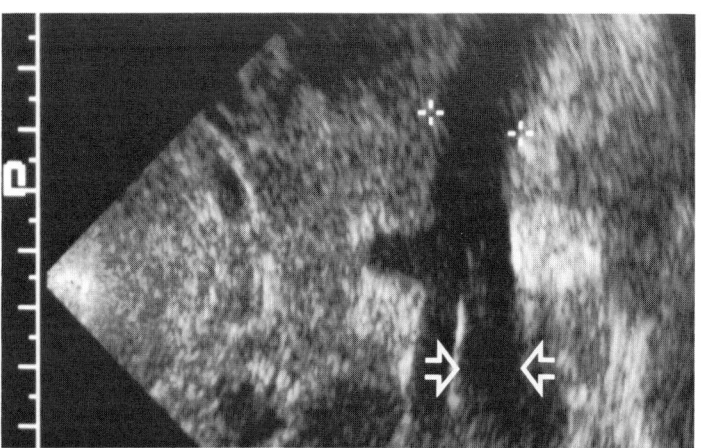

Figure 18–1. This is a coronal scan through the right flank in a 9-year-old boy whose liver disease was congenital hepatic fibrosis. Because of spontaneous splenorenal shunting, the left renal vein (open arrows) was hugely distended, and the increased flow also dilated the inferior vena cava (between crosses) above the renal vein. The figure is oriented so that the top is craniad and bottom is caudad.

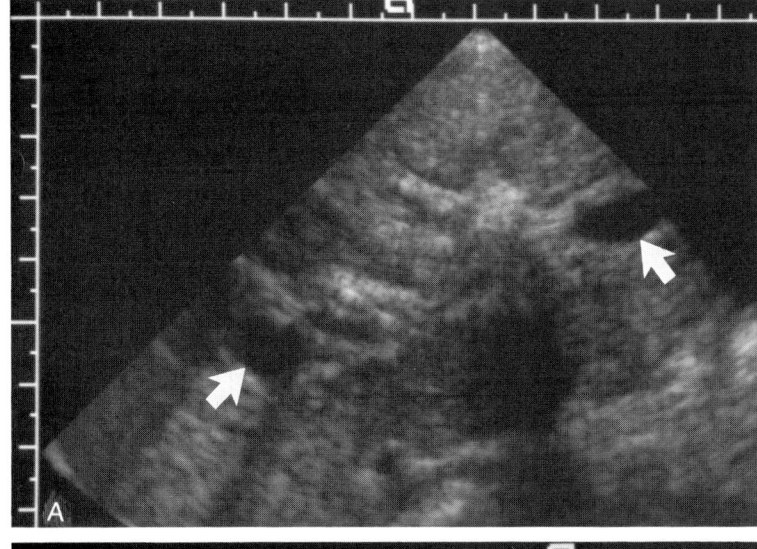
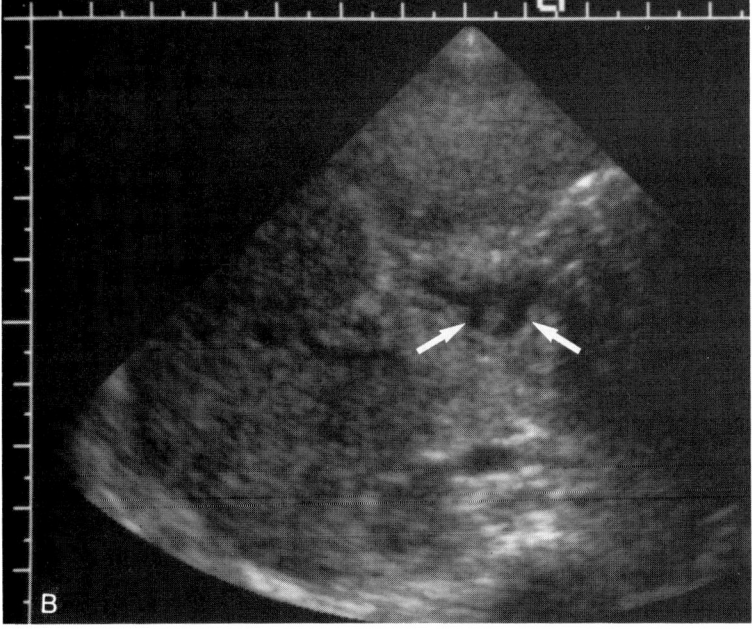

Figure 18–2. Transverse scans of the liver (**A**) show two bile lakes (arrows) in this child who has biliary atresia and who has undergone the Kasai procedure. Color-flow Doppler ultrasonography was used to make sure that neither of these echolucent areas was vascular. **B** is a scan at the level of the porta hepatis. There is fluid, presumably bile, in the loop of small bowel that is anastomosed to the hilum of the liver (arrows).

enlarge and become the major supplier of hepatic blood. Size (i.e., diameter) of the portal vein does not translate readily into measurements of intraluminal pressure or of blood flow. However, it is apparent from sequential scans that a child who is developing portal hypertension usually has a gradual diminution in size of the portal vein as cirrhosis progresses. The surgeon likes to be able to see a portal vein with a diameter of 4 mm at the porta hepatis. It must be emphasized that we tend to perform scans while children are fasting. The size and characteristics of blood flow in the portal vein change, depending on the splanchnic bed. Scans performed after feeding may be very different from those performed before feeding (Goyal et al., 1990).

The preoperative examination of vasculature must not be limited to the portal venous system. The transplantation involves anastomosis of the hepatic arterial supply and the hepatic venous drainage. Determination of the anatomy vis-à-vis branching of the celiac and superior mesenteric arteries, or the presence of a common celiac–mesenteric trunk or replaced right hepatic artery, are all useful mapping procedures. We remember with chagrin our failure to document, preoperatively, the presence of a normal inferior vena cava in the first baby to undergo hepatic transplantation at our hospital. Its absence, thereby making a difficult procedure even more difficult, was first recognized in the operating room. Since then we have looked for the inferior vena cava in *every* patient.

BILIARY TREE. In most children awaiting transplantation, biliary atresia is the reason for their hepatic failure, and most have already undergone a Kasai procedure or similar portoenterostomy for drainage of what little bile is produced and transported. Thus the gallbladder has already been removed, and a normal biliary tree is nonexistent. The liver may be flecked with bile lakes, and depending on the type of enterostomy, fluid may be present in the Roux-en-Y loop of small bowel at the porta hepatis (Fig. 18–2). In children for whom metabolic disease is the cause of hepatic failure, gallstones may be present.

POSTOPERATIVE EVALUATION

The fancy needlework required in order to fit a donated liver into a small child makes postoperative evaluation with ultrasonography dependent on good descriptions of the procedure—preferably from the person who performed the surgery. Placement of drainage tubes and catheters is evident from plain radiographs. Usually there are two Jackson-Pratt drains around the liver and a catheter in the biliary tree. This biliary catheter stints the anastomosis between the common bile duct of the donor liver and the efferent limb of the jejunal Roux-en-Y of the host. The catheter is brought through the intestinal and abdominal walls. This allows direct observation of the bile that is produced by the donor liver. All catheters generally create an echogenic focus and often a shadow (Fig. 18–3). Their presence, therefore, should be anticipated before the ultrasonographic examination.

Immediate postoperative scans are performed in semisterile conditions. The examiner wears a mask, gloves, and a nonsterile but clean gown over street clothes. The transducer is washed with germicidal cleanser and then sterile saline; the acoustic couplant is sterile. We have not used a plastic cover over the transducer as in intraoperative work, but this may be a requirement by some transplant units. The scans are performed through available windows on the anterior and lateral abdominal wall. The incision is chevron-shaped and extends across the abdomen under the costal margin. Stab wounds for drainage catheters are inferior to the incision. Our surgeons use staples to close the skin, but we avoid the incision line anyway in order to lessen the chance of infection, to reduce pain, and to avoid artifact. Most children remain intubated for 1 or 2 days after surgery or are heavily sedated. Extra medication for pain should be given before scanning if needed. If scans are performed immediately after surgery, air in the peritoneal cavity around the liver may interfere with scanning.

It is ideal if two people can collaborate in performing the immediate postoperative scans: one scanning and the other changing the settings on the ultrasound unit and labeling the films. Ultrasonographic studies are directed toward addressing the following issues.

PERIHEPATIC COLLECTIONS. Blood or bile (if a leak in the biliary anastomosis is present) may collect around the transplanted liver. The fissure formed by the falciform ligament seems to be a common site for accumulation of blood because it is anterior to the Jackson-Pratt drains (Fig. 18–4). De-

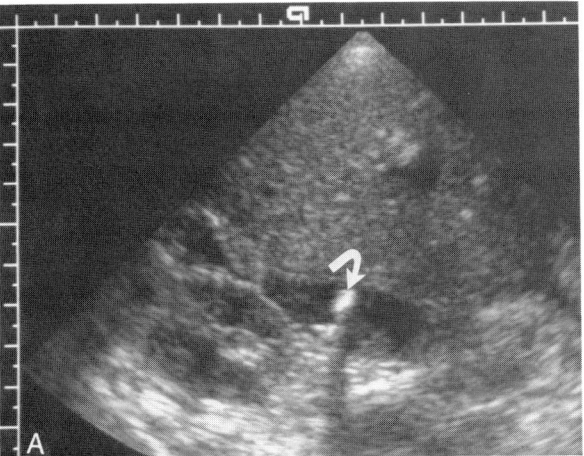
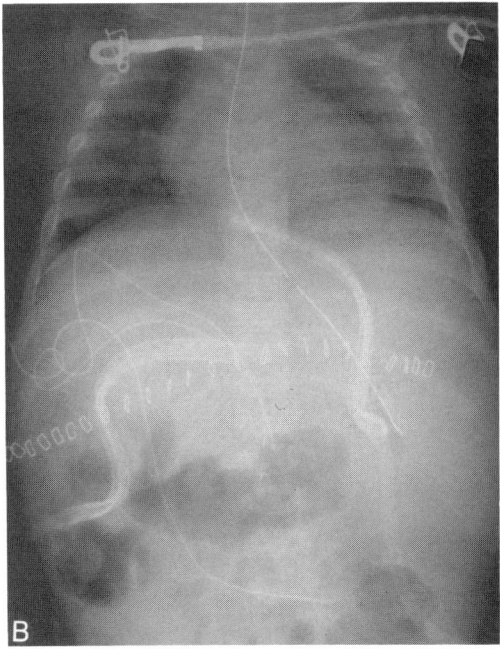

Figure 18–3. The shadowing echogenic focus (arrow, **A**) is a drainage catheter within a subhepatic collection. The catheter was intermittently draining bile. Connection between the common bile duct, the Roux-en-Y loop of small bowel, and the distal small bowel had been disrupted by infection after transplantation. This postoperative radiograph (**B**) is typical of most children who have undergone transplantation of the liver. The endotracheal tube, nasogastric tube, and cardiac leads are present over or in the chest. Jackson-Pratt drainage catheters, two biliary stents, and staples along the incision are present in the abdomen.

pending on how long the hemorrhage has been present, any collection may be echogenic, echolucent, or mixed in appearance. Bleeding is far more common when part of a liver, rather than a complete organ, has been transplanted. Biliary leakage, which is uncommon, may lead to accumulation of fluid in the porta hepatis or subhepatic space (Fig. 18–3).

HEPATIC PARENCHYMAL PATTERN. The hepatic parenchyma should be as uniformly echogenic as a normal liver. Immediately postoperatively there is often a fuzzy echogenic cuff around portal vasculature.

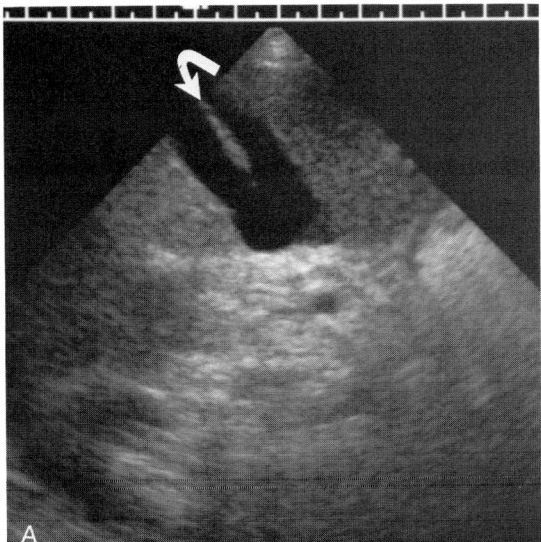
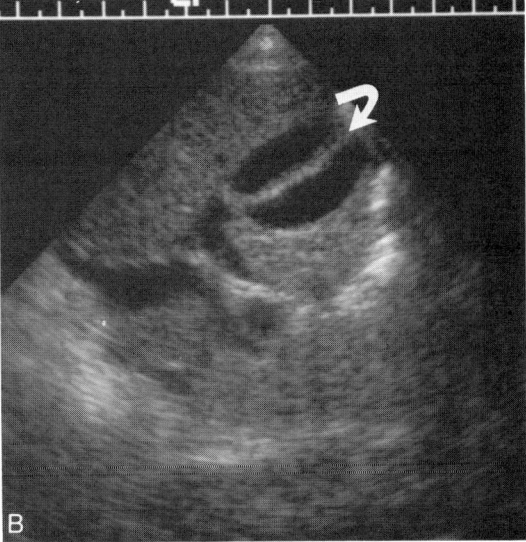

Figure 18–4. Transverse (**A**) and longitudinal (**B**) scans show fluid, presumably blood, around the falciform ligament (arrow) of the transplanted liver 3 days after the surgery.

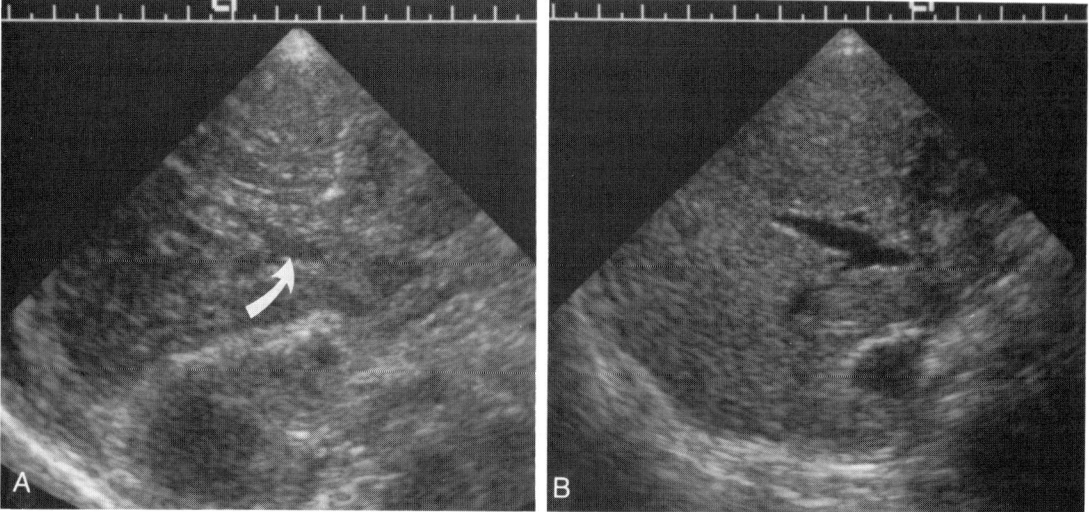

Figure 18–5. These two transverse scans were taken 1 month apart. The first, taken immediately after transplantation of the liver in this child who had biliary atresia, shows the portal vein (arrow) surrounded by an echogenic cuff (A), which disappeared 1 month later (B). Periportal echogenicity appears to represent edema, which clears with time.

This cuff correlates with edema on computed tomography (CT) scans, is fairly common, and seems to have no prognostic significance (Fig. 18–5). Air in the portal venous system of hepatic grafts has been identified in some adult patients. This results in a speckled pattern in the liver. We have encountered this in one child who, at the time, had gram-negative bacterial sepsis. Air in the biliary tree is not rare, inasmuch as most children have anastomosis between the bile duct of the graft to the Roux-en-Y limb of the small bowel (Fig. 18–6). Ischemia of the liver results from global or local lack of perfusion (Fig. 18–7). An ischemic liver tends to be echolucent, but because it then may become infected from bacteria that ascend through the anastomosis between biliary duct and bowel, abscess often ensues and the pattern becomes mixed. Ultrasonography can show no specific abnormality in the hepatic parenchymal pattern that signals acute or chronic rejection. Ultrasonography can be used to guide a biopsy, which is the best method by which to diagnose rejection.

VASCULATURE. The portal venous junction between graft and host is an oblique end-to-end anastomosis. The hepatic arterial

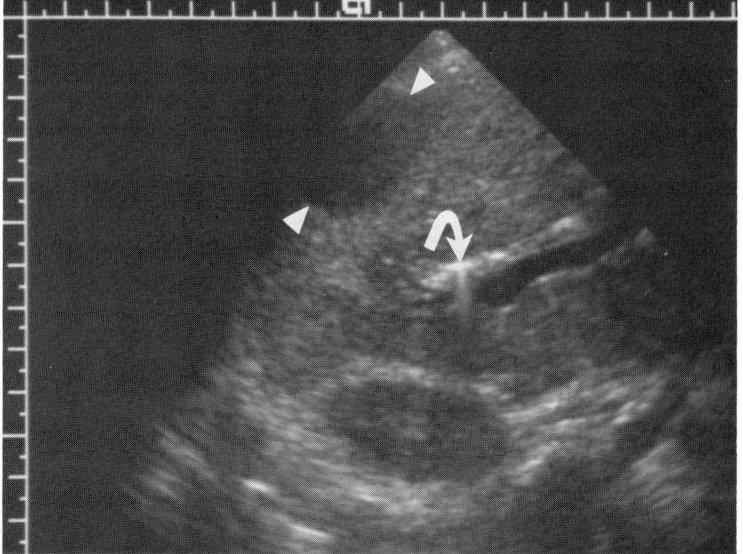

Figure 18–6. Air in the biliary tree presents as echogenic foci with dirty, "comet tail" shadowing (arrow). Air reaches the biliary tree via the Roux-en-Y limb of the small bowel in children who have had previous biliary atresia. Because these children have no common bile duct of their own available for anastomosis to the common bile duct from the graft, the small bowel is needed as a conduit for bile. Retrograde seeding, with enteric flora, is likely responsible for formation of abscesses in a child whose liver is poorly oxygenated. Note the subcapsular collection (arrowheads). This child, who had undergone transplantation 5 years previously, had had multiple episodes of gram-negative sepsis and required drainage of this abscess.

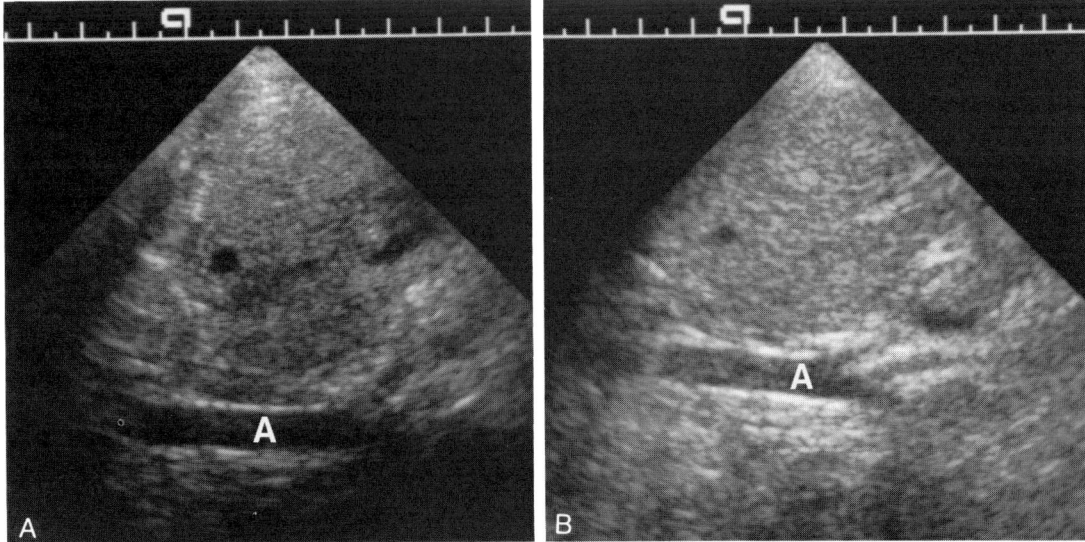

Figure 18–7. This boy was 18 months old when he underwent transplantation for liver disease secondary to ornithine-transcarbamylase deficiency. Ultrasonography performed several days after transplantation showed patchy inhomogeneity of the left lobe of the liver, anterior to the aorta, seen on the longitudinal scan (**A**). This was associated with no recognizable Doppler signal from the left hepatic artery. He was managed conservatively, and luckily, infection did not supervene. One month later, a longitudinal scan showed that the left lobe (**B**) was close to normal in appearance. This was associated with a reappearance of the left hepatic arterial signal. The presumption is that arterial flow to the left lobe was reestablished after a thrombus lysed or the artery was recanalized. A = aorta.

anastomosis may vary between patients, depending on the anatomy. A cuff of aorta is typically taken with the graft, which is then spliced into the crotch between the gastroduodenal and hepatic arteries of the host, in order that the anastomotic channel be as capacious as possible. This is of particular importance in babies who weigh less than 10 kg because hepatic arterial thrombosis is a major complication when vessels are very small. Between the vena cava of the graft and host, the anastomosis is end to end above the renal veins. The vena cava from the graft replaces that of the host throughout the intrahepatic course (Figs. 18–8, 18–9). For

Figure 18–8. Longitudinal scan of the cava after transplantation of the liver shows irregularity of the lumen at the level of the anastomosis (arrow) between the vessel of the host and the intrahepatic portion that accompanies the graft.

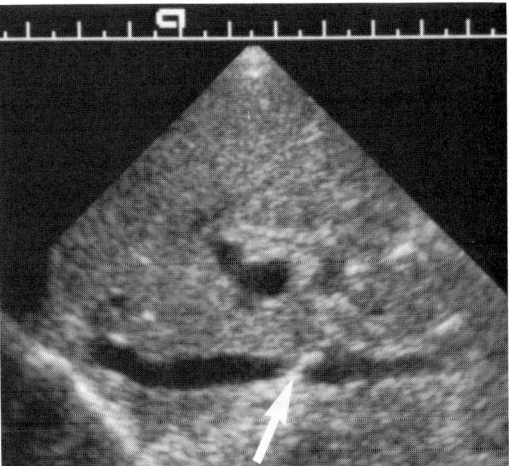

Figure 18–9. Occasionally, the anastomotic line between the two inferior venae cavae presents as an echogenic line across the lumen (arrow), as in this child.

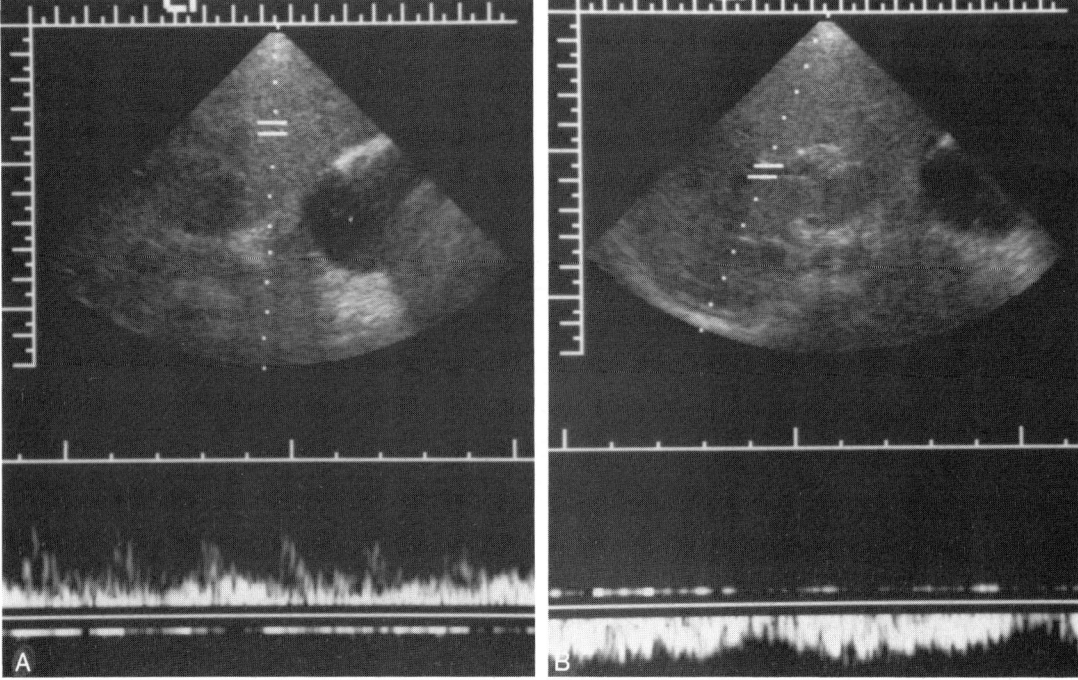

Figure 18-10. Pulsed Doppler ultrasonography is extremely useful for documenting the presence of arterial and portal venous flow. The transverse scan of the left lobe of the liver (A) shows superimposition of the left hepatic arterial and left portal venous signals, both appropriate in their hepatopetal direction. If one scans the right portal vein from the anterior approach (B), normal portal flow appears to be moving away from the transducer. Right hepatic arterial flow could also be documented in this patient, thereby establishing the fact that vascular anastomoses between graft and host were patent.

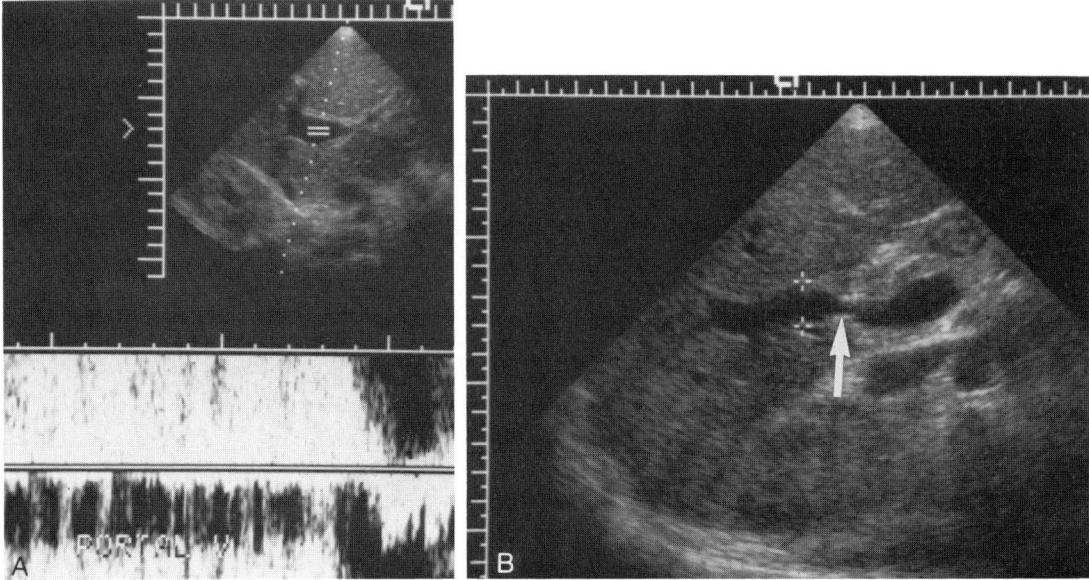

Figure 18-11. Turbulence just distal to the portal venous anastomosis (A) is associated with narrowing at the suture line (B). Crosses mark the portal vein of the graft, distal to the anastomotic narrowing (arrow). An oblique end-to-end anastomosis is now used to avoid the complication of circumferential narrowing that is evident in this patient.

evaluating the vasculature, color Doppler imaging has changed what used to be an hour's chore to several minutes' work. Color instantly demonstrates the hepatic vasculature, and the cursor of pulsed Doppler imaging can be placed on the colored vessels to identify them as venous or arterial. Because blood flow in both the portal vein and the hepatic artery is hepatopetal, their colored signals tend to blur together and present as one vessel. Pulsed Doppler imaging has to be used to discriminate between them (Fig. 18–10). We trace the hepatic artery and the portal vein from their respective anastomoses into each hepatic lobe. In order to be as parallel as possible to direction of flow, coronal scans are best for demonstrating right lobar vessels. Axial scans below the xiphoid process can be used to investigate left lobar vessels. Longitudinal or coronal scans can be used to view the inferior vena cava. Turbulence at the anastomotic sites is typical, but there should be blood flow beyond anastomoses (Fig. 18–11). Failure to demonstrate blood flow implies thrombosis of the affected vessel. Oxygen, as provided by the blood in the hepatic artery, is crucial to an already ischemic graft. It used to be thought that hepatic arterial thrombosis was an instant indication for retransplantation (Flint et al., 1988). The lack of available organs made surgeons at our hospital fathers of invention: They were able to nurse several babies through this complication by aggressive medical care, aided by percutaneous drainage of infected ischemic areas (Fig. 18–12; Hoffer et al., 1988). It appears that rearterialization of the graft may occur through collaterals provided by the

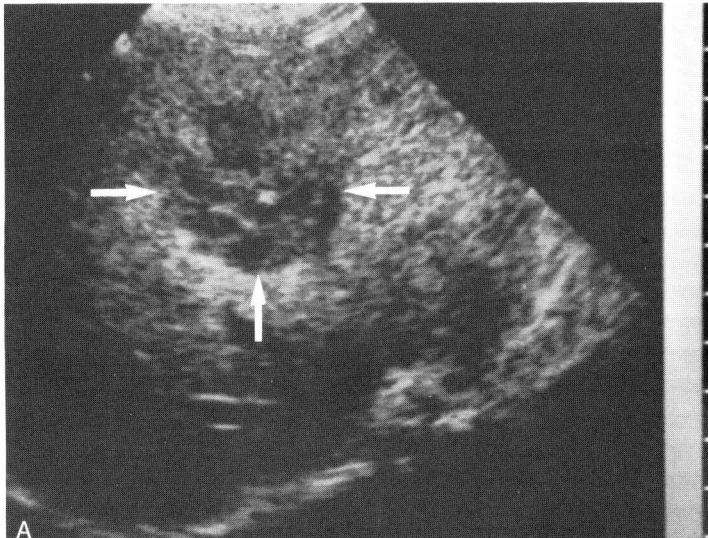

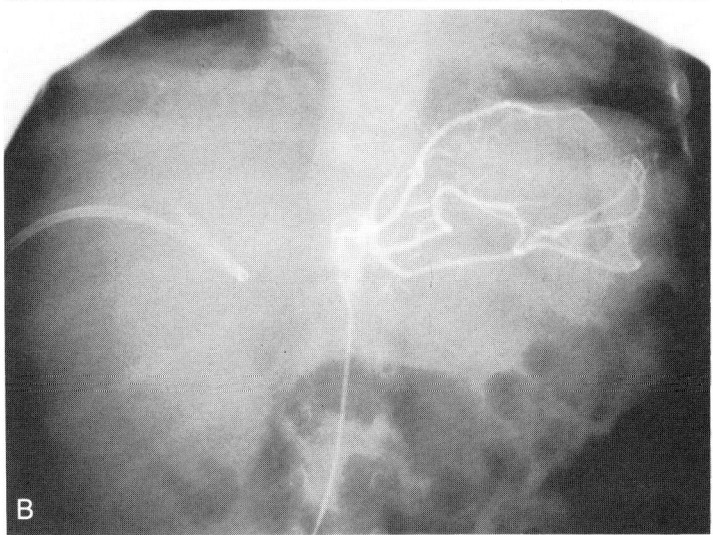

Figure 18–12. This transverse scan (A) was performed in 1984. It belongs to a little boy who was our first transplant patient. At the time the study was done, we had no Doppler equipment to aid us in assessing hepatic vasculature. The lucent mass within the liver (arrows) represented an abscess. We drained this percutaneously and then proceeded to angiography. The selective study of the celiac axis (B) showed no flow to the liver through the hepatic artery. Because no other liver was available for transplantation, this child was treated with antibiotics, oxygen, and percutaneous drainage of a second abscess in the right lobe that developed 1 week later. Gradually, he recovered and survived, which proved that hepatic arterial thrombosis is not a uniformly lethal situation requiring retransplantation.

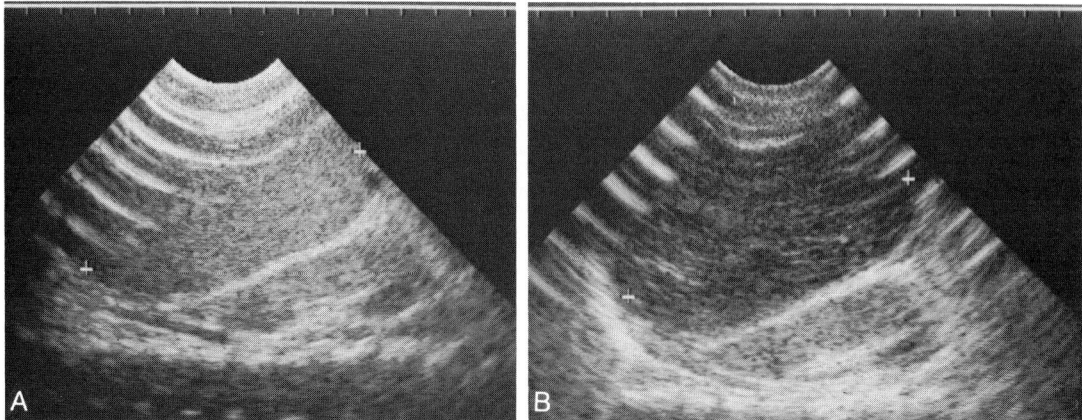

Figure 18–13. These coronal scans of the spleen were taken 5 days apart. In the interim, portal venous thrombosis, which followed hepatic transplantation, extended retrograde into the splenic vein. The first scan **(A)** is a limited coronal view of the spleen, but it shows normal splenic parenchymal pattern. Splenic infarction resulted in the ultrasonographic appearance of a diffusely lucent spleen **(B)**. This baby died shortly thereafter.

superior mesenteric artery via the Roux-en-Y loop of the jejunum (Hall et al., 1990). Thus an arterial signal within the liver has reemerged where previously there was none.

Portal venous thrombosis is less frequent a complication and less acutely serious than arterial obstruction. However, portal venous obstruction forces blood flow into the collateral pathways previously established when the host's liver failed. Variceal bleeding may result if collateral venous drainage is sparse. In addition, portal thrombosis may extend, retrograde, into the splenic vein and cause splenic infarction (Fig. 18–13; Plate XVII).

Abrupt damping of the normally pulsatile flow of hepatic veins has been associated both with cholangitis and with rejection (Coulden et al., 1990). It is worthwhile to

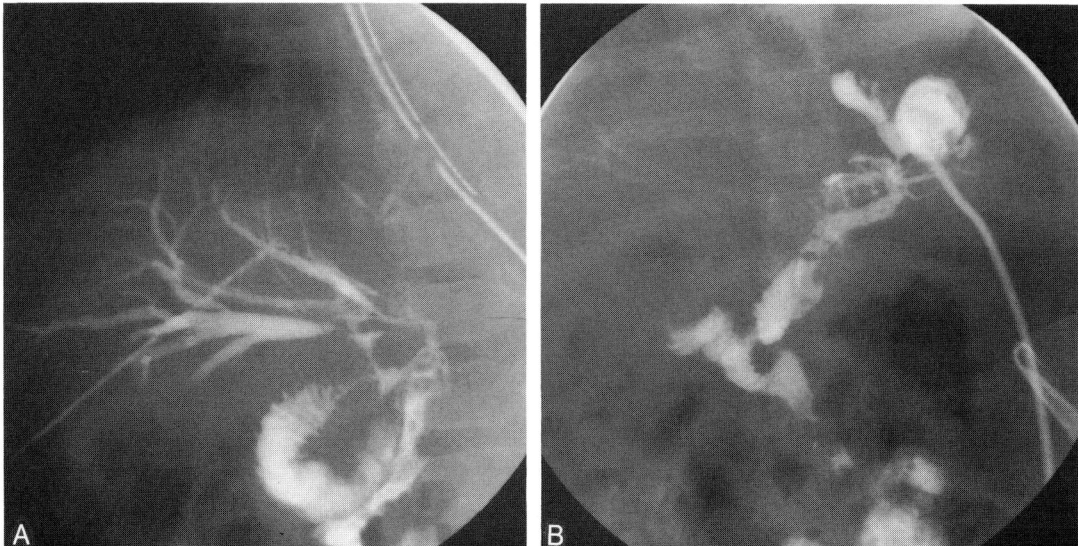

Figure 18–14. Notice the difference between the normal, regularly branching biliary tree in the right lobe of the liver **(A)**, in comparison with the abnormal biliary tree in the left lobe **(B)**. This patient had ischemia of the left lobe and chronic, resistant infection that resulted in cavitation of the liver extending out from the biliary tree. Unfortunately, this infection proved fatal. Attempted resection of the left lobe resulted in devascularization of the rest of the hepatic graft.

obtain a pulsed Doppler signal from hepatic veins during postoperative evaluation. It may provide useful ancillary information.

The biliary tree is very susceptible to ischemia. When the time between removal of the donated liver and its placement in the host has been prolonged or when hepatic arterial insufficiency or thrombosis complicates the surgery, the epithelium of the biliary tract is the weakest cellular link. Biliary lakes form as the epithelial lining becomes tattered and the liver cavitates. Infection complicates the whole process, but if treated and drained, the biliary tract can reconstitute and recover function. It does not return to normal, however. Its normal willowlike branching is replaced by saccular ectasia (Fig. 18-14).

REFERENCES

Bisset GS 3d. Strife JL, Balistreri WF: Evaluation of children for liver transplantation: Value of MR imaging and sonography. AJR 1990; 155:351-356.

Bowen AD, Keslar PJ, Newman B, et al: Adrenal hemorrhage after liver transplantation. Radiology 1990; 176:85-88.

Broelsch CE, Emond JC, Thistlethwaite JR, et al: Liver transplantation, including the concept of reduced-size liver transplants in children. Ann Surg 1988; 208:410-420.

Chezmar JL, Nelson RC, Bernardino ME: Portal venous gas after hepatic transplantation: Sonographic detection and clinical significance. AJR 1989; 153:1203-1205.

Coulden RA, Britton PD, Farman P et al: Preliminary report: Hepatic vein Doppler in the early diagnosis of acute liver transplant rejection. Lancet 1990; 336:273-275.

Dalen K, Day DL, Ascher NL, et al: Imaging of vascular complications after hepatic transplantation. AJR 1988; 150:1285-1290.

Flint EW, Sumkin JH, Zajko AB, et al: Duplex sonography of hepatic artery thrombosis after liver transplantation. AJR 1988; 151:481-483.

Gibson RN, Gibson PR, Donlan JD, et al: Identification of a patent paraumbilical vein by using Doppler sonography: Importance in the diagnosis of portal hypertension. AJR 1989; 153:513-516.

Goyal AK, Pokharna DS, Sharma SK: Ultrasonic measurements of portal vasculature in diagnosis of portal hypertension. A controversial subject reviewed. J Ultrasound Med 1990; 9:45-48.

Hall TR, McDiarmid SV, Grant EG, et al: False-negative duplex Doppler studies in children with hepatic artery thrombosis after liver transplantation. AJR 1990; 154:573-575.

Hoffer FA, Teele RL, Lillehei CW, et al: Infected bilomas and hepatic artery thrombosis in infant recipients of liver transplants. Interventional radiology and medical therapy as an alternative to retransplantation. Radiology 1988; 169:435-438.

Patriquin H, Tessier G, Grignon A, et al: Lesser omental thickness in normal children: Baseline for detection of portal hypertension. AJR 1985; 145:693-696.

Raby N, Karani J, Powell-Jackson P, et al: Assessment of portal vein patency: Comparison of arterial portography and ultrasound scanning. Clin Radiol 1988; 39:381-385.

Zonderland HM, Laméris JS, Terpstra OT, et al: Auxiliary partial liver transplantation: Imaging evaluation in 10 patients. AJR 1989; 153:981-985.

# CHAPTER 19

PARENCHYMAL RENAL DISEASE

Because ultrasonography is not affected by renal function and requires no intravenous injection of contrast, it is the study of choice for the child who presents in renal failure. Acute renal failure is defined as a rapid, severe decline in renal function with subsequent development of uremia. In most patients, it is reversible or self-limiting. Renal damage is initiated by a primary insult that leads to disruption of normal function of tubular cells. After a phase of established renal failure, structure and function recover, and renal microanatomy and physiology return to normal. Chronic renal failure is the irreversible loss of more than 50 percent of the glomerular filtration rate. Children with acute renal failure are much more likely to be referred for evaluation than are those with undiagnosed chronic disease, but the principles of ultrasonic examination apply to both groups. The checklist is as follows: (1) Is the bladder empty, partially filled, or hugely distended? We have seen children with "anuria" who had obstruction of the outlet of the bladder, rather than renal failure. One child had a rectal duplication cyst obstructing the bladder. Another was a premature baby who had physiologic obstruction resulting from morphine. If the bladder is empty, a bladder tap is futile. Echogenic silt in a partially filled bladder may be blood or cellular or crystalline debris. (2) Is hydronephrosis present? If so, is the dilatation likely obstructive in origin? Radiologic/surgical evaluation should follow in this situation (see section on hydronephrosis in Chapter 8). (3) If the collecting systems are not distended, is renal size normal for the patient's size and age? Small kidneys imply chronic renal disease; normal renal size suggests prerenal or acute renal causes for azotemia. (4) What is the parenchymal pattern? Are cortices echogenic, medullary pyramids echogenic, or both compartments abnormal? (5) Are renal arteries, veins, and inferior vena cava patent, and is blood flowing through them?

For this chapter, we assume that children with obstructive or reflux-associated hydronephrosis have been properly identified and consider only medical diseases of the kidney that result in renal dysfunction.

Increased renal parenchymal echogenicity strongly suggests medical renal disease. The mechanism of increased echogenicity is poorly understood. Changes in renal perfusion, cellular infiltrate of different types, change in interstitial fluid in relation to cellular fluid, and fibrosis may all be causal. Attempts have been made to classify diseases on the basis of their pattern of echogenicity (e.g., patchy, cortical only, medullary and cortical). There is a great deal of overlap between diseases, and so "histologic" results are just not available from the ultrasonic scans. It does seem that the greater the cortical echogenicity, the more severe or chronic the renal disease (Vergesslich et al., 1987; Brenbridge et al., 1986). The normal baby,

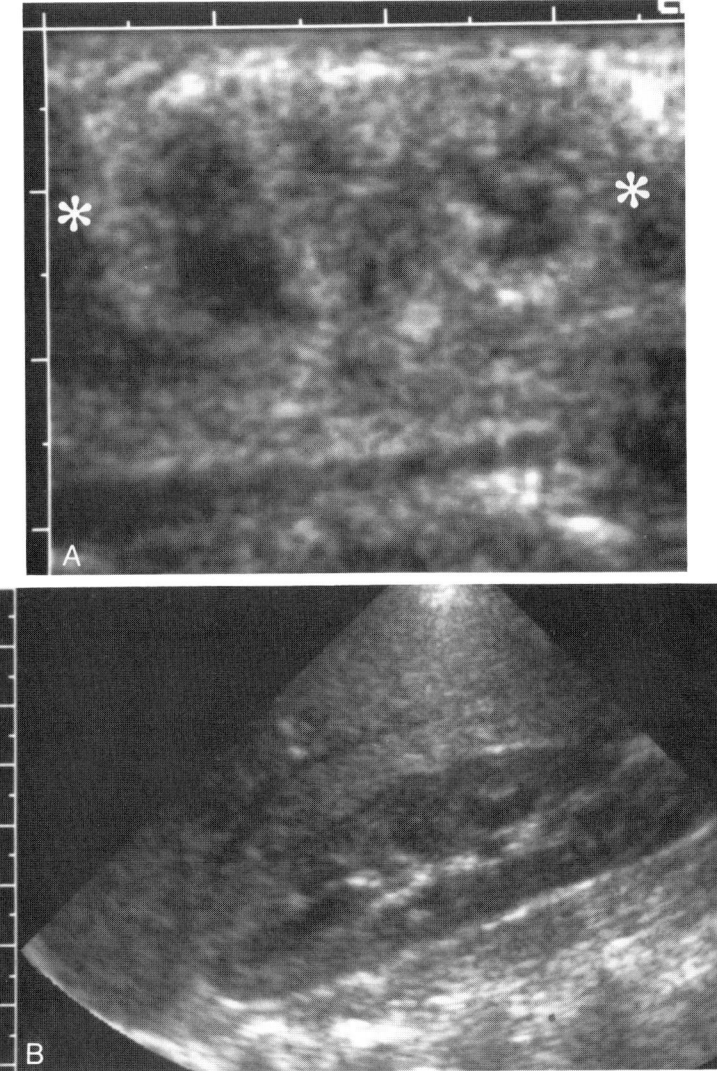

Figure 19–1. Coronal view of the left kidney of a baby who was born at only 28 weeks' gestational age shows a prominent, lucent medulla and marked echogenicity of the renal cortex (**A**). The cortex can remain echogenic throughout the first 6 months of life. (Here, as in other figures throughout this chapter, asterisks outline the kidney.) **B** is a longitudinal scan of a normal kidney in a 10-year-old.

from 0 to 6 months of age, has a more echogenic cortex than do older babies and children (Fig. 19–1). Diagnosis of superimposed renal parenchymal disease in neonates depends on noting inhomogeneity of cortex, changes in medullary-cortical relationship and interface, size of kidney, and other information such as ascites. Furthermore, the neonate has diseases peculiar to his or her age group. For these reasons, it is appropriate to consider neonatal medical renal disease as a discrete subset (Table 19–1).

Bilateral, diffusely echogenic kidneys that are markedly enlarged are typical of autosomal recessive polycystic renal disease. Be-

Table 19–1. CAUSES OF INCREASED RENAL PARENCHYMAL ECHOGENICITY IN NEONATES

Polycystic kidney
Transient renal dysfunction (possible result of tubular obstruction from Tamm-Horsfall protein)
Congenital nephrotic syndrome
Asphyxia
- cardiac related
- sepsis
- hypovolemia

Renal venous thrombosis
Renal arterial occlusion
Toxicity
- drugs

Infection
- bacterial
- fungal

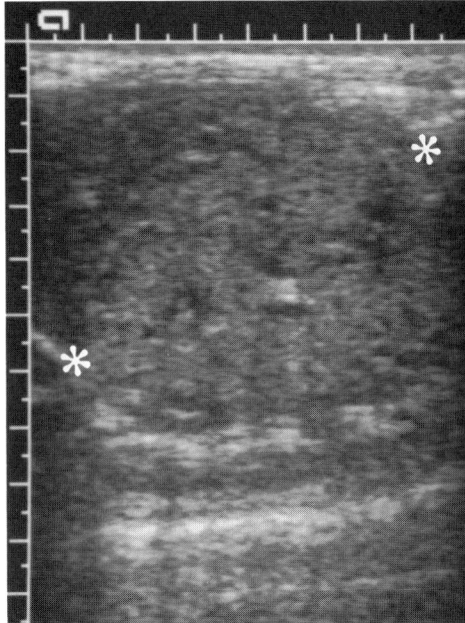

Figure 19–2. Recessive polycystic disease results in large kidneys, increased echogenicity from the multiple interfaces provided by small cysts, and obliteration of medullary-cortical borders.

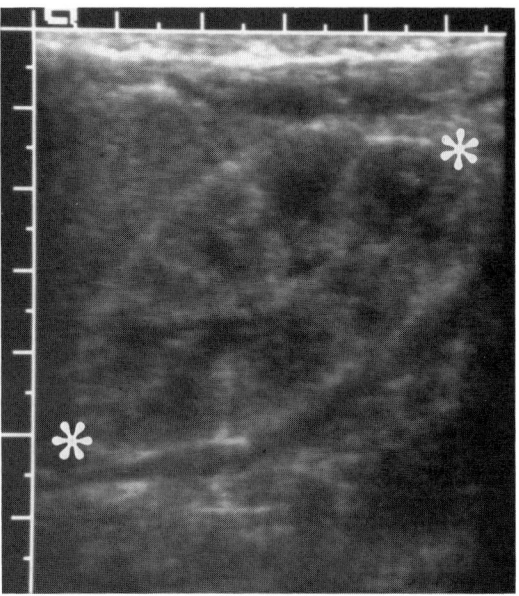

Figure 19–3. This 4-week-old patient has biopsy-proven Finnish-type congenital nephrotic syndrome. This is a longitudinal scan of the right kidney. Although his kidneys were larger than normal, there was still definition of the medullary-cortical border, and the cortex was not too echogenic.

cause of the size of the kidneys and the association of hepatic abnormality, there should be no confusion with other types of parenchymal disease (Fig. 19–2). Congenital nephrosis of the Finnish type has a histologic pattern of dilated tubules and Bowman spaces (Huttunen, 1976). The kidneys are larger than normal, but not huge; ascites and edema of soft tissues may be present. The reported ultrasonographic appearance is that of diffuse increased echogenicity which results in loss of distinction between cortex and medulla (Graif et al., 1982; Perale et al., 1988). Minimal change in parenchymal pattern may occur (Figs. 19–3, 19–4).

Transient renal dysfunction of an other-

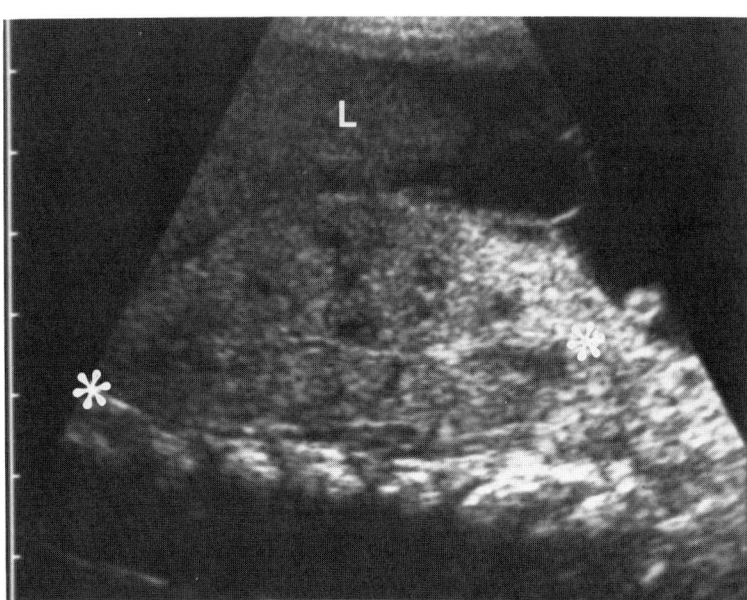

Figure 19–4. This 2-week-old also has biopsy-proven Finnish-type congenital nephrotic syndrome. Ascites surrounds the right lobe of liver (L). The kidney is slightly enlarged, measuring 6.4 cm, and there is poor delineation between cortex and medulla.

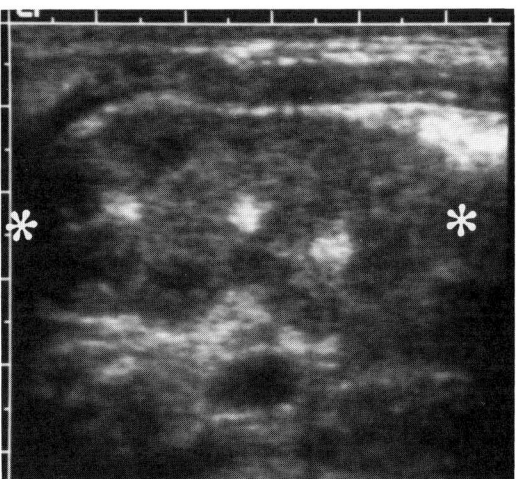

Figure 19–5. Note the increased echogenicity of medullary pyramids on the renal scan of this baby, who had been dehydrated for 2 days after birth. He was oliguric. Echogenicity probably represents proteinaceous precipitates in the tubules.

wise healthy neonate has been described (Avni, 1983; Hijazi et al., 1988), and we have encountered several such babies. It is possible that precipitation of protein in distal tubules is responsible for the clinical presentation of oliguria or anuria shortly after birth. Echogenicity of medullary pyramids supports this hypothesis, and both renal dysfunction and the medullary echoes usually clear within days (Fig. 19–5).

Anoxic damage of kidneys, secondary to perinatal asphyxia, may be underestimated in incidence as other systems—notably, the central nervous system and the cardiovascular system—are more dramatically affected. Furthermore, many affected babies die before the renal complications become manifest. In one study (Perlman and Tack, 1988), oliguria in the perinatal period was a sensitive indicator of infants at risk for neurologic deficits, if the infants survived. Acute tubular necrosis and, rarely, cortical necrosis are sequelae of renal ischemia, but the neonatal kidney maintains a remarkable capacity to recover (Fig. 19–6; Chevalier, 1984). Ischemia also results from cardiovascular anomalies that cause a decrease in renal arterial flow. Ischemia and toxic insult both result in increased echogenicity of the renal parenchyma, particularly the medullae. Aminoglycosides or other drugs that may have a direct nephrotoxic effect produce a tubulointerstitial nephropathy. For the baby of very low birth weight, one also has to consider renal candidiasis as a cause of diffuse renal echogenicity (see Chapter 7).

Although renal venous thrombosis has been considered "invariably bilateral" by some (Metreweli and Pearson, 1984), it has in our experience been typically unilateral. Investigation of future patients with color Doppler imaging will better show the extent of venous involvement (plates VI and VII). Thrombosis typically occurs in small vessels first and then extends into large veins. A preceding history of difficult delivery, anoxia, dehydration, sepsis, or maternal diabetes is common. Overt hematuria is virtually always present. Adrenal hemorrhage may coexist with renal venous thrombosis, especially on the left. The thrombosed kidney is larger than normal and patchily echogenic. Vascular streaks from perivascular hemorrhage have been described (Metreweli and Pearson, 1984; Lalmand et al., 1990). Previous unrecognized renal venous thrombosis is likely responsible for many "hypoplastic"

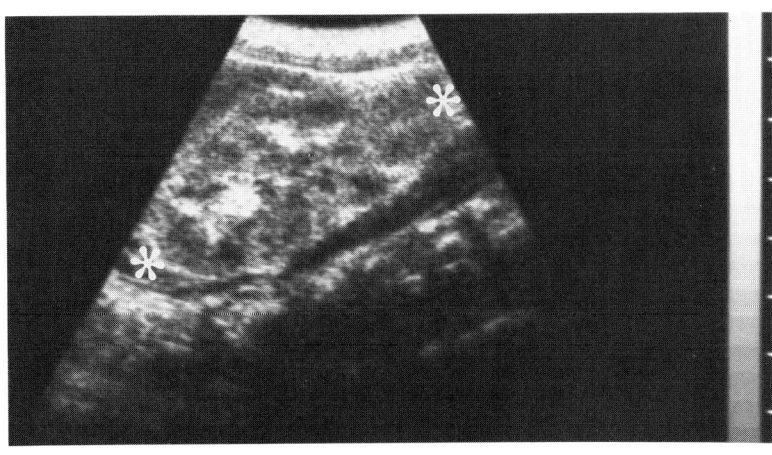

Figure 19–6. This 4-day-old had a history of birth anoxia and rising blood urea nitrogen (BUN) and creatinine levels. Longitudinal scans of both kidneys showed similar findings. Note on this longitudinal view of the left kidney the increased medullary echogenicity, which we assume is related to ischemia. Follow-up scan 6 days later showed resolution of these findings.

kidneys that are discovered later in life as an incidental finding on ultrasonography or intravenous urography. The process of evolving thrombosis and renal recovery takes weeks or months to complete. Hypertension is an uncommon complication, despite extensive renal damage (Fig. 19–7).

The baby with acute ischemia of the kidney from arterial occlusion may have a similar ultrasonographic picture of a swollen kidney

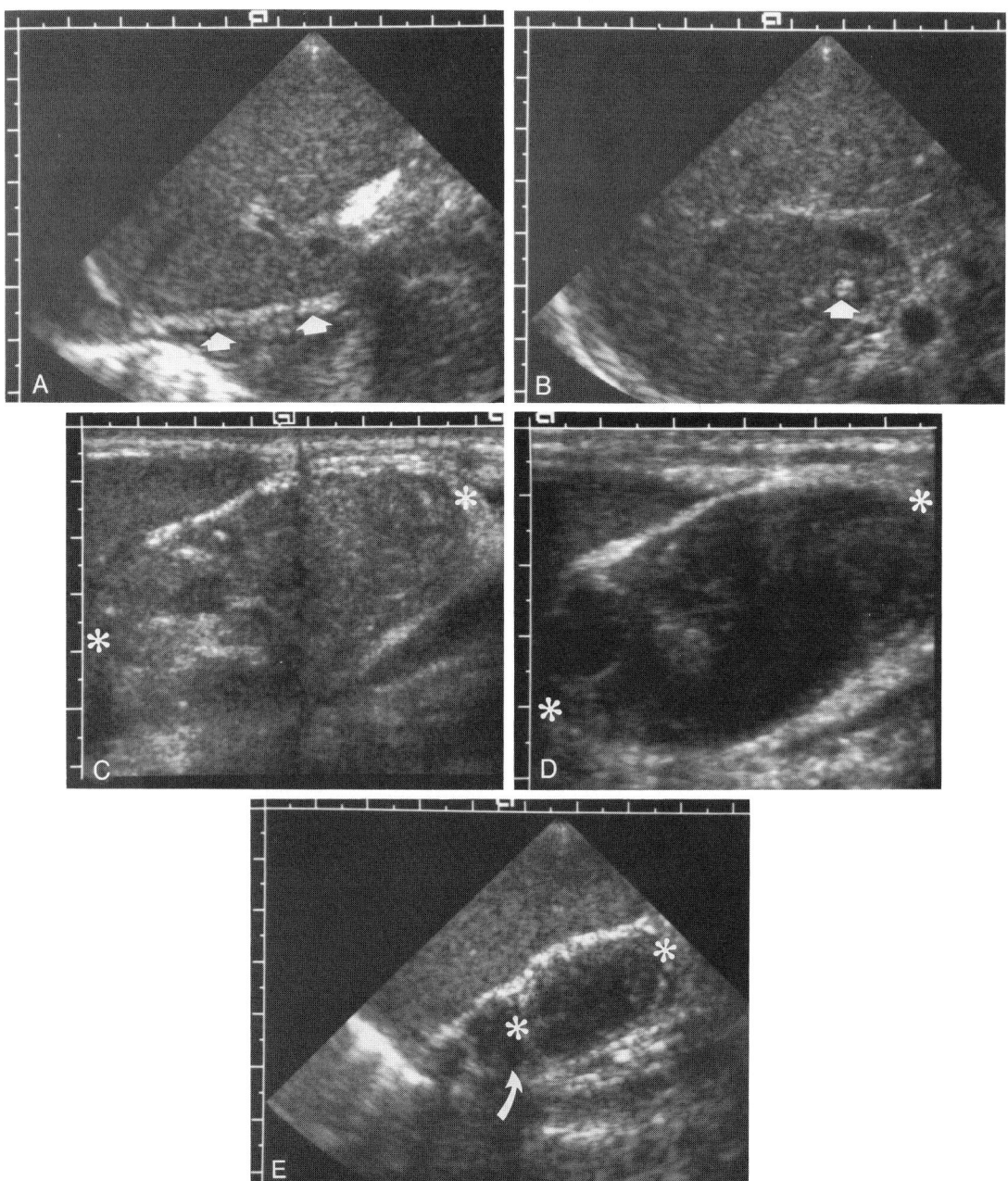

Figure 19–7. A series of scans shows the evolution of renal venous thrombosis in a baby who presented with gross hematuria. The longitudinal (**A**) and transverse (**B**) views of the right upper abdomen show a clot in the inferior vena cava (arrows). **C** is a longitudinal scan of the left kidney. The size of the kidney had increased so dramatically with its venous obstruction that it was close to 8 cm long. Longitudinal view of the left kidney 3 weeks later (**D**) showed that the kidney was more lucent and smaller. Five weeks later (**E**), the kidney had shrunk to 3 cm in length. Medullary-cortical differentiation is absent. Lucency superior to the kidney (arrow) is likely a resolving adrenal hemorrhage that was thought, in retrospect, to have accompanied the renal venous thrombosis on the left.

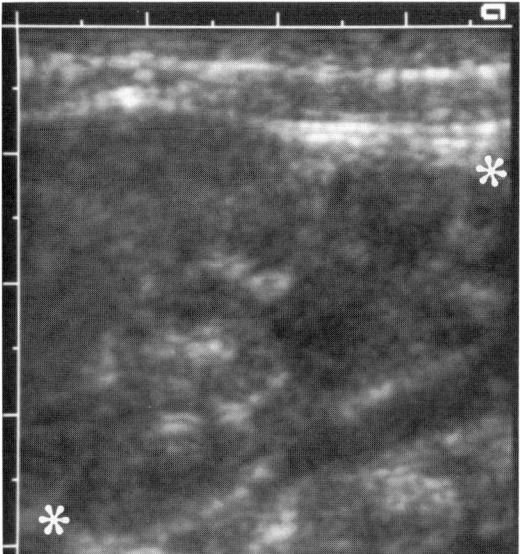

Figure 19-8. This is a coronal scan of the right kidney in a baby who had had unremitting hypertension after insertion of an umbilical artery catheter. This study was done when the infant was 12 days old. The renal outline is poorly defined, and echogenic tracks are readily apparent in the upper pole of the kidney. These likely represent thrombosed arteries or veins, or both. Color Doppler imaging revealed absolutely no blood flow to any portion of the kidney. The renal arterial signal ended at the renal hilum, which indicated complete thrombosis of the right renal artery.

and blurred medullary-cortical junction (Seibert et al., 1986). However, as opposed to venous thrombosis, which occurs in the immediate perinatal period, renal arterial occlusion tends to occur later in the baby's life, often in association with umbilical arterial catheters (Fig. 19-8). Acute hypertension and hematuria are clinical signs of renal compromise. Small size, increased echogenicity, and loss of function in the kidney may result if blockage of arterial flow has been complete. Doppler ultrasonography is indispensable in showing abnormalities of vascular flow in the kidneys. Any request from the neonatal nursery that indicates that a baby has severe renal dysfunction, hematuria, or hypertension results in our taking the unit equipped with Doppler scanning to the nursery. Coronal scans of the baby's abdomen are the most revealing because the main renal artery and vein can be instantly recognized with color Doppler imaging. The baby who is on the respirator is much easier to scan than the baby or child who is breathing spontaneously, simply because there is less artifact from motion. Arterial and venous flow should be evident in each section of the kidney, and the main vessels should be obviously patent and join with the inferior vena cava or the aorta (Plate VI).

Babies of very low birth weight (<1500 g) who are receiving furosemide are at risk for developing medullary nephrocalcinosis and, occasionally, discrete renal stones. Most who have been reported had had at least 10 days of therapy, and most were diagnosed after the age of 4 to 6 weeks (Ezzendeen et al., 1988; Jacinto et al., 1988; Kenney et al., 1988; Woolfield et al., 1988). Urinary function, as measured by serum creatinine and calculated rates of glomerular filtration, may be either normal or abnormal. Diuresis with thiazides can reverse nephrocalcinosis. Some degree of renal ischemia, immaturity, or other insult in the presence of hypercalciuria from the furosemide seems necessary for medullary calcinosis to occur. Although babies of low birth weight are primarily affected, children with congenital heart disease who are receiving furosemide have also developed medullary nephrocalcinosis (Reuter et al., 1985). The long-term implications of medullary deposition of calcium are as yet unknown.

The ultrasonographic appearance of medullary calcinosis is of variably dense medulla arrayed around the central sinus. Shadowing may or may not be present. Occasionally, a small echogenic shadowing focus is present when a discrete stone has formed. Ultrasonography is far more sensitive than plain radiographs in identifying the medullary calcinosis (Fig. 19-9).

In older babies and children, there are a multitude of glomerulonephritides, tubular abnormalities, and interstitial diseases that cause increased renal echogenicity. The most common are listed in Table 19-2. Renal cortical echogenicity has been divided into four groups: (1) The cortex has less echogenicity than the liver; (2) the cortex and the liver have equal echogenicity; (3) the cortex has greater echogenicity than the liver; and (4) the cortex and the central sinus have equal echogenicity. All reported studies have shown that the greater the echogenicity, the greater the severity of renal disease in general, as measured by functional studies (Brenbridge et al., 1986; Choyke et al., 1988; Hayden et al., 1984). However, the association is not strong enough to be a prognosticator of eventual outcome. There is no pattern that is specific for each type of medical renal disease. The most useful added information from the ultrasonograms is the size of the

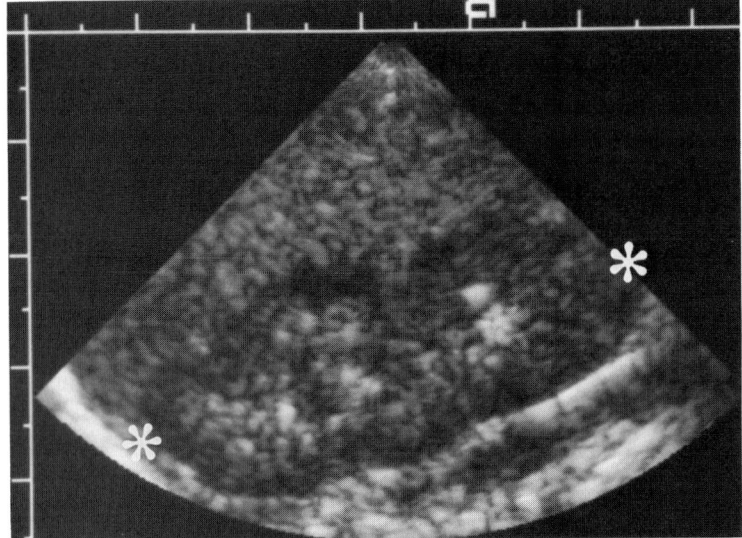

Figure 19–9. Hematuria prompted renal scans of this little baby, who had chronic pulmonary disease after premature birth at 25 weeks' gestational age. Longitudinal scan of the right kidney 4 months after birth shows parenchymal echogenicity limited to the medulla. This represents medullary calcinosis secondary to chronic therapy with furosemide.

kidneys. Small, echogenic kidneys indicate chronic disease (Figs. 19–10 to 19–13).

For all children with renal hyperechogenicity, it is valuable to look for ascites and pleural fluid during the ultrasonographic examination. Nephrotic syndrome, triggered by one of the glomerulopathies, is often associated with collections of fluid (Fig. 19–14). In children who present with hemolytic uremic syndrome, the colon commonly is affected by the same microangiopathic process as are the kidneys. Thickening of colonic wall may be a clue to the etiology of the renal disease. Coronal scans through the flanks, below the air-fluid level in the gut, are best for showing the wall of the bowel and luminal contents (Fig. 19–15).

Hyperperfusion injury to a solitary kidney may occur if fewer than a critical number of nephrons are present (Fig. 19–16). Focal segmental glomerulosclerosis, tubular atrophy, and interstitial fibrosis appear to be the pathologic correlates (Thorner et al., 1984). Follow-up of children who have had previous unilateral nephrectomy may reveal hyperechogenicity of the remaining kidney from this

Table 19–2. CAUSES OF INCREASED RENAL PARENCHYMAL ECHOGENICITY IN CHILDREN

Glomerular abnormality	Tubular toxicity (drug)
Nephrotic syndrome-associated	• aminoglycosides
Congenital (Finnish type)	• cephalosporin
Minimal change glomerulonephritis	• amphotericin
Focal glomerulosclerosis	• contrast media
Mesangiocapillary glomerulonephritis (also known as membranoproliferative)	Sickle cell disease
	Uric acid nephropathy
Postinfective glomerulonephritis (particularly streptococcal; also known as proliferative glomerulonephritis)	Acute and chronic pyelonephritis
	Interstitial fibrosis/nephritis
	• analgesics
IgA nephropathy	• erythromycin
Chronic glomerulonephritis	• sulfonamides
Nephropathy with Henoch-Schönlein purpura	• rifampicin
Hemolytic uremic syndrome	• methicillin, penicillin, ampicillin
Hyperperfusion injury	• irradiation
Tubulointerstitial abnormality	**Other**
Acute tubular necrosis	Alport, nail-patella, Laurence-Moon-Biedl, Bartter, and other syndromes associated with nephropathy
• hypotension (cardiac)	
• endotoxic shock	Dysplasia
• hypovolemia	Nephronophthisis
Hemoglobinuria/myoglobinuria	Glycogen storage disease
	Tyrosinemia
	Cystinosis
	Biliary atresia

Figure 19–10. The right kidney was large and poorly delineated from the liver in this 7-year-old girl, who had acute glomerulonephritis after streptococcal disease.

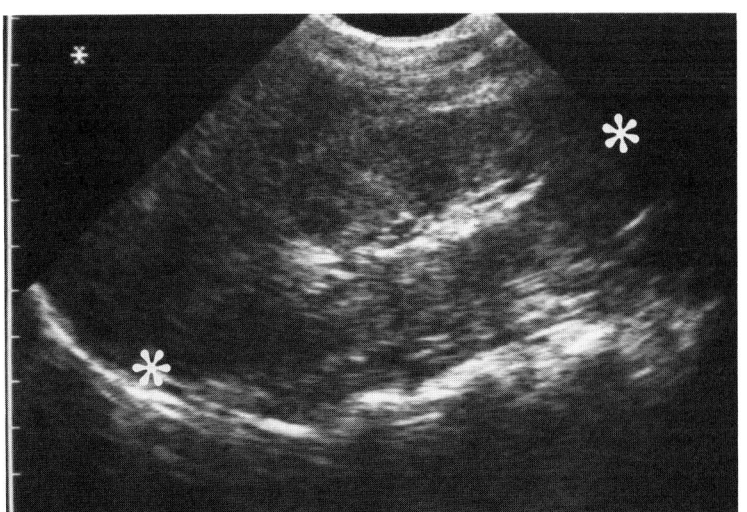

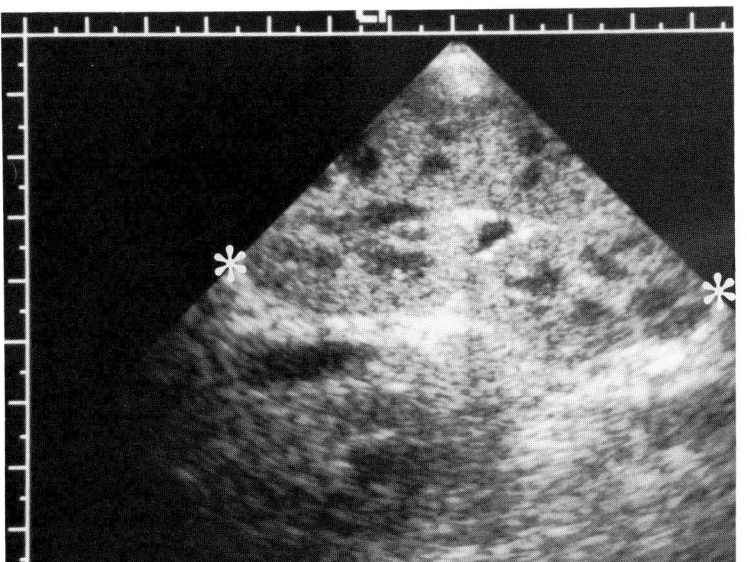

Figure 19–11. Hepatomegaly was the original presentation of this 10-year-old. Her kidneys were large and mildly echogenic. This longitudinal view of the right kidney shows unusually numerous medullary pyramids associated with cortical echogenicity. Endocrinologic workup revealed the presence of tyrosinemia. Patients with this metabolic defect may have large echogenic kidneys, as may children with glycogen storage disease, type I.

Figure 19–12. Ascites associated with a diffusely echogenic kidney is shown in this longitudinal scan of the right kidney in a patient with dense-deposit glomerular disease.

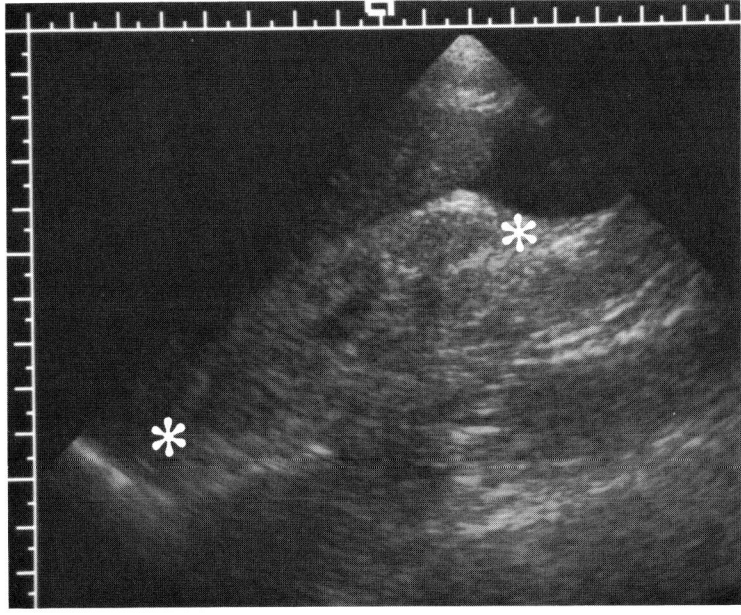

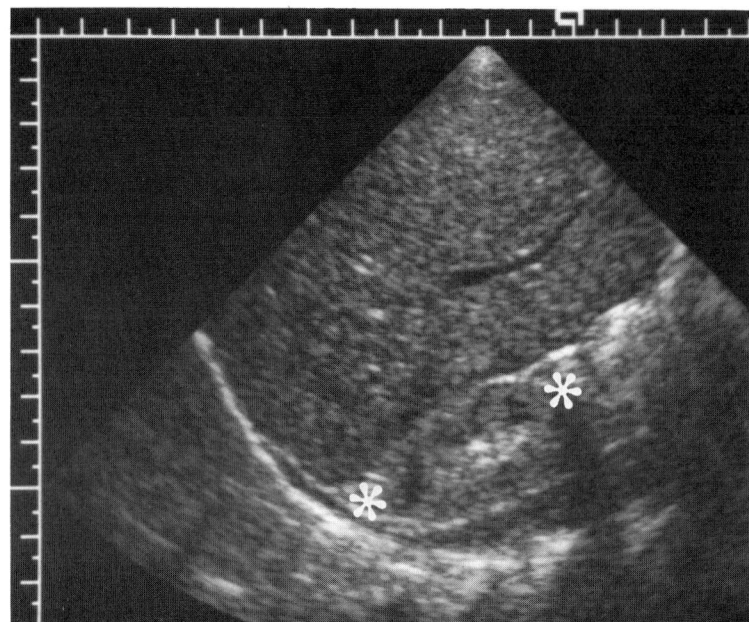

Figure 19–13. Bilateral renal dysplasia resulted in small size and increased echogenicity of the kidneys in this 8-year-old boy. Longitudinal view of the right kidney is shown. At the time, he had Fanconi's syndrome, a BUN level of 90, and a creatinine level of 0.9.

Figure 19–14. A 19-year-old was admitted to the hospital for clinical features of nephrotic syndrome, including edema, low levels of albumin and serum, and proteinuria. Ascites was diagnosed both on clinical examination and on ultrasonography. Views of the kidneys showed increased echogenicity of the renal cortex, as shown in this longitudinal scan of the right kidney. The etiology for the nephrotic syndrome was undefined; he had abused multiple drugs, including marijuana, heroin, and cocaine.

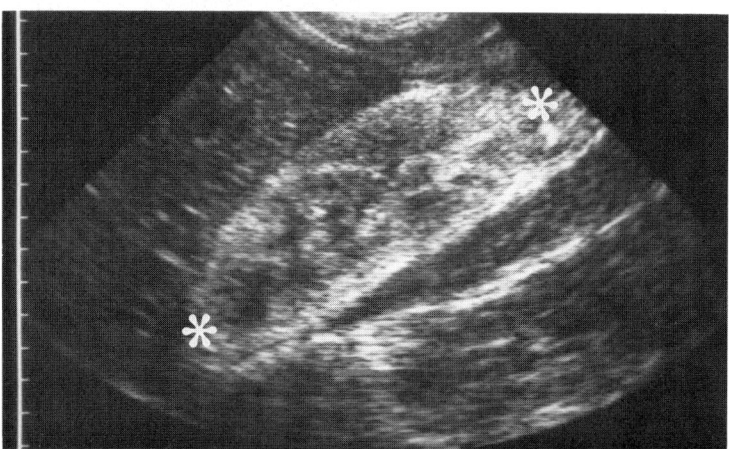

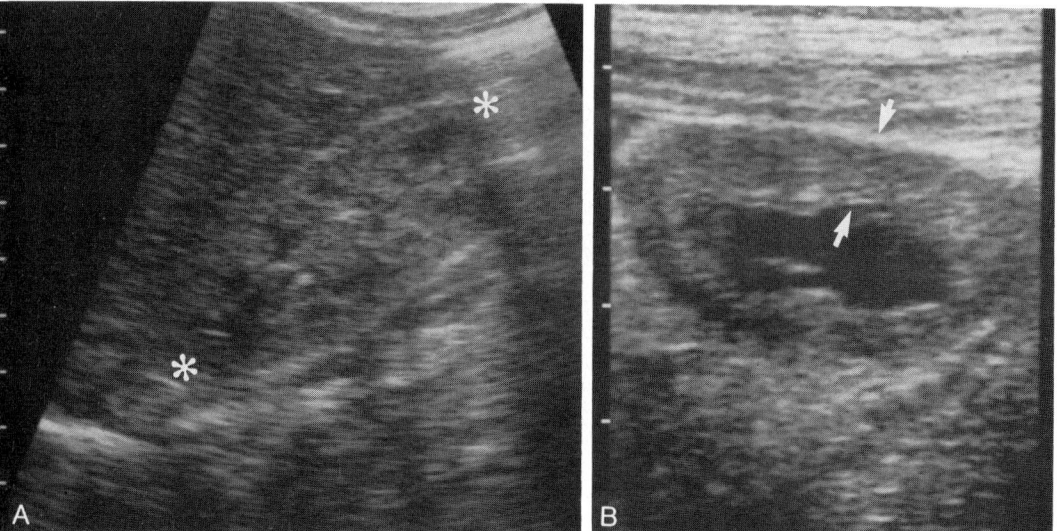

Figure 19–15. Hemolytic uremic syndrome is another of the medical renal diseases that cause increased parenchymal echogenicity (A). This little girl presented with bloody diarrhea and then developed renal failure. Transverse view of the colon (B) shows the thickened wall (arrows) from the microangiopathic process.

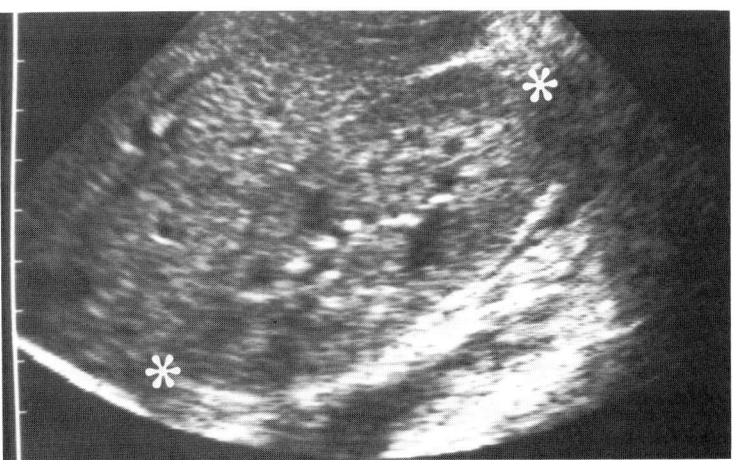

Figure 19–16. The cortex of this solitary right kidney seems unusually echogenic for a 5-year-old child. Hyperperfusion injury to a solitary kidney, either congenital or acquired, may occur and be manifested by increased cortical echogenicity. Normal vessels are responsible for the prominent tracks in the central portion of the kidney.

unusual injury (Avni et al., 1989). Hyperperfusion also seems to be the cause for the renal hyperechogenicity that is associated with biliary atresia but is not present in all patients (Fig. 19–17; Boechat et al., 1986).

Myoglobinuria is an unusual problem, but we have seen three children who developed renal failure after extreme physical exertion (Krensky et al., 1983). One had collapsed after the final event in a pentathlon. Another was a member of a steel band and had played to the point of exhaustion. Previous history of exertion, of course, clinches the diagnosis after the urinalysis has shown myoglobin.

The sickle cell trait is present in 8 percent of black Americans. Hematuria in patients with the trait is more common than in those who are homozygous for sickle cell disease. Sludging in arterioles of the kidney and subsequent effects on the interstitium (Tarry et al., 1987) are likely responsible for the renal hyperechogenicity that we often see as an incidental finding in patients undergoing biliary evaluation (Fig. 19–18). Repeated sickling in the papillary blood vessels results in areas of papillary necrosis. The necrotic tissue may slough, be absorbed, or calcify. Mesangiocapillary glomerulonephritis may complicate the renal abnormality. Interstitial damage results in release of antigen and autoimmune nephritis. Glomerulosclerosis has been described in homozygous patients; 25 percent of homozygous patients develop chronic renal failure by middle age (Davison, 1988).

Uric acid nephropathy is predominantly an obstructive uropathy resulting from crystals of uric acid that have been deposited in distal

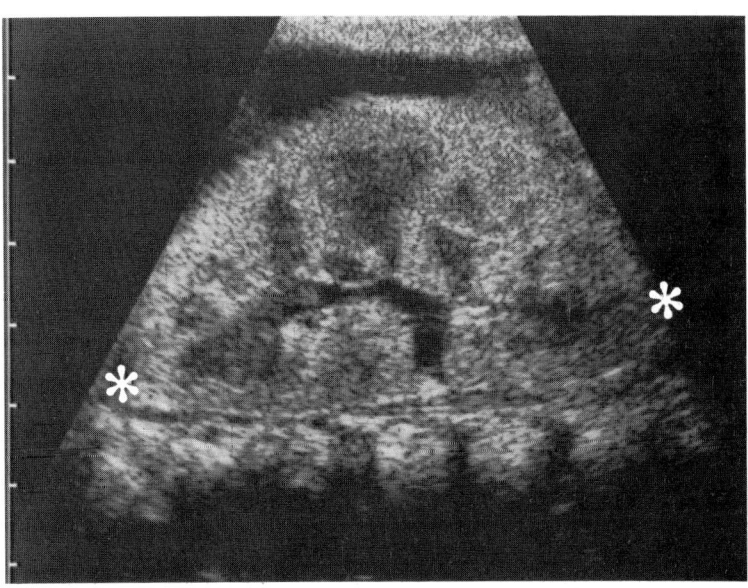

Figure 19–17. Large size and increased echogenicity of the kidneys have been associated with biliary atresia. This is a longitudinal scan of the left kidney in a baby who subsequently died of liver failure. Note the marked cortical echogenicity, which is out of proportion for her age of 10 months.

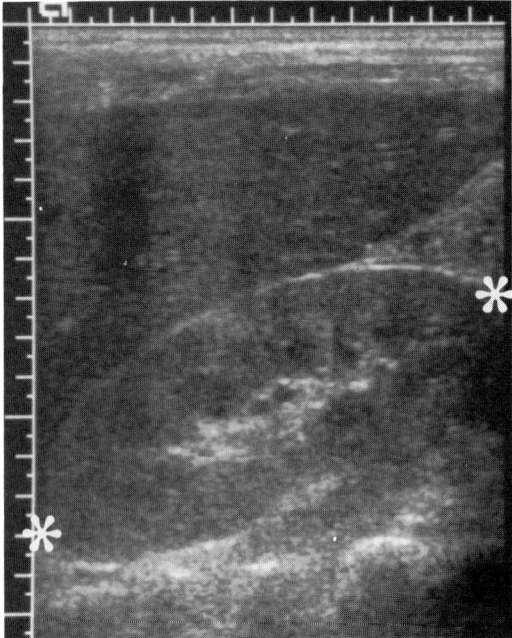

Figure 19–18. Sickle cell disease is responsible for the abnormal renal parenchymal echogenicity in this adolescent boy.

tubules and collecting ducts. However, the ultrasonographic picture is of increased parenchymal echogenicity, and the collecting systems are usually not distended. Children who are receiving cytotoxic therapy for neoplasms, especially the lymphoproliferative tumors, are at risk for uric acid nephropathy. The liberation of large amounts of nucleic acids, which are metabolized to uric acid, overwhelm the kidneys unless preventive measures, such as administration of allopurinol and hydration, are taken. Leukemic infiltrates in the kidney also may increase its echogenicity; we often are unable to distinguish between the disease itself and complications of therapy (Figs. 19–19, 19–20).

Certain drugs that are commonly used in pediatric practice are also associated with nephrotoxicity, and many very sick, hospitalized children have been given such medication. It is often impossible to know which of many insults delivered to their kidneys is or are responsible for the ultrasonographic appearance of hyperechogenicity.

When needed, renal biopsy should be done with a biopsy attachment on the transducer. This allows more specific placement of biopsy needle at the medullary-cortical junction or cortex, depending on the situation and nephrologist's wishes (Fig. 19–21). Some recommend use of a biopsy gun (Poster et al., 1990). Before biopsy, screening of patient's coagulation and platelets is routine. It is common after biopsy for small intrarenal or perirenal hematoma to be seen on follow-up ultrasonography (Fig. 19–22). This rarely causes any problem except for flank pain, which can be managed with simple analgesia. Intrarenal arteriovenous aneurysm is a rare, late complication of biopsy.

In the situation of acute renal failure, renal biopsy is reserved for very few patients. Indications include (1) diagnosis when no underlying cause for renal failure is evident; (2) confirmation of underlying glomerular disease; (3) suspicion of underlying systemic disease when diagnosis can be made most easily with renal biopsy (e.g., systemic lupus erythematosus); (4) when chronic renal failure, instead of an expected return of renal function, ensues. In children with chronic

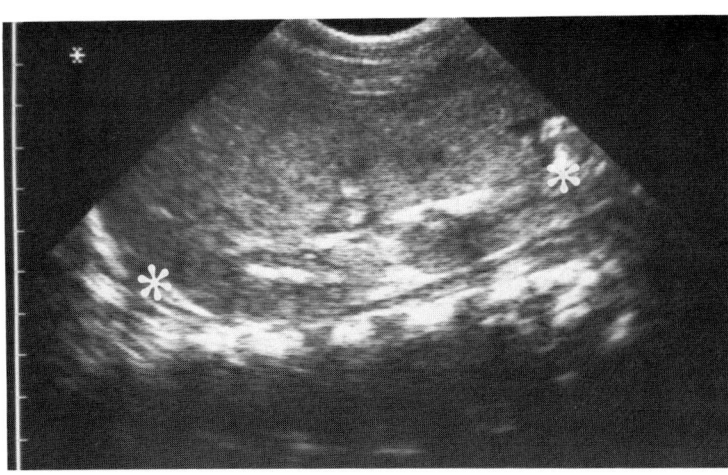

Figure 19–19. The kidney is very large and echogenic in this 2-year-old, who has acute lymphocytic leukemia in relapse. He died 6 weeks after this scan. Massive organomegaly was present; enlargement of the kidney likely represents diffuse leukemic infiltration.

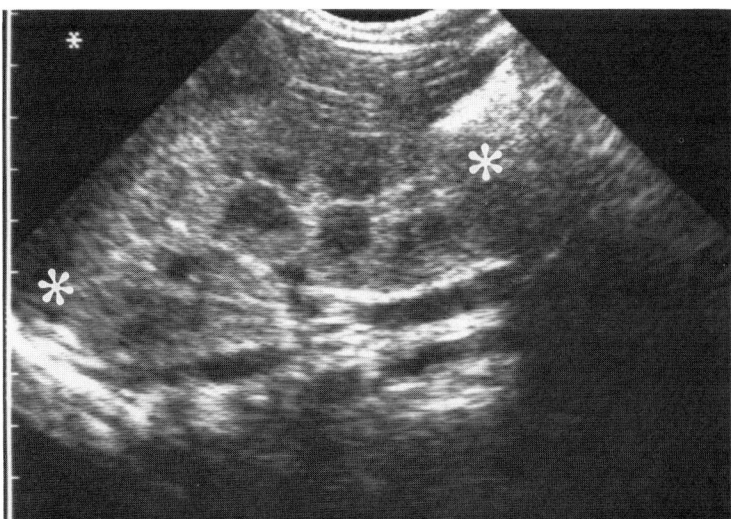

Figure 19-20. Longitudinal scan of the right kidney shows diffuse increase in cortical echogenicity, which was either secondary to the patient's known promyelocytic leukemia or secondary to hyperuricemia induced by chemotherapy.

renal failure and established disease, biopsy is used (1) to refine the diagnosis, especially in regard to possible therapy; (2) to establish the prognosis; and (3) to document the patient's natural history, specifically in response to therapy.

In a review of chronic renal failure in infants and children, Foreman and Chan (1988) compiled data from large studies that had previously been published. Of the children studied, 33 percent had glomerular abnormalities, 25 percent had urologic etiologies (obstructive or reflux), 16 percent had hereditary nephropathies, 11 percent had hypoplasia/dysplasia, 5 percent had vascular disorders, and 10 percent had other or unknown causes of their chronic renal failure. These numbers reflect a combined European–North American experience only, but it gives an idea of relative frequencies of problems affecting a pediatric population.

Overt hyperechogenicity is characteristic of crystalline deposition within renal parenchyma (Fig. 19-23). This is usually calcium and the result of severe or protracted hypercalcemia. Causes of nephrocalcinosis are listed in Table 19-3. Calcification begins in the medullary pyramids and, with time, becomes more diffuse. Erosion of conglomerates of calcium into the collecting system

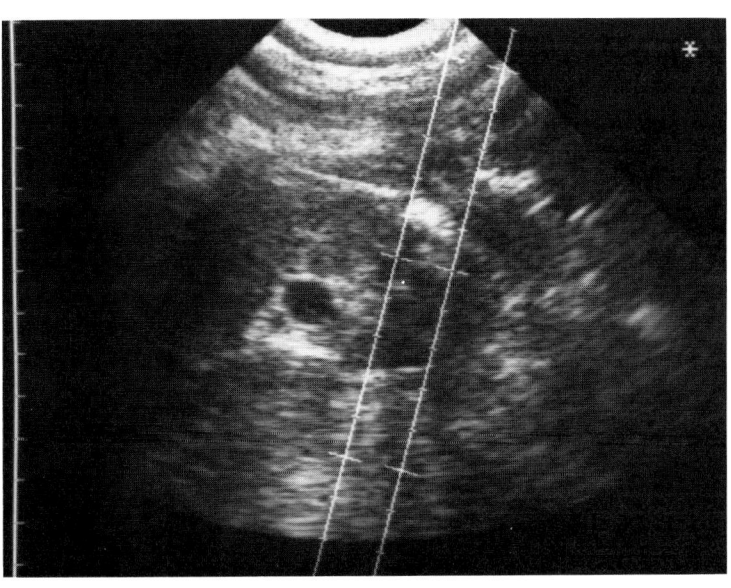

Figure 19-21. Longitudinal scan shows the markers for placement of the biopsy needle in this 15-year-old patient, who subsequently was shown to have focal segmental glomerulosclerosis. The lower pole of the right kidney is the usual and preferred site for biopsy.

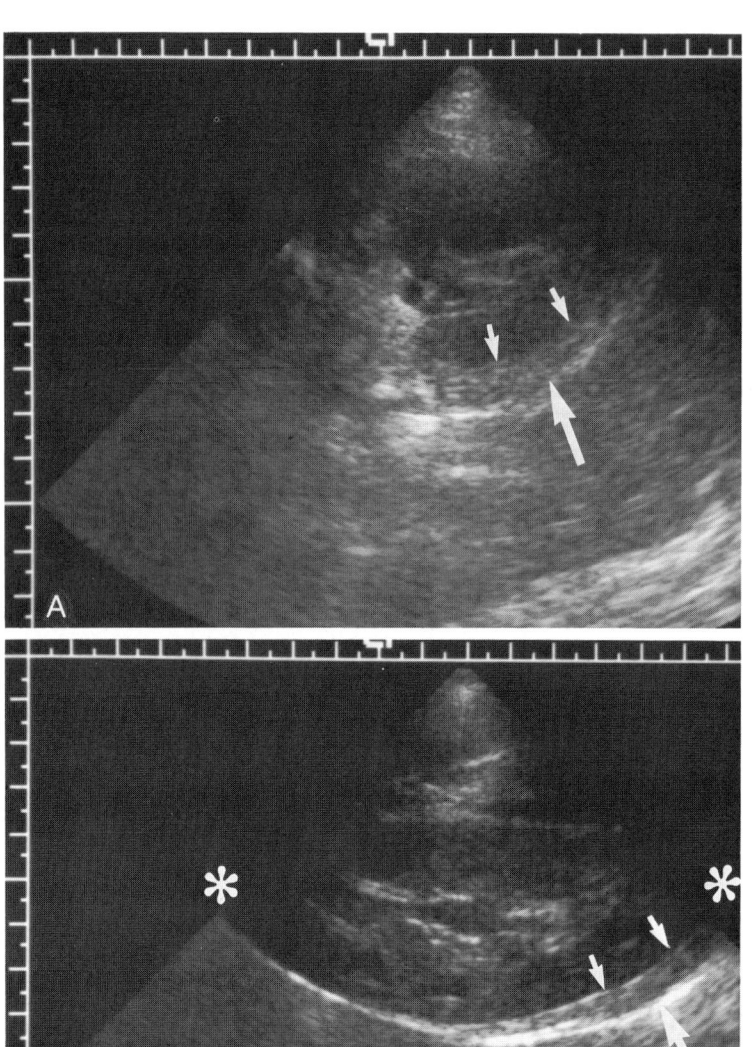

Figure 19–22. Transverse (A) and longitudinal (B) scans of this teenager's right kidney show perinephric hematoma (between arrows) anterior to the kidney 2 days after renal biopsy.

Figure 19–23. Urinary tract infection led to renal ultrasonography in this 14-month-old. The longitudinal scan of the right kidney shows markedly echogenic medullary pyramids. This was also true on the left. Final diagnosis was that of renal tubular acidosis, type 1. The baby had metabolic acidosis and increased levels of calcium in the urine, and the ratio of urinary calcium to creatinine was abnormal.

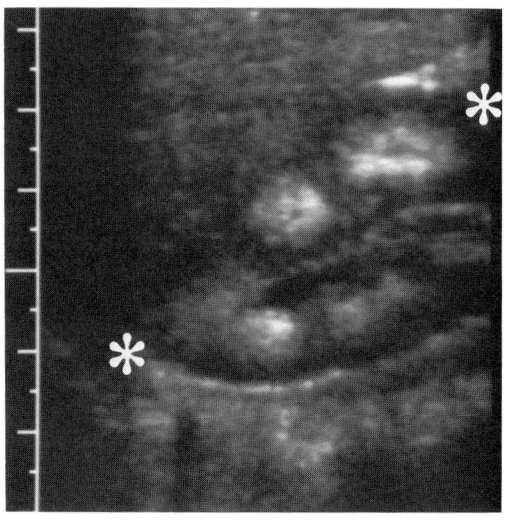

Table 19–3. CAUSES OF NEPHROCALCINOSIS IN CHILDREN

Renal tubular acidosis
Oxalosis
Primary hyperparathyroidism
Sarcoid
Hypervitaminosis D
Milk-alkali syndrome
Malignancy
Primary or secondary increase in steroids
Hyperthyroidism
Williams syndrome
Infection
Tuberculosis
Mycoses
Tumors
Medullary sponge kidney
Tubular necrosis
Infarction
Furosemide
Idiopathic

causes hematuria, pain, and variable degrees of obstruction. Therefore, the list of diseases associated with nephrocalcinosis overlaps that associated with nephrolithiasis (Chapter 6).

REFERENCES

Avni EF, Van Sinoy ML, Hall M, et al: Hypothesis: Reduced renal mass with glomerular hyperfiltration, a cause of renal hyperechogenicity in children. Pediatr Radiol 1989; 19:108–110.

Boechat MI, Querfeld U, Dietrich RB, et al: Large echogenic kidneys in biliary atresia. Ann Radiol 1986; 29:660–662.

Brenbridge ANAG, Chevalier RL, Kaiser DC: Increased renal cortical echogenicity in pediatric renal disease: Histopathologic correlations. JCU 1986; 14:595–600.

Brill PW, Jagannath A, Winchester P, et al: Adrenal hemorrhage and renal vein thrombosis in the newborn: MR imaging. Radiology 1989; 170:95–98.

Chevalier RL, Campbell F, Brenbridge ANAG: Prognostic factors in neonatal acute renal failure. Pediatrics 1984; 74:265–272.

Choyke PL, Grant EG, Hoffer FA, et al: Cortical echogenicity in the hemolytic uremic syndrome: Clinical correlation. J Ultrasound Med 1988; 7:439–442.

Cote G, Jequier S, Kaplan P: Increased renal medullary echogenicity in patients with Williams syndrome. Pediatr Radiol 1989; 19:481–483.

Davison AM: Nephrology (Mainstream Medicine). London: Heinemann Medical Books, 1988.

Evans JB, Shapeero LG, Roscelli JD: Infantile glomerulonephritis mimicking polycystic kidney disease. J Ultrasound Med 1988; 7:29–32.

Ezzendeen F, Adelman RD, Ahlfors CE: Renal calcification in preterm infants: Pathophysiology and long-term sequelae. J Pediatr 1988; 113:532–539.

Foreman JW, Chan JCM: Chronic renal failure in infants and children. J Pediatr 1988; 113:793–800.

Graif M, Lison M, Strauss S, et al: Congenital nephrosis: Ultrasonographic features. Pediatr Radiol 1982; 12:154–155.

Hayden CK Jr, Santa-Cruz FR, Amparo EG, et al: Ultrasonographic evaluation of the renal parenchyma in infancy and childhood. Radiology 1984; 152:413–417.

Hijazi Z, Keller MS, Gaudio KM, et al: Transient renal dysfunction of the neonate. Pediatrics 1988; 82:929–930.

Huttunen NP: Congenital nephrotic syndrome of Finnish type. Study of 75 patients. Arch Dis Child 1976; 51:344–348.

Jacinto JS, Modanlou HD, Crade M, et al: Renal calcification incidence in very low birth weight infants. Pediatrics 1988; 81:31–35.

Jantarasami T, Larew M, Kao SC, et al: Ultrasound demonstration of nephrocalcinosis in William's syndrome. JCU 1989; 17:533–534.

Jayogapal S, Cohen HL, Brill PW, et al: Calcified neonatal renal vein thrombosis demonstration by CT and US. Pediatr Radiol 1990; 20:160–162.

Kenney IJ, Aiken CG, Lenney W: Furosemide-induced nephrocalcinosis in very low birth weight infants. Pediatr Radiol 1988; 18:323–325.

Krensky AM, Reddish JM, Teele RL: Causes of increased renal echogenicity in pediatric patients. Pediatrics 1983; 72:840–846.

Lalmand B, Avni EF, Nasr A, et al: Perinatal renal vein thrombosis: Sonographic demonstration. J Ultrasound Med 1990; 9:437–442.

Lanning P, Uhari M, Kouvalainen, et al: Ultrasonic features of the congenital nephrotic syndrome of the Finnish type. Acta Paediatr Scand 1989; 78:717–720.

McLaughlin MG, Swayne LC, Rubinstein JB, et al: Transient acute tubular dysfunction in the newborn: CT findings. Pediatr Radiol 1990; 20:363–364.

Metreweli C, Pearson R: Echographic diagnosis of neonatal renal venous thrombosis. Pediatr Radiol 1984; 14:105–108.

Myracle MR, McGahan JP, Goetzman BW, et al: Ultrasound diagnosis of renal calcification in infants on chronic furosemide therapy. JCU 1986; 14:281–287.

Nybonde T, Mortensson W: Ultrasonography of the kidney following renal biopsy in children. Acta Radiol 1988; 29:151–153.

Patriquin HB, O'Regan S, Robitaille P, Paltiel H: Hemolytic-uremic syndrome: Intrarenal arterial Doppler patterns as a useful guide to therapy. Radiology 1989; 172: 625–628.

Perale R, Talenti E, Lubrano G, et al: Late ultrasonographic pattern in congenital nephrotic syndrome of Finnish type. Pediatr Radiol 1988; 18:71.

Perlman JM, Tack ED: Renal injury in the asphyxiated newborn infant: Relationship to neurologic outcome. J Pediatr 1988; 113:875–879.

Poster RB, Jones DB, Spirt BA: Percutaneous pediatric renal biopsy: Use of the biopsy gun. Radiology 1990; 176:725–727.

Reuter K, Kleinman PK, De Witt T, et al: Unsuspected medullary nephrocalcinosis from furosemide administration: Sonographic evaluation. JCU 1985; 13:357–359.

Ricci MA, Lloyd DA: Renal venous thrombosis in infants and children. Arch Surg 1990; 125:1195–1199.

Seibert JJ, Lindley SG, Corbitt SS, et al: Clot formation in the renal artery in the neonate demonstrated by ultrasound. JCU 1986; 14:470–473.

Sluysmans T, Vanoverschelde JP, Malvaux P: Growth failure associated with medullary sponge kidney, due to incomplete renal tubular acidosis type I. Eur J Pediatr 1987; 146:78–80.

Stevens SK, Parker BR: Renal oxypurine deposition in Lesch-Nyhan syndrome: Sonographic evaluation. Pediatr Radiol 1989; 19:479–480.

Tarry WF, Duckett JW Jr, Snyder HMcC III: Urological complications of sickle cell disease in a pediatric population. J Urol 1987; 138:572–574.

Thorner PS, Arbus GS, Celermajer DS, et al: Focal segmental glomerulosclerosis and progressive renal failure associated with a unilateral kidney. Pediatrics 1984; 73:806–810.

Toyoda K, Miyamoto Y, Ida M, et al: Hyperechoic medulla of the kidneys. Radiology 1989; 173:431–434.

Vergesslich KA, Sommer G, Wittich GR, et al: Acute renal failure in children. An ultrasonographic-clinical study. Eur J Radiol 1987; 7:263–265.

Wong SN, Lo RN, Yu EC: Renal blood flow pattern by noninvasive Doppler ultrasound in normal children and acute renal failure patients. J Ultrasound Med 1989; 8:135–141.

Woolfield N, Haslam R, LeQuesne G, et al: Ultrasound diagnosis of nephrocalcinosis in preterm infants. Arch Dis Child 1988; 63:86–88.

CHAPTER 20

RENAL TRANSPLANTATION

Techniques in hemodialysis and peritoneal dialysis have progressed to the point that infants and small children in renal failure can survive and grow. Therefore, more and smaller children are coming to renal transplantation than in the past. It is still true that the highest percentage of children who need a kidney have primary glomerular disease. It seems, however, that the percentage of children who have end-stage pyelonephritis is dropping. Other children who come to transplantation are those with hypoplasia-dysplasia, obstruction (typically from posterior urethral valve), polycystic disease, and metabolic diseases such as oxalosis and cystinosis. A child's pretransplantation evaluation is usually a follow-up ultrasonogram of the primary renal disease. Occasionally a child presents in renal failure, and our role is to help in diagnosing the underlying renal abnormality (see Chapter 19). The primary renal diagnosis is important for two reasons: (1) nephrectomy is done before transplantation when there is hydronephrosis, history or evidence of previous chronic infection, hypertension, or massive proteinuria; and (2) some renal diseases recur in the transplanted kidney. Oxalosis is a disorder of glyoxylate metabolism secondary to enzymatic deficiency and has a very high rate of recurrence (Fig. 20–1). Henoch-Schönlein purpura, focal segmental glomerulosclerosis, IgA nephropathy, and dense deposit disease (membranoproliferative glomerulonephritis, type II) also have high rates of recurrence in the grafts (Sheldon et al., 1987).

The pretransplantation evaluation of the child is primarily the work of the immunologist, microbiologist, and pediatrician. The radiologist has only one other role: that of evaluating the patient's bladder and urethra by voiding cystourethrogram.

Most programs in renal transplantation accept kidneys from living, related donors and

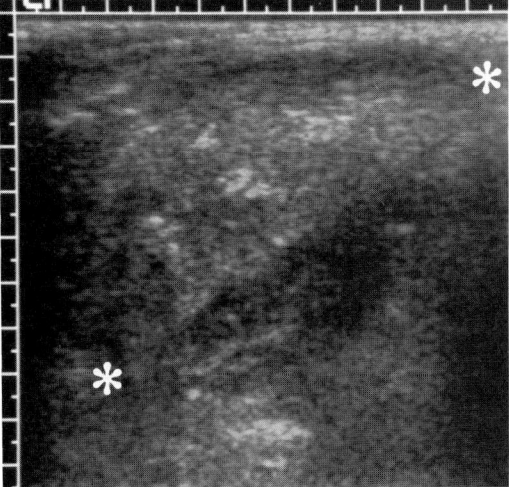

Figure 20–1. Oxalosis is a systemic disease that results in renal failure, and treatment involves a subsequent renal graft. This longitudinal scan shows patchy echogenicity of a transplanted kidney from deposition of crystalline oxalate. (Here, as in other figures throughout this chapter, asterisks outline the kidney.)

cadaveric donors. All of the evaluation of a living, related donor, who is usually a parent, is done at an "adult" institution. This includes renal ultrasonography, intravenous urography, and arteriography. Radionuclide scanning is performed 2 days before the transplantation to provide a baseline study for comparison later. The evaluation of the donor is carried out separately from that of the recipient because radiologists who have expertise in the imaging of adults can provide a better service. Also, the donor is removed from the pediatric environment, where subliminal pressure on the potential donor might introduce bias in interpretation or be considered coercive.

Children often are accompanied to the postoperative evaluations by a parent or parents. The ultrasonographer should be aware of the surgical history of the transplanted kidney. Emotions can run high if a parent's donated kidney is being rejected or if a cadaveric kidney—used because a parent, for whatever reason, could not be a donor—fails.

The type of operative procedure for renal transplantation depends on the size of the recipient. In large children and adolescents, the kidney is placed by a retroperitoneal approach through the anterior abdominal wall. The renal artery and vein are anastomosed to external iliac vessels or to the hypogastric artery and external iliac vein. In small children, generally those weighing less than 15 kg, the surgeons use an intraperitoneal approach and the vascular anastomoses are to the inferior vena cava or common iliac vein and to the distal aorta or common iliac artery. The ureter is implanted into the bladder by an antireflux technique (Figs. 20–2, 20–3).

Immediate postoperative complications in-

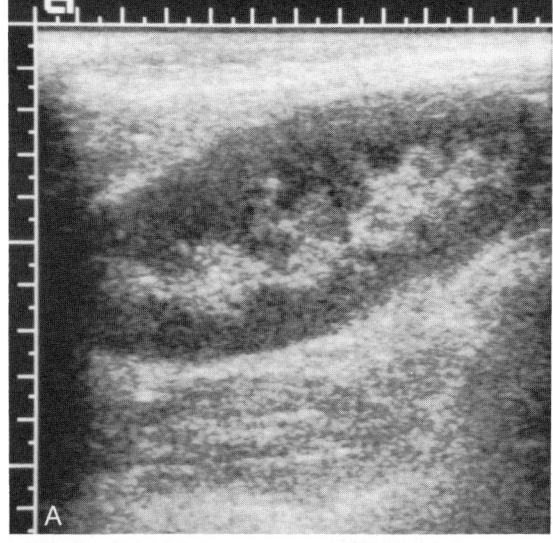

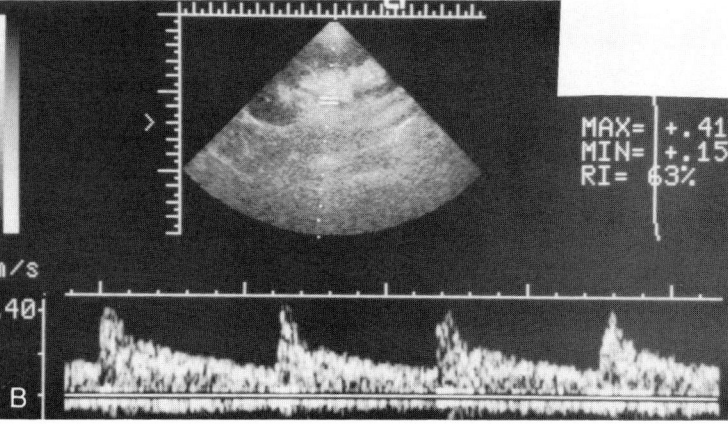

Figure 20–2. Longitudinal scan of the normal transplant kidney (**A**) shows delineation between medulla and cortex. The medullary pyramids are slightly more lucent than the cortex. The size of the kidney is unchanged from its baseline measurements before transplantation. This kidney is 12.7 cm long; the patient received the transplant from her father. **B** shows Doppler tracing from the hilar renal artery with a small component of an adjacent renal vein below the baseline. The renal arterial tracing shows a resistive index of 63 percent, which is within the normal range. Notice that throughout diastole, there is forward blood flow into the kidney.

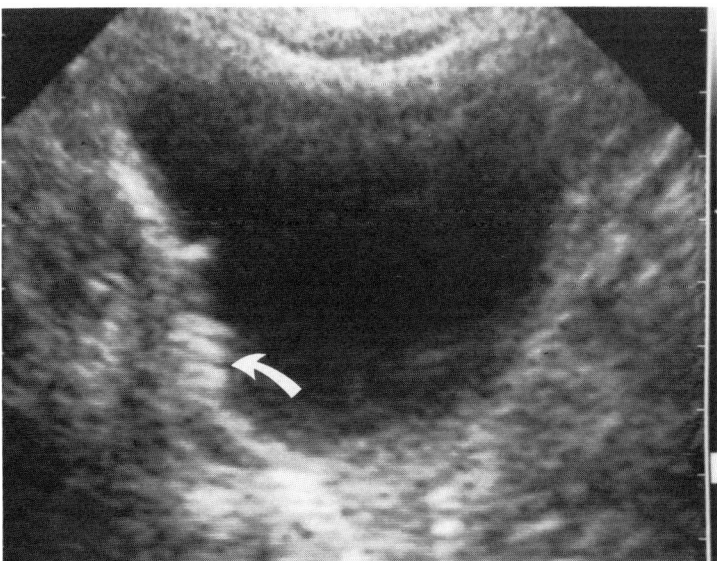

Figure 20–3. The ureter from the donated kidney is tunneled through the wall of the host's bladder. This transverse scan shows the irregular surface of the bladder (arrow) associated with implantation of the ureter.

clude bleeding around the graft, urinary leak, lymphatic leak, vascular thrombosis, hyperacute rejection, and acute tubular necrosis. Our protocol calls for expedient postoperative scans, which have to be done at the patient's bedside. A semisterile technique is used. A mask, gloves, and a gown over street clothes are worn. The dressing is taken down by the nurse. Sterile gel is used on a transducer that has been rinsed in germicidal cleanser and sterile saline. The transducer is placed lateral and medial to the longitudinal J-shaped incision, and scans are performed in semicoronal and axial planes. We generally follow the same routine for all studies of children who have had renal transplantation, although the emphasis changes the longer the postoperative interval is. Our checklist includes comments pertaining to immediate postoperative scans.

1. Perinephric and other collections: there is usually a drain around the kidney, and this is identified by its striped echogenicity. Blood may be lucent or echogenic. A maturing clot may be difficult to recognize (Fig. 20–4). Urinary leakage may occur at the site of ureteral implantation or above the ureterovesical junction. Surprisingly, renal scintigraphy has been reported as less sensitive than ultrasonography in diagnosing urinary leakage (Smith et al., 1988). Antegrade pyelography is the most definitive study when this complication is suspected. Lymphatic leaks are uncommon; our surgeons meticulously tie off lymphatic channels to prevent this complication. Some blood, pooling in the pelvis behind the bladder, may be evident if an intraperitoneal approach was used. Usually, the Foley catheter in the bladder keeps the bladder empty, thus preventing a good view of the cul-de-sac. However, the area of the bladder should always be scanned; poor urinary output may be due to a plugged Foley catheter.

2. Vascular supply: color Doppler ultrasonography is worth its purchase price after one appreciates how easy it is to evaluate blood flow in the transplanted kidney with one flick of a switch. We routinely use the 5-MHz linear array probe and scan the kidney from top to bottom. Color representing arterial and venous blood flow should be apparent in all sections. Its focal absence is easy to detect (Plate XVIII). Color also points us to specific vessels that can be sampled with pulsed Doppler ultrasonography. We track the main vessels, both arterial and venous, back to their anastomoses by following the color path with pulsed Doppler imaging. There is always turbulent blood flow at the anastomotic sites. Markedly increased velocity of flow implies anastomotic narrowing, which may or may not be transient and should be documented carefully on follow-up studies. We routinely measure resistive indices in arteries throughout the kidney, using them as a baseline for the particular patient (Fig. 20–2). Further discussion of this topic follows later.

3. Renal parenchymal pattern: as part of

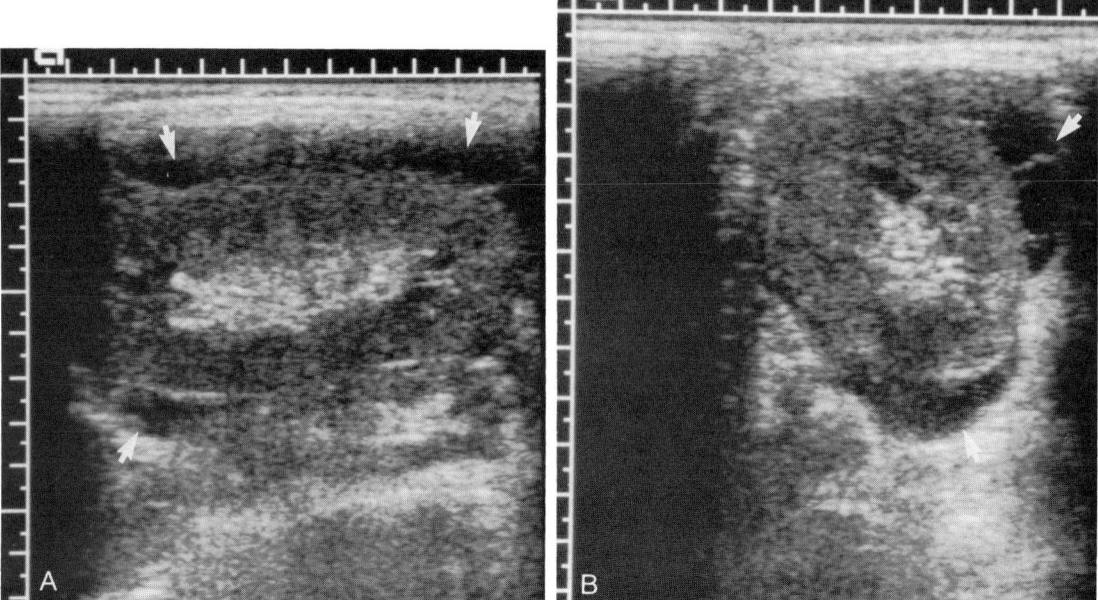

Figure 20–4. Longitudinal (**A**) and transverse (**B**) scans of this little girl 2 days after renal transplantation show blood (arrows) around the transplanted kidney. Fibrinous strands are beginning to form within the collection.

the ultrasonographic survey, we measure the length of the kidney; the postoperative scan serves as a baseline. We do not routinely measure volume although other researchers have advocated volumetric studies in the evaluation of rejection and acute tubular necrosis (ATN). Local ischemia resulting from an acutely obstructed vessel causes the affected parenchyma to become more echolucent. Over time, the region shrinks in size, the infarcted parenchyma becomes more echogenic, and the associated calix or calices dilate to fill in the void (Martin et al., 1988). The renal cortex and medulla should be distinguishable in the normal transplanted kidney. The fat around the renal sinus of an adult's kidney may be quite dramatic in contrast to the usual child's anatomy; it is not pathologic. It tends to increase in prominence after administration of steroids (Fig. 20–5).

4. Collecting system: diuresis causes mild separation of the walls of the collecting sys-

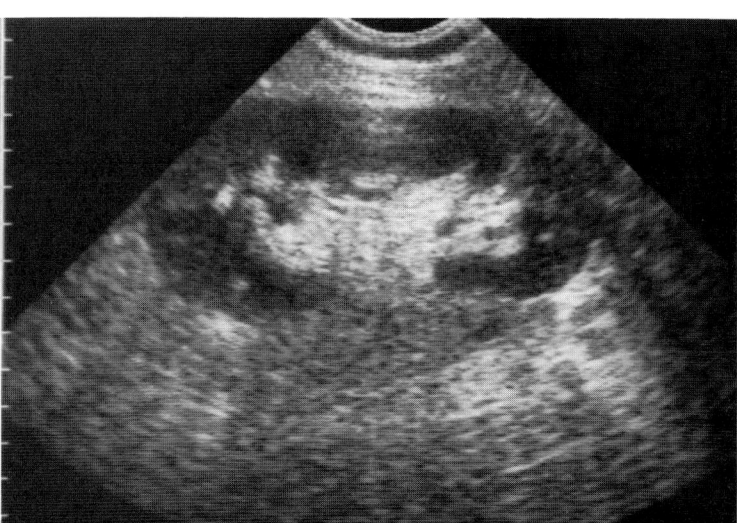

Figure 20–5. This patient's scan was performed 1 year after renal transplantation. His own kidneys had failed as a secondary result of chemotherapy for a tumor of the brain. His renal transplant was working very well. Note the rather obvious central echogenicity caused by fat around renal vessels and calices, in part secondary to the steroids taken for immunosuppression.

tem, but obvious dilatation is abnormal. In the postoperative phase, an intraureteral blood clot, tight ureterovesical anastomosis, and distal ureteral ischemia all may cause obstruction. A full bladder may cause pseudohydronephrosis.

Although we noted at the beginning of this chapter that many more young, small children are coming to renal transplantation, there is no question that this group has the lowest rates both of patient survival and of graft survival. Patients younger than 5 years of age have the lowest rates of survival. In a study from Toronto only 50 percent of patients who were 2 years old or younger at the time of surgery survived longer than 4 years (Churchill et al., 1988). Thrombosis of the vessels is a major factor in failure of the graft; the child's lower cardiac output in relation to a much larger kidney leads to inefficient renal perfusion and vascular thrombosis. Other poor prognostic variables include a cadaveric kidney from a young donor (less than 4 years old) and preceding obstructive uropathy. Of these two factors, the mechanism of failure with obstructive uropathy is better understood. The reduction in compliance of the bladder, which persists years after an obstructing valve has been fulgurated, results in compromise of ureteral transport of urine into the bladder. The high pressure in the bladder is transmitted to the grafted kidney and results in lower renal blood flow and glomerular filtration rate. In the study from Toronto, 60 percent of transplanted kidneys failed in the group of boys who had had obstruction from posterior urethral valve (Churchill et al., 1988).

Technical factors (i.e., smaller vessels to anastomose) obviously play a role in poorer prognosis when young kidneys are transplanted into young patients. However, there are other factors, which include the apparent increased vascular resistance in young cadaveric kidneys if they are stored for any length of time before grafting and the younger child's increased tendency toward rejection (Sheldon et al., 1987; Churchill et al., 1988).

Rejection is a complex interactive mechanism between host and graft mediated primarily by the T cells of the immune system. Classification of rejection follows:

1. Hyperacute rejection is almost always immediate and necessitates removal of the graft. Adequate immunologic screening prevents this complication.

2. Accelerated acute rejection occurs in the first week after transplantation; prognosis is poor, and destruction of the graft appears to result from both antibody and cell-mediated mechanisms.

3. Acute rejection occurs in the first year, typically presenting as pain, fever, and oliguria. Mononuclear infiltrate and vascular rejection are the histologic features, and it can be reversed with aggressive therapy.

4. Chronic rejection is insidious, usually asymptomatic loss of renal function months or years after transplantation. This appears histologically as glomerular and vascular injury.

ATN occurs after the graft has been ischemically damaged. Ischemia is more common in cadaveric grafts; it generally occurs in the week following transplantation. The drugs used to treat rejection are themselves nephrotoxic. This is particularly true for cyclosporine. Rejection, ATN, and drug toxicity have similar clinical presentations but obviously require different therapy. Early reports on duplex sonography of renal transplantations suggested that measurements derived from the waveform of the intrarenal arteries could discriminate among these three diagnoses. Our experience and that of others (Genkins et al., 1989; Keller, 1989; Allen et al., 1988) has not supported the early optimistic reports (Fig. 20–6). However, we make measurements and document the resistive index of the allograft at each examination. The patient is his or her best control subject, and a sudden or sustained gradual change in measurements suggests that histologic change is occurring within the graft. The resistive index (RI) is calculated as follows:

$$\frac{\text{peak velocity of systolic flow } - \text{ minimum velocity at end diastole}}{\text{peak velocity of systolic flow}}$$

Top normal value is considered to be 0.75, or 75 percent. When one reads the literature on Doppler ultrasonography, one should be aware that there are several measurements in use to characterize the waveform. Unfortunately, the RI has sometimes been termed the Pourcelot index, or "PI." This term then gets confused with the pulsatility index (also PI), which is calculated as follows:

$$\frac{\text{peak velocity of systolic flow } - \text{ minimum velocity at end diastole}}{\text{mean velocity during one cardiac cycle}}$$

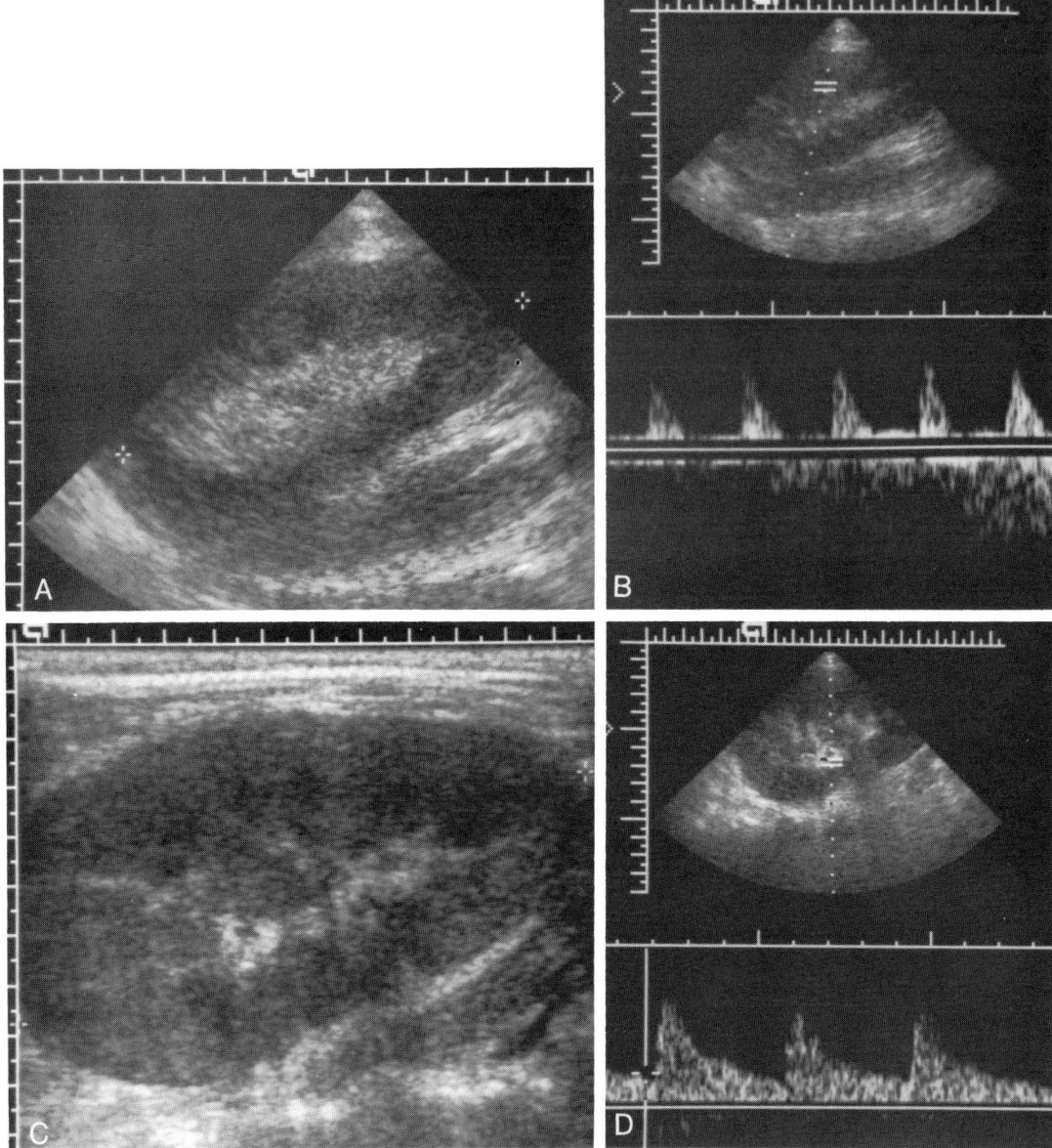

Figure 20–6. Longitudinal scan of the kidney immediately after renal transplantation from a parental donor shows the kidney to be slightly swollen but otherwise normal (**A**). The resistive index measured at the same time was 86 percent. Note the minimal forward blood flow during diastole (**B**). The patient had a clinical diagnosis of acute tubular necrosis. She recovered uneventfully, but 1 month later she had an episode in which creatinine and blood urea nitrogen (BUN) levels rose. The longitudinal scan of the kidney at this time (**C**) shows swelling of the graft and less distinct central echoes. It is 2 cm longer than the baseline measurement shown in **A**. The resistive index however was normal, measuring between 66 and 69 percent in different areas of the kidney (**D**). A biopsy at this time showed interstitial rejection; the patient received treatment with steroid pulse.

Top normal value for pulsatility index is 1.8. Other measurements, infrequently used but mentioned in the literature, include systolic/diastolic ratio (SDR, whose normal value is 4) and diastolic/systolic ratio (DSR, whose normal value is 0.25; Allen et al., 1988). It appears that the use of one or another measurement depends on the type of equipment available. Some manufacturers have programmed their units to calculate the resistive index; others, the pulsatility index.

Decrease in the forward velocity of diastolic flow correlates with increased renovascular resistance. Thus as intrarenal resistance rises, diastolic velocity falls, and RI rises. However, an abnormally high RI is not specific for rejection, as once thought. An increase in RI is a nonspecific sign of intrarenal pathology and has been noted in rejection, ATN, toxicity from cyclosporine, pyelonephritis, renal venous obstruction, and extrarenal compression of the graft (Warshauer et al., 1988; Genkins et al., 1989). A normal RI suggests that significant intrarenal pathology is absent. Of course, one would need biopsies on all patients who have normal ultrasonographic examinations in order to support that statement, and such a study is not appropriate. It apparently does not matter which vessel is chosen for measurements (Allen et al., 1988). We have found it easiest to use interlobar or segmental arteries because they are sharply defined with color Doppler ultrasonography for sampling with pulsed Doppler ultrasonography. Before Doppler scanning was available, there was great interest in diagnosing rejection on the basis of parenchymal pattern. Although neither completely specific for nor sensitive to the presence of rejection, the combination of three or more of the following findings is very suggestive of rejection: increased renal volume (more than 30 percent over baseline); abnormal medullary pyramids (prominent and rectangular rather than pyramidal); altered parenchymal echogenicity (mottled or increased); and reduction or absence of echoes from the central sinus (because of infiltration of fat by edema; Fig. 20–7; Slovis et al., 1984). These ultrasonographic findings can be combined with results from radionuclide studies before a decision regarding empiric treatment or biopsy is made.

Although delayed complications of transplantation may be silent, more often they are heralded either by symptoms reported by the patient or by a rising level of creatinine in blood. The following is a discussion of the most common problems other than rejection.

About one third of children who undergo renal transplantation have a minor or major postoperative urologic complication (Zaontz et al., 1988). Urinary leakage typically occurs immediately after surgery. Ureteral stricture is a less dramatic sequel to ischemic injury (Fig. 20–8). Hydronephrosis may result from obstruction (ureteral stricture, stone, blood clot), from vesicoureteral reflux, and from dysfunctional voiding in patients who have physiologic abnormalities of the bladder

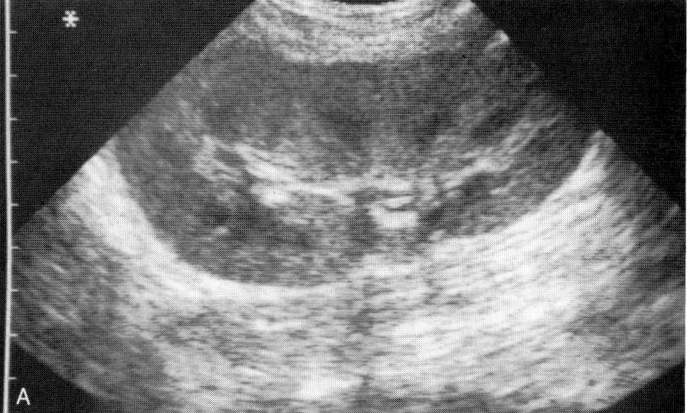
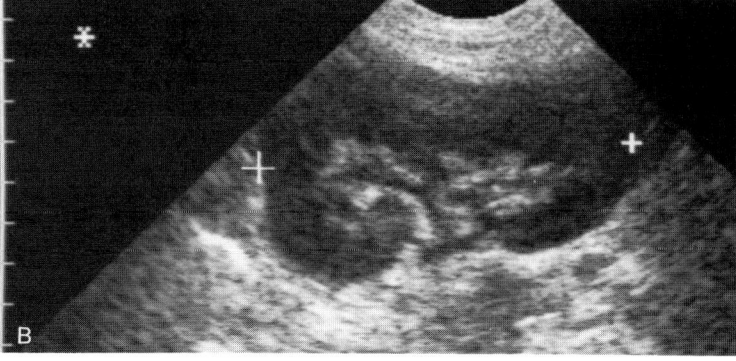

Figure 20–7. An episode of acute rejection produced this ultrasonographic picture of a swollen graft, slightly increased parenchymal echogenicity throughout the cortex, prominent medullary pyramids, and reduction of echoes from the central sinus (**A**). After therapy, a follow-up scan (**B**) shows a return to the normal baseline appearance of the transplanted kidney in this 12-year-old, who had undergone cadaveric transplantation. Crosses mark upper and lower edges of the kidney.

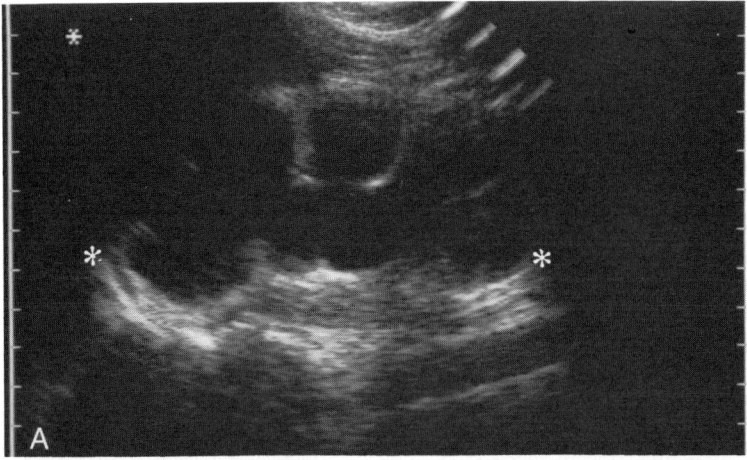
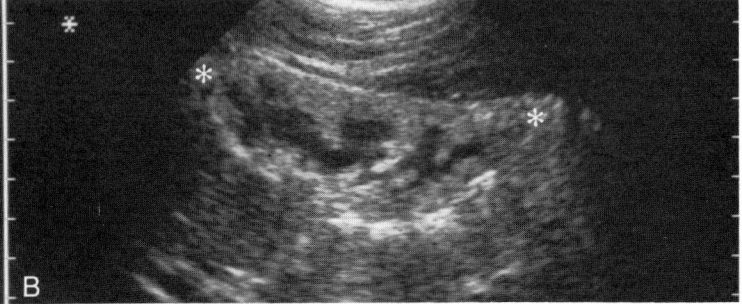
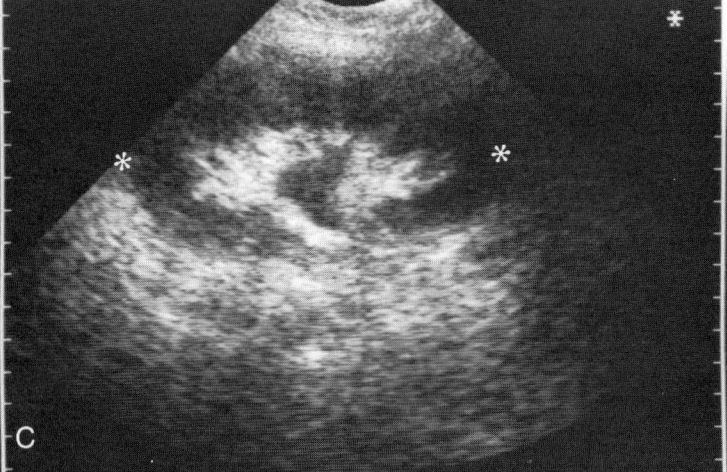

Figure 20–8. Longitudinal scans of the native kidneys in this adolescent girl show almost no cortex around the left hydronephrotic collecting system (**A**) and echogenic parenchyma surrounding an ectatic right renal collecting system (**B**). This patient had a neurogenic bladder with reflux and pyelonephritis. **C** shows her baseline renal scan after cadaveric renal transplantation to an ileal conduit.

(Figs. 20–9, 20–10). Dilatation of the collecting system also occurs ex vacuo as renal parenchyma shrivels from chronic rejection. Scans should always be repeated after the bladder has been fully emptied if there is any dilatation of the collecting system.

Not only are renal or vesical stones uncommon; their diagnosis is also difficult. Because the transplanted kidney is denervated, the child does not have the typical symptoms of renal colic when a stone is obstructing the ureter. Hypercalciuria, surgical stents or sutures, hyperoxaluria, and infection of the urinary tract are all predisposing situations for patients in whom nephrolithiasis has been reported (Fig. 20–11; Cho et al., 1988; Caldwell and Burns, 1988).

Urinary infection typically affects children who have undergone transplantation and in whom obstructive uropathy or reflux was the cause of renal failure. Thickening of the uroepithelial surface of the renal collecting sys-

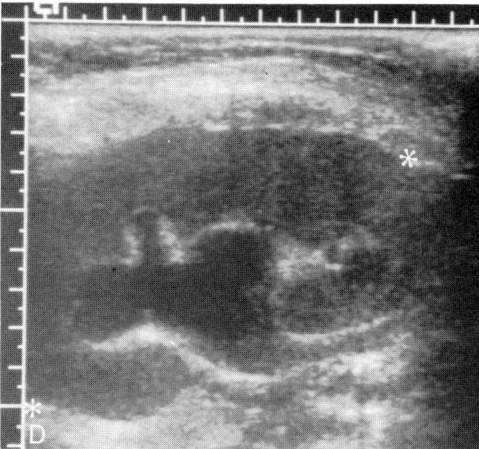
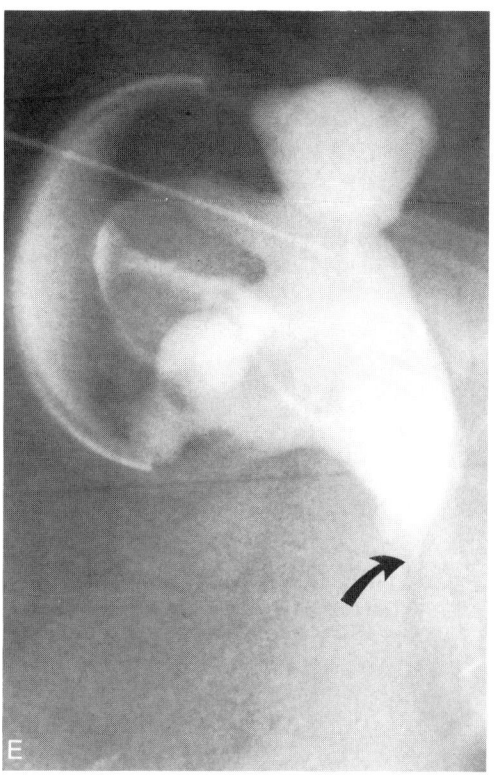

Figure 20–8 *Continued* Eight months later, creatinine levels increased to 1.4 from 1.2. Pelvic, infundibular, and mild caliceal dilation is now evident in the transplanted kidney (D). A nephrostomy tube was placed after antegrade study (E) showed stricture (arrow) of the ureter from the graft. One month later she underwent reconstruction of the ureteroileostomy after resection of the stricture.

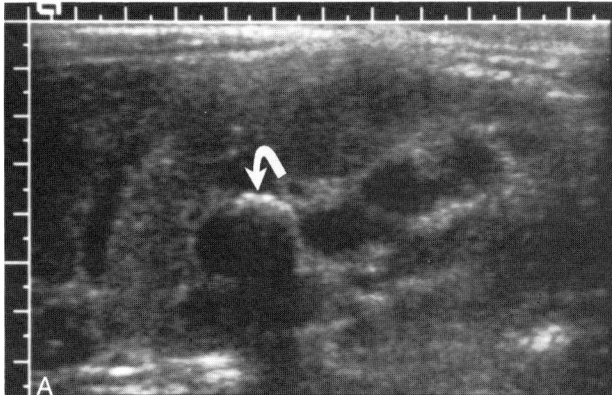
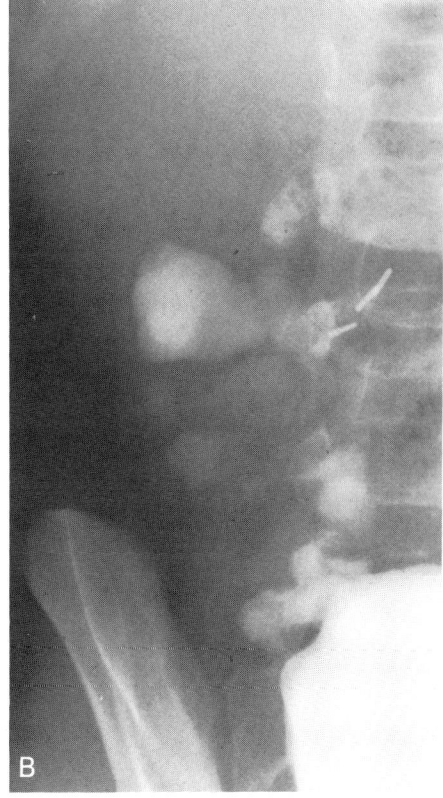

Figure 20–9. This 2-year-old girl had a Wilms tumor in her only kidney. She received one of her father's kidneys after a period of renal dialysis. A postoperative ureteral stricture necessitated reconstruction of the ureter with a piece of ileum. Subsequent sonogram (A) showed stones (arrow) in the upper calix of a mildly dilated collecting system. Cystogram (B) showed reflux into both the ileal ureter and the transplanted kidney as a cause for the stones and dilatation.

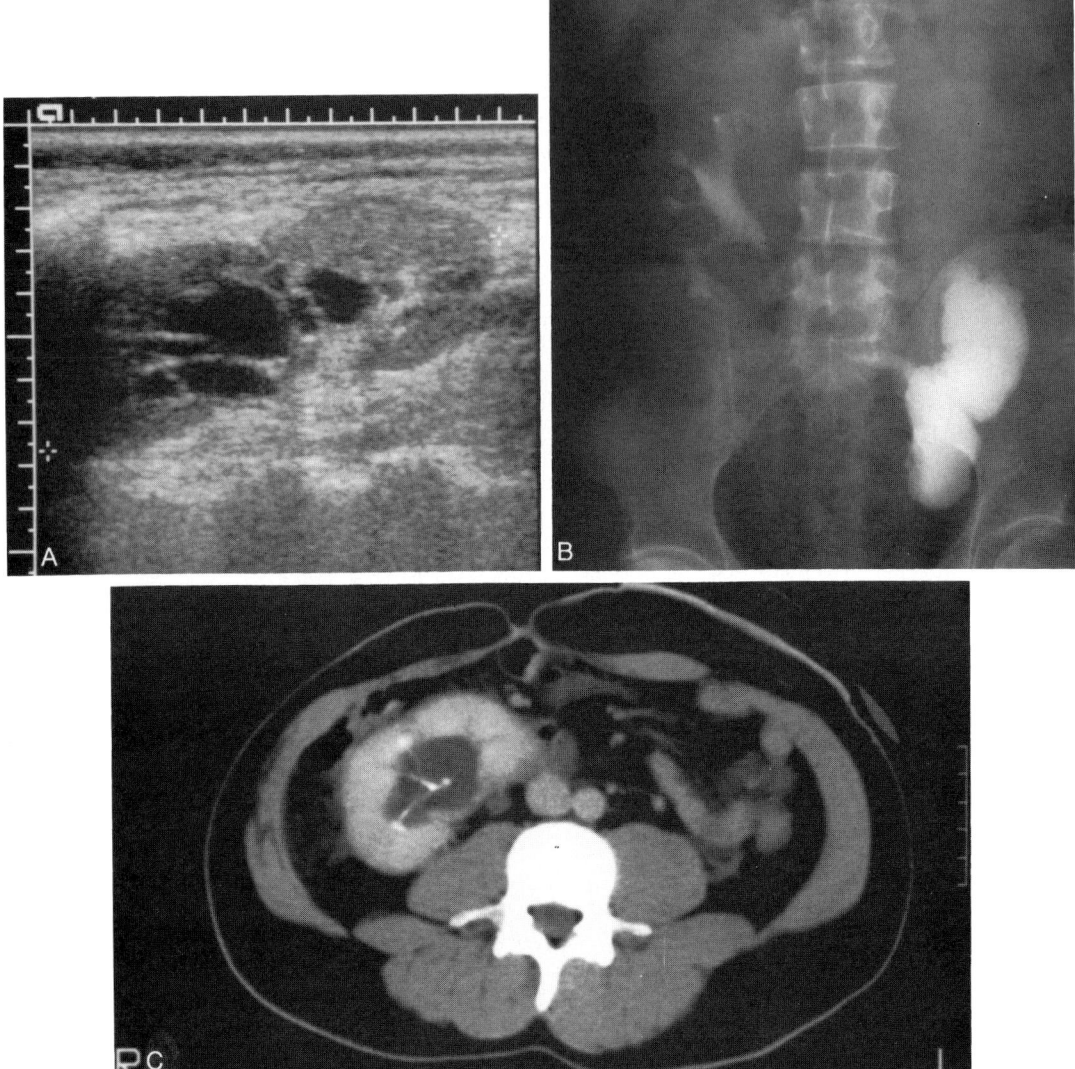

Figure 20–10. This patient has been followed for years at our institution since renal transplantation with ureteral implantation into an ileal loop. Echolucencies that gradually appeared within the transplanted kidney were diagnosed as hydronephrosis (**A**). The loopogram (**B**), however, showed a normal collecting system with attenuation of the infundibula. Computed tomography (CT) scan (**C**) shows the lucencies to be around the collecting system, and these undoubtedly represent lymphatic cysts in the renal hilum. We present this as a case of "pseudohydronephrosis." When an abnormality is identified on ultrasonography, it is always helpful to have a confirmatory physiologic study as well.

tem, once thought specific for rejection, may also be seen with infection (Nicolet et al., 1988).

When we see a child who presents after transplantation with hematuria as a primary complaint, we consider infection, stones, and vascular abnormality as possible causes. For any urologic symptom, however, it is important to remember that the transplanted kidney may not be the culprit. The patient's own kidneys, if still present, or the unused portions of his or her own urinary tract may be causing problems (Fig. 20–12).

Renovascular disease may present any time after transplantation, and it is usually heralded by hypertension. Damage to vessels, specifically the arteries, may result from poor surgical technique during creation of the arterial anastomosis, trauma from the perfusion catheters, intimal tears from trac-

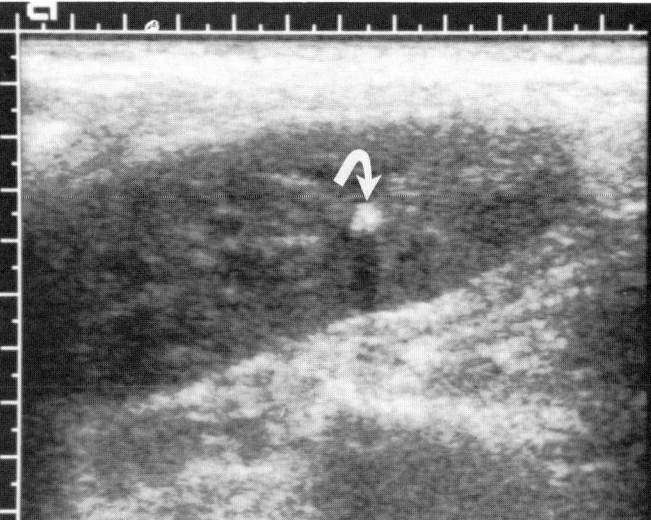

Figure 20–11. Two years after transplantation, routine follow-up ultrasonographic study showed shadowing stones (arrow) in this kidney transplanted from a parent. No etiology for the stones was apparent. Lithotripsy is a therapeutic option, but because this child is asymptomatic and uninfected, she is being managed conservatively at present.

tion, hemodynamic injury from end-to-side anastomoses, and vascular rejection. Cyclosporine is associated with a higher rate of vascular thrombosis (Fine, 1988). Therefore, although the anastomosis is the major area of interest, evaluation of the patient's entire arterial supply is necessary when he or she has acute onset of hypertension. Hypertension is not specific for renovascular disease. After transplantation, 85 percent of children may have hypertension, and a renovascular cause accounts for only a small percentage of all cases (Barth et al., 1989). A frequency shift greater than 7 kHz and associated distal turbulence within the artery have been used as criteria for diagnosing stenosis (Snider et al., 1989). When arterial narrowing is shown by Doppler imaging, angiography follows (Fig. 20–13). Angioplasty has been used to treat arterial stenosis and in some studies has been very successful in decreasing blood pressure by widening the arterial lumen

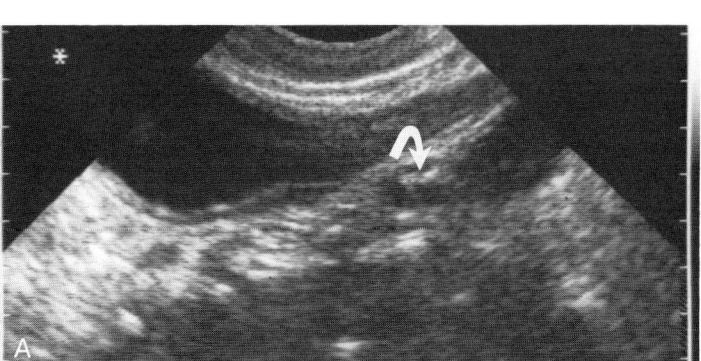
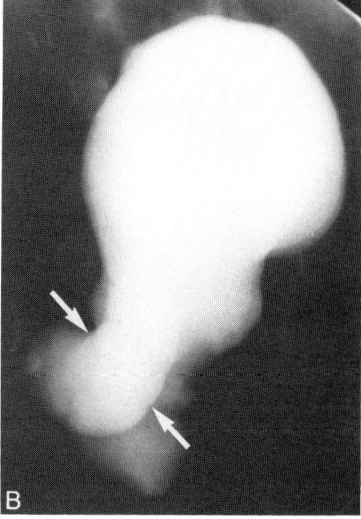

Figure 20–12. This little boy had had multiple ultrasonograms of his transplanted kidney, and no cause for his chronic hematuria had been identified. At each visit, however, he had always had an empty bladder. Finally, when he was kept in the ultrasonographic room until his bladder had filled, it was apparent that an unusual lucency adjacent to the bladder had two small foci representing stones (arrow) within it **(A)**. Voiding cystourethrogram **(B)** immediately followed and demonstrated reflux into an unused ureter (arrows). The resulting stasis in the unused ureter likely contributed to formation of stones.

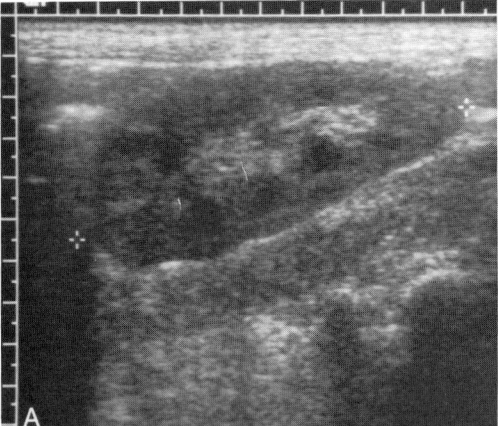
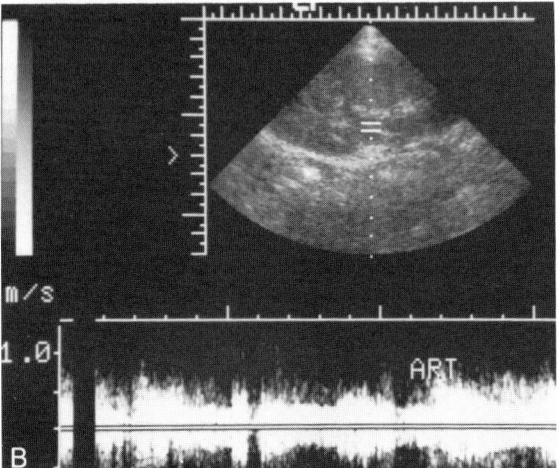
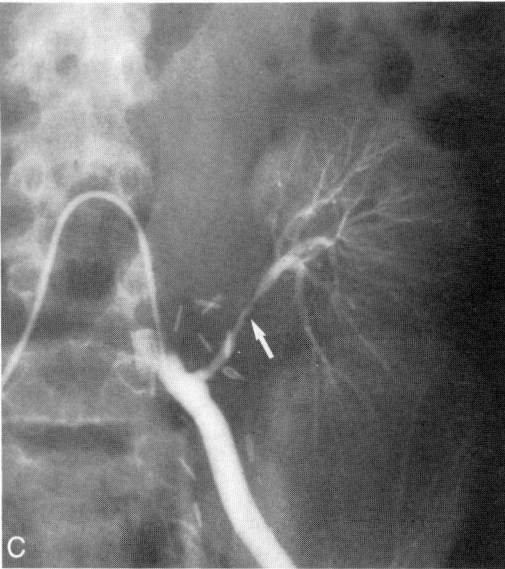

Figure 20–13. The longitudinal scan of this transplanted kidney **(A)** looks completely normal. On Doppler ultrasonography **(B)**, however, there was markedly turbulent blood flow in the renal artery at the hilum of the kidney. Angiography **(C)** followed for this child, who was hypertensive. Note the marked narrowing of the renal artery (arrow) beyond its anastomosis with the external iliac artery. Because of the degree, length, and position, the stenosis was not considered surgically accessible, and thus the patient underwent several angioplastic procedures in an attempt to alleviate the stenosis. Blood pressure dropped after each procedure. However, gradual restenosis resulted in recurrent hypertension.

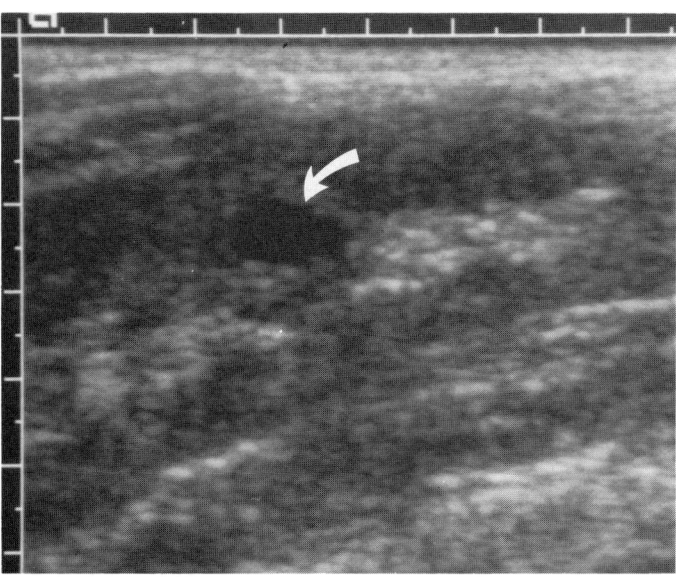

Figure 20–14. This renal cyst (arrow) was discovered in a transplanted kidney several months after the patient received the kidney from her father. Preoperative studies on the donated kidney had all yielded normal results. It is possible that this cyst is the result of a vascular accident involving a small segmental artery. However, it is not unusual to see a cyst develop in a transplanted kidney and be completely asymptomatic.

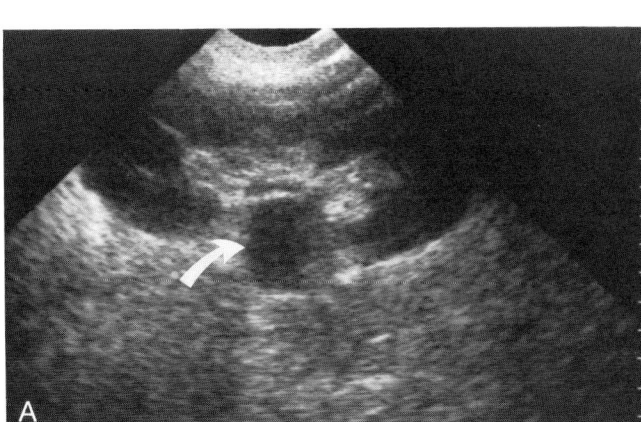 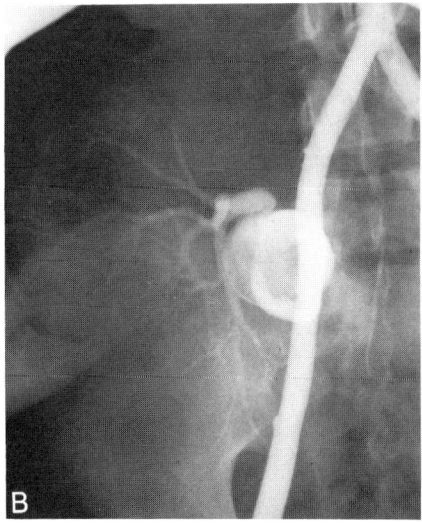

Figure 20–15. The lucency (arrow) adjacent to the transplanted kidney but apparently related to the hilum was interpreted as an extrarenal pelvis **(A)**. However, on multiple scans, this lucency never could be "joined" to the rest of the intrarenal collecting system. Doppler ultrasonography, if available at the time, would have immediately shown this cystic mass to be a pseudoaneurysm, as shown in the subsequent angiographic study **(B)**. An intimal tear in the vessel from the graft was likely responsible for this complication. Any lucency in or around the transplanted renal graft should be investigated with Doppler ultrasonography.

(Barth et al., 1989). Pseudoaneurysms within the kidney are virtually always a result of previous biopsy. Arteriovenous fistula can also result from biopsy (Stringer et al., 1989).

The parenchymal pattern of the transplanted kidney may change if the kidney is beset by multiple episodes of rejection, if the patient's original renal disease attacks the graft, if the kidney is infected, or if additional nephrotoxic drugs (e.g., amphotericin) are added to the already toxic cyclosporine. A renal cyst may occur in the transplanted kidney, possibly as a sign of accelerated aging (Fig. 20–14). Any echolucency within the kidney should be investigated with Doppler imaging so as to exclude pseudoaneurysm (Fig. 20–15; Tobben et al., 1988).

REFERENCES

Allen KS, Jorkasky DK, Arger PH, et al: Renal allografts: Prospective analysis of Doppler sonography. Radiology 1988; 169:371–376.

Barth MO, Gagnadoux MF, Mareschal JL, et al: Angioplasty of renal transplant artery stenosis in children. Pediatr Radiol 1989; 19:383–387.

Caldwell TC, Burns JR: Current operative management of urinary calculi after renal transplantation. J Urol 1988; 140:1360–1363.

Cho DK, Zackson DA, Cheigh J, et al: Urinary calculi in renal transplant recipients. Transplantation 1988; 45:899–902.

Churchill BM, Sheldon CA, McLorie GA, et al: Factors influencing patient and graft survival in 300 cadaveric pediatric renal transplants. J Urol 1988; 140 (Part 2):1129–1133.

Drake DG, Day DL, Letourneau JG, et al: Doppler evaluation of renal transplants in children: A prospective analysis with histopathologic correlation. AJR 1990; 154:785–787.

Fine RN: Renal transplantation of the infant and young child and the use of pediatric cadaver kidneys for transplantation in pediatric and adult recipients. Am J Kidney Dis 1988; 12:1–10.

Genkins SM, Sanfilippo FP, Carroll BA: Duplex Doppler sonography of renal transplants: Lack of sensitivity and specificity in establishing pathologic diagnosis. AJR 1989; 152:535–539.

Keller MS: Renal Doppler sonography in infants and children. Radiology 1989; 172:603–604.

Keown PA, Stiller CR, Wallace AC: Effect of cyclosporine on the kidney. J Pediatr 1987; 111:1029–1033.

Martin KW, McAlister WH, Shackelford GD: Acute renal infarction: Diagnosis by Doppler ultrasound. Pediatr Radiol 1988; 18:373–376.

Najarian JS, Ascher NL, Mauer SM: Kidney transplantation. In Welch KJ, Randolph JG, Ravitch MM, et al (eds): Pediatric Surgery (4th ed). Chicago: Year Book Medical Publishers, Inc., 1986, 360–373.

Nicolet V, Carignan L, Dubuc G, et al: Thickening of the renal collecting system: A nonspecific finding at US. Radiology 1988; 168:411–413.

Sheldon CA, McLorie GA, Churchill BM: Renal transplantation in children. Pediatr Clin North Am 1987; 34:1209–1232.

Slovis TL, Babcock DS, Hricak H, et al: Renal transplant rejection: Sonographic evaluation in children. Radiology 1984; 153:659–665.

Smith TP, Hunter DW, Letourneau JG, et al: Urine leaks after renal transplantation: Value of percutaneous pyelography and drainage for diagnosis and treatment. AJR 1988; 151:511–513.

Snider JF, Hunter DW, Moradian GP, et al: Transplant renal artery stenosis: Evaluation with duplex sonography. Radiology 1989; 172:1027–1030.

Stringer DA, O'Halpin D, Daneman A, et al: Duplex Doppler sonography for renal artery stenosis in the post-transplant pediatric patient. Pediatr Radiol 1989; 19:187–192.

Surratt JT, Siegel MJ, Middleton WD: Sonography of complications in pediatric renal allografts. Radiographics 1990; 10:687–699.

Tobben PJ, Zajko AB, Sumkin JH, et al: Pseudoaneurysms complicating organ transplantation: Roles of CT, duplex sonography, and angiography. Radiology 1988; 169:65–70.

Vergesslich KA, Khoss AE, Balzar E, et al: Acute renal transplant rejection in children: Assessment by Duplex Doppler sonography. Pediatr Radiol 1988; 18:474–478.

Waltzer WC, Shabtai M, Anaise D, et al: Usefulness and limitations of Doppler ultrasonography in the evaluation of post-operative renal allograft dysfunction [Abstract]. J Urol 1988; 139 (Part 4, No. 2):232A.

Wan SK, Ferguson CJ, Cochlin DL, et al: Duplex Doppler ultrasound in the diagnosis of acute renal allograft rejection. Clin Radiol 1989; 40:573–576.

Warshauer DM, Taylor KJ, Bia MJ, et al: Unusual causes of increased vascular impedance in renal transplants: Duplex Doppler evaluation. Radiology 1988; 169:367–370.

Zaontz MR, Hatch DA, Firlit CF: Urological complications in pediatric renal transplantation: Management and prevention. J Urol 1988; 140 (Part 2):1123–1128.

INDEX

Note: Page numbers in *italics* refer to illustrations; page numbers followed by t refer to tables.

Abdomen, aneurysm in, 385, *386*
  approach to evaluation of, 214–215
  heterotaxia of, splenic anomaly and, 414, *414*
  inflammation in, acquired immunodeficiency syndrome and, 355, *355–356*
    appendicitis and, 346–353, *347–354*. See also *Appendicitis*.
    fever and, 354–355, *355*
  mass in, 214–309. See also names of specific conditions.
    anterior, 274–309
      abdominal wall tumor as, 274–275
      carcinoma as, 275–276
      chronic granulomatous disease and, 279, *280*
      Crohn disease and, 277–278, *277–279*
      doughnut lesion as, 276
      edematous intestinal wall and, 279–280
      general considerations for, 274–281
      hemorrhagic intestinal wall and, 279–280
      lymphoma as, 275, *276*, 276–278
      Ménétrier disease and, 279
      mesenteric solid tumor as, 274, *275*
      peptic disease and, 279, *281*
      teratoma as, 274–275
      typhlitis and, 280–281
      ulcer and, 279, *281*
      ulcerative colitis and, 278, *279*
    cyst as, 283–285, *284, 285*
    hematoma as, 281
    hepatic mass as, 261–274. See also *Liver, mass in*.
    in presence of ventriculoperitoneal shunt, 285
    intussusception and, 281–282, *282*
    pelvic mass as, 285–309. See also *Pelvis, mass in*.
    retroperitoneal, 215–260
      abscess as, 257, *258*
      acquired immunodeficiency syndrome and, 259–260, *260*
      adrenal mass as, 240–250. See also *Adrenal gland, mass in*.
      hemorrhage and, 258

Abdomen *(Continued)*
      hydronephrosis and, 215–239. See also *Hydronephrosis*.
      lipoblastoma as, 257
      lipoma as, 257
      lymphangioma as, 258
      lymphoma as, 258–259, *259*
      neurogenic tumor as, 257, *257*
      other than hydronephrosis, 239–260
      psoas muscle, 257
      renal mass as, 250–256. See also *Kidney, mass in*.
      rhabdomyosarcoma as, 257
      teratoma as, 256–257
      trauma and, 364–371. See also *Trauma, abdominal, blunt*.
  pain in, as indication for renal ultrasonography, 137t
    intussusception and, 281
    recurrent, 343–345
      in adolescence, 344–345
      intermittent renal obstruction and, 344, *344*
      malrotation and, 344, *345*
      role of ultrasonography in, 343–344, *345*
    renal disorder and, 157, *157*
  vasculature in, 385, *385, 386*, 387
Abscess, adrenal, 242
  appendicitis and, *352*, 353
  hepatic, 272, *272*
  in acute pyelonephritis, 202, *203, 204*
  psoas, 257–258
    Crohn disease and, 354
  retroperitoneal, 257, *258*
  splenic, 411, *412, 413*
  testicular, 333
Achilles tendon, ruptured, 114
Acquired immunodeficiency syndrome. See also *Human immunodeficiency virus*.
  abdominal involvement in, 259–260, 355, *355*
  precautions with, 356
  retroperitoneal mass and, 259–260, *260*
Acrocephalosyndactyly, renal cystic disease and, 147t

Acute tubular necrosis, in native kidney, 465, 468t
  renal transplantation and, 480, 481, 482
Adenoma, adrenal, 249–250
  hepatic, 266, 267, 267–268
  parathyroid, 80
  thyroid, 80, 81
Adenopathy, cervical, 73–76, 74–77
  causes of, 74t
  infection and, 73–74, 77
  neoplastic, 74, 77
  node aspiration and, 74
Adolescence, abdominal pain in, recurrent, 344–345
  breast disease in, 106, 107, 107
  fatty liver in, 438
  pelvic mass in, 299–309. See also *Pelvis, mass in.*
  spleen in, 405
  urinary tract infection in, 200, 201
ADPD. See *Autosomal dominant polycystic kidney disease.*
Adrenal gland, hemorrhagic, 241–242, 242, 243
  hypertrophied, 240–241, 242
  in abdominal trauma, 371
  in renal agenesis, 146, 148
  mass in, 240–250
    adenoma as, 249–250
    carcinoma as, 249, 249–250
    neuroblastoma as, 242–244, 246–248, 248. See also *Neuroblastoma.*
    pheochromocytoma as, 248–249, 249
  neonatal, 318
  normal, 240, 240
Adrenarche, normal age for, 336
  premature, 318–319, 320
Agenesis, adrenal, 146
  renal, 146–149, 148–150
    familial theme in, 148
    syndromes associated with, 146, 146t
AIDS. See *Acquired immunodeficiency syndrome.*
Alpha-fetoprotein level, as sign of malignancy, 263, 264, 267
Alport syndrome, renal abnormality and, 146t
Alvarado score, in appendicitis, 346, 346t
Amebic disease, 273
Amenorrhea, 336–340
  primary, 336–338, 337–339
    chemotherapy in, 338
    general considerations for, 340
    gonadal dysgenesis in, 336–337, 337
    radiotherapy in, 338, 338, 339
    testicular feminization in, 338
    Turner syndrome in, 336–337, 337
  secondary, 338–340, 340
    ovarian tumor in, 340
    polycystic ovaries in, 339–340, 340
    pregnancy in, 338
    weight loss in, 340
Anemia, cholelithiasis and, 426, 427
  Fanconi, renal abnormality and, 146t
Aneurysm, abdominal, 385, 386
  extremity, 122, 122–124
  of vein of Galen, 50, 51, 52
Angiography, in hepatic mass, 268
Angiomatosis, cerebelloretinal, renal cystic disease and, 147t
Aniridia, Wilms tumor and, 137t, 157

Anorectal malformation, spinal dysraphism and, 61
Anorexia, amenorrhea and, 340
  appendicitis and, 346t, 349
Antibiotic therapy, appendicitis and, 349
Anticoagulant therapy, hemorrhagic ovarian cyst and, 304
Antimicrobial therapy, urinary tract infection and, 197
Anus, imperforate, 387, 387–388
  renal abnormality and, 146t
Apert syndrome, renal cystic disease and, 147t
Apgar score, 19, 20
Aplasia, renal, 146t
Appendicitis, 346–353, 347–354
  abscess and, 352, 353
  antibiotic therapy and, 349
  bladder distention and, 348, 349, 349, 350
  clinical examination in, 346, 346t
  diagnosis in, 350, 350–351
  differential diagnosis in, 346–347
  false-negative in, 350, 351, 351
  false-positive in, 350–352, 351
  pelvic free fluid in, 349, 349, 350
  perforated appendix and, 352–354, 353
  role of ultrasonography in, 346–347, 347
  rupture in, 347, 348, 349
Appendix testis, 334, 334
Aqueductal stenosis, ventriculomegaly and, 39–40, 40
Arachnoidal cyst, 46–47, 47, 48
Arnold-Chiari malformation, in premature infant, 8, 10
  meningomyelocele and, 59
  micropolygyria and, 33
  spinal ultrasonography in, 58
  ventriculomegaly and, 40, 42, 43, 44
ARPD. See *Autosomal recessive polycystic kidney disease.*
Artery(ies). See also *Vasculature.*
  carotid, ultrasonography of, 84, 85
  face and neck, ultrasonography of, 84, 85
  hepatic, 440, 440, 441, 443
    in hepatic transplantation, postoperative evaluation for, 456–457, 457–460, 459–461
      biliary tree in, 460, 461
      hepatic arterial thrombosis in, 459, 459
      portal venous thrombosis in, 460, 460
    preoperative evaluation for, 454
  renal, 139, 140, 387
    in hypertension, 159, 160, 161
    occlusion of, 466–467, 467
  splenic, malformation of, 414
  umbilical, single, 143
Ascariasis, in etiology of pancreatitis, 396–398
Ascites, 372–373, 375–377, 379–382, 384
  aspiration of, 384
  bile, 373
  causes of, 374t, 378t
  cerebrospinal fluid and, 373
  childhood, 373, 378t, 379–383
  chylous, 374t
  clinical information in, 373, 384
  fetal, 374t
  iatrogenic, 375
  laboratory studies in, 373, 384
  malignancy and, 374t, 378t, 382, 383
  neonatal, 373, 374t, 375, 377

Ascites (Continued)
  ovarian, 297
  volume of, in hepatic transplantation preoperative evaluation, 452
Asphyxia neonatorum, 19–25
  Apgar score as marker of, 19, 20
  computed tomography in, 23
  definition of, 19
  hypoxic-ischemic injury and, 19–21, 20–23
  incidence of, 19
  magnetic resonance imaging in, 23
  risk factors for, 19
  subdural hemorrhage and, 21–22, 23
  ultrasonography in, 20–23, 20–23
Ataxia, cerebellar, renal cystic disease and, 147t
ATN. See Acute tubular necrosis.
Atresia, biliary, choledochal cyst and, 418
  hepatic transplantation and, 452, 454
  jaundice and, 417–419, 418
  kidney involvement in, 419
  vaginal, 300
Autosomal dominant polycystic kidney disease, 181, 182, 183
Autosomal recessive polycystic kidney disease, 182–183, 184, 185

Bacterial infection. See also Meningitis, bacterial.
  adenopathy and, 73–74, 77
  hepatic abscess and, 272, 272
  in pneumonia, 93–94
  muscle mass and, 111, 112
  of urinary tract, 193–211. See also Urinary tract, infection of.
Baker cyst, 111–112
Barlow maneuver, 125, 125, 127, 129
Basal cell nevus syndrome, 178, 180
Beckwith-Wiedemann syndrome, renal cystic disease and, 147t
  other tumors and, 157
  Wilms tumor and, 156, 157, 157
"Bell-clapper" deformity, 333
Bertin, columns of, 141, 144
Bile, operative drainage of, 417
Bile duct, common, cholelithiasis in, 430, 432
Biliary atresia, choledochal cyst and, 418
  hepatic transplantation and, 452, 454
  jaundice and, 417–419, 418
  kidney involvement in, 419
Biliary tract, tumor of, 271–272
Biliary tree, anomaly of, 418, 420–422, 422–424, 425
  cholelithiasis in, 425–426
  in hepatic transplantation, 453, 454, 460, 461
  in pancreatitis, 398
Biopsy, fine needle, of neuroblastoma, 248
  renal, 472–473, 474
Bladder. See also Urinary tract.
  diseases simulating, 138
  hydronephrosis and, 228
  neurogenic, 169–171, 170, 171
  normal, 138, 139
  postoperative, 171–172, 172–175, 174–176
  reconstruction of, 174–176, 174–176
  tumor in, 294, 294–295
Blood pressure, measurement of, 158
Bowel, evaluation of, 278–279, 280

Brachio-oto renal syndrome, renal abnormality and, 146t
Branchial cleft, cyst in, 86
Breast, premature development of. See Thelarche, premature.
  tumors of, 107
  ultrasonography of, in adolescence and childhood, 106, 107, 107
Budd-Chiari syndrome, hepatic venous obstruction and, 447, 448
Burkitt lymphoma, 259, 275, 276, 276–278

Caliectasis, in acute pyelonephritis, 208, 209
Candidal infection, hepatic, 272–273, 273
  meningitis and, 27
  splenic, 409, 409–410
  urinary tract, 209–210, 211
Carcinoma, abdominal, 275–276
  adrenal, 249, 249–250
  colonic, 276
  fibrolamellar, 263
  hepatocellular, 263, 264
  ovarian, 303, 304
  pancreatic, 401–402, 401–402
  renal, 255–256, 256
  testicular, 329–330, 330
Cardiac disorder, ascites and, 374t, 378t, 379
  chest ultrasonography in. See Chest, ultrasonography of.
  congenital heart disease as, 143
  splenic infection and, 411, 412
  tumor as, 100, 101, 101
  unexplained cardiac failure and, 50, 51, 52
Caroli disease, 182, 421–422, 424, 425
Carotid artery, ultrasonography of, 84, 85
Cartilage, disorders of, 114, 115
Cast, hip ultrasonography in presence of, 132, 134
Cataract, congenital, renal abnormality and, 146t
Cat-scratch disease, splenic, 410
Cavum vergae, 44, 45
CDH. See Congenital dysplasia of hip.
Cerebellar vermis, absence of, 36–37, 38
Cerebelloretinal angiomatosis, renal cystic disease and, 147t
Cerebellum, hemorrhagic, 14, 16, 16
Cerebral edema, in asphyxiated infant, 20, 21
Cerebral palsy, intraparenchymal echogenicity and, 14
Cerebrohepatorenal syndrome, renal cystic disease and, 147t
Cerebrospinal fluid, infection of, 27. See also Meningitis.
  pseudocyst of, 285
  ventricular dilatation and, 18
Chemotherapy, amenorrhea and, 338
Chest, ultrasonography of, 91–107
  diaphragm in, 98–100, 98–100
  heart in, 91, 92
  in intrathoracic mass, 100–101, 105
    cardiac tumor and, 100, 101
    cystic adenomatoid malformation and, 100
    mediastinal mass and, 101, 103, 104, 105
    pulmonary sequestration and, 100–101, 102
    thymic mass and, 101, 104, 105

Chest *(Continued)*
　in pleural effusion, 91, 93–98. See also *Pleural effusion*.
　superficial mass and, 105, *106, 107, 107*
　technique in, 91
Childhood, ascites in, 373, *379–383*, 384
　causes of, 378t
　breast disease in, *106, 107*, 107
　causes of ventriculomegaly in, 43t
　chronic granulomatous disease of, abdominal mass in, 279, *280*
　　spleen in, 410, *410*
　Hodgkin disease in, 74, *75*
　pelvic mass in, 294–299. See also *Pelvis, mass in*.
　renal parenchymal disease in, 467–475. See also *Renal parenchymal disease, in childhood*.
　urinary tract infection in, 197–198, *199–201*, 200
Cholangiocarcinoma, 421
Cholangiography, in choledochal cyst, 421
Cholangiopancreatography, in choledochal cyst, 421
Cholecystitis, 430–434
　acalculous, 430, 433, *433*
　ascites and, 430, *431*
　cholelithiasis and, 430–434
　gallbladder wall thickening and, 430, *431*
Cholecystomegaly, 430, *432–434*, 433
Choledochal cyst, *418*, 420–421
Cholelithiasis, 425–429
　anemia and, 426, *427*
　biliary atresia and, 426
　cholecystitis and, 430–434
　cystic fibrosis and, 426, *427, 428*
　development of, 425
　diseases associated with, 425t
　floating, 429, *429*
　follow-up in, 426, *427*, 429
　in common bile duct, 430, *432*
　metabolic liver disease and, 426
　neonatal, 425, *426*
　parenteral nutrition and, 426, *428*
　postoperative, 426, *428, 429*
Cholestasis, 417
Choroid plexus, in premature infant, 8, *10*
　hemorrhage of, 8
Choroidal cyst, 45, *45*
Chromosome 13, trisomy of, 146t, 147t
Chromosome 18, trisomy of, 146t, 147t
Chromosome 19 translocation, renal cystic disease and, 147t
Chromosome 21, trisomy of, 146t, 147t
Chromosome 45x, abnormality of, 146t
Chronic granulomatous disease of childhood, abdominal mass in, 279, *280*
　spleen in, 410, *410*
Circumcision, urinary tract infection and, 194
Cloacal exstrophy, pelvic kidney and, 151
　renal abnormality and, 146t
　spinal anomalies and, 65, 68, *68*
Cockayne syndrome, renal abnormality and, 146t
Collecting system, of ectopic kidney, 149, 151
　of horseshoe kidney, 152, *153, 154*
　of malrotated kidney, 152, *155*
Colloid cyst, of third ventricle, 47
Colon, carcinoma of, 276

Computed tomography, in abdominal trauma, 365, *366*
　in asphyxia neonatorum, 23
　in deep sacral dimple, 61
　in dysmorphia, 45–46
　in gluteal mass, 111, *111*
　in hydranencephaly, 39
　in hypertension, 159
　in mediastinal mass, 101, *104*
　in meningitis, 28
　in neuroblastoma, 244
　in superficial thoracic mass, 105, *105*
　spinal ultrasonography *v*, 59–60, 61
Congenital dysplasia of hip, 123–134
　classification in, 126
　clinical signs in, 124–126, *125*
　incidence of, 126
　laxity in, 126–127
　maneuvers in, *125*, 125, 127, 129
　measured angles in, 130, *130*
　plaster or plastic cast and, 132, 134
　risk factors in, 126
　screening in, 126, 134
　secondary adaptive changes in, 130, *132, 133*
　stress view in, 129, 132
　teratologic dislocation in, 126
　ultrasonography in, 126–130, *127–133*, 132, 134
Congenital heart disease, as indication for ultrasonography, 143
Congenital intracranial neoplasm, 46–47, *46–49*
Congenital scoliosis, renal abnormality and, 146t
Conus medullaris, in spinal ultrasonography, 57, 58, *58, 59*
Corpus callosum, absence of, 34, *35–37*, 36, 49
　lipoma of, *36*, 46
　normal, 34, *34*
Cortical heterotopia, absence of corpus callosum and, 34
Cranial ultrasonography, 1–52
　coronal scans in, 2, *3*
　Doppler, 25–27
　　asphyxia neonatorum and, 26–27
　　intracranial hemorrhage and, 26
　　unexplained cardiac failure and, 50, *51*, 52
　feeding time and, 1
　in congenital neoplasm, 46–47, *46–49*
　in craniomegaly, 49–50, *50*
　in dysmorphia, 30–46. See also *Dysmorphia*.
　in ischemic injury to brain, 7
　in meningitis, infants and, 27–28, *29*, 30
　in periventricular leukomalacia, 7
　in unexplained cardiac failure, 50, *51*, 52
　intracranial hemorrhage and, 6–19, *17, 18*. See also *Premature infant, intracranial hemorrhage in*.
　normal scans in, 2, *3, 4, 5*
　of premature infant, 7–19. See also *Premature infant, cranial ultrasonography of*.
　of term infant, asphyxia neonatorum and, 20–23, *20–23*
　　Doppler ultrasonography and, 26–27
　　extracorporeal membrane oxygenation and, 24, *24–25*, 25
　parents' presence at, 4–5
　preparation for, 1
　sagittal scans in, 3, *4*
　technique in, 1, 2, *3–5*, *4, 5*

Cranial ultrasonography *(Continued)*
  terminology in, 7
Craniomegaly, 49–50, *50*
  cranial ultrasonography in, 49–50, *50*
Cranium, ultrasonography of. See *Cranial ultrasonography.*
Crohn disease, 354
  abdominal mass and, 277–278, *277–279*
  thickening of colonic wall in, 278
Cryptorchidism, ultrasonography in, 143, 323–325, *324, 325*
Cyclophosphamide, hematuria and, 163
Cyclosporine, vascular thrombosis and, 487
Cystic adenomatoid malformation, congenital, 100
Cystic encephalomalacia, in premature infant, 7
Cystic fibrosis, cholelithiasis and, 426, *427, 428*
  echogenic pancreas and, 391, *391*
  intussusception and, 282
  pancreatic cyst and, *400*, 401
Cystic hygroma. See also *Lymphangioma.*
  in extremity, Doppler image and, 117
  thoracic, 105, *106*
  ultrasonography in, 84, *86*
Cystitis, hematuria and, 163, *163*
Cystography, in perforation, 176
  in urinary tract infection, 197, 198, 200
Cystosarcoma phylloides, 100
Cyst(s), abdominal, 283–285, *284, 285*
  arachnoidal, 46–47, *47, 48*
  as scrotal mass, 328–329, *329*
  branchial cleft, 86
  choledochal, *418*, 420–421
  choroidal, 45, *45*
  colloid, of third ventricle, 47
  dermoid, 86, 292
  duplication, 283, *284*
  epidermoid, *329*, 329, 410–411, *412*
  epididymal, 328–329
  gastric, vomiting and, 360, *361*
  hepatic, 268, *268*, 269
    congenital, 271, *271*
  hydatid, 411
  multilocular cystic nephroma as, 250–251, *251*
  ovarian, hemorrhagic, 303, *305*
    in adolescence, 301, *301–305*, 303
    pelvic mass and, 292, *293, 294*, 294
    septated, 301, *302, 303*, 303
  pancreatic, *400*, 401
  pelvic, *291*, 291–292
    in adolescent boy, 309, *309*
  popliteal, 111–112, *113*
  renal, 137t, 146, 146t, 176–188
    chromosomal abnormality and, 187
    classification in, 177
    general considerations in, 176–177
    hypertension and, 178
    juvenile nephronophthisis as, 185–187, *186, 187*
    medullary cystic disease as, 186
    medullary sponge kidney as, 186–187
    multiple cysts as, 178–179, 181
      renal dysplasia in, 178–179, *181*, 181
    polycystic kidney disease as, 181–185, *182–185.* See also *Polycystic kidney disease.*
    single, 177–178, *178–180*

Cyst(s) *(Continued)*
  syndromes associated with, 147t, 187–188
  splenic, 410–411, *411, 412*
  testicular, 329
  thymic, 105
  thyroglossal, 79–80, *80*
  thyroid, 79–80, *80–82*
  urachal, 284, *285*
Cytomegalovirus, meningitis and, 30, *32*

Dandy-Walker malformation, 36–37, *38*
  absence of corpus callosum and, 34
  arachnoid cyst v, *47*, 48
  renal cystic disease and, 147t, 185
Deafness, congenital, renal abnormality and, 146t
Dermoid cyst, of neck, 86
  ovarian, 292
Developmental disorder, intraparenchymal echogenicity and, 14
Developmental dysplasia of hip. See *Congenital dysplasia of hip.*
Diandry, 146t
Diaphragm, cystic mass in, 101
  excursion of, 98–99
  hernia through, *98–100*, 99–100
    renal agenesis and, 152, *155*
  ultrasonography of, 98–100, *98–100*
    delayed, 99
Diastematomyelia, 61
Digyny, renal abnormality and, 146t
Diuretic ultrasonography, 223
Diverticulum, bladder, ureterocele v, 229
  pyelocaliceal, 178, *179*
Doppler ultrasonography, cranial, 25–27
  asphyxia neonatorum and, 26–27
  intracranial hemorrhage and, 26
  unexplained cardiac failure and, 50, *51, 52*
  in deep venous thrombosis, 118, *120*, 120, 121
  in hepatic transplantation, *458*, 459
  in hypertension, 159, *160*, 160
  in malformation of extremity, 117
  in painful scrotal mass, 332
  in portal hypertension, 446, 447
  in postoperative splenorenal shunt follow-up, 447
  in renal arterial occlusion, 467, *467*
  in renal mass, 250
  in renal transplantation, 479, 481–483
  in watershed infarct, 21
  of portal system, 446–447
Doughnut kidney, 152
Down syndrome. See *Trisomy 21.*
Drash syndrome, renal abnormality and, 146t
Dubowitz score, 1
Duodenum, trauma to, 367–368, *370, 371*
Duplication cyst, 283, *284*
Dwarfism, renal abnormality and, 146t
Dysmorphia, 30–46
  absence of corpus callosum in, 34, *34–37*, 36, *49*
  absence of septi pellucidi in, 36, *37*
  computed tomography in, 45–46
  Dandy-Walker malformation in, 36–37, *38*
  general considerations for, 30–31, 33–34, 45–46
  holoprosencephaly in, 37–39, *38, 39*
  hydranencephaly in, 39, *40*

Dysmorphia (Continued)
  lissencephaly in, 34
  magnetic resonance imaging in, 45–46
  micropolygyria in, 31, 33
  pachygyria in, 33, 33
  ventriculomegaly in, 39–42, 40–45, 43t, 44–46
Dysplasia, cervical, renal abnormality and, 146t
  choledochal cyst and, 421
  congenital, of hip. See *Congenital dysplasia of hip.*
  glomerular, syndromes associated with, 146t
  renal, 147t, 176, 177, 179, 181, 181
    as response to chronic obstruction, 232, 233
    syndromes associated with, 146t
  renal-retinal, renal cystic disease and, 147t
  skeletal, renal cystic disease and, 147t
Dystrophy, thoracic, asphyxiating, renal cystic disease and, 147t

Ear, abnormal, as indication for ultrasonography, 143
Echinococcus, 273–274
Echogenicity, cerebral intraparenchymal, 7
  asphyxia neonatorum and, 20, 20–21
  renal parenchymal disease and, 467–468, 469, 470
    in neonate, 462–463, 463
  cerebral palsy and, 14
  cranial ultrasonography of, intraventricular hemorrhage and, 14
  developmental disorder and, 14
  in premature infant, 13–14, 15
  intraventricular hemorrhage and, 14
ECMO. See *Extracorporeal membrane oxygenation.*
Edema, cerebral, in asphyxiated infant, 20, 21
  intestinal, 279–280
  scrotal swelling and, 335, 335
Edwards syndrome. See *Trisomy 18.*
Effusion, in joints, 115, 115, 116
  pleural. See *Pleural effusion.*
Ehlers-Danlos syndrome, renal cystic disease and, 147t
Empyema, bacterial infection in, 94
Encephalocele, renal cystic disease and, 147t
Encephalomalacia, cystic, in premature infant, 7
Endocrinologic ultrasonography, 317–340
  in ambiguous genitalia, 317–318
  in amenorrhea, 336–340. See also *Amenorrhea.*
  in Leydig tumor, 320, 322, 322
  in ovarian cyst, 319–320, 320
  in ovarian tumor, 320
  in precocious puberty, 318, 318
    female, 318–320, 319–321
    male, 318–320, 319–321
  scrotal ultrasonography as, 322–335. See also *Scrotum, ultrasonography of.*
  voiding urethography and, 318, 318
Endoscopic retrograde cholangiopancreatography, in pancreatitis, 398
Entamoeba histolytica, 273
Enterocolitis, necrotizing, 386, 387
Epidermoid cyst, of spleen, 410–411, 412
  of testis, 329, 329

Epididymis, cyst of, 328–329
  inflammation of, 332–333, 333, 334
  tumors of, 329
Epididymitis, 333, 334
Escherichia coli, adrenal hemorrhage and, 242
  in urinary tract infection, 193, 200, 204
  meningitis and, 29
Exomphalos, renal cystic disease and, 147t
Exstrophy, cloacal, pelvic kidney and, 151
  renal abnormality and, 146t
  spinal anomalies and, 65, 68, 68
Extracorporeal membrane oxygenation, 23–25
  chest ultrasonography and, 98, 99
  indications for, 23–24
  intracranial hemorrhage and, 23–24
  surgical reconstruction after, 84, 85
  technique in, 23–24
  ultrasonography in, 24, 24–25, 25
Extremity(ies), ultrasonography of, 109–134
  general considerations in, 109–110
  in congenital dysplasia of hip, 123–134. See also *Congenital dysplasia of hip.*
  in effusion, 115, 115, 116
  in fracture, 116, 117
  in infection, 111, 112
  in joint injury, 114–115
  in ligament injury, 114–115
  in mass, identification of, 111–112, 111–113
  in neuromuscular disease, 110
  in penetrating wound, 122–123, 123
    foreign body and, 112, 113, 114, 123
  in popliteal cyst, 111–112, 113
  in pseudoaneurysm, 122–123, 122–124
  in soft tissue neoplasm, 111, 112
  in subcutaneous fat measurement, 109–110, 110
  in tendon injury, 114–115
  in vascular abnormality, 116–123
    congenital abnormality of vessel and, 117, 118
    deep venous thrombosis and, 117–121
      Doppler imaging in, 118, 120, 120, 121
      previous intravenous catheter and, 121, 122
      risk factors in, 117
      technique in, 117–119

Face and neck, ultrasonography of, 73–89
  connective tissue and, 84, 86, 86–89
  in adenopathy, 73–76, 74–77
    causes of, 74t
    infection and, 73–74, 74–77
    neoplastic, 74, 77
    node aspiration and, 74
  in parathyroid disease, 80, 84, 84
  in sinus disease, 78–79
  in thyroid disease, 79–80, 80–83
  larynx and, 86, 89
  salivary glands and, 78, 78, 79
  vessels and, 84, 85
  vocal cords and, 86, 89
Falciform ligament, 441
Familial juvenile nephronophthisis, renal cystic disease and, 147t
Fanconi anemia, renal abnormality and, 146t

Fat, subcutaneous, ultrasonography in measurement of, 109–110, *110*
Feeding, cranial ultrasonography and, 1
Femoral vein, examination of, 118–119, *119–120*
Fetus, abdominal mass in, 214, 216–218, *216–219*
  ascites in, causes of, 374t
  cranial abnormality in, 44–45
  cystic adenomatoid malformation in, 100
  hydronephrosis in, 214, 216, 217
  spinal cord abnormality in, 60
Fever of unknown origin, 354–355, *355*
Fibroadenoma, breast, 107, *107*
Fibrolamellar carcinoma, 263
Fibromatosis colli, 86, *89*
Fibrosis, cystic. See *Cystic fibrosis.*
  hepatic, 422, 425
Fontanelle, 5
Foreign body, in extremity, 112, *113*, 114
Furosemide, 221
  urolithiasis and, 165

Galen, vein of, 50, *51*, 52
Gallbladder, anomaly of, 416, *417*
  contraction of, 418
  enlargement of, *422–434*, 430, *433*
  hydropic, 430
  in biliary atresia, 417–419, *418*
  in pancreatitis, 398
  inflammation of. See *Cholecystitis.*
  length of, 416, *417*
  location of, 416
  neonatal, biliary atresia and, 417–418, *418*
  shape of, 416
  wall thickening in, 430, *431*
Gallstone. See *Cholelithiasis.*
Gastroduodenal ultrasonography, in neonate, 357–362. See also *Vomiting, neonatal.*
Gastroesophageal reflux, vomiting and, 361
Gastrointestinal disorder, ascites and, 374t, *376*, 378t, *380, 381*
Genital anomaly, renal agenesis and, 146
Genital tract, ambiguous, 317–318
  duplication of, *300*, 300–301, *321*
  mass in, 292, *293*
Genitourinary disorder, ascites and, 374t, *375*, 378t
  tumor as, 294, *294–295*
Germinal matrix, hemorrhage in, in term infant, 22
  in premature infant, 8, *9*
Gestational age, determination of, 1
Gigantism, renal cystic disease and, 147t
GKD. See *Glomerulocystic kidney disease.*
Glomerular dysplasia, syndromes associated with, 146t
Glomerulocystic kidney disease, 147t, 183–185, *185*
Glomerulonephritis, hematuria and, 163, 163t
Glomerulonephropathy, syndromes associated with, 146t
Glycogen storage disease, 438
  hepatic adenoma and, 266, *267*
Goldenhar syndrome, 46
Goldston syndrome, 37
  renal cystic disease and, 147t

Gonad, dysgenetic, 336–337, *337*
  neonatal, 318
Gonadotropin-releasing hormone analog, in precocious puberty, 319, 320, *321*
Gynecologic anomaly, renal agenesis and, 146

Haemophilus influenzae, meningitis and, 27, *28*
Hair, pubic, premature appearance of. See *Adrenarche, premature.*
Hamartoma, hepatic, mesenchymal, *268*, 268–269, *269*
  renal mass as, 250, *251*
Harness, hip ultrasonography in presence of, 130, *131*
  Pavlik, *131*
Hashimoto thyroiditis, 80, *83*
Heart, disorders of. See *Cardiac disorder.*
  ultrasonography of, 91, *92*. See also *Chest, ultrasonography of.*
Hemangioendothelioma, hepatic, 269, *269*, *270*, 271
Hemangioma, face and neck, 84, *87*
  hepatic, 269, *270*, 271
  parotid, 78
  vascular birthmark as, 117, *118*
Hematoma, of bowel, 281
  trauma and, 281
Hematometrocolpos, 300, *301*
Hematuria, 163, *163*, 163t, *164*
  painless, 137t
  renal transplantation and, 486, *487*
  renal tumor and, 163
  renal ultrasonography in, 137t, 163, *163*, 163t, *164*
  urolithiasis and, 164, 168, *169*
Hemolytic uremic syndrome, 468, *470*
Hemorrhage, abdominal, 279–280
  adrenal, 241–242, *242*, *243*
  into ovarian cyst, 303, *305*
  intracerebellar, in premature infant, 14, 16, *16*
  intracranial, extracorporeal membrane oxygenation and, 23–24
  intraperitoneal, ascites and, 374t, *377*, 378t, *381*, *382*
  intraventricular, 7
    grading in, 8, 11, *12*, *13*
    hypoxic-ischemic insult and, 22
    intraparenchymal echogenicity and, 14
  retroperitoneal, 258
  subdural, asphyxia neonatorum and, 21–22, *23*
Henoch-Schönlein purpura, 279–280
  intussusception and, 282
Hepatic artery. See *Artery(ies), hepatic.*
Hepatic fibrosis, 422, 425
Hepatic vein. See *Vein(s), hepatic.*
Hepatitis, acute, causes of, 436, 436t
Hepatization, in pneumonia, 93
Hepatoblastoma, 263, *264*, *265*
Hepatocarcinoma, 263, *264*
Hepatoma. See *Hepatocarcinoma.*
Hepatosplenomegaly, acquired immunodeficiency syndrome and, 355
Hernia, as scrotal mass, 327, *327*
  diaphragmatic, *98–100*, 99–100
  renal agenesis and, 152, *155*

Hernia (Continued)
   hiatal, 99, 99
   hydrocele and, in male, 326, 327
Heterotaxia, abdominal, splenic anomaly and, 414, 414
Heterotopia, cortical, absence of corpus callosum and, 34
Hiatal hernia, 99, 99
Hip, congenital dysplasia of, 123–134. See also Congenital dysplasia of hip.
   fracture of, 116, 117
   infection of, 115–116, 116
Hodgkin disease, 258, 259
   in childhood, 74, 75
Holoprosencephaly, 37–39, 38, 39
   alobar, 38, 39, 40
   lobar, 38–39, 39
   semilobar, 39
Horseshoe kidney, 152, 153, 154
   Wilms tumor and, 157
Human immunodeficiency virus. See also Acquired immunodeficiency syndrome.
   abdominal lymphadenopathy and, 259–260
   cranial ultrasonography and, 30
   parotid abscess and, 78, 79
Hydatid cyst, 411
Hydatid disease, 273–274
Hydatid of Morgagni, 334, 334
Hydranencephaly, 39, 40
   computed tomography in, 39
   hydrocephalus v, 39, 40
Hydrocele, scrotal, 325–326, 326, 327
Hydrocephalus, 18–19
   hydranencephaly v, 39, 40
   ventriculomegaly and, 41, 41
Hydrometrocolpos, 292
Hydromyelia, 60–61
   definition of, 61
   intraoperative neurosonography in, 71, 71–72
Hydronephrosis, 137t, 139
   abdominal pain and, 157
   hematuria and, 163, 164
   postoperative, 172, 173, 174
   prenatal diagnosis in, 156, 216–218, 216–219, 237, 239
   renal transplantation and, 483–484, 485, 486
   retroperitoneal mass and, 215–239
      bilateral, 217, 218, 228, 234
      condition(s) associated with. See also names of specific conditions.
         chronic wetting as, 234–235, 236
         dilated collecting system as, 221
         duplex systems as, 233–234, 236–239
         multicystic dysplastic kidney as, 218–220, 219, 220
         posterior urethral valve as, 228, 230, 232, 232, 233
         postoperative edema as, 225, 226, 227
         primary megaureter as, 224–225, 225, 226
         prune-belly syndrome as, 236, 239, 239
         reflux as, 216–217, 217, 227–228, 231
         ureteral dilatation as, 220, 220–221, 223, 225, 226
         ureterocele as, 225, 226, 227, 228, 229
         urethral polyp as, 232, 234
         urinoma as, 230, 232, 233
      differential diagnosis in, 236
      follow-up in, 224

Hydronephrosis (Continued)
   furosemide in diagnosis of, 221
   general considerations for, 215–216, 235–236, 239
   neonatal, 216–218, 217–219
   nonobstructive causes of, 215, 236, 239, 239
   syndromes associated with, 146t
Hydrosyringomyelia, 61
Hydroureter, syndromes associated with, 146t
Hygroma, cystic. See also Lymphangioma.
   in extremity, Doppler image and, 117
   thoracic, 105, 106
   ultrasonography in, 84, 86
Hyperelastica, renal cystic disease and, 147t
Hyperparathyroidism, 80, 84, 84
Hyperplasia, nodular, focal, 266, 267
Hypertension, 137t
   blood pressure values in, 158
   causes of, 159, 159t
   incidence of, 158
   portal, 445, 446–447
      in hepatic transplantation, 452
   renal cystic disease and, 178
   renal transplantation and, 487–488, 488
   renal ultrasonography in, 158–159, 160–162
      neonate and, 159, 160
      pheochromocytoma and, 159–160, 162
      reflux nephropathy and, 160, 162
      renal anomaly and, 162–163
      renal parenchymal disease and, 160, 162
      renovascular disease and, 160
   Wilms tumor and, 162
Hypogenitalism, renal cystic disease and, 147t
Hypoglycemia, pancreatic disease and, 402–403
Hypospadias, as indication for ultrasonography, 143
Hypoxia, ischemia v, 19
Hypoxic-ischemic encephalopathy, 19
   in premature infant, 7
Hypoxic-ischemic injury, patterns in, 19–21, 20–23

Ileal conduit, 174
Iliac vein, examination of, 118
Imperforate anus, 387, 387–388
Infarction, splenic, 411, 413, 414
   watershed, 19, 21, 21, 22
Infection, adenopathy and, 73–74, 74–77, 77
   in etiology of ascites, 374t
   in pneumonia, 93–94
   muscle mass and, 111, 112
   urinary tract, 193–211. See also Urinary tract, infection of.
Insulinoma, pancreatic, 403
Intensive care nursery, cranial ultrasonography in, 1. See also Cranial ultrasonography.
Intussusception, 281–283, 282–285, 285
Ischemia, hypoxia v, 19

Jaundice, neonatal, 416–419
   biliary atresia and, 417–418, 418
   biliary tree anomaly and, 418, 420–422, 422–424, 425

Jaundice *(Continued)*
  cholangiography in, 419, *419*
  cholestatic, *418*, 421
  laboratory studies in, 417
  obstruction and, 419, *419*
  percutaneous hepatic biopsy in, 418
  perforation and, 419, *420*
  role of ultrasonography in, 417–418
  scintigraphy in, 418
  specific areas of interest in, 419
Jejunum, blunt trauma to, *368*, 371
Jeune syndrome, renal cystic disease and, 147t
Joint, ultrasonography in evaluation of, 114–115
Jugular vein, anomaly of, 84, *85*
  examination of, 121
Jumper's knee, 114
Juvenile nephronophthisis, 185–187, *186*, *187*
  familial, renal cystic disease and, 147t

Kallmann syndrome, 336
Kidney. See also *Renal* entries.
  absence of, 146–149, *148–150*
    familial theme in, 148
    hypertrophy of remaining kidney in, 148, *150*
    syndromes associated with, 146, 146t
  acute pyelonephritis and. See *Pyelonephritis, acute.*
  anomaly of, 145–154
    duplex kidney as, 152–154, *156*
    hypertension and, 162–163
    renal agenesis as, 146–149, *148–150*
      familial theme in, 148
    renal ectopia as, 149, 151–152, *151–155*
    syndromes associated with, 145, 146t
  blunt trauma to, 365, 367, *367*, 369–370, *370*
  candidal infection of, 209–210, *211*
  cystic. See *Cyst(s), renal; Glomerulocystic kidney disease; Multicystic dysplastic kidney; Polycystic kidney disease.*
  doughnut, 152
  duplex, 152–154, *156*, 233–234, *236–239*
  dysplastic, multicystic, 176, *177*
  ectopic, 149, 151–152, *151–155*
  horseshoe, 152, *153*, 154
    Wilms tumor and, 157
  in abdominal trauma, 369–370, *370*
  malrotated, 152, *155*
  mass in, 250–256. See also names of specific conditions.
    carcinoma as, 255–256, *256*
    general considerations for, 250
    mesoblastic nephroma as, 250, *251*
    multilocular cystic nephroma as, 250–251, *251*
    nephroblastomatosis as, 251–252
    Wilms tumor as, 252–255. See also *Wilms tumor.*
  normal, ultrasonography of, 137–144
    bladder in, 138, *139*
    collecting system in, 139, *140*, *144*
    columns of Bertin in, 141, *144*
    cortex in, 140, *141*
    fetal lobulation in, 141, *142*
    in childhood, 141, *144*

Kidney *(Continued)*
    in neonate, 137–141, *138*, *141*, *142*. See also *Neonate, normal kidneys in.*
    in prepubertal female, *138*
    medulla in, 140, *141*
    papilla in, 140–141, *141*
    parenchyma in, 140, *144*
    pelvis in, 139
    renal arteries in, 139, *140*
    renal length in, 141–142, *145*
    renal veins in, 139–140
    ureter in, 138
  obstruction in, transient, 465, *465*
  pelvic, 151
    dysplastic, 148, *150*
    pain and, 157
  renal scarring in, 197–198
  single, syndromes associated with, 146t
  sponge, medullary, 147t, 186–187
  supernumerary, 154
  transplantation of, 477–489. See also *Transplantation, renal.*
  ultrasonography of, 137–188. See also names of specific disorders.
    after normal voiding cystourethrogram, 208
    in renal cystic disease, 176–188. See also *Cyst(s), renal.*
    normal kidney in, 137–144. See also *Kidney, normal, ultrasonography of.*
    screening with, 137, 137t, 143–145
      in abdominal pain, 157, *157*
      in hematuria, 137t, 163, *163*, 163t, *164*
      urolithiasis and, 164, 168, *169*
    in hypertension. See *Hypertension.*
    in myelodysplasia, 169–171, *170*, *171*
      embryology and classification in, 60
    in neurogenic bladder, 169–171, *170*, *171*
    in postoperative evaluation, 171–172, 174–176
    in renal tumor, 137t, 154, *156*, 157
    in urolithiasis. See *Urolithiasis.*
    VATER association in, 143, 145, 146, 146t
Klippel-Trenaunay syndrome, 413
  portal vein irregularity in, 446, *446*
Knee, articular cartilage of, 115
  effusion in, 115, *115*

Laryngocele, 86
Larynx, ultrasonography of, 86, *89*
Laurence-Moon-Biedl syndrome, renal cystic disease and, 147t
Leiomyoma, uterine, in adolescence, 307, *307*
Leukemia, hepatic involvement in, 262
  renal involvement in, 472
  scrotal mass and, 331, *331*
  splenic involvement in, 405, *407*
Leukomalacia, periventricular, asphyxia neonatorum and, 19–20
  in premature infant, 7
Leydig tumor, precocious puberty and, 320, 322, *322*
Ligament, ultrasonography in evaluation of, 114–115
Ligamentum teres, 441, *443*
Ligamentum venosum, 441, *443*
Lipoblastoma, retroperitoneal, 257

Lipoma, corpus callosum, 36, 46
  lumbosascral, 62–63, 65, 66, 67
  retroperitoneal, 257
Lipomeningomyelocele, 62, 65, 67
  definition of, 60
Lipomyelocele, 65
Lissencephaly, in dysmorphia, 34
Liver, 416–418. See also *Biliary tree; Gallbladder; Hepatic fibrosis.*
  ascites and, 374t, 377, 378t, 379
  biliary atresia and, 417–419, 418, 419
    kidney involvement and, 419
  blunt trauma to, 365, 366, 368–369, 369
  chronic disease of, 439, 439t, 439–440, 440
  fatty, 436–438, 436–438
  general consideration for, 416
  in acute hepatitis, 436, 436t
  in hepatic parenchymal disease, 434–440. See also names of specific diseases.
  in severe asphyxia, 436, 436
  jaundice and, neonatal, 416–419. See also *Jaundice, neonatal.*
  left lobe of, 434–435, 435
  length of, 434
  mass in, 261–274
    adenoma as, 266–267, 267–268
    benign, epithelial, 263, 266, 267
      mesenchymal, 269, 270
    biliary tract tumor as, 271–272
    cyst as, 268, 268, 269, 271, 271
    differential diagnosis in, 263, 264, 268
    general considerations for, 261–262
    hydatid disease as, 273–274
    inflammatory, 272–273
    metastatic disease as, 261, 261–262, 262
    primary, epithelial derivatives as, 263, 264–267, 267–268
      mesenchymal derivatives as, 268–269, 268–271, 271
    technique in evaluation of, 262–263
    vascular, 269, 270, 271
  right lobe of, 435, 435
  transplantation of. See *Transplantation, hepatic.*
  vasculature in. See also *Artery(ies); Vein(s).*
    abnormality of, 440–446, 440–448, 448
Lymphangioma. See also *Cystic hygroma.*
  mesenteric, 284, 285
  pancreatic, 402
  retroperitoneal, 258
  splenic, 413, 414
  ultrasonography in, 84, 86
Lymphoma, Burkitt, 275, 276, 276–278
  classification of, 258
  colonic, 275, 276, 276–278
  hepatic involvement in, 262
  Hodgkin, 74, 75, 258, 259
  incidence of, 258
  lymphoblastic, 258–259, 259
  non-Hodgkin, 258, 259
  ovarian, 298
  retroperitoneal, 258–259, 259
Lymphosarcoma, bowel, 282

Macrocrania, benign, 49, 50
Macroglossia, renal cystic disease and, 147t
Magnetic resonance imaging, coronal, 100

Magnetic resonance imaging *(Continued)*
  in abdominal testis, 325
  in asphyxia neonatorum, 23
  in deep sacral dimple, 61
  in dysmorphia, 45–46
  in gluteal mass, 111, 111
  in hepatic mass, 268
  in neuroblastoma, 244
  spinal ultrasonography v, 59–60, 61
Mainzer-Saldino syndrome, renal cystic disease and, 147t
Male, cryptorchid, 323–325, 324, 325
Malrotation, vomiting and, 361–362, 362
Mayer-Rokitansky-Küster-Hauser syndrome, 300
  amenorrhea and, 337–338
Meckel-Gruber syndrome, renal cystic disease and, 147t, 185, 186
Medulla, renal, calcinosis and, 467, 467
  cystic disease and, 147t
Medullary sponge kidney, 186–187
Megacalicosis, 239
Megaureter, primary, 224–225, 225, 226
Menarche, normal age for, 336
Ménétrier disease, abdominal mass and, 279
Meningitis, bacterial, in infant, complications of, 27, 28
  computed tomography in, 28
  congenital infection and, 28, 30, 32
  etiology of, 27, 28, 29
  extra-axial fluid collection in, 28, 30
  in utero infection and, 30, 32
  pathophysiology of, 27
  TORCH infections and, 30, 32
  ultrasonography in, 27–28, 28–32
  deep sacral dimple as risk factor in, 61
Meningocele, 60, 62, 63, 64
Meningococcemia, 242
Meningomyelocele, 61–62. See also *Myelodysplasia.*
  Arnold-Chiari malformation and, 59
  definition of, 60
Mental retardation, renal cystic disease and, 147t
Mesenchymoma, malignant, 271
Mesentery, lymphangioma of, 284, 285
  tumors of, 274, 275
Microlithiasis, testicular, 335, 336
Micropolygyria, in dysmorphia, 31, 33
Morgagni, foramen of, hernia through, 99
  hydatid of, 334, 334
Müllerian duct, 322, 322
  aplasia of, renal abnormality and, 146t
Multicystic dysplastic kidney, hydronephrosis and, 218–220, 219, 220
  unilateral, incidence of, 219
Muscle, of extremity, mass in, 111, 111
  measurement of, 110
  psoas, 257
Mycobacterial infection, in adenopathy, 73–74, 74–77
Myelocystocele, definition of, 60
Myelodysplasia, 137t. See also *Meningomyelocele.*
  embryology and classification in, 60
  renal ultrasonography in, 169–171, 170, 171
  spinal ultrasonography in, 59
Myoglobinuria, 461

Nail-Patella syndrome, renal abnormality and, 146t
Necrotizing enterocolitis, 386, 387
Needle aspiration, in cervical adenopathy, 74
  thyroidal abscess, 80
Neonate. See also *Premature infant*.
  abdominal ultrasonography of, abdominal mass and, 214–215. See also *Abdomen, mass in*.
  adrenal gland in, 318
  ambiguous genitalia in, 317–318
  ascites in, 373, 375, 377
    causes of, 374t
  asphyxia neonatorum and, 19–25. See also *Asphyxia neonatorum*.
  congenital dysplasia of hip in, 124–127, 125
  cranial ultrasonography of, 1–52. See also *Cranial ultrasonography*.
  diaphragmatic hernia in, 98, 99
  dysmorphic, 30–46. See also *Dysmorphia*.
  fibromatosis colli in, 86, 89
  fracture and deformity in, 116
  gonad in, 318
  hepatic hematoma in, 365, 366
  hypertension in, 159, 160
  jaundice in, 416–419. See also *Jaundice, neonatal*.
  normal kidneys in, 137–138, 138. See also *Kidney, normal*.
    appearance of renal cyst in, 140–141, 141
    central sinus in, 139
    cortical echogenicity in, 140
    fetal lobulation in, 141, 142
    medulla in, 140, 141
  pelvic mass in, 289–292, 290–294, 294
    abscess as, 292
    cystic, 291, 291–292, 293, 294, 294
    genital tract anomaly and, 292, 293
    ovarian cyst as, 292, 293, 294, 294
    prerectal mass as, 292
    rectal mass as, 292
    retrorectal mass as, 291, 291–292
    sacrococcygeal teratoma as, 289–291, 290, 291
  perinatal asphyxia of, 19–25. See also *Asphyxia neonatorum*.
  renal agenesis in, 146–148, 148
  renal cortical echogenicity in, 462–463, 463
  renal mass in, 250
  renal parenchymal disease in, 462–467. See also *Renal parenchymal disease, in childhood*.
  shunt placement in, intraoperative neurosonography and, 71
  spinal ultrasonography of, 59
  urinary anomaly in, incidence of, 217
  urinary tract infection in, 195–197, 196–198
Nephrectomy, in Wilms tumor, 255
Nephroblastomatosis, 157
  Wilms tumor and, 251–252
Nephrocalcinosis, 473, 474, 475, 475t
Nephrolithiasis, renal transplantation and, 484, 487
Nephroma, cystic, multilocular, 250–251, 251
  mesoblastic, 250, 251
Nephronophthisis, juvenile, 185–187, 186–187
  familial, renal cystic disease and, 147t
Nephropathy, syndromes associated with, 146t
Nephropathy reflex, 194

Nephrosis, congenital, 464, 464
Nephrostomy, in multicystic dysplasia of kidney, 219
Nephrotic syndrome, 464, 468
  congenital, Finnish-type, 464, 464
  scrotal mass and, 326, 326
Nesidioblastosis, 402–403
Neuroblastoma, 242–244, 246–248, 248
  as scrotal mass, 331, 331
  calcification in, 244, 246
  computed tomography in, 244
  connective tissue, 86, 88
  cystic, 244, 245
  Evans staging system in, 244, 244t
  fine-needle biopsy of, 248
  follow-up in, 248, 248
  intrathoracic mass as, 103
  kidney and, 244, 248
  laboratory tests in, 244
  magnetic resonance imaging in, 244
  metastatic, 244, 246–248, 261, 261–262, 262
  myoclonic encephalopathy of infancy and, 243–244
  paraspinal, in infant, 68–69, 69
  prenatal diagnosis in, 262
  radionuclide scan in, 244
  retroperitoneal, 244
Neuroectodermal tumor, 46, 46
  pleural effusion in, 97
Neurofibromatosis, hypertension and, 160
  pleural effusion in, 96
Neurogenic bladder, 169–171, 170, 171
Neurogenic tumor, as retroperitoneal mass, 257, 257
Neurologic examination, abnormal, spinal abnormality and, 65
Neuromuscular disease, ultrasonography in, 110
Neurosonography, intraoperative, 69–71, 69–72
  for shunt placement in neonate, 71
  in hydromyelia, 71, 71–72
  of spinal cord, 71, 71–72
  preparation in, 69–70
  uses for, 69
Nipples, supernumerary, 143
Nodular renal blastema. See *Nephroblastomatosis*.
Non-Hodgkin lymphoma, 258, 259
Nuclear scintigraphy, in painful scrotal mass, 335

Obesity, fatty liver and, 436, 437, 437
  renal cystic disease and, 147t
Omphalocele, repair of, renal agenesis and, 152
Oral-facial-digital syndrome, type I, renal cystic disease and, 147t
Orchiopexy, 324
Orchitis, 333
Ortolani maneuver, 124–125, 125
Osteochondritis dissecans, 115
Osteochondroma, thoracic, 105
Osteomyelitis, 115
Osteosarcoma, pleural effusion in, 96
Ovary, cystic, 286, 286
  amenorrhea and, 339–340, 340
  hemorrhagic, 303, 305

Ovary (Continued)
  in adolescence, 301, 301–305, 303
    rhabdomyosarcoma and, 304
    pelvic mass and, 292, 293, 294, 294
    septated, 301, 302, 303, 303
  lymphoma of, 298
  metastatic disease in, 297, 299
  neoplasm in, adolescence and, 303
  torsion of, 296–297, 298
  tumor in, 295–296, 295–297
    amenorrhea and, 340
    ascites associated with, 217
Oxalosis, renal transplantation and, 477, 477

Pachygyria, in dysmorphia, 33, 33
Pain, abdominal, intussusception and, 281
  recurrent, 343–345
    in adolescence, 344–345
    intermittent obstruction and, 344, 344
    malrotation and, 344, 345
    role of ultrasonography in, 343–344, 345
  renal disorder and, 157, 157
  renal ultrasonography in, 137t, 157, 157
  scrotal, 331–335, 332–335. See also *Scrotum, ultrasonography of, in unilateral scrotal mass.*
Pancreas, 389–403
  aberrant, 398
  annular, 360–361, 398
  blunt trauma to, 367–368
  dimensions of, age, 389, 390, 390t
  ductal anomaly in, 398
  in abdominal trauma, 371
  in childhood, 389, 390
  mass in, 400–402, 401–403
    benign lymphangioma as, 402
    cyst as, 400, 401
    insulinoma and, 403
    multiple endocrine neoplasia and, 403
    neoplasm as, 401, 401–402, 402
    nesidioblastosis and, 402–403
    pseudocyst as, 400, 401
Pancreas divisum, in pancreatitis, 398
Pancreatitis, 389–399
  abdominal trauma and, 281
  aberrant pancreatic tissue and, 398
  annular pancreas in, 398
  ascariasis in etiology of, 396–398
  biliary tree in, 398
  cystic fibrosis and, 398–399
  drug-related, 396
  ductal anomaly and, 398
  ductal diameter in, 389, 390
  echogenic pancreas and, 389, 391, 391, 392, 396
  etiology of, 391
  exogenous secretin in, 399
  fibrosing, chronic, 399, 399
  follow-up in, 398–399, 399
  gallbladder in, 398
  gallstone-associated, 398
  general considerations for, 389
  hereditary, 396
  in endoscopic retrograde cholangiopancreatography, 398
  infectious, 396
  pancreas divisum in, 398

Pancreatitis (Continued)
  peptic disease and, 396
  recurrent, 398
  Schistosomiasis in etiology of, 396, 398
  splenic venous thrombosis and, 399
  trauma and, 391–392, 394, 394
    follow-up in, 394, 394–396, 395–397
    pseudocyst in, 394–396, 395–397
  ultrasonography in, 389, 391, 393
  vomiting and, 361
Parathyroid disease, ultrasonography in, 80, 84, 84
Parent, presence of, at cranial scan of infant, 4–5
Parotid gland, ultrasonography of, 78, 78, 79
Patau syndrome. See *Trisomy 13.*
Patellar tendinitis, 114
Patent ductus arteriosus, 26, 26
Pavlik harness, 131
Pelvic inflammatory disease, in adolescence, 303, 305, 305–306, 306
  simulating appendicitis, 352
Pelvic kidney, pain and, 157
Pelvis, in renal ultrasonography, 139
  mass in, 285–309. See also *Ovary, cystic.*
    ectopic pregnancy and, 286
    embryonal rhabdomyosarcoma as, 294, 294–295, 295
    general considerations for, 285–286
    genitourinary tumor as, 294, 294–295, 295
    in adolescence, 299–309
      bicornuate uterus and, 307, 308, 309
      chronic obstruction of vas deferens and, 309
      Gartner cyst and, 308, 309
      genital tract duplication and, 300, 300–301
      imperforate hymen and, 299, 299–300
      incidental cyst and, 308, 309
      leiomyoma and, 307, 307
      males and, 309, 309
      ovarian cyst and, 301, 301–305, 303
        hemorrhagic, 303, 305
        septated, 301, 301–305, 303
      ovarian neoplasm and, 303, 304
      ovarian torsion and, 303
      pelvic inflammatory disease and, 303, 305, 305–306, 306
      pregnancy diagnosis and, 299, 303
      seminal vesicle cyst and, 309
      surgery in etiology of, 309
      tubo-ovarian abscess and, 305, 305–306
    in childhood, 294–299
    in neonate, 289–292, 290–294, 294. See also *Neonate, pelvic mass in.*
    ovarian ascites as, 297
    ovarian torsion as, 296–297, 298
    ovarian tumor as, 295–296, 295–297
  normal, 286, 287–289, 289
Peptic disease, abdominal mass and, 279, 281
  pancreatitis and, 396
Pericardium, cyst of, 101
Peritoneal lavage, in abdominal trauma, 364
Pheochromocytoma, 248–249, 249
  hypertension and, 159–160, 162
  malignancy in, 249
  syndromes associated with, 249
PID. See *Pelvic inflammatory disease.*
Pilonidal sinus, 61

Pleural effusion, 91, 93–98
  conditions associated with, 93–94, 96
  connective tissue disorder and, 94, 95
  laboratory studies in, 98
  malignant condition and, *96*, 96–98, *97*
  pneumonia and, *93*, 93–94, *94*, 97
  postoperative, 94, *95*
  thoracentesis in, 91, 93, 97–98
  tubes and catheters as causes of, 93
Pneumonia, *93*, 93–94, *94*
  bacterial infection in, 93–94
  hepatization in, 93
Pneumothorax, acute, in premature infant, intracranial hemorrhage and, 6
Polycystic kidney disease, 181–185, *182–185*
  dominant, autosomal as, 181, *182*, *183*
  general considerations in, 184–185
  glomerulocystic kidney disease as, 147t, 183–185, *185*
  neonatal, 463–464, *464*
  recessive, autosomal as, 182–183, *184*, *185*
Polydactyly, renal cystic disease and, 147t
Polyorchidism, 329
Polyp, urethral, 232, *234*
Polysplenia, abdominal heterotaxia with, 414, *414*
  biliary atresia and, 418
Popliteal cyst, 111–112, *113*
Popliteal vein, examination of, 119–120, *120*
Portal vein, aneurysmal, *446*
  anomaly of, 443, *444*, 445
  cavernous transformation of, *408, 409, 444*, 445
  development of, 440
  enlargement of, 446
  gas in, 385, *386*, 387
  general considerations for, 447
  idiopathic occlusion of, 445
  normal, 440–441, *442, 443*
  obstruction of, 445, *445*
  portal hypertension and, *445*, 446–447, 452
  preduodenal, 445
  thrombosis of, *408, 409, 444*, 445–446
  tumor invasion in, 446
Pourcelot index, 481
Precocious puberty, in boys, 320, 322, *322*
  in girls, 318–320, *319–321*
Pregnancy, amenorrhea and, 338
Premature infant, choroid plexus in, 8, *10*
  cranial ultrasonography of, 7–19
    areas of interest in, 7–8, *8*
    choroid plexus and, 8, *10*
    data worksheet for, 11, *12*
    germinal matrix and, 8, *9*, *10*, 16–17, *17*
    indications for, 8
    intracerebellar hemorrhage and, 14, 16, *16*
    intraparenchymal echogenicity and, 13–14, *15*
    intraventricular hemorrhage and, 8, 11, *12, 13*
      intraparenchymal echogenicity and, 14
    peritrigonal blush and, 13, *14*
    periventricular blush and, 13
    pitfalls in, 8, *10, 11*
    technique in, 1, *2*, 3–5, *4, 5*
    ventricular dilatation and, *16–18*, 16–19
  cystic encephalomalacia in, 7
  germinal matrix in, 8, *9*
  gestational age of, 1

Premature infant *(Continued)*
  hypoxic-ischemic injury in, 7
  intracranial hemorrhage in, acute pneumothorax and, 6
    clinical background for, 5–6
    cranial ultrasonography in, 16–19, *17, 18*, 26
    Doppler ultrasonography in, 26–27
    extracorporeal membrane oxygenation and, 23–25, *24, 25*
    periventricular leukomalacia and, 7
    risk factors for, 6
    ventricular dilatation and, *16–18*, 16–19
      hydrocephalus and, 18
  intraparenchymal echogenicity in, 13–14, *15*
  ventriculomegaly in, *16–18*, 16–19
Probst, bundles of, 34, *35*
Prosthesis, urinary, 176, *176*
Proteus, in urinary tract infection, 193
Prune-belly syndrome, 236, *239*, 239
  renal abnormality and, 146t
Pseudoaneurysm, in extremity, 122, *122–124*
  renal transplantation and, *489*, 489
Pseudocyst, cerebrospinal fluid, 285
  pancreatic, 400, *401*
  splenic, 411
Pseudohermaphroditism, renal abnormality and, 146t
Pseudomonas, in urinary tract infection, 193
Psoas abscess, 257–258
  Crohn disease and, 354
Pubic hair, premature appearance of. See *Adrenarche, premature.*
Pyelonephritis, 201–209
  acute, abscess in, 202, *203, 204*
    caliectasis in, 208, *209*
    complications in, 202, *203*
    indications in, 201, *203*
    pyonephrosis and, 202–203, *204*, 205, *205*
    renal growth and, 208
    ultrasonography of kidney in, 208
  scarring in, 197–198, 205, *206–208*, 207–208
  xanthogranulomatous, 209, *210*
Pylephlebitis, 446
Pyloric stenosis, 357, *358*, 359–360, *360*, 360t
Pyomyositis, 111, *112*
Pyonephrosis, 202–203, *204*, 205, *205*

Radionuclide scan, in neuroblastoma, 244
Radiotherapy, amenorrhea and, 338, *338, 339*
Rectum, abnormal, spinal abnormality and, 65, *67, 68*, 68
  as origin of pelvic mass, 292
Reflux, gastroesophageal, vomiting and, 361
  neonatal, 217, *217*
  nephropathy, 194
  sterile, 217, *217*
  urinary tract infection and, 197, *199*, 201, *202*
  urolithiasis and, 168, *168*
  vaginal, 197, *199*
  vesicoureteral. See *Vesicoureteral reflux.*
Reflux nephropathy, 194
Renal. See also *Kidney.*
Renal agenesis, 146–149, *148–150*
  familial theme in, 148
  syndromes associated with, 146, 146t

Renal anomaly(ies), 145–154
  duplex kidney as, 152–154, *156*
  hypertension and, 162–163
  renal agenesis as, 146–149, *148–150*
    familial theme in, 148
  renal ectopia as, 149, 151–152, *151–155*
  syndromes associated with, 145, 146t
Renal artery, 139, *140*, 387
  in hypertension, 159–160, *161*
  occlusion of, 466–467, *467*
Renal failure, acute, 462
  chronic, 473
  general considerations for, 462
  hyperparathyroidism and, 80, 84, *84*
  idiopathic, in adolescence, 185
  renal biopsy in, 472–473, *474*
Renal mass. See *Kidney, mass in.*
Renal medullary cystic disease, 186
Renal parenchymal disease, 462–475
  causes of, 463t, 468t
    cortical echogenicity and, 467–468, *469,*
      470
    drug-related, 472
    hemolytic uremic syndrome as, 468, *470*
    hyperperfusion injury as, 468, *471*, 471
    myoglobinuria as, 471
    nephrocalcinosis as, 473, *474, 475*, 475t
    nephrotic syndrome as, *464*, 468
    sickle cell trait as, 471, *472*
    uric acid nephropathy as, 471–472, *472,*
      473
  neonatal, 462–467
    anoxic damage as, 465, *465*
    arterial occlusion as, 466–467, *467*
    congenital nephrosis as, 464, *464*
    cortical echogenicity and, 462–463, *463*
    drug-related, 467, *467*
    medullary calcinosis as, 467, *467*
    polycystic disease as, 463–464
    renal venous thrombosis as, 465–466, *466*
    transient renal obstruction as, 465, *465*
  renal biopsy in, 472–473, *474*
Renal tuberculosis, urinary tract infection and,
  211
Renal vein, 139–140
  thrombosis of, *385*, 385, 465–466, *466*
Retina, atrophy of, renal abnormality and, 146t
  renal-retinal dysplasia and, 147t
Retinitis pigmentosa, renal cystic disease and,
  147t
Retroperitoneal mass, 215–260. See also
  Abdomen, mass in, retroperitoneal.
Reye syndrome, fatty liver and, 438
Rhabdomyosarcoma, botryoid, 271–272
  embryonal, *294*, 294–295, *295*
    as scrotal mass, 330
  hepatic involvement in, 262, *262*
  of neck, 86
  ovarian, in adolescence, 304
  retroperitoneal, 257
  thoracic, 105
Rotator cuff, injury of, 114–115

Sacral dimple, deep, computed tomography in,
  61
  magnetic resonance imaging in, 61
  spinal ultrasonography in, 59, 61, 62, *63*

Sacrococcygeal teratoma, 68, 289–291, *290, 291*
Salivary gland, ultrasonography of, 78, *78, 79*
Sarcoma, breast, 107
Schistosoma haematobium, 210–211, *211*
Schistosomiasis, in chronic hepatic fibrosis, 439,
  439t
  in etiology of pancreatitis, 396, 398
  in etiology of portal hypertension, 447
  in etiology of urinary tract infection, 210–211
Schizencephaly, absence of septi pellucidi and,
  36
Scintigraphy, in choledochal cyst, 421
  in multicystic dysplasia of kidney, 219
  nuclear, in painful scrotal mass, 335
Scoliosis, congenital, renal abnormality and,
  146t
Scrotum, ultrasonography of, 322–335
  general considerations for, 322–323
  in bilateral scrotal swelling, 335, *335*
  in cryptorchidism, 143, *323*–325, *324, 325*
  in unilateral scrotal mass, 325–335
    painful, 331–335, *332–335*
      abscess as, 333
      "bell-clapper" deformity and, 333
      causes of, 332t
      epididymitis as, 333, *334*
      epididymo-orchitis and, 332, *334*
      orchitis as, 333
      torsion and, *332*, 332–333, *333*
      trauma and, *334*, 334–335, *335*
    painless, 325–331
      benign, 326–329, *326–329*
        adrenal rest as, 329
        bilobed testis as, 329
        cyst as, 328–329, *329*
        hernia as, 326, 327, *327*
        hydrocele as, 325–326, *327*
        teratoma as, 329
        varicocele as, 327–328, *328*
      causes of, 325t
      malignant, 329–331, *330, 331*
  indications for, 323
  normal scrotal anatomy and, *322*, 322–323,
    323
  technique in, 322
Secretin, exogenous, 399
Septi pellucidi, absence of, 36, *37*
Serologic testing, in amebic disease, 273
Shunt, vascular, in extremity, complications of,
  122, *122*
  ventricular, intraoperative neurosonography
    in placement of, 69, 71
  ventriculomegaly and, 40, 41, *41, 42*
Shwachman-Diamond syndrome, 391, *391*
Sickle cell trait, 471, *472*
Sinus disease, ultrasonography in, 78–79
Spinal cord, diameter of, 61–62
  fat on surface of, 65
  intraoperative scans of, *71*, 71–72
  malformation of, embryology and classifica-
    tion in, 60
  normal, in spinal ultrasonography, 57–59,
    58, 59
Spine, ultrasonography of, 57–62
  abnormal neurologic examination and, 65
  abnormal rectum and, 65, *67, 68*, 68
  computed tomography *v,* 59–60, 61
  general considerations for, 57
  in absent or abnormal vertebra, 60–61

Spine (Continued)
   in anorectal malformation, 61
   in Arnold-Chiari II malformation, *58*
   in deep sacral dimple, 59, 61, *62, 63*
   in intramedullary and extramedullary tumors, 68–69, *69*
   in meningomyelocele, 61–62
   in myelodysplasia, 59
   in sacrococcygeal teratoma, 68
   in skin-covered soft tissue mass, 62–63, *63–67,* 65
   indications for, 60
   intraoperative, *69–71,* 69–72
     for shunt placement in neonate, 69, 71
     in hydromyelia, *71,* 71–72
     of spinal cord, *71,* 71–72
     preparation for, 69–70
     uses for, 69
   magnetic resonance imaging *v,* 59–60, 61
   of conus medullaris, 57, *58, 58, 59*
   of normal spine, 57–59, *58, 59*
Spleen, 405–415
   abscess in, 411, *412, 413*
   absence of, 415
   accessory, 414–415, *415*
   anomaly of, 414–415
   arteriovenous malformation of, 414
   cyst in, 410–411, *411, 412*
   ectopic, 414
   enlargement of, 405–406, *407, 408, 409*
   focal calcification in, 410, *410*
   general considerations for, 405
   in abdominal trauma, 369, *369*
   in adolescence, 405
   in candidiasis, *409,* 409–410
   in cat-scratch disease, 410
   in chronic hepatic disease, 406, *407*
   in hepatic transplantation preoperative evaluation, 452
   in portal vein thrombosis, *408,* 409
   in viral illness, 409
   infarction in, 411, *413,* 414
   lymphangioma in, *413,* 414
   multiple, 414, *415,* 418
   pseudocyst in, 411
   size of, 405, *406*
   trauma to, 405, *406*
   venous thrombosis in, pancreatitis and, 399
Splenic artery, malformation of, 414
Splenic vein, malformation of 414
   thrombosis of, 411, *413,* 414
Splenomegaly, fever and, 355
Splint, hip ultrasonography in presence of, 130, *131*
Status marmoratus, 19, 20, *20*
Stein-Leventhal syndrome, amenorrhea and, 339
Steroid therapy, hepatic adenoma and, 268
Streptococcus, meningitis and, 27, *29*
Subclavian vein, examination of, 121, *122*
Syringomyelia, *71*
   definition of, 61

Task Force on Blood Pressure Control in Children (1987), 158
Teflon, intramural injection of, 174, *174*

Tendon, ultrasonography in evaluation of, 114–115
Teratoma, abdominal wall, 274
   connective tissue, 86
   gastric, 274–275
   mediastinal, 105
   ovarian, 296, *296, 297*
   retroperitoneal, 256–257
   sacrococcygeal, 68, 289–291, *290, 291*
   scrotal, 329
Testicular feminization, 338
Testis. See also *Scrotum, ultrasonography of.*
   abdominal, 325
   abscess of, 333
   bilobed, 329
   cryptorchid, 143, 323–325, *324, 325*
   cystic mass in, 329
   impalpable, 324
   inflammation of, 333
   intra-abdominal, in female, 338
   microlithiasis in, 335, *336*
   multiple, 329
   normal, *322,* 322–323, *323*
   size variation in, 323
   torsion of, *332,* 332–333, *333*
   trauma to, *334,* 334–335
   undescended. See *Cryptorchidism.*
Thelarche, normal age for, 336
   premature, 318–319, *319,* 320
Thoracentesis, ultrasonic-guided, 91, 93, 97–98
Thrombosis, arterial, hepatic, retransplantation and, 459, *459*
   cyclosporine and, 487
   portal vein, *408, 409, 444,* 445–446
   venous, deep, 117–121
     Doppler imaging in, 118, 120, *120, 121*
     previous catheter placement and, 121, *122*
     risk factors in, 117
     technique in, 117–119
     renal, 385, *385*
       neonatal, 465–466, *466*
     splenic, pancreatitis and, 399
Thymus, cyst in, 105
   ectopic, 86, *88*
   mass in, 101, *104,* 105
   normal, 105
Thyroglossal cyst, 79–80, *80*
Thyroid disease, ultrasonography in, 79–80, *80–83*
Thyroid mass, 79–80
Thyroiditis, Hashimoto, 80, *83*
TORCH infection, meningitis and, 28, 30, *32*
Transplantation, hepatic, 452–461
   postoperative evaluation in, 454–457, *455–460,* 459–461
     general considerations for, 454
     parenchymal pattern in, 455–456
     perihepatic collections in, 454–455, *455*
     vasculature in, 456–457, *457–460,* 459–461
   preoperative evaluation in, 452, *453,* 454
     biliary tree in, *453,* 454
     liver size and shape in, 452
     parenchymal pattern in, 452
     spleen in, 452
     varices in, 452, *453*
     vasculature in, 452, 454
     volume of ascites in, 452

Transplantation *(Continued)*
  renal, 477–489
    complications in, 478–479
    donor selection in, 477–478
    general considerations for, 477
    indications for, 477
    operative procedure for, *478, 479*
    oxalosis and, 477, *477*
    parenchymal pattern in, 489
    postoperative complications in, 478–489
      acute tubular necrosis and, 480, 481, *482*
      checklist for, 479–480
      hematuria as, 486, *487*
      immediate, 479
      nephrolithiasis as, 484, *487*
      pseudoaneurysm as, 489, *489*
      pulsatility index and, 481–482
      rejection classification and, 481–483
      renal cyst as, *488*, 489
      renovascular disease as, 486–487, 489
      resistive index and, 481–483
      urologic, 483–484, *484–487*, 486
    postoperative scans in, 479–481
    preoperative evaluation in, 477
    prognostic variables in, 481
Trauma, abdominal, blunt, 364–371
  computed tomography in, 365, *365*
  general considerations for, 364
  hepatic injury and, 365, *366*, 368–369, *369*
  jejunal injury and, *368*, 371
  laboratory studies in, 364, 365
  pancreatoduodenal injury and, 367–368, *370*, 371
  peritoneal lavage in, 364
  physical examination in, 364
  radiographic examination in, 365
  renal injury and, 365, 367, *367*, 369–370, *370*
  ultrasonography in, 365–371
    adrenal gland in, 371
    duodenum in, *370*, 371
    free fluid and, *368, 369*
    hepatic injury and, 368–369, *369*
    kidney in, 369–370, *370*
    spleen in, 368–369, *369*
  urography in, 365
  duodenal, 367–368, *370*, 371
  pelvic, 301
  splenic, 405, *406*
Triploidy, renal abnormality and, 146t
  renal cystic disease and, 147t
Trisomy 13, renal abnormality and, 146t
  renal cystic disease and, 147t
Trisomy 18, renal abnormality and, 146t
  renal cystic disease and, 147t
Trisomy 21, gyral anomaly in, 34
  intrathoracic mass and, *104*
  renal abnormality and, 146t
  renal cystic disease and, 147t
Tuberculosis, renal, urinary tract infection and, 211
Tuberous sclerosis, 46, *47*, 101, *187*, 187–188, *188*
  renal cystic disease and, 147t
Tubular necrosis, acute, renal transplantation and, 480, 481, *482*
Turner syndrome, 336–337, *337*
  renal abnormality and, 146t, 151, *152*
Typhlitis, 280–281

Tyrosinemia, fatty liver and, 438, *438*

Ulcer, abdominal mass and, 279, *281*
Ulcerative colitis, abdominal mass and, 278, 279
Ultrasonography. See under specific anatomic sites and disorders.
Umbilical artery, single, 143
Umbilical vein, 441, *444*, 445, 446
Urachal cyst, 284, *285*
Uremic syndrome, infection in, 163, *163*, 163t
Ureter, 138
  ectopic, duplex kidney and, 153, 154, *156*
  obstructed, 235, *237*
  in duplex system, 233–234
  reimplantation of, 171–172, *172, 173*
  retrocaval, syndromes associated with, 146t
Ureterocele, 235, *238*
  diverticulum of bladder v, *229*
  ectopic, 233–234, 235, *237*
Ureterosigmoidostomy, complications of, 174
Urethra, obstruction at, 216
  polyp in, 232, *234*
Urethral valve, posterior, hydronephrosis and, 228, 230, 232, *232, 233*
Uric acid nephropathy, 471–472, *472, 473*
Urinary tract, decompression of, 230
  infection of, 163, *163*, 163t, 193–211
    acute pyelonephritis and. See *Pyelonephritis, acute.*
    antimicrobial therapy in, 197
    bacterial, 210–211, *211*
    candidal, 209–210, *211*
    circumcision and, 194
    cystography in, 197, 198, 200
    focal inflammation and, 197–198, *200*
    imaging techniques in, 194–195, 198, 200
    in adolescence, 200, *201*
    in childhood, 197–198, *199–201*, 200
    in neonate, 195–197, *196–198*
    intravenous urography in, 194, 198
    pathogens in, 193–194
    reflux and, 197, *199*, 201, *202*
    renal transplantation and, 484, 486
    renal tuberculosis and, 211
    scarring and, 194, 197–198, *206–208*
    schistosomal, 210–211
    specimen collection in, 193
    urolithiasis and, 164–165, *165, 166*
    vesicoureteral reflux and, 194, 197, *199*
    voiding studies in, 194, *196*
  reconstruction of, 174–176, *174–176*
Urinoma, 230, 232, *233*
Urography, excretory, 234–235, *236*
  in abdominal trauma, 301
  intravenous, 194, 198
Urolithiasis, 164–166, *165–169*, 168–169
  anatomic abnormality and, 164–165, *165, 166*
  calcification in, 168, *168*
  furosemide and, 165
  hematuria and, 164, 168, *169*
  metabolic disease and, 165–166, 166t, *167*
  myelodysplasia and, 169–171, *170, 171*
  reflux of air and, 168, *168*
  urinary infection and, 164–165, *165, 166*
Uterus, absence of, amenorrhea and, *337*, 337–338

Uterus *(Continued)*
    bicornuate, 307, *308*, 309
    hypoplastic, 337
    normal, 138, *139*
    tumor in, 295, *295*
    unicornuate, 318

Vagina, atresia of, 300
    reflux in, 197, *199*
    tumor in, 295, *295*
Valsalva maneuver, in ultrasonography of extremity, deep venous thrombosis and, 119
Varicocele, scrotal, 327–328, *328*
Vascular shunt, in extremity, complications of, 122, *122*
Vasculature. See also *Artery(ies); Vein(s).*
    abdominal, 385, *385*, *386*, 387
    absent, 39, *40*
    hepatic, abnormality of, 440–447, *442–446*, *448*
VATER complex, 143, 145, 146t
    renal agenesis and, 146
Vein(s). See also *Vasculature.*
    drainage of, in neonatal brain, 26
    face and neck, ultrasonography of, 84, *85*
    femoral, examination of, 118–119, *119–120*
    hepatic, 440–447, *442–446*, *448*
        in hepatic transplantation, postoperative evaluation for, 456–457, *457–460*, 459–461
            preoperative evaluation for, 452, *453*, 454
        inferior vena cava vein as, 441, *442–444*
        obstruction in, Budd-Chiari syndrome, 447, *448*
    iliac, examination of, 118
    jugular, examination of, 121
        popliteal, examination of, 119–120, *120*
        portal triad, 443
        portal. See *Portal vein.*
    renal, 139–140
    splenic, malformation of, 414
        thrombosis of, 411, *413*, 414
    subclavian, examination of, 121, *122*
    thrombosis of, 117–121
        deep, 117–121. See also *Thrombosis, venous, deep.*
        Doppler imaging in, 118, 120, *120*, *121*
        previous catheter placement and, 121, *122*
        risk factors in, 117
        technique in, 117–119
    umbilical, 441, *444*, *445*, *446*
Vein of Galen, 50, *51*, *52*
Vena cava, inferior, joining hepatic vein, 441, *442–444*
    thrombosis of, imaging of, 117–118
Ventricular shunt, intraoperative neurosonography in placement of, 69, 71
    ventriculomegaly and, 40, 41, *41*, *42*
Ventriculomegaly, aqueductal stenosis and, 39–40, *40*
    Arnold-Chiari II malformation and, 40, *42*, *43*, 44
    causes of, 43t
    hydrocephalus and, *41*, 41

Ventriculomegaly *(Continued)*
    in benign macrocrania, 49, *50*
    in dysmorphia, 39–42, *40–45*, 43t, 44–46
    in premature infant, *16–18*, 16–19
        hydrocephalus and, 18
    ventricular shunting in, 40, 41, *41*, *42*
Vesicoureteral reflux, 194, 197, *199*
    diagnosis in, 227–228, *231*
    prenatal diagnosis in, 216–217
    urinary tract infection and, 194, 197, *199*
Viral infection, in cervical adenopathy, 73–74, *74–77*
    spleen in, 409
Vocal cord, ultrasonography of, 86, *89*
Vomiting, neonatal, 357–362
    annular pancreas in, 360–361
    antral web in, 360
    duodenal web in, 360
    gastric duplication cyst in, 360, *361*
    gastritis in, 360, *361*
    gastroesophageal reflux in, 361
    malrotation in, 361–362, *362*
    pancreatitis in, 361
    pyloric stenosis in, 357, *358*, 359–360, *360*, 360t
von Hippel-Lindau disease, pancreatic cyst and, *400*, 401
    renal cystic disease and, 147t

Waterhouse-Friderichsen syndrome, 242
Watershed infarct, 21, *21*, *22*, 29
Weight loss, amenorrhea and, 340
Wilms tumor, 137t, 252–255
    bilateral, 253
    calcification in, 253
    computed tomography and ultrasonography in, 253, *254*, 255
    congenital malformations associated with, 252–253
    cystic, 251
    differential diagnosis in, 202
    extrarenal, 253, *254*
    general considerations for, 252
    genetic research in, 252–253
    grouping system in, 252t, 253
    hypertension and, 162
    incidence of, 250–252
    metastatic, 253
    nephrectomy in, 255
    nephroblastomatosis and, 251–252
    predisposition for, syndromes associated with, 146t
    prognosis in, 253
    size of, 255, *255*
    ultrasonography in, 154, *156*, 157
Wolffian duct, in duplex system, 233
Wolman disease, 241

Xanthogranulomatous pyelonephritis, 209, *210*

Zellweger syndrome, renal cystic disease and, 147t